Pediatric Cardiac Intensive Care

Pediatric Cardiac Intensive Care

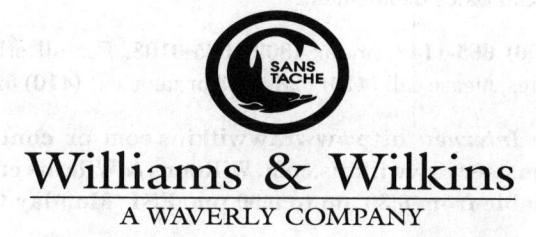

Editors

Anthony C. Chang, MD
Medical Director
Cardiac Intensive Care Program and
Cardiac Intensive Care Unit
Miami Children's Hospital
Miami, Florida

Frank L. Hanley, MD
Professor and Chief of Cardiothoracic Surgery
University of California, San Francisco, School of Medicine
San Francisco, California

Gil Wernovsky, MD
Associate Professor of Pediatrics
University of Pennsylvania School of Medicine
Director, Cardiac Intensive Care Unit
Children's Hospital of Philadelphia
Philadelphia, Pennsylvania

David L. Wessel, MD
Associate Professor of Pediatrics
Harvard Medical School
Director, Cardiac Intensive Care Unit
Children's Hospital
Boston, Massachusetts

**Illustrations by
Charles W. Hoffman, MA**

Williams & Wilkins
A WAVERLY COMPANY

BALTIMORE • PHILADELPHIA • LONDON • PARIS • BANGKOK
HONG KONG • MUNICH • SYDNEY • TOKYO • WROCLAW

Editor: Jonathan W. Pine, Jr.
Managing Editor: Leah Ann Kiehne Hayes
Marketing Manager: Daniell T. Griffin
Project Editor: Ulita Lushnycky
Design Coordinator: Mario Fernandez

Copyright © 1998 Williams & Wilkins

351 West Camden Street
Baltimore, Maryland 21201-2436 USA

Rose Tree Corporate Center
1400 North Providence Road
Building II, Suite 5025
Media, Pennsylvania 19063-2043 USA

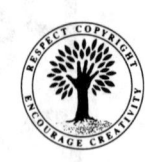

All rights reserved. This book is protected by copyright. No part of this book may be reproduced in any form or by any means, including photocopying, or utilized by any information storage and retrieval system without written permission from the copyright owner.

Accurate indications, adverse reactions, and dosage schedules for drugs are provided in this book, but it is possible that they may change. The reader is urged to review the package information data of the manufacturers of the medications mentioned.

Printed in Canada

Library of Congress Cataloging-in-Publication Data

Pediatric cardiac intensive care / editors, Anthony C. Chang . . . [et al.].
    p.   cm.
    Includes bibliographical references and index.
    ISBN 0-683-01508-7
    1. Pediatric cardiology. 2. Pediatric intensive care.   I. Chang, Anthony C.
    [DNLM: 1. Heart Diseases—in infancy & childhood. 2. Heart Diseases—therapy. 3. Intensive Care—in infancy & childhood.   WS 290 P3708 1998]
    RJ421.P398 1998
    618.92′12028—dc21
    DNLM/DLC
    for Library of Congress   97-39558
                                                                        CIP

The publishers have made every effort to trace the copyright holders for borrowed material. If they have inadvertently overlooked any, they will be pleased to make the necessary arrangements at the first opportunity.

To purchase additional copies of this book, call our customer service department at **(800) 638-0672** or fax orders to **(800) 447-8438**. For other book services, including chapter reprints and large quantity sales, ask for the Special Sales department.

Canadian customers should call **(800) 665-1148**, or fax **(800) 665-0103**. For all other calls originating outside of the United States, please call **(410) 528-4223** or fax us at **(410) 528-8550**.

Visit Williams & Wilkins on the Internet: http://www.wwilkins.com or contact our customer service department at custserv@wwilkins.com. Williams & Wilkins customer service representatives are available from 8:30 am to 6:00 pm, EST, Monday through Friday, for telephone access.

                                                                                               97 98 99 00 01
                                                                        1 2 3 4 5 6 7 8 9 10

This book is dedicated to all those who devote their lives
to the care of critically ill children with heart disease and
also to these families and children, who continue to
inspire us all with their courage and forbearance.

Foreword

In the beginning of pediatric cardiac surgery, denoted by the first successful ligation of a patent ductus arteriosus by Dr. Gross (1938), Crafoord's coarctation repair (1944), and by Blalock and Taussig's systemic artery-to-pulmonary artery shunt (1944), surgeons were mostly responsible for the postoperative management of patients. The same was still true after the early efforts of open heart surgery, be it caval inflow occlusion under moderate (30°C) hypothermia by Lewis and Taufic (1952), the first successful use of an artificial heart lung machine by Gibbon (1953), or after controlled cross-circulation by Lillehei (1954). A stormy and complicated postoperative course was the rule, rather than the exception in those days. For example, hyperkalemia secondary to red blood cell destruction, before the use of hemodilution was a dreaded and often lethal complication. Younger colleagues may be surprised to learn that as late as 1958 it took approximately 5 hours to obtain the results of a serum potassium determination by the clinical laboratory. Cardiologists, both adult and pediatric, rarely ventured into the surgical recovery room (where most of the patients spent their first and sometimes second postoperative week) or into the Intensive Care Unit (ICU). With very few exceptions, anesthesiologists were quite eager to deliver their patients, as soon as possible to the recovery room with a prevailing attitude of *aprés moi le deluge*.

However, as the number of operations increased and, more importantly, as the surgical procedures became more complex, we all realized that both the surgical manpower and more glaringly, our expertise, proved inadequate to provide optimal comprehensive care for these critically ill patients. Soon, pediatric anesthesiologists and cardiologists began to join in postoperative care. During the early 1960s, pediatric cardiology trainees and often also anesthesia residents began to rotate for several months in the Cardiac Intensive Care Unit. As a consequence, some of the pediatric cardiology junior staff developed special interest in the area of intensive care and started to dedicate themselves full time to intensive care work while it emerged as a multidisciplinary entity. These developments varied somewhat from institution to institution; in some, the intensivists developed through the ranks of anesthesia; elsewhere, pediatric cardiologists dominated Pediatric ICU programs.

I must admit to a bias concerning the need for pediatric cardiology training along with the development of intensive care skills for those involved in the care of critically ill children with heart disease. At least a thorough understanding of congenital heart disease, its anatomy and pathophysiology, is required for individuals entrusted with the care of children before and after cardiac surgery. This includes the pediatric cardiac surgeons who I am convinced must continue to play an important role in the perioperative management of their patients. Hence, surgical training must include a profound understanding of all aspects of postoperative care, the effects of cardiopulmonary bypass (with or without hypothermia or circulatory arrest) on the various organs or sub-systems, and a hands-on involvement with defined responsibilities in the ICU. It is mainly through this very special and intense interdisciplinary experience in which nurses, intensive care cardiologists, surgeons, anesthesiologists, and other para-medical personnel work closely together and develop a lasting team spirit; through direct and shared clinical responsibility they learn to appreciate each other's expertise and contribution to the ultimate goal of their endeavor—fully recovered patients.

One cannot overemphasize the important role played by the nurses. They not only provide superb professional care around the clock, but in addition and most importantly, establish a humane link between the patients, their parents, family, and the medical staff. Surgeons in particular, perhaps overly preoccupied by the technical-scientific aspects of patient care, often tend to varying degrees to neglect somewhat our humane obligations of our profession. The need for compassion and human contact is particularly great in an ICU setting.

In reviewing the many chapters and the list of contributors to this excellent book on "Pediatric Cardiac Intensive Care," I immediately detected a shared philosophy of care, a team spirit, and multiple examples of an all important interdisciplinary collaboration. I have the good fortune of knowing most co-authors personally quite well and to have worked with many of them in Boston during various times of their professional development. Their vast experience and their important individual contributions to this field are reflected in the excellence of this book. I am certain that this effort will soon have an impact worldwide and improve the perioperative care of children with congenital heart disease. It is hoped that this book will also provide a stimulus to a new generation of colleagues to contribute new ideas to the development of this fascinating and rapidly advancing field.

Aldo R. Castañeda, MD, PhD
William E. Ladd Professor of Surgery, Emeritus
Harvard Medical School
Children's Hospital

Preface

There is only one good, knowledge, and one evil, ignorance.
- Socrates

Since the first description of a congenital heart defect by Leonardo da Vinci in 1531, numerous advances have been made in the fields of pediatric cardiology, cardiac surgery, and intensive care. The new subspecialty of pediatric cardiac intensive care has recently emerged as a well-defined clinical area that demands expertise from all these subspecialties. Despite the rapid expansion of knowledge in pediatric cardiac intensive care, little has been written specifically for this new subspecialty and information has to be culled from many separate sources.

This textbook is especially designed for all physicians, nurses, and support personnel who are involved in the care of critically ill neonates and children with heart disease. The multidisciplinary contributors are world renowned experts from the largest pediatric cardiac centers in the subspecialties of cardiology, intensive care, cardiac surgery, cardiac anesthesia, neurology, neonatology, and nursing. We are forever indebted to these distinguished contributors for their work.

The first part of this book provides a primer on cardiology and intensive care to serve as a scientific foundation for the remainder of the book. The second part focuses on lesion-specific perioperative care. The remainder of the book discusses other issues in cardiac intensive care, such as transplantation and mechanical cardiopulmonary support as well as topics in cardiac evaluation and management, acquired and chronic heart disease, and socioeconomic issues.

A myriad of recent advances have been made in pediatric cardiac intensive care. Nitric oxide, as a modulating biomolecule in the pulmonary vasculature, has attained a prominent role as a selective pulmonary vasodilator in perioperative care of children with congenital heart disease. In addition, technologic developments in mechanical cardiopulmonary support systems have evolved into more sophisticated equipment that is better suited for resuscitation of critically ill neonates. New drugs such as milrinone and propafenone have been successfully added to the pharmacologic armamentarium in the cardiac intensive care setting. Proliferation of point-of-care bedside laboratory testing has also contributed to efficiency of intensive care. Lastly, new innovations in imaging such as three-dimensional echocardiography and magnetic resonance imaging as well as intraoperative cardioscopy have improved accuracy of diagnosis.

Many challenges remain for pediatric cardiac intensive care. In the treatment of pulmonary hypertension, new agents such as magnesium sulfate, lipo-prostaglandin I_2 analog, aerosolized prostacyclin, and partial liquid ventilation need to be assessed as potential therapies. In addition, with the increasing emphasis from the health care industry that demands specialized intensive care at lower cost, database management systems will be essential to improve efficiency and control cost while monitoring quality of care. Additional challenges involve the emergence of new types of patients, including adults with congenital heart disease and patients with complex heart disease who require new techniques in interventional cardiac catheterization. Finally, in the not too distant future, fetal surgery and fetal transumbilical cardiac catheterization will evolve into reality and demand specific perioperative intensive care. All of these new developments require acquisition of new knowledge and clinical know-how, and this new subspecialty continues as one of the most exciting fields in medicine.

—The Editors

Acknowledgment

I would like to acknowledge Ms. Theola Ray, Mr. Oscar Ordenana, Mr. Roque Ventura, and Dr. Alejandra Avilla for their technical assistance with the echocardiographic figures. I would also like to acknowledge the secretarial assistance and consistent support of my assistant Ms. Miriam Gonzalez. Lastly, I would like to express my deep gratitude to my colleagues at Miami Children's Hospital, particularly Mr. Bill McDonald and Drs. Ana Maria Rosales, Abdulwahab Aldousany, Evan Zahn, Jeffrey Jacobs, and Redmond Burke, as well as the nursing staff in the cardiac intensive care unit, who have continued to provide encouragement throughout this process.

—Anthony C. Chang, MD

I would like to thank my wife, Lauren, and two children, Simon and Jenna, who supported me through the many hours of work necessary to complete this text, and my patients and their families, from whom I learn something new every day. Finally, I would like to thank my parents for not allowing me to become a musician.

—Gil Wernovsky, MD

I would like to thank all members of the Cardiovascular Program in Boston who contributed their collective experience and expertise to the philosophy of care that grounds this book.

—David L. Wessel, MD

List of Contributors

Ian Adatia, MB, ChB, MRCP (UK), FRCP (C)
Assistant Professor of Cardiology and Critical Care
 Medicine
University of Toronto Faculty of Medicine
Hospital for Sick Children
Toronto, Ontario, Canada

Abdul Aldousany, MD
Director
Echocardiography Laboratory
Miami Children's Hospital
Miami, Florida

Teresa Atz, BSN, RN
Staff Nurse
Cardiovascular Intensive Care Unit
Children's Hospital
Boston, Massachusetts

Desmond Bohn, MB, BCh, FRCPC
Associate Professor of Anaesthesia and Pediatrics
University of Toronto Faculty of Medicine
Associate Chief of Critical Care Medicine
The Hospital for Sick Children
Toronto, Ontario, Canada

Edward L. Bove, MD
Professor of Surgery
Director, Pediatric Cardiovascular Surgery
University of Michigan Medical Center
Ann Arbor, Michigan

Redmond P. Burke, MD
Chief, Cardiovascular Division
Miami Children's Hospital
Miami, Florida

Anthony C. Chang, MD
Medical Director, Cardiac Intensive Care Program
Cardiac Intensive Care Unit
Miami Children's Hospital
Miami, Florida

Steven D. Colan, MD
Associate Professor of Pediatrics
Harvard Medical School
Director, Noninvasive Laboratories
Department of Cardiology
Children's Hospital
Boston, Massachusetts

Peter N. Cox, MB, ChB, FFARCS, FRCP (C)
Assistant Professor of Anaesthesia
University of Toronto Faculty of Medicine
Clinical Director, Critical Care Unit
The Hospital for Sick Children
Toronto, Ontario, Canada

Ralph E. Delius, MD
Assistant Professor of Surgery
Division of Cardiothoracic Surgery
University of Iowa Hospitals and Clinics
Iowa City, Iowa

Adre J. du Plessis, MB, ChB, MPH
Assistant Professor of Neurology
Harvard Medical School
Children's Hospital
Boston, Massachusetts

Martin J. Elliott, MD, FRCS
Consultant in Cardiothoracic Surgery
Great Ormond Street Hospital for Children, N.H.S. Trust
London, United Kingdom

Kenneth E. Fellows, MD
Professor of Radiology
University of Pennsylvania Medical School
Radiologist-in-Chief
The Children's Hospital of Philadelphia
Philadelphia, Pennsylvania

Jeffrey R. Fineman, MD
Associate Professor of Pediatrics
Division of Pediatric Critical Care Medicine
University of California, San Francisco, School of
 Medicine
San Francisco, California

Eva Nozik Grayck, MD
Assistant Professor of Pediatrics
Duke University Medical Center
Durham, North Carolina

Barbara P. Gross, RN, MSN
Cardiothoracic Surgery Program
Heart Institute
Children's Hospital of Los Angeles
Los Angeles, California

Jurg Hammer, MD
Chief, Pediatric Intensive Care Unit
Children's Hospital
University of Basel
Basel, Switzerland

Frank L. Hanley, MD
Professor and Chief of Cardiothoracic Surgery
University of California, San Francisco, School of Medicine
San Francisco, California

Patricia Hickey, MS, RN
Director, Cardiovascular Patient Services
Department of Nursing
Children's Hospital
Boston, Massachusetts

Paul R. Hickey, MD
Professor of Anaesthesia
Harvard Medical School
Anesthesiologist-in-Chief
Children's Hospital
Boston, Massachusetts

Henry J. Issenberg, MD
Associate Professor of Pediatrics and Cardiothoracic Surgery
Director, Pediatric Heart Station
Albert Einstein College of Medicine
Montefiore Medical Center
Bronx, New York

Jeffrey Jacobs, MD
Attending Cardiovascular Surgeon
Director, Extracorporeal Membrane Oxygenation Program
Miami Children's Hospital
Miami, Florida

Richard A. Jonas, MD
William E. Ladd Professor of Surgery
Harvard Medical School
Cardiovascular Surgeon-in-Chief
Children's Hospital
Boston, Massachusetts

Frank Kern, MD
Associate Professor of Anesthesiology and Pediatrics
Chief of Pediatric Anesthesia
Duke University Medical Center
Duke Children's Hospital
Durham, North Carolina

Thomas J. Kulik, MD
Associate Professor of Pediatrics
University of Michigan Medical School
Medical Director, Pediatric Cardiothoracic Intensive Care Unit
C.S. Mott Children's Hospital
University of Michigan Hospitals
Ann Arbor, Michigan

Peter C. Laussen, MBBS, FANZCA
Assistant Professor of Anaesthesia
Harvard Medical School
Co-Director, Cardiac Anesthesia Service
Assistant Director, Cardiac Intensive Care Unit
Children's Hospital
Boston, Massachusetts

Alan B. Lewis, MD
Professor of Pediatrics
University of Southern California, School of Medicine
Associate Director of Cardiology
Children's Hospital of Los Angeles
Los Angeles, California

James E. Lock, MD
Alexander S. Nadas Professor of Pediatrics
Harvard Medical School
Cardiologist-in-Chief
Chairman of Cardiology
Children's Hospital
Boston, Massachusetts

Duncan J. Macrae, MB, FRCA, FRCPCH
Director, Cardiac Intensive Care Unit
Great Ormond Street Hospital for Sick Children
London, United Kingdom

Barry Marcus, MD
Director
Echocardiography Laboratory
Children's Hospital of Los Angeles
Los Angeles, California

Bradley S. Marino, MD, MPP
Fellow in Pediatric Cardiology
The Children's Hospital of Philadelphia
Philadelphia, Pennsylvania

Richard I. Markowitz, MD
Professor of Radiology
University of Pennsylvania School of Medicine
Deputy Radiologist-in-Chief
The Children's Hospital of Philadelphia
Philadelphia, Pennsylvania

John E. Mayer, Jr., MD
Professor of Surgery
Harvard Medical School
Senior Associate in Cardiac Surgery
Children's Hospital
Boston, Massachusetts

Jon N. Meliones, MD, FCCM
Professor of Pediatrics and Anesthesia
Chief, Division of Critical Care Medicine
Duke University Medical Center
Durham, North Carolina

David Paul Nelson, MD, PhD
Assistant Professor of Pediatrics
Co-Director, Cardiac Intensive Care Unit
Children's Hospital Medical Center
Cincinnati, Ohio

Christopher J.L. Newth, MB, FRCP (C)
Professor of Pediatrics
University of Southern California School of Medicine
Division of Pediatric Critical Care Medicine
Children's Hospital of Los Angeles
Los Angeles, California

James C. Perry, MD
Director, Electrophysiology and Pacing
Cardiology Division
Children's Heart Institute
San Diego, California

Mohan Reddy, MD
Assistant Professor of Surgery
University of California, San Francisco, School of Medicine
San Francisco, California

Andrew Redington, MD, FRCP
Professor of Congenital Heart Disease
National Heart and Lung Institute
Imperial College
Royal Brompton Hospital
London, United Kingdom

Jonathan J. Rome, MD
Assistant Professor of Pediatrics
University of Pennsylvania School of Medicine
Director, Cardiac Catheterization Laboratory
The Children's Hospital of Pennsylvania
Philadelphia, Pennsylvania

Anthony F. Rossi, MD
Assistant Professor of Pediatrics
Director, Pediatric Cardiac Intensive Care Unit
Mount Sinai Medical Center
New York, New York

Stephen J. Roth, MD, MPH
Assistant Professor of Pediatrics
Harvard Medical School
Assistant Director, Cardiac Intensive Care Unit
Associate in Cardiology
Children's Hospital
Boston, Massachusetts

Leslie Schoenberg, RN, MN, CPNP
Pediatric Clinical Coordinator
Lifetime Homecare and Kangaroo Kids
Marina Del Rey, California

Lara S. Shekerdemian, MD
National Heart and Lung Institute
Imperial College
Royal Bromptom Hospital
London, United Kingdom

Scott J. Soifer, MD
Professor and Vice Chair of Pediatrics
Director, Division of Pediatric Cardiac Intensive Care Medicine
Cardiovascular Research Institute
University of California, San Francisco, School of Medicine
San Francisco, California

Thomas L. Spray, MD
Chief, Cardiothoracic Surgery
The Children's Hospital of Philadelphia
Philadelphia, Pennsylvania

Vaughn A. Starnes, MD
Professor of Surgery
University of Southern California School of Medicine
Head, Division of Cardiothoracic Surgery
Childrens Hospital of Los Angeles
Los Angeles, California

David F. Teitel, MD
Professor of Pediatrics
Chief, Division of Pediatric Cardiology
Cardiovascular Research Institute
University of California, San Francisco, School of Medicine
San Francisco, California

Robert D. Truog, MD
Associate Professor of Anaesthesia and Pediatrics
Harvard Medical School
Director, Multidisciplinary Intensive Care Unit
Children's Hospital
Boston, Massachusetts

Richard Van Praagh, MD
Professor of Pathology
Harvard Medical School
Director of Cardiac Registry
Children's Hospital
Boston, Massachusetts

Edward P. Walsh, MD
Associate Professor of Pediatrics
Harvard Medical School
Director, Electrophysiologic Labs
Department of Cardiology
Children's Hospital
Boston, Massachusetts

Winfield Wells, MD
Associate Professor of Surgery
University of Southern California School of Medicine
Cardiothoracic Surgeon
Children's Hospital of Los Angeles
Los Angeles, California

Gil Wernovsky, MD, FACC
Associate Professor of Pediatrics
University of Pennsylvania School of Medicine
Director, Cardiac Intensive Care Unit
The Children's Hospital of Philadelphia
Philadelphia, Pennsylvania

David L. Wessel, MD
Associate Professor of Pediatrics and Anaesthesia
Harvard Medical School
Director, Cardiac Intensive Care Unit
Senior Associate in Cardiology
Children's Hospital
Boston, Massachusetts

Pierre C. Wong, MD
Assistant Professor of Pediatrics
University of Southern California School of Medicine
Director, Echocardiology and Transplant Cardiology
Children's Hospital Los Angeles
Los Angeles, California

Howard Alan Zucker, MD, FACC
Assistant Professor of Pediatrics and Anesthesiology
Columbia University College of Physicians and Surgeons
Pediatric Director, Intensive Care Unit
Babies and Children's Hospital of New York
New York, New York

Contents

Dedication v
Foreword by Aldo R. Castañeda vii
Preface ix
Acknowledgement xi
List of Contributors xiii
Color Plate xxi

Section I   Basic Principles in Cardiology

Chapter 1: Cardiac Anatomy
            Richard Van Praagh 3

Chapter 2: The Fetal and Neonatal Circulations
            Jeffrey R. Fineman and Scott J. Soifer 17

Chapter 3: Cardiac Physiology—Selected Topics in Normal Hearts
            David F. Teitel 25

Chapter 4: Cardiac Diagnostic Evaluation
            Anthony F. Rossi 37

Chapter 5: Cardiovascular Pharmacology
            Lara S. Shekerdemian and Andrew Redington 45

Chapter 6: Normal Physiology of the Respiratory System
            David Paul Nelson and David L. Wessel 67

Section II   Basic Principles in Intensive Care

Chapter 7: Principles of Sedation and Analgesia
            Peter C. Laussen and Paul R. Hickey 85

Chapter 8: The Airway and Mechanical Ventilation
            Howard Alan Zucker 95

Chapter 9: Cardiopulmonary Interactions
            Desmond Bohn 107

Chapter 10: Cardiopulmonary Resuscitation
            Duncan J. Macrae 127

Chapter 11: Invasive and Noninvasive Monitoring
            Ian Adatia and Peter N. Cox 137

Chapter 26:	Perioperative Issues in Other Organ Systems Eva Nozik Grayck, Jon N. Meliones, and Frank Kern 397	

Section IV Special Cardiac Evaluation and Management in Cardiac Intensive Care

Chapter 27: Perioperative Radiographic Studies
Richard I. Markowitz and Kenneth E. Fellows 407

Chapter 28: Echocardiography

    28.1 Principles of Echocardiography
           Steven D. Colan 425

    28.2 Perioperative Echocardiographic Examination in the Intensive Care Setting
           Abdul Aldousany and Barry Marcus 440

Chapter 29: Cardiac Catheterization in the Critically Ill Cardiac Patient
Jonathan J. Rome and James E. Lock 447

Chapter 30: Diagnosis and Management of Cardiac Arrhythmias
James C. Perry and Edward P. Walsh 461

Section V Diagnosis and Management of Acquired and Chronic Heart Disease

Chapter 31: The Failing Myocardium
Alan B. Lewis 483

Chapter 32: Pulmonary Hypertension
Thomas J. Kulik 497

Chapter 33: Miscellaneous Topics
Henry J. Issenberg 507

Section VI Issues in Cardiac Intensive Care

Chapter 34: Nursing Perspective in the Cardiac Intensive Care Unit
Patricia Hickey and Teresa Atz 519

Chapter 35: The Role of the Advanced Practice Nurse
Leslie Schoenberg and Barbara P. Gross 525

Chapter 36: Ethical and Legal Issues
Robert D. Truog 531

Appendix: Drugs 543

Index 549

Color Plate Section

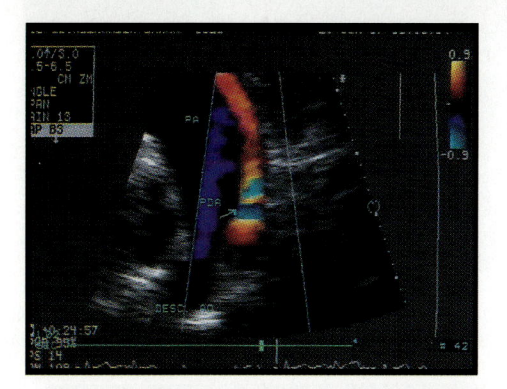

Figure 15.2.2. High parasternal view of an infant with a patent ductus arteriosus (PDA) (*arrow*) more clearly delineated with the aid of color Doppler flow mapping. The high velocity flow causes the color mapping to be mosaic colored. PA, pulmonary artery. DESC. AO, descending aorta.

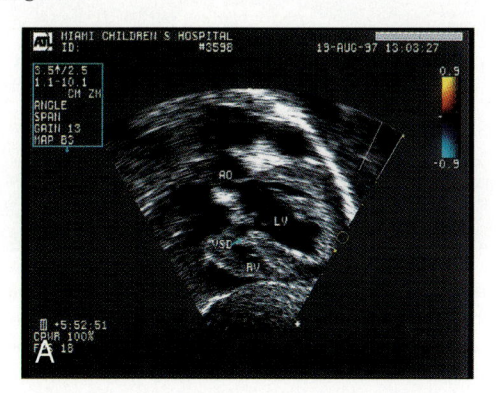

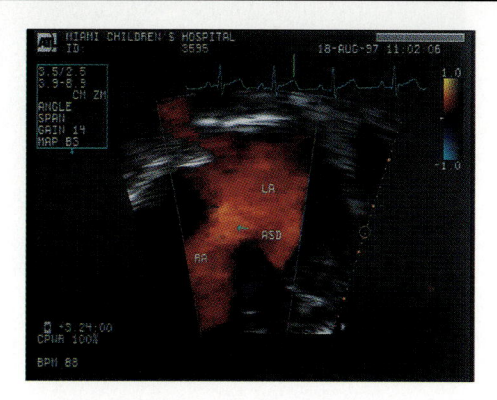

Figure 15.3.2. Subcostal view from a child with an atrial septal defect, secundum type. Left-to-right shunting is demonstrated by color Doppler flow mapping via a defect in the atrial septum (ASD) between the right (RA) and left atria (LA).

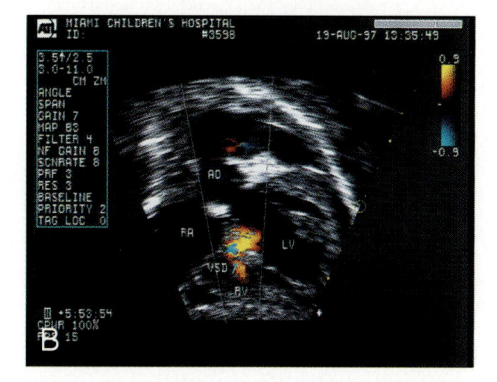

Figure 15.4.2. Subcostal four-chamber view from a child with membranous type of ventricular septal defect (VSD). In figure A, the VSD is visualized as a defect between the left ventricle (LV) and right ventricle (RV). There is tricuspid valve tissue as septal aneurysm (arrow) protruding into the RV and thus partially closing the defect. In figure B, color Doppler mapping shows left to right shunt (arrow) via the VSD.

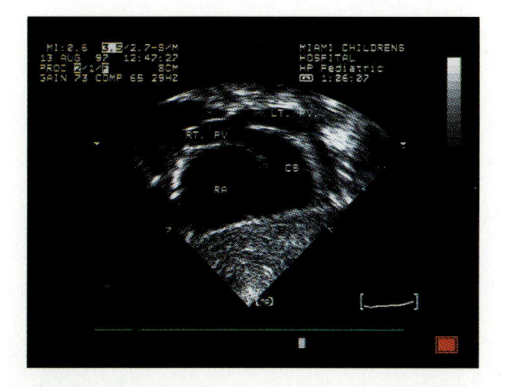

FIGURE 15.6.2. Subcostal view of an infant with total anomalous pulmonary venous return to the coronary sinus. This view shows a dilated coronary sinus (CS) into which the right pulmonary veins (RT.PV) and left pulmonary veins (LT.PV) drain. The right atrium (RA) also appears to be dilated.

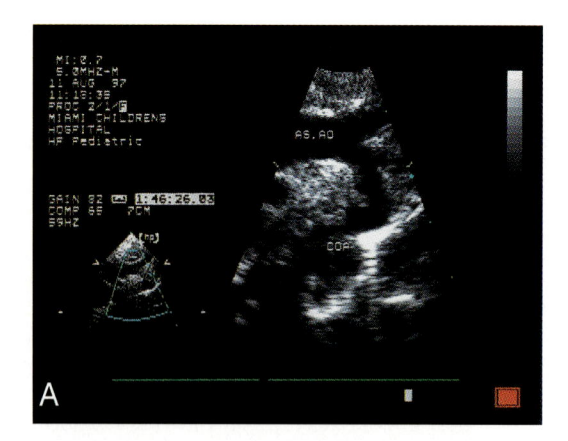

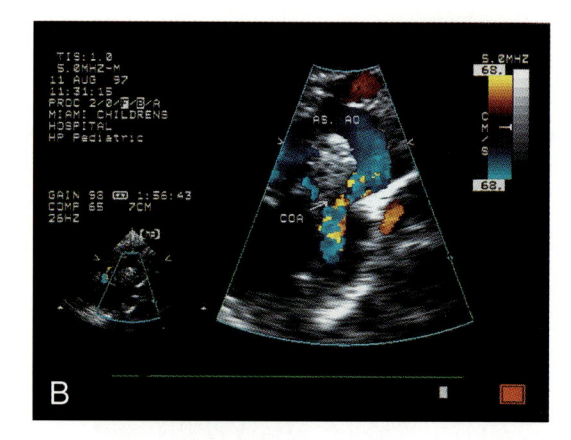

Figure 16.3.2. (**A**) Suprasternal long-axis view from an infant with coarctation of the aorta. AS. AO, ascending aorta. COA, coarctation. With color Doppler flow mapping (**B**), turbulence (*arrow*) is seen secondary to high velocity blood coursing through the area of coarctation.

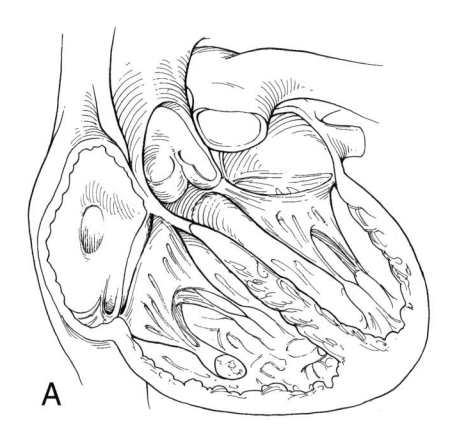

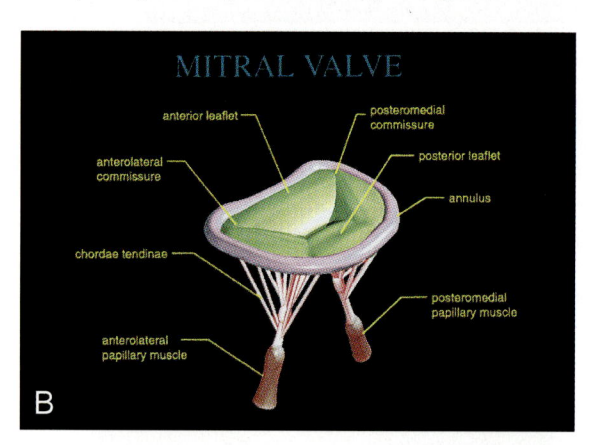

Figure 20.1.1. (**A**), Anatomy of the atrioventricular valves. Note that both the mitral and tricuspid valves are in fibrous continuity with the aortic annulus. The mitral valve has two distinct and well-developed papillary muscles with no cordal attachments to the interventricular septum, whereas the tricuspid valve has multiple small papillary muscles with major attachments to the interventricular septum. Congenital mitral valve abnormalities can occur at multiple sites along the entire mitral valve annulus, excessive thickening or redundancy of the mitral valve leaflet tissue itself, failure of development of the valve commissurae, elongation or shortening of the cordal structure, and abnormal development and positioning of the papillary muscles including solitary papillary muscle. These abnormalities can result in mitral valve stenosis, regurgitation, or both. (**B**), The mitral valve apparatus is composed of five parts: the valvular leaflets, the annulus, the chordae tendineae, the papillary muscles, and the left ventricular wall. This figure is a computer-generated image of the mitral valve (produced by Jeffrey A. White, MS).

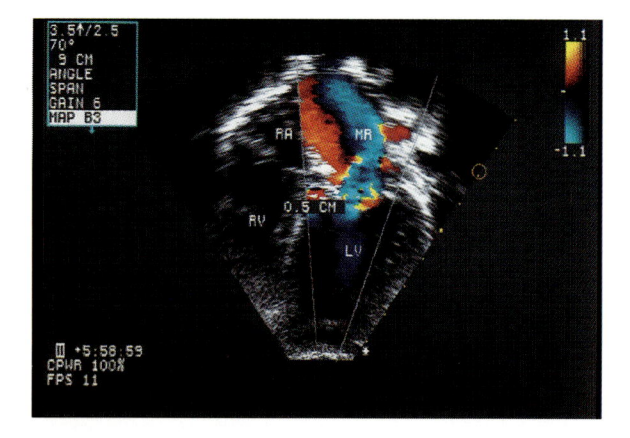

Figure 20.1.2. Apical four-chamber view from a child with mitral regurgitation (demonstrated by blue color Doppler jet and labelled MR).

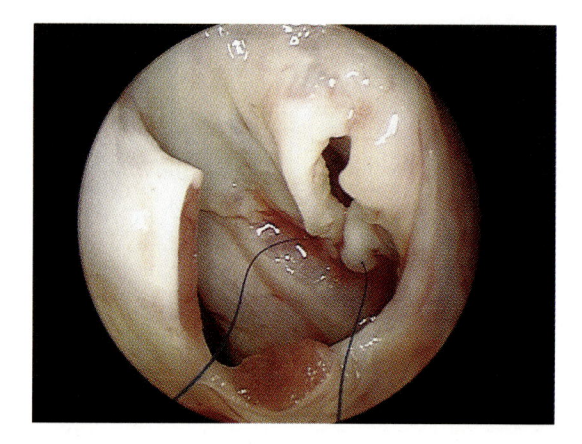

Figure 20.1.3. This intraoperative photograph demonstrates a cleft of the anterior mitral valve leaflet.

Color Plate   xxiii

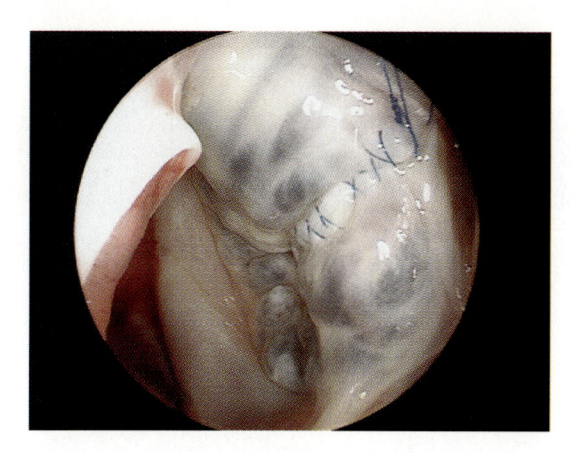

Figure 20.1.4. This intraoperative photograph demonstrates the cleft from Figure 20.1.3. after mitral valvuloplasty. The leaflets are suspended with saline and appear competent.

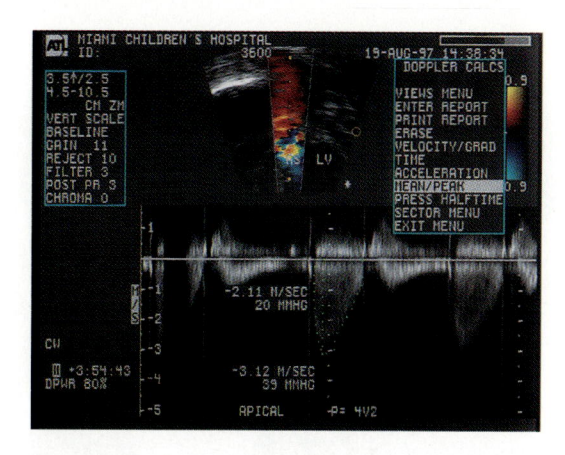

Figure 28.1.8. Aortic stenosis. From an apical view, the systolic gradient in a child with aortic stenosis (AS) is calculated using the Bernoulli equation (see text). The velocity of flow is measured at 3.12 M per second and the calculated gradient is 39 mm Hg. The color Doppler flow is used for localization of the stenotic region. LV, left ventricle.

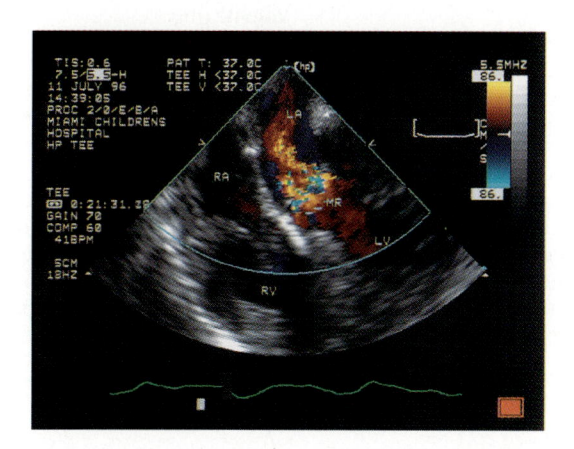

Figure 28.2.3. Mitral regurgitation. This transesophageal echocardiogram shows significant mitral regurgitation (labeled MR) after repair for primum atrial septal defect. RA, right atrium; RV, right ventricle; and LV, left ventricle.

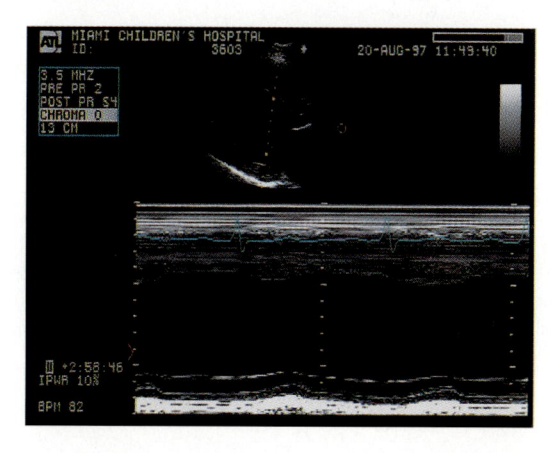

Figure 28.2.1. Shortening fraction. The M-mode echocardiogram of a child with cardiomyopathy and a dilated left ventricle shows gross appearance of diminished shortening fraction with little change in left ventricular dimensions. The shortening fraction is calculated by measurement of the left end-diastolic and end-systolic dimensions (see text).

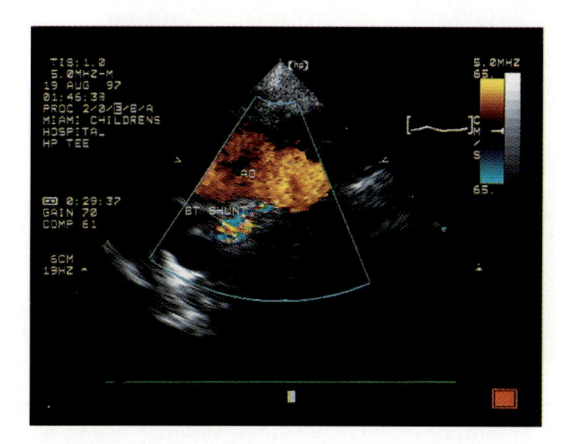

Figure 28.2.5. Aortopulmonary shunt. This color Doppler study from a patient with tetralogy of Fallot and Blalock-Taussig shunt at the suprasternal position shows mosaic-colored (high-velocity) shunt flow (BT SHUNT) arising from the aorta (AO).

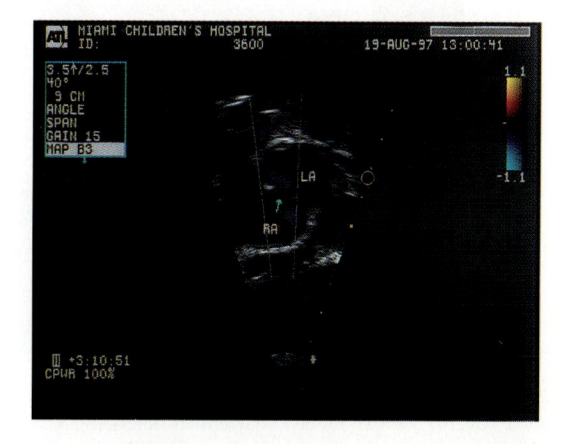

Figure 28.2.4. Right-to-left atrial shunt. This color Doppler flow study from subxiphoid position demonstrates right-to-left atrial level shunting (arrow pointing to blue-colored flow away from the transducer) via an atrial septal defect. RA, right atrium; LA, left atrium.

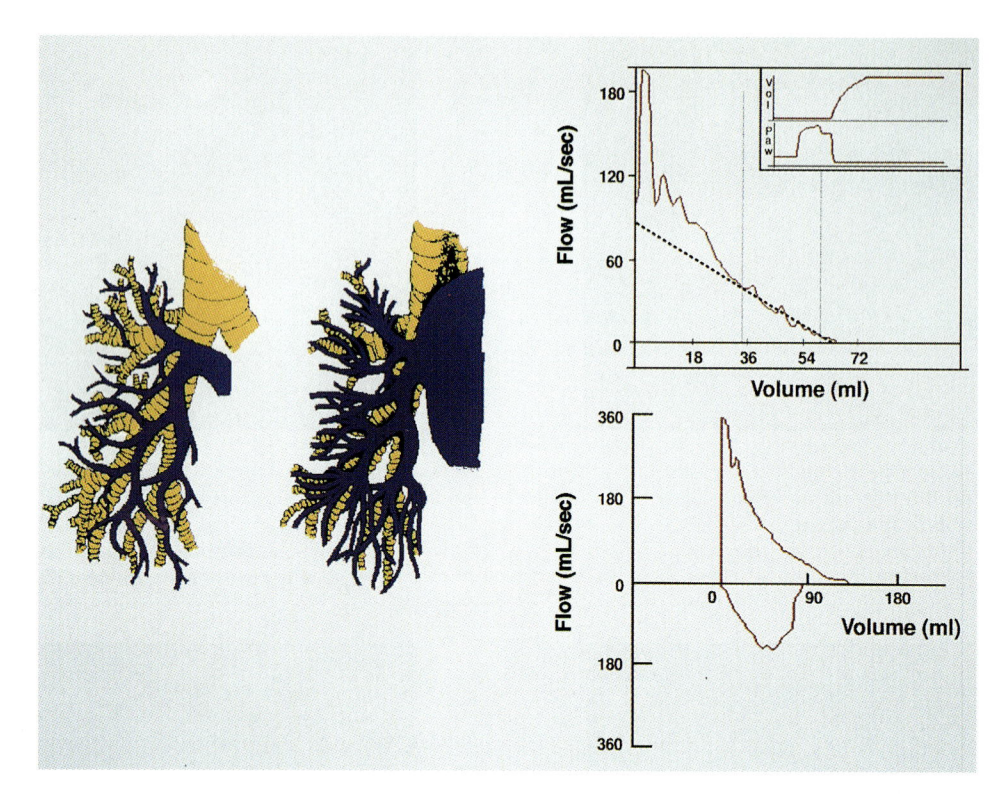

Figure 23.3. Pulmonary function in absent pulmonary valve syndrome. **Left.** Vascular compression by engorged pulmonary arteries and abnormal pulmonary artery branching in the absent pulmonary valve syndrome on the right compared with the normal anatomy on the left. **Upper right.** The concave passive flow-volume loop measured by single breath occlusion demonstrates obstructive airways disease in a 1-month-old child with absent pulmonary valve syndrome (APVS) with a markedly elevated respiratory resistance of 0.55 cm H_2O/mL/sec (normal: 0.04–0.10 cm H_2O/mL/sec). **Lower right.** The forced deflation flow-volume loop demonstrates small airway obstruction in the same infant. The forced vital capacity is within normal limits (55 mL/kg), but the maximal expiratory flow values are reduced (MEF_{25} = 12.3 mL/kg/sec).

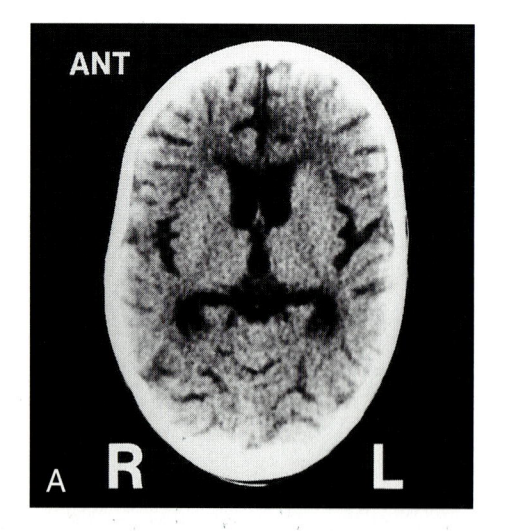

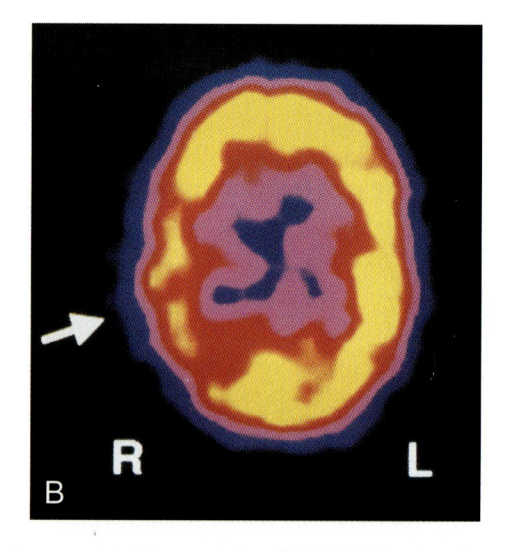

Figure 24.4. Brain computed tomography (CT) (**A**) and single photon emission computed tomography (SPECT) (**B**) scans in a patient who developed severe, persistent choreoathetosis following repair of pulmonary atresia. Brain CT scan shows moderate degree of global atrophic change but no focal area of injury. SPECT at an equivalent horizontal level shows decreased perfusion in the right temporoparietal and basal ganglia regions (arrow). (Reprinted with permission from du Plessis AJ, Treves ST, Hickey PR, et al. Regional cerebral perfusion abnormalities after cardiac operations. J Thorac Cardiovasc Surg 1994;107:1036–1043).

Section I:

Basic Principles in Cardiology

Cardiac Anatomy

Richard Van Praagh, MD

Morphologic anatomy and segmental anatomy are two of the most important keys to the diagnostic understanding and surgical management of congenital heart disease.

MORPHOLOGIC ANATOMY

In congenital heart disease, cardiac chambers are diagnosed in terms of their myocardial morphology, not in terms of relative position (such as right-sided or left-sided), nor in terms of the vessel or valve of entry or exit (such as aortic ventricle or pulmonary ventricle), and not in terms of the type of blood conveyed by the chamber (such as arterial, or venous, or mixed). The latter are variables in congenital heart disease, whereas the myocardial morphology is relatively constant (1–12).

Morphologically Right Atrium

The morphologically right atrium (RA) receives the inferior vena cava (IVC) and has a large, triangular, anterior atrial appendage (Fig. 1.1A). Normally, the RA also receives the superior vena cava (SVC); however, the SVC is not a highly reliable diagnostic marker of the RA, whereas the IVC is the medial venous component of the RA and the appendage is a sulcus known as the sulcus terminalis or the sinoatrial sulcus. Sulcus terminalis (terminal sulcus or depression) indicates that this sulcus marks the termination of the medial venous component of the RA and the beginning of the lateral muscular portion of the RA. Sinoatrial sulcus means that this mild depression lies at the junction of the sinus venosus medially and the right atrium (appendage) laterally. The significance of the sinoatrial sulcus (sulcus terminalis) is that this is where the pacemaker—the sinoatrial (SA) node—is located. The head of the SA node lies lateral to the SVC, immediately subepicardially, and its tail extends downward in the sulcus terminalis toward the IVC. The SA node is supplied in approximately 55% of people by the right coronary artery, and in approximately 45% by the left coronary artery. The sulcus terminalis (or sinoatrial sulcus) externally corresponds to the crista terminalis (terminal crest) internally.

The interior of the RA (Fig. 1.1B) is characterized by the ostium of the IVC. Another highly reliable diagnostic feature of the RA is the ostium of the coronary sinus (CoS); abnormally, however, the ostium of CoS is not always present, and when unroofed, the CoS can open into the morphologically left atrium (LA). Normally, the SVC opens into the RA; but abnormally, the SVC also can open into the LA.

The RA is that atrium which displays on its septal surface septum secundum (Sept II). The superior limbic band of Sept II lies medial to the entry of the SVC (to the left of the SVC in situs solitus, or to the right of the SVC in situs inversus). The inferior limbic band of Sept II lies inferior and somewhat anterior to septum primum (Sept I).

The superior limbic band (limbus = border, Latin) of Sept II consists of atrial musculature; it is the crista dividens (dividing crest, Latin) of the prenatal cardiovascular physiologists. The superior limbic band is the crest on which the returning blood from the placenta divides into the via sinistra (left road) and via dextra (right road). Normally, about 60% of the oxygenated inferior vena caval return takes the via sinistra to the left atrium, left ventricle, ascending aorta, and thence to the brain, whereas about 40% takes the via dextra to the right ventricle, main pulmonary artery, ductus arteriosus, and thence to the organs below the diaphragm.

The superior limbic band of Sept II is the limbic ledge, a useful landmark for those who perform cardiac catheterizations. When doing a Brockenbrough atrial septostomy to catheterize the LA, coming from the leg, the catheter is advanced into the right superior vena cava. Then with the tip of the catheter pointing toward the LA, the catheter is retracted, the tip pulled downward into the right atrium until the limbic ledge can be seen or felt. Just beneath the superior limbic band of Sept II, the catheter tip goes a little further leftward, indicating that it is just beneath the superior limbic band, and against the sealed septum primum. This is where the trans-septal catheter passage is performed.

The inferior limbic band of Sept II is a venous structure. Confusingly, the inferior limbic band of Sept II is the tissue from which Sept I and the left venous valve both develop. In other words, septum secundum of the anatomists is a composite structure when viewed with developmental understanding: the superior limbic band of Sept II is a muscular structure, the anterior interatrial plica; but the inferior limbic band of Sept II, as classically defined, is venous tissue—the sinus venosus tissue from which the left venous valve and septum primum both develop.

In view of its composite structure, when using the term septum secundum, we use it to mean the superior limbic

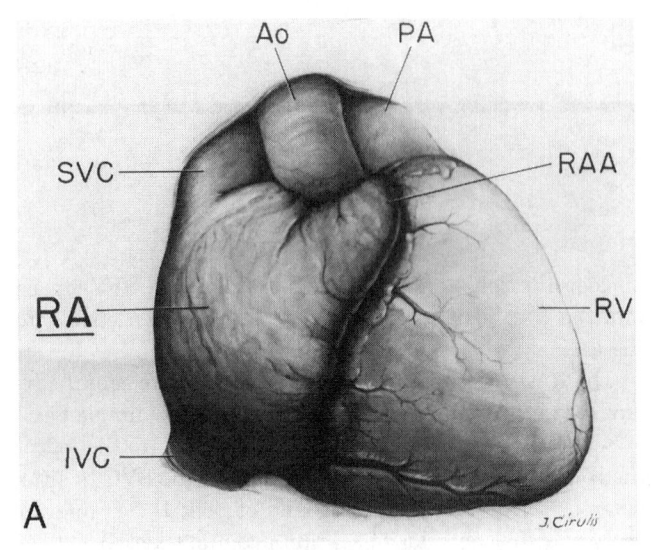

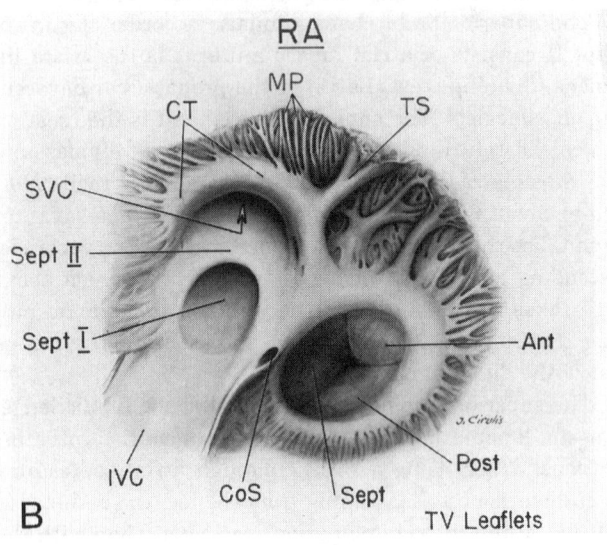

Figure 1.1. **A**. Exterior of the morphologically right atrium (*RA*), seen from the front. **B**. Interior of RA. *Ant*, anterior; *Ao*, aorta; *CoS*, coronary sinus; *CT*, crista terminalis (terminal crest); *IVC*, inferior vena cava; *MP*, musculi pectinati (pectinate muscles); *PA*, pulmonary artery; *post*, posterior; *RAA*, right atrial appendage; *RV*, morphologically right ventricle; *Sept*, septal; *Sept I*, septum primum; *Sept II*, septum secundum; *SVC*, superior vena cava; *TS*, tinea sagittalis (sagittal worm); *TV*, tricuspid valve. Reprinted with permission from Van Praagh R, Vlad P. Dextrocardia, mesocardia, and levocardia: the segmental approach to diagnosis in congenital heart disease. In: Keith JD, Rowe RD, Vlad P, eds. Heart disease in infancy and childhood, 3rd ed. New York: Macmillan Publishing Co, 1978;638–695.

Septum primum (Sept I), the flap valve of the foramen ovale, lies on the left atrial side of the atrial Sept II: to the left of Sept II in visceroatrial situs solitus (usual or normal atrial pattern, with RA right-sided), and to the right of Sept II in visceroatrial situs inversus (mirror-image pattern of the viscera and atria, in which the RA is left-sided).

Prenatally, the atrial septum is a unidirection flap valve or monocusp valve: septum primum is the valve or "door" that opens into the LA; and septum secundum is the "door jamb" against which Sept I closes (valva = door, Latin).

There are seven cardiac valves, not just four. In addition to the four obvious ones (tricuspid, mitral, pulmonary, and aortic), there are three more: the eustachian valve (of the IVC), the thebesian valve (of the CoS), and the atrial septum (Sept I and Sept II).

Sept I normally attaches on the left atrial side of the superior limbic band of Sept II. Normally, therefore, only the superior limbic band of Sept II is well seen from within the RA (Fig.1.1), because the left atrial attachments of Sept I normally cannot be seen from the RA aspect. Rarely, however, the attachments of Sept I can be seen from the RA aspect—when Sept II is absent or deficient, as can occur with visceral heterotaxy and polysplenia.

The ridge of muscle lateral to the entry of the SVC (to the right in situs solitus, to the left in situs inversus) is the crista terminalis (terminal crest) (Fig. 1.1B). The crista terminalis corresponds internally to the sulcus terminalis externally. From the surgical standpoint, deep sutures should not be placed in the crista terminalis, to avoid the sick sinus syndrome. In the Mustard procedure for D-transposition of the great arteries, the SVC part of the Mustard baffle often was attached to the crista terminalis, leading to thrombosis of the SA nodal artery (that runs through the SA node like a shishkabob skewer). Thrombosis of the SA nodal artery led to ischemic necrosis of the SA node, and hence to sick sinus syndrome. This same lesson concerning the surgical and conduction system significance of the crista terminalis (and the sulcus terminalis) can also apply to the modified Fontan-Kreutzer procedure, and particularly when a lateral tunnel is sutured into the right atrial orifice of the SVC (i.e., into the crista terminalis) (Fig. 1.1B).

The tinea sagittalis runs at right angles into the crista terminalis (Fig. 1.1A). The practical significance of the tinea sagittalis is that it is a favorite place for catheter tips to get stuck and lodged, just behind the tinea sagittalis. The catheter tip may appear far to the left, yet be very anterior. A little injudicious push of the catheter at this point can perforate the RA.

Musculi pectinati or pectinate muscles are prominent in the RA, because the right atrial appendage is incorporated into the cavity of the RA to a major degree. Musculi pectinati means comblike muscles (pecten = comb, Latin). Pectinate muscles, like the teeth of a comb, are unusually

band only—because the inferior limbic band appears in fact to be part of the origin of septum primum. To avoid confusion, we call the *inferior limbic band* just that; we do not call it the inferior limbic band of septum secundum, because we know that the inferior limbic band is intimately related to septum primum (not septum secundum).

parallel and do not crisscross. Hence, the right atrial appendage is like an accordion. It is compliant or distensible, and thin. This is why blood can be seen swirling around inside the RA in the operating room. The thin and compliant nature of the RA appendage is important for the diastolic function of the RA, which is to aspirate or suck the systemic venous blood back into the RA. Negative intrathoracic pressure can be conveyed to the venous blood via a normally thin-walled RA, but probably much less well via a markedly hypertrophied RA free wall.

The atrioventricular node and His bundle unfortunately are invisible; so it is important to know where these structures are. One of the better ways of localizing the AV node and the proximal unbranched portion of the His bundle is as follows (Fig. 1.1B): First, find the ostium of the coronary sinus. Then find pars membranacea septi (the membranous portion of the septum), which lies at the junction of the anterior and septal leaflets of the tricuspid valve. Remember that the membranous septum lies between the ventricles (the interventricular portion of the membranous septum) and between the left ventricle and the right atrium (the atrioventricular portion of the membranous septum). Then mentally draw a line between these two structures (the RA ostium of CoS and the membranous septum): this is exactly where the AV node and His bundle are. Even minor trauma to this region can result in permanent complete heart block; the AV node and bundle are immediately subendocardial.

Another way of localizing the AV node and His bundle is to use the triangle of Koch, within which these AV conduction tissues lie. The triangle of Koch is formed by (*a*) the tendon of Todaro (the invisible anterior extension of the eustachian valve of the IVC); (*b*) the thebesian valve of the CoS; and (*c*) the origin of the septal leaflet of the tricuspid valve. Because the tendon of Todaro is grossly invisible (but well seen histologically), the location of this tendon can be found by gently pulling on the eustachian valve. When pulling the eustachian valve gently inferiorly, its anterior extension—the tendon of Todaro—appears as a line or elevation. Even if the thebesian valve is poorly formed, the plane of the coronary sinus ostium can be seen. The origin of the septal leaflet of the tricuspid valve usually is easy to see. One of the problems with using the triangle of Koch to localize the AV node and bundle is that this triangle is too large. The coronary sinus—membranous septum line is more precise.

From anatomic and developmental standpoints, three main components make up the RA: (*a*) the sinus venosus (i.e., SVC, IVC, and CoS ostium), which lie medial to the crista terminalis; (*b*) the primitive atrium, the muscular atrial appendage; and (*c*) the AV canal (i.e., the AV canal septum, which is missing in common AV canal) plus a contribution to the leaflets of the TV, or the MV (depending on which type of ventricular loop is present).

Morphologically Left Atrium

The external appearance of the morphologically left atrium (LA) (Fig. 1.2A) is entirely different from that of the RA (Fig. 1.1A). The left atrial appendage is long and thin, as well as relatively small and posterior—like a pointing finger, or a windsock at an airport. Normally, the left atrial appendage remains an appendix—essentially not incorporated into the cavity of the LA. Normally, the pulmonary veins also connect with the LA.

The left atrium interior of the LA (Fig. 1.2B) confirms that the musculi pectinati of the LA are barely visible from within the LA cavity. Lack of incorporation of the appendage into the cavity of the LA has several consequences.

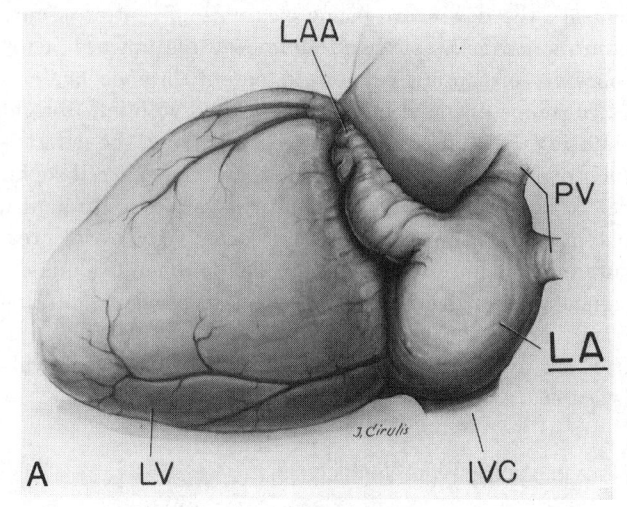

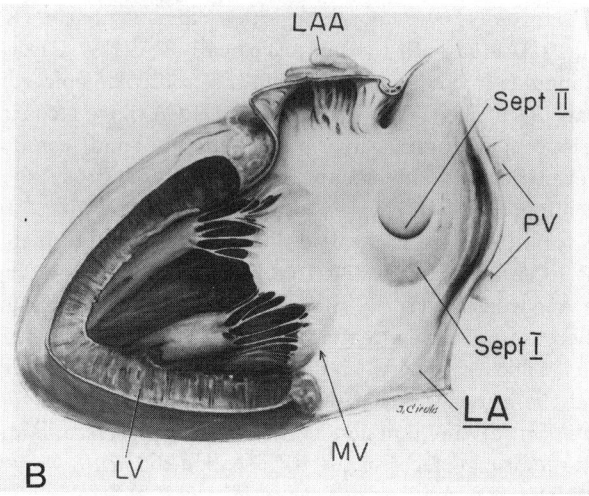

Figure 1.2. **A.** Exterior of morphologically left atrium (*LA*), left lateral view. **B.** Interior of LA. *LAA*, left atrial appendage; *LV*, morphologically left ventricle; *MV*, mitral valve; *PV*, pulmonary veins. Reprinted with permission from Van Praagh R, Vlad P. Dextrocardia, mesocardia, and levocardia: the segmental approach to diagnosis in congenital heart disease. In: Keith JD, Rowe RD, Vlad P, eds. Heart disease in infancy and childhood, 3rd ed. New York: Macmillan Publishing Co, 1978;638–695.

First, the LA is therefore less compliant, less distensible, than is the RA. Less compliance is appropriate for the LA because it has to eject into the thicker-walled and less compliant morphologically left ventricle (LV), whereas the RA has to eject into a thinner-walled and more compliant RV. Hence, form follows function. However, if and when atrial fibrillation occurs, the appendixlike shape of the appendage of the LA appears to predispose to the development of thrombi, which can be associated with strokes.

The ostium secundum is the space above septum primum. It is on the left atrial side of, and parallel to the atrial septum. The plane of ostium secundum is vertical and usually does not pass across the atrial septum.

The foramen ovale is an oval foramen that has right-left length. It passes horizontally across the atrial septum beneath the downward-facing concavity of septum secundum's superior limbic band and above the upward-facing concavity of septum primum. A patent foramen ovale is valve competent, and it is not associated with left-to-right shunting. If a left-to-right shunt is occurring, the defect is then regarded as an ostium secundum type of atrial septal defect. Rarely, right-to-left shunting can occur through a patent foramen ovale if, for any reason, right atrial pressure exceeds left atrial pressure. The foramen ovale is designed to open from RA to LA, but to prevent shunting from LA to RA.

Fossa ovalis (oval fossa) means that the foramen ovale is sealed. (A "fossa ovalis defect" is an oxymoron.)

Morphologically Right Ventricle

Externally, the morphologically right ventricle (RV) (Fig. 1.3A)–as with the morphologically RA (Fig. 1.1A)–is triangular in shape, as seen from the front. The epicardial branches of the right coronary artery (RCA) have a characteristic appearance. Superiorly, relatively small conal or preventricular branches are seen (Fig. 1.3A). Inferiorly, a prominent branch courses along the acute margin of the RV, and therefore it is called the acute marginal branch of the RCA (M in Fig. 1.3A). In anatomy (and in geometry), an angle less than 90° degrees is called an acute angle, whereas an angle greater than 90° is called an obtuse angle. The angle between diaphragmatic surface of the RV and the anterior surface of the RV typically is less than 90°. Hence, the junction between the anterior and diaphragmatic surfaces of the RV is called the *acute margin*, and the coronary artery running along this margin is therefore known as the *acute marginal branch* (as mentioned above). The acute marginal branch of the RCA supplies the anterior papillary muscle of the RV and the adjacent RV free wall. The anterior descending coronary artery (AD in Fig. 1.3A) indicates the location of the interventricular septum. Hence, by external inspection and palpation, the surgeon can tell where the RV stops and the LV (the morphologically left ventricle) begins. Hence, by external inspection and palpation, in addition to identifying the RV, its size and wall thickness (hypertrophy or hypoplasia) can also be assessed by palpation.

Internally, the morphologic features of the RV are highly characteristic (Fig. 1.3B)—and different from those of the LV. The tricuspid valve (TV, Fig. 1.3B) is the atrioventricular (AV) valve that opens into the RV; the TV may or may not open out of the RA; when discordant L-loop ventricles coexist, the TV opens out of the LA. The morphology of the AV valves corresponds to that of the ventricles of entry, not to that of the atria of exit. The tricuspid valve has been described as "septophilic" (i.e., it attaches to the right ventricular septal surface, as well as to the right ventricular free wall).

The number of tricuspid valve leaflets is variable. In infancy, the TV often appears only to have two leaflets, parietal and septal. But throughout most of adolescent and adult life, the TV has three leaflets because the parietal (free wall) leaflet is subdivided into anterior and posterior portions by the chordal insertions from the anterior papillary muscle (AP, Fig. 1.3B). In old age, particularly after several bouts of congestive heart failure, an infundibular leaflet appears—just beneath the conal septum and between the anterior and septal leaflets of the TV. Because the number of TV leaflets varies from two to four, the TV cannot be identified reliably by counting leaflets. The depths of the TV leaflets are all approximately the same, although the anterior leaflet usually is somewhat deeper than the others.

The papillary muscles of the TV are numerous, small, and arise both from the septal and the free wall surfaces. Some of these small papillary muscles are little more than trabeculae carneae. Because the papillary musculature of the TV is relatively small, a right ventriculotomy can readily be performed. The situation in the LV is very different.

The trabeculae carneae (fleshy ridges) of the RV are coarse, few, and straight (different from those of the LV).

The conal septum, just beneath the pulmonary valve in the normal heart, is also called the *parietal band* (PB in Fig. 1.3B) because it runs onto the parietal or free wall of the RV.

The septal band (SB in Fig. 1.3B), also regarded as a conal structure, runs along the anterosuperior portion of the right ventricular septal surface. The septal band continues into the moderator band (MB in Fig. 1.3B), which bridges the RV cavity and inserts into the right ventricular free wall (FW in Fig. 1.3B) via the anterior papillary muscle of the RV.

The subpulmonary conus consists of the conal septum and the adjacent subpulmonary free wall. The conal septum has also been called the *parietal band* because it ex-

Cardiac Anatomy 7

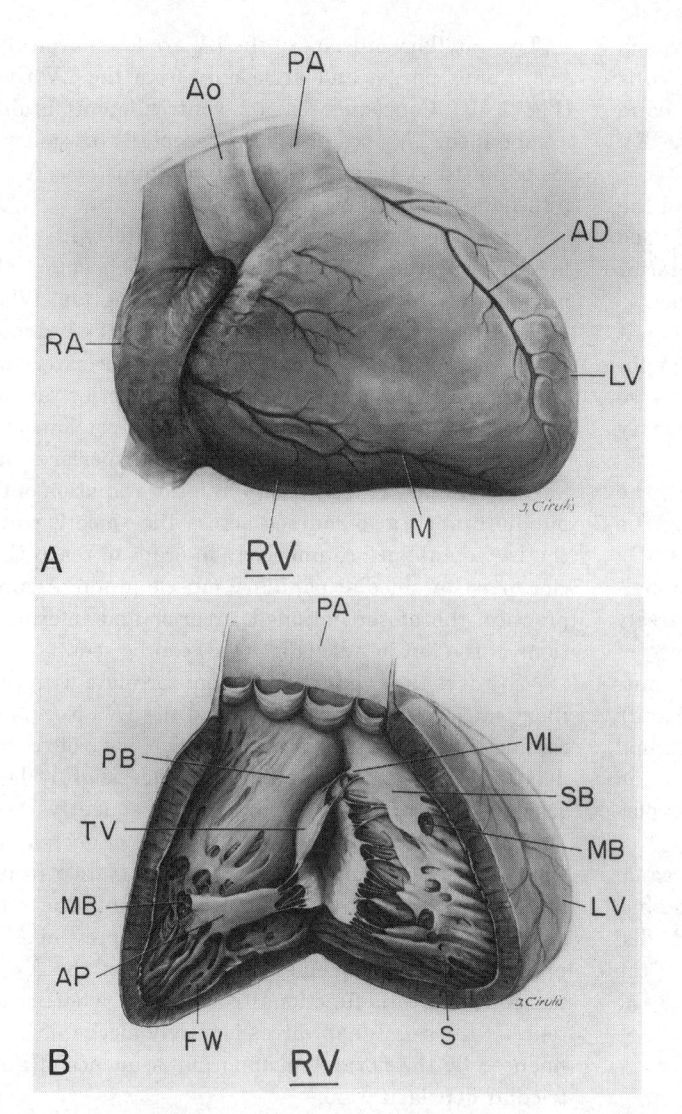

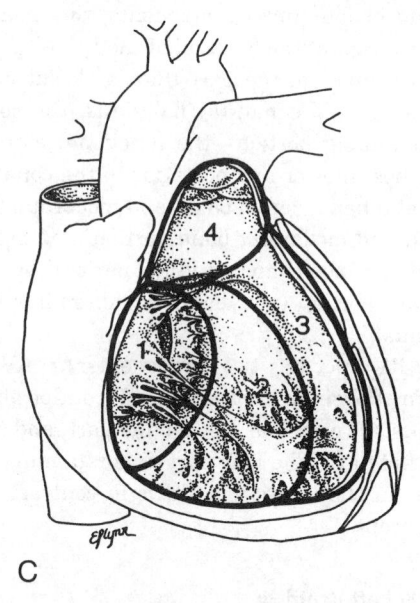

Figure 1.3. A. Exterior of morphologically right ventricle (RV), viewed from the front. B. Interior of RV. AD, anterior descending coronary artery; Ao, aorta; AP, anterior papillary muscle; FW, free wall; LV, morphologically left ventricle; M, acute marginal branch of right coronary artery; MB, moderator band; ML, muscle of Lancisi; PA, pulmonary artery; PB, parietal band; RA, right atrium; S, septum; SB, septal band; TV, tricuspid valve. Reprinted with permission from Van Praagh R, Vlad P. Dextrocardia, mesocardia, and levocardia: the segmental approach to diagnosis in congenital heart disease. In: Keith JD, Rowe RD, Vlad P, eds. Heart disease in infancy and childhood, 3rd ed. New York: Macmillan Publishing Co, 1978;638–695. C. The four main anatomic and developmental components of the RV: (1) atrioventricular canal; (2) sinus; (3) septal band (proximal conus); and (4) parietal band (distal subsemilunar conus). Components 1 and 2 = RV inflow tract. Components 3 and 4 = RV outflow tract. Reprinted with permission from Van Praagh R, Geva T, Kreutzer J. Ventricular septal defects: how shall we describe, name, and classify them? J Am Coll Cardiol 1989;14:1298–1299.

tends onto the parietal or free wall of the RV. The central subsemilunar portion, beneath the septal commissures of the semilunar valves (at the aortopulmonary septum), is the conal septum, accurately speaking; whereas the parietal or free wall extension is not really the conal septum. Interposition of the subpulmonary conus prevents pulmonary valve-AV valve direct fibrous continuity.

The right bundle branch of the AV conduction system passes immediately beneath the membranous septum, which is located behind and slightly below the muscle of Lancisi (ML in Fig. 1.3B). (The muscle of Lancisi is also known as the muscle of Lushka, or the medial papillary muscle, or the papillary muscle of the conus.) The right bundle passes just beneath this papillary muscle of the conus and proceeds down the septal band, paralleling the inferior margin of the septal band and being located approximately one third of the distance from the inferior to the superior margin of the septal band. With a little practice, it is usually possible to see the right bundle branch grossly. It is a linear yellowish-white structure that runs down the septal band and across on the moderator band to the anterior papillary muscle and thence into the RV free wall.

The correlation between the conduction system and the papillary musculature is noteworthy. The RV has only one really well-formed papillary muscle group—the anterior papillary muscle (Fig. 1.3B). The right bundle branch is the superior radiation. The RV has no inferior radiation, it is thought, because it has no other sizeable inferior papillary muscle group (as there is in the LV). The RV is also regarded as a one coronary ventricle (the right coronary artery).

From an anatomic and developmental standpoint, the RV is made up of four main components, this being the quadripartite concept of the RV (and of the LV) (Fig. 1.3C): (a) AV canal or junction, the part that is absent or malformed in common AV canal; (b) RV sinus, the coarsely trabeculated pumping portion—the functional essence of the RV—that lies inferior and posterior to the conal musculature (parietal band, septal band, and moderator band); (c) septal band and moderator band portion (i.e., proximal or apical portion of the conus); and (d) parietal band and related free-wall portion (i.e., distal or subsemilunar portion of the conus).

Hence, the RV inlet has two components: (a) AV canal portion, and (b) RV sinus portion. The RV outlet also has two components: (a) proximal septal band part, and (b) distal parietal band part. The four-part understanding of the RV helps explain the location of VSDs in contrast to the "tripartite" concept.

Morphologically Left Ventricle

Externally, the morphologically left ventricle (LV) displays a conical configuration, reminiscent of a torpedo or a bullet. The margin of the LV free wall is described as obtuse, meaning that it describes an angle of greater than 90°. The obtuse marginal or diagonal arteries (D in Fig. 1.4A) are highly characteristic, and they supply the anterolateral and posteromedial papillary muscles and the adjacent LV free wall myocardium.

Internally, the morphologic features of the LV (Fig. 1.4B) are distinctive and different from those of the RV (Fig. 1.3B). The mitral valve (MV) has been described as "septophobic," meaning that it never normally attaches to the LV septal surface, but arises only from the LV free wall surface. The anterior leaflet of the MV is deep and curtainlike, being well designed to occlude an approximately circular systemic AV orifice. The posterior leaflet, by contrast, is a shallow fringe. The anterior leaflet of the MV is the "door," and the posterior leaflet is the "door jamb."

The papillary muscles of the LV are few—typically only two groups, large, and arise only from the LV free wall (Fig. 1.4B). Consequently, left ventriculotomy is difficult, except at the LV apex or high paraseptally (coronary arteries permitting), because the LV free wall is largely covered internally by papillary muscles.

Again, the conduction system correlates with the papillary musculature. The left bundle branch enters the LV immediately beneath the membranous septum. When the great arteries are normally related, the membranous septum lies immediately beneath the right coronary-noncoronary commissure of the aortic valve. Superior radiation of the left bundle courses across the smooth portion of the left ventricular septal surface to reach the superior or anterolateral papillary muscle group. Inferior radiation of the left bundle branch also courses across the smooth portion of the LV septal surface inferiorly in order to reach the inferior or posteromedial papillary muscle group. Again, with practice, the aforementioned superior and inferior radiations of the left bundle (Fig. 1.4B) can be seen.

Why does the conduction system correlate with the papillary muscles, in both the RV and the LV? Normally, the conduction system brings the accession wave of ventricular depolarization to the papillary muscles slightly before it reaches the ventricular free walls. Consequently, the papillary muscles normally go into a state of increased tone slightly before the onset of ventricular systole to prevent the AV valve leaflets from being blown into the atria, resulting in AV valve regurgitation (i.e., to prevent AV valve prolapse and its sequelae). Competence of the AV valves has an important functional component, whereas competence of the semilunar valves is purely mechanical—not influenced by the normal or abnormal sequence of atrioventricular depolarization.

The trabeculae carneae of the LV are distinctive (Fig. 1.4B) and different from those of the RV (Fig. 1.3B). The superior one half to two thirds of the LV septal surface is smooth, whereas the inferior one third to one half of the LV septal surface has numerous, fine, oblique trabeculae carneae that form a latticelike mesh. Hence, from a diagnostic standpoint, the LV typically appears finely or minimally trabeculated (Fig. 1.4B), whereas the RV appears coarsely trabeculated (Fig. 1.3B).

Normal absence of the subaortic conal free-wall myocardium permits aortic-mitral direct fibrous continuity (Fig. 1.4B). The conal septum lies beneath the right coronary leaflet of the aortic valve.

The subaortic landmarks are surgically important for transaortic surgical procedures. When the great arteries are normally related (Fig. 1.4B), the right coronary-noncoronary commissure of the aortic valve sits right above the membranous septum and the left bundle branch of the conduction system. The noncononary-left coronary commissure is located directly above the anterior leaflet of the mi-

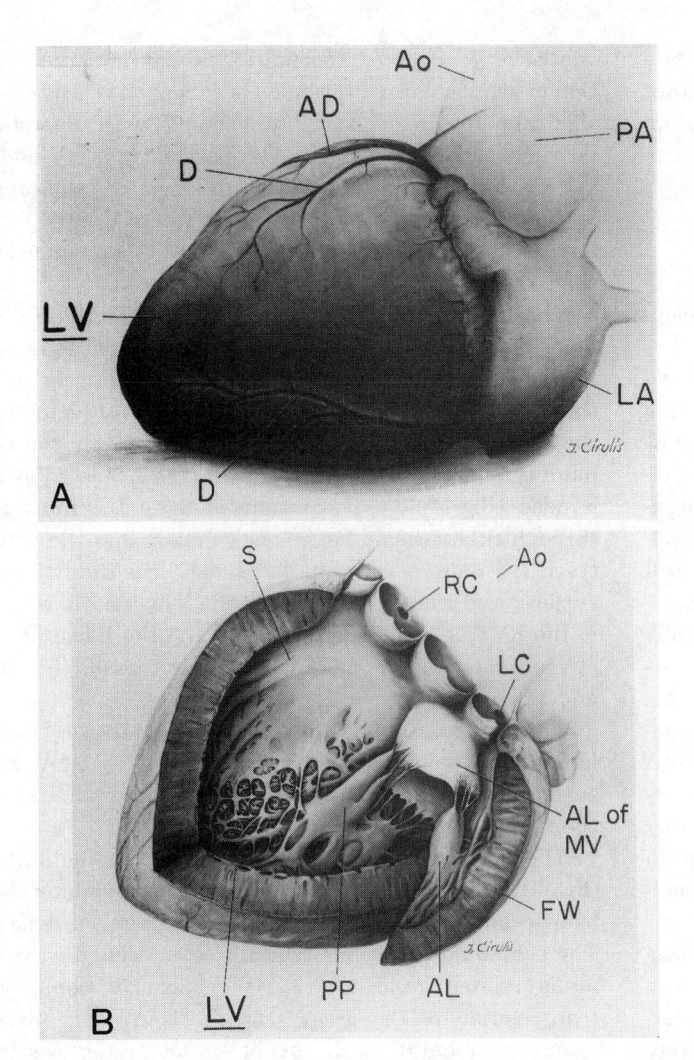

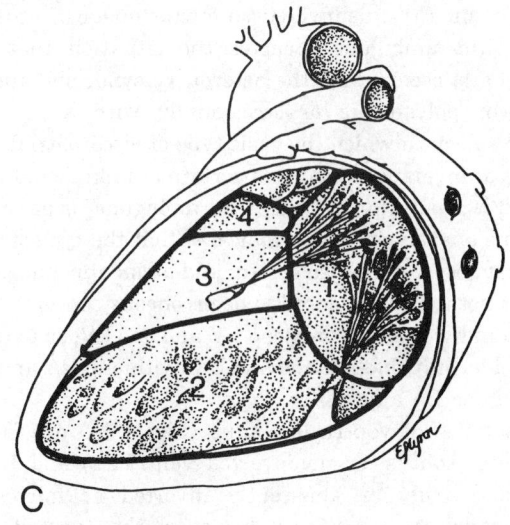

Figure 1.4. A. Exterior of morphologically left ventricle (*LV*), left posterolateral view. **B.** Interior of LV. *AD*, anterior descending coronary artery; *AL*, anterolateral (papillary muscle); *AL of MV*, anterior leaflet of mitral valve; *Ao*, aorta; *D*, diagonal or obtuse marginal branches of the left coronary artery; *FW*, free wall; *LA*, left atrium; *LC*, left coronary (ostium); *MV*, mitral valve; *PP*, posteromedial papillary (muscle); *RC*, right coronary (ostium); *S*, septum. Reprinted with permission from Van Praagh R, Vlad P. Dextrocardia, mesocardia, and levocardia: the segmental approach to diagnosis in congenital heart disease. In: Keith JD, Rowe RD, Vlad P, eds. Heart disease in infancy and childhood, 3rd ed. New York: Macmillan Publishing Co, 1978;638–695. **C.** The four main anatomic and developmental components of the LV: (**1**) atrioventricular canal; (**2**) sinus; (**3**) proximal conus; and (**4**) distal or subsemilunar conus. Components 1 and 2 = LV inflow tract. Components 1, 3 and 4 = LV outflow tract. Reprinted with permission from Van Praagh R, Geva T, Kreutzer J. Ventricular septal defects: how shall we describe, name, and classify them? J Am Coll Cardiol 1989;14:1298–1299.

tral valve. The intercoronary commissure is right above the conal septum.

Again, the LV is composed of four main component parts (Fig. 1.4C): (*a*) AV canal component, that is so abnormal in common AV canal; (*b*) finely trabeculated LV sinus; (*c*) smooth superior portion of the LV septal surface that is the proximal part of the conus (and is trans-septally continuous with the septal band on the RV side); and (*d*) distal or subsemilunar part of the conus, beneath the right coronary leaflet and the intercoronary commissure with normally related great arteries.

The LV is the ancient systemic pump of the Chordates (humans belong to Phylum Chordata, which includes all animals with a notochord). From the functional standpoint, the LV is a thing of beauty. Phylogenetically, it is about 500 million years old, dating back to our ancient fish ancestors.

The RV is equally beautiful from a functional standpoint, but probably only about 200 million years old, dating from the evolution of mammals. The RV sinus is the lung pump. The conus performs an "arterial switch operation" during embryogenesis. Both the lung pump (RV sinus) and the arterial switch mechanism (conus) are adaptations to air-breathing and land-living. Most of what we call congenital heart disease are developmental errors in these adaptations to our terrestrial, air-breathing lifestyle: anomalies of septation, malformations of conotruncus (infundibulum and great arteries), and anomalies of the tricuspid valve and RV sinus.

SEGMENTAL ANATOMY

The cardiac segments are the anatomic and developmental components out of which all human hearts are made. The three main segments are (a) atria, (b) ventricles, and (c) great arteries. The two connecting segments are the AV canal (junction) and the conus (infundibulum).

The two types of visceroatrial situs (Fig. 1.5) are (a) situs solitus, the usual or normal pattern of anatomic organization, and (b) situs inversus, a mirror-image of situs solitus. "Situs ambiguus" denotes the situation that still occasionally occurs with the heterotaxy syndrome and asplenia or polysplenia or occasionally with a normally formed spleen in which the basic type of visceroatrial situs (solitus or inversus) remains uncertain or unknown. In this respect, it is noteworthy that "situs ambiguus" is not a specific type of situs; it merely indicates that the type of situs is undiagnosed. Atrial isomerism and atrial appendage isomerism both are considered to be erroneous concepts. Just as each individual has only one RV and one LV, so too each person has only one RA and one LA (with one RA appendage and one LA appendage).

Two types of ventricular situs (Fig. 1.6A) are D-loop ventricles (solitus, or noninverted ventricles) and L-loop ventricles (truly or apparently inverted or mirror-image ventricles). Sometimes, however, the type of ventricular situs may not be clear, as with superoinferior ventricles, crisscross atrioventricular relations, and single ventricle. With these anomalies, the conventional definition of ventricular noninversion or inversion relative to the sagittal plane breaks down. For example, with superoinferior ventricles and crisscross AV relations, both RV and LV are right-sided and left-sided. With single RV and no vestige of an LV, how can one identify where the LV should have been? The brief answer is: chirality or handedness (Fig. 1.6B and 1.6C).

The D-loop RV is right-handed (Fig. 1.6B). Literally or figuratively, with a D-loop RV, the thumb of one's right hand goes through the tricuspid valve, one's fingers go into the RV outflow tract, the palm of only the right hand faces the RV septal surface, and the dorsum of only the right hand is adjacent to the RV free wall. The L-loop RV is left-handed (Fig. 1.6C). The thumb of one's left hand goes through the tricuspid valve, one's fingers into the outflow tract, the palm of only the left hand faces the RV septal surface, and the dorsum of only the left hand is adjacent to the RV free wall. The D-loop RV and the L-loop RV are stereoisomers, as are one's right and left hands (Fig. 1.6B and 1.6C).

Chirality also applies to the LV. The D-loop LV is left-handed: the palm of only the left hand faces the LV septal surface. The L-loop LV is right-handed: the palm of only the right hand faces the LV septal surface.

The four anatomic types of conus (infundibulum) are (Fig. 1.7): (a) subpulmonary, (b) subaortic, (c) bilateral (subaortic and subpulmonary), and (d) absent or deficient. The subpulmonary conus typically is associated with normally related great arteries; the subaortic conus with transposition of the great arteries (TGA); the bilateral conus frequently with double-outlet right ventricle (DORV); and the absent or deficient subsemilunar conus rarely can be associated with double-outlet left ventricle

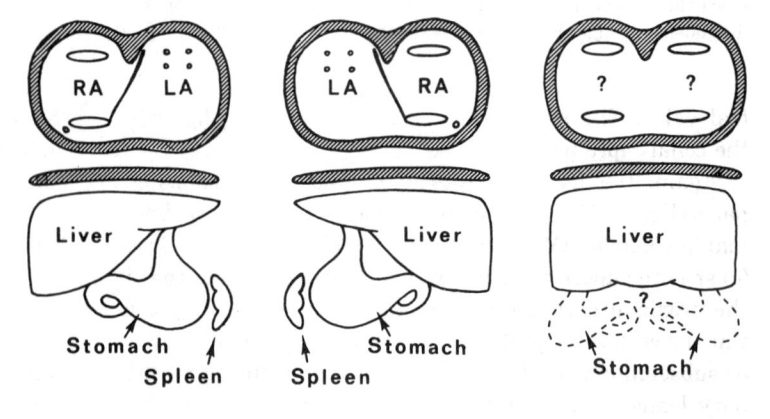

Figure 1.5. The two types of visceroatrial situs, diagnostically important for atrial localization. In "situs ambiguus" with visceral heterotaxy, the situs of the viscera and the atria may be undiagnosed(?). Situs ambiguus (undiagnosed situs) is not a specific third type of visceroatrial situs. *LA*, left atrium; *RA*, right atrium. Reprinted with permission from Van Praagh R. The segmental approach to diagnosis in congenital heart disease. In Bergsma D, ed. Birth Defects: Original Article Series 1972;8:4–23.

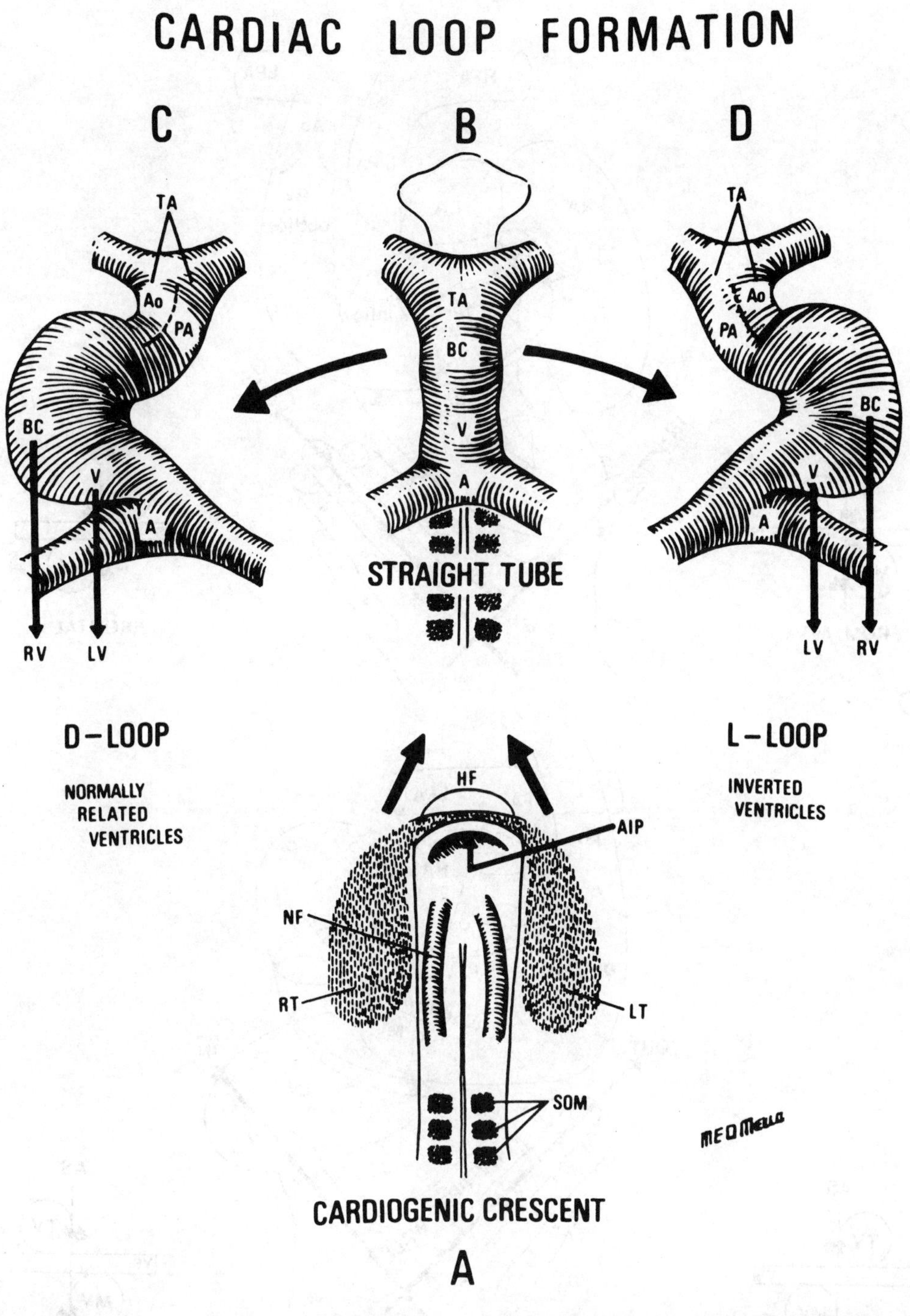

CARDIAC LOOP FORMATION

Figure 1.6. **A.** Cardiac loop formation, viewed from ventral aspect. The cardiogenic crescent of precardiac mesoderm resembles an upside-down horseshoe. The left (*LT*) and right (*RT*) halves migrate cephalad and medially on the foregut endoderm (*arrows*), forming a straight heart tube. Normally, the straight heart tube loops or folds in a rightward (dextro = right, Latin) direction, forming a D-loop with solitus or normally related ventricles. The morphologically right ventricle (*RV*), derived from the proximal portion of the bulbus cordis (*BC*), lies to the right of the morphologically left ventricle (*LV*), which is derived from the ventricle (*V*) of the bulboventricular loop. Abnormally, the straight heart tube loops or folds in a leftward (levo = left, Latin) direction, forming an L-loop. L-loop formation is associated with ventricular inversion, RV lying to the left of the LV. Reprinted with permission from Van Praagh R. The segmental approach to understanding complex cardiac lesions. In: Eldridge WJ, Goldberg H, Lemole GM, eds. Current problems in congenital heart disease. New York: SP Medical and Scientific Books, 1979:1–18.

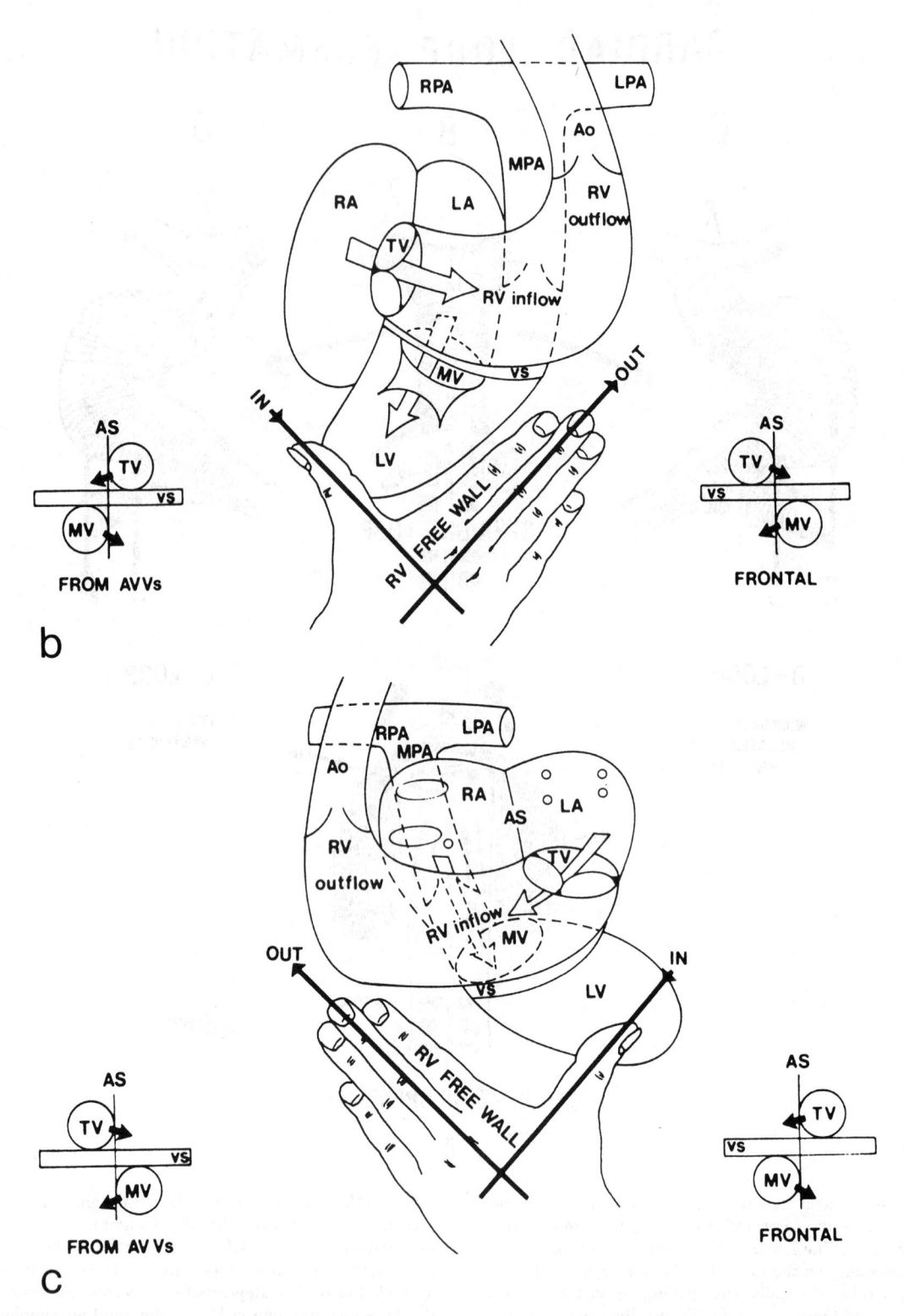

Figure 1.6 (*Continued*). **B.** The D-loop RV is right-handed. **C.** The L-loop RV is left-handed. *A*, primitive atrium; *AIP*, anterior intestinal portal; *Ao*, aorta; *AS*, atrial septum; *AVVs*, atrioventricular valves; *HF*, head fold; *NF*, neural fold; *LPA*, left pulmonary artery; *MPA*, main pulmonary artery; *MV*, mitral valve; *PA*, pulmonary artery; *RPA*, right pulmonary artery; *SOM*, somites; *TA*, truncus arteriosus; *TV*, tricuspid valve; *VS*, ventricular septum. Reprinted with permission from Van Praagh S, LaCorte M, Fellows KE, et al. Superoinferior ventricles, anatomic and angiocardiographic finding in 10 postmortem cases. In: Van Praagh R, Takao A, eds. Etiology and morphology of congenital heart disease. Mt Kisco, NY: Futura, 1980:317–378.

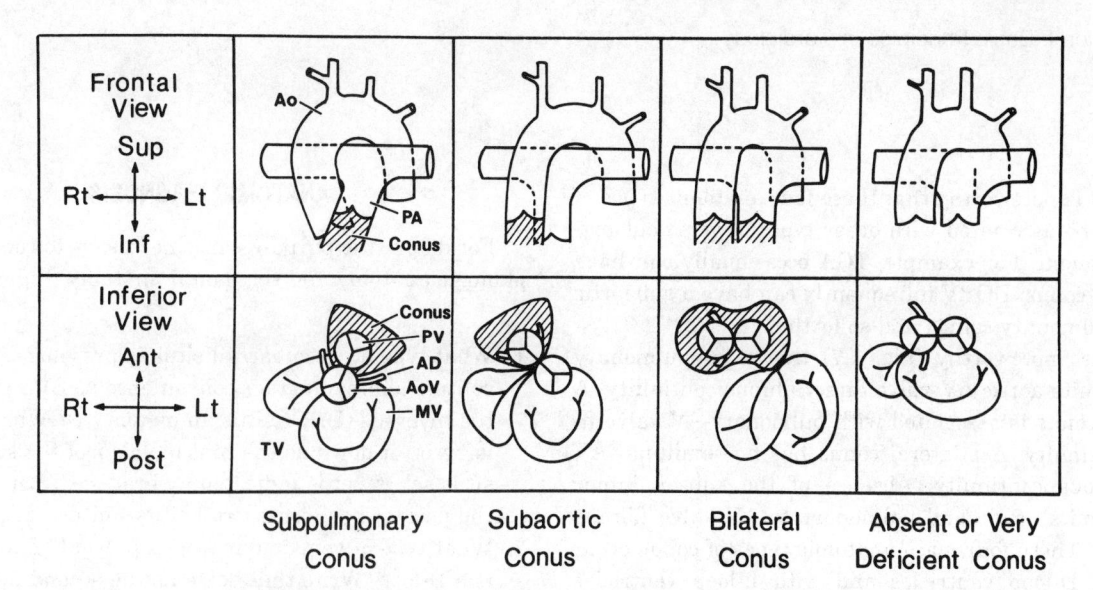

Figure 1.7. Anatomic types of subsemilunar infundibulum (conus arteriosus). *AD*, anterior descending coronary artery; *Ant*, anterior; *Ao*, aorta; *AoV*, aortic valve; *Inf*, inferior; *Lt*, left; *MV*, mitral valve; *PA*, main pulmonary artery; *Post*, posterior; *PV*, pulmonary valve; *Rt*, right; *Sup*, superior; *TV*, tricuspid valve. Reprinted with permission from Van Praagh R, Vlad P. Dextrocardia, mesocardia, and levocardia: the segmental approach to diagnosis in congenital heart disease. In: Keith JD, Rowe RD, Vlad P, eds. Heart disease in infancy and childhood, 3rd ed. New York: Macmillan Publishing Co, 1978;638–695.

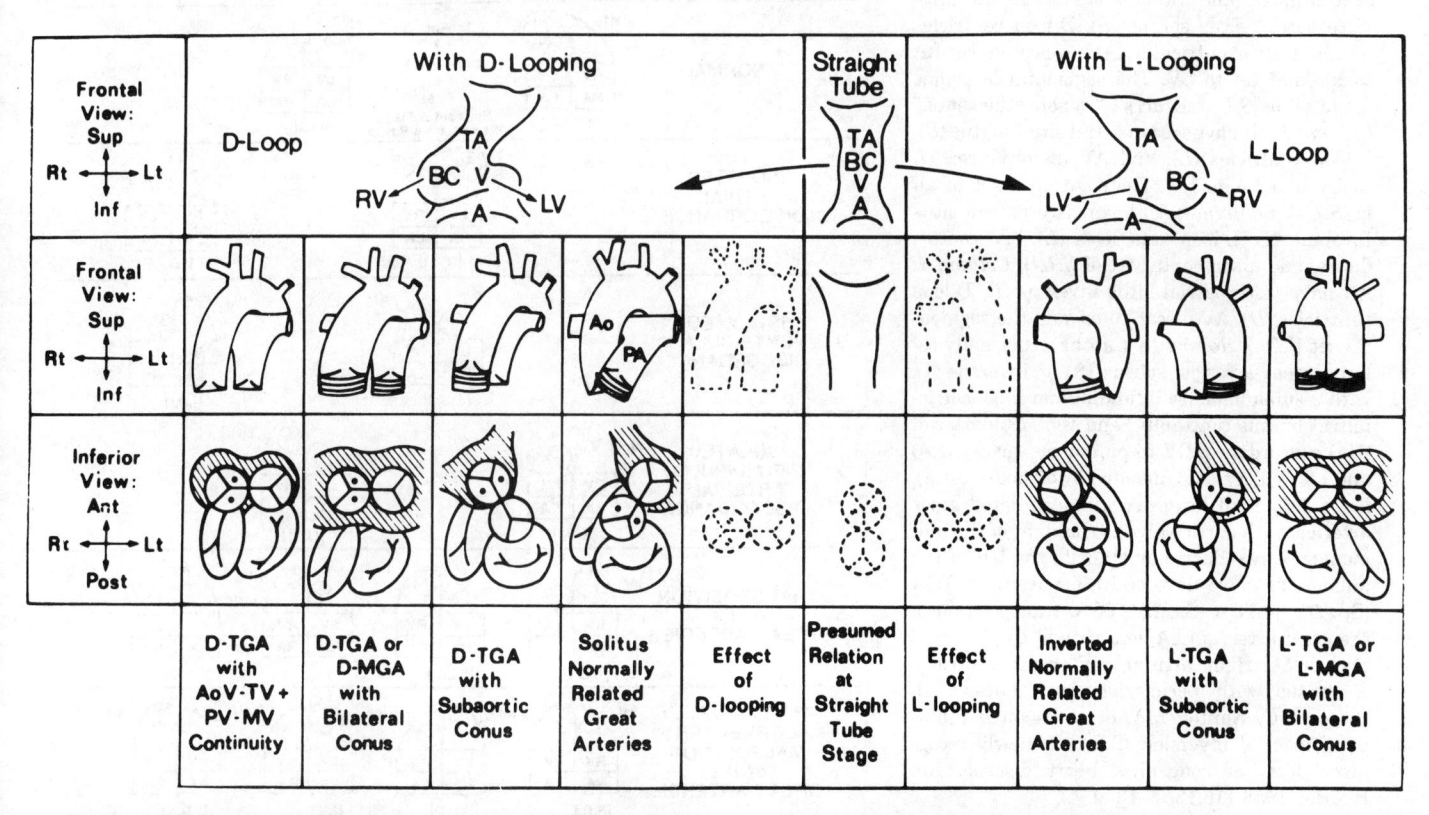

Figure 1.8. Variations in conotruncal (infundibuloarterial) anatomy with D-loop and L-loop ventricles. A subpulmonary conus with aortic-mitral fibrous continuity occurs with solitus normally related great arteries and D-loop ventricles, and with inverted normally related great arteries and L-loop ventricles. A subaortic conus with pulmonary-mitral fibrous continuity is typical of D-transposition of the great arteries (*D-TGA*) with D-loop ventricles, and of the L-transposition of the great arteries (*L-TGA*) with L-loop ventricles. A bilateral conus (subaortic and subpulmonary) with no semilunar-atrioventricular fibrous continuity can occur with D-TGA and D-malposition of the great arteries (*D-MGA*), with double-outlet right ventricle, double-outlet left ventricle, and anatomically corrected malposition of the great arteries and D-loop ventricles, and with L-TGA and L-malposition of the great arteries (*L-MGA*) and L-loop ventricles. A bilaterally absent conus can rarely occur with D-TGA and aortic-tricuspid fibrous continuity and pulmonary-mitral fibrous continuity with D-loop ventricles. We have never observed L-TGA with bilaterally absent conus with L-loop ventricles; hence this possibility is not diagramed. *A*, atrium; *BC*, bulbus cordis; *Inf*, inferior; *Lt*, left; *LV*, morphologically left ventricle; *Post*, posterior; *Rt*, right; *RV*, morphologically right ventricle; *TA*, truncus arteriosus; *V*, ventricle. Reprinted with permission from Van Praagh R, Van Praagh S. Isolated ventricular inversion, a consideration of the morphogenesis, definition, and diagnosis of nontransposed and transposed great arteries. Am J Cardiol 1966;17:395–406.

(DOLV). It is noteworthy that these four anatomic types of conus can be associated with other types of ventriculoarterial alignment. For example, TGA occasionally can have a bilateral conus; DORV infrequently can have a subaortic or a subpulmonary conus, and so forth.

It is also noteworthy (Fig. 1.7) that a subpulmonary conus permits aortic-AV valve direct fibrous continuity. A subaortic conus is associated with pulmonary-AV valve fibrous continuity. A bilateral conus has no semilunar-AV valve fibrous continuity. Absence of the subsemilunar conus permits aortic and pulmonary to AV valve fibrous continuity. These four main anatomic types of conus occur both with D-loop ventricles and with L-loop ventricles (Fig. 1.8).

ANATOMIC DIAGNOSIS

For diagnostic purposes, it is necessary to combine morphologic anatomy and segmental anatomy (Fig. 1.9).

1. What type of visceroatrial situs is present? Is it situs solitus (abbreviated for convenience as S)? Or is it situs inversus (I)? Or situs ambiguus (A)? Whatever it is, write it down as the first member of the segmental situs set. A set is indicated by braces: {}. Let us say the patient has viseroatrial situs solitus: {S,-,-}.
2. What type of ventricular loop is present? Let us say it is a D-loop. Write that down as the second member of the segmental situs set: {S,D,-}.

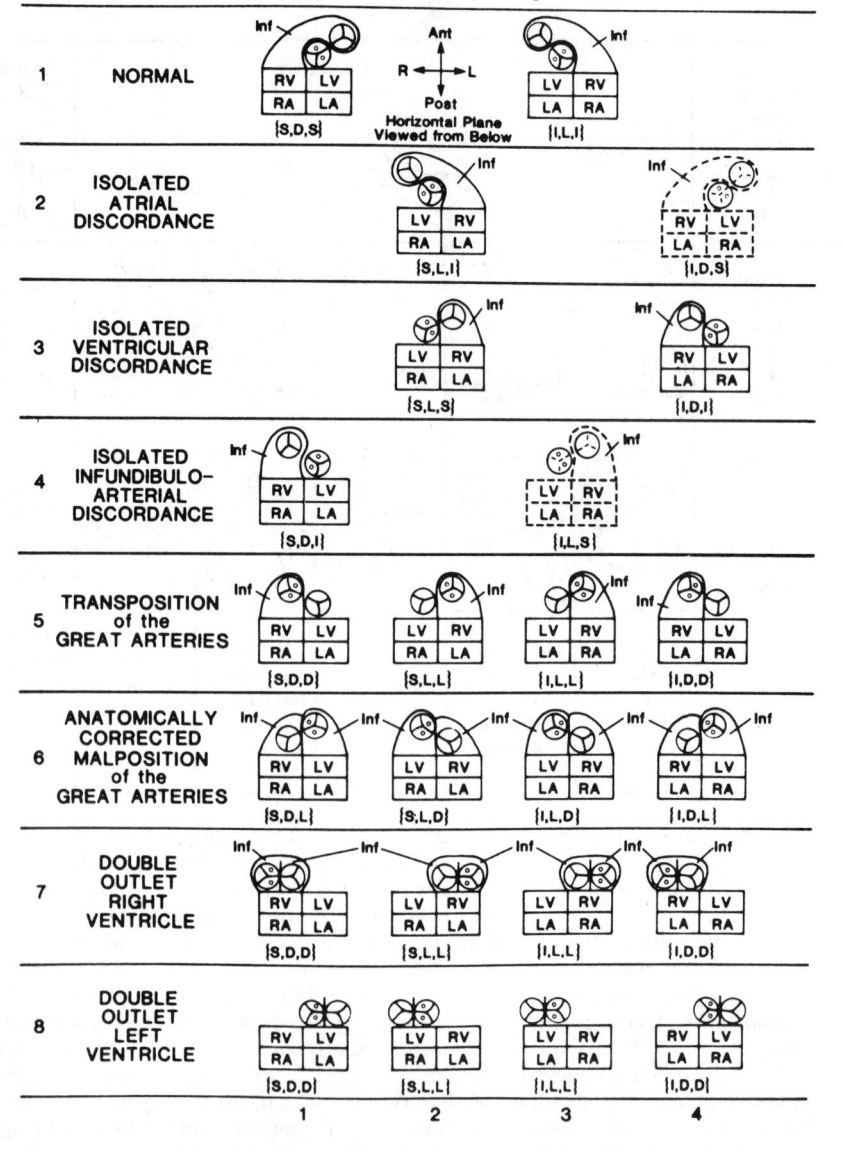

Figure 1.9. Types of human heart, anteroinferior view (similar to subxiphoid two-dimensional echocardiographic view). *Column 1*: All have visceroatrial situs solitus (S), D-loop ventricles (*D*), and atrioventricular (*AV*) concordance: RA to RV and LA to LV. The segmental anatomic set in all is {*S,D,-*}. Braces { } denote "the set of." *Column 2*: all have visceroatrial situs solitus (*S*), L-loop ventricles (*L*), and AV discordance: RA to LV and LA to RV. The segmental set in all is {*S,L,-*}. *Column 3*: All have visceroatrial situs inversus (*I*), L-loop ventricles (*L*), AV concordance, and a segmental set of {*I,L,-*}. *Column 4*: All have visceroatrial situs inversus (*I*), D-loop ventricles (*D*), AV discordance, and the segmental set {*I,D,-*}. *Rows 1 to 4* all have normally related great arteries: solitus (*S*) or inversus (*I*), with a subpulmonary infundibulum (*Inf*), aortic-mitral fibrous continuity, and ventriculoarterial (*VA*) concordance: RV to pulmonary artery (*PA*) and LV to aorta (*Ao*) (denoted by coronary ostia). *Rows 5 to 8* all have abnormally related great arteries, with aortic valve to the right of the pulmonary valve (dextro or D) or to the left of the pulmonary valve (levo or L), for example, TGA {S,D,*D*}, or TGA {S,L,*L*}. (TGA, transposition of the great arteries.) *LA*, left atrium; *LV*, left ventricle; *RA*, right atrium; *RV*, right ventricle. Reprinted with permission from Foran RB, Belcourt C, Nanton MA, et al. Isolated infundibuloarterial inversion {S,D,I}: a newly recognized form of congenital heart disease. Am Heart J 1988;116:1337–1350.

3. What is the status of the great arteries? Let us say that the aortic valve is anterior and to the right of the pulmonary valve. So, some sort of D-malposition of the great arteries is present. Write that down as the third member of the segmental situs set: {S,D,D}.
4. What are the ventriculoarterial alignments? Is TGA present (aorta from RV and pulmonary artery from LV)? Or is DORV present (aorta and pulmonary artery both from RV)? Let us say it is TGA. Write the ventriculoarterial alignments in front of the segmental situs set: TGA {S,D,D}. (It should be understood that TGA is one type of ventriculoarterial malalignment; others include DORV, DOLV, and so forth.)
5. What type of conus is present? Let us say that a subaortic conus is present. Write that down, if you wish, after the segmental situs set: TGA {S,D,D} with subaortic conus. One may choose to omit the anatomic type of conus, because a subaortic conus is so frequent with D-TGA.
6. What associated malformations, if any, are present? Let us say that the patient has a ventricular septal defect (VSD), with posterior malalignment of the conal septum resulting in pulmonary outflow tract stenosis (PS). Add these associated malformations to your diagnosis: TGA {S,D,D} with subaortic conus, VSD, and PS.
7. Are there any acquired changes of significance, including therapeutic procedures? Let us say the patient has had a Rastelli procedure with a right ventricular-to-pulmonary artery conduit, and has been experiencing some chest pains recently. So now the diagnosis becomes: TGA {S,D,D} with subaortic conus, VSD, PS, and status post Rastelli procedure, with chest pain.
8. Now the physician is ready to act. Diagnosis never stops. A two-dimensional echocardiogram or an MRI is obtained, revealing that a neo-pseudointima has partly detached from the wall of the dacron conduit. A "peel" dissection or thromboembolus may be imminent. The medical team and the family may well decide to proceed with surgery, to exchange the old dacron conduit for a new homograft conduit. But in the never-ending "chess game" of clinical medicine, the physician must already be looking ahead, wondering what the next move will be. Follow-up with vigilant diagnosis and timely management will continue.

SUMMARY

Morphologic anatomy (Figs. 1.1 to 1.4) and segmental anatomy (Figs. 1.5 to 1.9) are basic parts of patient diagnosis and management.

REFERENCES

1. Lev M. Pathologic diagnosis of positional variations in the cardiac chambers in congenital heart disease. Lab Invest 1954;3:71–82.
2. Van Praagh R, Ongley PA, Swan HJC. Anatomic types of single or common ventricle in man, morphologic and geometric aspects in sixty autopsied cases. Am J Cardiol 1964;13:367–386.
3. Van Praagh R, Van Praagh S, Vlad P, et al. Anatomic types of congenital dextrocardia, diagnostic and embryologic implications. Am J Cardiol 1964;13:510–531.
4. Melhuish BPP, Van Praagh R. Juxtaposition of the atrial appendages, a sign of severe cyanotic congenital heart disease. Br Heart J 1968;30:269–284.
5. Van Praagh R. The segmental approach to diagnosis in congenital heart disease. In: Bergsma D, ed. Birth Defects: Original Article Series 1972;8:4–23.
6. Kirklin JW, Pacifico AD, Bargeron LM, et al. Cardiac repair in anatomically corrected malposition of the great arteries. Circulation 1973;48:153–159.
7. Shinebourne EA, Macartney FJ, Anderson RH. Sequential chamber localization–logical approach to diagnosis in congenital heart disease. Br Heart J 1976;38:327–339.
8. Otero Coto E, Quero Jiménez M. Aproximación segmentaria al diagnóstico y clasificación de las cardiopatías congènitas, fundamentos y utilidad. Rev Esp Cardiol 1977;30:557–566.
9. Stanger P, Rudolph AM, Edwards JE. Cardiac malpositions, overview based on study of sixty-five necropsy specimens. Circulation 1977;56:159–172.
10. Rao PS. Systematic approach to differential diagnosis. Am Heart J 1981;102:389–403.
11. Van Praagh R, Van Praagh S. Morphologic anatomy. In: Fyler DC, ed. Nadas' pediatric cardiology. Philadelphia: Hanley & Belfus, 1992:17–26.
12. Van Praagh R. Segmental approach to diagnosis. In: Fyler DC, ed. Nadas' pediatric cardiology. Philadelphia: Hanley & Belfus, 1992:27–35.
13. Van Praagh R, Vlad P. Dextrocardia, mesocardia, and levocardia: the segmental approach to diagnosis in congenital heart disease. In: Keith JD, Rowe RD, Vlad P, eds. Heart disease in infancy and childhood, 3rd ed. New York: Macmillan Publishing Co, 1978:638–695.
14. Van Praagh R, Geva T, Kreutzer J. Ventricular septal defects: how shall we describe, name, and classify them? J Am Coll Cardiol 1989;14:1298–1299.
15. Van Praagh R. The segmental approach to understanding complex cardiac lesions. In: Eldridge WJ, Goldberg H, Lemole GM, eds. Current problems in congenital heart disease. New York: SP Medical and Scientific Books, 1979:1–18.
16. Van Praagh S, LaCorte M, Fellows KE, et al. Superoinferior ventricles, anatomic and angiocardiographic finding in 10 postmortem cases. In: Van Praagh R, Takao A, eds. Etiology and morphogenesis of congenital heart disease. Mt Kisco, NY: Futura, 1980:317–378.
17. Van Praagh R, Van Praagh S. Isolated ventricular inversion, a consideration of the morphogenesis, definition, and diagnosis of nontransposed and transposed great arteries. Am J Cardiol 1966;17:395–406.
18. Foran RB, Belcourt C, Nanton MA, et al. Isolated infundibuloarterial inversion {S,D,I}: a newly recognized form of congenital heart disease. Am Heart J 1988;116:1337–1350.

The Fetal and Neonatal Circulations

Jeffrey R. Fineman, MD, and Scott J. Soifer, MD

Dramatic changes occur in the cardiovascular system at birth. The fetal circulation is characterized by parallel circulations, intracardic shunts, high pulmonary vascular resistance, and relatively low cardiac output. Gas exchange occurs in the placenta. The neonatal circulation is characterized by series circulations, no intracardiac shunts, low pulmonary vascular resistance, and relatively high cardiac output. Gas exchange occurs in the lungs. An understanding and appreciation of these different circulations with their transition and the clinical relevance of these principles are essential for caretakers in the intensive care setting who care for critically ill newborns and infants with congenital heart disease.

FETAL CIRCULATION

Fetal Blood Flow Patterns

Fetal circulation has large shunts between the right and left atria (the foramen ovale) and between the pulmonary artery and the aorta (the ductus arteriosus) (Fig. 2.1, Panel A). There is nonuniform blood flow in the fetus produced by these central shunts as well as by the anatomic structures.

Visualization of the inferior vena cava in fetal sheep demonstrates the interesting streaming pattern of fetal blood flow. Less oxygenated blood appears to run along the lateral wall of the inferior vena cava. A large proportion of this stream crosses the tricuspid valve and enters the right ventricle. More oxygenated blood appears to run along the medial wall of the inferior vena cava. A large proportion of this stream is directed into the left atrium, crosses the mitral valve, and enters the left ventricle. Because of the streaming pattern of fetal blood, the right ventricle receives relatively desaturated blood with decreased substrate concentration when compared with the left ventricle. Right ventricular output is then directed to the umbilical-placental circulation (for oxygen and substrate uptake), and left ventricular output is directed to the fetal body (for oxygen and substrate delivery).

Cardiac output of the two ventricles is in parallel in the fetus, whereas it is in series after birth. In the late gestation fetal lamb, total combined output of the right and left ventricles is approximately 400 mL/min.kg, with about 60% distributed to the fetal body and 40% distributed to the umbilical-placental circulation. In the late gestation fetal lamb, PaO_2 and oxygen saturation are 23–25 mm Hg and 60 to 65% in the left ventricle and 20–22 mm Hg and 55 to 60% in the right ventricle. The right ventricle receives poorly oxygenated blood from the superior vena cava (from the brain and upper fetal body) and coronary sinus (from the heart), and more highly oxygenated blood from the inferior vena cava, which is a mixture of highly oxygenated blood from the umbilical-placental circulation (from the ductus venosus and left hepatic veins) and poorly oxygenated blood from the lower fetal body (Fig. 2.1, Panel B). It then ejects this blood (approximately two thirds of combined ventricular output, CVO) into the main pulmonary trunk, through the ductus arteriosus into the descending aorta (87% of right ventricular output or 57% of CVO), and to the lower fetal body (27% of right ventricular output) and the placenta (60% of right ventricular output).

Because of the high pulmonary vascular resistance, only a small percentage of blood (13% of right ventricular output or 8% of CVO) enters the pulmonary circulation (see below). The left ventricle receives more highly oxygenated blood via the inferior vena cava from the ductus venosus, which is directed by the eustachian valve across the foramen ovale, and a small amount of poorly oxygenated blood from the lungs. The left ventricle then ejects this blood (approximately one third of CVO) into the ascending aorta to supply the heart (8% of left ventricular output or 3% of CVO), brain, and upper fetal body (63% of left ventricular output or 22% of CVO). A smaller percentage of left ventricular output (29% of left ventricular output or 10% of CVO) crosses the aortic isthmus to the descending aorta (1–5).

Fetal Vascular Pressure

Because of the foramen ovale, the right and left atrial pressures are equal. In the late gestation fetal lamb, vena caval and left atrial pressures are 3–5 mm Hg and 2–4 mm Hg higher than amniotic cavity pressure. This pressure gradient ensures right-to-left atrial shunting of blood and filling of the left ventricle. In the late gestation fetal lamb, right and left ventricular systolic pressures are similar (65–70 mm Hg). Pulmonary arterial and aortic systolic and diastolic pressures are also similar (65–70 mm Hg/ 30–35 mm Hg).

Afterload of the fetal ventricles is different: In the right ventricle it is low because it ejects most of its blood into the low resistance umbilical-placental circulation, whereas

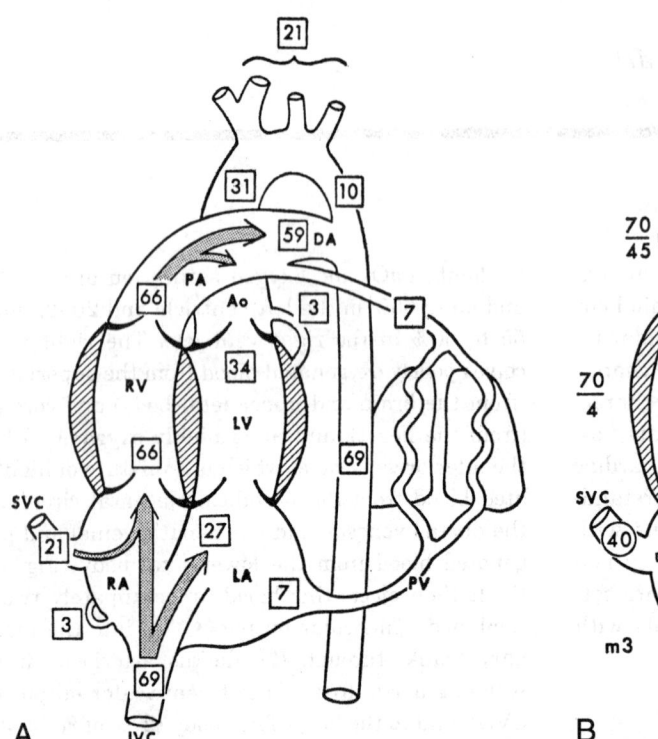

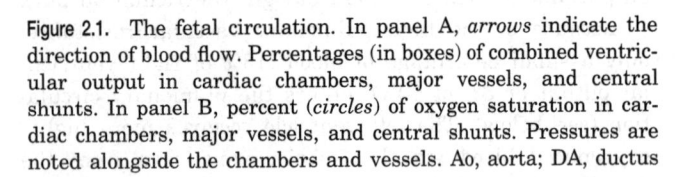

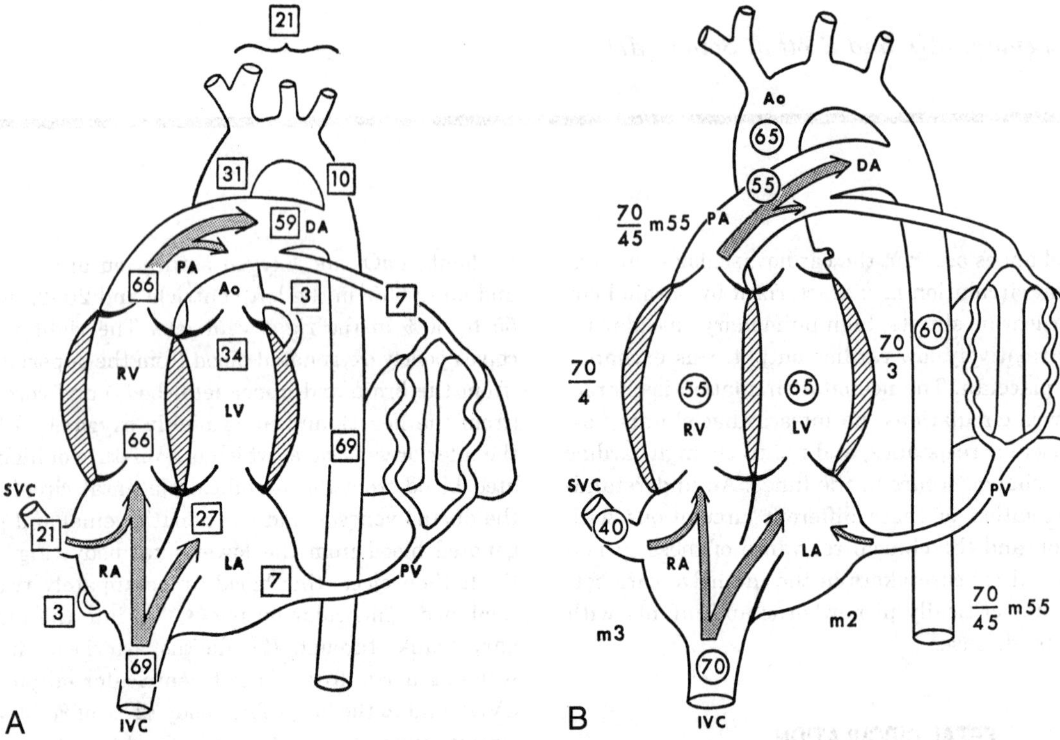

Figure 2.1. The fetal circulation. In panel A, *arrows* indicate the direction of blood flow. Percentages (in boxes) of combined ventricular output in cardiac chambers, major vessels, and central shunts. In panel B, percent (*circles*) of oxygen saturation in cardiac chambers, major vessels, and central shunts. Pressures are noted alongside the chambers and vessels. Ao, aorta; DA, ductus arteriosus; IVC, inferior vena cava; LA, left atrium; LV, left ventricle; PA, pulmonary artery; PV, pulmonary vein; RA, right atrium; RV, right ventricle; SVC, superior vena cava. (Modified from Rudolph AM. In: Congenital diseases of the heart. Chicago: Year Book, 1974.)

afterload is high in the left ventricle because it ejects its blood into the high resistance upper body circulation. Because preload of the right and left ventricles is similar but the afterload is different, the output of the ventricles may be different. In the fetal lamb, the right ventricle ejects nearly twice as much blood as the left ventricle. In the human fetus, the right ventricle ejects more blood than the left ventricle even though the increased brain blood flow is supplied by the left ventricle.

Fetal Pulmonary Vascular Resistance

Morphologic development of the pulmonary circulation affects the physiologic changes that occur in the perinatal period. In the fetus, pulmonary arteries have a thicker medial smooth muscle coat relative to the external diameter of the artery than do similar size pulmonary arteries in the adult. Small pulmonary arteries (20–50 μm in external diameter) have the thickest medial smooth muscle coat. This greater muscularity accounts, in part, for the higher pulmonary vascular resistance in the near-term fetus (6, 7).

These small pulmonary arteries can be identified by their relationship to airways. Preacinar pulmonary arteries are proximal to, or course with, the terminal bronchioli, whereas intra-acinar pulmonary arteries course with the respiratory bronchioli and alveolar ducts, or are within the alveolar walls. In the late gestation fetus, only about 50% of the pulmonary arteries associated with respiratory bronchioli are muscularized (either partially or completely). The pulmonary arteries within the alveolar wall are not muscularized (8, 9). The partially and not muscularized pulmonary arteries contain pericytes and intermediate cells (intermediate in position and structure between pericytes and smooth muscle cells), which are the precursors of smooth muscle cells. In a variety of clinical conditions including fetal hypoxemia, hypertension, and altered fetal blood flow patterns in congenital heart disease, these cells can differentiate into smooth muscle cells, completely muscularizing most of the small pulmonary arteries within alveolar walls (10). This increases fetal pulmonary vascular resistance and can affect the transition to extrauterine life (see below).

In the fetus, pulmonary blood flow is low, supplying only nutritional requirements for lung growth and performing some metabolic functions. In young fetuses, pulmonary blood flow is approximately 3 to 4% of the total combined left and right ventricular outputs of the heart.

This value increases to about 6% near gestation, corresponding temporally with the onset of the release of surface active material into lung fluid. This is followed by another progressive slow rise in pulmonary blood flow, reaching about 8 to 10% near term (1).

Fetal pulmonary arterial pressure increases with advancing gestation. At term, mean pulmonary arterial pressure is about 50 mm Hg, generally exceeding mean descending aortic pressure by 1–2 mm Hg (2). Pulmonary vascular resistance early in gestation is extremely high relative to that in the infant and adult, probably because of the few small arteries present. Pulmonary vascular resistance falls progressively during the last half of gestation, new arteries develop, and cross-sectional area increases; however, baseline pulmonary vascular resistance is still much higher than after birth (11).

Many factors, including mechanical effects, oxygenation state, and production of vasoactive substances, regulate the tone of the fetal pulmonary circulation (Fig. 2.2) (12). In unventilated fetal lungs, fluid filling the alveolar space compresses the small pulmonary arteries, which increases pulmonary vascular resistance. The normally low O_2 tension in pulmonary and systemic fetal arterial blood also increases pulmonary vascular resistance (13). The exact mechanism and site of hypoxic pulmonary vasoconstriction in the fetal pulmonary circulation remains unclear. In isolated fetal pulmonary arteries, oxygen modulates production of both prostacyclin and endothelium-derived nitric oxide (NO), two potent vasoactive substances that may in part underlie the responses of the developing pulmonary circulation to changes in oxygenation (14, 15). Oxygen-related changes in pulmonary vascular resistance are also affected by pH; acidemia increases pulmonary vascular resistance and accentuates hypoxic vasoconstrictor responses.

In addition to mechanical factors and the hypoxic environment, the fetal pulmonary circulation actively and continuously produces vasoactive substances, which modulate the degree of vasoconstriction under normal conditions, and which may play a more active role during periods of fetal stress. These substances are mainly endothelial-derived and include metabolites of arachidonic acid and endothelial-derived NO. *Prostacyclin* produces vasodilation by activating adenylate cyclase via receptor G protein-coupled mechanisms. Activation of adenylate cyclase results in increased adenosine 3′,5′-cyclic monophosphate (cAMP) concentrations, thus initiating a cascade that results in smooth muscle relaxation. A maturational increase in prostacyclin production occurs throughout gestation, which parallels the decrease in pulmonary vascular resistance in the fetal third trimester (14). However, in vivo, prostaglandin inhibition does not change resting pulmonary vascular resistance, which questions the importance of basal prostacyclin activity in mediating resting fetal pulmonary vascular tone (16). *Nitric oxide,* produced by vascular endothelium of all blood vessels including the pulmonary arteries, may be the most important regulator of vascular tone. NO is synthesized by the oxidation of the quanidino nitrogen moiety of L-arginine by the activation of nitric oxide synthase (17). Once released from endothelial cells, NO diffuses into vascular smooth muscle cells and activates soluble guanylate cyclase, the enzyme that catalyzes the production of guanosine-3′-5′-cyclic monophosphate (cGMP) from guanosine-5′-triphosphate. Activation of guanylate cyclase increases the concentrations of cGMP, thus initiating a cascade that results in smooth muscle relaxation (18). In fetal lambs, exogenous NO decreases fetal pulmonary vascular resistance, whereas endogenous NO synthesis inhibition increases pulmonary vascular resistance, suggesting that basal NO production, in part, mediates fetal pulmonary vascular tone (19). *Endothelin-1* (ET-1), a 21 amino acid polypeptide also produced by vascular endothelial cells, has potent vasoactive properties (20). The hemodynamic effects of ET-1 are mediated by at least two distinctive receptor populations: ET_a receptors, which are located on vascular smooth muscle cells, are likely responsible for the vasoconstricting effects of ET-1, whereas the ET_b receptors located on vascular endothelial cells are likely responsible for the vasodilating effects of ET-1 (21, 22). In the pulmonary circulation, exogenous ET-1 increases pulmonary vascular resistance in adult animals, but decreases pulmonary vascular resistance in fetal and

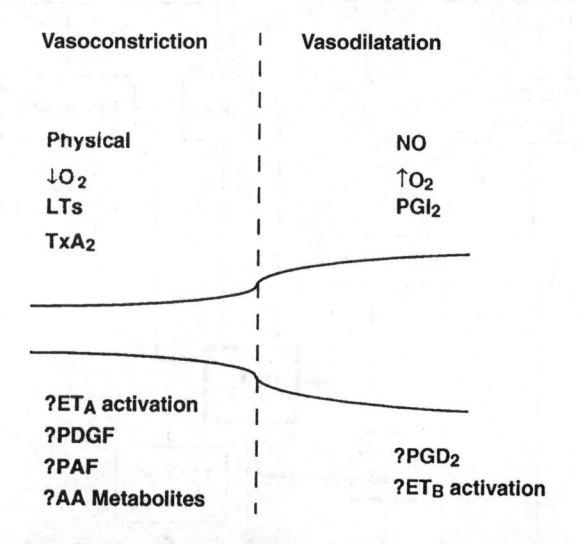

Figure 2.2. Factors considered to be involved in the control of pulmonary vascular resistance in the fetus. AA, arachidonic acid; ET, endothelin; LTs, leukotrienes; NO, nitric oxide; PAF, platelet activating factor; PDGF, platelet-derived growth factor; TXA_2, thromboxane A_2; ET_A, ETA receptor; ET_B, ETB receptor. (Modified from Soifer SJ, Fineman JR, Heymann MA. The pulmonary circulation. In: Gluckman PA, Heymann MA, eds. Pediatrics and perinatology: the scientific basis. Kent, United Kingdom: Edward Arnold, 1996:749–755.)

neonatal lambs (23, 24). In addition, selective ET_a receptor blockade decreases fetal pulmonary vascular resistance (25). *Leukotrienes (LT)* are synthesized from arachidonic acid by the 5'-lipoxygenase enzyme in pulmonary arterial tissue, mast cells, and alveolar macrophages. Exogenous LTC_4 and LTD_4 increase pulmonary vascular resistance in newborn and adult animals. In the fetal lamb, inhibition of endogenous leukotriene synthesis or action decreases pulmonary vascular resistance. In addition, leukotrienes have been isolated from the lung lavage fluid of newborn infants with persistent pulmonary hypertension (26–29).

Therefore, maintenance of the high fetal pulmonary vascular resistance most likely reflects a balance of mechanical influences and the release of a variety of vasoactive substances; those that produce vasoconstriction (low O_2, LTs, ET-1) and those that produce vasodilation (high O_2, prostacyclin, NO).

CIRCULATORY CHANGES AT BIRTH

Changes in Pulmonary Vascular Resistance at Birth

The decrease in pulmonary vascular resistance with ventilation and oxygenation at birth is regulated by a complex and incompletely understood interplay between mechanical and metabolic factors (Fig. 2.3).

At least two components cause the decrease in pulmonary vascular resistance with the initiation of ventilation and oxygenation. First, is partial pulmonary vasodilation caused by physical expansion of the lung and production of prostacyclin. This probably is independent of fetal oxygenation, and results in a modest increase in pulmonary blood flow and decrease in pulmonary vascular resistance (30, 31). Next, is a further pulmonary vasodilation associated with fetal oxygenation and NO production that is not dependent on the production of prostacyclin (19). This results in an increase in pulmonary blood flow and decrease in pulmonary vascular resistance to newborn values. Both components are necessary for the successful transition to extrauterine life.

Rhythmic distention of the lung with a gas mixture that does not change fetal blood gases decreases pulmonary vascular resistance and increases pulmonary blood flow. This results from a combination of mechanical and humoral factors. By replacing alveolar fluid with gas, rhythmic distention of the lung may decrease compression on the small pulmonary arteries, thereby decreasing pulmonary vascular resistance. In addition, a gas-liquid interface

Figure 2.3. Factors likely to be responsible for the changes of pulmonary vascular resistance and pulmonary blood flow with ventilation with oxygen at birth. A II, angiotension II; NO, nitric oxide; O_2, oxygen; PGD_2, prostaglandin D_2; PGI_2, prostacyclin; Q_p, pulmonary blood flow. (Modified from Soifer SJ, Fineman JR, Heymann MA. The pulmonary circulation. In: Gluckman PA, Heymann MA, eds. Pediatrics and perinatology: the scientific basis. Kent, United Kingdom: Edward Arnold, 1996: 749–755.)

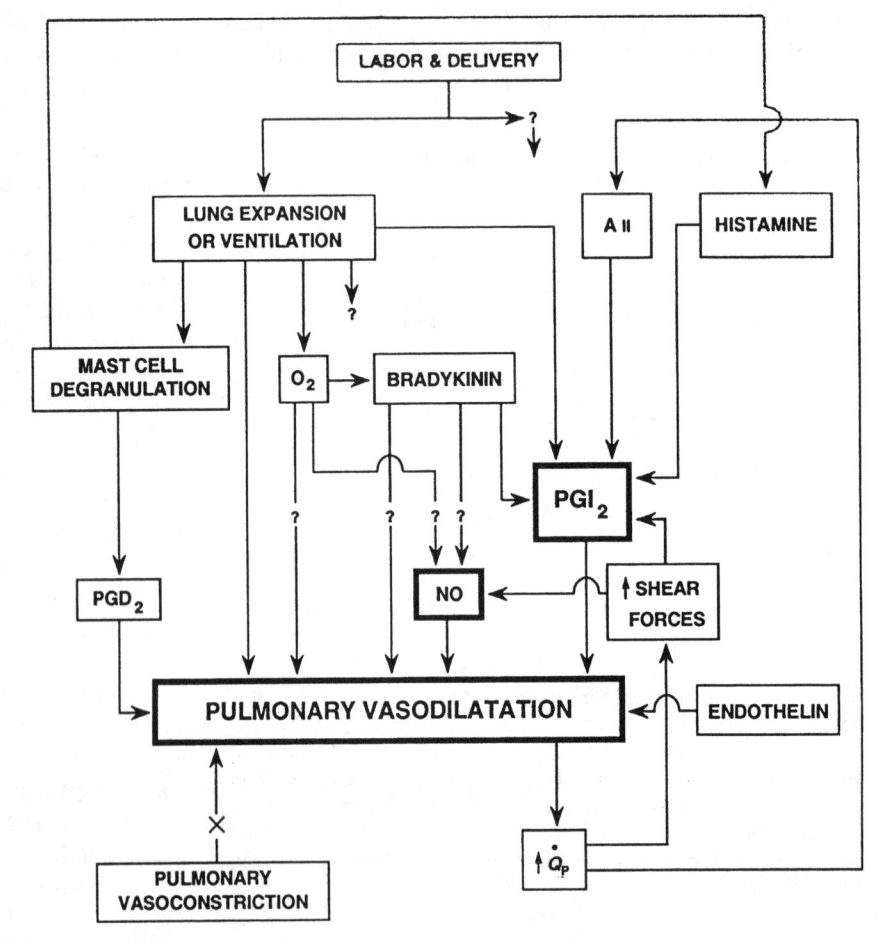

is produced in the alveoli and the resulting change in surface tension can exert a negative pressure on the small pulmonary arteries, dilating them and maintaining their patency (19). Prostacyclin production by the lung is also increased by mechanical distention, which results in further pulmonary vasodilation. Ventilation of fetal lungs with air or O_2 to increase O_2 tension increases pulmonary blood flow and decreases pulmonary vascular resistance to newborn levels. However, ventilation of the fetus without oxygenation produces only partial pulmonary vasodilation. The increase in alveolar or arterial O_2 tension can decrease pulmonary vascular resistance either directly by dilating the small pulmonary arteries, or indirectly by stimulating the production of other vasodilator substances such as NO.

In the fetus, pulmonary and systemic pressures are equal because the pulmonary artery and aorta are connected by the large ductus arteriosus. By 24 hours of age, with closure of the ductus arteriosus, pulmonary arterial pressure decreases to half systemic arterial pressure, and then decreases slowly to reach adult levels by 4 weeks of age. Pulmonary arterial pressure continues to decrease over the next 3 to 6 months. This decrease in pulmonary arterial pressure is associated with a thinning of the medial smooth muscular layer of the small pulmonary arteries. Pulmonary vascular resistance reaches adult levels by 3 to 6 months of age (11).

Two clinically important pathologic conditions are associated with an altered decrease in pulmonary vascular resistance at birth: persistent pulmonary hypertension of the newborn (PPHN) and congenital heart defects with large communications at the ventricular or great vessel level. PPHN is characterized by failure to achieve and/or maintain the decrease in pulmonary vascular resistance that normally occurs at birth. In a number of clinical conditions (e.g., respiratory distress syndrome, meconium aspiration, or sepsis) pulmonary vascular resistance does not decrease normally at birth. The ultimate pathophysiologic effects are reduced pulmonary blood flow and reduced systemic oxygen delivery. The pathophysiologic mechanisms preventing the normal pulmonary vasodilation and fall in pulmonary vascular resistance with ventilation and oxygenation at birth are not known. Pathologic changes in the pulmonary circulation of some infants who die of PPHN indicate that prolonged in utero events have altered the pulmonary circulation. Recent in vitro and in vivo data suggest that in utero events resulting in endothelial dysfunction and impaired NO and ET-1 activity may be a potential cause for PPHN (32, 33).

Pulmonary vascular resistance also does not decrease normally in newborns with large communications at the ventricular or great vessel level (34). The exact mechanisms for the delayed fall in pulmonary vascular resistance in the presence of increased pulmonary blood flow or pressure remain unclear. However, recent data also suggest that endothelial injury secondary to increased pulmonary blood flow or pressure, may participate in these alterations in pulmonary vascular resistance, and the development of pulmonary hypertension (35).

Closure of Central Shunts and the Systemic Circulation

At birth, major circulatory changes occur. With ligation of the umbilical cord, the removal of the placenta and separation of the newborn from the umbilical-placental circulation, a decrease in inferior vena caval blood flow occurs, resulting in decreased right atrial pressure. With the establishment of the lungs as the site of gas exchange, pulmonary blood flow increases. The resulting increase in pulmonary venous return increases left atrial pressure. Coupled with the decrease in right atrial pressure, this leads to closure of the foramen ovale. In newborns with congenital heart disease, if the foramen ovale does not close, then a left-to-right or right-to-left atrial shunt persists, depending on atrial pressures.

At birth, exposure of the ductus arteriosus to the increase in oxygenation and decreased plasma concentrations of prostaglandin E_2 (PGE_2) results in rapid constriction. The decrease in the plasma concentration of PGE_2 (which maintains ductus arteriosus patency in utero) after birth, is caused by the removal of the placenta as a source of PGE_2 and the increased metabolism in the lung (secondary to increased pulmonary blood flow). These changes contribute to closure of the ductus arteriosus by 24 hours of age. A higher incidence of persistent patency of the ductus arteriosus in preterm as compared with full-term newborns is caused by the decreased responsiveness of the ductus arteriosus to increased arterial PO_2 and to increased plasma concentrations of PGE_2 (36). If the ductus arteriosus remains patent after birth, the decrease in pulmonary vascular resistance that occurs with ventilation and oxygenation results in left-to-right shunting of blood. If pulmonary vascular resistance is increased by hypoxia or other factors, or if the pulmonary circulation is underdeveloped as in certain congenital heart diseases, right-to-left shunting of blood through the ductus arteriosus occurs.

Closure of the foramen ovale and ductus arteriosus results in separation of the right and left sides of the heart and the establishment of series circulations. Cardiac output (the output of each ventricle) increases immediately after birth (in the sheep to 300–425 mL/min·kg or a combined ventricular output of 600–850 mL/min·kg). This increase in cardiac output is necessary to meet the newborn's increased oxygen consumption due to increased cardiorespiratory and thermoregulatory work. Factors producing this increase in cardiac output include the increased production and release of thyroid hormone, cortisol, and catecholamines (37).

The increase in cardiac output at birth is associated with increases in myocardial, renal, and gastrointestinal blood flow with a decrease in adrenal and cerebral blood flows. Both reflex and humoral factors play a role in controlling these changes in organ blood flows. In the adult, local control of blood flow is closely related to oxygen availability and demand. The mechanisms responsible for this autoregulation include intrinsic modulation of local vascular resistance and alterations in tissue oxygen extraction. The autoregulatory capacity in the fetus and newborn is not well understood. Fetal systemic arterial pressure increases with increasing size and age. Systemic vascular resistance also increases at birth and continues to increase relative to body surface area for several weeks postnatally. The organs involved in these changes in vascular resistance are not completely understood.

NEONATAL MYOCARDIAL FUNCTION

The fetal heart demonstrates immaturity of structure, function, and innervation when compared with the newborn or adult heart. Myocardial cell diameter is smaller and contractile elements are fewer in the fetal myocardium than in that of the adult. A low concentration of contractile elements is present in newborn cardiac myocytes compared with adults, although individual sarcomeres are functionally equivalent (38). Fetal myocardium also has a decrease in sarcoplasmic reticulum and a poorly developed or absent T-tubule system when compared with the adult myocardium. The immature myocardium has a greater dependency on trans-sarcolemmal calcium influx for the generation of contraction than the adult myocardium (39, 40). Therefore, this structural and functional immaturity of the perinatal myocardium can explain, in part, the greater sensitivity to the negative inotropic effects of calcium channel blockers in infancy, and the greater calcium requirements of the newborn to maintain an adequate inotropic state in the perioperative period (41).

Determinants of Cardiac Output

In both the immature and mature myocardium, systolic function is primarily determined by the rate of contraction (heart rate), the amount of blood distending the ventricles immediately before contraction (preload), the intrinsic ability of the myocardial fibers to contract (contractility), and the resistance against which the myocardium must eject (afterload). The ability of the fetal myocardium to increase cardiac output in response to these determinants is greatly limited compared with the postnatal myocardium.

Heart Rate

In the immature heart, spontaneous changes in heart rate are associated with small changes in ventricular output. In the fetal lamb, spontaneous increases in heart rate increase combined ventricular output, whereas decreases in heart rate decrease combined ventricular output. Stroke volume is greater at the slower rates but not sufficiently to compensate for the decrease in heart rate. In the human, sustained fetal bradycardia (less than 100 beats per minute) or tachycardia (more than 250 beats per minute) produce congestive heart failure (hydrops fetalis). In the mature heart, changes in heart rate over a broad physiologic range do not produce significant changes in output. At slower rates, the Frank-Starling mechanism allows for increases in stroke volume secondary to increased end-diastolic volumes. At rapid heart rates, some increase is seen in output secondary to an intrinsic increase in myocardial contractility caused by changes in Ca^{2+} availability. The greater rate dependency of the fetal heart compared with the mature heart is probably related to greater ventricular interactions and lesser compliance of the fetal heart.

Preload

In the fetus, an intact Frank-Starling mechanism has been demonstrated: changes in preload are associated with small changes in combined ventricular output in the fetal sheep. However, the ability to increase output by recruiting the Frank-Starling mechanism is greatly limited in the fetus. This limitation is multifactorial, and it may be due to the immaturity of the myocardium and the increased stiffness of myocardial fibers. However, it must be kept in mind that preload studies in the fetus are difficult to interpret because of the affected fetal circulatory environment. For example, the umbilical-placental circulation absorbs much of the increase in volume in response to volume infusions, limiting the associated change in preload; the near-maximally dilated vascular bed of the fetus causes an increase in afterload when volume is infused to increase preload, and the diastolic ventricular interaction of the fetus limits the filling of each ventricle as atrial pressures increase simultaneously. The newborn heart has a greater ability to recruit the Frank-Starling mechanism, but it is still limited compared with the adult. This limitation is related, in part, to a higher resting cardiac output, greater myocardial stiffness, and afterload mismatch.

Contractility

Developmental changes are found in resting contractile state and contractile reserve. In the fetal myocardium, an increase is seen in resting tension, but a significant decrease in the active tension developed at all muscle lengths along the length-tension curve. Causes of this impairment are multiple, and they include decreased sympathetic innervation, decreased β-adrenoceptor concentration, immaturity of the sarcoplasmic reticulum, and decreased concentration and function of myofibrils. Immediately after birth, an increase in contractile state is induced by the increased production and release of thyroid hormone, cortisol, and catecholamines (38, 39). Over the first month of life in the lamb, a decrease is found in the contractile state, but an increase in contractile reserve. The newborn heart has higher resting indices of myocardial performance than the adult heart. However, the newborn heart is unable to increase its contractile state or significantly improve ventricular performance. Clinically, this may explain why higher concentrations of inotropic drugs are required in newborns than in older children and adults to achieve similar hemodynamic effects.

Afterload

Afterload is the resistance the ventricles have to overcome to eject blood into the circulation. In isolated muscle strips, afterload is measured as the rate of muscle shortening versus the load on the muscle. Fetal and newborn hearts are more sensitive to changes in afterload than is the adult heart. Small increases in afterload decrease cardiac output more in fetal and newborn animals than in the adult. In the intact heart, arterial pressure is the major determinant of afterload. Because arterial pressure increases during fetal life, afterload also increases. Changes in afterload contribute to the increase in cardiac output at birth. With pulmonary vasodilation and closure of the ductus arteriosus, right ventricular afterload decreases. With the establishment of series circulations, the left ventricle ejects blood to both the upper and lower bodies. The cross-sectional area of these vascular beds is increased; therefore, left ventricular afterload decreases. In the newborn, the increases in afterload associated with aortic stenosis or coarctation of the aorta are poorly tolerated as congestive heart failure rapidly develops. In the adult, only severe obstruction to left ventricular output produces symptoms.

Myocardial Adaptations

In the fetal heart, biventricular mass increases with development. In the postnatal heart, differential growth of the left and right ventricular myocardium occurs in response to both the increase in left ventricular work and the decrease in right ventricular work during the transitional circulation. Left ventricular weight increases relative to body weight, whereas right ventricular weight is unchanged or decreases.

Clinically, the relationship between ventricular work load and ventricular mass in the developing heart is well demonstrated in the infant with transposition of the great vessels. Banding of the pulmonary artery in preparation for the arterial switch procedure results in a marked increase in left ventricular mass shortly after the increase in afterload (42). The developmental increase in ventricular mass is both a function of increases in number and size of the ventricular myocytes. In the fetus and newborn, cell division is the major contributor to the increase in ventricular mass. By 2 months of age, physiologic hypertrophy is prominent (39). Mechanisms that regulate these processes are not well established.

The effects of hypoxemia and asphyxia on the function of the immature and mature myocardium have been widely studied. In general, the ability of the fetal and neonatal heart to tolerate acute hypoxemia and acidosis is superior to that of the adult (43). In the newborn lamb heart studied in situ, isolated hypoxemia (PO_2 less than 25 mm Hg) or isolated acidosis (pH = 6.8) did not decrease ventricular performance as long as adrenergic support was intact (44). However, hypoxemia and acidosis in combination resulted in significant decreases in ventricular performance. With sympathetic nervous system blockade or calcium flux blockade, hypoxemia or acidosis alone resulted in profound myocardial depression, suggesting a role of the adrenergic nervous system and calcium ions in the adaptation to these acute stresses.

SUMMARY

In the fetus, pulmonary blood flow is low, as gas exchange occurs in the placenta. Central shunts and streaming patterns produce parallel circulations, with the left ventricle ejecting more highly oxygenated blood (to the brain and heart) than the right ventricle. Although filling and arterial pressures are similar, right ventricular afterload is less than left ventricular afterload. The fetal myocardium is structurally and functionally immature when compared with the adult. Little reserve is present to increase cardiac output, as the fetal heart appears to function at the top of the ventricular function curve. Changes in heart rate and afterload are important. At birth, cardiac output is increased due, in part, to an increased contractile state and to the decrease in the afterload of both ventricles. Cardiac output decreases over the first months of life and a contractile reserve develops. With pulmonary vasodilation, the increase in pulmonary blood flow and the removal of the placenta as the site of gas exchange, the central shunts close and serial circulations are established. Factors maintaining pulmonary vasoconstriction in the fetus and producing pulmonary vasodilation with ventilation are not completely understood. Mechanical factors, the oxygen environment, and vasoactive substances are all important. A continued understanding of the fetal circulation, its transition, and aberrations associated with congenital heart disease remains essential for those who care for these critically ill newborns, infants, and children.

REFERENCES

1. Rudolph AM, Heymann MA. Circulatory changes during growth in the fetal lamb. Circ Res 1970;289–299.
2. Rudolph AM. Fetal and neonatal pulmonary circulation. Ann Rev Physiol 1979;41:383–395.
3. Rudolph AM. Hepatic and ductus venosus blood flows during fetal life. Hepatology 1983;3:254.

4. Anderson DF, Bissonnette JM, Farer JJ, et al. Central shunt flows and pressures in the mature fetal lamb. Am J Physiol 1981;241:H60.
5. Teitel DF, Iwamoto HS, Rudolph AM. Effects of birth-related events on central blood flow patterns. Pediatr Res 1987;22:557.
6. Levin DL, Rudolph AM, Heymann MA, et al. Morphological development of the pulmonary vascular bed in fetal lambs. Circulation 1976;53:144–151.
7. Hislop A, Reid LM. Intra-pulmonary arterial development during fetal life-branching pattern and structure. J Anat 1972;113:35–48.
8. Reid LM. Structure and function in pulmonary hypertension. New perceptions. Chest 1986;89:279–288.
9. Hislop A, Reid LM. Pulmonary arterial development during childhood: branching pattern and structure. Thorax 1973;28:129–135.
10. Meyrick B, Reid L. The effect of continued hypoxia on rat pulmonary arterial circulation: an ultrastructural study. Lab Invest 1978;38:188–200.
11. Heymann MA, Soifer SJ. Control of the fetal and neonatal pulmonary circulation. In: Weir EK, Reeves JT, eds. Pulmonary vascular physiology and pathophysiology. New York: Marcel Dekker, 1989:33.
12. Fineman JR, Soifer SJ, Heymann MA. Regulation of pulmonary vascular tone in the perinatal period. Annu Rev Physiol 1995;57:115–134.
13. Parker HR, Purves MJ. Some effects of maternal hyperoxia and hypoxia on the gas tension and vascular pressures in the fetal sheep. Quarterly Journal of Experimental Physiology 1967;52:205.
14. Shaul PW, Farrar MA, Magness RR. Oxygen modulation of pulmonary arterial prostacyclin synthesis is developmentally regulated. Am J Physiol 1993;265:H621–H628.
15. Shaul PW, Farrar MA, Zellers TM. Oxygen modulates endothelium-derived relaxing factor production in fetal pulmonary arteries. Am J Physiol 1992;262:H355–H364.
16. Morin FC, Egan EA, Norfleet WT. Indomethacin does not diminish the pulmonary vascular response of the fetus to increased oxygen tension. Pediatr Res 1988;24:696–700.
17. Palmer RMJ, Ashton DS, Moncada S. Vascular endothelial cells synthesize nitric oxide from L-arginine. Nature 1988;333:664–666.
18. Fiscus RR. Molecular mechanisms of endothelium-mediated vasodilation. Semin Thromb Hemost 1988;14:12–22.
19. Abman SH, Chatfield BA, Hall SL, et al. Role of endothelium-derived relaxing during transition of pulmonary circulation at birth. Am J Physiol 1990;259:H1921–H1927.
20. Yanagisawa M, Kurihara H, Kimura S, et al. A novel potent vasoconstrictor peptide produced by vascular endothelial cells. Nature 1988;332:411–415.
21. Arai H, Hori S, Aramori I, et al. Cloning and expression of a cDNA encoding an endothelin receptor. Nature 1990;348:730–732.
22. Sakurai T, Yanagisawa M, Takuwa Y, et al. Cloning of a cDNA encoding a non-isopeptide-selective subtype of the endothelin receptor. Nature 1990;348:732–735.
23. Chatfield BA, McMurtry IF, Hall SL, et al. Hemodynamic effects of endothelin-1 on ovine fetal pulmonary circulation. Am J Physiol 1991;261:R182–R187.
24. Wong J, Vanderford PA, Fineman JR, et al. Developmental effects of endothelin-1 on the pulmonary circulation in sheep. Pediatr Res 1994;36:2141–2148.
25. Ivy DD, Kinsella JP, Abman SH. Physiologic characterization of endothelin A and B receptor activity in the ovine fetal pulmonary circulation. J Clin Invest 1994;93:2141–2148.
26. Le Bidios J, Soifer SJ, Clyman RI, et al. Piripost: a putative leokotriene synthesis inhibitor increases pulmonary blood flow in fetal lambs. Pediatr Res 1987;22:350–354.
27. Soifer SJ, Loitz RD, Roman C, et al. Leukotriene end organ antagonists increase pulmonary blood in fetal lambs. Am J Physiol 1985;249:H570–H576.
28. Velvis H, Krussel J, Roman C, et al. Leukotrienes C4, D4, and E4 in fetal lamb tracheal fluid. J Dev Phys 1990;14:37–41.
29. Stenmark KR, James SL, Voelkei NF, et al. Leukotriene C4 and D4 in neonates with hypoxemia and pulmonary hypertension. N Engl J Med 1983;309:77–80.
30. Velvis H, Moore P, Heymann MA. Prostaglandin inhibition prevents the fall in pulmonary vascular resistance as a result of rhythmic distension of the lungs in fetal lambs. Pediatr Res 1991;30:62–68.
31. Lefler CW, Hessler JR, Green RS. The onset of breathing at birth stimulates pulmonary vascular prostacyclin synthesis. Pediatr Res 1984;18:938–942.
32. Fineman JR, Wong J, Morin FC, et al. Chronic nitric oxide inhibition in utero produces persistent pulmonary hypertension in newborn lambs. J Clin Invest 1994;93:2675–2683.
33. Ivy DD, Ziegler JW, Dubus MF, et al. Chronic intrauterine pulmonary hypertension alters endothelin receptor activity in the ovine fetal lung. Pediatr Res 1996;39:435–442.
34. Hoffman JIE, Rudolph AM. The natural history of ventricular septal defects in infancy. Am J Cardiol 1965;16:634–653.
35. Reddy VM, Wong J, Liddicoat JR, et al. Altered endothelium-dependent vasoactive responses in lambs with pulmonary hypertension and increased pulmonary blood flow. Am J Physiol 1996;271:H562–H570.
36. Clyman RI. Ductus arteriosus. In: Gluckman PA, Heymann MA, eds. Pediatrics and perinatology: the scientific basis. Kent, United Kingdom: Edward Arnold, 1996:755–761.
37. Teitel DF. Physiologic development of the cardiovascular system in the fetus. In: Polin RA, Fox WW, eds. Fetal and neonatal physiology. Philadelphia: WB Saunders, 1992:609–619.
38. Anderson PAW. Physiology of the fetal, neonatal, and adult heart. In: Polin RA, Fox WW, eds. Fetal and neonatal physiology. Philadelphia: WB Saunders, 1992:722–758.
39. Boucek RJ Jr, Shelton M, Artman M, et al. Comparative effects of verapamil, nifedipine and diltiazem on contractile function in the isolated immature and adult rabbit heart. Pediatr Res 1984;18:948–952.
40. Artman M, Graham TP Jr, Boucek RJ Jr. Effects of postnatal maturation on myocardial contractile responses to calcium antagonists and changes in contraction frequency. J Cardiovasc Physiol 1985;7:850–855.
42. Boutin C, Wernovsky G, Sanders SP, et al. Rapid two-stage arterial switch operation. Evaluation of left ventricular systolic mechanics late after an acute pressure overload stimulus in infancy. Circulation 1994;90:1294–1303.
43. Talner NS, Lister G, Fahey JT. Effects of asphyxia on the myocardium of the fetus and newborn. In: Polin RA, Fox WW, eds. Fetal and neonatal physiology. Philadelphia: WB Saunders, 1992:759–769.
44. Downing SE, Talner NS, Gardner TH. Influences of arterial oxygen tension and pH on cardiac function in the newborn lamb. Am J Physiol 1966;211:1203.

Cardiac Physiology

Selected Topics in Normal Hearts

David F. Teitel, MD

BASIC CARDIAC MECHANICS

Cardiac Output

The heart fills and empties one to two times a second, circulating blood to the microcirculation for metabolic activities. Although this is a simple task, it requires a complex interplay of active and passive processes, involving the heart itself, the central and peripheral circulations, and the neurohormonal axis. All the mechanisms controlling these processes function by finely adjusting systemic blood flow on a beat-by-beat basis within a narrow range, determined primarily by the oxygen demands of the body. In the absence of intracardiac and extracardiac shunts, the left and right ventricular outputs are the same, each being equal to "cardiac output."

Classic teaching has considered the four determinants of cardiac output (heart rate, preload, afterload, and contractility) as independent factors, each of which can be measured and manipulated independently to alter output. Recent studies have demonstrated complex interrelationships exist among these determinants. This has necessitated the development of a more sophisticated approach to cardiac mechanics, in which each determinant is not considered in isolation but as it affects some or all of the others.

This chapter presents an approach to cardiac mechanics from a clinical viewpoint that incorporates these concepts, but in a practical way to be clinically relevant to the cardiac intensivist. To this end, the basic physiology of systolic and diastolic mechanics are reviewed first, and then a practical approach is presented to evaluating and altering function using pressure-volume loop analysis.

Systolic Mechanics

The four primary determinants of systolic function of the heart are (*a*) preload, or the initial volume of the left ventricle prior to ejection; (*b*) afterload, or the combined resistance to ejection of blood by heart and blood inertia, impedance of the central vasculature, and resistance of the peripheral microvasculature; (*c*) heart rate; and (*d*) contractility, defined as the intrinsic ability of the myocyte to contract, changing when the metabolic or hormonal milieu alters systolic performance independent of the three other determinants. Over the last several decades, studies have focused on describing indices of contractility, which by this classic definition must be independent of preload, afterload, and heart rate. All of these efforts have failed to varying degrees, not because these indices were inadequate descriptors of contractility, but rather because the primary assumption that these determinants are independent was invalid.

Recent studies have focused on the contractile apparatus of the heart from both cellular and subcellular perspectives. From these studies, it is clear that the ability of the individual contractile elements to generate force is determined by the amount of activator calcium available to the sarcomere and its sensitivity to calcium. Using this concept, it has become clear that not only are the four determinants of systolic performance interdependent, but that the other three determinants alter systolic performance to a large extent by directly altering the intrinsic contractility of the myocyte.

Defining and quantifying systolic function of the heart has therefore been an elusive investigative goal. A simple approach to systolic function is based on the classic studies of muscle, which describe three basic properties of muscle function: (*a*) the length-tension relationship, which states that the force generated by a contracting muscle is dependent on the initial length, or preload, of the muscle fiber; (*b*) the force-velocity relationship, which states that the velocity of shortening of a muscle fiber is dependent on the load against which it shortens, or afterload; and (*c*) the force-frequency relationship, which states that the force generated by a contraction is dependent on the rate of contraction of the muscle fiber.

It has long been known that the force-frequency relationship exists because a faster rate of depolarization of a muscle decreases the time for sequestration of free, intracellular calcium into the sarcoplasmic reticulum and its transport back across the sarcolemma during diastole. This increases activator calcium availability for the next depolarization, and thus the force of contraction is greater and it is achieved more rapidly. The other two basic properties of muscle, the length-tension and force-velocity relationships, define the effects of preload and afterload, respectively, on pump performance, and they have been considered to be independent of contractility (1, 2). However, direct preload effects on contractility have been shown in the intact heart and in the sarcomere itself—this length-dependent activation of the myofibril is likely secondary to increased calcium sensitivity at longer initial lengths (3–7). This can be secondary either to a variation in calcium affinity of troponin C over different lengths (8–10) or to a greater exposure of the myosin head to troponin C as stretch displaces the troponin C molecules from the tropomyosin framework (11). The afterload dependence of contraction also has been demonstrated: recent studies in the intact circulation and isolated heart have shown that acute increases in afterload acutely increase contractility independent of indirect effects of β-adrenergic stimulation (12, 13). It has been hypothesized that some of this afterload dependence is on the basis of beat-to-beat changes in calcium flux related to shortening deactivation (14, 15), but it has also been demonstrated using indices of contractility in the pre-ejection phase of systole (12). Recently it has also been shown that ejecting beats can actually generate greater rather than lesser pressures than isovolumic beats (13), so that there appear to be subcellular processes that act in a direction opposite to shortening deactivation.

Thus, as one attempts to evaluate contractility in the clinical setting, and alter systolic performance by manipulation of load, heart rate, and contractility, it is important to consider that these four determinants of cardiac performance are not independent variables that can be separately manipulated, but are instead interdependent physiologic variables.

Diastolic Mechanics

Diastolic mechanics can be separated into two distinct but temporally overlapping components, active relaxation and the passive stiffness of the myocardium. At the end of ejection, most sarcomeres have shortened to their fullest extent and begin to lengthen. Active relaxation (myofilament deactivation) occurs rapidly, although it is not yet complete when the mitral valve opens and filling begins. The passive stiffness of the left ventricle is determined primarily by nonmyocytic elements, including extracellular matrix, cellular support structures, and the coronary vascular bed. Passive stiffness of these components does not allow the sarcomere to overstretch, so that cross bridge formation can always occur with the next depolarization. In addition, the ventricle's geometry affects its passive stiffness: changing its shape or wall thickness independent of changes in composition of the ventricle significantly alters local stresses and thus diastolic filling.

Stiffness, or elastance, of any structure can be measured by the amount of stress generated in the wall of that structure when it is stretched from its resting, nonstressed length to a defined length. The model of time-varying elastance has been used to describe the ventricle throughout the cardiac cycle. In this model, the ventricle is represented as a single elastic element, without viscous forces. Thus, its elastance at any time in the cardiac cycle can be calculated from the equation:

$$(1) \quad E_t = \frac{P_t}{(V_t - V_0)}$$

where E_t is the elastance at that point in time, P_t is the pressure and V_t is the volume at that time, and V_0 is the unstressed volume, when the pressure is zero. Elastance at end-diastole is a good representation of the passive property of the chamber because relaxation is complete and contraction has not yet begun. Once contraction begins, the sarcomere shortens and thus the elastance of the ventricle is determined not by its passive elements but by its contractile element (discussed below).

In addition to the intrinsic passive stiffness of the left ventricle, external factors affect its diastolic mechanics. Left atrial pressure is an important determinant of the flow across the mitral valve, as it significantly affects the transmitral pressure gradient (16). Both the right ventricle and pericardium can significantly constrain filling of the left ventricle during diastole; the former is particularly important in pulmonary hypertension, the latter in acute ventricular dilation. Lastly, surrounding thoracic structures and intrathoracic pressure can constrain left ventricular filling, which can be a critically important factor in the intensive care setting in which positive pressure ventilation often is used, and the intrathoracic structures may be constrained in a recently closed chest with an enlarged heart and/or excessive fluid.

Evaluation of the relaxation characteristics of the heart is difficult because it occupies only a small portion of the cardiac cycle. Isovolumic relaxation occurs in the few milliseconds between aortic valve closure and mitral valve opening, and thus its evaluation by indices such as the half-time of pressure decay, or γ, requires exact, rapid measurement of pressure. Relaxation, as with contraction, is affected by the processes that alter the amount of calcium linked to the myofilament and the sensitivity of the myofilament to that calcium. Therefore, relaxation rate is shortened by increases in both contractility and afterload (17). Not only is the extent of afterload important to relaxation, but the events of contraction also play a major role: the later the afterload is placed on the ventricle during ejection, the longer the relaxation rate (18). Preload also affects relaxation, as increases in end-diastolic pressure prolong the relaxation rate independent of aortic pressure (19).

Pressure-Volume Analysis

Because the role of the intact heart is to generate pressure and eject blood, many investigators have recently studied cardiac performance in the pressure-volume phase. If left ventricular pressure and volume are measured simultaneously, the resulting pressure-volume loop provides information about the systolic and diastolic performance of the heart. Moreover, acquisition of simultaneous pressure and volume measurements allows for the calculation of elastance throughout the cardiac cycle (Eq. 1), and thus the model of time-varying elastance as it characterizes ventricular function can be used in both systole and diastole.

A typical pressure volume loop for a 5-year-old child is shown in Figure 3.1. Starting at point 1, the end-diastolic volume is about 75 mL, achieved at an end-diastolic pressure of 5 mm Hg. End-diastolic pressure for a given end-diastolic volume is determined by the passive stiffness, or elastance, of the heart, and it is determined by the passive elastic elements. Isovolumic contraction then begins, as the sarcomeres shorten rapidly, but without a change in ventricular volume. During this phase, pressure within the ventricle increases rapidly, and it is determined no longer by the passive elastic elements in the chamber but almost entirely by the contractile elements (sarcomeres) as they shorten. Thus the elastance of the heart throughout systole is now a function of the contractile element itself. During isovolumic contraction, pressure increases rapidly, and the maximal rate of this pressure increase (dP/dt_{max}) has been extensively used as an index of systolic performance. This index is primarily determined by preload and the intrinsic contractility of the myocyte, which, as discussed above, is rate dependent. If afterload is low, ejection begins while the rate of pressure development is still increasing and thus decrease $dPdt_{max}$ independent of changes in preload or contractility.

Once the pressure within the ventricle begins to exceed the pressure in the proximal aorta, the aortic valve opens and ejection begins (point 2). The aorta fills with blood and the ventricle empties, generating a peak pressure of about 100 mm Hg. End-systole occurs at maximal systolic elastance (Eq. 1), at a pressure just below peak pressure, and at a volume just above the minimal volume of 25 mL.

The aortic valve then closes (point 4), and the volume changes from point 2 to point 4 is the stroke volume of the cycle (50 mL). Dividing stroke volume by the end-diastolic volume yields a normal ejection fraction of 67%. Pressure profile during ejection is an excellent descriptor of afterload (Fig. 3.2), and it is reflected in the aortic pressure tracing, which is monitored in the intensive care unit. Arterial elastance (E_a) (Fig. 3.2) is a recently used index of the combined afterload of the central impedance and peripheral resistance vessels. Mean arterial elastance throughout ejection is the pressure generated to eject blood divided by the stroke volume. By incorporating central impedance, it is a more accurate estimate of the afterload of the arterial bed on ventricular ejection than is calculation of peripheral resistance alone.

From point 4 to point 5 (Fig. 3.1), the heart is actively and rapidly relaxing but not changing volume, and thus is in the phase of diastole called "isovolumic relaxation." This

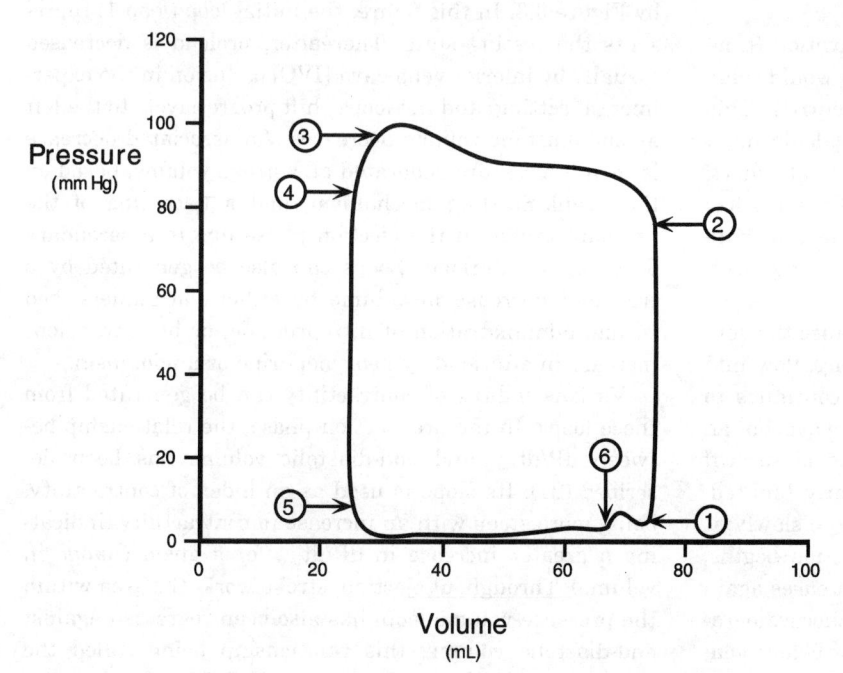

Figure 3.1. Idealized pressure-volume loop. The contraction begins at end-diastole (point 1), and isovolumic contraction proceeds until the aortic valve opens (point 2). Ejection then continues through maximal elastance ("end-systole," point 3) until the aortic valve closes (point 4). Isovolumic relaxation occurs until the mitral valve opens (point 5). Passive filling of the ventricle occurs until the atrium contracts (point 6) and generates active filling until end-diastole, when the next contraction begins (point 1).

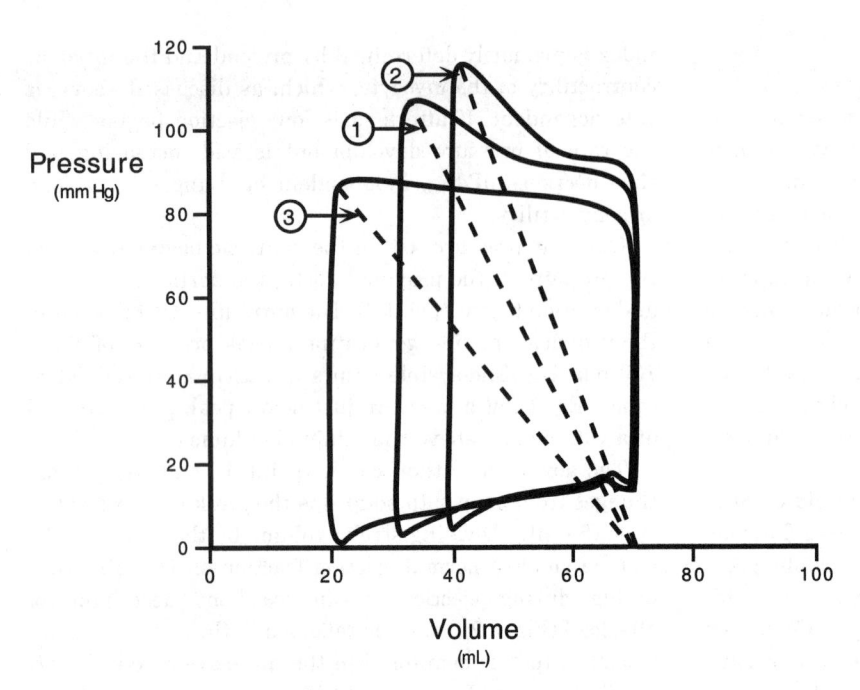

Figure 3.2. Arterial elastance. *Dotted line 1* represents a normal arterial elastance, calculated by dividing peak pressure by stroke volume. An increase in arterial elastance (*line 2*) changes the profile of the pressure during ejection to a more prolonged and steeper shape, as it is harder to eject the stroke volume into a less compliant arterial system. *Line 3* represents a decrease in arterial elastance, with a flatter pressure profile throughout ejection, as blood runs off more easily into the distal vascular bed, preventing an increase in pressure as blood is pumped into the central arterial system.

phase is primarily dependent on the ability of the myofilament to release activator calcium and of the sarcoplasmic reticulum to actively sequester most of it, the rest being transported back across the sarcolemma by the Na^+–Ca^+ exchanger. The best descriptor of this phase is τ, which is the half-time of pressure decay from the equation

$$(2) \quad P_t = P_0^{e^{\frac{-t}{\tau}}} - P_\infty$$

where P_0 is the pressure at the onset of relaxation (time zero) and P_∞ is the pressure that the ventricle would relax to if no filling or subsequent contraction occurred. This pressure is often assumed to be zero when calculating τ (20). This phase of diastole, however, is exceedingly short, comprising approximately 10% of the time of the cardiac cycle. Thus, it is often difficult to acquire an adequate number of data points in the rapidly beating young heart to reliably measure τ.

At point 5, the mitral valve opens, and, because the ventricle is still relaxing while the atrium is filling, flow into the ventricle is initially rapid and pressure continues to fall. This rapid flow corresponds to the E wave on an M-mode echocardiography. If the ventricle is more stiff than normal, this E wave may be significantly blunted. Thereafter, flow into the ventricle proceeds more slowly; it is called "diastasis." At point 6 atrial contraction begins, and the flow of blood into the left ventricle increases again (corresponding to the A wave on M-mode echocardiography). At the end of atrial contraction and just before ventricular contraction is point 1, or end-diastole.

Pressure-Volume Analyses over Changing Load

Because of a complex interaction of load on both systolic and diastolic function, single beat indices of both are exceedingly difficult to interpret. To take into account this interaction, most indices of systolic and diastolic function are best considered over changing load. This is represented by Figure 3.3. In this figure, the initial loop (loop 1) represents the resting state. Thereafter, preload is decreased (usually by inferior vena cava [IVC] occlusion in the experimental setting) and the loops shift progressively to the left as end-diastolic volume decreases. An associated decrease is seen in pressure generated and stroke volume, based on the Frank-Starling mechanism, and a flattening of the pressure profile in the ejection phase due to a secondary decrease in afterload. Loops can also be generated by a transient decrease in volume by either tourniquets, bed tilting, administration of nitroprusside, or by a transient increase in afterload by neosynephrine or angiotensin.

Various indices of contractility can be generated from these loops. In the pre-ejection phase, the relationship between dP/dt_{max} and end-diastolic volume has been described (21). Its slope is used as an index of contractility, being more steep with an increase in contractility (indicating a greater increase in dP/dt_{max} for a given change in volume). Throughout ejection, stroke work (the area within the pressure-volume loop) has also been regressed against end-diastolic volume, this relationship being called the "preload-recruitable stroke work index" (22). This has also

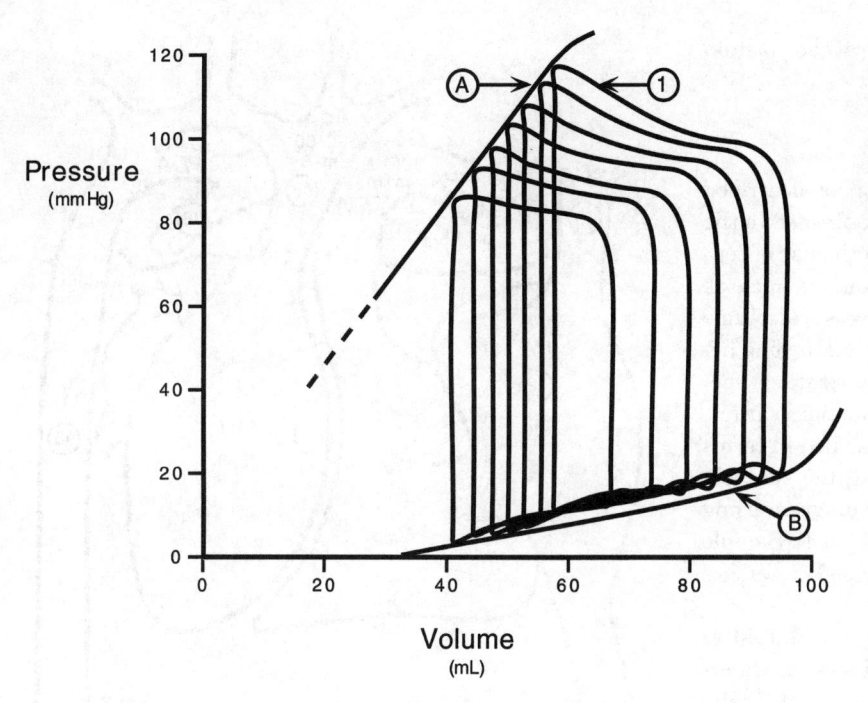

Figure 3.3. Pressure-volume loops during IVC occlusion. From the initial loop (1), pressure and volume decrease as IVC occlusion decreases filling of the left ventricle. From the end-systolic points, the end-systolic pressure-volume relationship (A) can be defined by the slope and intercept of a linear description of the curve. From the end-diastolic points, a non-linear end-diastolic pressure-volume relationship (B) can also be described.

been found to be linear over a physiologic range and sensitive to increases in contractility. Perhaps the most widely used index is the end-systolic pressure-volume relationship, which is also relatively linear over a physiologic range and increases in steepness with increases in contractile state (23, 24). This, in conjunction with the end-diastolic pressure-volume relationship, forms the boundaries within which all loops generated by a ventricle within a given contractile state are constrained. End-diastolic pressure-volume relationship is an index of the passive stiffness of the ventricle, and it can be fitted to a nonlinear regression equation.

Many other indices of ventricular performance and circulatory interactions can be derived from these pressure-volume loops. For example, coupling of ventricle output with the elastance of the arterial bed has become a major area of interest, particularly because many pathologic states are associated with "afterload-preload mismatch" (25) that leads to inefficient ventricular function. By plotting end-systolic elastance (E_{es}) against arterial elastance (E_a) (26–28), it can be shown that the most efficient mechanical work of the ventricle occurs when the E_{es}/E_a ratio is approximately 1:1. A ratio of 1.1 has been found to exist in the normal dog (27), with ratios much less than 1 occurring in adult humans with ventricular dysfunction secondary to ischemic heart disease (29). In the adult dog is found a large plateau over which stroke work is maintained: it does not begin to fall until E_{es}/E_a ratio is less than about 0.4–0.5 or until E_{es}/E_a increases beyond about 2.0 (27).

Not only can indices of performance be derived from pressure-volume loops, indices of myocardial oxygen consumption and energy efficiency also can be calculated and the effects of changing load can be assessed. This will be presented in detail below.

CARDIAC CATHETERIZATION

Overview

Indications for cardiac catheterization have changed dramatically over the past decade. Previously, most patients in whom surgery was being considered first underwent a detailed diagnostic catheterization, which focused on careful delineation of anatomic detail and hemodynamic profile. With the rapid improvement of echocardiographic techniques such as two-dimensional echocardiography, standard and color Doppler, and three-dimensional reconstructions, as well as other noninvasive methodologies such as magnetic resonance imaging, anatomic and physiologic information can be adequately acquired without cardiac catheterization. Thus, catheterizations are now primarily being performed in (a) patients for therapeutic interventions either instead of or in conjunction with surgical procedures, (b) patients whose anatomic or hemodynamic information is not adequately defined by noninvasive studies, and (c) patients who have other diagnostic or therapeutic indications (electrophysiologic studies or ablations and myocardial biopsy). This section reviews the hemodynamic information available in the catheterization laboratory.

Physiologic Diagram

Complex analysis of cardiac mechanics as described above (Basic Cardiac Mechanics) is rarely performed in the catheterization laboratory. With progress in the use of conductance catheter (30, 31) and other techniques such as radionuclide imaging (32), ventricular pressure-volume loops can be generated continuously without disturbing hemodynamic stability. Most diagnostic catheterizations specifically evaluate the heart in terms of its function (cardiac output and oxygen delivery) and the vascular bed in terms of peripheral resistance. Within this context, the simplest way to view these data is with a physiologic diagram using an anatomic representation of the heart (Fig. 3.4). Sample calculations of pulmonary and systemic blood flows are presented in the figure legend.

To consider cardiovascular hemodynamics, it is best to follow the diagram in terms of lines of blood flow, considering hemoglobin oxygen saturation, pressures, and finally outputs, shunts, and resistances. Saturations in vessels and chambers are obtained to demonstrate levels of shunting and to measure pulmonary and systemic blood flows, the latter in conjunction with measurement of hemoglobin concentration and oxygen consumption. To calculate systemic blood flow, saturations representative of systemic arterial and mixed venous saturation must be measured; to calculate pulmonary blood flow, representative pulmonary arterial and pulmonary venous saturations are needed.

Oxygen Saturation

Mixed venous saturation is best represented by the most distal, well-mixed sample that is still proximal to any left-to-right shunt. In the absence of any shunt, mixed venous and pulmonary arterial saturations are identical, and thus pulmonary arterial saturation should be used to represent both. If an arterial level shunt such as a patent ductus arteriosus is present, mixed venous saturation should be represented by the saturation obtained in the right ventricle (RV). If an atrial or a ventricular level shunt is present, mixed venous saturation is best approximated by the saturation in the superior vena cava (SVC). Inferior vena caval (IVC) blood is not well mixed because of streaming patterns of the highly oxygenated renal venous blood and the less oxygenated hepatic venous and lower body blood. Sampling in the IVC should thus be performed primarily to consider specific diagnoses (such as total anomalous pulmonary venous connection or hepatic arteriovenous malformations). Similarly, right atrial (RA) blood is not well mixed: SVC, coronary sinus, and IVC streams of very different oxygen saturations are present.

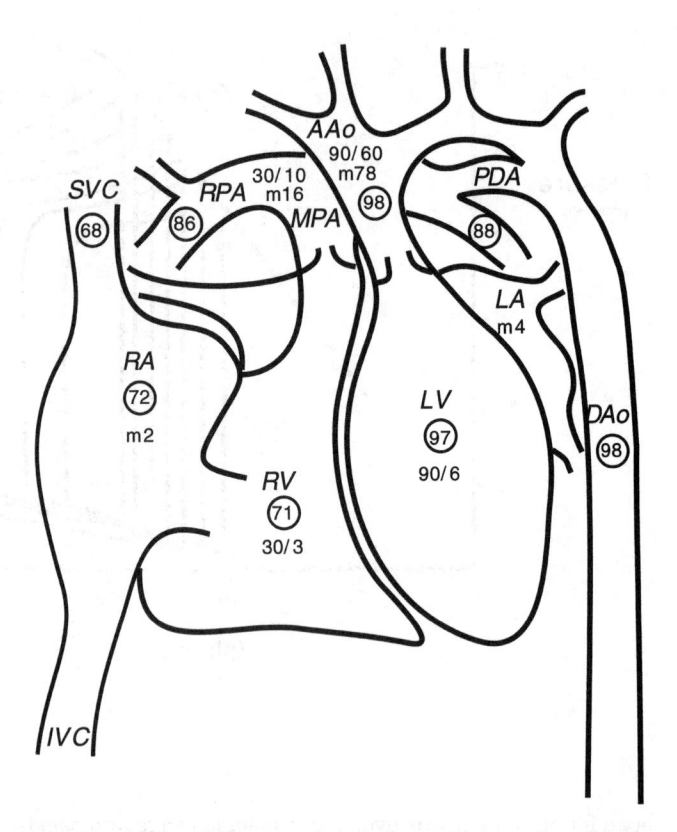

Figure 3.4. Anatomic diagram for cardiac catheterization. Saturations are in the circles, pressures are not circled, and m represents mean pressures. The anatomic diagram presents hemodynamic data for a patient with a patent ductus arteriosus (PDA). For blood flow calculations, the most distal well mixed venous sample proximal to the shunt is 71%, in the right ventricle (RV). The pulmonary arterial saturation is difficult to ascertain but may be considered as the average value between the right (RPA) and left (LPA) pulmonary arterial saturations, or 87%. The pulmonary venous and systemic arterial saturations are the same because there is no right-to-left shunt, and are thus best represented by the most distal arterial saturation, that being 98% in the descending aorta (DAo). If oxygen consumption is 150 mL/min/m² and hemoglobin concentration is 12.0 g/L, pulmonary blood flow is 8.4 mL/min/m² and systemic blood flow is 3.4 mL/min/m², yielding a pulmonary to systemic blood flow ratio of 2.5:1. From the flows and the transpulmonary and transystemic pressure gradients of 12 mm Hg and 76 mm Hg, respectively, pulmonary vascular resistance is 1.4 RU and systemic vascular resistance is 22.3 RU (see the text for explanation of the calculations). AAo, ascending aorta; LA, left atrium; LV, left ventricle; MPA, main pulmonary artery; RA, right atrium; SVC, superior vena cava.

For pulmonary blood flow calculations, pulmonary arterial saturation can be obtained in either branch, except in the presence of aortopulmonary communications, which can cause different saturations in the right and left branches. In this situation, it is difficult to estimate mixed pulmonary arterial saturation, and either both branch values can be used to yield a range of pulmonary blood flows or an average value can be calculated.

On the left side, pulmonary venous and systemic arterial saturations should be identical in the absence of a right-to-left shunt. The principle of obtaining the most distal, well-mixed sample should be used in this case, and they are both best represented by aortic saturation. Samples from the pulmonary veins and left atrium (LA) may not accurately represent mixed pulmonary venous blood if local differences are seen in pulmonary venous saturations. With a right-to-left atrial shunt, pulmonary venous saturations must be obtained. In the case of a right-to-left ventricular shunt, LA saturations can be used as representative of the mixed pulmonary venous blood. Sampling from the aorta in any location should yield similar values for systemic arterial saturation, except with coarctation or interruption of the aorta with right-to-left ductal shunting. This situation makes calculation of systemic blood flow impossible.

Pressure Measurements

When measuring vascular pressures, it is important to use consistently the same phase of the respiratory cycle. Large fluctuations in phasic and mean pressures can be seen in those areas with compliant walls (such as the RA and pulmonary veins) when even modest airway obstruction exists. As with saturation measurements, vascular pressures are best considered along lines of flow as well.

Superior vena cava and IVC pressures are recorded only in the rare situations of venous-atrial obstruction. RA pressure tracings show a dominant 'a' wave, similar to right ventricular end-diastolic pressure. Right ventricular systolic pressure is measured in the body and outflow areas if outflow obstruction is likely, such as in tetralogy of Fallot. Similarly, pressures in the main pulmonary artery are measured not only immediately above the valve but also just proximal to the right and left branches if supravalvar obstruction is considered possible. Branch pulmonary artery pressures are measured wherever a natural or surgical obstruction is considered possible. Pulmonary capillary wedge pressures are compared with left atrial pressures to exclude pulmonary venous stenoses. In the absence of such pulmonary venous stenoses, venous wedge 'a' wave pressures can be compared with LV end-diastolic pressure to evaluate the mitral valve for stenosis.

Left atrium pressures demonstrate a dominant 'v' wave, except with mitral stenosis or a noncompliant LV. The 'a' wave should approximate the LV end-diastolic pressure. As with the RV, LV systolic pressure is measured in both the body and outflow portions of the ventricle if intracavitary obstruction is considered possible, as can occur in subaortic stenosis. Ascending aortic pressures are measured immediately above the valve and more distally with supravalvar stenosis. Pressures are also measured in the descending aorta when the diagnosis of a hypoplastic aortic arch or a coarctation of the aorta is considered. Generally, systolic pressures increase and diastolic pressures decrease as the catheter is advanced from the heart because of stiffness of the central vessels and the presence of reflected waves. Also, local flow disturbances can alter pressures. A high-velocity jet directed toward a blood vessel (such as occurs in the innominate artery with supravalvar aortic stenosis) can allow kinetic energy to be converted to potential energy in the wall of the vessel and increase measured pressure (Coanda effect), whereas a high-velocity stream of blood perpendicular to a vessel decreases pressure (Bernoulli effect).

Basic Calculations

Systemic, pulmonary, and effective pulmonary flow can be calculated using the Fick principle from hemoglobin concentration, saturations, and oxygen consumption. Blood flow across any vascular bed can be calculated from knowing the concentration of a substance (in this situation, oxygen) on both sides of the bed and the amount of uptake or release of that substance by that vascular bed.

Therefore, pulmonary blood flow can be calculated from the equation:

$$(3) \quad Q_p = \frac{\dot{V}_{O_2}}{C_{O_2}(PV - PA)}$$

where Q_p is pulmonary blood flow (usually indexed to m² and measured per minute), $\dot{V}_{O_2}$ is oxygen uptake (equal to oxygen consumption), and $C_{O_2}(PV-PA)$ is the arterial oxygen content difference between the pulmonary veins (PV) and pulmonary arteries (PA).

Similarly, systemic blood flow can be calculated from the same equation by substituting systemic arterial (SA) oxygen content for PV content, and systemic venous (SV) oxygen content for PA content. Effective pulmonary blood flow is the amount of blood going to the lung that is effectively oxygenated so that SV oxygen content is used instead of PA oxygen content in the above equation.

Oxygen consumption is the amount of oxygen taken up by the body. It can be measured in the catheterization laboratory in the spontaneously breathing patient using the flow-through method (33, 34), it or can be estimated from nomograms based on surface area or age, and heart rate. Oxygen content can be calculated by multiplying the hemoglobin oxygen carrying capacity (about 13.6 mL O_2/L) and the hemoglobin oxygen saturation. Adding oxygen dissolved in blood to the calculation of content usually is important only if the arterial oxygen concentration is well above 100 mm Hg. This is because only 3 mL O_2 is directly dissolved per 100 mm Hg of oxygen tension. In a patient with a hemoglobin concentration of 15.0 g/L and an arterial PO_2 of 100 mm Hg, this would add only 3 mL O_2 dissolved in the blood to 204 mL O_2 bound to hemoglobin.

Oxygen delivery can be calculated by multiplying systemic blood flow by the content of oxygen in the blood. From oxygen consumption and delivery data, the fraction of oxygen extracted can be calculated, and is approximately 25 to 30% in the normal situation. Fractional extraction of oxygen is perhaps one of the best parameters of how well the heart is doing its job of delivering adequate oxygen and substrate for metabolic stability. Short of measuring fractional extraction, the single most useful index of metabolic stability is mixed venous saturation, which is being monitored with more and more frequency in the intensive care setting using indwelling oximeter catheters.

Other methodologies like dye dilution and thermodilution techniques can also be used to measure blood flow. A known quantity of a substance (iodocyanide green for dye dilution) or a known temperature of saline is injected into a central vein, and complete mixing is assumed by the time it reaches the systemic or pulmonary arterial bed.

For dye dilution curves, dye concentration is usually recorded in a systemic artery over the time for a single circulation. Integrated concentration over that time (Fig. 3.5A) is used to calculate systemic blood flow. With a left-to-right shunt, an early recirculation phase is apparent (Fig. 3.5B), which represents the quantity of blood that returns directly to the pulmonary circulation without going through the peripheral systemic bed. Thus the sum of the two phases represents pulmonary blood flow. For thermodilution studies, the thermistor for measuring pressure is usually in the pulmonary artery, on the same catheter through which the cold saline is injected. Integrated change in temperature can be used in a similar fashion to that of the dye dilution curve to calculate systemic blood flow but not to determine a left-to-right shunt.

Vascular resistances are calculated from the mean pressure difference across the vascular bed of interest, divided by the amount of flow crossing that bed, from the equation:

(4) $$R = \frac{\overline{P}_a - \overline{P}_v}{Q}$$

where R is the resistance, $\overline{P}$ is the mean pressure in the arterial (a) or venous (v) side of the bed, and Q is flow. When pressure and flow are measured in their standard units (mm Hg and $mL \cdot min^{-1} \cdot m^2$, respectively), resistance is in Wood, or resistance (RU), units.

Pulmonary vascular resistance is usually less than 3 RU, whereas systemic vascular resistance is more variable, ranging from about 15 to as high as 30 RU in the normal child. Frequently, if pulmonary vascular resistance is elevated, various maneuvers are performed in the catheterization laboratory to dilate the pulmonary vascular bed, thus determining its reactivity. These maneuvers are discussed elsewhere (see Chapter 32, *Pulmonary Hypertension*). It is important to note that vascular resistance is an index of the cross-sectional bed of the arteriolar-capillary-venule complex, and it does not include impedance of the central vessels. With any central obstructions (such as coarctation of the aorta on the systemic side, or branch pulmonary artery stenosis on the pulmonary side), resistance cannot be accurately calculated, because the perfusion pressures of all sites of the vascular bed are not equal.

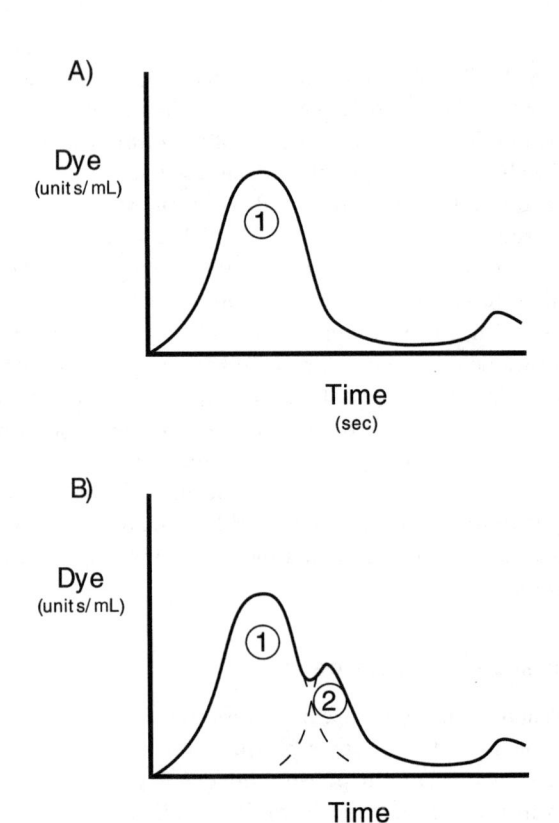

Figure 3.5. Dye dilution curves. **A.** A normal curve in the absence of shunting. There is a first pass of dye recorded by the sensor (*curve 1*), with late recirculation after the dye passes through the systemic and pulmonary vascular beds. Blood flow can be calculated from the area under the curve, the amount of dye injected, and the sampling rate. **B.** A curve in the presence of a left-to-right shunt. After the initial curve, there is an early recirculation curve (*2*) representing early return of dye as it passes through the defect/shunt, through the pulmonary vascular bed, and to the sensor early. The recirculation phase represents the left-to-right shunt, so that pulmonary blood flow can be calculated from the sum of curves 1 and 2, and the pulmonary to systemic blood flow ratio can be calculated by dividing this sum by curve 1.

MYOCARDIAL OXYGEN PHYSIOLOGY

Overview

Uninterrupted flow of large quantities of oxygenated blood to the myocardium is critical to its normal function.

Unique to the heart is that this flow must be maintained despite regular forceful contractions, which only abolishes flow to the capillary bed during systole, but can also reverse flow (toward the epicardial vessels). Blood must flow from epicardium to endocardium, from low to high intramyocardial pressure, in a relative proportion to meet the metabolic demands of each layer. Such flow must be regulated in such a way that areas of high demand can immediately increase their blood supply.

Coronary Circulatory Physiology

The myocardium extracts about 60 to 75% of oxygen from the blood that passes through it, a much larger percentage than other organs, which average about 30% oxygen extraction. Because of this high level of extraction, coronary sinus oxygen tension is low, generally around 20–25 mm Hg. This low level of oxygen tension requires that any increase in oxygen demand is met by an increase in blood flow rather than an increase in extraction. The left ventricle can normally increase its work up to fourfold, and coronary flow must likewise increase. Although the vascular bed is innervated and can respond to sympathetic stimulation and to a wide variety of circulating vasoactive substances, the primary mechanisms controlling myocardial flow are autoregulation and metabolic regulation.

Autoregulation describes local pressure regulation of the resistance vessels of the myocardium such that, at a constant oxygen consumption, blood flow remains constant over a fairly wide range of perfusion pressures (Fig. 3.6). At pressures above and below the autoregulatory range, flow is linearly related to perfusion pressure. Autoregulation protects the subendocardium from ischemia during vasodilatory stresses, as long as aortic diastolic pressure remains above 30 mm Hg and 40 mm Hg in the immature and mature heart, respectively. Vasodilatory drugs that maximally dilate the coronary resistance vessels allow determination of the coronary reserve, which is the difference in flow between the autoregulatory and dilated states at a given perfusion pressure. The mechanisms that control autoregulation are not fully known, but the primary candidates include myogenic activity of vascular smooth muscle, tissue pressure (35, 36), and local metabolic control. Myogenic control of autoregulation is based on the theory that increased intravascular pressure stimulates vasoconstriction of vascular smooth muscle (36). A venous-arterial reflex has also been described where an increase in venous pressure causes arteriolar constriction, probably by a neurally mediated mechanism (36). Autoregulation can also be affected by tissue pressure. Coronary circulation accounts for up to 15% of the volume of the myocardium, so that changes in its blood volume can profoundly affect local tissue pressure and alter blood flow (36).

The central concept in metabolic regulation is the metabolic hypothesis, which states that blood flow is closely linked to tissue metabolism. Reduction of blood inflow would cause an accumulation of vasodilator substances, which would in turn cause vasodilation and increased blood flow. Adenosine is a prime candidate for this vasodilator substance because it is a potent vasodilator produced locally by the breakdown of adenosine triphosphate (ATP) when oxygen delivery is reduced. In addition, it has recently been shown that ATP-dependent potassium channels are important modulators of vascular tone in many high-flow vascular beds. Ischemia activates these channels in the myocardium, and their inhibition reduces maximal coronary flow. Lastly, other chemical mediators include carbon dioxide and hydrogen ion.

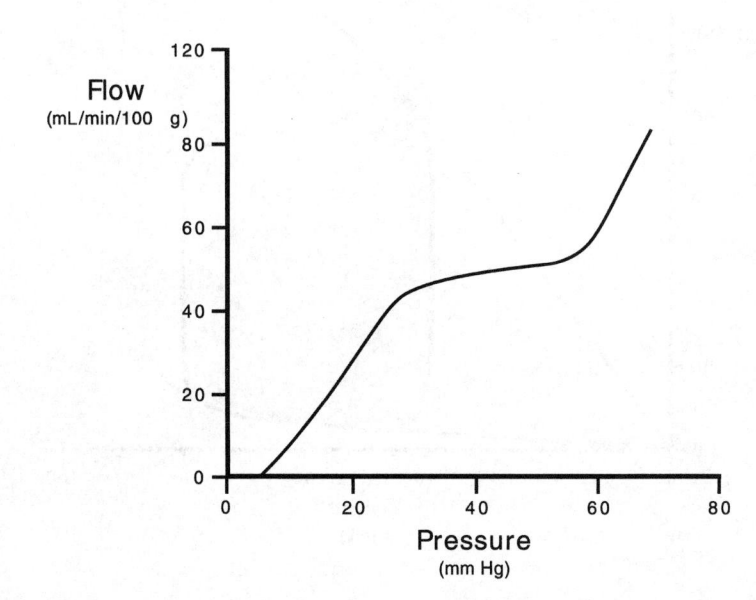

Figure 3.6. Autoregulation curve. A typical pressure-flow relationship of the coronary circulation. At low and high perfusion pressures and in the setting of constant myocardial oxygen consumption, coronary blood flow varies directly with perfusion pressure. In the autoregulatory range (from about 30 to 60 mm Hg), any change in perfusion pressure is counterbalanced by a change in vascular resistance, so that flow remains relatively constant.

Myocardial Oxygen Consumption

Myocardial oxygen consumption is directly linked to myocardial work, and it can be broken down into three components. First, a small amount of energy is required for basal metabolism, which does not appear to change across contractile states but is heart rate dependent (37). Second, a somewhat greater amount of energy is required for excitation-contraction coupling, which is thought to represent the energy utilization of the sarcoplasmic reticulum. This component is dependent on the contractile state of the heart, increasing with increasing contractility independent of changes in actual mechanical performance (38). This has been called the "oxygen wasting effect" of increasing contractile state (39). Lastly, the largest component of energy requirements is that needed for the mechanical performance of the heart. This component is determined by many factors, but primarily by the wall stress that the heart generates during systole and by its frequency of contraction (40).

Thus, a frequently used index of myocardial oxygen consumption is the double product, which is simply the product of the peak systolic pressure and heart rate. Because the double product does not consider energy utilization for excitation-contraction coupling, the relationship of the double product and oxygen consumption only holds within a given contractile state. In addition, it does not consider the pressure profile during ejection and the volume of blood ejected, changes that alter the integrated stress throughout systole. Thus, although clinically useful, it is only a rough estimate of oxygen consumption.

Using the time-varying elastance model described above, a much better understanding of the relationship between mechanical work and oxygen consumption can be derived. From the pressure-volume loop, the mechanical work of the heart can be divided into two parts, which combined are termed the "pressure-volume area" (PVA) (Fig. 3.7) (41–43). External work of the heart (EW), calculated as the area within the loop itself, represents the functional work of the heart as it ejects blood against a varying pressure. Mechanical efficiency of the heart is the ratio of this external work to total myocardial oxygen consumption, which is generally about 30%.

In addition to this external work, stress is still seen in the myocardium at the end of systole. This component of the mechanical work of the heart is termed "potential energy," because it is not dissipated by the external work of ejection. This energy is afterload dependent; at high afterload, little ejection has occurred, the end-systolic elastance is still high, and a great deal of potential energy remains. With lower afterload, little energy remains in the heart, potential energy is low, and the ratio of EW to total work increases, representing increased efficiency of the heart from an ejection standpoint.

In summary, myocardial oxygen delivery is finely regulated, primarily by alterations in coronary blood flow, which are under local autoregulatory and other metabolic factors. Because resistance to flow exists not only in the resistance vessels themselves but also in the myocardium due to intramyocardial stresses caused by contraction, a relatively high perfusion pressure must be maintained during diastole. A fairly constant 65 to 70% of oxygen de-

Figure 3.7. Myocardial work and pressure-volume area (*PVA*). The total work of the heart is represented by the PVA, which can be divided into that which generates output, or *external work* (*area 1*, within the pressure-volume loop) and the *potential energy* remaining within the wall of the ventricle after ejection (*area 2*). PVA closely correlates with myocardial oxygen consumption at a constant contractile state, and its components determine the mechanical efficiency of the heart, as described in the text.

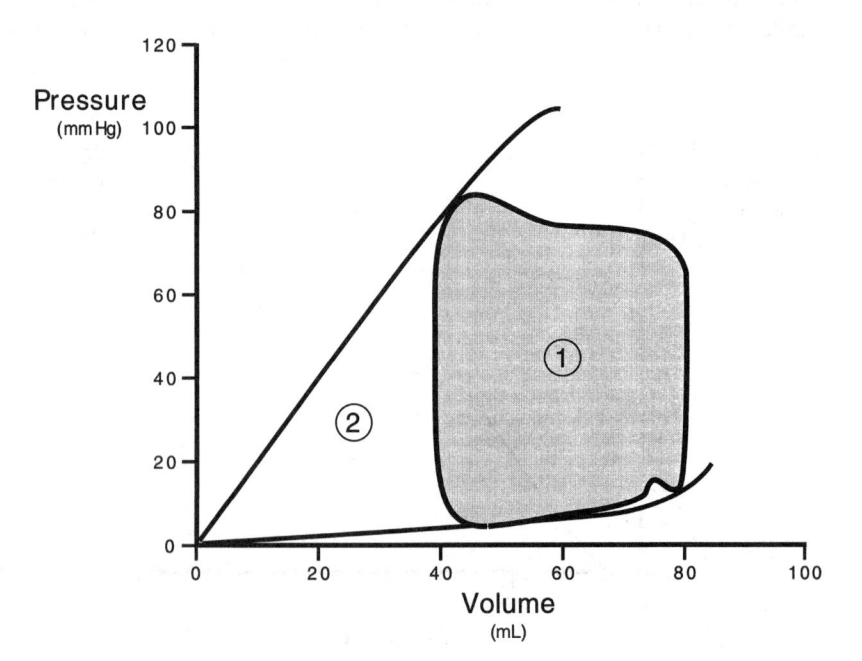

livered to the myocardium is consumed. That consumption is directed toward basal metabolism, energy required for excitation contraction coupling independent of cross bridge linking, and mechanical work of cross bridge linking. The latter incorporates both external work of the heart, as it ejects blood, and potential energy remaining in its wall at end-systole, which represents the remaining stiffness, or elasticity, in the wall secondary to residual cross bridge links.

REFERENCES

1. Van den Bos GC, Elzinga G, Westerhof N, et al. Problems in the use of indices of myocardial contractility. Cardiovasc Res 1973;7:834–848.
2. Elzinga G, Westerhof N. How to quantify pump function of the heart. Circ Res 1979;44:303–308.
3. Hibberd MG, Jewell BR. Calcium- and length-dependent force production in rat ventricular muscle. J Physiol (Lond) 1982;329(527):527–540.
4. Kentish JC, ter Keurs HE, Ricciardi L, et al. Comparison between the sarcomere length-force relations of intact and skinned trabeculae from rat right ventricle. Influence of calcium concentrations on these relations. Circ Res 1986;58(6):755–768.
5. Lakatta EG. Starling's law of the heart is explained by an intimate interaction of muscle length and myofilament calcuim activation. J Am Coll Card 1987;10:1157–1164.
6. Parmley WW, Chuck L. Length-dependent changes in myocardial contractile state. Am J Physiol 1973;224(5):1195–1199.
7. ter Keurs HE, Rijnsburger WH, van Heuningen R, et al. Tension development and sarcomere length in rat cardiac trabeculae. Evidence of length-dependent activation. Circ Res 1980;46(5):703–714.
8. Allen DG, Kurihara S. The effects of muscle length on intracellular calcium transients in mammalian cardiac muscle. J Physiol (Lond) 1982;327(79):79–94.
9. Allen DG, Kentish JC. Calcium concentration in the myoplasm of skinned ferret ventricular muscle following changes in muscle length. J Physiol (Lond) 1988;407(489):489–503.
10. Babu A, Sonnenblick E, Gulati J. Molecular basis for the influence of muscle length on myocardial performance. Science 1988;240(4848):74–76.
11. Murray JM, Weber A. Competition between tropomyosin and myosin and cooperativity of the tropomyosin-actin filament. In: Frinell AD, Brazier MAB, eds. The regulation of muscle contraction. New York: Acadmic Press, 1981:261–275.
12. van der Velde ET, Burkhoff D, Steendijk P, et al. Nonlinearity and load sensitivity of end-systolic pressure-volume relation of canine left ventricle in vivo. Circulation 1991;83(1):315–327.
13. Burkhoff D, de Tombe PP, Hunter WC, et al. Contractile strength and mechanical efficiency of left ventricle are enhanced by physiological afterload. Am J Physiol 1991:H569–578.
14. van der Linden LP, van der Velde ET, Bruschke AV, et al.J. Identifiablity of left ventricular end-systolic pressure-volume relationships. Am J Physiol 1988;254(6 P. 2):H1113–1124.
15. Hunter WC. End-systolic pressure as a balance between opposing effects of ejection. Circ Res 1989;64:265–275.
16. Ishida Y, Meisner JS, Tsujioka K, et al. Left ventricular filling dynamics: influence of left ventricular relaxation and left atrial pressure [published erratum appears in Circulation 1986;74(3):462]. Circulation 1986;74(1):187–196.
17. Hori M, Inoue M, Fukunami M, et al. An increase in afterload augments ventricular relaxation rate in isolated perfused canine hearts. Cardiovasc Res 1985;19(10):649–654.
18. Hori M, Inoue M, Kitakaze M, et al. Loading sequence is a major determinant of afterload-dependent relaxation in intact canine heart. Am J Physiol 1985;249(4 P. 2):H747–754.
19. Raff GL, Glantz SA. Volume loading slows left ventricular isovolumic relaxation rate. Evidence of load-dependent relaxation in the intact dog heart. Circ Res 1981;48(6 P. 1):813–824.
20. Yellin EL, Hori M, Yoran C, et al. Left ventricular relaxation in the filling and nonfilling intact canine heart. Am J Physiol 1986;250(4 P. 2):H620–629.
21. Little WC. The left ventricular dP/dtmax-end-diastolic volume relation in closed-chest dogs. Circ Res 1985;56(6):808–815.
22. Glower DD, Spratt JA, Snow ND, et al. Linearity of the Frank-Starling relationship in the intact heart: the concept of preload recruitable stroke work. Circulation 1985;71(5):994–1009.
23. Sagawa K. The ventricular pressure-volume diagram revisited. Circ Res 1978;43(5):677–687.
24. Suga H, Sagawa K. Instantaneous pressure-volume relationships and their ratio in the excised, supported canine left ventricle. Circ Res 1974;35:117–126.
25. Ross J Jr. Afterload mismatch and preload reserve: a conceptual framework for the analysis of ventricular function. Prog Cardiovasc Dis 1976;28:255–264.
26. Sunagawa K, Maughan WL, Burkhoff D, et al. Left ventricular interaction with arterial load studied in isolated canine ventricle. Am J Physiol 1983;245(5 P. 1):H773–780.
27. Little WC, Cheng CP. Left ventricular-arterial coupling in conscious dogs. Am J Physiol 1991;261(1 P. 2):H70–76.
28. Burkhoff D, Sagawa K. Ventricular efficiency predicted by an analytical model. Am J Physiol 1986;250(6 P. 2):R1021–1027.
29. Asanoi H, Sasayama S, Kameyama T. Ventriculoarterial coupling in normal and failing heart in humans [published erratum appears in Circ Res 1990;66(4):1170]. Circ Res 1989;65(2):483–493.
30. Baan J, Van der Velde ET, De Bruin HG, et al. Continuous measurement of left ventricular volume in animals and humans by conductance catheter. Circulation 1984;70(5):812–823.
31. Kass DA, Midei M, Brinker J, et al. Influence of coronary occlusion during PTCA on end-systolic and end-diastolic pressure-volume relations in humans. Circulation 1990;81(2):447–460.
32. McKay RG, Aroesty JM, Heller GV, et al. Assessment of the end-systolic pressure-volume relationship in human beings with the use of a time-varying elastance model. Circulation 1986;74(1):97–104.
33. Lister G Jr, Hoffman JI, Rudolph AM. Measurement of oxygen consumption: assessing the accuracy of a method. J Appl Physiol 1977;43(5):916–917.
34. Lister G, Hoffman JI, Rudolph AM. Oxygen uptake in infants and children: a simple method for measurement. Pediatrics 1974;53(5):656–662.
35. Little RC, Little WC. Local control of peripheral circulation. Physiology of the heart and circulation. 4th ed. Chicago: Year Book Medical Publishers, 1989:267–283.
36. Johnson PC. Autoregulation of blood flow. Circ Res 1986;59(5):483–495.

37. Klocke FJ, Braunwald E, Ross J Jr. Oxygen cost of electrical activation of the heart. Circ Res 1966;18(4):357–365.
38. Suga H, Hisano R, Goto Y, et al. Effect of positive inotropic agents on the relation between oxygen consumption and systolic pressure volume area in canine left ventricle. Circ Res 1983;53(3):306–318.
39. Rooke GA, Feigl EO. Work as a correlate of canine left ventricular oxygen consumption, and the problem of catecholamine oxygen wasting. Circ Res 1982;50(2):273–286.
40. Braunwald E. Control of myocardial oxygen consumption: physiologic and clinical considerations. Am J Cardiol 1971;27(4):416–432.
41. Khalafbeigui F, Suga H, Sagawa K. Left ventricular systolic pressure-volume area correlates with oxygen consumption. Am J Physiol 1979;237(5):H566–569.
42. Suga H. Total mechanical energy of a ventricle model and cardiac oxygen consumption. Am J Physiol 1979;236(3):H498–505.
43. Suga H, Hayashi T, Shirahata M, et al. Regression of cardiac oxygen consumption on ventricular pressure-volume area in dog. Am J Physiol 1981;240(3):H320–325.
44. Huxley AF. Muscular contraction. J Physiol (Lond) 1974;243(1):1–43.

Cardiac Diagnostic Evaluation

Anthony F. Rossi, MD

Evaluation of the infant with suspected heart disease has evolved in the last two decades into one that is heavily reliant on biomedical technology. Undiagnosed, the critically ill infant with suspected heart disease was once solely dependent on the astute clinician for accurate diagnosis. Nowadays, it is not uncommon to witness the echocardiographer's transducer on an infant's chest before the clinician's stethoscope. The current role of the physical examination in defining a cardiac anomaly, once imperative for accuracy is perhaps less clear. Nonetheless, the clinician still plays a crucial function in formulating a differential diagnosis, as well as in discerning which technology is best suited for optimal management of the critically ill neonate with suspected heart disease. Early recognition, prompt noninvasive diagnosis, and medical stabilization of critically ill infants with congenital heart disease has resulted in a significantly lower mortality rate over the last two decades.

Infants with heart disease may present with one or more of the following signs and symptoms. Most commonly, the cardiologist is consulted to evaluate the neonate with a heart murmur. Although most of these consultations are not urgent, evaluation should be carried out in a timely fashion because ductal-dependent congenital heart disease may present with an "innocent-sounding" heart murmur. Infants with hypoplastic left heart syndrome often present with little more than a nonspecific murmur. More urgent indications for cardiac evaluation include respiratory distress and cyanosis or shock (Table 4.1). Cyanosis in the absence of respiratory distress in a newborn, as well as circulatory collapse in the first few weeks of life, should be considered heart disease until proved otherwise. The most common group of structural heart diseases causing shock in the newborn are the left-sided obstructive lesions, although severe arrhythmias (both bradycardias and tachycardias) or cardiomyopathies are occasionally responsible. If the cardiovascular evaluation of a newborn in shock will be delayed, such as for transport, it is not unreasonable to begin prostaglandin E_1 pending evaluation (1, 2).

TRANSITIONAL CIRCULATION

Proper clinical evaluation of the newborn infant requires detailed understanding with respect to changes of the transitional circulation. Evaluation of every newborn with suspected heart disease requires the basic knowledge that (*a*) systemic vascular resistance increases dramatically with clamping of the umbilical cord; (*b*) pulmonary vascular resistance begins to fall with the infant's first breath, decreases most notably in the first day of life, and continues to do so for the first month of life; and (*c*) the ductus arteriosus will begin to close, typically within 24 to 48 hours of birth. Metamorphosis from fetal to neonatal circulation occurs rapidly at first and then continues for weeks following delivery (see also Chapter 18, *Single Ventricle Lesions*) (3).

Implications of the transitional circulation are most important in the newborn with a left-to-right shunt lesion. In infants with congenital heart defects, the rate of fall in pulmonary vascular resistance is much less predictable than in the normal newborn. Neonates with large left-to-right shunts may have persistently elevated pulmonary vascular resistance levels for weeks after birth. Persistence of high pulmonary vascular resistance, by virtue of its profound effect on the physiology of many congenital heart lesions, can mask the presentation of significant congenital heart disease early in life. For example, an infant with a large ventricular septal defect will have little or no shunting until the pulmonary vascular resistance begins to fall. Under these circumstances, symptoms and signs of a large left-to-right shunt (e.g., tachypnea, poor feeding, hepatomegaly, and murmur) can not be obvious until the infant's 6-week check-up, or even later (3–6).

PHYSICAL EXAMINATION

Inspection

Evaluation of the infant with suspected heart disease begins with a careful observation of the infant's general appearance. Initial clinical assessment is crucial and helps dictate the rapidity with which the evaluation is conducted. It is best to observe the infant undressed and under a radiant warmer. The child's activity is of paramount importance. An active, vigorously crying child indicates a much lower level of acuity than a listless child who barely reacts to noxious stimuli such as blood drawing. Cyanosis, if present, should be characterized as generalized, central, or restricted to the upper or lower extremities. Peripheral perfusion, respiration pattern, and dysmorphic features must be evaluated (Table 4.2).

Table 4.1. Congestive Heart Failure Presenting in the First Two Months of Life

In utero (hydrops fetalis)	Anemia	Hemolytic disease secondary to Rh sensitization, fetal-maternal transfusion, hypoplastic anemia
	Tachycardia	SVT, atrial flutter, ventricular tachycardia
	Bradycardia	Congenital heart block
	Volume overload	Ebstein's anomaly with TR, AVC with severe AV valve regurgitation, Arteriovenous malformation
	Ventricular dysfunction	Myocarditis, cardiomyopathy
Day 1	Noncardiac	Asphyxia, sepsis, hypoglycemia, hypovolemia
Weeks 1–2	LV obstructive lesions	AS, coarctation, HLHS, IAA
	Left-to-right shunt lesions	PDA, AP window, truncus arteriosus
Weeks 2–8	Left-to-right shunt lesions	AVC, VSD, TAPVR, single ventricle without PS
	Decreased pump performance	Anomalous left coronary artery, endocardial fibroelastosis, glycogen storage disease, myocarditis

AP, aortopulmonary; AS, aortic stenosis; AVC, atrioventricular canal; HLHS, hypoplastic left heart syndrome; IAA, interrupted aortic arch; PDA, patent ductus arteriosus; PS, pulmonic stenosis; SVT, supraventricular tachycardia; TAPVR, total anomalous pulmonary venous return; TR, tricuspid regurgitation; VSD, ventricular septal defect.

Table 4.2. Cardiovascular Anomalies Associated with Common Pediatric Syndromes

Syndrome	Anomaly
Trixomy 21	AVC, ASD primum, VSD, TOF
Trisomy 18	VSD, PDA, DORV
Trisomy 13	VSD
Turner's (45:XO)	Coarctation of the aorta, HLHS
Cat's Eye	TAPVR, TOF
Mucopolysaccharidoses	HCM, CHF
Pompe	HCM, CHF, L-G-L
Williams	Supravalvular AS, branch PS, diffuse and/or discrete arterial stenosis
Noonan	PS, ASD
Holt-Oram	ASD
Di George, Catch 22	Aortic arch anomalies, IAA, TOF, TA
Goldenhar	TOF
Tuberous sclerosis	Rhabdomyomas, W-P-W

AS, aortic stenosis; ASD, atrial septal defect; AVC, atrioventricular canal; CHF, congestive heart failure; DORV, double outlet right ventricle; HCM, hypertrophic cardiomyopathy; HLHS, hypoplastic left heart syndrome; IAA, interrupted aortic arch; L-G-L, Lown-Ganong-Levine; PS, pulmonic stenosis; TA, truncus arteriosus; TAPVR, total anomalous pulmonary venous return; TOF, tetralogy of Fallot; VSD, ventricular septal defect; W-P-W, Wolff-Parkinson-White.

Inspection of the thorax with attention to the precordial area may yield important findings. Chest symmetry and location of the maximal cardiac impulse should be evaluated. Although a somewhat hyperactive precordium may be present in the first few hours of life, by 6 to 12 hours the precordium should be quiet. The temptation to limit the physical examination to those areas relevant to the cardiovascular system must be resisted. Once the infant has been stabilized, attention should be directed to screening for associated anomalies such as cleft palate, esophageal or anal atresia, facial and skeletal deformities, in addition to the many other anomalies associated with the cardiovascular system (7–10).

Assessment of Peripheral Perfusion

In patients with low cardiac output or congestive heart failure, pallor is secondary to peripheral vasoconstriction, caused by high circulating endogenous catecholamines. In this setting, the infant's skin color is usually pale gray, with mottling and cyanosis of the distal extremities and delayed capillary refill. Extremities are cool and pulses may be weak and thready. Neonates with left heart obstructive lesions (such as hypoplastic left heart syndrome, coarctation of the aorta, or critical aortic stenosis) often present in this manner (see Chapter 18). As the ductus begins to close, systemic cardiac output becomes compromised. Decreased systemic perfusion leads to the development of metabolic acidosis and decreased coronary perfusion, which further diminishes cardiac function. Early recognition of this condition is crucial, as this vicious cycle may only be reversed with the administration of prostaglandin E_1.

A careful evaluation of an infant's pulses is essential in the assessment of suspected heart disease (Table 4.3). The ability to palpate a patient's pulse is related to the pulse pressure (i.e., difference between the systolic and diastolic blood pressure) and stroke volume. Patients with low cardiac output normally have weak thready pulses (secondary to narrow pulse pressure). Patients with systemic artery to pulmonary artery connections (such as a patent ductus arteriosus, aortopulmonary window, arteriovenous malformation, or excessive aortopulmonary collaterals) may have

Table 4.3. Pulse Patterns in Patients with Congenital Heart Disease

Upper Extremity	Lower Extremity	Anomaly and Comments
++	++	Normal, cyanotic heart disease without AP collaterals, ASD, VSD
+++	+++	PDA, AP window, AP collaterals, "duct-dependent" lesions with nonrestrictive ductus (e.g., HLHS, IAA, PA/IVS)
+	+	Aortic stenosis, HLHS (restrictive ductus)
++	+/0	Coarctation of the aorta, IAA (restrictive ductus)

AP, aortopulmonary; ASD, atrial septal defect; HLHS hypoplastic left heart syndrome; IAA, interrupted aortic arch; PA/IVS, pulmonary atresia with intact ventricular septum; VSD, ventricular septal defect.

"bounding" pulses secondary to a widened pulse pressure. Pulses should be palpated in both upper and lower extremities. Weak or thready pulses in all four extremities can be present in patients with poor systemic cardiac output secondary to hypoplastic left heart syndrome or critical aortic stenosis. Palpable upper extremity pulses with diminished or absent lower extremity pulses is diagnostic of coarctation of the aorta or interrupted aortic arch. Bounding pulses do not exclude left ventricle obstructive disease: the baby with hypoplastic left heart syndrome or coarctation and a widely patent ductus arteriosus may have significant pulmonary "run-off" and easily palpable "bounding" pulses (see also Chapter 12, *Preoperative Care*).

Respiratory Effort

Observation of an infant's respiratory effort is crucial in distinguishing cardiac from noncardiac causes of cyanosis. It is essential to note rate and pattern of breathing. Respiratory rates are higher in the first few hours of life and fall to less than 45 per minute in term infants and less than 60 in preterm infants by 24 hours. Variations in rate can also normally occur. So-called "periodic breathing" patterns, with short periods of apnea, are not uncommon in normal newborn infants. In neonates, the predominant work of breathing is borne by the diaphragm. Accessory muscles of respiration are not typically used by normal neonates. Their use or severe retractions suggests pulmonary disease as the cause of hypoxemia or hypercarbia. Respiratory rates of infants with congenital heart defects are typically at the upper limits of normal. Respiratory patterns of infants with heart disease differ from normal infants not so much in the effort but rather by the regularity of the tachypnea and lack of normal variation in the respiratory rate.

Heart Rate

Heart rate variability is common in the first few weeks of life. A resting heart rate of 120 to 130 beats per minute (bpm) is normal in newborn infants. A resting heart rate of less than 90 or more than 160 warrants investigation. Although sinus tachycardia is a common finding in patients with congenital heart disease and low cardiac output or congestive heart failure, heart rate is typically in the normal range in most patients with uncomplicated cyanotic heart disease. Sinus bradycardia in a full-term infant is present when the heart rate is less than 90 bpm. Normal infants can exhibit short, transient decreases in heart rate to 70 bpm during bowel movements, eating, or hiccupping, and these decreases are secondary to enhanced vagal tone. More prolonged periods of bradycardia are abnormal. Heart rates of less than 60 bpm require immediate attention. In intubated mechanically ventilated infants, bradycardia can be secondary to hypoxia or hypercarbia related to a ventilator malfunction or inadvertent extubation. In a quiet, nondistressed infant bradycardia can be secondary to congenital complete heart block.

Edema

Edema of the limbs, although a common finding in older patients with congestive heart failure, is unusual in infants. Limb edema in infants can be associated with congenital heart disease in patients with Noonan or Turner syndrome. In those instances, edema is usually present in the dorsum of the hands or feet, and it is related to local factors rather than to congestive heart failure. Edema secondary to congestive heart failure in neonates and infants is more commonly noted in the eyelids or dependent areas such as the sacrum.

Heart Auscultation

Properly performed auscultation of the newborn's heart requires considerable patience and an optimal examining environment. A calm infant whose heart rate is in the normal range provides optimal auscultation. The infant should be disturbed as little as possible during the examination—a cold stethoscope will certainly startle the infant. Placing the stethoscope on the infant's chest and allowing the infant to become accustomed to its presence before beginning the examination is helpful; it may be useful to perform the preliminary examination through the shirt. It should be stressed that cardiovascular auscultation does not involve only the thorax but should include abdomen (especially over the liver) and cranium. Arteriovenous malformations although uncommon, are often diagnosed late as a cause of congestive heart failure in newborns.

The first heart sound (produced by mitral and tricuspid valve closure) is normally single in newborns. The second heart sound (aortic and pulmonic closure) is single in most newborns during the first 6 hours of age. By 48 hours the second heart sound is audibly split in most infants. An examiner's ability to discern splitting of S2 depends on a slow heart rate, and it is therefore best heard during sleep. Feeding will calm an infant but may result in an increased heart rate, thereby obscuring the splitting. A single second heart sound is associated with many simple and complex cardiac defects including any defect that results in equalization of pulmonic and aortic pressures. Other lesions such as aortic or pulmonary atresia, hypoplastic left heart syndrome, truncus arteriosus, and transposition of the great arteries also present with a single S2. Quality of the second heart sound must also be noted. A loud pulmonary component occurs in patients with pulmonary hypertension, but this may be normal in the first few days of life. A systolic ejection click is often noted in normal babies in the first few hours of life. After 24 hours, an ejection click should be considered pathologic. Ejection clicks are most often associated with either dilation of a great artery or malformation of a semilunar valve (11).

Soft murmurs are frequently noted in newborn infants; most of these are innocent in nature. These innocent murmurs can be divided into two varieties: those associated with the normal changes occurring in the transitional circulation, and those that are not. "Innocent" systolic murmurs of the newborn are typically soft and nonspecific, becoming audible during the first few days of life. For instance, murmurs secondary to a patent ductus arteriosus are common. The ductal murmur may change, as the caliber of the ductus changes or pulmonary vascular resistance falls (12, 13). A soft blowing systolic murmur heard best at the lower left sternal border is often noted in patients with mild tricuspid regurgitation; a history of a difficult delivery is consistent with transient neonatal myocardial ischemia, which can result in transient mitral or tricuspid regurgitation (14). This murmur can be confused with a small ventricular septal defect, but it is transient and often absent after a few days of life. Loud, harsh murmurs present in the delivery room are usually pathologic; they typically represent semilunar valve stenosis or atrioventricular valve regurgitation and require further investigation.

Cyanosis

A diagnosis of cyanosis made by inspecting the newborn infant can be difficult. A number of factors including lighting, reflected light from wall paint, skin pigmentation, and the examiner's experience can impede the detection of cyanosis. Newborns are often noted to be dusky; peripheral cyanosis of the hands and feet can be present in normal infants. Polycythemic infants (often secondary to cord stripping) appear ruddy and cyanotic (15). Severely anemic infants may not appear cyanotic at all, because approximately 3 to 5 g of reduced hemoglobin per deciliter of arterial blood must be present before cyanosis becomes clinically detectable in most patients. Inspection of the oral mucosa or tongue is helpful to determine cyanosis. Once cyanosis is detected, evaluation should begin with pulse oximetry. Oximetry of both upper and lower extremities (pre and postductal) can lead to a rapid clinical diagnosis. It is recommended that oximetry of both the right and left arms and one lower extremity be performed so not to be misled in situations such as juxtaductal left subclavian artery in coarctation of the aorta; anomalous origin of either the right or left subclavian artery from the descending aorta (which is postductal) in many heart defects; and transposition associated with coarctation of the aorta (16).

When hypoxemia has been confirmed by pulse oximetry (pulse oximetry saturation of less than 90%), further evaluation is mandated. Infants who are desaturated but in no respiratory distress are much more likely to have cyanotic heart disease than pulmonary disease as a cause of hypoxemia. In patients with congenital heart disease "differential cyanosis" may be present. Differential cyanosis refers to the appearance of cyanosis limited only to either the upper or lower extremities. Congenital heart disease may or may not be the cause of cyanosis of the lower extremities with normal oxygen saturation in the upper extremities. Patients with interrupted aortic arch or coarctation of the aorta may present in this manner, as well as those with pulmonary hypertension of the newborn (PPHN) (17). Birth history may give important clues to the diagnosis of infants with desaturated lower extremities. Infants with traumatic delivery, birth asphyxia, low Apgar scores, or infants with meconium aspiration all are at risk for the development of PPHN and right-to-left ductal shunting. However, a birth history that is often associated with PPHN does not exclude the possibility of structural congenital heart disease, and the presence of differential cyanosis alone warrants a full cardiac evaluation including an echocardiogram (Table 4.4) (18, 19). Cyanosis of the upper extremities associated with normal oxygen saturation of the lower extremities ("reverse differential cyanosis") in newborn patients is pathognomonic for transposition of the

Table 4.4. Indication for Emergent Echocardiographic Evaluation of an Infant

1. Po_2 on arterial blood gas <50 torr with inspired oxygen content of 1.0
2. Differential cyanosis
3. Murmur associated with cyanosis
4. Cyanosis without respiratory distress

great arteries associated with either coarctation of the aorta, interruption of the aortic arch, or suprasystemic pulmonary vascular resistance.

HYPEROXIA CHALLENGE

Change in arterial P_{O_2} in response to breathing 100% oxygen is perhaps the most useful screening tool in the evaluation of infants with generalized cyanosis. This hyperoxic challenge ("hyperoxia test") is not without pitfalls and must be performed properly to ensure optimal sensitivity. The advent of routine pulse oximetry has resulted in some physicians performing this test incorrectly without measuring arterial P_{O_2}, relying instead on changes in oxygen saturation to rule out cyanotic heart disease. However, infants with cyanotic heart disease often achieve oxygen saturations of 100% when breathing an F_{IO_2} of 1.0. The hyperoxia test should therefore be performed as follows. Infants with oxygen saturations of less than 90% by pulse oximetry should receive 100% oxygen for at least 10 minutes. An arterial blood gas should then be performed. Infants with a P_{O_2} of greater than 200 torr almost never have congenital heart disease as a cause of cyanosis. At the other end of the spectrum, infants whose P_{O_2} fails to rise above 70 torr in the presence of a normal P_{CO_2} are very likely to have congenital heart disease and an echocardiogram should be performed promptly. If the P_{O_2} is in the range of 150 to 200 torr, congenital heart disease is unlikely, but it cannot be excluded. Results in this range may indicate a need for further diagnostic testing including echocardiography, depending on the clinical situation (see also Chapter 12, *Preoperative Care*).

SUMMARY

A few simple rules apply when evaluating the newborn with suspected heart disease. A murmur associated with significant cyanosis warrants echocardiographic evaluation of the heart (2). Absence of a murmur does not rule out congenital heart disease. Significant structural cyanotic heart disease can present with no heart murmur (such as transposition of the great arteries or tetralogy of Fallot with pulmonary atresia). Finally, murmurs of significant (but noncritical) congenital heart disease such as a small ventricular septal defect can be absent in the first few days of life and only become apparent in the next few weeks as the pulmonary vascular resistance begins to fall (3).

ELECTROCARDIOGRAM

Despite recent advances in the echocardiographic evaluation of patients with suspected congenital heart disease, the electrocardiogram remains an important screening tool. It is invaluable in the emergent treatment of electrolyte emergencies. Although emergent rhythm disturbances sometimes dictate management of life-threatening problems based on rhythm strips, the scalar 12-lead ECG is pivotal in the management of most rhythm disturbances in infants and children (see also Chapter 30, *Diagnosis and Management of Cardiac Arrhythmias*). With the exception of ventricular fibrillation or hemodynamically significant ventricular tachycardia, most arrhythmias are stable enough to allow careful evaluation of the rhythm disturbance prior to treatment.

ECG Interpretation

The electrocardiogram should be examined in a systematic fashion. An ECG that is grossly abnormal often has valuable information missed if a systematic approach is not employed. Typically, measurement would begin with that of intracardiac conduction intervals. This should include duration of the P wave, QRS complex, and QT interval corrected for rate. PR and RP intervals should also be measured. Next should come rate determination, followed by that of rhythm. If the P wave-QRS association is not readily apparent on the 12-lead electrocardiogram, it can be performed at faster paper speeds or with the gain increased. The P wave axis should next be determined; it should be calculated in much the same manner as the QRS axis. In normal sinus rhythm, the P wave is upright in lead I and aVF, giving an axis of between 0 and 90°. The QRS axis is calculated next. Evidence of atrial and ventricular hypertrophy is now evaluated. Finally, attention is turned to the ST segments and T waves.

Normal Electrocardiogram

A normal heart beat begins with depolarization of the sinoatrial node. Adjacent atrial muscle tissue is then depolarized in a wavelike fashion. This wave is propagated across the atria and arrives in the area of the atrioventricular node in approximately 30 to 40 milliseconds. The wave continues through the left atrium and is terminated in the lateral left atrium approximately 80 milliseconds after it had begun. This activity is noted on the surface ECG as the P wave. Repolarization of the atria is not readily apparent on the ECG. Once the waveform reaches the specialized conduction tissue of the AV node, the impulse is slowed. Impulse propagation through the AV node is not apparent on the surface ECG. Intracardiac electrophysiologic recording is required to record conduction through the AV node. The impulse continues through the bundle of His. Impulse propagation increases velocity in the bundle of His and continues through the specialized conduction tissue of the left and right bundle branches. The PR interval is the sum of all the events that have occurred to this point. Finally the impulse exits from the

Purkinje fibers. HV interval of the His bundle recording is a measure of His-Purkinje conduction time. The QRS is complete when all the ventricular cells have depolarized. Repolarization, and generation of the T wave and ST intervals, are less organized. In general, repolarization occurs in just the opposite sequence as depolarization, and from the epicardium toward the endocardium.

Maturational Changes in the Electrocardiogram

Knowledge of normal variations in the electrocardiogram and maturational changes that occur is crucial in interpreting the pediatric ECG. Also, significant differences exist in the ECG of the premature and full-term infant. Resting heart rates change with age, as well as most intervals and duration of the P wave and QRS complexes. The QRS axis changes, shifting gradually leftward beginning shortly after birth, and the ST-T wave axis changes. A heart rate of 130 bpm in an 18-year-old patient represents tachycardia, but is normal for a 1-week-old newborn. A tachycardia with a QRS duration of 0.12 seconds would be considered a narrow complex tachycardia in an adolescent, but would be a wide complex tachycardia (suggestive of ventricular tachycardia) in a 1-week-old infant. Likewise, although a QRS axis of +120° is normal in a 1-week-old, it represents right axis deviation in an 18-year-old.

Changes in ECG morphology occur from the first day of life through adolescence. The most significant changes, however, occur at three distinct time periods. These are the first few days of life, years 1 to 2, and childhood to adolescence. In general, with advancing age, changes include:

1. A decrease in heart rate
2. An increase in P wave and QRS duration
3. An increase in QRS voltage
4. An increase in the PR interval
5. A leftward shift in the frontal plane QRS axis
6. A right ventricular dominant pattern which converts to a left ventricular dominant pattern.

This transition from RV dominance to LV dominance is related to changes that occur in the ventricular mass ratios secondary to changes in afterload occurring during the transition from the fetal circulation (RV dominant) to the mature circulation (decreasing pulmonary vascular resistance and increasing systemic vascular resistance with age). ECG changes lag behind the changes in pulmonary vascular resistance. In addition, the T wave exhibits characteristic changes in the precordial leads over time. The T wave is normally upright in the right precordial leads on day 1 of life. By 48 to 72 hours of age, the T wave will become inverted in V_1 in normal infants. This pattern remains constant until 8 to 10 years of age in most children, and occasionally into adolescence in some, when the T wave once again becomes upright in V_1 and remains so. This T wave change begins early in childhood and the progression of T wave changes from inverted to an upright position begins in the left precordium and marches through the right precordium with increasing age, concluding with upright T waves in V_1 (20–23).

Hypertrophy

Hypertrophy is often inferred from the surface ECG despite the fact that ECG patterns are often similar whether the heart is truly thickened (hypertrophied) or dilated. Nevertheless, criteria are readily available for the diagnosis of left and right atrial enlargement, and left and right ventricular "hypertrophy." As with other aspects of the pediatric ECG interpretation, these criteria are age specific.

Right and Left Atrial Enlargement

Right atrial depolarization is recorded in the initial portion of the P wave. A narrow P wave in lead II of greater than 0.3 mV in height is indicative of right atrial enlargement. Depolarization of the left atrium occurs in the terminal portion of the P wave. A biphasic P wave, with a duration of more than 0.10 seconds is suggestive of left atrial enlargement. Because biphasic P waves are often seen in normal pediatric ECGs, it is important to document prolonged depolarization. A P wave with a negative terminal deflection of greater than 0.1 mV and duration of more than 0.04 seconds in lead V_1 is confirmatory.

Right Ventricular Hypertrophy

Signs suggesting right ventricular hypertrophy are particularly important in pediatric patients because congenital heart lesions often impose abnormal volume or pressure demands on the right ventricle. Height of the R in the right precordial leads (V3R and V_1) and the depth of the S in V_6 are important indicators of possible right ventricular hypertrophy (RVH). These rules are age dependent. An R wave in lead V_1 of greater than the 98% for age outside the newborn period is specific for RVH. An upright T wave in lead V_1 at greater than 7 days of age is also indicative of RVH. The T wave direction, combined with an abnormal R wave amplitude, increases the precision in diagnosing RVH. Right axis deviation, a QR pattern in lead V_1 or a RSR′ pattern in lead V_1 all are suggestive of RVH and can be used to support voltage or T wave criteria.

Left Ventricular Hypertrophy

Diagnosis of LVH from the surface ECG is neither 100% specific nor sensitive. Voltage criteria include R wave amplitudes of greater than 95% in leads V_5 and V_6. Inverted T waves in the left precordial and inferior leads (II, II, aVF) along with depression of the ST segment is considered an LV strain pattern and often noted in patients with aortic stenosis. An abnormal ratio of the R and S waves in V_1 and an abnormally increased Q wave in lead V_6 are suggestive of LVH.

Myocardial Ischemia

The ECG is an important tool in the diagnosis of myocardial ischemia. Myocardial ischemia is most clearly demonstrated as changes in the T wave or ST segments. Appearance of abnormal Q waves is thought to signify cell death. In contrast to the adult patient, localized myocardial ischemia is rare in pediatric patients. An exception would include the patient with anomalous origin of the left coronary artery from the pulmonary artery (see also Chapter 20, *Miscellaneous Lesions*). More commonly, myocardial ischemia as indicated by distorted peaked T waves, T wave inversion, and ST segment depression or elevation is part of a global process indicative of an imbalance of myocardial oxygen delivery to demand.

REFERENCES

1. Scott DJ, Rigby ML, Miller GAH, et al. The presentation of symptomatic heart disease in infancy based on 10 years' experience (1973–82). Implications for the provision of services. Br Heart J 1984;52:248–257.
2. Emmanouilides GC, Baylen BG. Structural congenital heart disease in the newborn: its differentiation from nonstructural heart disease. Paediatrician 1981;10:46.
3. Rudolph A. The changes in the newborn circulation after birth: the importance in congenital heart disease. Circulation 1970;41:343.
4. Emmanouilides GC, Moss AJ, Duffie ER Jr, et al. Pulmonary artery pressure changes in newborn infant from birth to three days of age. J Pediatr 1964;65:327.
5. Hoffman J, Rudolph A. Natural history of ventricular septal defects in infancy. Am J Cardiol 1965;16:634.
6. Heymann MA, Soifer SJ. Persistent pulmonary hypertension of the newborn. In: Fishman AP, ed. The pulmonary circulation: normal and abnormal. Philadelphia: University of Pennsylvania Press, 1990:371.
7. Alagille D, Odievre M, Gautier M, et al. Hepatic ductular hypoplasia associated with characteristic facies, vertebral malformations, retarded physical, mental and sexual development and cardiac murmur. J Pediatr 1975;86:63–71.
8. Pierpont ME, Moller JH. The genetics of cardiovascular disease. Boston: Martinus Nijhoff Publishing, 1987.
9. Cullum L, Lieberman J. The association of congenital heart disease with Down's Syndrome (mongolism). Am J Cardiol 1969;24:1349–1355.
10. Nora JJ, Torres FG, Sinha AK, et al. Characteristic cardiovascular anomalies of XO Turner syndrome, XX and XY phenotype and XO-XX Turner mosaic. Am J Cardiol 1970;25:639–641.
11. Braudo M, Rowe RD. Auscultation of the heart-early neonatal period. Am J Dis Child 1961;101:575–577.
12. Lyon RA, Rauh LW, Stirling JW. Heart murmurs in newborn infants. J Pediatr 1940;16:310–317.
13. Taylor WC. The incidence and significance of systolic cardiac murmurs in infants. Arch Dis Child 1953;28:52–54.
14. Berry TE, Muster AJ, Paul MH. Transient neonatal tricuspid regurgitation: possible relation with premature closure of the ductus arteriosus. J Am Coll Cardiol 1983;2:1178.
15. Gatti RA, Muster AJ, Cole RB, et al. Neonatal polycythemia with transient cyanosis and cardiorespiratory abnormalities. J Pediatr 1963; 69:1063–1072.
16. Goldman HI, Maralit A, Sun S, et al. Neonatal cyanosis and arterial oxygen saturation. J Pediatr 1973;82:319–324.
17. Goetzman B, Riemenschneider T. Persistence of the fetal circulation. Pediatr Rev 1980;2:37.
18. Lees MH. Cyanosis of the newborn infant. J Pediatr 1970;77:484–498.
19. Yabek SM. Neonatal Cyanosis. Reappraisal of response to 100% oxygen breathing. Am J Dis Child 1984;138:880–884.
20. Davigon A, Rautaharju R, Boiselle F, et al. Normal ECG standards for infants and children. Pediatr Cardiol 1980;1:123–131.
21. Hait G, Gasul BM. The evolution and significance of T-wave changes in the normal newborn during the first seven days of life. Am J Cardiol 1963;12:494–504.
22. Liebman J. The normal electrocardiogram. In: Liebman J, Plonsey R, Gillette PC, eds. Pediatric electrocardiography. Baltimore: Williams & Wilkins, 1982:144–171.
23. Walsh SZ. The electrocardiogram during the first week of life. Br Heart J 1963;25:784–794.

Cardiovascular Pharmacology

Lara S. Shekerdemian, MD, MRCP, and Andrew Redington, MD, FRCP

Since William Withering observed that the foxglove helped patients with dropsy (1), dramatic advances have been made in cardiovascular pharmacology. Successful cardiac intensive care primarily depends on "anticipating" potential problems with prompt intervention. To achieve this end, thorough clinical assessment must be combined with meticulous noninvasive and invasive monitoring and strategic pharmacologic support.

This chapter first introduces several basic concepts of cardiac pharmacology, and then discusses the mechanism of action, metabolism, guidelines for clinical use, and adverse effects of the most commonly used cardiovascular drugs in the cardiac intensive care setting. Antidysrhythmic agents are covered in Chapter 30, *Diagnosis and Management of Cardiac Arrhythmias*.

BASIC PRINCIPLES

Drug Bioavailability

Whereas t $(1/2)\alpha$ is the rapid *distribution* phase, t $(1/2)\beta$ is the slower *elimination* half-life. The bioavailability or plasma concentration of an exogenously administered drug depends on its (a) absorption, (b) volume of distribution, and (c) metabolism and elimination. These factors are heavily influenced by the patient's age.

Absorption

Absorption of an enteral drug is unreliable, particularly in critically ill children and during the first months of life (2–4). The gastrointestinal tract presents a drug with both favorable and unfavorable stimuli in terms of pH, motility, and enzyme secretion, all of which can influence absorption, degradation, and thus availability of the drug.

At birth, gastric pH is nearly neutral, but the presence of hydrochloric acid in the lumen of the stomach gives its contents a pH of between 1.5 and 3 within a few hours of life. Gastric secretions (acid, pepsin, and intrinsic factor) reach adult levels by the third month, and pancreatic exocrine activity attains adult levels by the end of the first year of life. Peristalsis in neonates is also variable and somewhat erratic, with transit times reaching adult rates by about 8 months of age.

Volume of Distribution

Distribution of most drugs within the body is strongly influenced by a number of age-dependent factors. Among the most important of these are (a) relative ratio of body water to fat and (b) drug-protein binding (2–5).

Neonates and infants have a greater body *water:fat ratio* than adults; in addition, the water concentration of neonatal adipose tissue is approximately double that of adults. Following administration of a drug, the infant's total plasma concentration (C) is related to the total amount of the drug in the body (A) and the volume of distribution (Vd) by the equation: $A = Vd \times C$. Pediatric patients, therefore, have a greater volume of distribution for water-soluble drugs than adults.

Drug-protein binding is influenced by many factors, including nutritional state of the child; presence of fetal albumin; total serum albumin, globulin, and protein concentrations; number of binding sites; and affinity of the binding sites for the drugs. Levels of serum albumin and protein as well as their binding capacity do not approach adult levels until the child is 1 year of age.

Metabolism and Elimination

Liver is the primary organ of drug metabolism, with additional sites being the lung, kidney, and gastrointestinal tract.

Hepatic drug metabolism can transform an active drug into inactive metabolites, as in the case of catecholamines, or alter a parent drug into active metabolites, as with some phosphodiesterase inhibitors. Hepatic enzymes can also convert a parent drug into its active counterpart, as observed with propranolol and theophylline. Enzyme systems display different rates of maturation (2, 4), with phase I enzyme reactions–oxidation, reduction, hydrolysis, and hydroxylation–reaching adult capacity within a few months of birth; however, some of the phase II (or conjugation) reactions–glucuronidation, sulphation, and acetylation–remain immature until around 5 years of age.

Many cardiovascular drugs (e.g., digoxin, furosemide, and dobutamine) undergo *renal excretion*. Maturation of renal function does not follow a uniform pattern, with rates of development varying between the different components (2–4). Although tubular reabsorption does not appear to be limited in neonates, glomerular filtration rate and renal blood flow do not reach adult levels until 6 months and 1 year of age, respectively.

Pharmacotherapy of Heart Failure

Low-output cardiac failure with transient or prolonged impairment of myocardial function is commonly encountered in the pediatric cardiac intensive care setting. In the period following cardiopulmonary bypass for cardiac surgery, for instance, myocardial function is often reversibly depressed with transient elevation of both preload and afterload. Low-output failure is also seen in other myocardial dysfunction states, which can be primary (as in dilated cardiomyopathy) or secondary (as in metabolic disturbance or arrhythmias [see Chapter 31, *The Failing Myocardium*]).

Cellular Basis for Manipulation of Cardiac Output

Cellular mechanisms controlling contraction and relaxation of the myocardium and the vascular smooth muscle form the molecular basis for contractility and systemic and pulmonary vascular resistance; to a great extent, these interactions determine cardiac output. A basic understanding of these mechanisms is essential for full appreciation of the physiology of heart failure and the modes of action of cardiovascular drugs.

Myocardial Contraction

Myocardial contractility increases over the first few months of life, as do the numbers of sympathetic nerve fibers within the myocardium and the total concentration of endogenous noradrenaline (6). This explains in part the greater dependence of cardiac output on heart rate (rather than contractility) in the neonatal heart. The immature heart has limited responsiveness to cardiotonic medications for several reasons, including (*a*) relatively high noncontractile content, (*b*) decreased availability of releasable norepinephrine, (*c*) less mature sympathetic system, (*d*) underdeveloped intracellular calcium regulatory mechanisms, and (*e*) decreased functional reserve capacity.

Ionized calcium plays a central role in the maintenance of myocardial contractility, and its effects are mediated via the intracellular concentration, calcium requirements of the muscle cell, and sensitivity of the myofilaments to calcium (7, 8). Deficiencies in the intracellular calcium homeostasis contribute significantly to myocardial dysfunction (9, 10), and therapeutic manipulation of these parameters directly can influence the force of myocardial contraction. Membrane depolarization of the myocardial sarcolemma allows the influx of "trigger" calcium across the voltage-gated calcium channels of the transverse tubule (see Fig. 5.1). This then activates the so-called "calcium-induced calcium release" across the ryanodine receptor (RyR)–mediated calcium release of the sarcoplasmic reticulum. Cytosolic calcium then binds to the troponin C of the myofilaments, allowing the contractile process to begin. Dissociation of calcium from this complex initiates relaxation, and released calcium is then sequestered by the Ca^{2+} adenosine diphosphate (ATPase) within the sarcoplasmic reticulum.

A number of *cyclic-adenosine monophosphate (AMP)-dependent protein kinases* exist in mammalian myocardial cells. Phosphorylation of sites on the sarcolemma, sarcoplasmic reticulum, and troponin complex results in an influx of calcium across the sarcolemma, acceleration of calcium uptake by the sarcoplasmic reticulum, and an increased rate of dissociation of calcium from troponin C. By increasing intracellular cyclic AMP, therefore, myocardial contractility is improved.

Inosityl 1, 4, 5 triphosphate (IP_3) and diacyl glycerol (DAG) are two additional myocardial second messengers that have been shown in vitro to increase contractility by modulating intracellular calcium. Their role in the physiology of heart failure is currently being widely investigated, which may provide a key to its future management.

Vascular Smooth Muscle

Although intracellular calcium also plays an important role in regulation of vascular smooth muscle tone, the mechanisms by which it does so are rather different (7). Calcium appears to trigger vascular smooth muscle contraction, but it does not influence force, duration, or termination of contraction. On entering the vascular smooth muscle cytoplasm, calcium initiates phosphorylation of myosin light chains by myosin light chain kinase, thus promoting myosin-actin cross bridge formation. Relaxation, or termination of contraction, depends either on dephosphorylation of the light chain by a calcium-independent phosphatase, or on a reduction in sensitivity to calcium. Agents that increase intracellular cyclic-AMP appear to increase intracellular calcium requirements for contraction, thus encouraging smooth muscle relaxation with resultant vasodilation (11).

Calcium-independent contractile mechanisms also exist in vascular smooth muscle. G protein-mediated activation of phospholipase C results in the breakdown of phosphatidylinositol biphosphate into IP_3 and DAG. IP_3 releases calcium from the sarcoplasmic reticulum, initiating contraction, and DAG activates protein kinase C with subsequent phosphorylation of intracellular proteins.

Contractile activity of the vascular smooth muscle can be modified either directly by pharmacologic agents such as the sympathomimetic amines or indirectly by the overlying endothelium (12). The response can either be vasoconstriction or vasodilation, and it changes with age (13). An example of endothelium-dependent vasorelaxation is the nitric oxide (NO) pathway, by stimulation of nitric oxide synthase (14). Increased formation of NO requires the cofactors magnesium, calcium and L-arginine. NO or a nitrosothiol then diffuses through to the underlying smooth muscle, increases the activity of guanyl cyclase, and hence the formation of cyclic 3'-5"-guanosine monophosphate (15). This indirectly decreases the intracellular concentration of calcium and hence enhances relaxation of the smooth muscle.

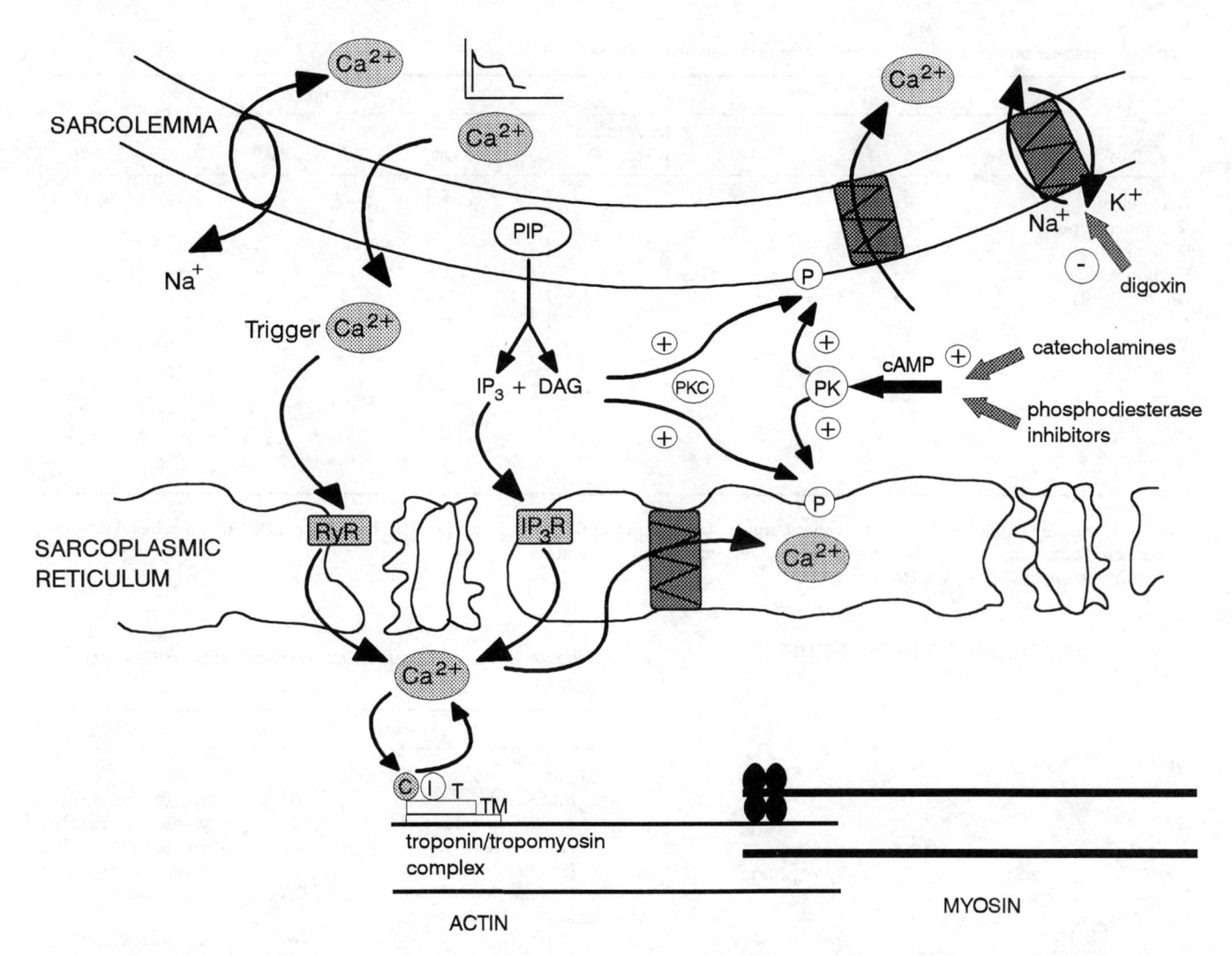

Figure 5.1. Myocardial cell showing the contractile process and sites of action of cardiovascular drugs. cAMP, adenosine 3'5'-cyclic monophosphate; C,I,T, troponin C,I,T; DAG, diacyl glycerol; IP$_3$, inositol 1,4,5 triphosphate; IP$_3$R, IP$_3$ calcium-release channel; P, sites of phosphorylation; PIP, phosphoinosityl phosphate; PK, cyclic-AMP dependent protein kinase; PKC, protein kinase C; RyR, ryanodine calcium-release channel; TM, tropomyosin.

In summary, two chief sites of action exist for cardiovascular drugs: myocardium and vascular smooth muscle. Pharmacologic agents can be used to improve the myocardial contractility by increasing intracellular cyclic AMP or to manipulate the systemic or pulmonary vascular resistance by their effects on vascular smooth muscle. Sites of action and hemodynamic effects of the common cardiovascular drugs used to treat heart failure are summarized in Table 5.1.

CATECHOLAMINES

Catecholamines are sympathomimetic amines that contain O-dihydrobenzene. The pathways of endogenous catecholamine synthesis are shown in Figure 5.2. Commonly used endogenous catecholamines are dopamine, epinephrine, and norepinephrine, whereas dobutamine and isoproterenol are synthetic catecholamines.

Effector cells' response to endogenous and exogenous catecholamines is related primarily to their interaction with α and β-adrenergic (originally classified by Ahlquist in 1948 (16) and dopaminergic receptors (see Table 5.2). Stimulation of α_1 receptors increases calcium influx into the postsynaptic effector cell, and α_2, β_1, and β_2 activation stimulates adenylate cyclase, giving rise to an increase in levels of intracellular cyclic AMP. Following this, cyclic AMP-dependent enzymatic activity leads to recruitment of calcium channels to allow calcium entry into the cell.

It is important to understand that antecedent congestive heart failure and sustained use of catecholamines can

Table 5.1. Inotropes and Vasodilators—Their Sites of Action and Hemodynamic Effects

Drug	Receptor					Hemodynamic Effects					
	α	β_1	β_2	DA[a]	Na$^+$/K$^+$ ATPase	CO	Contr.	SVR	MAP	PCWP	HR
Epinephrine	+++	+++	+++			↑↑	↑	↑↔↓	↑↔	↑↔	↔/↑/↑↑
Norepinephrine	+++	+				↑↔↓	↑	↑↑↑	↑↑	↑↔	↑/↑↑
Dopamine	++	++	+	++*		↑↑	↑	↑↔↓	↑↔	↑↔	↑
Dobutamine	+	+++	+			↑↑	↑↔	↓	↓↔	↔	↑↔
Isoproterenol		+++	+++			↑↑	↔	↓↓	↓	↓	↑↑
Amrinone						↑↑	↑↔↓	↓↓	↓↔	↑↔↓	↑↔
Milrinone						↑↑	↑	↓↓	↓↔	↓↔	↑↔
Enoximone						↑↑	↑↔	↓↓	↓↔	↓↔	↑↔
Nitroprusside						↑	↔	↓↓	↓	↓	↑↔
Nitroglycerin						↑	↔	↓	↓	↓↔	↑↔
Captopril						↑	↔	↓	↓	↓↔	↓↔
Digoxin					+++	↑	↑				

ATPase, adenosine triphosphatase; CO, cardiac output; Contr., contractility; DA, dopamine; HR, heart rate; MAP, mean arterial pressure; PCWP, pulmonary capillary wedge pressure; SVR, systemic vascular resistance
[a] Dopamine stimulates DA_1 and DA_2 receptors.

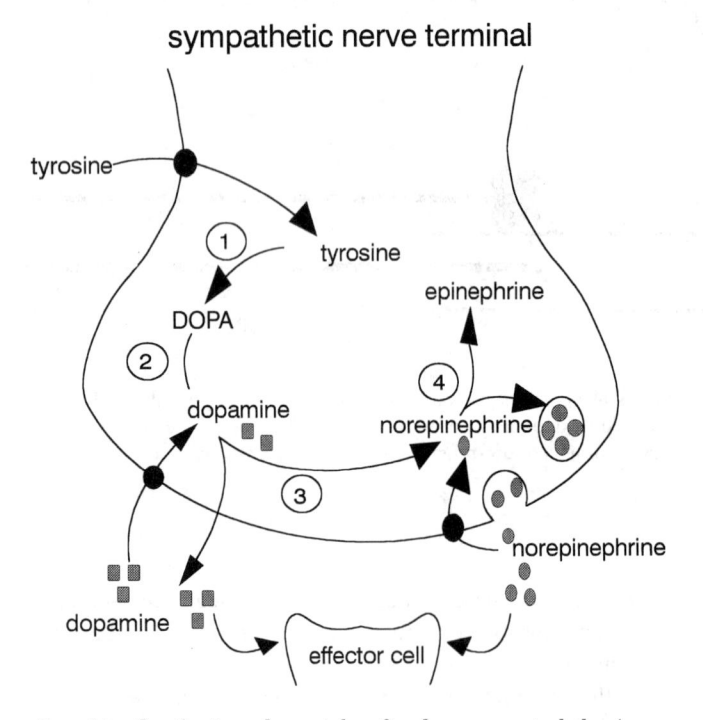

Figure 5.2. Synthesis and reuptake of endogenous catecholamines. Enzymatic steps: 1. Tyrosine-hydroxylase; 2. DOPA-decarboxylase; 3. Dopamine-hydroxylase; 4. Phenylethanolamine-methyl-transferase.

Table 5.2. Sites of Endogenous Catecholamine Receptors and Effects of Activation

Site	Receptor Type	Stimulation
Heart		
Sinus node	β_1	Increased heart rate
Atrioventricular node	β_1	Increased heart rate
Atria + ventricles	β_1	Increased contractility
Coronary circulation	α	Vasoconstriction
Coronary circulation	DA	Vasodilatation
Peripheral Vasculature		
Skin	α	Vasoconstriction
Pulmonary	α	Vasoconstriction
Renal	DA	Vasodilatation
Mesenteric + splanchnic	β_2, DA	Vasodilatation
Skeletal muscle	β_2	Vasodilatation
Nonvascular		
Renal tubule	DA	Diuresis
Bronchial tree	β_2	Bronchodilatation

DA, dopamine

lead to down-regulation of β-receptors and, therefore, decrease the efficacy of catecholamines. In addition, maturational differences in receptor density and affinity to β-agonists between immature and older animals affect inotropic therapy response (17).

The main adverse effects of catecholamines in general are (a) excessive chronotropy with increase in myocardial oxygen consumption and possible myocardial ischemia, (b) tachydysrhythmias, and (c) increase in afterload from activation of peripheral α-receptors, which can lead to tissue and end-organ ischemia.

Epinephrine

Epinephrine, the end product of endogenous catecholamine synthesis, which is released from the adrenal medulla, is a potent direct agonist of both α and β receptors.

An infusion of low dose epinephrine results predominantly in β-adrenoreceptor activation with an increase in heart rate, contractility, and lowering of the systemic vascular resistance caused by dilation of splanchnic and skeletal muscle vascular beds. Higher doses stimulate α-receptors, with an increased systemic vascular resistance and mean arterial pressure; at such doses, increased myocardial oxygen demand is almost inevitable. In addition to cardiovascular effects, increased plasma epinephrine has important metabolic effects including increased glycolysis and hyperglycemia. It has been demonstrated that epinephrine at high doses (1 μg/kg/min) can also cause *irreversible* myocardial damage in the neonatal myocardium consisting of sarcolemmal rupture and loss of mitochondrial architecture that is independent of its induced tachycardia effects (18).

Metabolism

The half-life of epinephrine is 2 to 3 minutes. It undergoes rapid metabolism by two routes: (*a*) renal and hepatic catecholamine orthomethyl transferase (COMT) converts epinephrine to metanephrine, and (*b*) neuronal monoamine oxidase (MAO) deaminates epinephrine. The products then undergo hepatic sulfation or glucuronidation to end in renal elimination.

Guidelines for Clinical Use

Epinephrine is administered as a continuous central intravenous infusion to the critically ill child with systemic hypotension, myocardial dysfunction, or low cardiac output. In combination with a vasodilator such as nitroprusside, it has been demonstrated to be of benefit in children with low cardiac output after cardiac surgery (19). It is also used for septic shock.

In its use as a drug in cardiopulmonary resuscitation, a much larger (10 times) dose (20) can be given via the endotracheal route. Evidence indicates that the standard dose of 0.01 mg/kg may be too low for effective cardiac resuscitation (21).

It should be noted that decrease in renal perfusion leading to oliguria can be observed with epinephrine that is not necessarily observed with dopamine or dobutamine (22). In addition, hyperglycemia and leukocytosis can be associated with epinephrine use. Lastly, tissue extravasation can lead to necrosis; this complication should be treated with local administration of the α-adrenergic blocker phentolamine.

Norepinephrine

Norepinephrine, a precursor of epinephrine, is a potent adrenergic agent that acts primarily on α-receptors.

Norepinephrine causes a significant increase in systemic vascular resistance as well as arterial blood pressure and myocardial oxygen consumption, with little change in contractility or in cardiac output. Norepinephrine levels are found to be increased in children with congestive heart failure (23) as well as following cardiopulmonary bypass for cardiac surgery (24).

Metabolism

Norepinephrine has a short half-life of 1 to 2 minutes, and it is rapidly metabolized, as epinephrine, by COMT and MAO (see above).

Guidelines for Clinical Use

Norepinephrine is rarely indicated as an inotropic agent in low cardiac output states, and in the pediatric cardiac intensive care unit it is most often used in combination with agents such as dopamine and epinephrine in situations with septic shock or cardiogenic shock associated with persistent hypotension and low systemic vascular resistance.

Norepinephrine can also be used in the treatment of hypercyanotic spells in tetralogy of Fallot (or similar pathophysiology) that are refractory to the conventional treatment of high inspired oxygen, intravenous morphine, and β-blocker. The presumed mode of action is systemic vasoconstriction (effect similar to administration of phenylephrine) sufficient to divert blood to the pulmonary vessels through the right ventricular outflow tract, thus increasing pulmonary blood flow.

Dopamine

Dopamine (3-hydroxy tyramine), a precursor of norepinephrine, mediates its effects directly on α- and β-adrenergic as well as dopamine receptors and indirectly via norepinephrine release from presynaptic sympathetic terminals.

With a perfusion pressure within the autoregulatory range, renal effects of dopamine are achieved by stimulation of the tubular (i.e., nonvascular) dopamine (DA_1) receptors (25). By reducing the sensitivity of vascular smooth muscle to intracellular calcium, stimulation of postsynaptic DA_1 receptors causes relaxation of the cerebral, renal, coronary, mesenteric, and pulmonary vasculature (25, 26). DA_2 receptors are pre- and postsynaptic in location, and they can be both vascular and nonvascular as well. Stimulation of these DA_2 receptors results in dilation of renal and mesenteric vascular beds by inhibition of adenylate cyclase activity and phosphatidylinositol turnover (25).

Low dose dopamine exerts its effects by stimulation of only the DA receptors, with a resulting increase in renal, mesenteric, and coronary blood flow without an appreciable change in myocardial oxygen consumption or in cardiac output (27, 28). Dopaminergic receptor activation either lowers or has no effect on the systemic vascular resistance.

At a medium dose, activation of β-adrenergic receptors stimulates an increase in contractility, heart rate, and norepinephrine release. At a high dose, α effects usually predominate with peripheral vasoconstriction, increases in systemic and pulmonary vascular resistances, heart rate, and blood pressure.

In the pediatric population, a great deal of individual variability is found in the dose response of dopamine, relationship between dose and plasma level, and degree of α, β, and DA receptor activation (29, 30). Intravenous dopamine is taken up by the sympathetic nerve ending for conversion to norepinephrine (31), which subsequently can be used either to replenish depleting stores in the sick child or for its inotropic properties. It is important to note that 30% of plasma dopamine is protein bound (30) so that the degree of nourishment and liver function of the critically ill child contribute to the level of unbound drug. Because of the varying rates of adrenergic receptor maturation, α-effects of dopamine may precede some of its β effects in neonates; in addition, the immature heart has decreased norepinephrine stores.

Metabolism

Exogenous dopamine is either peripherally metabolized by COMT or taken up by the sympathetic nerve endings where it is converted to norepinephrine, stored, or metabolized by MAO. A fraction of the drug is excreted unchanged by the kidneys. Interestingly, dopamine clearance appears to be dose-related if dobutamine is simultaneously administered (29).

Guidelines for Clinical Use

Dopamine is the most widely used catecholamine to treat systemic hypotension and low cardiac output in neonates, infants, and children, and it is a particularly good single agent for children with low cardiac output after cardiac surgery (32). Dopamine has also been used effectively in myocardial dysfunction, such as in neonates who had postasphyxia myocardial dysfunction (33).

Low dose dopamine suits best the normotensive child with oliguria and normal pulmonary capillary wedge pressure. Although low dose dopamine (5 μg/kg/min) was demonstrated to increase renal blood flow, a lower dose (2.5 μg/kg/min) increased renal plasma flow only in children older than 5 years of age (34). Increasing hypotension and a decreasing cardiac output with suboptimal heart rate can be treated by a dose increase to medium levels. Larger doses (more than 10 μg/kg/min) may be necessary in preterm infants less than 30 weeks gestation (35) to achieve the same effects. High dose dopamine should be used cautiously because of the potential unwanted α effects; in these circumstances, combination with a vasodilator (such as nitroprusside) is preferable (36).

Because of its potential to *increase* pulmonary artery pressure and pulmonary vascular resistance, dopamine should be used with caution in children with elevated pulmonary artery pressure or pulmonary vascular resistance. When compared with dobutamine, dopamine (at a dose of 7 μg/kg/min) had a greater effect in increasing pulmonary vascular resistance (37).

Dobutamine

The primary effect of dobutamine is to improve myocardial contractility primarily by β_1 stimulation, with additional β_2-mediated vasodilation and α-agonist effects.

Dobutamine's biochemical structure is a modified form of isoproterenol, and its actions are mediated by direct β-adrenergic stimulation without influence on norepinephrine release. Dobutamine is a synthetic catecholamine developed as a selective β-adrenergic agent to increase myocardial contractility, cardiac output, and blood pressure in the presence of myocardial failure (38, 39).

When compared with dopamine, intravenous dobutamine has been shown to similarly increase myocardial oxygen demand, but this is coupled with a significantly greater increase in coronary blood flow (40, 41). Dobutamine was demonstrated, however, to be less effective than dopamine in raising systemic arterial pressure (42). Comparison between dopamine and dobutamine at a low dose (2.5 μg/kg/min) failed to show a significant difference in the urine output and renal function in children after cardiopulmonary bypass (43).

Animal studies have suggested a blunted response by the immature cardiovascular system to intravenous dobutamine (44, 45), and this hypothesis has been supported by some studies suggesting a decreased responsiveness in neonates and infants (46, 47). Others have shown, however, a convincing increase in cardiac output at doses as low as 0.5 μg/kg/min without a significant change in systolic and diastolic blood pressures or heart rate (48).

Metabolism

Dobutamine has a half-life of 2 minutes, and it is rapidly methylated by COMT with subsequent hepatic glucuronidation. It is excreted both in the bile and by the kidneys.

Guidelines for Clinical Use

Dobutamine is a good agent for increasing inotropy without increasing heart rate in patients with myocardial dysfunction (49). Dobutamine at doses of 2 to 8 μg/kg/min was demonstrated to increase cardiac output and stroke volume while decreasing capillary wedge pressure with *no* effect on heart rate or systemic or pulmonary vascular resistances (50). Although certain lesions with small and noncompliant left ventricles may not respond adequately to dobutamine after surgery (51), dobutamine has been demonstrated to improve diastolic relaxation in children even at low doses (52).

Dobutamine is also a preferred agent for patients with pulmonary hypertension because it does not appear to increase pulmonary vascular pressure and resistance in pediatric patients after cardiac surgery (53).

Isoproterenol

Isoproterenol is a synthetic β_1 and β_2 agonist with virtually no α effects. Isoproterenol has positive chronotropic and inotropic effects, peripheral and pulmonary vasodilation, and bronchodilation. Low diastolic pressure from peripheral vasodilation in combination with induced tachycardia can compromise myocardial oxygen delivery with resulting myocardial ischemia.

Metabolism

The principal route of metabolism is by hepatic and renal COMT with subsequent hepatic conjugation; elimination is by the renal route.

Guidelines for Clinical Use

Adverse effects of isoproterenol on myocardial oxygen balance (54) limit its use in the pediatric cardiac intensive care setting because it can lead to myocardial ischemia. It can, however, be useful in those patients with bradycardia or atrioventricular block, even in the setting of the transplanted heart. In addition, isoproterenol can help to maintain heart rate and inotropic properties in patients after surgery that has led to right ventricular myocardial dysfunction, such as for tetralogy of Fallot (55). Lastly, isoproterenol has also been demonstrated to have a therapeutic role in the treatment of pulmonary hypertension (56).

Isoproterenol should be *avoided* in children with subaortic stenosis or lesions with similar pathophysiology (such as hypertrophic cardiomyopathy or single ventricle lesions with subaortic stenosis) as it increases the outflow tract gradient (57) because of its inotropic and vasodilatory properties. Isoproterenol should also be *avoided* in patients with tetralogy of Fallot as it may potentiate hypercyanotic spells. Lastly, because isoproterenol significantly decreases diastolic blood pressure, it should be used only with caution in patients with lesions and surgeries with low diastolic pressure (such as those with systemic to pulmonary shunts or aortic regurgitation).

Digoxin

Digoxin increases the availability of intracellular calcium for myocardial contraction by inhibiting the sarcolemmal Na^+-K^+ATPase (see Chapter 30, *Diagnosis and Management of Cardiac Arrhythmias* for antidysrhythmic uses).

In adults with congestive cardiac failure, there appear to be responders and nonresponders to digoxin therapy (58). Enhancement of parasympathetic activity seen with digoxin can have negative inotropic effects, and by producing a reduction in heart rate can potentially limit cardiac output.

Although pediatric literature on the efficacy of digoxin is scanty, a recent study of infants with congestive cardiac failure secondary to left-to-right shunting concluded that when added to a diuretic regimen, digoxin improved contractility without any significant improvement of symptoms (59).

Metabolism

Less than 25% of circulating digoxin is protein bound, the remainder being free. About 60 to 90% of digoxin is eliminated unchanged by the kidney (60).

Guidelines for Clinical Use

For myocardial dysfunction, intravenous digoxin used concomitantly with other intravenous inotropic agents is of questionable benefit. In some cardiac intensive care units digoxin is routinely initiated after certain surgeries (e.g., corrective surgery for tetralogy of Fallot) to maintain pharmacologic support after cessation of intravenous agents. Enteral absorption of digoxin can be affected by congestive heart failure and presence of antacids so that the parenteral form may be preferred in the intensive care unit.

Contraindications to its use include hypertrophic cardiomyopathy.

Adverse Effects

A number of factors can potentiate digoxin toxicity. By increasing myocardial digoxin concentration, hypokalemia is one of the most common and avoidable conditions. Other factors that can increase likelihood for digoxin toxicity include myocardial ischemia or myocardial inflammation (such as myocarditis or the postoperative myocardium), hypoxia, alkalosis, renal failure, prematurity, hypothyroidism, and interactions with other drugs (e.g., furosemide, verapamil, spironolactone, amiodarone, indomethacin, quinidine, and certain antibiotics such as erythromycin).

Care must be taken to monitor serum digoxin levels as toxicity is not uncommon (61) and life-threatening arrhythmias may be the first manifestation. These arrhythmias include (*a*) bradycardia due to depression of sinoatrial or atrioventricular nodes, (*b*) atrioventricular block, (*c*) ventricular bigeminy, and (*d*) tachycardias of either atrial or ventricular origin. In addition, gastrointestinal symptoms such as nausea, vomiting, and anorexia are not uncommon.

PHOSPHODIESTERASE INHIBITORS

Phosphodiesterase (PDE) is the enzyme responsible for the breakdown of 3'5' cyclic adenosine monophosphate (cAMP). Commonly used PDE inhibitors are specific for "fraction-III" PDE, which is the predominant form in cardiac muscle, and is also present in vascular smooth muscle. By increasing intracellular cyclic-AMP, PDE-III inhibitors increase the intracellular calcium availability for myocardial contraction, and promote relaxation of vascular smooth muscle (62). Advantages of PDE inhibitors over catecholamines include their independent action from β-receptor activation, particularly when these receptors are downregulated (as observed in congestive heart failure and chronic catecholamine use).

At a physiologic level, phosphodiesterase inhibition increases the rate of attainment of peak left ventricular systolic pressure, increases the rate of myocardial diastolic relaxation, reduces left ventricular end-diastolic pressure, induces peripheral arterial and venous vasodilation, and reduces myocardial oxygen consumption. Thus, the three hemodynamic effects of PDE inhibitors are (a) increased inotropy as a result of cAMP-mediated increase in transsarcolemmal calcium flux; (b) vasodilation secondary to cAMP-mediated increase in calcium uptake and decrease in calcium available for contraction; and (c) increased lusitropy, or improved relaxation of the myocardium during diastole. Lastly, platelet PDE III is also inhibited by phosphodiesterase inhibitors, and the possible antithrombotic effect of these drugs is of clinical importance in patients after cardiac surgery.

Amrinone

Amrinone, a bipyridine derivative, was the first PDE III inhibitor to be investigated, and its pharmacologic effects—an increase in cyclic AMP, cAMP-specific PDE, and cAMP protein kinase—have remained undisputed since they were originally demonstrated (63). Furthermore, amrinone was shown to produce a dose-dependent increase in developed tension in isolated mammalian atrial and papillary muscles (64, 65).

Since its introduction into clinical practice in 1984, amrinone has been widely used both orally and as an intravenous infusion in the management of low-output cardiac failure. In adults who have undergone cardiopulmonary bypass, amrinone increases cardiac index by causing peripheral vasodilation and lowering the systemic vascular resistance, with a concomitant decrease in myocardial oxygen consumption (66, 67).

In the neonatal piglet myocardium, amrinone produces a reversible negative inotropic effect, evidenced by a fall in peak systolic pressure, increased left ventricular end-diastolic pressure, reduced rate of peak tension attainment, and increased coronary sinus blood flow (68). These findings indicate that probably a lower level of adenylate cyclase activity or a reduced sensitivity to cyclic-AMP is found in the immature myocardium. In isolated perfused lungs and in animal models, amrinone has been shown to lower elevated pulmonary artery pressure and pulmonary vascular resistance in a dose-related fashion (69–72).

Metabolism

About 10 to 40% of amrinone is excreted unchanged in the urine. The remainder is acetylated, glucuronidated, or conjugated with glutathione in the liver to enable renal elimination. The drug should therefore be used with caution in slow acetylators.

The half-life of amrinone progressively diminishes over the first few months of life, from 12 hours at 1 week to around 6 hours at the age of 6 months (73). It has been demonstrated, however, that infants may require a larger dose to achieve similar therapeutic levels compared with adults (74).

Guidelines for Clinical Use

Amrinone has been shown to significantly improve cardiac index in children with low cardiac output and myocardial dysfunction secondary to dilated cardiomyopathy or following cardiac surgery (75). When administered to children as a continuous infusion after cardiac surgery, amrinone has been demonstrated to increase cardiac index and decrease systemic vascular resistance without a significant increase in heart rate (76). Amrinone may be of particular benefit to children after cardiopulmonary bypass who are normotensive with a low cardiac output and an elevated left ventricular afterload, and also in children with coexisting pulmonary hypertension (77). Lastly, amrinone has been recently demonstrated to increase cardiac index significantly in children after the Fontan operation (78).

Adverse Effects

Significant hypotension can be associated with intravenous administration of amrinone, particularly if the infusion is preceded by a bolus dose; this undesired effect can be avoided by administration of volume and maintenance of adequate preload (79). Thrombocytopenia is often seen in adults on long-term oral therapy, and it is occasionally seen in pediatric patients receiving infusions (80). Tachyarrhythmias have not been reported in children receiving the doses outlined above.

Milrinone

Milrinone, a 2-methyl, 5-carbonitrile congener of amrinone, is a potent bipyridine phosphodiesterase inhibitor that has been investigated extensively in adults. Its positive effect on myocardial contractility appears to be well complemented by its peripheral vasodilatory properties, and thus an increase in cardiac output without an increase in myocardial oxygen demand follows its administration (81). In adults with congestive cardiac failure, intravenous milrinone increases the diastolic relaxation rate of myocardial fibers and reduces ventricular preload (81–83). In addition, both a bolus dose and a continuous infusion of intravenous milrinone significantly lower pulmonary arterial pressure and pulmonary vascular resistance in animal models and in adults after cardiac surgery (84–86). Oral milrinone has been used in adults with severe congestive cardiac failure with questionable results. The recent PROMISE (Prospective Randomized Milrinone Survival Evaluation) trial showing reduced survival without improvement in quality of life has introduced a note of caution in its long-term use (87). Unlike amrinone, milrinone has *not* been shown to have negative inotropic effects on the neonatal myocardium (88).

A comparison between milrinone and dobutamine suggested that milrinone was superior in lowering systemic vascular resistance for any given increase in dP/dt (89), whereas comparison between milrinone and nitroprusside showed that in equally hypotensive doses, milrinone was superior in increasing the peak dP/dt (90).

Metabolism

Milrinone has an elimination half-life of approximately 3 hours. It circulates approximately 70% plasma protein bound, and is excreted unchanged by the kidney. Dose reductions should be made in cases of renal impairment.

Guidelines for Clinical Use

Clinical uses for milrinone are the same as those indicated for amrinone (see above). Milrinone administration in neonates with low cardiac output after cardiac surgery was demonstrated to lower filling pressures, systemic and pulmonary arterial pressures, and resistances, while improving cardiac index; milrinone did not increase myocardial oxygen consumption (91) (see Fig. 5.3).

Adverse Effects

The main reported side-effects of intravenous milrinone in adults have included hypotension and ventricular or supraventricular tachyarrhythmias, which were not observed with use in children.

Enoximone

Enoximone, an imidazole derivative, is a newer peak III phosphodiesteras inhibitor that is not yet widely applied in the United States.

In a study comparing the effects of enoximone and dobutamine in adults after cardiac surgery, both similarly increased cardiac index, stroke volume, and stroke work index while reducing pulmonary capillary wedge pressure and systemic vascular resistance. Myocardial oxygen consumption, however, was significantly lower in the patients who received enoximone (92). In neonates and in children after cardiopulmonary bypass, intravenous enoximone increased cardiac index and lowered systemic vascular resistance and right and left atrial pressures similarly to the more traditional combination of dobutamine and phenoxybenzamine (93, 94).

Enoximone undergoes extensive hepatic metabolism to its sulphoxide, also hemodynamically active, which undergoes renal elimination. Renal and liver function should be monitored daily, as in cases of impaired organ function the highly variable half-life of enoximone (1–20 hours) may be increased.

VASODILATORS

Pure arterial and venous vasodilators can be used either alone or in combination with other cardiovascular drugs to improve cardiac output by reducing ventricular preload and afterload. In general, vasodilators are useful adjunctive therapy for (*a*) myocardial dysfunction secondary to dilated cardiomyopathy, coronary insufficiency, or cardiac surgery; (*b*) systemic or pulmonary hypertension; and (*c*) valvular regurgitation leading to volume overload.

Vasodilators most commonly used in the cardiac intensive care setting include nitroglycerin, sodium nitroprusside, hydralazine, calcium antagonists, and the orally available angiotensin-converting enzyme inhibitors captopril and enalapril.

Nitroglycerin

Nitroglycerin is a potent venous vasodilator, but it is also an effective vasodilator of systemic and pulmonary arteries. In the vascular endothelial cell, nitroglycerin is converted to nitric oxide (NO). This in turn activates guanylate cyclase and thus increases intracellular cyclic guanosine monophosphate (GMP), a potent relaxant of vascular smooth muscle.

Intravenous nitroglycerin lowers myocardial oxygen consumption; by reducing the preload and afterload, it also lowers the right and left atrial pressures, left ventricular end-diastolic pressure and volume, and systemic and pulmonary arterial pressures. Nitroglycerin also has an important additional effect on the coronary vasculature with dilation of both epicardial and collateral coronary arteries (95).

Metabolism

Nitroglycerin's half-life is less than 5 minutes. It undergoes rapid hepatic and vascular endothelial conversion to

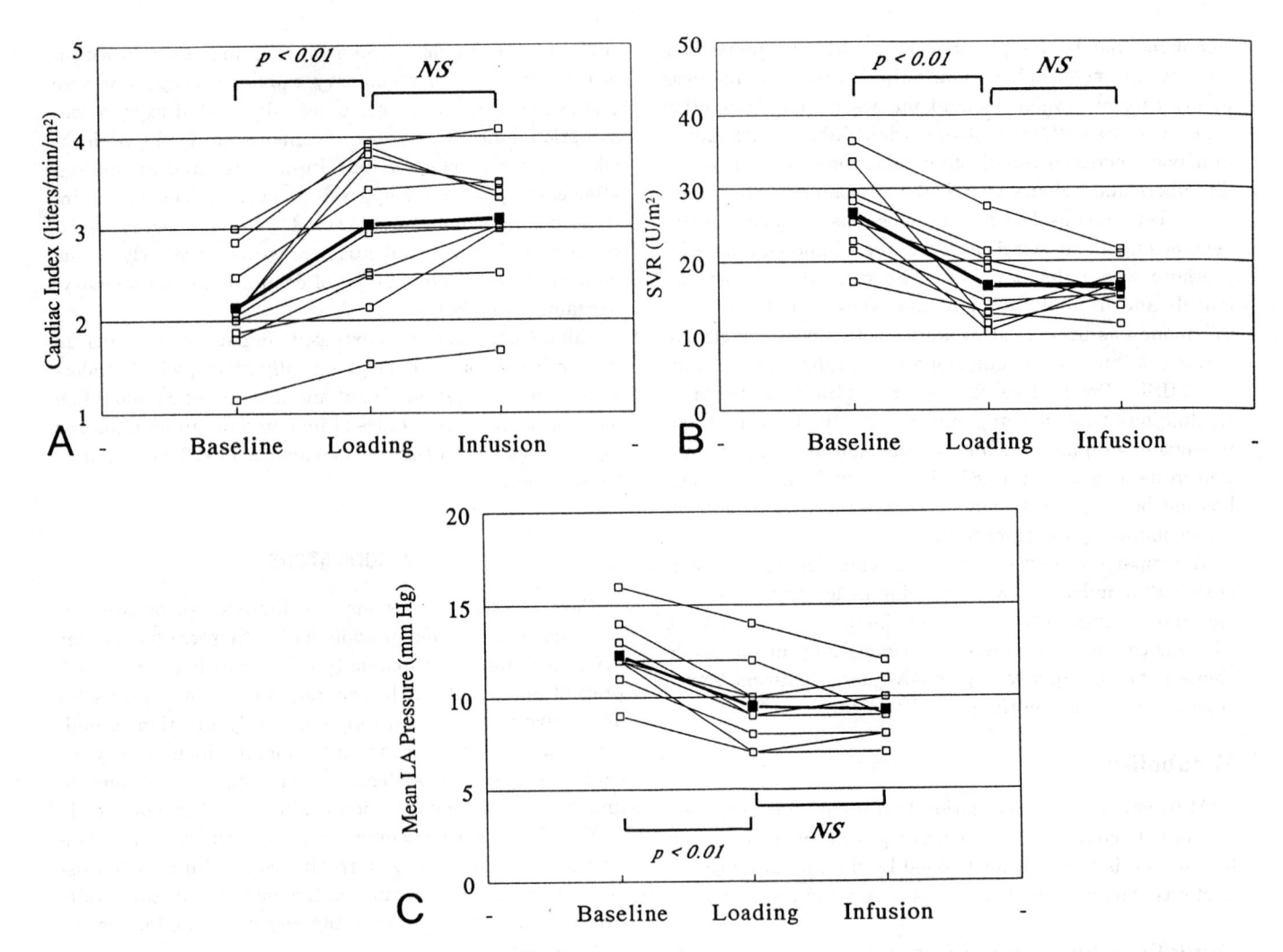

Figure 5.3. Hemodynamic effects of milrinone in 10 neonates with low (<3.0 L/min/m^2) cardiac index after repair of transposition of the great arteries (n = 6), tetralogy of Fallot (n = 2), total anomalous pulmonary venous return (n = 1), and truncus arteriosus (n = 1). After baseline measurements of right and left atrial pressures, systemic blood pressure, and thermodilution cardiac output, 50 μg/kg for 30 minutes. Cardiac index (A) rose significantly following the loading dose and was maintained during continuous infusion. Improved cardiac index was associated with a significant fall in systemic vascular resistance (SVR) (B) and left atrial pressure (C). NS, not significant. (Modified from Chang AC, Atz AM, Wernovsky G, et al. Milrinone: evaluation of hemodynamic effects in neonates after cardiac surgery [Abstract]. Circulation 1993; 88:335.)

the inactive 1, 2 and 1, 3 dinitrates, which are subsequently excreted by the kidney.

Guidelines for Clinical Use

When infused intravenously to children, nitroglycerin augments cardiac output by significantly reducing systemic vascular resistance in those with myocardial dysfunction and low cardiac output after cardiopulmonary bypass (96, 97). Intravenous nitroglycerin is also an effective pharmacologic agent in the treatment of systemic and pulmonary hypertension (96).

Ample experience with nitroglycerine has been acquired in treating adults with coronary ischemia. Some centers have prophylactically used nitroglycerine for postoperative patients in whom coronary artery manipulation was involved (such as arterial switch operation for transposition of the great arteries or the Ross operation); evidence indicates that increased endothelin-1 and resultant coronary arterial spasm can be reversed by nitroglycerin administration (98).

Adverse Effects

The most common unwanted effect of intravenous nitroglycerin is dose-dependent hypotension with associated reflex tachycardia. This adverse effect responds rapidly to discontinuation of the intravenous infusion and/or administration of fluids. In older children, headache and even increased intracranial pressure can occur, but they usually respond to dose reduction.

Sodium Nitroprusside

Sodium nitroprusside is a nonreceptor stimulant of guanulate cyclase, and it increases intracellular cyclic GMP in a manner similar to nitroglycerin; it therefore acts as a nitric oxide donor. Its clinical effect is a significant reduction in preload and afterload due to dilation of both venous and arteriolar beds.

Sodium nitroprusside produces a greater reduction in systemic and pulmonary arterial pressures than does nitroglycerin, and it is usually used in combination with an inotropic agent; this strategy has been demonstrated to increase cardiac output and decrease systemic vascular resistance (99). An age-dependent response and sensitivity to nitroprusside is also found (100).

Metabolism

Nitroprusside has a plasma half-life of less than 10 minutes and on contact with red blood cells, it rapidly forms methemoglobin and cyanide. Cyanide is slowly released from the erythrocyte into the plasma and, in the presence of hepatic thiosulphate and rhodanase, it is transformed to thiocyanate which then undergoes renal excretion.

Effective clearance of cyanide is rarely a problem at an infusion rate of below 2 μg/kg/min because its accumulation is partially buffered by methemoglobin. In cases of normal renal function, elimination half-life of thiocyanate is about 7 days.

Guidelines for Clinical Use

By lowering systemic vascular resistance, sodium nitroprusside improves cardiac output of children with myocardial dysfunction secondary to postoperative heart failure, dilated cardiomyopathy, or mitral and aortic valve regurgitation (101, 102). It is also an effective agent in children with systemic hypertension crisis (103) or systemic hypertension after coarctation repair (104); treatment for hypertension should probably be accompanied by β-blockade to minimize reflex tachycardia. Nitroprusside also has an important role in the treatment of pulmonary hypertension (105), although its use in neonates with persistent pulmonary hypertension and clinical shock had varied responses (106).

Nitroprusside has been used after surgery to the aortic root, aortic valve, or aortic arch to reduce even mild hypertension to minimize the likelihood of bleeding at the anastomotic sites. In addition, nitroprusside has also been shown to improve cardiac output and lower filling pressures following the Fontan operation (107). Lastly, nitroprusside has been demonstrated to improve diastolic function after coarctation repair (108).

Adverse Effects

Similar to nitroglycerine, the most common side effect of intravenous sodium nitroprusside is hypotension accompanied sometimes by excessive tachycardia.

Prolonged infusion of sodium nitroprusside can cause cyanide and thiocyanate toxicity, and the latter can escalate significantly in cases of renal failure. Symptoms and signs of toxicity include tissue hypoxia, convulsions, vomiting, muscle spasms, and bone marrow suppression. Cyanide toxicity can be monitored by following mixed venous oxygen tension (which is increased in cyanide toxicity); pH (toxicity leads to metabolic acidosis); and for plasma levels of cyanide and thiocyanate in patients on continuous nitroprusside infusions (109). Whereas toxicity can be treated with sodium thiosulfate, it is not likely to occur in children with normal hepatic and renal function (110).

Lastly, it should also be noted that nitroprusside, as with other vasodilators, can attenuate hypoxic pulmonary vasoconstriction and lead to significant intrapulmonary right-to-left shunting and hypoxemia.

Hydralazine

Hydralazine has its main effect on the precapillary arterioles without much influence on the venous capacitance vessels. Vasodilation is most prominent in renal, coronary, cerebral, and splanchnic beds.

Metabolism

Peak effect of hydralazine can be observed in minutes and elimination occurs in 2 to 4 hours. Hydralazine is metabolized in the liver via hepatic acetylation.

Guidelines for Clinical Use

Hydralazine can be used in children with myocardial dysfunction. An earlier study showed that hydralazine is beneficial in treating children with primary myocardial disease (111) and useful in children with large ventricular septal defect (112). One study also reported on the use of hydralazine for severe myocardial dysfunction observed during extracorporeal membrane oxygenation (113).

Although hydralazine can be used to treat systemic hypertension (such as postcoarctectomy hypertension), other pharmacologic therapy such as labetalol and nitroprusside may be less prone to causing hypotension (114).

Adverse Effects

In addition to hypotension, the vasodilating effect of hydralazine is further limited by reflex tachycardia; concomitant use of β-blockers is sometimes necessary to minimize this undesired effect. Lupuslike syndrome with positive antinuclear antibodies can also occur.

CALCIUM ANTAGONISTS

Calcium-channel antagonists bind to the voltage-sensitive calcium channels, reducing inward calcium flux to vascular smooth muscle as well as coronary and conducting tissue.

The most commonly used calcium antagonists in the pediatric population are nifedipine and verapamil. Although calcium antagonist use in neonates and infants is generally considered contraindicated, its therapeutic role as a vasodilator and a negative inotropic agent in certain clinical situations will be discussed briefly below.

Nifedipine

Nifedipine causes a fall in systemic and pulmonary arterial blood pressure and their respective resistances; it also has a reflex-positive chronotropic effect. It undergoes extensive hepatic metabolism, and the free drug and its metabolites are excreted in urine.

Nifedipine can be administered intravenously, orally, or sublingually. Little clinical data are found on nifedipine use in infants. In older children, nifedipine can be used to treat systemic hypertension (a) observed after surgery to the aorta, (b) associated with cyclosporin-induced hypertension after organ transplantation (see Chapter 21, *Pediatric Heart and Lung Transplantation*), or (c) secondary to a renovascular cause (115, 116). Nifedipine also lowers the pulmonary vascular resistance and increases pulmonary blood flow in children with established pulmonary hypertension secondary to a left-to-right shunt, thus providing a degree of palliation to children with inoperable congenital heart defects (117). A potential role appears to be seen in nifedipine for the treatment of pulmonary hypertension seen in children with bronchopulmonary dysplasia (118). Its use in primary pulmonary hypertension is promising, but treatment must be carefully monitored and individualized (119).

Verapamil

Verapamil is metabolized in the liver. As with nifedipine, verapamil should be used with caution in cases of heart block, and it should be avoided in use with β-blockers or digoxin. Verapamil can lead to cardiac arrest or asystole in neonates. Calcium should be readily available to treat cardiac decompensation.

Verapamil is primarily used in children for the acute termination and long-term prophylaxis of supraventricular tachyarrhythmias (see Chapter 30). It also has a role in the treatment of hypertrophic cardiomyopathy, as it has been shown to improve left ventricular diastolic filling (120).

ANGIOTENSIN-CONVERTING ENZYME INHIBITORS

The renin-angiotensin-aldosterone system is activated in congestive heart failure. Reduced renal perfusion pressure coupled with an increased sympathetic drive enhances renin release from the renal juxtaglomerular apparatus. Renin converts inactive angiotensinogen to angiotensin I. Angiotensin-converting enzyme (ACE) transforms angiotensin I to angiotensin II in the liver. Angiotensin II has a number of important physiologic effects, including direct and indirect effects on the systemic vascular resistance. It is a potent vasoconstrictor that also augments the endogenous sympathetic output and inhibits the action of bradykinin, an endogenous vascular smooth muscle relaxant. Finally, angiotensin II increases sodium retention by aldosterone activation. Angiotensin-converting enzyme inhibitors act by decreasing formation of vasoconstrictor angiotensin II and concomitantly inhibit aldosterone secretion.

Captopril

Captopril, the first orally available ACE inhibitor, lowers systemic vascular resistance and systemic blood pressure without a concomitant increase in heart rate. It is a highly effective afterload reducing agent, and it improves left ventricular compliance with symptomatic relief and improved exercise tolerance in patients with ventricular dysfunction (121, 122). In children with myocardial failure, captopril improves cardiac output by lowering systemic vascular resistance and increasing left ventricular stroke volume (123).

Metabolism

Captopril's half-life is 2 hours, but it can be much prolonged in cases of renal impairment. About 60% of captopril undergoes hepatic metabolism to captopril cysteine disulphide and captopril disulphide, which are then excreted both in to the bile and by the renal route. The remaining 40% is excreted unchanged by the kidney.

Guidelines for Clinical Use

In the pediatric cardiac intensive care setting, captopril is an effective oral "continuation" therapy for children who have been receiving intravenous infusions of dobutamine, phosphodiesterase inhibitors, or sodium nitroprusside.

Captopril is considered by many to be the enteral drug of choice for children with myocardial dysfunction with impaired ventricular performance and an elevated left ventricular end-diastolic pressure (e.g., in the setting of primary or secondary dilated cardiomyopathy) (124); captopril, however, should *not* be used for patients with restrictive cardiomyopathy (123). In addition, in children with congestive cardiac failure secondary to a left-to-right shunt with a normal or low pulmonary vascular resistance, captopril increases systemic perfusion, reduces the degree of shunt, and thus reduces left ventricular volume overload (125, 126). Lastly, captopril can be a good agent for systemic hypertension secondary to postcoarctation surgery or renal disease in the absence of renal artery stenosis (127).

Adverse Effects

Hypotension is a relatively common first-dose phenomenon, but to a large extent it is avoidable if a small test dose is followed by a gradually increasing dose. Renal failure has also been reported as a complication. Captopril is an aldosterone antagonist, and its combination with potassium-sparing diuretics should be avoided. Neutropenia can occur with prolonged high dosage of captopril. Other reported side effects include cough and loss of taste perception.

Doses should be reduced in cases of renal impairment and in neonates (because of apparent increased antihypertensive effect and duration of action in this age group).

Enalapril

Inhibition of ACE with enalapril has been established in infants with congestive heart failure (128). In children with dilated cardiomyopathy, enalapril use has been demonstrated to improve long-term survival (129). In addition, enalapril has been used in children with congestive heart failure secondary to left-to-right shunt, ventricular dysfunction, valvular regurgitation, or after cardiac surgery. Renal failure, however, is more commonly seen in younger children and neonates with low weight, and renal function should be monitored (130). Intravenous use of enalapril in neonates and enteral use for older children for renovascular hypertension have been reported (131, 132).

A parenteral form of enalapril is available. It should be noted that enalapril has been observed to suppress normal accumulation of elastin and collagen in cardiovascular tissues of growing rats (133).

DIURETICS

Diuresis in the critically ill child can be accomplished in two ways: (*a*) by improving renal perfusion and (*b*) by influencing tubular function. Renal perfusion is intimately related to cardiac output, and methods of manipulating this have been discussed above.

Structure and function of the nephron together with sites of action of commonly used diuretic drugs are illustrated in Figure 5.4. The *proximal tubule* is the major site of reabsorption of sodium, bicarbonate, glucose, and amino acids, accounting for approximately 60% of the filtered load. The proximal tubule also has secretory capacity—in the latter portion urea and organic acids are secreted into the urine. No diuretic agents act primarily on the proximal tubule. In the *loop of Henle*, the thin descending limb is the site where water is reabsorbed, and the ascending limb is where sodium, chloride, and potassium are reabsorbed, leaving only 20% of the filtered water and 10% of the filtered sodium in the lumen. The loop diuretics, furosemide, bumetanide, and ethacrynic acid, block ion reabsorption by cortical and medullary portions of the ascending limb. In the *distal tubule* and *collecting ducts*, potassium and hydrogen ions are secreted in the urine with reabsorption of sodium, which is influenced by aldosterone. In the collecting ducts, water reabsorption is antidiuretic hormone dependent. Thiazide diuretics cause a poorly defined inhibition of salt transport at the distal tubule. Triamterene and amiloride inhibit sodium and water reabsorption with a potassium-sparing effect at the distal tubule and collecting ducts. Spironolactone inhibits aldosterone action at both sites with resulting sodium loss and potassium retention. Mannitol is a powerful osmotic diuretic that acts on all parts of the nephron.

Furosemide

Furosemide, the prototype of the loop diuretic agents, is the most commonly employed diuretic in the cardiac intensive care setting. It appears to have favorable hemodynamic effects that include reducing pulmonary and renal vascular resistances while increasing blood flows in these organs.

The potent effect of a bolus dose of furosemide can be sufficient to necessitate volume administration for hypotension and also cause a significant disturbance in electrolyte balance—clearly an unwanted scenario in the critically ill child. Recent research has focused on administering furosemide as a *continuous* infusion in an attempt to avoid the undesired effects of intermittent boluses (134). A study in children following cardiac surgery showed that total urinary sodium and chloride losses were significantly higher in the group receiving intermittent boluses, but no significant difference was seen in serum electrolyte values. Total daily urine output did not significantly differ between the two groups, but the hourly variability did, thus illustrating the brisk "intermittent" response to boluses of the drug (135).

Metabolism

Furosemide is excreted primarily via the kidney by glomerular filtration and tubular secretion. Half-life of furosemide can be 2 to 10 times longer in the neonate compared with the adult.

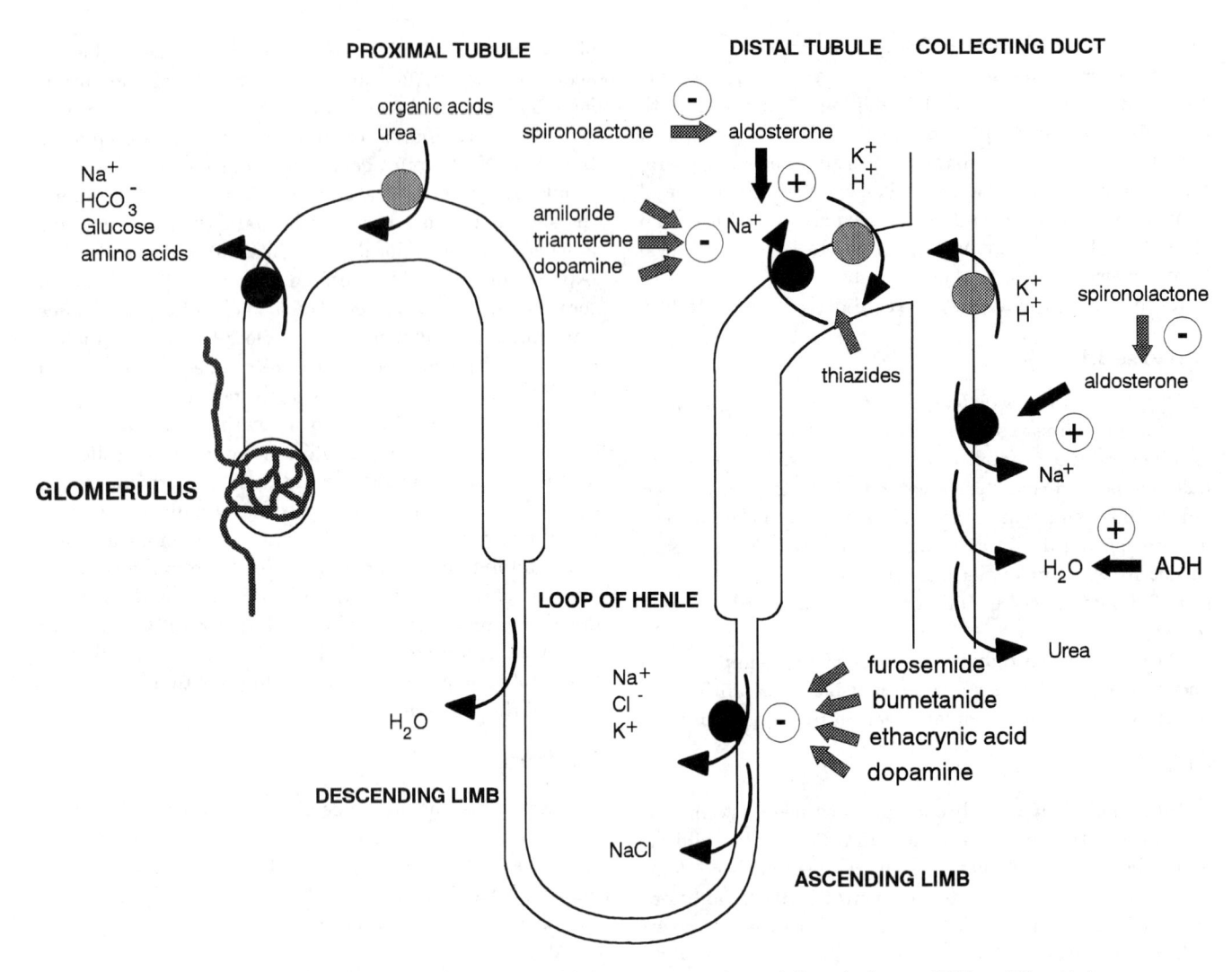

Figure 5.4. The nephron: structure, function, and sites of action of commonly used diuretic drugs. ADH, antidiuretic hormone.

Guidelines for Clinical Use

Furosemide is an effective diuretic agent in children with fluid overload secondary to myocardial failure, following cardiopulmonary bypass, or in those with a poor urine output without severe renal impairment. A continuous infusion of furosemide stimulates a more physiologic and controlled diuresis than does the administration of intermittent intravenous boluses. It is also noteworthy that furosemide is more effective in cases of adequate plasma proteins because it is transported to the nephrons via plasma proteins. Lastly, in furosemide nonresponders, bumetamide or ethacrynic acid can be used.

Other less common clinical indications for furosemide use include hyperkalemia.

Adverse Effects

Hypovolemia and metabolic alkalosis with electrolyte disturbances–hyponatremia, hypokalemia, and hypochloremia–are the most common side effects, but these are less likely to occur with a continuous infusion than with intermittent boluses of furosemide. Ototoxicity and cholelithiasis and renal calcifications are also infrequently observed complications of furosemide therapy, especially in cases of renal impairment and in the premature neonate. Supraventricular tachycardia (without serum electrolyte disturbance) has been reported in pediatric patients receiving an infusion at a starting dose of 1 mg/kg/h–a higher dose than usually recommended (136). Lastly, furosemide has been demonstrated to increase the incidence of patent ductus arteriosus (137).

MISCELLANEOUS

BETA BLOCKERS

Esmolol

Esmolol is a short-acting specific β_1 antagonist. Clinical uses in the cardiac intensive care setting for intravenous esmolol include (a) treatment of systemic hypertension after coarctation of the aorta repair (138); (b) therapy to alleviate dynamic right or left sided outflow tract obstruction, such as for tetralogy of Fallot or for hypertrophic cardiomyopathy, respectively; (c) tachydysrhythmias (such as junctional ectopic tachycardia) (see Chapter 30).

Adverse effects of esmolol include bradycardia, hypotension, and bronchospasm. It should be used with caution in conjunction with calcium channel blockers and should also be avoided in cases of sinus bradycardia or atrioventricular block.

Labetalol

Labetalol is both an α- and β-blocker. It has been used successfully in the treatment of systemic hypertension (139) with minimal decrease in heart rate. Systemic hypertension after coarctation repair has also been successfully treated with labetalol (140).

As with esmolol, adverse effects of labetalol include hypotension, bradycardia, and bronchospasm. It should also be avoided in cases of sinus bradycardia or atrioventricular block. A reversible but generalized myopathy secondary to rhabdomyolysis has been reported (141).

VASOCONSTRICTOR

Phenylephrine

Phenylephrine is a pure α-agonist with vasoconstrictive properties. Indications for use of intravenous phenylephrine include (a) tetralogy of Fallot hypercyanotic spell and also other clinical situations in which the pathophysiology dictates that an increase in systemic vascular resistance is needed to increase pulmonary blood flow (such as Blalock-Taussig shunt stenosis or thrombosis); and (b) termination of supraventricular tachycardia (142).

Phenylephrine use is contraindicated in severe hypertension. Side effects of phenylephrine include severe vasoconstriction and decrease in urine output secondary to reduced renal blood flow.

DUCTUS MANIPULATION

Medical manipulation of the arterial duct depends on control of its muscle tone by endogenous prostaglandin production. Early in vitro studies demonstrated marked relaxation in the presence of prostaglandin E (PGE) and a low oxygen tension, but intense contraction in the presence of blockers of PGE synthesis and increased arterial oxygen tension. Prostaglandin E has been widely applied to maintain ductal patency, whereas indomethacin is used for medical closure of the ductus arteriosus.

Prostaglandin E_1

In 1975, the effectiveness of E-type prostaglandins in maintaining patency of the arterial duct was demonstrated in neonates with cyanotic congenital heart disease (143). Since then, intravenous prostaglandin E_1 has played a vital role in the initial management and stabilization of infants with "ductal-dependent" circulation (144).

A patent ductus arteriosus can supply blood to the pulmonary circulation if pulmonary blood flow from the right ventricle is reduced (such as critical pulmonary stenosis) or support systemic circulation when outflow is restricted from the left ventricle (such as hypoplastic left ventricle syndrome). In neonates with transposition of the great arteries and suboptimal mixing, a patent ductus arteriosus can potentially improve oxygenation and hemodynamic status. Although prostaglandin administration can be effective in neonates up to 4 weeks of life (145), it is most effective in neonates less than 3 days of life.

Prostaglandin use in certain lesions can lead to deterioration; these include (a) obstructive type of total anomalous pulmonary venous connection (as increased pulmonary blood flow can lead to worsening of pulmonary edema), (b) tetralogy of Fallot with pulmonary atresia and aortopulmonary collaterals (as excessive vasodilation secondary to prostaglandin can decrease perfusion pressure from the collaterals to the pulmonary bed), and (c) transposition of the great arteries before atrial septotomy (because increased pulmonary blood flow and venous return can close a previously patent foramen ovale and decrease interatrial mixing with resultant cyanosis) or even after atrial septotomy (as prostaglandin infusion can maintain patency of a large ductus arteriosus and result in excessive pulmonary blood flow, thus creating a "steal" from the systemic circulation).

Adverse effects of prostaglandin E_1 are apnea (particularly in neonates less than 2 kg and in neonates with cyanosis), seizures, cutaneous flushing, hypotension, and temperature elevation. In addition, less common side effects include cortical hyperostosis and soft tissue swelling (146). Recently, gastric outlet obstruction secondary to antral mucosal hyperplasia has been reported as a side effect associated with prolonged (more than 120 hours) prostaglandin infusion (147). Lower dose of intravenous prostaglandin infusion has not been demonstrated to decrease the incidence of complications (148).

Indomethacin

Patency of the arterial duct is not always an advantage, and it can cause signs and symptoms of excessive pulmonary blood flow, which are poorly tolerated in the premature neonate. Contraction of the arterial duct has been demonstrated by inhibiting prostaglandin synthesis using nonsteroidal anti-inflammatory drugs.

Indomethacin inhibits cyclo-oxygenase, a key enzyme in prostaglandin syntheses, and over the past two decades it has been used in neonatal care to pharmacologically close the ductus arteriosus. Plasma half-life of indomethacin is long because it is not well excreted by the kidney. Among contraindications to its use are elevated blood urea nitrogen (BUN) and creatinine (30 and 1.8 mg/dL, respectively), thrombocytopenia (less than 50,000), evidence of bleeding (intraventricular hemorrhage or gastrointestinal bleeding), or active necrotizing enterocolitis.

The most notable adverse effect of indomethacin use is reduced renal function and urine output, most likely secondary to reduced renal prostaglandin. Another complication of indomethacin therapy includes decreased platelet function, although indomethacin use has actually been associated with a decrease in neonatal intraventricular hemorrhage (149). Concerns about reduced cerebral blood flow, sometimes with resultant ischemia, have stimulated a search for an alternative (150, 151). Ibuprofen appears to have a similar effect to indomethacin on the arterial duct without compromising cerebral perfusion, and so it may be a better option in the premature neonate.

ANTICOAGULANTS

Warfarin

Warfarin inactivates vitamin K and therefore interferes with the vitamin K-dependent coagulation factors (II, VII, IX, and X) as well as prothrombin.

Clinical indications for warfarin in the cardiac intensive care setting include anticoagulation for (a) patients with prosthetic valves (152), (b) certain patients who may be at higher risk for thrombosis after surgery, particularly patients who had cavopulmonary anastomoses (bidirectional cavopulmonary shunt or Fontan), and (c) patients with stasis of blood in the heart (dilated cardiomyopathy or atrial flutter and fibrillation).

Doses are adjusted to achieve a prothrombin time 1 to 1.5 times normal value. More recently, INR (international normalized ratio, based on a international reference thromboplastin) between 2.5 and 4.5 is considered a goal of therapy for anticoagulation. Children less than 1 year of age seem to require a higher maintenance dose (0.3 mg/kg) than older children (0.1 mg/kg) (153). Warfarin can cause multiple anomalies in the fetus if administered during pregnancy.

Heparin

Heparin is a glycosaminoglycuran that accelerates the process in which antithrombin III inhibits factors X, IX, XI, and XIII as well as thrombin.

Heparin is metabolized in the reticuloendothelial system with a half-life of 1 to 2 hours. Clinical indications include (a) prophylaxis against thrombosis in patients who had placement of a systemic-pulmonary artery shunt; (b) deep vein thrombosis (infants seem to require a higher maintenance infusion–28U/kg/h–than older children (154); (c) femoral artery thrombosis (up to 71% response to therapy) (155).

Heparin can also be used for those clinical indications listed above for warfarin prior to initiation of enteral warfarin (prosthetic valves, cavopulmonary anastomoses, and dilated cardiomyopathy or atrial dysrhythmias). Recent evidence suggests that heparin-bonded catheters have a reduced incidence of thrombotic complications and catheter-related blood cultures (156).

During heparin therapy, activated partial thromboplastin time (PTT) is maintained at about 1.5 to 2.5 times normal (usually checked 4 to 8 hours after the initial bolus dose). Severe bleeding can be reversed by protamine sulfate (1 mg/100 U heparin) administration. Heparin-induced thrombocytopenia can occur.

Aspirin

Aspirin derives its antiplatelet activities via inhibition of the enzyme cyclo-oxygenase by acetylation, leading to inhibition of thromboxane A_2, a platelet aggregator.

Aspirin is degraded by hepatic microsomal enzymes. The more common indications for aspirin use includes a) prophylaxis for certain postoperative patients (systemic-pulmonary artery shunt and cavopulmonary anastomoses) and b) for children with Kawasaki disease and coronary artery aneurysm and/or thrombosis. A therapeutic role is also seen for aspirin in prosthetic valve anticoagulation.

Aspirin has several side effects that include ulcer and gastrointestinal bleeding.

THROMBOLYTIC AGENTS

Thrombolytic agents incur enzymatic degradation of existing thrombus by conversion of endogenous plasminogen to plasmin, the endogenous fibrinolytic substance. Clinical indication for these agents is dissolution of large intravascular or intracardiac venous or arterial thromboses. A role is also seen for these agents in maintaining patency of central venous catheters.

Recent (within 1 to 2 weeks) surgery or major procedure is a contraindication to thrombolytic agent use. Other contraindications include intracerebral bleeding and severe hypertension. As with anticoagulant therapy, the major complication with antithrombotic therapy is bleeding. Status of the thrombus being treated by these agents should be assessed every 8 to 12 hours to minimize duration of therapy.

Streptokinase

Streptokinase, a protein from the streptococcal bacteria, converts plasminogen to plasmin. Streptokinase is metabolized by the liver with a half-life of about 30 minutes or less. During therapy, monitoring for thrombin clotting time, or prothrombin time, fibrinogen, fibrinolytic split products (because fibrinogen is degraded), platelet count, plasminogen, and antithrombin III is indicated.

Many studies report on the successful use of streptokinase in the treatment of thromboses, including: arterial thromboses (157, 158) and even venous thrombosis after the Fontan operation (159). Lower doses (1000 U/kg/h) have also been found to be effective in treating arterial thromboses (160).

Side effects of streptokinase therapy include fever, which is not uncommon as streptokinase can induce an antigenic reaction. Hypotension can also occur with rapid administration of streptokinase. Lastly, bronchospasm has been reported as a complication of therapy.

Urokinase

Urokinase, derived from human renal cells, is a proteolytic enzyme that converts plasminogen to plasmin.

Its advantage over streptokinase is that it is less antigenic, but compared with streptokinase, it is considerably more expensive. Monitoring during its use is similar to that for streptokinase.

Clinical experience with urokinase has been extensive. Use in central venous catheter thromboses (161), even at low doses (200 U/kg/h), can be effective (162). Urokinase has also been used to treat arterial thromboses in neonates (163). Important to note is that thromboses of greater than 3 weeks duration may not respond to therapy with urokinase (164).

Tissue-Type Plasminogen Activator (tPA)

Tissue-type plasminogen activator accelerates activation of plasminogen to plasmin in the presence of fibrin. Tissue plasminogen activator was initially produced from human melanoma cells, but it can now be synthesized by recombinant DNA techniques. The advantage of tPA over streptokinase or urokinase is that it has less systemic effects at low doses; in addition, it has little effect on fibrinogen. Tissue-type plasminogen activator is, however, much more expensive than the other thrombolytic agents. With the use of tPA, simultaneous heparin infusion is recommended because reocclusion can be higher than observed with other thrombolytic agents. As with other antithrombin agents, the major serious complication of tPA use is bleeding, which may be less at a lower dose (0.1 mg/kg/h) (165).

The most common usage for tPA has been in the treatment of myocardial infarction in adults. Reported uses for this relatively new agent in pediatric patients include (a) treatment for coronary arterial thromboses in Kawasaki disease (166); (b) thrombosed Blalock-Taussig shunts (167); (c) arterial occlusion after cardiac catheterization (168); (d) right atrial thrombus associated with central venous catheters in children (169); and (e) vena caval thrombosis in children following cardiac surgery (170).

REFERENCES

1. Withering W. An account of the foxglove and some of its medical uses with practical remarks on dropsy and other diseases. In: Willins FA, Keyes TE, eds. Classics of cardiology. New York: Henry Schumann 1941;231–252.
2. Kearns GL, Reed MD. Clinical pharmacokinetics in infants and children. A reappraisal. Clinical Pharmacokinetics 1989;17(Suppl 1):29–67.
3. Steinberg C, Notterman DA. Pharmacokinetics of cardiovascular drugs in children. Clinical Pharmacokinetics 1994;27(5):345–367.
4. Besunder JB, Reed MD, Blumer JL. Principles of drug biodisposition in the neonate. A critical evaluation of the pharmacokinetic-pharmacodynamic interface. Clinical Pharmacokinetics 1988;28:189–216.
5. Friis-Hansen B. Body water compartments in children. Changes during growth and related changes in body composition. Pediatrics 1961;28:169–174.
6. Legato MJ. Cellular mechanisms of normal growth in the mammalian heart. Qualitative features of ventricular architecture in the dog from birth to 5 months of age. Circ Res 1979;44:250–262.
7. Morgan J, Perreault C, Morgan K. The cellular basis of contraction and relaxation in cardiac and vascular smooth muscle. Am Heart J 1991;121 (3 Part 1):961–968.
8. Morgan J, Morgan K. Calcium and cardiovascular function intracellular calcium levels during contraction and relaxation of mammalian cardiac and vascular smooth muscle as detected with aequorin. Am J Med 1984;77(Suppl A):33–46.
9. Gwathmey W, Copelas L, MacKinnon R. Abnormal intracellular calcium handling in myocardium from patients with end-stage heart failure. Circ Res 1987;75:331–339.
10. Go LO, Moschella MC, Watras J, et al. Differential regulation of two types of intracellular calcium release channels during end-stage heart failure. J Clin Invest 1995;95(2):888–894.
11. Morgan JP, Morgan KG. Alteration in cytoplasmic ionized calcium levels in smooth muscle by vasodilators in the ferret. J Physiol 1984;357:539.
12. Furchgott RF, Zawadzki JV. The obligatory role of endothelial cells in the relaxation of arterial smooth muscle by acetylcholine. Nature 1980;288:373–376.
13. Palmer R, Ferrige A, Moncada S. Nitric oxide accounts for the biological activity of endothelium derived relaxing factor. Nature 1987;327:524–526.
14. Levy M, Tulloh RMR, Komai H, et al. Maturation of the contractile response and its endothelial modulation in newborn porcine intrapulmonary arteries. Pediatr Res 1995;38:25–29.
15. Rapoport RM, Murad F. Agonist-induced endothelium dependent relaxation in rat thoracic aorta may be mediated through c-GMP. Circ Res 1983;52:352–357.
16. Ahlquist RP. A study of adrenotropic receptors. Am J Physiol 1948;153:586.
17. Tanaka H, Shigenobu K. Role of beta-adrenoceptor adenylate cyclase system in the developmental decrease in sensitivity to isoprenaline in fetal and neonatal rat heart. Br J Pharmacol 1990;100:138–142.
18. Caspi J, Coles JG, Benson LN, et al. Heart rate indepen-

dence of catecholamine induced myocardial damage in the newborn pig. Pediatr Res 1994;36:49–54.
19. Benzing G, Helmsworth JA, Schreiber JT, et al. Nitroprusside and epinephrine for treatment of low output in children after open heart surgery. Ann Thorac Surg 1979;27:523–528.
20. Emergency Cardiac Care Committee and Subcommittees. American Heart Association Guidelines for cardiopulmonary resuscitation and emergency cardiac care. JAMA 1992;268:2172–2299.
21. Goetting MG, Paradis NA. High dose epinephrine in refractory pediatric cardiac arrest. Crit Care Med 1989;17:1258–1262.
22. Sato Y, Matsuzawa H, Eguchi S. Comparative study of effects of adrenaline, dobutamine and dopamine on systemic hemodynamics and renal blood flow in patients following open heart surgery. Jpn Circ J 1982;46:1059–1072.
23. Wu JR, Chang HR, Huang TY, et al. Reduction in lymphocyte beta adrenergic receptor density in infants and children with heart failure secondary to congenital heart disease. Am J Cardiol 1996;77:170–174.
24. Anad KJ, Hansen DD, Hickey PR. Hormonal metabolic stress responses in neonates undergoing cardiac surgery. Anesthesiology 1990;73:661–670.
25. Loc MF, Heafe SS. Cardiovascular dopamine receptors. Role of renal dopamine and dopamine receptors in sodium excretion. Pharmacol Toxicol 1990;66:237–243.
26. Polak MJ, Drummond WH. Systemic and pulmonary vascular effects of selective dopamine (DA1) receptor blockade in lambs. Pediatr Res 1993;33:181–184.
27. Beregovich J, Bianchi C, Rubler S. Dose-related hemodynamic and renal effects of dopamine in congestive heart failure. Am Heart J 1974;87:550–557.
28. Murphy MB, Elliot WJ. Dopamine and dopamine receptor agonists in cardiovascular therapy [review]. Crit Care Med 1990;18(Suppl:1);S14–18.
29. Eldadah MK, Schwartz PH, Harrison R, et al. Pharmacokinetics of dopamine in infants and children. Cri Care Med 1991;19(8):1008–1011.
30. Banner W, Vernon DD, Dean M. Nonlinear dopamine pharmacokinetics in pediatric patients. J Pharmacol Exp Ther 1989;248:131–133.
31. Goodall MC, Alton H. Metabolism of 3-hydroxytyramine (dopamine) in human subjects. Biochem Pharmacol 1968;17;905.
32. Lang P, Williams RG, Norwood WI, et al. The hemodynamic effects of dopamine in infants after correcitve cardiac surgery. J Pediatr 1980;96:630–637.
33. DiSessa TG, Leitner M, Ti CC, et al. The cardiovascular effects of dopamine in the severely asphyxiated neonate. J Pediatr 1981;99:772–776.
34. Girardin E, Berner M, Rouge JC, et al. Effect of low dose dopamine on hemodynamic and renal function in children. Pediatr Res 1989;26:200–203.
35. Miall-Allen VM, Whitelaw AG. Response to dopamine and dobutamine in the preterm infant less than 30 weeks gestation. Crit Care Med 1989;17:1166–1169.
36. Stephenson LW, Edmunds LH, Raphaely R, et al. Effects of nitroprusside and dopamine on pulmonary arterial vasculature in children after cardiac surgery. Circulation 1979;60:104–110.
37. Booker PD, Evans C, Franks R. Comparison of the hemodynamic effects of dopamine and dobutamine in young children undergoing cardiac surgery. Br J Anaesthesiol 1995;74:419–423.

38. Tuttle R, Mills J. Development of a new catecholamine to selectively increase cardiac contractility. Circ Res 1975;35:185–196.
39. Beregovich J, Bianchi C, D'Angelo R, et al. Haemodynamic effects of a new inotropic agent (dobutamine) in chronic cardiac failure. Br Heart J 1975;37(6):629–634.
40. Butterworth J. Selecting an inotrope for the cardiac surgery patient. Journal of Cardiothoracic and Vascular Anesthesia 1993;7(4 Suppl 2);26–32.
41. Fowler MB, Alderman EL, Oesterle SN, et al. Dobutamine and dopamine after cardiac surgery: greater augmentation of myocardial blood flow with dobutamine. Circulation 1984;70(I):103–111.
42. Miall-Allen VM, Whitelaw AG. Response to dopamine and dobutamine in the preterm infant less than 30 weeks gestation. Crit Care Med 1989;17:1166–1169.
43. Wenstone R, Campbell JM, Booker PD, et al. Renal function after cardiopulmonary bypass in children. Comparison of dopamine with dobutamine. Br J Anaesth 1991;67(5):591–594.
44. Driscoll D, Gillette P, Lewis R, et al. Comparative hemodynamic effects of isoproterenol, dopamine and dobutamine in the newborn dog. Pediatr Res 1979;13:1006–1009.
45. Driscoll D, Gillette P, Lewis R, Fukushige J, et al. Comparison of the cardiovascular action of isoproterenol, dopamine and dobutamine in the neonatal and mature dog. Pediatr Cardiol 1980;1:307–314.
46. Martinez A, Padbury J, Thio S. Dobutamine pharmacokinetics and cardiovascular responses in critically ill neonates. Pediatrics 1992;89(1):47–51.
47. Perkin R, Levin D, Webb R, et al. Dobutamine. A hemodynamic evaluation in children with shock. J Pediatr 1982;100:977–983.
48. Berg R, Donnerstein R, Padbury J. Dobutamine infusions in children pharmacokinetics and hemodynamic actions. Crit Care Med 1993;21:768–686.
49. Habib DM, Padbury JF, Anas NG, et al. Dobutamine pharmacokinetics and pharmacodynamics in pediatric intensive care patients. Crit Care Med 1992;20:601–608.
50. Driscoll DJ, Gillette PC, Duff DF, et al. Hemodynamic effects of dobutamine in children. Am J Cardiol 1979;43:581–585.
51. Berner M, Rouge JC, Friedli B. The hemodynamic effect of phentolamine and dobutamine after open heart operations in children: influence of the underlying heart defect. Ann Thorac Surg 1983;35:643–650.
52. Harada K, Tamura M, Ito T, et al. Effects of low-dose dobutamine on left ventricular diastolic filling in children. Pediatr Cardiol 1996;17:220–225.
53. Booker PD, Evans C, Franks R. Comparison of the haemodynamic effects of dopamine and dobutamine in young children undergoing cardiac surgery. Br J Anaesth 1995;74(4):419–423.
54. Matson JR, Loughlin GM, Strunk RC. Myocardial ischemia complicating the use of isoproterenol in asthmatic children. J Pediatr 1978;92:776–778.
55. Jaccard C, Berner M, Touge JC, et al. Hemodynamic effect of isoprenaline and dobutamine immediately after correction of tetralogy of Fallot: relative importance of inotropic and chronotropic action in supporting cardiac output. J Thorac Cardiovasc Surg 1984;87:862–869.
56. Hopkins RA, Bull C, Haworth SG, et al. Pulmonary hypertensive crises following surgery for congenital heart defects in young children. Eur J Cardiothorac Surg 1991;5:628–634.
57. Razzouk AJ, Freedom RM, Cohen AJ, et al. The recognition, identification of morphologic substrate, and treatment of su-

baortic stenosis after a Fontan operation. J Thorac Cardiovasc Surg 1992;104:1750–1753.
58. de Bono D. Digoxin in eurhythmic heart failure: PROVED or "not proven"? Lancet 1994;343:128–129.
59. Kimball TR, Daniels SR, Meyer RA, et al. Effect of digoxin on contractility and symptoms in infants with a large ventricular septal defect. Am J Cardiol 1991;68(13):1377–1382.
60. Steiner E. Renal tubular secretion of digoxin. Circulation 1974;50;103.
61. Smith TW, Antman EM, Friedman PL, et al. Digitalis glycosides. Mechanisms and manifestations of toxicity. Prog Cardiovasc Dis 1984;26:413–458 and 27:21–56.
62. Honerjager P. Pharmacology of bipyridine phosphodiesterase III inhibitors. Am Heart J 1991;121:6(Part 2);1939–1944.
63. Levine SD, Jacoby M, Satriano JA, et al. The effects of amrinone on transport and cyclic AMP metabolism in toad urinary bladder. J Pharmacol Exp Ther 1981;262(2):220–224.
64. Wilmshurst PT, Walker JM, Fry CH, et al. Inotropic and vasodilator effects of amrinone on isolated human tissue. Cardiovas Res 1984;18(5):302–309.
65. Alousi AA, Farah AE, Lesher GY, et al. Cardiotonic activity of amrinone –Win 40680 (5-amino-3, 4′-bipyridine-6 (1H0-one). Circ Res 1979;45(5):666–677.
66. Wilmshurst PT, Thompson DS, Juul SM, et al. Comparison of the effects of amrinone and sodium nitroprusside on haemodynamics, contractility and myocardial metabolism in patients with cardiac failure due to coronary artery disease and dilated cardiomyopathy. Br Heart J 1984;52(1):38–48.
67. Butterworth JF. Use of amrinone in cardiac surgery patients. J Cardiothorac Vasc Anesth 1993;7(Suppl 2):1–7.
68. Ross-Asciutto N, Asciutto R, Chen V, et al. Negative inotropic effects of amrinone in the neonatal piglet heart. Circ Res 61(6):847–852.
69. Berger JI, Gibson RL, Clarke W, et al. Effect of amrinone on group B streptococcus-induced pulmonary hypertension in piglets. Pediatr Pulmonol 193;16:303–310.
70. Clarke WR, Morray JP, Powers K, et al. Amrinone reduces pulmonary vascular resistance by U46619 in isolated perfused lungs. J Cardiovasc Pharmacol 1991;18:85–94.
71. Hill NS, Rounds S. Amrinone dilates pulmonary vessels and blunts hypoxic vasoconstriction. Proc Soc Exp Biol Med 1983;173:205–212.
72. Mammel MC, Einzig S, Kulik TJ, et al. Pulmonary vascular effects of amrinone in conscious lambs. Pediatr Res 1983;17:720–724.
73. Allen-Webb EM, Ross MP, Pappas JB, et al. Age-related amrinone pharmacokinetics in a pediatric population. Crit Care Med 1994;22(6):1016–1024.
74. Lawless S, Burckart G, Diven W, et al. Amrinone in neonates and infants after cardiac surgery. Crit Care Med 1989;17:751–754.
75. Berner M, Jaccard C, Oberhansli I, Rouge J-C, et al. Hemodynamic effects of amrinone in children after cardiac surgery. Int Care Med 1990;16:85–88.
76. Jaccard C, Berner M, Oberhansli I. Dose response curve of amrinone immediately after cardiac surgery in children. Pediatr Cardiol 1987;8:220A.
77. Robinson BYW, Gelbrand H, Mas MS. Selective pulmonary and systemic vasodilator effects of amrinone in children. New therapeutic implications. J Am Coll Cardiol 1993;21:1461–1465.
78. Sorensen GK, Ramamoorthy C, Lynn AM, et al. Hemodynamic effects of amrinone in children after Fontan surgery. Anesth Analg 1996;82:241–246.
79. Lynn AM, Sorensen GK, Williams GD, et al. Hemodynamic effects of amrinone and colloid administration in children following cardiac surgery. J Cardiothorac Vasc Anesth 7(5);1993;560–565.
80. Ross MP, Allen-Webb EM, Pappas JB, et al. Amrinone associated thrombocytopenia: pharmacokinetic analysis. Clin Pharmacol Ther 1993;53:661–667.
81. Colucci WS. Cardiovascular effect of milrinone [review]. Am Heart J 1991;121(6 Part 2);1945–1947.
82. Krams R, McFalls E, van der Giessen WJ, et al. Does intravenous milrinone have a direct effect on diastolic function. Am Heart J 1991;121(6 Part 2):1951–1955.
83. Monrad S, McKay RG, Baim DS, et al. Improvement in indexes of diastolic performance in patients with congestive heart failure treated with milrinone. Circulation 1984;70:1030–1037.
84. George M, Lehot JJ, Estanove S. Haemodynamic and biological effects of intravenous milrinone in patients with a low cardiac output syndrome following cardiac surgery. Eur J Anaesth 1992;Suppl 5:31–34.
85. Feneck RO. Milrinone and postoperative pulmonary hypertension. J Cardiothorac Vasc Anesth 1993;7(2 Suppl 1):21–23.
86. Harris MN, Daborn AK, O'Dwyer JP. Milrinone and the pulmonary vascular system. Eur J Anaesth 1992;(Suppl)5:27–30.
87. Packer M, Carver MD, Rodaheffer RJ, et al. Effect of oral milrinone on mortality in severe chronic heart failure. N Engl J Med 1991;325:1468.
88. Ross-Ascuitto NT, Ascuitto RJ, Ramage D. Positive inotropic, vasodilatory, and chronotropic effects of milrinone on the postischemic neonatal pig heart. Am J Cardiol 1989;64:414.
89. Colucci WS, Wright RF, Jaski BE. Milrinone and dobutamine in severe heart failure: differing hemodynamic effects and individual patient responses. Circulation 1986;73:175–183.
90. Jaski BE, Fifer MA, Wright RF. Positive inotropic and vasodilator actions of milrinone in patients with severe congestive heart failure: dose-response relationships and comparison to nitroprusside. J Clin Invest 1985;75:643–649.
91. Chang AC, Atz AM, Wernovsky G, et al. Milrinone: systemic and pulmonary hemodynamic effects in neonates and infants after cardiac surgery. Crit Care Med 1995;23:1907–1914.
92. Lancon JP, Caillard B, Volot F, et al. Comparaison de l'enoximone et de la dobutamine dans le traitement du bas debit cardiaque apres chirurgie cardiaque. Annales Francaises d'Anesthesie et de Reanimation 1990;9:289–294.
93. Innes PA, Frazer RS, Booker PD, et al. Comparison of the haemodynamic effects of dobutamine with enoximone after open heart surgery in small children. Br J Anaesth 1994;71(1):77–81.
94. Hausdorf G. Experience with phosphodiesterase inhibitors in paediatric cardiac surgery. Eur J Anaesth 1993;(Suppl)8:25–30.
95. Conti CR, Feldman RL, Pepine CJ, et al. Effect of glyceryl trinitrate on coronary and systemic hemodynamics in man. Am J Med 1984;(Suppl)74:28.
96. Ilbawi MN, Idriss FS, Deleon SY, et al. Hemodynamic effects of intravenous nitroglycerin in pediatric patients after heart surgery. Circulation 1985;72(3 Part 2) II:101–107.
97. Benson LN, Bohn D, Edmonds JF, et al. Nitroglycerine therapy in children with low cardiac index after heart surgery. Cardiovasc Med 1979;4:207–215.
98. McGowan FX, Davis PJ, Siewers RD, et al. Coronary vaso-

constriction mediated by endothelin-1 in neonates: reversal by nitroglycerin. J Thorac Cardiovasc Surg 1995;109:88–97.
99. Benzig G, Helmsworth JA, Schreiber JT, et al. Nitropruside and epinephrine for treatment of low output in children after open heart surgery. Ann Thorac Surg 1979;27:523–528.
100. Balaraman V, Kullama LK, Robillard JE, et al. Developmental changes in sodium nitroprusside and atrial natriuretic factor mediated relaxation in the guinea pig aorta. Pediatr Res 1990;27:392–395.
101. Beekman RH, Rocchini AP, Dick M, et al. Vasodilator therapy in children. Acute and chronic effects in children with left ventricular dysfunction or mitral regurgitation. Pediatrics 1984;73:43–51.
102. Applebaum A, Blackstone EH, Kouchoukos NT, et al. Afterload reduction and cardiac output in infants early after intracardiac surgery. Am J Cardiol 1977;39:445–451.
103. Deal JE, Barratt TM, Dillon MJ. Management of hypertensive emergencies. Arch Dis Child 1992;67:1089–1092.
104. Will RJ, Walker OM, Traugott RC, et al. Sodium nitroprusside and propranolol therapy for management of postcoarctectomy hypertension. J Thorac Cardiovasc Surg 1978;75:722–724.
105. Rubis LJ, Stephenson LW, Johnston MR, et al. Comparison of effects of prostaglandin and nitroprusside on pulmonary vascular resistance in children after open heart surgery. Ann Thorac Surg 1981;32:563–570.
106. Benitz WE, Malachowski N, Cohen RS, et al. Use of sodium nitroprusside in neonates: efficacy and safety. J Pediatr 1985;106:102–110.
107. Williams DB, Kiernan PD, Schaff HV, et al. The hemodynamic response to dopamine and nitroprusside following right atrium to pulmonary artery bypass (Fontan procedure). Ann Thorac Surg 1982;34:51–57.
108. Krogmann ON, Rammos S, Jakob M, et al. Left ventricular diastolic dysfunction late after coarctation repair in childhood: influence of left ventricular hypertrophy. J Am Coll Cardiol 1993;21:1454–1460.
109. Linakis JG, Lacouture PG, Woolf A. Monitoring cyanide and thiocyante concentrations during infusion of sodium nitroprusside in children. Pediatr Cardiol 1991;12:214–218.
110. Kunathai S, Sholler GF, Celermajer, et al. Nitroprusside in children after cardiopulmonary bypass: a study of thiocyanate toxicity. Pediatr Cardiol 1989;10:121–124.
111. Rao PS. Chronic afterload reduction in infants and children with primary myocardial disease. J Pediatr 1986;108:530–534.
112. Nakazawa M, Takao A, Chon Y, et al. Significance of systemic vascular resistance in determining the hemodynamic effects of hydralazine on large ventricular septal defects. Circ 1983;68:420–424.
113. Hirschl RB, Heiss KF, Bartlett RH. Severe myocardial dysfunction during extracorporeal membrane oxygenation. J Pediatr Surg 1992;27:48–53.
114. Deal JE, Barratt TM, Dillon MJ. Management of hypertensive emergencies. Arch Dis Child 1992;67:1089–1092.
115. Sinaiko AR. Treatment of hypertension in children. Pediatr Nephrol 1994;8:603–609.
116. Lopez-Herce J, Albajara L, Cagigas P, et al. Treatment of hypertensive crisis in children with nifedipine. Int Care Med 1988;14:519–521.
117. Wimmer M, Schlemmer M. Long-term hemodynamic effects of nifedipine on congenital heart disease with Eisenmenger's mechanism in children. Cardiovasc Drugs Ther 1992;6(2):183–186.
118. Johnson CE, Beekman RH, Kostyshak DA, et al. Pharmacokinetics and pharmacodynamics of nifedipine in children with bronchopulmonary dysplasia and pulmonary hypertension. Pediatr Res 1991;29:500–503.
119. Houde C, Bohn DJ, Freedom RM, et al. Profile of pediatric patients with pulmonary hypertension judged by responsiveness to vasodilators. Br Heart J 1993;70:461–468.
120. Shaffer EM, Rocchini AP, Spicer Rl, et al. Effects of verapamil on left ventricular diastolic filling in children with hypertrophic cardiomyopathy. Am J Cardiol 1988;61:413–417.
121. Ader R, Chatterjee K, Ports T, et al. Immediate and sustained hemodynamics and clinical improvement in chronic heart failure by an oral angiotensin converting enzyme inhibitor. Circulation 1980;61:931.
122. Kramer BL, Massie BM, Topic N. Controlled trial of captopril in chronic heart failure. A rest and exercise hemodynamic study. Circulation 1983;67:807.
123. Begur AR, Beekman RH, Rocchini AP, et al. Acute hemodynamic effects of captopril in children with a congestive or restrictive cardiomyopathy. Circulation 1991;83(2):523–527.
124. Stern H, Weil J, Genz T, et al. Captopril in children with dilated cardiomyopathy: acute and long term effects in a prospective study of hemodynamic and hormonal effects. Pediatr Cardiol 1990;11:22–28.
125. Montigny M, Davignon A, Fouron J-C, et al. Captopril in infants for congestive heart failure secondary to a large ventricular left to right shunt. Am J Cardiol 1989;63:631–633.
126. Webster MW, Neutze JM, Calder AL. Acute hemodynamic effects of converting enzyme inhibition in children with intracardiac shunts. Pediatr Cardiol 1992;13(3):129–135.
127. Morsi MR, Madina EH, Anglo AA, et al. Evaluation of captopril versus reserpine and furosemide in treating hypertensive children with acute post-streptococcal glomerulonephritis. Acta Pediatr 1992;81:145–149.
128. Dutertre JP, Billaud EM, Autret E, et al. Inhibition of angiotensin converting enzyme with enalapril maleate in infants with congestive heart failure. Br J Clin Pharmacol 1993;35:528–530.
129. Lewis AB, Chabot M. The effect of treatment with angiotensin-converting enzyme inhibitors on survival of pediatric patients with dilated cardiomyopathy. Pediatr Cardiol 1993;14:9–12.
130. Leversha AM, Wilson NJ, Clarkson PM, et al. Efficacy and dosage of enalapril in congenital and acquired heart disease. Arch Dis Child 1994;70:335–339.
131. Mason T, Polak MJ, Pyles L, et al. Treatment of neonatal renovascular hypertension with intravenous enalapril. Am J Perinatol 1992;9:254–257.
132. Miller K, Atkin B, Rodel PV, et al. Enalapril: a well tolerated and efficacious agent for the pediatric hypertensive patient. J Cardiovasc Pharmacol 1987;7:S154–156.
133. Keeley FW, Elmoselhi A, Leenen FH. Enalapril suppresses normal accumulation of elastin and collagen in cardiovascular tissues of growing rats. Am J Physiol 1992;262:H1013–1021.
134. Lahav M, Regev A, Ra'anani P, et al. Intermittent administration of furosemide vs continuous infusion preceded by a loading dose for congestive heart failure. Chest 1992;102(3):725–731.
135. Singh NC, Kissoon N, Al Mofada A, et al. Comparison of continuous versus intermittent furosemide administration in postoperative pediatric cardiac patients. Crit Care Med 1991;20(1):17–21.

136. Wilson NJ, Adderley RJ, McEniery JA. Supraventricular tachycardia associated with continuous furosemide infusion. Can J Anaesth 1991;38(4 Pt 1):502–505.
137. Green TP, Thompson TR, Johnson D, et al. Furosemide promotes patent ductus arteriosus in premature infants with respiratory distress syndrome. N Engl J Med 1983;308:743–750.
138. Vincent RN, Cllick LA, Williams HM, et al. Esmolol as an adjunct in the treatment of systemic hypertension after operative repair of coarctation of the aorta. Am J Cardiol 1990;65:941–943.
139. Bunchman TE, Lunch RE, Wood EG. Intravenously administered labetalol for treatment of hypertension in children. J Pediatr 1992;120:140–144.
140. Jones SE. Coarctation in children. Controlled hypotension using labetalol and halothane. Anesthesia 1979;34:1052–1055.
141. Willis JK, Tilton AH, Harkin JC, et al. Reversible myopathy due to labetalol. Pediatr Neurol 1990;6:275–276.
142. Garson A, Gillette PC, McNamara DG. Supraventricular tachycardia in children: clinical features, response to treatment, and long term followup in 217 patients. J Pediatr 1981;98:875–882.
143. Olley PM, Coceani F, Bodach E. E-type prostaglandins a new emergency therapy for certain cyanotic congenital heart malformations. Circulation 1976;53(4):728–731.
144. Teixeira OH, Carpenter B, MacMurray SB, et al. Long term prostaglandin E1 therapy in congenital heart defects. J Am Coll Cardiol 1984;3:838–843.
145. Freed MD, Heymann MA, Lewis AB, et al. Prostaglandin E1 in infants with ductus arteriosus-dependent congenital heart disease. Circulation 1981;64:899–905
146. Jureidini S, Chase NA, Alpert BS, et al. Soft tissue swelling in two neonates during prostaglandin E1 therapy. Pediatr Cardiol 1986;7:157–160.
147. Peled N, Dagan O, Babyn P, et al. Gastric outlet obstruction induced by prostaglandin therapy in neonates. N Engl J Med 1992;327:505–510.
148. Singh GK, Fond LV, Salmon AP, et al. Study of low dosage prostaglandin–usages and complications. Eur Heart J 1994;15:377–381.
149. Ment LR, Duncan CC, Ehrenkranz RA, et al. Randomized indomethacin trial for prevention of intraventricular hemorrhage in very low birth weight infants. J Pediatr 1985;107:937–943.
150. Liem KD, Hopman JC, Kollee LA, et al. Effects of repeated indomethacin administration on cerebral oxygenation and haemodynamics is preterm infants. Combined near infrared spectrophotometry and Doppler ultrasound study. Eur J Pediatr 1994;153(7):504–509.
151. Ment LR, Oh W, Ehrenkranz RA, et al. Low-dose indomethacin therapy and extension of intraventricular hemorrhage. A multicenter randomized trial. J Pediatr 1994;124(6):952–955.
152. Ibrahim M, Cliland J, O'Kane H, et al. St Jude medical prosthesis in children. J Thorac Cardiovasc Surg 1994;108:52–56.
153. Andrew M, Marzinotto V, Brooker LA, et al. Oral anticoagulation therapy in pediatric patients: a prospective study. Thromb Haemost 1994;71:265–269.
154. Andrew M, Marzinotto V, Massicotte P, et al. Heparin therapy in pediatric patients: a prospective cohort study. Pediatr Res 1994;35:78–83.
155. Ino T, Benson LN, Freedom RM, et al. Thrombolytic therapy for femoral artery thrombosis after pediatric cardiac catheterization. Am Heart J 1988;115:633–639.
156. Krafte-Jacobs B, Sivit CJ, Mejia R, et al. Catheter related thrombosis in critically ill children: comparison of catheters with and without heparin bonding. J Pediatr 1995;126:50–54.
157. Evans DJ, Pizer BL, Moghal NE, et al. Neonatal aortic arch thrombosis. Arch Dis Child 1994;71:125–127.
158. Kothari S, Varma S, Wasir HS. Thrombolytic therapy in infants and children. Am Heart J 1994;127:651–657.
159. Fyfe DA, Kline CH, Sade RM, et al. Transesophageal echocardiography detects thrombus formation not identified by transthoracic echcoardiography after the Fontan operation. J Am Coll Cardiol 1991;18:1733–1737.
160. Kirk CR, Qureshi SA. Streptokinase in the management of arterial thrombosis in infancy. Int J Cardiol 1989;25:15–20.
161. Barzaghi A, DellOrto M, Rovelli A, et al. Central venous catheter clots: incidence, clinical significance and catheter care in patients with hematologic malignancies. Pediatr Hematol Oncol 1995;12:243–250.
162. Bagnall HA, Gumperts E, Atkinson J. Continuous infusion of low dose urokinase in the treatment of central venous catheter thrombosis in infants and children. Pediatrics 1989;83:936–969.
163. Giacoia GP. High dose urokinase therapy in newborn infants with major vessel thrombosis. Clin Pediatr (Phila) 1993;32:231–237.
164. Ryan CA, Andrew M. Failure of thrombolytic therapy in four children with extensive thromboses. Am J Dis Child 1992;146:187–193.
165. Levy M, Benson LN, Burrows PE, et al. Tissue plasminogen activator for the treatment of thromboembolism in infants and children. J Pediatr 1991;118:467–472.
166. Tsubata S, Ichida F, Hamamichi Y, et al. Successful thrombolytic therapy using tissue-type plasminogen activator in Kawasaki disease. Pediatr Cardiol 1995;16:186–189.
167. Klinge J, Hofbeck M, Ries M, et al. Thrombolyse von modifizierten Blalock-Taussig im Kindesalter mit rekombinantem Gewebeplasminogenaktivator. Z Kardiol 1995;84:476–480.
168. Ries M, Singer H, Hofbeck M, et al. Tissue plasminogen activator treatment for femoral artery thrombosis after cardiac catheterization in infants and children. Br Heart J 1993;70:382–385.
169. Wacker P, Oberhansli I, Didier D, et al. Right atrial thrombosis associated with central venous catheter in children with cancer. Med Pediatr Oncol 1994;22:53–57.
170. Asante A, Sreeram N, McKay R, et al. Thrombolysis with tissue-type plasminogen activator following cardiac surgery in children. Int J Cardiol 1992;35:317–322.

Normal Physiology of the Respiratory System

David Paul Nelson MD, PhD, and David L. Wessel MD

Alterations in respiratory physiology can have significant impact on cardiac performance through cardiorespiratory interactions. These interactions are often magnified in patients with congenital heart disease (1). Patients with congenital heart disease often present with respiratory symptoms, and they are markedly more susceptible to respiratory compromise (2, 3). In addition, respiratory physiology becomes uniquely important in the management of cardiac patients with abnormal circulation (4) (i.e., single ventricle, intracardiac shunting, and so forth). In these patients, variations in cardiac physiology result in alterations of pulmonary mechanics (5–8), gas exchange (9–11), fluid flux (12, 13) and O_2 transport (14).

This chapter reviews the normal physiology of the respiratory system to lay a groundwork to discuss respiratory failure of cardiac origin. Because the essence of respiratory physiology is oxygen delivery and carbon dioxide elimination, this review is organized according to the steps necessary for the transport of oxygen from the atmosphere to the cell (15), including (a) pulmonary mechanics and the mechanics of gas flow into the alveoli, (b) gas exchange in the lung, (c) pulmonary circulation and distribution of pulmonary blood flow, and (4) matching of ventilation and perfusion. In each section, alterations in respiratory physiology common to patients with acquired and congenital heart diseases will be discussed.

PULMONARY MECHANICS: STATICS

Gas exchange in the lung requires movement of gas into and out of the lung, which in turn depends on multiple factors: the compliance of the lungs and chest wall, respiratory muscles, pressure or force differential applied across the lung, and resistance to gas flow in and out of the lung. Interactions of these factors determine physiologic lung volumes.

Lung Volumes

Figure 6.1 schematically illustrates lung volumes as would be measured by a spirometer (16). Total lung capacity (TLC) is the volume of gas contained in the lung at the end of maximal inspiration. After inspiration to TLC, the maximal amount of gas that can be forcefully expired from the lungs is termed the vital capacity (VC). After maximal expiration, the amount of gas still remaining in the lung is the residual volume (RV). Functional residual capacity (FRC), the gas volume in the lung at the end of a passive expiration, is the lung volume at which the outward force of the chest wall is equivalent to the inwardly opposing elastic force of the lung parenchyma. In normal physiology, tidal volume (V_T) is the volume of gas moved in and out of the lungs during spontaneous tidal ventilation.

Closing capacity (CC) is a theoretic lung volume, below which airway closure can occur, leading to relative or total hypoventilation in dependent parts of the lung (16–18). The relationship between CC and FRC is important, because when FRC falls below the CC, dependent areas of the lung are likely to collapse, worsening gas exchange (17). CC is typically lower than FRC, but FRC is age dependent, and it can be reduced by pulmonary edema, increased pulmonary blood volume, and supine positioning, all of which are common in critically ill patients with congenital heart disease. Similarly, CC can be altered by enlarged great arteries or cardiac chambers and by increases in pulmonary arterial pressures or flow. The relationship between FRC and CC is at least partially responsible for the observation that prone positioning improves regional lung collapse and thus gas exchange in both experimental animals and patients. This effect can be magnified in infants because FRC is lower in infants than adults because of the highly compliant newborn chest wall (19). Most tidal breathing in infants takes place in the range of the CC, which may explain why regional lung collapse is relatively common in critically ill infants (20).

Lung volumes are routinely measured by spirometry, either directly using a classic water seal spirometer or by integrating inspiratory and expiratory flows to obtain lung volumes (21). RV, and thus TLC and FRC, cannot be measured spirometrically, so they are measured by gas dilution techniques, body plethysmography, or radiographic planimetry (22). Evaluation of pulmonary function in infants and children is covered in depth in Chapter 23, *Pulmonary Issues*.

Pulmonary Compliance

Compliance is a mechanical characteristic that relates a change in volume of a system to a change in the distending pressure of the system (23). Pulmonary compliance (C_L) is therefore change in lung volume relative to the change in transmural pressure distending the lung:

$$C_L = \Delta V \text{ (in liters)}/\Delta P \text{ (in cm } H_2O)$$

Figure 6.1. Lung volumes as measured by a spirometer.

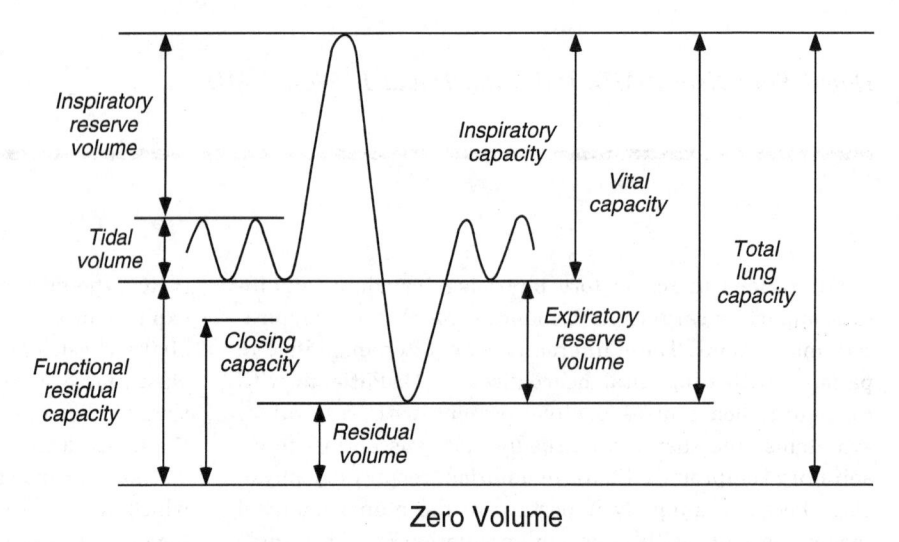

Figure 6.2. Mechanical characteristics of the chest wall, lungs, and total respiratory (lung-chest wall) system. FRC, forced residual capacity; TLC, total lung capacity; RV, residual volume. (Adapted with permission from Leff AR, Schumacker PT. Respiratory physiology. Philadelphia: WB Saunders, 1993.)

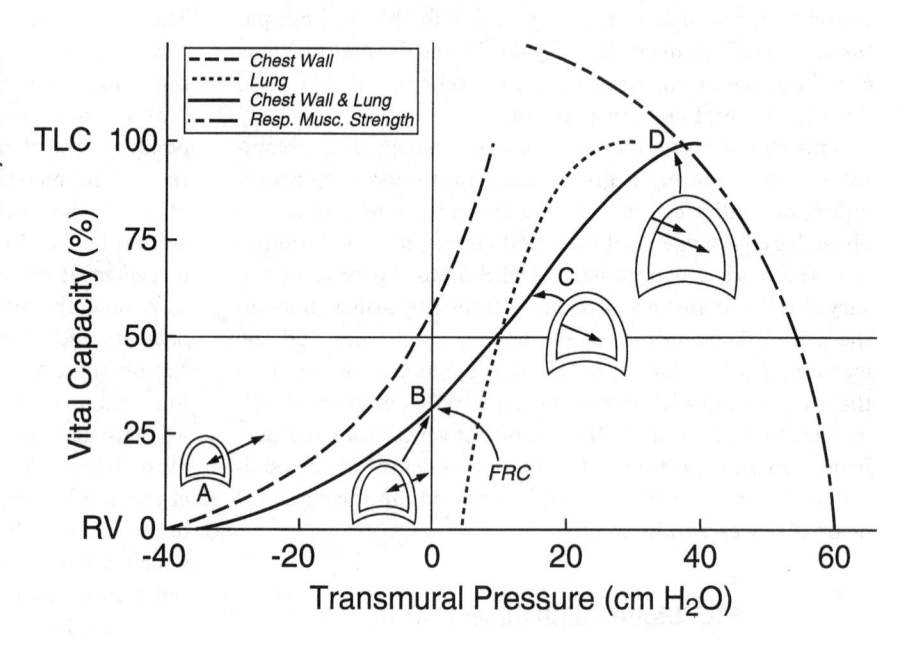

Compliance is a volume-dependent measurement, and thus does not necessarily indicate intrinsic elastic properties of lung tissue. For example, following a pneumonectomy pulmonary compliance will be half the preoperative value even though the elastic character of the lung tissue is unchanged (23). Similarly, the low lung volume of an infant would correspond to low pulmonary compliance (19). Volume-dependent differences in compliance can be normalized by dividing compliance by FRC to obtain the specific compliance.

Pressure-Volume Relations of the Lung and Chest Wall

Distension of the lung requires a positive transmural distending pressure. Because the lung and chest wall act together as one system (24), the transmural pressure of the lung alone (transpulmonary pressure, P_{tp}) is defined as the pressure differential between the lung airspaces (alveolar pressure, P_{alv}) and lung pleura (pleural pressure, P_{pl}). Figure 6.2 illustrates the mechanical characteristics of the chest wall alone, lung alone, and lung-chest wall system (25). Consider first the properties of the chest wall alone. In the absence of the lung's inward elastic recoil, the chest wall will tend to expand to a larger volume so that the natural resting volume of the chest wall alone is approximately 60% TLC. Only a small amount of positive pressure is required to distend the chest wall to TLC, whereas a large negative transmural pressure is necessary to reduce the chest wall volume to RV.

In contrast to the chest wall, the inwardly elastic force

of the lung parenchyma would tend to reduce lung volume in the absence of the chest wall. The natural resting volume of the lung alone would be much less than FRC (not shown in Fig. 6.2).

The mechanics of the total lung-chest wall system comprise the sum of the pressure-volume characteristics of the lung and chest wall separately. The properties of the system at RV are predominantly determined by the chest wall, because the lung is minimally distended. RV is therefore largely determined by the ability of the expiratory muscles to oppose the outward recoil forces of the chest wall (point A, Fig. 6.2). Expiratory muscle force decreases at lower lung volumes because of reduced muscle length. RV can therefore be altered by changes in chest wall mechanics or weakened expiratory muscle strength.

Functional residual capacity occurs when the outward recoil force of the chest wall is balanced by the inward elastic force of the lung, and it is thus the lung volume associated with a total transmural pressure of zero (point B, Fig. 6.2). FRC is an equilibrium point, which can be altered by reduced lung compliance or changes in chest wall mechanics (e.g., kyphoscoliosis, open chest, abdominal ascites). This can be an important factor in critically ill patients because maintenance of an adequate FRC is important to avoid regional lung collapse and to avoid increases in pulmonary vascular resistance caused by low lung volumes (17, 18).

Volumes greater than FRC require a positive total transmural pressure. At TLC, the elastic recoil forces of the lung and chest wall are additive and must be balanced by the ability of the inspiratory muscles to expand the lung-chest wall system. Figure 6.2 illustrates how inspiratory muscle force decreases at higher lung volumes. TLC is therefore determined by the balance of the respiratory muscle strength and the inward elastic recoil of the lung-chest wall system. Respiratory muscle weakness or diaphragmatic paresis can lead to reductions in TLC and other lung volumes (26–28). Newborn infants have extremely compliant chest walls, however, pressure-volume relationships of the respiratory system change with growth throughout infancy and childhood (20, 29).

Congenital heart lesions often result in changes in pulmonary compliance and the pressure volume relationship of the respiratory system. Acute pressure or volume overload often causes a reduction in pulmonary compliance (5–8), which contributes to the increased work of breathing common in these patients. The changes in compliance in these patients is thought to be caused by increases in lung fluid secondary to left atrial hypertension. Excessive pulmonary blood flow can also lead to changes in pulmonary compliance because of increases in pulmonary blood volume or pressures. Elevated pulmonary arterial pressures also contribute to reductions in pulmonary compliance (30).

Surface Tension and Surfactant

The pressure-volume relationships discussed above assume inflation of the lung with gas. If a lung is inflated with saline, less distending pressure is required for inflation, and the lung will appear to be more compliant. The explanation of this is that alveolar surface is liquid lined, forming an air-liquid interface, which contributes alveolar surface tension forces to lung compliance. During air inflation, alveolar surface tension forces increase the effective lung elastic recoil pressure generated at any lung volume. In contrast, the alveolar air-liquid interface is abolished during liquid inflation and surface tension forces are canceled so that only the elastic structural elements of the lung contribute to elastic lung recoil (24).

Surface tension at air-liquid interfaces is reduced in the presence of detergents, because detergents interrupt the polar attraction of water molecules at the surface of the interface. The alveolar surface tension at the alveolar air-liquid interface is reduced by the presence of surfactant, a mixture of endogenous lipids and proteins that is the most effective detergent ever found (30). Surfactant increases lung compliance by reducing the force necessary to overcome alveolar surface tension. Surfactant also accounts for lung hysteresis, the fact that the inflation and deflation pressure-volume curves are not identical; less pressure is required at each lung volume during deflation because of the physical properties of surfactant (31).

In addition to improving lung compliance, surfactant helps keep the lungs dry. This occurs because surfactant reduces transmural pressure keeping alveoli inflated. The relationship between wall tension and transmural pressure is a consequence of Laplace's law:

$$P = 2T/r$$

where P is transmural pressure, T is total wall tension and r is the radius of the alveolar sphere. This means that the pressure differential between alveolar gas and the surrounding interstitial space is reduced, which in turn reduces the interstitial pressure and thus the hydrostatic pressure force for fluid to leave the pulmonary capillaries.

A third role for surfactant is to provide stability for alveolar lung units. In the absence of surfactant, the law of Laplace would dictate that the transmural pressure necessary to inflate an alveoli would decrease as the alveoli become larger. The consequence of this is that smaller alveoli would tend to collapse into larger alveoli. The presence of surfactant ameliorates this effect because in addition to reducing surface tension in all alveoli, surface tension will be reduced most in the smallest alveoli, which will help to stabilize alveoli of various sizes. The other factor that contributes to alveolar stability is termed "pulmonary interdependence" (32, 33), the fact that all alveoli are interconnected by the structural architecture of the lung. Each alveolus, as well as pulmonary vessels and airways, is tethered by the surrounding lung architecture and thus ultimately linked to the distending pleural pressure.

Respiratory distress syndrome of the premature infant is a well-described condition resulting from deficiency of surfactant. As would be anticipated, infants with this condition have stiff, edematous lungs, with diffuse regions of lung collapse (34). Surfactant appears to play a role in other causes of acute respiratory failure (35). Cardiopulmonary bypass has been shown to diminish surfactant activity, which may contribute to changes in pulmonary compliance and respiratory function in the postoperative cardiac patient (36).

Regional Lung Compliance and Ventilation

As discussed, static lung volume is set by the transmural pressure gradient. Because of gravity and the weight of the lung itself, a gradient in pleural pressure is found from the top of the lung to the bottom so that Ppl is more negative near the top and less negative at the bottom of the lung. Because transpulmonary pressure is dependent on pleural pressure, the pleural pressure gradient leads to a gradient in transpulmonary pressure. Consequently, when Palv is atmospheric, Ptp will be lower in the more dependent areas of the lung, resulting in regional differences in lung distension (23, 37, 38). Figure 6.3 illustrates the regional differences in lung distension caused by gravity. At FRC, alveoli in the more dependent areas of the lung will be less distended than alveoli in nondependent areas. On inflation to TLC, the dependent and nondependent alveoli will both be inflated near maximally, because both areas of the lung reach the flat noncompliant part of the pressure-volume curve. Because the dependent alveoli were initially smaller in volume, the net volume change is greater for the dependent compared with the nondependent alveoli. The overall effect of gravity therefore is to cause regional variations in pulmonary ventilation. These variations may be amplified in patients with congenital heart disease because of airway obstruction and changes in pulmonary compliance.

DYNAMIC MECHANICS OF GAS FLOW

Movement of gas into and out of the lung requires a transpulmonary pressure gradient to overcome the frictional resistance to gas flow in the airways (39–41) (airway resistance) and the frictional resistance of the lung and chest wall to displacement (31, 42) (tissue resistance). Airway resistance makes up most (65 to 75%) of the total resistance of the respiratory system, but tissue resistance is rate-dependent and at higher respiratory rates may become significant.

Airway Resistance

Movement of air through the airways is determined by the principles of fluid mechanics (39). Air flow into and out of the lung requires the generation of a pressure gradient to overcome airway resistance. The pressure gradient required will depend on flow rate, flow characteristics, and airway size (41). Flow patterns can have a marked effect on the resistance to airflow in airways. In laminar flow, the gas particles travel in an organized energy-efficient manner so that gas movement is parallel to the axis of the airway (38). Poiseuille's law defines the relationship between pressure and flow during laminar flow:

$$\Delta P = \dot{V} * (8\eta L)/\pi r^4$$

where $\dot{V}$ is flow, η is fluid viscosity, L is length of the airway, and r is the airway radius. Note that during laminar flow, the radius of the airway is the predominant determinant of airway resistance, so that small changes in airway caliber effects resistance markedly. In contrast to laminar flow, turbulent flow is a disorganized flow pattern. Although the net movement of gas occurs parallel to the airway axis, turbulent eddies and vortices generate flows perpendicular to the airway, leading to an inefficient use of energy. This disrupted flow pattern leads to a steeper drop in pressure along the airway than in laminar flow. The pressure-flow relationship in turbulent flow is nonlinear; the driving pressure is proportional to the gas density, the square of the gas flow rate and inversely proportional to the fifth power of the airway radius (16).

It is possible to predict flow patterns in a system by calculating the Reynolds number:

$$Re = (D * u * \rho)/\eta$$

where D is the airway diameter, u is the average velocity of flow, ρ is the density of the fluid, and η is the fluid or

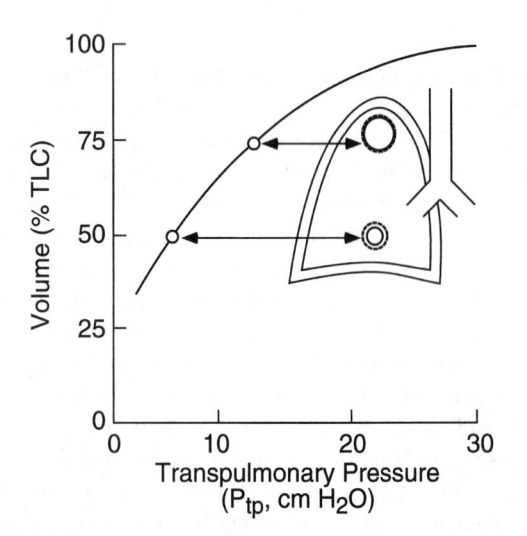

Figure 6.3. Gravitational effects dictate that alveoli in the more dependent areas of the lung are less distended. TLC, total lung capacity. (Adapted with permission from Gibson GJ, Pride NB. Lung distensibility: the state pressure-volume curve of the lungs and its use in clinical assessment. British Journal of Diseases of the Chest 1976;70:143–183.)

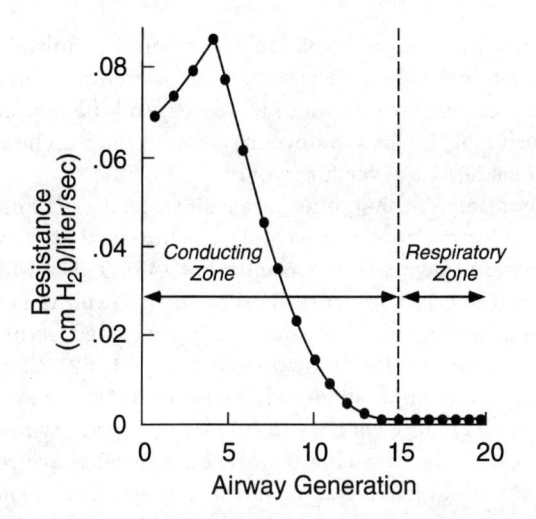

Figure 6.4. In contrast to the infant, airways greater than 2 mm and less than the ninth generation in adults contribute most of total airway resistance. (Adapted with permission from Pedley TJ. The prediction of pressure drop and variation of resistance within the human bronchial airways. Respir Physiol 1970;9:387–393.)

gas viscosity (16). Flow tends to be turbulent for a Re of approximately 2000 or greater and laminar below this level. Gas velocities in the trachea and larger airways are large and calculation of Re indicates that flow in these larger airways is turbulent even during quiet tidal breathing. Laminar flow becomes prevalent in smaller, peripheral airways because gas velocity and airway diameter are dramatically reduced, which results in a lower calculated Re.

Because of turbulent flow in larger airways, the upper airway contributes nearly half of the total airway resistance. Figure 6.4 illustrates that airways greater than 2 mm and less than ninth generation contribute more than 80% of the total airway resistance in the adult lung (43). By contrast, smaller airways account for as much as half of the total airway resistance in infants and young children, which explains why children are so susceptible to diseases that alter small airway measurement resistance (e.g., congestive heart failure, pulmonary hypertension, or bronchiolitis) (44, 45).

Airway Reactivity

A major determinant of the caliber of the conducting airways is bronchial smooth muscle tone. Airway smooth muscle tone is modulated by neurohumoral innervation and by local mediators in the airway epithelium in response to airway irritants. Airways are innervated by several different components of the autonomic nervous system (46). Parasympathetic innervation provides a baseline level of airway smooth muscle tone, and it plays a role in reflex parasympathetic bronchoconstriction in response to airway irritants. Airway smooth muscle is not innervated directly by sympathetic innervation, but bronchodilation occurs in response to increases in circulating endogenous or exogenous catecholamines or inhaled β-agonists. The nonadrenergic-noncholinergic (NANC) inhibitory innervation of the airways leads to relaxation of the airway smooth muscle. Finally, the NANC-stimulatory system can lead to mild bronchoconstriction in response to certain airway stimuli (e.g., cold and exercise). Pulmonary C-fibers appear to have a role in the afferent limb of the NANC-stimulatory response.

The parasympathetic nervous system provides some degree of bronchomotor tone at all times (47). Further bronchoconstriction can result from local airway irritants that stimulate mast cell degranulation and the consequent release of local bronchoactive mediators and activation of reflex parasympathetic bronchoconstriction. This "triggered" bronchoconstriction is exaggerated in individuals with reactive airways disease and asthma.

Airway edema, which is common in children with congenital heart diseases with elevated left-atrial pressure or increased pulmonary blood flow, also plays a significant role in bronchomotor tone (2). The most obvious effect of airway edema is physical narrowing of the airways, which is most significant in the peripheral, small caliber airways. In addition, the law of Laplace predicts that increases in wall tension caused by smooth muscle constriction will have a greater effect in airways with smaller caliber. Therefore, once the airway is narrowed by edema formation, changes in smooth muscle tone will have an exaggerated effect. Finally, edema in lung parenchyma surrounding the airways may interfere with the tethering effect of the lung architecture that helps distend airways, blood vessels, and alveoli (48).

Flow-Volume Relationships and Expiratory Flow Limitation

As illustrated in Figure 6.5, airway resistance can be altered by changes in lung volume (47). Airway resistance is decreased as lung volumes exceed FRC. As lung volume

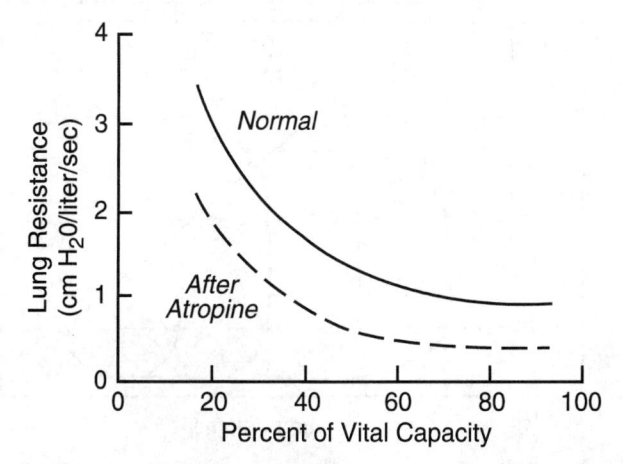

Figure 6.5. Airway resistance decreases as lung volumes exceed functional residual capacity (FRC). (Adapted with permission from Vincent NJ, Knudson R, Leith DE, et al. Factors influencing pulmonary resistance. J Appl Physiol 1970;29(2):236–243.)

increases, airway caliber increases because of tethering of airways by surrounding lung architecture and by inhibition of parasympathetic-induced bronchomotor tone (Hering-Breuer reflex). Below FRC, airway resistance can increase dramatically as a result of airway collapse and flow limitation (38).

Maximal inspiratory flow rate is effort-dependent, and it is influenced by respiratory muscle strength and the elastic recoil of the lung. By contrast, forced maximal expiratory flow is a function of lung volume and is effort-independent (Fig. 6.6). During forced expiration, pleural pressure and intrathoracic pressure become positive, which would narrow the airways if not for the opposing force of intrabronchial pressure and the tethering effect of lung interdependence (38, 49, 50). Intrabronchial pressure falls progressively from alveoli to trachea because of resistive losses and the Bernoulli effect. At a point where transmural airway pressure becomes negative, airway collapse and thus flow limitation will occur. Maximal expiratory flow limitation is volume-dependent for multiple reasons: as lung volume decreases lung static recoil pressure decreases, airway resistance increases, and the mechanical tethering of the airways by surrounding lung architecture becomes less at lower lung volumes (38, 50).

Acute and chronic lung disease can lead to changes in the expiratory flow-volume relationship so that maximal expiratory flows are abnormally low (45). This results in the characteristic concave pattern to the expiratory flow-volume loop in which expiration is prolonged because of the slow rate of flow-limited expiration (51, 52). Lung pathology can lead to abnormal expiratory flows for multiple reasons including changes in (a) airway reactivity and airway resistance, (b) reduced static lung recoil pressures, (c) loss of mechanical tethering of the airways, and (d) abnormalities in airway structural rigidity (i.e., tracheomalacia, bronchomalacia).

Patients with congenital heart disease have abnormal expiratory flow-volume curves, demonstrating the presence of lower airway obstruction (53). The cause of this is presumably multifactorial, and it includes airway edema, changes in airway reactivity, and reduced tethering of the airways secondary to pulmonary interstitial edema. Pulmonary hypertension can also play a role in increasing airway resistance. In addition to lower airway obstruction, congenital heart disease also predisposes patients to upper airway obstruction due to compression by vascular structures or enlarged cardiac chambers. The combination of upper and lower airways obstruction explains why patients with congenital heart disease often present with wheezing, retractions, and patchy areas of lobar collapse.

Work of Breathing

A certain amount of energy is necessary to overcome the pressure-volume relations of the lung and chest wall (elastic work) and to overcome the frictional resistance to gas flow in the airways (resistive work). The amount of energy needed for tidal ventilation as a function of time is the work of breathing. Work of breathing will be increased by conditions of increased airway resistance, decreased compliance, or increased respiratory frequency. Work of breathing can be dramatically increased in patients with congenital heart disease because of increases in both resistive and elastic work, and this must be anticipated when determining a child's nutritional requirements.

GAS EXCHANGE IN THE LUNG

Pulmonary gas exchange requires movement of gas in and out of the lung and then diffusion of gases across the alveolar-capillary surface to allow equilibration between alveolar air and pulmonary capillary blood. Optimal pulmonary gas exchange requires matching the ventilation of each alveoli to perfusion of the associated pulmonary capil-

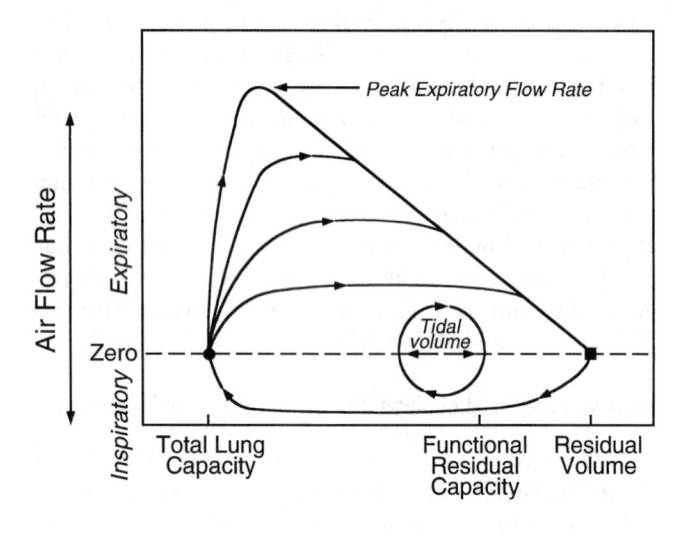

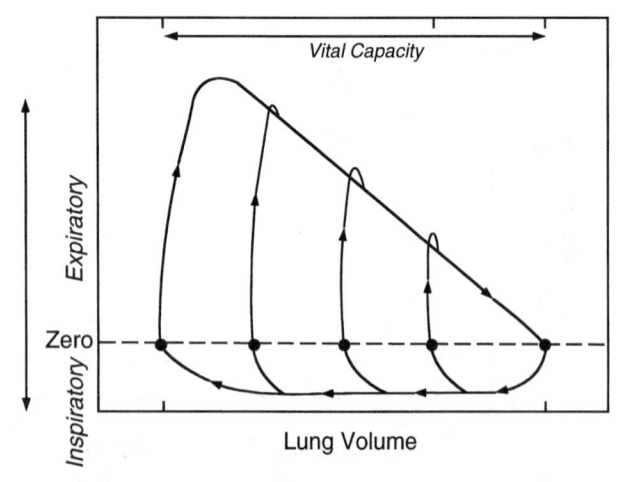

Figure 6.6. Inspiratory and forced maximal expiratory flow rates. (Adapted with permission from Nunn JF. Nunn's applied repsiratory physiology. 4th ed. Cambridge: Butterworth-Heinemann Ltd, 1993.)

laries (54, 55). This section first covers ventilation and perfusion separately and then considers factors that provide optimal matching of ventilation to perfusion.

Ventilation

Gas Properties

The physical properties of gases are important components to alveolar ventilation (16, 56). Ambient air is composed of a mixture of oxygen, nitrogen, and trace amounts of carbon dioxide and other inert gases. The composition of a gas mixture is specified by the individual gas fractions that determine the corresponding partial pressures of each gas in the mixture. The partial pressure of a specific gas in a mixture is the fraction of the total pressure that is exerted by that gas, and it is thus calculated as the product of the dry gas fraction and barometric pressure. Alveolar gas is fully humidified by the upper airways, so that it has a constant water vapor pressure determined by body temperature (47 torr at 37°C). This effectively reduces the partial pressures of the gases present in the alveoli. Alveolar partial pressure of a specific gas X is therefore:

$$P_X = (P_B - 47) * F_X$$

where P_X is the partial pressure of gas X, P_B is total ambient barometric pressure, and F_X is the dry gas fraction of gas X.

Diffusion

All movement of gases from one locale to another, including gas exchange in the lung and systemic circulation, is ultimately dependent on diffusion (16, 56). Respiratory gases must diffuse through the alveolar-capillary membrane, plasma, and red blood cell membrane during pulmonary gas exchange. Diffusion of oxygen or carbon dioxide across a barrier obeys Fick's law of diffusion:

$$\dot{V}_{gas} = (DA/T)(\Delta P)$$

The volume of gas per unit time ($\dot{V}_{gas}$) moving through a tissue is directly proportional to the diffusion coefficient (D) and the surface area of the tissue (A), and it is inversely proportional to the tissue thickness (T). Diffusion is also dependent on the partial pressure gradient for the gas. The diffusion coefficient is related to the solubility of the gas in the tissue and inversely proportional to the square root of its molecular weight (16).

It is estimated that blood passing through the lung usually spends about 0.75 seconds in the pulmonary capillaries (57). Mixed-venous blood enters the pulmonary capillaries with P_{CO_2} and P_{O_2} of approximately 47 and 40 torr, respectively (54, 55). Gas diffusion for both oxygen and carbon dioxide proceeds rapidly so that equilibrium with alveolar gas is achieved within about one third of its available time in the pulmonary capillary; the P_{CO_2} and P_{O_2} of typical end-capillary blood will thus be approximately 40 and 100 torr, respectively. The equilibration time for oxygen and carbon dioxide are similar even though carbon dioxide will diffuse through water 20 times more rapidly because of its greater solubility in water. This is explained because diffusion across the alveolar-capillary membrane is also dependent on the ratio of the gas solubility in the alveolar-capillary membrane to the gas solubility in the blood (54). If the solubility in the membrane is significantly less than that of the blood, the net effect is that it will take much longer for the gas to reach equilibrium. Carbon dioxide and oxygen equilibrate at similar rates because the larger diffusion coefficient of carbon dioxide is offset by its lower membrane:blood solubility ratio (54).

One of the consequences of the rapid equilibration between alveolar gas and pulmonary capillary blood is that oxygen and carbon dioxide exchange is almost never limited by diffusion. Diffusion limitation has been demonstrated only in a few extraordinary physiologic conditions, such as world class athletes performing strenuous exercise and healthy subjects exercising at very high altitude (58). Diffusion limitation has almost never been shown to contribute significantly to gas exchange abnormalities in patients with acute and chronic lung disease.

Dead Space and Alveolar Ventilation

During tidal breathing, lung volume increases by the V_T during inspiration. Most tidal volume will be distributed to alveoli, but a small fraction will remain in the conducting airways (the volume in milliliters of the conducting airways is approximately equal to body weight in pounds). The gas contained in the conducting airways does not contribute to gas exchange, and it is therefore termed "anatomic dead space" ($V_{Danatomic}$). In ideal lungs all alveoli participate in gas exchange, but in real lungs and especially in diseased lungs some alveoli receive ventilation but do not participate in effective gas exchange (56). The volume of each tidal volume that enters alveoli but does not participate in gas exchange is termed "alveolar dead space" ($V_{Dalveolar}$). The total volume of the respiratory system that does not participate in gas exchange is thus the sum of the anatomic and alveolar dead space, which is known as physiologic dead space (V_D). The physiologic dead space is subtracted from the tidal volume to calculate the volume of each breath that participates in gas exchange (V_A). Under normal conditions, alveolar dead space is negligible and physiologic dead space is essentially equivalent to anatomic dead space. Because physiologic dead space does not contribute to expired concentrations of carbon dioxide, physiologic dead space can be calculated by measuring the amount of carbon dioxide in mixed expired and alveolar air ($P_A CO_2$):

$$V_D/V_T = (P_A CO_2 - P_E CO_2)/P_A CO_2$$

This relationship is known as the Bohr equation; thus physiologic dead space is sometimes referred to as the "Bohr dead space" (16).

Ventilation is designated as volume of gas per minute. The product of V_T and respiratory frequency is the minute volume or minute ventilation (V_E). The portion of the minute volume that participates in effective gas exchange is the alveolar ventilation (V_A), and that portion that does not contribute to alveolar gas exchange is physiologic dead space ventilation (V_D). Because the minute volume is the sum of the alveolar and dead space ventilation, note that:

$$\dot{V}_A = \dot{V}_E - \dot{V}_D$$

Carbon Dioxide Elimination

Alveolar ventilation must be adequate to allow elimination of carbon dioxide from pulmonary capillary blood. Under normal steady state conditions, the quantity of carbon dioxide produced by the body tissues ($\dot{V}CO_2$) will be equivalent to the amount of carbon dioxide eliminated from the lungs during alveolar ventilation (15). Because inspired gas contains essentially no carbon dioxide, the exhaled flow of carbon dioxide is the product of alveolar ventilation and the alveolar carbon dioxide gas fraction:

$$\dot{V}CO_2 = \dot{V}_A * F_ACO_2$$

This relationship is defined as the alveolar carbon dioxide equation (54). Because a gas fraction is proportionate to the partial pressure for the gas, the equation can be solved for alveolar $PaCO_2$:

$$P_ACO_2 = \dot{V}CO_2 * (P_B - P_{H_2O})/\dot{V}_A$$

The fact that alveolar PCO_2 is directly related to alveolar ventilation is an extremely important concept for management of mechanically ventilated patients, because it indicates that doubling the alveolar ventilation will half the alveolar and thus arterial PCO_2.

Alveolar Gas Equation

Because exchange of oxygen occurs by diffusion, the driving force for this process is the alveolar PO_2 (P_AO_2). Because each alveoli takes up carbon dioxide and transfers oxygen, alveolar PO_2 is less than the inspired PO_2 by an amount proportionate to the alveolar PCO_2 (P_ACO_2):

$$P_AO_2 = FIO_2 * (P_B - 47) - P_ACO_2/R$$

where FIO_2 is the inspired gas fraction for oxygen, P_B is barometric pressure, and R is the respiratory exchange ratio. The respiratory exchange ratio is the ratio of carbon dioxide eliminated ($\dot{V}CO_2$) relative to oxygen uptake ($\dot{V}O_2$). This formula is known as the "alveolar gas equation" (54). It is important to be able to calculate alveolar PO_2 in the cardiac intensive care unit, to determine the cause of arterial hypoxia. For example, infants with single ventricle physiology are often ventilated with atmospheric or subatmospheric levels of oxygen and PCO_2 is often elevated because of contraction alkalosis from vigorous diuresis (59). When FIO_2 is relatively low and PCO_2 is elevated, alveolar PO_2 can become critically low, resulting in pulmonary venous and systemic arterial desaturation (60).

Pulmonary Circulation and Distribution of Pulmonary Blood Flow

The pulmonary circulation and manipulation of pulmonary vascular resistance is an area of particular interest for the pediatric cardiac intensivist. Congenital heart lesions manifesting large left-to-right shunts often result in pulmonary hypertension and changes in pulmonary vascular reactivity. Manipulation of pulmonary vascular resistance is essential in patients with Fontan and single ventricle physiology. It is essential to understand the basic principles of the pulmonary circulation, because manipulations to change pulmonary pressures or flows can alter pulmonary gas exchange by changing the distribution of perfusion within the lung.

These examples illustrate situations where the intensivist would like to manipulate the pulmonary circulation separate from the systemic circulation. The function of the two circulations are different, which is reflected in several physiologic differences (61). In contrast to the systemic circulation, the pulmonary circulation is a low resistance vascular bed. Physiologically, this is appropriate because the pulmonary circulation is required to accept the entire cardiac output at all times. The pulmonary circulation is also a relatively low pressure and highly pulsatile circulation; compared with the systemic circulation, hydrostatic pressures in the pulmonary circulation can be as low as is consistent to direct blood only to the top of the lung. Despite receiving the entire cardiac output, the volume of blood in the pulmonary circulation is smaller than that of the systemic circulation by a factor of about 10. Because of these differences, normal pulmonary arteries contain much less smooth muscle than systemic arteries of equivalent size.

Pulmonary Pressure-Flow Relationships

Because of the differences noted above, pressure-flow relationships in the pulmonary vascular bed are unique in several ways. Pulmonary arterial branches follow the course of the airway bronchioles until reaching the terminal respiratory bronchioles, at which point they branch off to give rise to the capillary networks within the alveolar walls (15). The various pulmonary vessels have been differentiated physiologically into extra-alveolar and alveolar vessels (62). Extra-alveolar vessels include all the small arteries and veins that course through the lung parenchyma extending to the terminal respiratory units. They are subjected to the pleural pressure by way of the tethering forces of the surrounding lung architecture. Alveolar vessels are highly susceptible to the shape, size, and pressure of the alveoli that are in direct proximity to them. Hence, the transmural pressure of alveolar vessels will depend on the hydrostatic pressure within each vessel relative to surrounding alveolar pressures.

The simplest way to consider pressure-flow relationships in the pulmonary circulation is to calculate pulmonary vascular resistance from the mean flow and pressure in the entire pulmonary bed:

$$R_p = (P_{pa} - P_{la})/\dot{Q}_p$$

where R_p is the pulmonary vascular resistance, P_{pa} and P_{la} are mean pulmonary arterial and left atrial pressures, respectively, and $\dot{Q}_p$ is mean pulmonary blood flow. This value is used most often clinically to describe the pulmonary circulation, but it is not really a complete description of the pressure-flow properties of the pulmonary bed (61, 63, 64). For example, this calculation implies that the pulmonary pressure-flow relationship is linear, which is inaccurate. The pulmonary pressure-flow relationship is a nonlinear relationship that depends on such factors as magnitude of blood flow, absolute magnitude of pulmonary arterial and venous pressures, alveolar pressures, lung volume, gravity, and, of course, various vasoactive mediators (61–64).

The pressure-flow relationship of a lung can be assessed by progressively increasing the pulmonary arterial driving pressure and measuring the corresponding lung blood flow (64). Figure 6.7 shows the normal pressure-flow relationships of an isolated lung at different static alveolar pressures (note that these measurements represent zone 2 conditions, i.e., $P_{pv} < P_A$). It is obvious that this relationship is nonlinear; as driving pressure increases, increases in flow become incrementally greater (64). In addition, in the absence of a vasodilating agent, the calculated pulmonary vascular resistance at higher pressures and flows will be lower. This is demonstrated graphically in Figure 6.8, which shows that isolated increases in either pulmonary arterial or venous pressure causes pulmonary vascular resistance to fall. The explanation of this phenomenon is that pulmonary arteries are more compliant than systemic vessels, and thus they are more susceptible to changes in transmural pressure. As driving pressure rises, the pulmonary arteries become more distended, thus increasing vessel caliber and contributing toward the decreased vascular resistance at higher pressures. In addition, some vascular channels remain closed at lower driving pressures, but reopen as the intravascular pressure rises. This vascular recruitment also contributes toward the decrement in vascular resistance as transmural pressure is increased.

A clinically relevant consequence of the nonlinearity of the pulmonary circulation is that calculations of pulmonary vascular resistance can vary depending on mean pul-

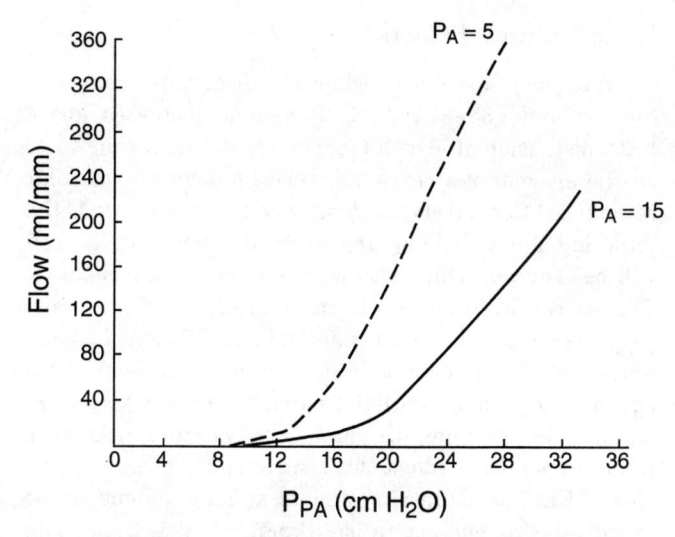

Figure 6.7. Normal pressure-flow relationships of an isolated lung at different static alveolar pressures. P_A, alveolar pressure; P_{pa}, pulmonary arterial pressures. (Adapted with permission from Graham R, Skoog C, Oppenheimer L, et al. Critical closure in the canine pulmonary vasculature. Circ Res 1982;50:566–572.)

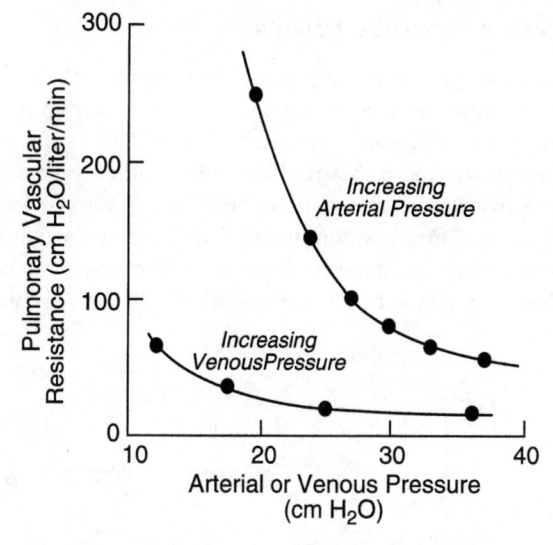

Figure 6.8. Pulmonary vascular resistance decreases in the isolated lung as arterial or venous pressure increases. (Adapted with permission from West JB. Respiratory Physiology, Baltimore: Williams & Wilkins, 1995.)

monary arterial pressure and total pulmonary blood flow. Accurate assessment of changes in pulmonary vascular resistance therefore requires determination of the pressure-flow relationship and not isolated calculations of pulmonary vascular resistance. The two exceptions to this rule that allow accurate assessment of pulmonary vascular resistance changes without complete determination of pressure-flow relationships include (a) changes in the pulmonary pressure gradient in the absence of changes in pulmonary blood flow and (b) changes in pulmonary blood flow while the pressure gradient remains constant. These are the criteria used to assess efficacy of pulmonary vasodilator trials in patients with pulmonary hypertension.

Lung Volume Effects

Pulmonary vascular resistance is affected by changes in lung volume (65–67). As lung volume increases above FRC, distension of alveoli tends to exert a distorting force on the alveolar vessels, which raises pulmonary vascular resistance. Conversely, at lung volumes below FRC, the tethering forces holding the extra-alveolar vessels open will be reduced, which also increases vascular resistance. The net result, as illustrated in Figure 6.9, is that pulmonary vascular resistance is minimal at FRC. This has significant clinical relevance for determining ventilator strategy in mechanically ventilated patients. Optimal ventilator management to minimize pulmonary vascular resistance would thus aim to adjust the positive end-expiratory pressure (PEEP) to maintain patients at lung volumes close to FRC during end-expiration. Practically it is difficult to measure FRC in intubated patients, but this is usually done empirically by adjusting the PEEP and other ventilatory parameters to prevent lung collapse while avoiding overdistension.

Alveolar Pressure Effects

Alveolar pressure is another determinant of the pulmonary pressure-flow relationship. As shown in Figure 6.7, when alveolar pressure is raised, flow will be reduced for any given driving pressure, thus indicating an increase in pulmonary vascular resistance (67). This occurs because alveolar pressure is communicated to the alveolar vessels, thus exerting a collapsing force to reduce alveolar vessel caliber. The clinical relevance of this is obvious: increases in alveolar pressure caused by PEEP or positive pressure ventilation can influence pulmonary vascular resistance.

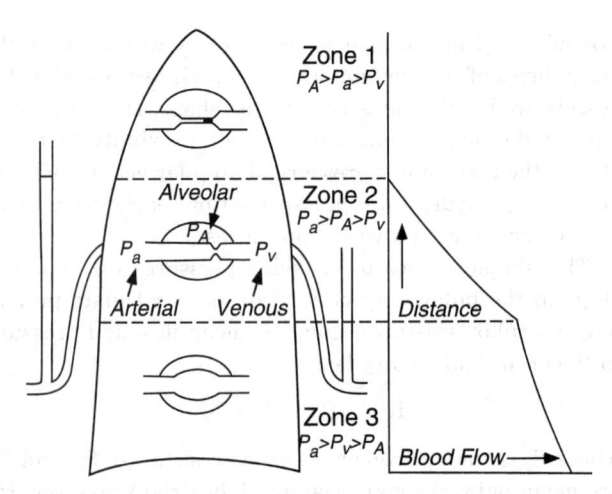

Figure 6.10. Distribution of blood flow in the upright lung showing the gravitational effects on the distribution of pulmonary blood flow. P_A, alveolar pressure; Ppa, pulmonary arterial pressure; Pp_V, pulmonary venous pressure. (Adapted with permission from West JB. Respiratory Physiology, Baltimore: Williams & Wilkins, 1995.)

Regional Pulmonary Blood Flows

As illustrated in Figure 6.10, dependent alveoli at the bottom of the lung tend to be much better perfused than nondependent alveoli (62, 67, 68). Alveolar pressure plays a role in these regional differences in pulmonary blood flow distribution because blood flow to various regions of the lung depends on interaction of three different pressures: the effective inflow and outflow pressures (P_{pa} and P_{pv}) and alveolar pressure (P_A). Intravascular pressures are routinely measured relative to the right atrium so that absolute P_{pa} and P_{pv} of each particular lung region will differ by 1 cm H_2O per centimeter vertical distance relative to the right atrium. Consequently, P_{pa} and P_{pv} will be greatest at the bottom and least at the top of the lung, while P_A remains constant throughout the lung.

Under certain circumstances, absolute pulmonary arterial pressure may be less than alveolar pressure so that alveolar vessels are completely collapsed, resulting in no regional blood flow (61, 62). This lung region, where $P_A > P_{pa} > P_{pv}$, is referred to as "zone 1" (see Fig. 6.10). Zone 1 conditions do not normally occur in healthy individuals, but they can occur if alveolar pressure is increased (during positive pressure ventilation or high-frequency oscillatory ventilation), in situations of hypovolemia, or in patients with diminished pulmonary blood flow where P_{pa} is reduced.

In regions of the lung where alveolar pressure is greater than pulmonary arterial pressure but less than pulmonary venous pressure, the effective pressure gradient for regional blood flow will be the arterial-alveolar pressure dif-

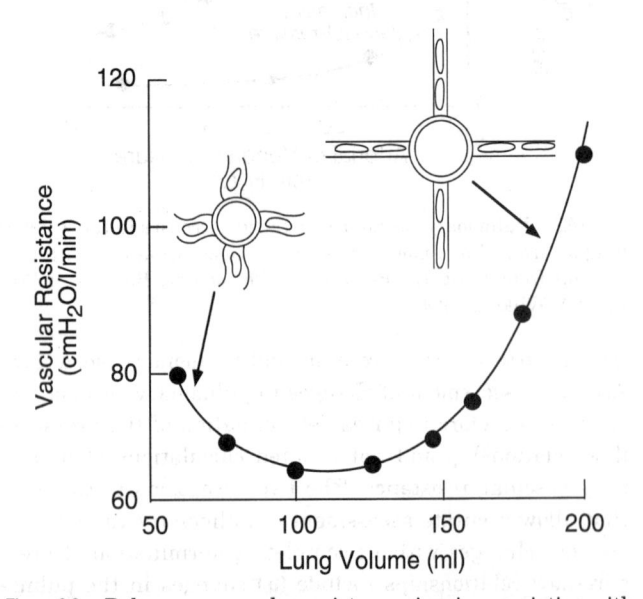

Figure 6.9. Pulmonary vascular resistance rises in association with very large or very small lung volumes. Pulmonary vascular resistance is lowest at functional residual capacity (FRC). (Adapted with permission from West JB. Respiratory Physiology, Baltimore: Williams & Wilkins, 1995.)

ference (61, 62). These conditions describe the "zone 2" region of the lung, which has been described as a vascular waterfall, because flow is not dependent on "downstream" pressure (64). Note that the absolute pressure gradient increases in the more dependent regions of zone 2, which corresponds to increased flow. Vascular distension and recruitment within zone 2 also contributes to this increase.

In the most dependent regions of the lung, both pulmonary arterial and venous pressures will be greater than alveolar pressure and the driving force for blood flow will be the arterial-venous pressure gradient. This region of the lung, which receives the greatest blood flow, is referred to as "zone 3" (61, 62). Flow also increases moving down the zone 3 region, although the pressure gradient remains constant because absolute arterial and venous pressure becomes greater so that vascular resistance is reduced by distension and recruitment (see Fig. 6.8).

When lungs become congested with fluid because of excess lung fluid flux, fluid accumulation in the interstitial spaces surrounding the extra-alveolar vessels can increase vascular resistance analogous to the way airway edema increases airway resistance. If lung fluid flux exceeds lymphatic clearance, the interstitial pressure (P_{is}) will build up and eventually exceed pulmonary venous pressure. This condition, where $P_{pa} > P_{is} > P_{pv} > P_A$, is termed "zone 4." Regional blood flow in zone 4 is reduced because of physical narrowing of the pulmonary vessels and because interstitial fluid interferes with the tethering effect, which distends the extra-alveolar vessels (69). Although zone 4 conditions do not normally occur in healthy children, they are not uncommon in patients with congenital heart disease who commonly have excess lung fluid flux (e.g., patients with increased pulmonary blood flow or increased left-atrial pressure).

Hypoxic Pulmonary Vasoconstriction and Pulmonary Vasoreactivity

A variety of physiologic stimuli and pharmocologic mediators result in pulmonary vasoreactivity (61). Important vasoactive physiologic stimuli include oxygen (vasodilation), carbon dioxide (vasoconstriction), and reduced pH (vasoconstriction). Many of these stimuli and mediators are discussed in greater detail in other chapters. Here, we discuss only the effect of hypoxia on pulmonary vascular tone, because it plays a major role in pulmonary gas exchange by contributing to the matching of ventilation to perfusion.

Hypoxia is one of the most potent pulmonary vasoactive substances (70, 71). Hypoxia results in hypoxic pulmonary vasoconstriction (HPV) even at an alveolar P_{O_2} of 80, which is only slightly less than that of normal ideal alveolar gas. As alveolar P_{O_2} falls further, the pressor response becomes dramatic. Reduced P_{O_2} in both alveolar gas and mixed venous blood contributes to hypoxic pulmonary vasoconstriction, so that a reduced mixed-venous P_{O_2} augments the usual HPV response. The mechanism for HPV is not well understood, but it is known that the site of vasoconstriction is within alveolar vessels (61, 71).

Hypoxic pulmonary vasoconstriction functions to direct blood flow away from hypoxic regions of the lung, and by doing so it therefore contributes to better gas exchange. If the entire lung becomes hypoxic, for example at high altitudes, vasoconstriction will be more generalized and lead to an overall increase in pulmonary vascular resistance (58). Intravenous vasodilators may override hypoxic pulmonary vasoconstriction and increase the intrapulmonary shunt fraction in patients with severe pulmonary parenchymal disease.

Lung Fluid Balance

To preserve efficient gas exchange, it is essential that the pulmonary airspaces be kept free of excessive fluid. Fluid flux across the pulmonary capillary bed obeys Starling's law (72, 73):

$$\text{Fluid flux} = K_{fc}[(P_c - P_{is}) - \sigma_d(\pi_c - \pi_{is})]$$

where K_{fc} is the capillary filtration coefficient, P_c and P_{is} are pulmonary capillary and pulmonary interstitial hydrostatic pressures, σ_d is the reflection coefficient, and π_c and π_{is} are pulmonary capillary and pulmonary interstitial colloid oncotic pressures. Net fluid flux reflects a balance of the forces influencing fluid filtration out of the vessels (the hydrostatic pressure gradient, $P_c - P_{is}$) and the forces promoting fluid reabsorption (the colloid-osmotic pressure gradient, which draws water back into the vascular spaces, $\pi_c - \pi_{is}$). The reflection coefficient, σ_d, is a measure of the permeability of the capillary membrane to the osmotically active proteins. A high reflection coefficient (close to 1.0) indicates a highly impermeable membrane where a protein concentration gradient will exert its maximal osmotic effect.

The small flux of fluid out of the vascular spaces initially enters the interstitial spaces surrounding the capillaries. It then travels to the peribronchial interstitial spaces that surround the bronchi and small arteries, from where it can enter the lymphatic system and be cleared back to the vascular system. When lung fluid flux exceeds the capacity for lymphatic clearance, interstitial edema fluid begins to accumulate (16, 74) (stage 1 edema formation). Interstitial fluid alone does not hinder gas exchange, but as interstitial edema further accumulates, the edema fluid will spill into the alveoli. Alveolar edema will initially fill the rims of the alveoli (stage 2), but then it will flood and collapse alveoli, resulting in gas exchange impairment (stage 3).

Pulmonary edema is normally classified as hydrostatic

or cardiogenic pulmonary edema (75) (corresponding to an elevated left-atrial pressure), and high permeability pulmonary edema (caused by increased permeability and a decreased σ_d of the pulmonary capillaries) (74). High flow pulmonary edema, which is commonly seen after pulmonary arterial balloon-dilation procedures, is probably a form of hydrostatic pulmonary edema, although the mechanism is not well understood. Recent investigations indicate that chronic elevation of left atrial pressure secondary to congestive heart failure or mitral stenosis results in vascular remodeling and thickening of the alveolar-capillary basement membrane (12). Animal studies suggest that this thickening may reduce lung liquid flux and help prevent cardiogenic edema by reducing the capillary filtration coefficient (K_{fc}) (13).

VENTILATION-PERFUSION RELATIONSHIPS

Matching of ventilation to perfusion must occur in each alveoli to ensure optimal gas exchange (54, 55). The ventilation-perfusion ratio (V_A/Q) is the ratio of alveolar ventilation to capillary blood flow for a single alveoli, group of alveoli, or entire lung (76). If the entire lung were one big ideal alveolus, the V_A/Q ratio would approximate unity, because alveolar ventilation and cardiac output are usually approximately equal. Ventilation and perfusion are not distributed homogeneously, however. Both ventilation and pulmonary blood flow increase from the top to the bottom of the lungs due to gravity effects (36, 37, 65–68), but blood flow increases more rapidly so that V_A/Q will not be homogeneous across the lung. Many other factors can lead to ventilation-perfusion inhomogeneity, such as pulmonary edema, airway plugging, or atelectasis.

Ventilation-Perfusion Inequality

Mucus plugging, regional inhomogeneity of airway resistance, pulmonary edema, or atelectasis can lead to perfusion of alveoli in a region without adequate ventilation (the extreme of this would be shunt). Conversely, regional inhomogeneity in pulmonary vascular resistance or a pulmonary emboli will lead to ventilation of regional alveoli without adequate perfusion (the extreme of this is deadspace ventilation). Blood from alveoli that are adequately perfused, but poorly ventilated ($V_A/Q < 1.0$), tends to have slightly increased P_{CO_2} but markedly reduced P_{O_2}. Blood from relatively overventilated alveoli ($V_A/Q > 1.0$) will have slightly reduced P_{CO_2} but the P_{O_2} will be normal and not increased because of the flat upper portion of the oxyhemoglobin dissociation curve. In conditions associated with ventilation-perfusion abnormalities, Pa_{CO_2} may be normal because carbon dioxide can be eliminated from the overventilated alveoli to compensate for underventilated alveoli; however, the alveolar-arterial P_{O_2} gradient can be large because of the venous admixture of desaturated blood from poorly ventilated alveoli (54). Note that hypoxic pulmonary vasoconstriction helps counteract ventilation-perfusion inequalities by reducing flow to poorly ventilated alveoli vis á vis reduced alveolar P_{O_2} levels (70, 71).

Calculation of the alveolar-arterial P_{O_2} gradient can be a useful clinical exercise to estimate the degree of ventilation-perfusion inequality (16, 54). Alveolar P_{O_2} is calculated assuming an ideal lung using the alveolar gas equation discussed previously. The alveolar-arterial P_{O_2} gradient is the difference between the calculated ideal alveolar P_{O_2} and the measured arterial P_{O_2}. Another estimate of the extent of ventilation-perfusion inhomogeneity is the shunt fraction (16, 54). This equation calculates the fraction of the cardiac output (Qs/Qt) distributed to a hypothetical region of the lung that has perfusion but no ventilation.

$$Qs/Qt = (Cc'_{O_2} - Ca_{O_2})/(Cc'_{O_2} - Cmv_{O_2})$$

Cc'_{O_2} is the calculated O_2 content of blood leaving an ideal alveolus, and Ca_{O_2} and Cmv_{O_2} are measured arterial and mixed-venous O_2 content. Cc'_{O_2} is calculated using the alveolar gas equation to calculate the P_{O_2} and O_2 content of blood from an ideal alveoli. The shunt fraction can be calculated even if the gas exchange abnormality is V_A/Q inequality and not absolute shunt because the equation takes into account the contribution of low V_A/Q regions that contribute to arterial blood desaturation. The shunt fraction so determined for a lung with V_A/Q inequality is termed the "venous admixture," to thus acknowledge that the value is a hypothetical shunt.

Mixed-Venous Oxygen Content

Blood leaving alveoli with low ventilation-perfusion ratios will have a P_{O_2} close to the value of the mixed-venous blood entering the alveoli. This blood then admixes with well-oxygenated blood coming from normally ventilated alveoli. Hence, the lower the oxygen content of the mixed venous blood, the lower will be the oxygen content of systemic arterial blood for a given amount of shunt or V_A/Q mismatch (77). Thus, in patients with arterial oxygen desaturation caused by V_A/Q inequality, interventions that increase mixed venous oxygen content (60, 77) (e.g., increased cardiac output, increased hematocrit) will improve arterial oxygen content.

Therapies Used to Improve Ventilation-Perfusion Inequality

Most of the routine respiratory interventions common to the intensive care unit are intended to counter shunt or V_A/Q mismatch. Various modes of positive pressure ventilation are available, and the intensivist seeks to choose a ventilatory mode and pattern that will improve the distribution of ventilation in lungs with altered compliance and resistance. PEEP aims to maintain lung volume near FRC and to prevent atelectasis. Pharmacologic agents are used to reduce airway resistance and improve the distribution of alveolar ventilation.

Oxygen is the most common therapy used in patients with respiratory compromise and ventilation-perfusion mismatch. Increasing the concentration of inspired oxygen helps overcome the alveolar-arterial O_2 gradient by increasing alveolar P_{O_2} in poorly ventilated alveoli. Oxygen therapy is also used routinely to determine the cause of arterial desaturation. Ventilation-perfusion inequality is improved significantly by oxygen therapy, whereas an intracardiac or intrapulmonary right-to-left shunt is not.

Congenital heart disease often leads to abnormalities of gas exchange. Patients with excessive pulmonary blood flow often have abnormally elevated alveolar-arterial O_2 gradients, which can lead to pulmonary venous desaturation (10). The increased venous admixture in these patients is caused by a low ventilation:perfusion ratio for the entire lungs, which leads to alveoli that are well perfused, but poorly ventilated. Gas exchange is further aggravated by the presence of pulmonary edema and airway obstruction, which disturbs the homogeneity of alveolar ventilation. Similarly, acute pressure overload in infants or children leads to ventilation-perfusion mismatch on the basis of pulmonary edema and airway obstruction.

Cyanotic congenital cardiac lesions associated with diminished pulmonary blood flow also result in abnormalities in pulmonary gas exchange (78). In these patients, the arterial hypoxemia leads to hyperventilation, with increases in both tidal volume and respiratory rate. The excessive ventilation results in an increase in the physiologic dead space ventilation because some areas of the lung are well ventilated but poorly perfused. This increases the work of breathing in cyanotic patients. In addition, positive pressure mechanical ventilation in these patients may further increase physiologic dead space by increasing zone 1 conditions when mean airway (alveolar) pressure increases (2).

Respiratory physiology is an essential foundation of critical care medicine, especially in the critical care of patients with cardiac disease. Respiratory abnormalities frequently reflect the type and extent of underlying heart disease. The pattern of breathing and efficiency of gas exchange are often targets of treatment in the cardiac patient that prove to be just as important as heart rate, blood pressure, and other hemodynamic variables. It is therefore essential that medical specialists caring for critically ill children with heart disease recognize the essential role of basic respiratory physiology in the cardiac intensive care unit.

REFERENCES

1. Robotham JA, Peters J, Takata M, et al. Cardiorespiratory interactions. In: Rogers MC, ed. Textbook of pediatric intensive care. Vol 1, 2nd ed. Baltimore: Williams & Wilkins, 1992: 357–382.
2. Lister G, Talner NS. Management of respiratory failure of cardiac origin. In: Gregory GA, ed. Respiratory failure in the child, New York: Churchill Livingstone, 1981:67–87.
3. Dantzker MD. The influence of cardiovascular function on gas exchange. Clin Chest Med 1983;4(2):149–159.
4. Wernovsky G, Chang AC, Wessel DL. Intensive care. In: Emmanouilides GC, Allen HD, Riemenschneider TA, et al, eds. Heart disease in infants, children, and adolescents. Vol 1, 5th ed. Baltimore: Williams & Wilkins, 1995:398–439.
5. Bancalari E, Jesse MJ, Gelband H, et al. Lung mechanics in congenital heart disease with increased and decreased pulmonary blood flow. J Pediatr 1997;90:192–195.
6. Davies CJ, Cooper SG, Fletcher ME, et al. Total respiratory compliance in infants and young children with congenital heart disease. Pediatr Pulmonol 1990;8:155–161.
7. Griffin AJ, Ferrara JD, Lax JO, et al. Pulmonary compliance. An index of cardiovascular status in infancy. Am J Dis Child 1972;123:89–95.
8. Howlett G. Lung mechanics in normal infants and infants with congenital heart disease. Arch Dis Child 1972;47: 707–715.
9. Fletcher R. Relationship between alveolar dead space and arterial oxygenation in children with congenital cardiac disease. Br J Anaesth 1989;62:168–176.
10. Lees MH, Way RC, Ross BB. Ventilation and respiratory gas transfer of infants with increased pulmonary blood flow. Pediatrics 1967;40:259–271.
11. Levin AR, Ho E, Auld PA. Alveolar-arterial oxygen gradients in infants and children with left-to-right shunts. J Pediatr 1973;83:979–987.
12. West JB, Mathieu-Costello O. Vulnerability of pulmonary capillaries in heart disease. Circulation 1995;92:622–631.
13. Townsley MI, Fu Z, Mathieu-Costello O, et al. Pulmonary microvascular permeability: responses to high vascular pressure after induction of pacing-induced heart failure in dogs. Circ Res 1995;77:317–325.
14. Barnea O, Austin EH, Richman B, et al. Balancing the circulation: theoretic optimization of pulmonary/systemic flow ratio in hypoplastic left heart syndrome. J Am Coll Cardiol 1994;24:1376–1381.
15. Weibel ER. The pathway for oxygen. Cambridge, MA: Harvard University Press, 1984.
16. Nunn JF. Nunn's applied respiratory physiology. 4th ed. Cambridge: Butterworth-Heinemann Ltd, 1993.
17. Mansell A, Bryan C, Levison H. Airway closure in children. J Appl Physiol 1972;33:711–714.
18. Burger EJ Jr, Macklem P. Airway closure: demonstration by breathing 100 percent O_2 at low lung volumes and by N_2 washout. J Appl Physiol 1968;25:139–148.
19. Scarpelli EM. Pulmonary physiology of the fetus, newborn, and child. Philadelphia: Lea & Febiger, 1975.
20. Smith CA, Nelson NM. The physiology of the newborn infant. Springfield, IL: Charles C Thomas, 1976.
21. Eigen H. Pulmonary function testing: a practical guide to its use in pediatric practice. Pediatr Rev 1986;7(8):235–245.
22. DuBois AB, Botelho SY, Bedell GN, et al. A rapid plethysmographic method for measuring thoracic gas volume: a comparison with a nitrogen washout method for measuring functional residual capacity in normal subjects. J Clin Invest 1956; 35:322–326.
23. Comroe JH. Physiology of respiration. 2nd ed. Chicago: Year Book Medical Publisher, 1975.
24. Mead J. Mechanical properties of the lungs. Physiol Rev 1961;41(2):281–330.
25. Gibson GJ, Pride NB. Lung distensibility: the static pressure-volume curve of the lungs and its use in clinical assessment. British Journal of Diseases of the Chest 1976;70:143–183.

26. Watanabe T, Trusler GA, Williams WG, et al. Phrenic nerve paralysis after pediatric cardiac surgery. Retrospective study of 125 cases. J Thorac Cardiovasc Surg 1987;94:383–388.
27. Aubier M, Trippenbach T, Roussos C. Respiratory muscle fatigue during cardiogenic shock. J Appl Physiol 1981;51(2):499–508.
28. Roussos C, Macklem PT. The respiratory muscles. N Engl J Med 1982;307:786–797.
29. Thorsteinsson A, Larsson A, Jonmarker C, et al. Pressure-volume relations of the respiratory system in healthy children. Am J Respir Crit Care Med 1994;150:421–430.
30. Notter RH, Finkelstein JN. Pulmonary surfactant: an interdisciplinary approach. J Appl Physiol 1984;57(6):1613–1624.
31. Bachofen H. Lung tissue resistance and pulmonary hysteresis, J Appl Physiol 1968;24(3):296–301.
32. Macklem PT, Murphy B. The forces applied to the lung in health and disease. Am J Med 1974;57:371–377.
33. Mead J, Takishima T, Leith D. Stress distribution in lungs: a model of pulmonary elasticity. J Appl Physiol 1970;28(5):596–608.
34. Jobe A, Ikegami M. Surfactant for the treatment of respiratory distress syndrome. Am Rev Respir Dis 1987;136:1256.
35. Lachmann B. Surfactant treatment for lung diseases other than the infant respiratory distress syndrome. In: Jobe AH, Taeusch HW, eds. Surfactant treatment of lung disease. Columbus: Ross Laboratories, 1988.
36. McGowan FX Jr, Ikegami M, del Nido PJ, et al. Cardiopulmonary bypass significantly reduces surfactant activity in children. J Thorac Cardiovasc Surg 1993;106(6):968–977.
37. Hoppin FC, Green ID, Mead J. Distribution of pleural pressure in dogs. J Appl Physiol 1969;27:863–873.
38. Milic-Emili J, Henderson JA, Dolovich MB, et al. Regional distribution of inspired gas in the lung. J Appl Physiol 1966;21:749–759.
39. Pride NB. The assessment of airflow obstruction: role of measurements of airways resistance and of tests of forced expiration. British Journal of Diseases of the Chest 1971;65:135–169.
40. DuBois A, Botelho SY, Comroe JH Jr. A new method for measuring airway resistance in man using a body plethysmograph: values in normal subjects and in patients with respiratory disease. J Clin Invest 1956;35:327–335.
41. Wood, LDH, Engel LA, Griffin P, et al. Effect of gas physical properties and flow on lower pulmonary resistance. J Appl Physiol 1976;41(2):234–244.
42. Mead J. Measurement of the inertia of the lungs at increased ambient pressure. J Appl Physiol 1956;9:208.
43. Pedley TJ. The prediction of pressure drop and variation of resistance within the human bronchial airways. Respir Physiol 1970;9:387–393.
44. Hogg JC, Williams J, Richardson JB, et al. Age as factor in the distribution of lower airway conductance and in the pathologic anatomy of obstructive lung disease. N Engl J Med 1970;282:1283–1289.
45. Hogg JC, Macklem PT, Thurlbeck WM. Site and nature of airway obstruction in chronic obstructive lung disease. N Engl J Med 1968;278(25):1355–1360.
46. Leff A. State of the art: endogenous regulation of bronchomotor tone. Am Rev Respir Dis 1988;137:1198–1216.
47. Vincent NJ, Knudson R, Leith DE, et al. Factors influencing pulmonary resistance. J Appl Physiol 1970;29(2):236–243.
48. Leff AR. Toward the formation of a modern theory of asthma. Perspect Biol Med 1990;33:292–302.
49. Pedley TJ, Drazen JM. Aerodynamic theory. In: Handbook of physiology. Section 3. Vol III. Washington, DC: American Physiology Society 1986;4:41–54, 1986.
50. Rodarte JR, Rehder K. Dynamics of respiration. In: Handbook of physiology. Section 3. Vol III. Washington, DC: American Physiology Society 1986;10:131–144.
51. Ingram RH Jr, Pedley TJ. Pressure-flow relationships in the lungs. In: Handbook of physiology. Section 3. Vol III. Washington, DC: American Physiology Society 1986;18:277–296.
52. Hyatt RE, Black LF. The flow-volume curve: a current perspective. Am Rev Respir Dis 1973;107:191–199.
53. Motoyama EK, Laks H, Oh T, et al. Deflation flow-volume curves in infants with congenital heart disease: evidence for lower airway obstruction. Circulation 1978;58(4) (Suppl 2):107–111.
54. West JB. Ventilation/blood flow and gas exchange. Oxford: Blackwell Scientific Publications, 1977.
55. Rahn H, Farhi LE. Ventilation, perfusion, and gas exchange-the V_A/Q concept. In: Fern WO, Rahn H, eds. Handbook of physiology. Vol 1. Washington, DC: American Physiology Society 1986:735–765.
56. Engel LLA, Macklem PT. Gas mixing and distribution in the lung. In: Widdicombe JG. International review of respiratory physiology. Vol II. Baltimore: University Park Press, 1977:37–82.
57. Roughton FJ. Average time spent by blood in human lung capillary and its relation to the rates of CO uptake and elimination in man. Am J Physiol 1945;143:621–626.
58. Leff AR, Schumacker PT. Respiratory physiology. Philadelphia: WB Saunders, 1993.
59. Mayer JE Jr. Initial management of the single ventricle patient. Semin Thorac Cardiovasc Surg 1994;6(1):2–7.
60. Barnea O, Austin EH, Richman B, et al. Balancing the circulation: theoretic optimization of pulmonary/systemic flow ratio in hypoplastic left heart syndrome. J Am Coll Cardiol 1994;24:1376–1381.
61. Fishman AP. Pulmonary circulation. In: Handbook of physiology. Section 3. Vol 1. Washington, DC: American Physiologic Society, 1985:3.
62. West JB, Dollery CT, Naimark A. Distribution of blood pressure in isolated lung: relation to vascular and alveolar pressures. J Appl Physiol 1964;19:713–720.
63. Graham R, Skoog C, Oppenheimer L, et al. Critical closure in the canine pulmonary vasculature. Circ Res 1982;50:566–572.
64. Hakim TS, Chang HK, Michel RP. The rectilinear presssure-flow relationship in the pulmonary vasculature: zones 2 and 3. Respir Physiol 1985;61:115–123.
65. Howell JBL, Permutt S, Proctor DF, et al. Effect of inflation of the lung on different parts of pulmonary vascular bed. J Appl Physiol 1961;16(1):71–76.
66. Permutt S, Howell JBL, Proctor DF, et al. Effect of lung inflation on static pressure-volume characteristics of pulmonary vessels. J Appl Physiol 1961;16(1):64–70.
67. Hughes JMB, Glazier JB, Maloney JE, et al. Effects of lung volume on the distribution of pulmonary blood flow in man. Resp Physiol 1968;4:58–72.
68. Anthonisen NR, Milic-Emili J. Distribution of pulmonary perfusion in erect man. J Appl Physiol 1966;21(3):760–766.
69. West JB, Dollery CT, Heard BE. Increased pulmonary vascular resistance in the dependent zone of the isolated dog lung caused by perivascular edema. Circ Res 1965;17(3):191–206.
70. Marshall C, Marshall BE. Site and sensitivity for stimulation of hypoxic pulmonary vasoconstriction. J Appl Physiol 1983;55:711–718.
71. Rock P, Patterson GA, Permutt S, et al. Nature and distribu-

tion of vascular resistance in hypoxic pig lungs. J Appl Physiol 1985;59(6):1891–1901.
72. Taylor, AE. Capillary fluid filtration: Starling forces and lymph flow. Circ Res 1981;49(3):557–575.
73. Renkin EM. Some consequences of capillary permeability to macromolecules: Starling's hypothesis reconsidered. Am J Physiol 1986;250(19):H706–H710.
74. Crandall ED, Staub NC, Goldberg HS, et al. Recent developments in pulmonary edema. Ann Int Med 1983;99(6):808–822.
75. Guyton AC, Lindsey AW. Effect of elevated left atrial pressure and decreased plasma protein concentration on the development of pulmonary edema. Circ Res 1959;7:649–657.
76. Wagner PD, Saltzman HA, West, JB. Measurement of continuous distributions of ventilation-perfusion ratios: theory. J Appl Physiol 1974;36(5):588–605.
77. Sandoval J, Long GR, Skoog C, et al. Independent influence of blood flow rate and mixed venous P_{O_2} on shunt fraction. J Appl Physiol 1983;55(4):1128–1133.
78. Lees MH, Burnell RH, Morgan CL, et al. Ventilation-perfusion relationships in children with heart disease and diminished pulmonary blood flow. Pediatrics 1968;42:778–785.

Section II:

Basic Principles in Intensive Care

Principles of Sedation and Analgesia

Peter C. Laussen, MD, and Paul R. Hickey, MD

An essential component of patient management after congenital heart surgery is the maintenance of adequate analgesia and sedation. Besides relieving pain and anxiety after surgery and during procedures, attenuating the stress response and enabling synchrony with mechanical ventilation are important considerations. In both the acute and chronic setting, the drugs chosen and how they are used have a significant impact on patient management. Frequently a combination of drugs such as opioids and benzodiazepines are used, thereby keeping total drug dose to a minimum. Side effects, toxicity, tolerance, and dependency must always be considered and treatment strategies re-evaluated.

INDICATIONS

Preoperative Management

A number of patients, particularly newborns, require resuscitation and stabilization prior to surgery. Sedation and analgesia, with or without paralysis, is often required to minimize cardiorespiratory work, to assist with coordinated mechanical ventilation, and to relieve pain during procedures, such as line placement and balloon septostomy. Drug doses should be titrated to the desired effect; however, the potential for inducing tolerance, with subsequent increased dose requirements following surgery, must be considered.

Postoperative Management

Analgesia and Anxiolysis

Recovery following cardiac surgery and duration of mechanical ventilation depend on a number of factors, including preoperative clinical condition, type and duration of surgical repair, hemodynamic stability, and complications such as postoperative bleeding and dysrhythmias.

Patients who are stable clinically and undergo an uncomplicated surgical repair (e.g., atrial septal defect [ASD] or ventricular septal defect [VSD] repair) are usually weaned and extubated in the early postoperative period. Opioids are titrated to ensure analgesia without respiratory depression, and sedation with benzodiazepines may be indicated for restless or irritable patients who may dislodge transthoracic lines and chest drains. A similar approach is applicable to patients following a modified Fontan procedure when early resumption of spontaneous ventilation and extubation is preferable because of the deleterious effects of positive pressure ventilation on preload and pulmonary blood flow.

Stress Response Attenuation

Cardiac surgery and cardiopulmonary bypass induce a significant stress response that can be attenuated by high dose opiate anesthesia, continuing into the initial postoperative period (1, 2). A study from the Children's Hospital, Boston, compared two groups of neonates who received different anesthetic and sedation regimens. One group received high dose sufentanil, which was continued into the postoperative period, and a second group was managed with morphine and halothane in the operating room and then continued with morphine and diazepam postoperatively. The group that received high dose sufentanil had a significant attenuation of their stress response, which was associated with reduced morbidity and mortality. This study demonstrated the benefit of continuing deep sedation and analgesia, with or without paralysis, for the first 12 to 24 hours following surgery in neonates with minimal cardiorespiratory reserve.

Patients benefitting from this approach include those with limited myocardial reserve, labile pulmonary hypertension, and need of complex repairs.

Limited Myocardial Reserve Although surgical repair may relieve a pre-existing volume or pressure overload, the myocardium does not recover immediately, and its function may be worse secondary to ischemia and edema associated with aortic cross clamping and cardiopulmonary bypass. Myocardial work and oxygen demand is increased by tachycardia and increased ventricular wall tension. Deep sedation and analgesia reduce endogenous catecholamine release and therefore myocardial work. Paralysis with controlled positive pressure ventilation may be necessary to manage pulmonary edema, improve gas exchange, and reduce the oxygen debt associated with an increased work of breathing.

Labile Pulmonary Hypertension Patients with labile pulmonary artery pressures (e.g., total anomalous pulmonary connection and complete atrioventricular canal defect) are susceptible to pulmonary hypertensive crises when stimulated, particularly after surgery. Pulmonary vascular resistance and pressures can increase after cardiopulmonary bypass secondary to increased lung water, atelectasis, increased circulating inflammatory mediators, complement activation, and drug infusions. This is exacerbated in the intensive care unit (ICU) during procedures such as endotracheal suction or emergence from anesthesia and paralysis. Continued sedation and analgesia may be necessary for some days until pulmonary reactivity diminishes.

Complex Repairs Following complex repairs that have required prolonged cardiopulmonary bypass and aortic cross clamp times, total body water is increased, particularly in neonates and infants. Paralysis and sedation may be required to facilitate mechanical ventilation because of lung and chest wall edema and ascites. In some patients attempted closure of the sternum can result in significant hemodynamic and respiratory compromise. Delayed sternal closure can be undertaken in the cardiac intensive care unit (CICU); however, patients will need deep levels of sedation and analgesia, and usually paralysis, until closure is achieved.

Procedures in the Cardiac Intensive Care Unit

A number of procedures can be performed in the CICU with appropriate sedation and analgesia. Besides line placement, these include thoracocentesis, percardiocentesis, cardioversion, transesophageal echocardiography, bronchoscopy, and delayed sternal closure.

Induced mild hypothermia may be necessary to treat certain dysrhythmias such as junctional ectopic tachycardia. Deep sedation and paralysis is important to limit the hemodynamic response to hypothermia.

Mechanical Ventilation

Cardiorespiratory interactions in patients with congenital heart defects and in those postsurgery are frequently complex. Depending on the mode and pattern of ventilation, synchrony between patient and ventilator is important during both controlled ventilation and weaning. Sedation is often necessary to facilitate this and reduce both myocardial and respiratory work.

A small group of patients may require prolonged ventilation for residual hemodynamic or respiratory problems. Examples include persistent cardiac failure, recurrent pleural effusions, sepsis, phrenic nerve palsy with diaphragm paresis, and muscle weakness from inadequate nutrition and prolonged paralysis. Slow weaning from mechanical ventilation is necessary and a suitable analgesia and sedation management plan is essential. Commonly, a combination of a benzodiazepine and opiate is used; however, it is essential this be re-evaluated to avoid complications of drug toxicity, tolerance, and dependence.

ASSESSMENT

Analgesia requirements for young children can be difficult to assess, particularly when they are paralyzed and on a ventilator. Primarily, autonomic signs such as hypertension, tachycardia, pupillary size, diaphoresis, and tearing are used. Children not paralyzed will grimace and withdraw from a painful stimulus. If breathing spontaneously, changes in respiratory patterns such as tachypnea, grunting, and splinting of the chest wall may be evident. Guidelines for the sedation of pediatric patients have been published by the American Academy of Pediatrics (3, 4). Table 7.1 lists dosages for some of the drugs commonly used in pediatric cardiac intensive care.

However, changes in autonomic signs do not only reflect pain. Other causes include awareness as the patient emerges from anesthesia and sedation, seizures, fever, hypoxemia, hypercapnia, and changes in vasoactive drug infusions. Despite this, some patients may receive additional opioid or benzodiazepine doses when hypertensive and tachycardic, which will only contribute to early tolerance to these drugs and possible withdrawal symptoms.

Level of sedation produced by a drug is dependent on stimulus intensity. It is common for patients to receive additional sedation during a procedure (e.g., endotracheal tube suction or withdrawal of catheters); however, on completion of the stimulus, patients can remain deeply sedated. Titrating doses of drugs such as fentanyl and midazolam to a specific blood concentration and sedation level is impractical because of significant interpatient variability in drug metabolism and clearance.

SEDATIVES

Chloral Hydrate

Chloral hydrate is commonly used to sedate children prior to medical procedures and imaging studies. It can be administered orally or rectally in a dose ranging from 50 to 100 mg/kg (maximal dose 1 g). Onset of action is within 15 to 30 minutes with a duration of action between 2 to 4 hours. Onset and level of sedation are improved if the drug is administered near the normal nap time for a child and if the child has been fasting. Between 10 to 20% of children will have a dysphoric reaction to chloral hydrate, frequently being excitable and uncooperative. On the other hand, some children become excessively sedated with respiratory depression and potential inability to protect their airway. This is particularly the case when chloral hydrate is combined with other sedatives or opioids, or if a second dose has been administered because of inadequate sedation following the initial dose.

Regular administration of chloral hydrate to provide sedation for intensive care patients is controversial. Admin-

Table 7.1. Dosages of Drugs Commonly Used in Pediatric Cardiac Intensive Care

Drug	Dose
Sedatives	
Chloral hydrate	PO/PR 50–100 mg/kg
Diazepam	IV bolus 0.05–0.1 mg/kg
	PO 0.1–0.2 mg/kg
Midazolam	PO 0.5–0.75 mg/kg
	IV bolus 0.05–0.1 mg/kg
	IV infusion 0.05–0.2 mg/kg/h
Lorazepam	PO and IV bolus 0.05–0.1 mg/kg (maximal 2 mg)
	IV infusion 0.025–0.05 mg/kg/h (maximal 2 mg/kg)
Analgesics	
Morphine	IV bolus 0.1–0.2 mg/kg
	IV infusion 25–50 µg/kg/h
	Epidural bolus 50–75 µg/kg
Fentanyl	IV bolus for analgesia 0.5–1 µg/kg (max 4–5 µg/kg)
	IV bolus for intubation 10–15 µg/kg
	IV infusion 2–5 µg/kg/h
Sufentanil	IV bolus 0.1–0.2 µg/kg
	IV infusion 0.5–2 µg/kg/h
Methadone	IV or PO bolus 0.1–0.2 mg/kg
Ketamine	IV bolus 1–2 mg/kg
	IM bolus 5–10 mg/kg
	IV infusion 2 mg/kg/h
Anesthetic Agents	
Thiopental	IV bolus 3–5 mg/kg
Methohexital	IV bolus 1–2 mg/kg
Pentobarbital	IV bolus 1–2 mg/kg
Propofol	IV bolus 1.5–3 mg/kg
	IV infusion 100–150 µg/kg/min
Etomidate	IV bolus 0.3 mg/kg
Muscle Relaxants	
Succinylcholine	IV bolus (neonates and infants) 2 mg/kg. Combine with atropine 20 µg/kg or glycopyrolate 10 µg/kg.
	IV bolus (children to adults) 1 mg/kg
	IM bolus 3–4 mg/kg
Rocuronium	IV bolus 0.6–1.2 mg/kg
Mivacurium	IV bolus 0.2 mg/kg
Metocurine	IV bolus 0.3 mg/kg
Vecuronium	IV bolus 0.1 mg/kg
	IV infusion 0.05–0.2 mg/kg/h
Atracurium	IV bolus 0.5 mg/kg
Cisatracurium	IV bolus 0.2 mg/kg
	IV infusion 0.2 mg/kg/h
Pancuronium	IV bolus (intubating dose) 0.2 mg/kg
	IV bolus (maintenance dose) 0.1 mg/kg
Neostigmine	Reversal: IV bolus 0.05 mg/kg. Atropine 0.025 mg/kg or Glycopyrolate 0.02 mg/kg must be given concurrently.

IM, intramuscular; IV, intravenous; PO, orally; PR, per rectum.

istered intermittently, it can be used to supplement benzodiazepines and opioids, to assist during drug withdrawal, and it is useful as a nocturnal hypnotic when trying to establish normal sleep patterns.

The American Academy of Pediatrics has published guidelines for the use of chloral hydrate (5). Although the Academy noted chloral hydrate is often administered in repetitive doses to maintain prolonged sedation in infants and children, significant concerns were raised about this practice. Chloral hydrate is metabolized to trichloroethanol and trichloroacetic acid, both of which are pharmacologically active and can contribute to acute toxicity (6). These metabolites have long half-lives of over 24 hours, which leads to accumulation during repetitive dosing. Evidence indicates that chloral hydrate or its metabolites can increase the risk of both direct and indirect hyperbilirubinemia in newborns. Trichloroacetic acid is highly protein bound and could compete with bilirubin for albumin binding sites. High doses can also contribute to metabolic acidosis. Central nervous system depression can occur with chronic exposure to chloral hydrate, and it is worsened when combined with benzodiazepines or barbiturates. Physical dependence and tolerance have also been observed after chronic ingestion, as have withdrawal symptoms.

Benzodiazepines

Benzodiazepines are commonly used sedatives in the ICU, and they have anxiolytic, anticonvulsant, hypnotic, and amnestic properties. When given in appropriate doses, they provide excellent conscious sedation; however, they can cause dose-dependent respiratory depression, and their use may result in significant hypotension in patients with limited hemodynamic reserve. A significant problem with chronic administration in the ICU is the development of tolerance and withdrawal symptoms.

Diazepam

Diazepam is a long-acting benzodiazepine with a half-life of 24 hours. The major route of administration is oral, but it can also be given rectally. It is poorly absorbed after an intramuscular injection and causes significant pain when administered intravenously. Prolonged sedation can result from repeated administration because of its long half-life and active metabolites. Diazepam is metabolized primarily by the liver, and it should be used with caution in patients with liver dysfunction.

Midazolam

Midazolam is a short-acting, water-soluble benzodiazepine that can be administered intravenously, intramuscularly, orally, and rectally. It is a commonly prescribed premedicant prior to anesthesia and an effective sedative for procedures in the ICU (7). As a continuous infusion, midazolam is a useful drug for children following congenital heart surgery. However, if the cardiac output and splanchnic perfusion is diminished, hepatic metabolism of midazolam will be reduced and drug accumulation is likely.

The oral or rectal dose is 0.5 to 0.7 mg/kg, the increased dose necessary because of poor bioavailability from high first pass metabolism in the liver. Onset time is between 15 and 30 minutes with a duration of action of 2 to 4 hours. This route is commonly used for anesthesia premedication, mixing the intravenous form with a flavored syrup to mask the bitter taste.

Tachyphylaxis can occur within days of commencing a continuous midazolam infusion. Withdrawal symptoms of restlessness, agitation, and visual hallucinations can occur following prolonged administration, and they can be managed either by gradual reduction in infusion rate or regular administration of a longer acting benzodiazepine such as lorazepam. Following abrupt discontinuation of midazolam and fentanyl reversible encephalopathy characterized by movement disorders, dystonic posturing, and poor social interaction has been reported (15). Resolution generally occurs within 2 to 4 weeks without permanent sequela.

Lorazepam

Lorazepam has a long duration of action of between 4 and 8 hours, with an elimination half-life of approximately 18 hours. It is suitable for oral, intravenous, or intramuscular administration. It is metabolized in the liver via glucuronyl transferase rather than the P450 system, and it has no active metabolites. As with other benzodiazepines, tolerance and withdrawal symptoms can occur. Prescribed on a regular basis, lorazepam is useful for longer term sedation, as a supplement to an existing sedation regimen, and during opioid and midazolam infusion withdrawal.

ANALGESICS

Opioid Analgesics

Opioid analgesics are the mainstay of pain management in the CICU, and in high doses they can be used to provide anesthesia. They also provide sedation for patients while mechanically ventilated, and they blunt hemodynamic response to procedures such as endotracheal tube suction. Hypercyanotic episodes associated with tetralogy of Fallot and air hunger associated with congestive heart failure are also effectively treated with opioids.

Respiratory depression from opioids is dose related, and it varies with age, clinical condition, disease state, and pain severity. Opioids all cause a decrease in minute ventilation, with diminished responses to both hypoxemia and hypercapnia. They must be administered with caution in neonates and in infants aged younger than 3 months because of their heightened susceptibility to respiratory depression, and in patients with limited respiratory reserve, neurologic disorders, or airway compromise.

The most commonly used opioids in the CICU are morphine, fentanyl, sufentanil, and methadone, which are all pure agonists. Tolerance development is dose and time related, and it is a particular problem in postoperative cardiac patients who often receive large doses of opioids as part of their cardiac anesthetic technique.

Physical dependence is common and continued administration of opioids is frequently necessary to prevent withdrawal symptoms such as dysphoria, agitation, piloerection, tachypnea, tachycardia, and diaphoresis. Physical dependence can develop quickly following regular opioid use for as little as 2 weeks. It can be managed by gradually tapering the opioid dose as the patient's pain subsides, or administrating a longer acting opioid such as methadone.

Frequently opioids are administered as an intravenous or intramuscular bolus, which results in peaks and troughs in drug levels. Periods of oversedation and undermedication can occur, establishing an unacceptable pain cycle. It is more appropriate to use a continuous infusion so that a constant blood and analgesic level is maintained.

Alternative methods of opioid administration include patient-controlled analgesia (PCA) and epidural infusions. PCA is suitable in older patients, allowing them to administer a predetermined bolus of opioid according to their analgesic requirements. A continuous background infusion of opioid is sometimes used in conjunction with PCA and a "shut-off" period is set on the PCA device to limit overdosing.

Epidural opioid administration, either as a bolus or continuous infusion, binds to opioid receptors in the dorsal horn of the spinal cord, producing analgesia without motor nerve or sympathetic blockade. Rostral spread of morphine allows lumbar or even caudal administration of morphine to be effective for pain arising in thoracic dermatomes. However, rostral spread in the cerebrospinal fluid to the brain and brainstem can result in delayed respiratory depression, particularly if systemic opioids are also administered. Patients receiving epidural opioids need to be closely monitored for respiratory depression with pulse oximetry and respiratory monitoring. Side effects from epidural opioid administration include pruritus, nausea and vomiting, and urinary retention. These may be relieved with naloxone.

Morphine

Morphine is the *gold standard* against which other opioids are compared. It has a dose-dependent analgesic effect and better sedative properties than synthetic opioids such as fentanyl and sufentanil. Marked individual variation in dose requirements is found, and frequent reassessment of analgesic level is necessary. Intravenous morphine is best administered as a continuous infusion, resulting in a more constant analgesic level. Intermittent or continuous epidural morphine also provides effective pain relief after congenital heart surgery, with lower total opioid requirements and decreased nursing time; however, the incidence of postoperative vomiting can be increased. Care must be taken administering systemic opioids to patients who have received epidural morphine because of the risk of delayed respiratory depression. Continuous respiratory monitoring is essential.

Hydromorphine is five to seven times more potent than morphine, and it should be considered when adverse effects related to histamine release (e.g., pruritis) occur with morphine administration.

Morphine can cause hypotension in patients with limited hemodynamic reserve who are reliant on high endogenous catecholamine levels. It also causes histamine release, which will potentially increase pulmonary vascular resistance and pulmonary artery pressures, and decrease systemic vascular resistance. However, for most postoperative patients, morphine provides ideal analgesia and sedation.

Fentanyl

Fentanyl and its analogs, sufentanil and alfentanil, have a shorter duration of action than morphine, and they generate less histamine release, therefore causing less vasodilation and hypotension. It is approximately 100 times more potent than morphine, with a high degree of lipid solubility, allowing rapid penetration of the blood brain barrier. It therefore has a rapid onset and its termination of action is primarily determined by redistribution rather than by metabolism. Its opioid effects last for 30 to 45 minutes, although respiratory depression can last considerably longer.

Fentanyl blocks the stress response in a dose-related fashion, while maintaining both systemic and pulmonary hemodynamic stability (8). It is commonly used in the CICU during intubation with a bolus dose of 10 to 15 μg/kg effectively obtunding hemodynamic response to intubation (9). Endotracheal suction can cause intense pulmonary vasoconstriction and circulatory collapse in susceptible patients with a labile pulmonary vascular resistance. Fentanyl at a dose of 25 μg/kg in conjunction with a small dose of pancuronium 0.015 mg/kg has been demonstrated to suppress this response (10). However, patients with high circulating catecholamine levels (e.g. severe cardiac failure or critical aortic stenosis) can become hypotensive after a bolus induction dose, and fentanyl must be used with caution in these patients. Fentanyl is more appropriate in patients at risk for pulmonary hypertension because of lack of histamine release and beneficial effects on pulmonary vascular resistance.

Chest wall rigidity is an idiosyncratic and dose-related reaction that can occur with a rapid bolus, and it requires treatment with naloxone or paralysis. For this reason, it is preferable to confine the use of large fentanyl boluses and infusions to paralyzed or heavily sedated patients.

Synthetic opioids are potent analgesics, but they have limited sedative action. Combining them with a benzodiazepine is effective and will reduce the total opioid dose required. However, great interpatient variability in fentanyl clearance exists in children, making titration of an infusion difficult. Experience with extracorporeal membrane oxygenation (ECMO) patients indicates that tolerance and dependence to a fentanyl infusion develops rapidly and significant increases in infusion rates may be necessary (11, 12). Infants on ECMO who received fentanyl for more than 5 days or a total dose greater than 1.6 mg/kg were particularly at risk for developing neonatal opioid abstinence syndrome (13). Opioid withdrawal was also observed in a prospective study in critically ill children receiving fentanyl by continuous infusion after a total dose of 2.5 mg/kg or 9 days of continuous infusion (14). Following cardiac surgery using large doses of fentanyl, acute tolerance can rapidly occur, necessitating an increased initial infusion rate. Further, tolerance onset can be quicker when an infusion is used rather than intermittent boluses, possibly because of the increased duration of receptor occupancy.

Gastrointestinal and neurologic symptoms can be associated with fentanyl withdrawal, including poor feeding, vomiting, loose stools, tremor, and irritability. Overt withdrawal syndromes have been described in case reports of patients receiving prolonged infusions of fentanyl, either alone or in combination with midazolam. A movement disorder characterized by extreme irritability, myoclonus, ataxia, dystonic posturing, choreoathetosis, poor social interaction, and insomnia has been described in case reports; however, it is unclear whether this encephalopathy represents benzodiazepine or opioid withdrawal (15, 16).

Sufentanil

Sufentanil is a synthetic opioid that is 12 to 15 times more potent than fentanyl, although its effects are similar and it offers no specific advantage. If large doses of fentanyl are required because tolerance has developed, sufentanil should be considered as a reduced infusion volume can be used. One possible advantage of using a potent opioid such as sufentanil relates to tolerance development. More potent opioids occupy a smaller fraction of the total number of available receptors compared with less potent agents such as morphine. Therefore, the receptor reserve is greater for sufentanil and tolerance can develop later.

Methadone

Methadone is a synthetic opioid with a potency similar to morphine; however, it has a prolonged elimination half-life of between 18 to 24 hours. It can be given intravenously and is well absorbed orally. It is therefore particularly useful to treat patients with opioid withdrawal (17). Various withdrawal regimens can be used depending on the prior opioid dose and duration of treatment. A relatively quick withdrawal plan commences with 0.2 mg/kg methadone every 8 hours, tapering over 7 to 10 days. Larger methadone doses may be required for patients who have developed significant opioid tolerance. If morphine had been used, the previous total morphine requirement per day can be calculated and methadone prescribed on a milligram-for-milligram basis, administered in two or three divided doses per day. Similarly, following prolonged fentanyl administration, the appropriate daily dose of methadone would be equivalent to the total fentanyl dose per day. Once stable, the dose can then be slowly tapered and continued orally.

Ketamine

Ketamine is a phencyclidine derivative, classified as a "dissociative" anesthetic agent. It effectively dissociates the thalamic and limbic systems and provides intense analgesia. It has a rapid onset, short duration of action of between 10 and 15 minutes, and an elimination half-life of between 2 and 3 hours. Ketamine is effectively administered intravenously or intramuscularly. Bioavailability is poor when taken orally because of rapid hepatic clearance, and it is rarely administered this way. Ketamine provides adequate anesthesia for most ICU procedures including intubation, drainage of pleuropericardial effusions, and sternal wound exploration and closure. It can also be given by continuous intravenous infusion for analgesia and sedation (18).

Ketamine produces a type of catalepsy whereby the eyes remain open, usually with nystagmus and intact corneal reflexes. Occasionally nonpurposeful myoclonic movements can occur. It will dilate cerebral blood vessels and should be avoided in patients with intracranial hypertension.

Ketamine is a useful agent in the cardiac ICU. Heart rate and blood pressure usually increase through sympathomimetic actions resulting from central stimulation and diminished postganglionic catecholamine uptake. However, it does have direct myocardial depressant effects, and it should be used with caution in patients with limited myocardial reserve in whom the sympathomimetic effects may be inadequate to offset myocardial depression.

Conflicting reports have been made about the effect of ketamine on pulmonary vascular resistance. One study on a small number of children during cardiac catheterization, concluded that ketamine caused a significant increase in pulmonary vascular resistance in patients predisposed to pulmonary hypertension (19). However, earlier studies demonstrated minimal effects of ketamine on pulmonary artery pressure or vascular resistance in young children, either breathing spontaneously or during controlled ventilation (20, 21). On balance, ketamine alone has minimal effects on pulmonary vascular resistance, and it is safe to use in patients with pulmonary hypertension, provided secondary events such as hypoventilation and airway obstruction are avoided.

Dose-related respiratory depression can occur; however, after a 2 mg/kg bolus patients continue to breath spontaneously. Airway secretions are increased and, although airway reflexes seem intact, aspiration can occur. It is essential that patients fast prior to administration of ketamine and that complete airway management equipment is available. Increase in airway secretions can lead to laryngospasm during airway manipulation and antisialogogues such as atropine or glycopyrolate should be administered concurrently. It is also a bronchodilator and useful in patients with reactive airways.

Major side effects include emergence delirium, hallucinations, and nightmares. These can be ameliorated with concurrent use of benzodiazepines.

ANESTHETIC AGENTS

Barbiturates

Short-acting barbiturates, thiopental and methohexital, are rarely used in the CICU, and they should be administered only by those trained in anesthesia. They are primarily used as induction agents for anesthesia and may have significant side effects. Both agents are direct myocardial depressants and venodilators, causing severe hypotension in patients with limited cardiac reserve. They have a rapid onset with a short duration of action, due mainly to redistribution. High lipid solubility allows rapid brain penetration with loss of consciousness and apnea. However, little indication is seen for continuous infusions of barbiturates to provide sedation in the CICU. Drug accumulation occurs because of high lipid solubility, along with tolerance, dependency, and withdrawal symptoms.

The longer acting barbiturate, pentobarbital, has been used to sedate children for radiologic investigations, as well as in the ICU setting. Commonly it is used in patients who have become tolerant to benzodiazepine and opiate regimens, although its use in the CICU is limited because of potential cardiovascular side effects.

Propofol

Propofol is a phenol derivative, supplied in a soy emulsion and egg phospholipid to make an injectable emulsion. It is used primarily as an anesthetic agent either for induction or as part of a total intravenous anesthetic technique. A major disadvantage is pain on injection, although this can be overcome by the addition of lidocaine. Because propofol has a short duration of action and rapid clearance, it has been used by infusion or repeat bolus doses, with patients waking rapidly when it is discontinued (22).

Hypotension secondary to a decrease in systemic vascular resistance and direct myocardial depression limits propofol use in the CICU as an induction agent. Propofol has been used in adult ICUs for continuous sedation, although the infusions are costly. Currently propofol is not approved for longer term infusion in pediatric patients because of isolated case reports of metabolic acidosis and neurologic side effects (23). In the CICU, propofol is currently used for short procedures such as cardioversion and transesophageal echocardiography.

Etomidate

Etomidate is an anesthetic induction agent with the advantage of minimal cardiovascular and respiratory depression and rapid recovery. An intravenous dose of 0.3 mg/kg induces a rapid loss of consciousness with a duration of 3 to 5 minutes. It has a high volume of distribution and rapid clearance with an elimination half-life of between 1 and 5 hours. It causes pain on injection and may be associated with spontaneous movements, hiccoughing, and myoclonus. Upper airway reflexes are increased with potential laryngospasm.

Etomidate is commonly combined with opioids such as fentanyl, and it is a useful induction agent in patients with limited hemodynamic reserve. It is not approved for continuous infusion in the ICU setting because it depresses adrenal steroidogenesis (24).

MUSCLE RELAXANTS

Muscle relaxants are more commonly used in pediatric intensive care units compared with adult units. Besides being used to facilitate intubation and controlled mechanical ventilation, patients with limited cardiorespiratory reserve also benefit from paralysis by a reduction in myocardial work and oxygen demand. Paralysis and deep sedation are particularly important for patients with labile pulmonary hypertension. However, prolonged paralysis carries the concomitant risks of prolonged ventilatory support, delays establishment of enteral nutrition, may result in tolerance and prolonged muscle weakness after discontinuing the muscle relaxant, and increases total hospital stay and costs.

Depolarizing Muscle Relaxants

Depolarizing agents are noncompetitive antagonists acting at the motor end plate, initiating depolarization of the membrane and then blocking further transmission of impulses. They have a rapid onset, short duration of action, and are not reversible.

Succinylcholine is the only depolarizing agent in clinical use. It is structurally similar to two acetylcholine molecules and therefore has an effect on the sinoatrial node, causing bradycardia. This response is exaggerated in children, especially after multiple doses, and atropine (20 μg/kg) or glycopyrrolate (10 μg/kg) should be given at the same time. Succinylcholine has rapid onset within 60 seconds and duration of action of between 5 and 10 minutes. It is rapidly metabolized by the enzyme plasma cholinesterase, which is produced in the liver.

Because of its rapid onset and short duration, succinylcholine is primarily used to facilitate intubation, particularly during a rapid sequence induction in patients with a full stomach or those at risk of potential aspiration. Usual intravenous dose in older patients is 1 mg/kg; however, in children aged less than 1 year, a larger dose of 2 mg/kg is required, mainly because of the greater surface area:weight ratio in these patients. Succinylcholine can also be administered intramuscularly in urgent situations when no intravenous access is available, at a dose usually double the intravenous dose (i.e., 3 to 4 mg/kg).

Succinylcholine is not a benign drug, however, and it may be unnecessary for routine intubations in uncomplicated patients. Side effects include bradycardia, increased intraocular pressure, increased intracranial pressure, increased intragastric pressure, and muscle pains (particularly in older patients); it is also a trigger agent for malignant hyperpyrexia. Severe hyperkalemia can result following succinylcholine administration in patients recovering from major trauma, severe burns, spinal cord injuries, cerebral vascular accidents, and muscular dystrophy. Duration of action is also prolonged in patients with abnormal plasma cholinesterase.

Nondepolarizing Muscle Relaxants

Nondepolarizing drugs are competitive antagonists, competing with acetylcholine for binding at receptors on the motor end plate. This receptor has two alpha subunits, and an acetylcholine molecule must bind to each subunit to effect depolarization. Nondepolarizing agents block conduction by either binding to one or both of the alpha subunits.

A number of nondepolarizing muscle relaxants are available, classified according to duration of action. Long-acting muscle relaxants and paralysis are useful in patients with severe cardiorespiratory compromise, including severe cardiac failure requiring significant inotrope support, and in patients with reactive pulmonary hypertension; and to facilitate mechanical ventilation when tight control of gas exchange is necessary. For most patients, however, long-acting muscle relaxants are not necessary provided sedation is adequate and appropriate. These drugs have no analgesic or sedative properties and should never be administered alone to patients.

Duration of action of nondepolarizing relaxants is increased by acidosis, hypercapnia, hypothermia, and following certain drug interactions, particularly with aminoglycoside antibiotics.

Tachyphylaxis can also develop with chronic administration of nondepolarizing muscle relaxants. Cause for this is uncertain, but it may be related to the development of additional acetylcholine receptors along the muscle fibers separate to the motor end plate (25).

Prolonged weakness following long-term nondepolarizing administration can occur, lasting days to weeks, although the cause is unclear. One factor may be prolonged drug effect secondary to reduced clearance, active metabolites, or relative overdose, particularly in patients with renal disease and in those receiving steroids (26). Another cause may relate to a poorly characterized myopathy that has also been described after prolonged use of muscle relaxants. Coincident findings include elevated serum creatine kinase, myoglobinuria, and diminished evoked and compound action potentials. Nerve conduction studies have been reported as normal, although atrophy and muscle necrosis have been noted histologically. Slow, complete recovery occurs. It can be more common when steriod-based relaxants, such as pancuronium and vecuronium, are used for prolonged relaxation (27, 28).

Competitive block of nondepolarizing agents can be antagonized by antiacetylcholinesterase drugs such as neostigmine, edrophonium, and pyridostigmine. These drugs block the acetylcholinesterase enzyme at the motor end plate that is responsible for normal acetylcholine breakdown. Therefore, acetylcholine concentration at the motor end plate is increased and available to compete with residual neuromuscular blocking agents. It is essential to remember that this effect is not specific to the motor end plate and, in particular, it also increases acetylcholine levels at muscurinic sites such as the sinoatrial node, thereby resulting in bradycardia or even asystole. Atropine or glycopyrolate must always be administered concurrently.

Fast Onset, Intermediate Duration of Action

Rocuronium Rocuronium is an aminosteroid with the fastest onset time for all currently available nondepolarizing neuromuscular blocking agents. Time to complete neuromuscular blockade for an intubating dose of 0.6 mg/kg ranges from 30 to 180 seconds; however, adequate intubating conditions are usually achieved within 60 seconds (29). It may therefore be an alternative for succinylcholine if it is contraindicated during an emergent rapid sequence induction. Duration of action averages 25 minutes, although recovery is slower in infants. Rocuronium is a safe drug to administer to patients with limited hemodynamic reserve and it does not release histamine. Although heart rate can increase slightly from vagolytic effects, it is less than that with pancuronium use.

Intermediate Onset, Short Duration of Action

Mivacurium Mivacurium is a benzylisoquinolinium derivative metabolized by plasma cholinesterase. Its onset of action is slower than for succinylcholine and rocuronium and satisfactory intubating conditions can be achieved within 2 to 3 minutes after a dose of 0.2 to 0.3 mg/kg. Onset time may be shorter in neonates and infants, but further pharmacodynamic and pharmacokinetic studies are necessary.

Mivacurium has a short duration of action of 6 to 10 minutes, and it is useful for only short surgical procedures. A continuous infusion of 6 to 7 μg/kg/min in adults and 14 μg/kg/min in children is recommended for maintenance of muscle relaxation, with the only advantage being rapid spontaneous recovery of neuromuscular function once the infusion is discontinued (30). Little indication is seen for its use in the critical care setting. Prolonged neuromuscular blockade occurs in patients with atypical plasma cholinesterase.

Intermediate Onset, Intermediate Duration of Action

Metocurine Metocurine is an analog of d-tubocurine and at a dose of 0.3 mg/kg provides paralysis for 45 to 60 minutes. It also has minimal hemodynamic side effects; it causes less tachycardia than pancuronium, which is its major advantage.

Vecuronium Vecuronium (0.1 mg/kg) has an intermediate duration of action of approximately 30 minutes. In infants, however, vecuronium behaves as a longer acting agent. It is also a safe drug to administer to patients with limited hemodynamic reserve, resulting in minimal change in blood pressure or heart rate. However, when combined with fentanyl, significant bradycardia can occur, and atropine is often necessary. It is rarely indicated in the CICU because of its shorter duration of action and cost, although it is suitable as a continuous intravenous infusion.

Atracurium Atracurium (0.5 mg/kg) also has an intermediate duration of action of around 30 minutes. It has a unique metabolism, undergoing spontaneous pH-dependent hydrolysis without requiring hepatic metabolism. Its effects on the cardiovascular system are also relatively benign with minimal change in blood pressure and heart rate. However, histamine release can occur, with associated tachycardia and a small reduction in blood pressure. As with vecuronium, little indication is seen for atracurium in the ICU setting other than as a continuous intravenous infusion.

Cisatracurium Cisatracurium is a stereoisomer of atracurium. Its main advantage is lack of histamine release and, therefore, hemodynamic stability. Although more potent, it has a similar onset time and duration of action as atracurium (31).

Long Onset, Long Duration of Action

Pancuronium At a dose of 0.1 mg/kg, pancuronium has an onset of action between 2 to 3 minutes and a duration of action of approximately 1 hour. Pancuronium is safe to administer in patients with limited hemodynamic reserve as it causes a mild tachycardia and increase in blood pressure, which is caused by delayed re-uptake of norepinephrine at receptor sites, and pancuronium does not release histamine nor cause ganglionic blockade.

Pancuronium can also be used to facilitate intubation at a dose of 0.2 mg/kg; however, an airway needs to be maintained with bag and mask ventilation for 1 to 2 minutes before adequate intubating conditions are achieved.

REFERENCES

1. Annand KJS, Hansen DD, Hickey PR. Hormonal-metabolic stress responses in neonates undergoing cardiac surgery. Anesthesiology 1990;73:661–670.
2. Anand KJS, Hickey PR. Halothane-morphine compared with high dose sufentanil for anesthesia and post-operative analgesia in neonatal cardiac surgery. N Engl J Med 1992;326:1–9.
3. American Academy of Pediatrics, Committee on Drugs. Guidelines for monitoring and management of pediatric patients during and after sedation for diagnostic and therapeutic procedures. Pediatrics 1992;89:1110–1115.
4. Coté CJ. Sedation for the pediatric patient. Pediatr Clin North Am 1994;41(1):31–58.
5. American Academy of Pediatrics, Committee on Drugs and Committee on Environmental Health. Use of chloral hydrate for sedation in children. Pediatrics 1993;92:471–473.
6. Steinberg AD. Should chloral hydrate be banned? Pediatrics 1993;92:442–446.
7. Lloyd-Thomas AR, Booker PD. Infusion of midazolam in pediatric patients after cardiac surgery. Br J Anaesth 1986;58:1109–1115.
8. Hickey PR, Hansen DD, Wessel DL. Pulmonary and systemic hemodynamic responses to fentanyl in infants. Anesth Analg 1985;64:483–486.
9. Yaster M. The dose response of fentanyl in neonatal anesthesia. Anesthesiology 1987;66:433–435.
10. Hickey PR, Hansen DD, Wessel DL, et al. Blunting of stress responses in the pulmonary circulation of infants by fentanyl. Anesth Analg 1985;64:1137–1142.
11. Arnold JH, Truog RD, Scovone JM, Fenton T. Changes in the pharmacodynamic response to fentanyl in neonates during continuous infusion. J Pediatr 1991;119:639–643.
12. Katz R, Kelly HW. Pharmacokinetics of continuous infusions of fentanyl in critically ill children. Crit Care Med 1993;21:995–1000.
13. Arnold JH, Truog RD, Orav EJ, et al. Tolerance and dependence in neonates sedated with fentanyl during extracorporeal membrane oxygenation. Anesthesiology 1990;73:1136–1140.
14. Katz R, Kelly HW, Hsi A. A prospective study on the occurrence of withdrawal in critically ill children who receive fentanyl by continuous infusion. Crit Care Med 1994;22:763–767.
15. Bergman I, Steeves M, Burckart G, et al. Reversible neurologic abnormalities associated with prolonged intravenous midazolam and fentanyl administration. J Pediatr 1991;119:644–649.
16. Lane JC, Tennison MB, Lawless ST, et al. Movement disorder after withdrawal of fentanyl infusion. J Pediatr 1991;119:649–651.
17. Tobias JD, Schleien CS, Haun SE. Methadone as treatment for iatrogenic narcotic dependency in pediatric intensive care patients. Crit Care Med 1991;18:1292–1293.
18. Tobias JD, Martin LD, Wetzel RC. Ketamine by continuous infusion for sedation in the pediatric intensive care unit. Crit Care Med 1990;18:819–821.
19. Wolfe RR, Loehr JP, Schaffer MS, et al. Hemodynamic effects of ketamine, hypoxia and hyperoxia in children with surgically treated congenital heart disease residing 1200 meters above sea level. Am J Cardiol 1991;67:84–87.
20. Morray JP, Lynn AM, Stamm SJ, et al. Hemodynamic effects of ketamine in children with congenital heart disease. Anesth Analg 1984;63:895–899.
21. Hickey PR, Hansen DD, Stafford MM, et al. Pulmonary and systemic hemodynamic response to ketamine in infants with normal and elevated pulmonary vascular resistance. Anesthesiology 1985;62:287–293.
22. Smith I, White PF, Nathanson M, et al. Propofol: an update on its clinical use. Anesthesiology 1994;81:1005–1043.
23. Parke TJ, Stevens JE, Rice ASC, et al. Metabolic acidosis and fatal myocardial failure after propofol infusion in children: five case reports. BMJ 1992;305:613–616.
24. Wagner RL, White PF. Etomidate inhibits adrenocortical function in surgical patients. Anesthesiology 1984;60:647.
25. Coursin DB, Kelly JS, Prielipp RC. Muscle relaxants in critical care. Curr Opin Anesthesiol 1993;6:341–346.
26. Watling SM, Dasta JF. Prolonged paralysis in intensive care unit patients after the use of neuromuscular blocking agents: a review of the literature. Crit Care Med 1994;22:884–893.
27. Hansen-Flaschen J, Cowan J, Raps EC. Neuromuscular blockade in the ICU: more than we bargained for? Am Rev Resp Dis 1993;147:234–237.
28. Griffin D, Fairman N, Coursin DB, et al. Acute myopathy during treatment of status asthmaticus with corticosteroids and steroidal relaxants. Chest 1992;102:510–514.
29. Agoston S. Onset time and evaluation of intubating conditions: rocuronium in perspective. Eur J Anaesthesiol 1995;12(Suppl 1):31–37.
30. Meratoja OA, Taivainen T. Mivacurium chloride in infants and children. Acta Anaesthesiol Scand 1995; 39(Suppl 1):41–44.
31. Meratoja OA. Pharmacodynamics and safety of cisatracurium in children aged 2–12 years undergoing anesthesia. Curr Opin Anesthesiol 1996;9 (Suppl 1): 27–31.

The Airway and Mechanical Ventilation

Howard Alan Zucker, MD, FACC

Intubation of the trachea and support of respiration for the postoperative patient are key components of the critical care management of neonates, infants, and children with congenital heart disease. Appropriate equipment, pharmacologic agents, and skilled personnel are crucial to the successful placement of a tracheal tube as well as to the management of projected, impending, or existing respiratory failure. Inadequate or inappropriate cardiopulmonary support in the postoperative congenital heart disease patient often results in significant hemodynamic compromise including decreased cardiac output, metabolic disturbances, and arrhythmias, all of which can precipitate life-threatening events.

INTUBATION

Securing an artificial airway in the pediatric patient is indicated when either (a) adequate gas exchange can no longer voluntarily occur because of respiratory, cardiac, or neurologic failure, and/or (b) obstruction of the airway has occurred because of intrinsic or extrinsic pathology. Initial assessment of the airway is performed by examination for head, neck, and jaw mobility, and evaluation for oropharyngeal masses, and alignment of tracheal and oropharyngeal planes (1).

Equipment essential for tracheal tube placement includes (a) oxygen source, (b) suction and catheters, (c) bag-valve-mask, (d) laryngoscopes (Miller, MacIntosh, WisHipple blades), (e) endotracheal tubes appropriate for age, (f) Magill forceps for nasotracheal placement, (g) stylets, and (h) oral and nasal airways. The most useful adjunct when placing a tracheal tube is a second set of skilled hands capable of providing mechanical assistance and monitoring vital signs.

Oxygen provision via a high pressure in-line source to an ambu bag should be available. Preoxygenation for 5 minutes prior to administration of anesthetic agents often avoids rapid desaturation during laryngoscopy. Placement of the head in a "sniffing" position aligns the oropharynx and larynx to allow for optimal visualization (1). An evaluation for any dental abnormalities as well as mandibular or maxillary deformities is indicated prior to intubation. Airway abnormalities associated with congenital heart disease have been noted in patients with Cornelia de Lange syndrome, Pierre Robin syndrome, trisomy 21, Aperts disease, Pompe's disease, Treacher Collins syndrome, and Rubinstein Taybi syndrome.

Direct laryngoscopy is performed using either a Miller (straight) blade (2) or MacIntosh (curved) blade (3) with the former placed below the epiglottis and the latter placed in the valleculae. External application of cricoid pressure helps visualize the vocal cords in patients with an anterior airway. A direct correlation exists between tube size and age employing the formula:

$$\text{Endotracheal tube size (mm ID)} = \frac{(\text{age [years]} + 16)}{4}$$

For neonates to 6 months of age a 3.0 or 3.5 mm internal diameter (ID) endotracheal tube is used and from 6 months to 1 year a 3.5–4.0 mm ID tube is considered acceptable. In addition to tracheal diameter, tracheal length changes with age. The distance from the glottis to the bifurcation increases from 5.5 cm in the newborn to 3-month-old baby, to 7.5 cm in the 6 to 12 month old (4). By 12 to 18 months of age the tracheal length is approximately 8 cm. After 2 years of age the insertion distance can be determined by the formula (5, 6):

$$\frac{\text{Age (years)}}{2} + 12 \text{ or } \frac{\text{weight (kg)}}{5} + 12$$

Endotracheal tube position changes with head movement. Extension of the head raises the position of the tracheal tube, potentially causing dislodgment, whereas flexion lowers it, potentially causing a main stem intubation. It is imperative that tube position be determined after intubation. This is most easily accomplished by obtaining a chest roentgenogram. Bilateral breath sounds must be confirmed after placement of a tracheal tube. Use of capnometry or capnography can assist in assuring correct placement (7). The subglottic area remains the narrowest point in the pediatric airway, hence contributing to the child's increased propensity for stridor after extubation (8). To help alleviate this complication uncuffed endotracheal tubes are recommended in neonates, infants, and young children. It is advisable to maintain an air leak of approximately 15–30 cm H_2O pressure around the uncuffed tube. As the child grows the airway diameter increases and placement of a cuffed tube is recommended after 8 years of age. Gas diffusion into the cuff can cause unintentional inflation. Therefore, routine checks of the cuffs should be performed by the respiratory therapist. Overdistended cuffs can obstruct the right or left main stem bronchus.

Reintubation of the postoperative patient with a full stomach requires a rapid sequence technique. It is advisable to have available two laryngoscopes with different size blades, two suction catheters, and two styleted tracheal tubes of different sizes. Preoxygenation, followed by administration of anesthetic agents in rapid sequence, is performed with the help of an assistant who applies cricoid pressure (Sellick maneuver) to avoid aspiration of stomach contents after loss of airway reflexes (9). Although placement of the tracheal tube via the nasal route may be favored, safety dictates that patients intubated via the rapid sequence technique be initially intubated orally. After aspiration of stomach contents the orotracheal tube is electively changed to a nasotracheal one using a Magill forceps to facilitate placement. Prior to instrumenting the nares in the pediatric postoperative or postcatheterization patient consideration is given to the child's anticoagulation status to avoid posterior pharyngeal bleeding.

The risk of major physiologic changes, including diminished cardiac output, arrhythmias, and death, supports the contention that all neonatal and pediatric patients be intubated under general anesthetic conditions (10–12). Lability of the sympathetic nervous system in the neonate and young child can trigger sudden hemodynamic changes in response to painful stimulation. Intubation under controlled conditions involves the administration of amnestics, analgesics, neuromuscular blockers, and antisialogogues. Although atropine is administered prior to manipulation of the airway in an effort to avoid vagally mediated bradycardia and to diminish airway secretions, avoidance of this agent may be considered in cardiac patients with an underlying predisposition to arrhythmias. Amnestic agents, including barbiturates, etomidate, ketamine, and benzodiazepines, should be included in the pharmacologic armamentarium used at the time of intubation. The child's intravascular volume status and underlying cardiac function must be assessed prior to selection of sedative agents. Elevations in pulmonary and systemic vascular resistance occurring with laryngoscopy can be avoided with the use of intravenous opioids and intravenous or topical lidocaine prior to intubation.

Depolarizing or non-depolarizing neuromuscular blocking agents are useful in facilitating intubation. Succinylcholine, a depolarizing agent (noncompetitive blocker) provides rapid relaxation within 60 seconds. Although beneficial in rapid-sequence inductions, the potential risks of succinylcholine, including increased intracranial pressure, increased intragastric pressure, bradycardia, cardiac arrest, and malignant hyperthermia, must be considered prior to use. Non-depolarizing agents (competitive blockers) are classified by length of action with vecuronium, rocuronium, and atracurium among the shorter acting agents, and pancuronium and metacurine among the longer acting ones. Although longer acting agents are advantageous in the intensive care unit (ICU) setting, the adverse effect of tachycardia as seen with pancuronium may limit its use in the postoperative cardiac patient. Pharmacokinetics and pharmacodynamics of all neuromuscular blockers may be markedly altered in patients with transient or prolonged hepatic or renal injury. The effects of congestive heart failure, a prolonged cardiopulmonary bypass period, use of multiple vasoactive agents, and hypothermic circulatory arrest may cause elevations in blood urea nitrogen, creatinine, and transaminases. Therefore, a twitch monitor should be used to assess extent of neuromuscular blockade when administering non-depolarizing agents either as a bolus or continuous infusion in the cardiac intensive care unit.

Although infrequent, reintubation of the postoperative cardiac patient may be required prior to catheterization and prior to additional surgery. The cardiologist or other physician must be capable of providing bag-mask ventilation as the first line of respiratory support. If concerns are raised regarding the child's anatomy, choice of pharmacologic agents, or technical issues relating to intubation it may be advisable for the cardiac intensivist to obtain assistance from a pediatric anesthesiologist. The myocardium of the pediatric cardiac patient, preoperatively as well as postoperatively, may have limited reserve and all efforts should be directed at performing reintubations under controlled conditions (13–15).

MECHANICAL VENTILATION

The concept of a volume preset ventilator with a variable piston-cylinder force generator driven by an electric motor was initially introduced by Trendelenburg in Leipzig, Germany in 1910. Nearly 20 years later, in 1929, Drinker, Shaw, and McKhann mass produced an electrically powered negative-pressure body tank called an "iron lung" (16). However, it was not until the polio epidemic of the 1950s that significant improvements in respiratory support became available for clinical use. Tracheostomy placement with subsequent positive pressure volume ventilation using an Engstrom ventilator markedly reduced mortality from poliomyelitis in Copenhagen, Denmark (17). Development of critical care units in the 1960s followed by the recent advances by the microprocessing chip industry in the 1990s have led to expansive changes in mechanical ventilatory strategies for neonatal, pediatric, and adult patients (Table 8.1).

The basic principles of life support center on adequate gas exchange. Cardiopulmonary support in the preoperative and postoperative patient often requires mechanical ventilation. Although cardiac arrest in the general pediat-

Table 8.1. Pediatric Ventilator Technical Features

	Age Group		
	Neonate 0.5–5.0 kg	Infant 3.5–10.0 kg	Infant or Child 10–70 kg
Driven by	Pneumatic/Electrical	Electrical	Electrical/Pneumatic
Inspiratory factors			
Cycling	Time	Time	Time
Limit	Time or pressure	Volume or pressure	Volume or pressure
Flow-generated pattern	Constant square wave	Constant square wave	Constant square, decelerating, or sine
Pressure plateau ("pause")	Yes, if pressure limited	Yes, 0–2.0 sec	Yes, variable duration
Inspiratory time set	0.4–0.7 sec	0.7–1.0 sec	0.7–1.0 sec
I:E ratio	4:1–1:10	4:1–1:6	4:1–1:6
IMV modes	IMV only	IMV and SIMV	IMV and SIMV
IMV circuitry	Continuous flow	Demand valve and continuous flow	Demand valve and continuous flow
Circuit compressible volume	1 mL/cm H_2O	0.3–0.5 mL/cm H_2O	3–4 mL/cm H_2O
PEEP/CPAP range	0–20 cm H_2O	0–25 cm H_2O	0–50 cm H_2O
Pressure support	Yes	Yes	Yes
Tidal volume	Not preset	12–15 mL/kg	12–15 mL/kg
Rate (breaths/min)	25–40	15–40	8–20
Examples	Baby Bird	Bear LS 104–150	Bear 2 or 5
	Bear Cub	Infrasonics	Puritan Bennett 7200A
	Sechrist BP200	Infant Star	Siemens Servo 900C
			Siemens Servo 300

CPAP, continuous positive airway pressure; IMV, intermittent mandatory ventilation; PEEP, positive end-expiratory pressure.

ric population is preceded by respiratory failure, such is not the situation in patients with congenital heart disease. Therefore, immediate identification of the precipitating event with early intervention can result in a more favorable outcome.

The respiratory tract is divided into conducting, transitional, and respiratory zones. These various generations provide for either gas delivery or gas exchange. By the time a child is aged 2 years some 400,000,000 alveoli are available for oxygen delivery and carbon dioxide removal (18). The trachea originates at the inferior aspect of the cricoid cartilage opposite the fourth cervical vertebrae in the infant and opposite the sixth cervical vertebrae in the adolescent. Unlike in the adult, the child's larynx is in a more cephalad position, the epiglottis is floppy and "U" shaped, and the subglottic area is the narrowest part of the airway. These findings make visualization and placement of the tracheal tube somewhat more difficult in the pediatric patient. Poiseulle's Law defines resistance as an inverse relationship to the fourth power of the radius. Therefore, airways of children are more susceptible to increases in resistance secondary to edema and mucus. A compliant chest cavity in concert with fewer fatigue resistant fibers in the diaphragm can limit a critically ill child's ability to generate adequate negative intrathoracic pressure to entrain the appropriate tidal volume (Fig. 8.1) (1). Coupling the anatomic and histologic differences seen in the pediatric patient with an increased oxygen consumption (8 mL/kg/min in the child versus 4 mL/kg/min in the adult) potentially creates early development of hypoxemia and hypercarbia in the stressed neonate, infant, or child.

In the mechanics of breathing a synchronized active contraction of the diaphragm and intercostal muscles generates negative intrathoracic pressure, followed by a passive phase of chest wall relaxation and lung recoil. The compliant chest cavity limits a pediatric patient's ability to increase gas exchange (19). Increased work of breathing and increased oxygen consumption caused by inefficient use of energy often results in ventilation perfusion ($\dot{V}/\dot{Q}$) mismatch. These efforts may indicate respiratory failure secondary to fatigue. Assisted ventilation, utilized to reduce intrapulmonary shunt and minimize $\dot{V}/\dot{Q}$ mismatch, is the acceptable therapy when normal physiologic processes do not provide for adequate gas exchange. Unfavorable hemodynamic results secondary to ineffective oxygenation or ventilation suggest that mechanical ventilation

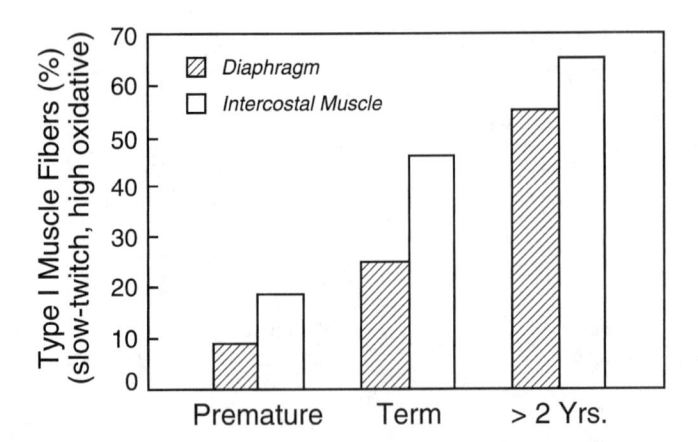

Figure 8.1. Muscle fiber composition of the diaphragm and intercostal muscles related to age. Note that a premature infant's diaphragm and intercostal muscles have fewer type I fibers compared with term newborns and older children. The data suggest a possible mechanism for early fatigue in premature and term infants when the work of breathing is increased. (Reprinted with permission from Coté CJ, Ryan JF, Todres ID, et al. A practice of anesthesia for infants and children. 2nd ed. Philadelphia: WB Saunders, 1993.)

Table 8.2. Indications for Positive-Pressure Mechanical Ventilation and Respiratory Support of the Pediatric Patient

1. Acute respiratory failure
   a. Inadequate ventilation
      Apnea
      Hypopnea
      Vd/Vt > 0.6
      VC < 15 mL/kg
      Rising $Paco_2$ or $Paco_2$ > 50 mm Hg (acutely)
   b. Inadequate oxygenation
      Pao_2 < 70 mm Hg or Sao_2 < 93% with Fio_2 > 0.6
      $AaDo_2$ gradient > 300 mm Hg with Fio_2 = 1.0
      Qs/Qt > 15–20%
2. To secure the airway
   a. Neurologic dysfunction (obtundation, coma, high spinal cord injury, intractable seizures)
   b. Upper gastrointestinal bleed/aspiration risk
   c. Toxic or foreign body ingestion
   d. Upper airway obstruction (i.e., croup, epiglottitis, vascular rings)
   e. Airway edema, trauma, or burns
3. To control ventilation
   a. Elevated intracranial pressure
   b. Neuromuscular disease
   c. Acute reactive airway disease or bronchospasm
   d. Pulmonary parenchymal processes
   e. Postoperative state
   f. Restrictive lung disease due to abdominal distension, obesity, kyphoscoliosis, flail chest, pleural disease, or tumor
4. To decrease work of breathing
   a. Sepsis
   b. Metabolic acidosis
   c. Chronic pulmonary disease
   d. Congestive heart failure
   e. Pulmonary edema
   f. Acute reactive airway disease
   g. Shock/circulatory failure

Reprinted with permission from Savarese A, Zucker H. The pediatric pulmonary system. In: Bell C, Hughes C, Oh T, eds. The pediatric anesthesia handbook. St. Louis: Mosby-Year Book, 1991.

be utilized in the early postoperative period for many patients undergoing palliative or reparative procedures. Indications for providing positive pressure ventilation are outlined in Table 8.2 (20). Inspired oxygen concentration and elevated mean airway pressure are key factors contributing to oxygenation in the patient supported by mechanical ventilation. The former can be provided through increased Fio_2 and the latter through adjustments in positive end-expiratory pressure (PEEP), intermittent mandatory ventilation (IMV), inspiratory time (i-time), and flow. Carbon dioxide elimination is determined by alveolar ventilation, which is defined as the difference between minute ventilation and dead space ventilation. The latter, dead space ventilation, can vary as Vd/Vt changes. PEEP, IMV, tidal volume, and peak inspiratory pressure can all affect Vd/Vt.

Ventilatory support can be categorized by three variables that determine assisted breaths: (a) what initiates the mechanical breath–trigger; (b) what determines the offset–cycling; and (c) what controls the gas volume delivered or pressure generated–limit.

Triggers to mechanical ventilation can be time, flow, or pressure. Sensitivity adjustments in these variables can initiate a breath with greater or less ease. Flow rate or time will terminate a positive pressure breath after a set cycle length. Termination of most breaths for pediatric patients are time-cycled. Inspiratory : expiratory ratios determine percentage of time gas is delivered during positive pressure ventilation. If unchecked, mechanical breaths would continue to expand alveoli until the end of the inspiratory period. The limit variable–volume, pressure, or pressure support–will prevent the potential detrimental effects of overdistension of the lung fields (21).

Mechanical ventilation in the adult requires opening of a demand valve triggered by the patient's spontaneous respiratory effort. However, pediatric and neonatal ventilators use a continuous flow IMV system to prevent the increased work of breathing required to trigger a breath (22). Newer ventilator circuitry allows for more versatile systems including flow-triggering and pressure-triggering mechanisms. With flow-triggering, a 0.5 L/min or 1.0 L/min flow must be generated in the neonate or pediatric patient, respectively, prior to delivery of a ventilator breath. Similarly, in pressure-triggering, 0.5 cm H_2O or 1.0 cm H_2O pressure must be created by the patient to initiate a mechanical breath. To create distension of the alveolus, gas must flow across a pressure gradient from the extrathoracic to the intrathoracic airway. Gas flow patterns that occur can either result in a square wave schematic (volume-limited breaths) secondary to constant delivery, or a decelerating wave schematic (pressure-limited breaths) secondary to variable flow.

Each alveolus will be distended to a variable extent based on its individual time constant. Time constant, defined as the product of resistance and compliance, measures the time to equilibrium for each alveolar unit (23). Sixty-three percent of the gas volume will be at equilibrium after one time constant, 87% after two, and 95% after three time constants. Pathologic states causing parenchymal disease and airway injury can result in marked discrepancies in time constants causing partial or complete atelectasis and/or hyperinflation. To avoid these abnormalities in lung expansion, normal inspiratory and expiratory times should allow for approximately four time constants. Procedures for initiating positive pressure mechanical ventilation are outlined in Table 8.3.

MODES OF VENTILATION

Volume Control

A set volume is delivered independent of lung compliance or resistance. Constant inspiratory flow is delivered during the inspiratory time (i-time), resulting in a square wave pattern. With tidal volume and minute ventilation set, the peak inspiratory pressure (PIP) becomes a dependent variable with potential for marked elevations. No inspiratory plateau is achieved and flow terminates at peak inspiratory pressure (Fig. 8.2). The patient may trigger the sensitivity variable (flow or pressure), resulting in the delivery of a volume-controlled breath. Volume control provides for fixed minute ventilation. Therefore $Paco_2$ and pH remain stable and are independent of changes in lung compliance or intravascular and extravascular volume (24). Flow volume loops (Fig. 8.3) help the intensivist assess both gas flow patterns during volume control and pressure control ventilation (24).

Pressure Control

In pressure control mode a peak airway pressure is determined prior to initiation of mechanical ventilation, and further adjustments are made to optimize chest expansion and gas exchange. Pressure remains constant throughout inspiration and tidal volume becomes a dependent variable. Therefore, lung compliance and airway resistance are critical factors in determining gas delivery. Flow is delivered in a decelerating pattern (Figs. 8.4 and 8.5) (25). The I:E ratio and the IMV are set by the physician or respira-

Table 8.3. Procedures for Initiating Positive Pressure Mechanical Ventilation

1. Select ventilator based on:
   Patient/disease characteristics
   Therapeutic goals
   Technical advantages of the specific ventilator
2. Ensure proper setup of the machine
   Correct wall-source connections for gases
   Cycling and flow rates
   Humidification and warming of gases
   Alarms activated (apnea, disconnect, low Vt, low pressure)
   Oxygen analyzer in circuit
3. Choose mode
   Volume or pressure limited
   IMV or SIMV
   CPAP with spontaneous ventilation
   Inspiratory pressure support
4. Choose inspiratory parameters
   Peak inspiratory pressure
   Inspiratory time
   Preset Vt (12–15 mL/kg)
   I:E ratio (typically 1:2) (for obstructive disease choose 1:3 or 1:4 to allow for prolonged expiratory time)
   Inspiratory flow generator pattern
5. Choose frequency (bpm)
   Use age-specific norms
6. Choose F_{IO_2}
   Aim for < 0.50 to avoid o_2 toxicity
7. Select end-expiratory distending pressure
   CPAP (usually 3–5 cm H_2O)
   PEEP (usually 3–5 cm H_2O)
8. Assess adequacy of ventilation and oxygenation
   Color and perfusion
   Chest excursion
   Breath sounds
   Arterial blood gas for Pao_2 (> 70 mm Hg) and $Paco_2$ (35–45 mm Hg)
   Pulse oximetry and capnometry
   Hemodynamics
9. Consider sedatives and muscle relaxants
   Narcotics
   Benzodiazepines
   Intermittent or long acting nondepolarizing muscle relaxants
10. Ensure good pulmonary toilet
    Endotracheal tube
    Change ventilator circuits at 48 h
    Chest physiotherapy
    Bronchodilator/nebulizer therapy
11. Maintain optimal matching of o_2 delivery to consumption
    Sedation/muscle relaxation
    Fever control
    Nutritional support
    Correct anemia
    30–45 degree head elevation to improve $\dot{V}/\dot{Q}$

CPAP, continuous positive airway pressure; IMV, intermittent mandatory ventilation; PEEP, positive end-expiratory pressure; SIMV, synchronized intermittent mandatory ventilation. (Reprinted with permission from Savarese A, Zucker H. The pediatric pulmonary system. In: Bell C, Hughes C, Oh T, eds. The pediatric anesthesia handbook. St. Louis: Mosby-Year Book, 1991.)

tory therapist. Similar to volume ventilation, sensitivity for either flow or pressure will trigger the ventilator to deliver a mechanical breath with a preset inspiratory pressure. Pressure control ventilation allows for better gas distribution, and it provides a tidal volume with lower PIPs than volume control ventilation. These two factors contribute to diminished barotrauma with this mode of respiratory support (26).

Pressure Support Ventilation

As with pressure control, a decelerating inspiratory flow pattern exists, but it requires triggering by the patient to deliver a breath. On initiation of this patient-triggered breath constant pressure is delivered during the inspiratory period. Termination of the breath occurs when flow decreases to 25% of peak flow (23). The decelerating flow pattern can vary in amount based on the inspiratory time. Because this mode of ventilation is initiated by the patient, the IMV, tidal volume, and I:E times can vary considerably between breaths (Fig. 8.6). Pressure support ventilation is a patient-triggered, pressure-limited mode of positive pressure ventilation (23). Better patient-ventilator synchrony with less tendency for development of pneumothoraces, atelectasis, hypoxemia, and hypercarbia occurs with patient-triggered mechanical ventilation. Furthermore, contribution from intrinsic respiratory muscle activity working in concert with mechanical ventilation often decreases work of breathing. Spontaneous respirations in the pure volume and pressure control modes are associated with ineffective gas exchange. Advantages and disadvantages of these three modes of ventilation are summarized in Table 8.4.

Volume Control plus Pressure Support

Volume control plus pressure support is a combination of controlled and supported breaths. Patient-triggered breaths are pressure supported; however, a fixed number of "backup breaths" in the volume control mode are programmed. The safety feature of a fixed synchronized intermittent mandatory ventilation (SIMV) allows for adequate gas exchange in the event of respiratory drive impairment secondary to the administration of opioids or other anesthetic agents. Patient-triggered breaths during the SIMV period result in delivery of a volume-controlled breath; however, breaths triggered after this period has passed result in delivery of a pressure-supported breath. As a failsafe feature, a mandatory volume-controlled breath is delivered if neither a patient-triggered volume-controlled breath nor a pressure-supported breath occurs within a fixed time period (25). One disadvantage to this mode of ventilation is the mixing of both square wave and decelerating wave flow patterns (Fig. 8.7).

Pressure Control plus Pressure Support

Similar to volume control and pressure support, pressure control plus pressure support ventilation provides for a combination of controlled and supported breaths for patients not receiving neuromuscular blockade. Unlike ventilatory modes previously discussed, all breaths are delivered with a decelerating inspiratory flow pattern. The patient triggers his/her own pressure-supported breaths and the ventilator provides a "backup" of pressure-con-

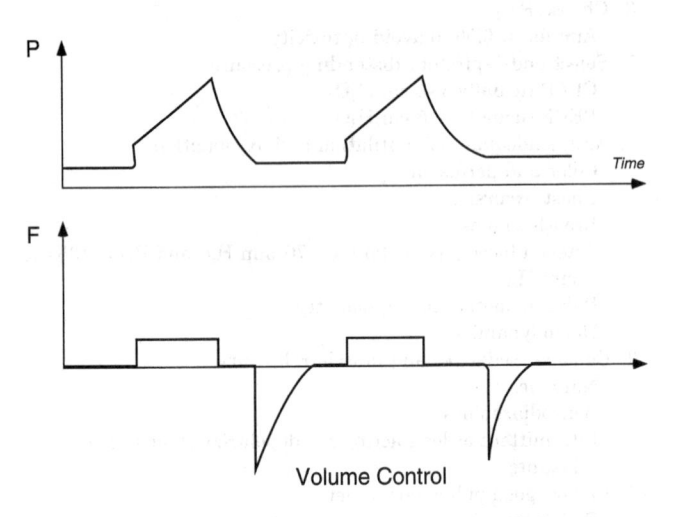

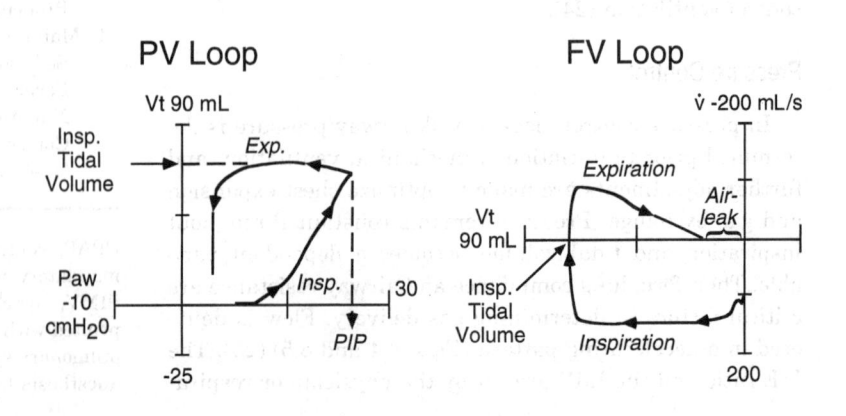

Figure 8.2. Graphic representation of pressure and flow versus time in volume control mode.

Figure 8.3. Pressure-volume and flow-volume loops in volume-limited, constant flow ventilation in normal lungs. Paw, airway pressure; PIP, peak inspiratory pressure. (Reprinted with permission from Wilson B, Cheifetz I, Meliones J. Optimizing mechanical ventilation in infants and children. Bird Products Corporation, Palm Springs, CA, 1995.)

trolled breaths. Although the inspiratory pressure is set in both modes, thereby limiting the amount of barotrauma, a potential exists for inadequate delivery of tidal volume if lung compliance is poor and/or airway resistance is high (22, 27). During the set SIMV period delivery of a pressure-controlled breath occurs if (a) the patient triggers the sensitivity setting of the ventilator, or (b) no respiratory activity occurs during the fixed SIMV time period. If the patient triggers the ventilator after the SIMV period then a pressure-supported breath is delivered (Fig. 8.8) (25). In both, volume control plus pressure support and pressure control plus pressure support ventilation, the ventilatory breaths are triggered by either flow or pressure changes.

Pressure Regulated plus Volume Control

With standard pressure or volume ventilation it is often necessary to sacrifice one variable for the other. The latest technologies provide for regulation of both pressure and volume delivered through adjustments in flow.

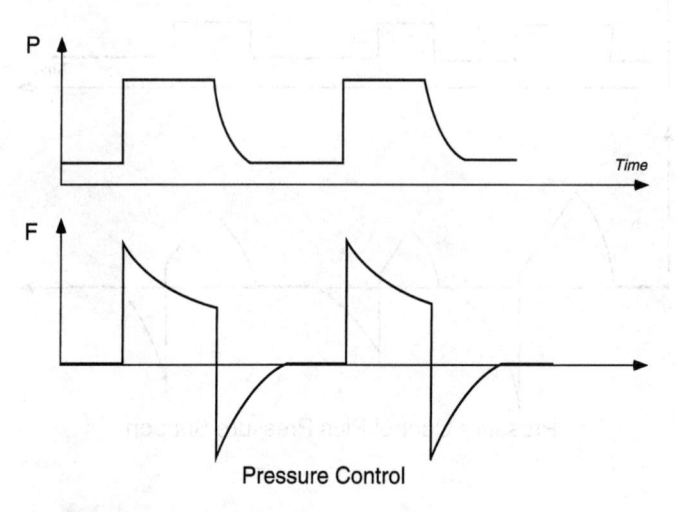

Figure 8.4. Graphic representation of pressure and flow versus time in pressure control mode.

Inverse Ratio Ventilation

In either volume-controlled or pressure-controlled ventilation the I:E ratio can be set to provide a shorter percentage of time in the inspiratory cycle. Presumably this mode, known as "inverse ratio ventilation" (IRV), offers better gas distribution during the inspiratory period of ventilation and favors increased alveolar recruitment (23). This latter finding increases functional residual capacity and improves ventilation to perfusion matching. With shorter inspiratory times, a tendency is seen for increased mean airway pressure and resultant barotrauma. Unlike pressure support where spontaneous respiratory effort is instrumental in the ventilatory strategy, IRV is not physiologic and suppression of intrinsic respiratory drive is advantageous. In all modes of ventilation it is important to allow adequate time for expiration. Elevation in expiratory resistance as a result of intrinsic airway disease (e.g., bronchospasm) or extrinsic processes (e.g., airway compression) can result in gas trapping (28).

High Frequency Ventilation

High frequency ventilation utilizes small tidal volumes at nonphysiologic rates to provide effective gas exchange. High frequency ventilation is subdivided into three modes of delivery: high frequency positive pressure ventilation (HFPPV), high frequency jet ventilation (HFJV), and high frequency oscillation (HFO), the former uses standard ventilator equipment at tidal volumes of 3–4 mL/kg with IMVs of 60 to 150 per minute, whereas the latter two invoke the use of specialized technology. With HFJV flow is delivered through noncompliant tubing at 0–50 psi with an interrupter providing for rates of 60–600 per minute. Directly proportional to driving pressure and "i-time," tidal volumes range between 2–5 mL/kg (29). As a result of lower mean airway pressure, HFJV has been shown to improve cardiac output in single ventricle patients who have undergone the Fontan procedure (30). HFO uses pistons to generate frequencies of 60–3600 cpm and tidal volumes of

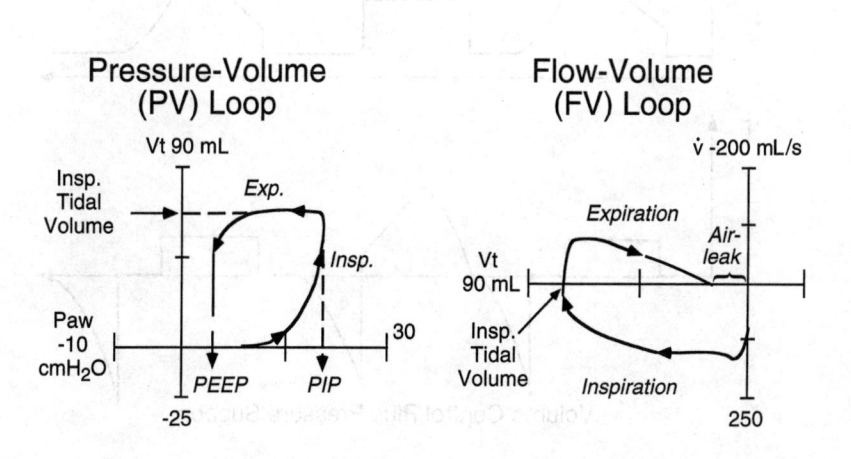

Figure 8.5. Graphic representation of pressure-volume loop and flow-volume loop in pressure control ventilation. Paw, airway pressure; PEEP, positive end-expiratory pressure; PIP, peak inspiratory pressure.

Figure 8.6. Graphic representation of pressure and flow versus time in pressure support mode.

Pressure Support

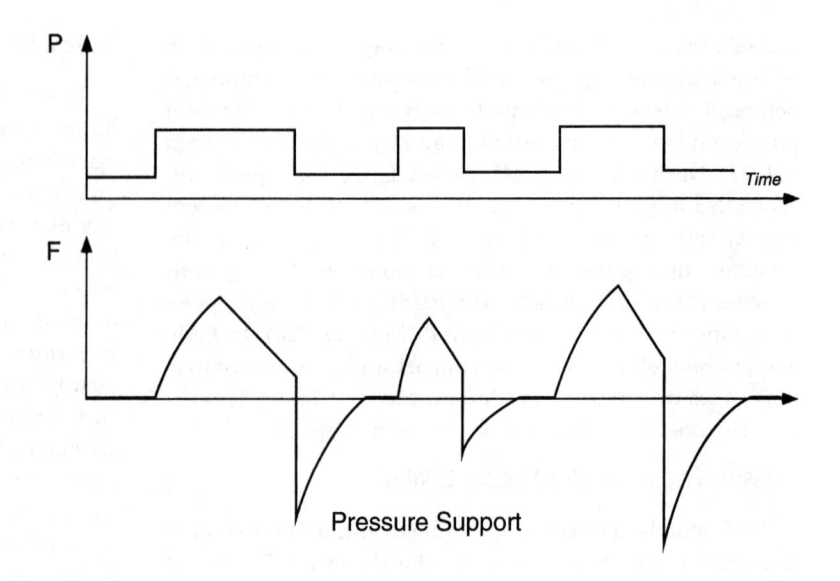

Figure 8.7. Graphic representation of pressure and flow in volume control plus pressure support mode.

Pressure Control Plus Pressure Support

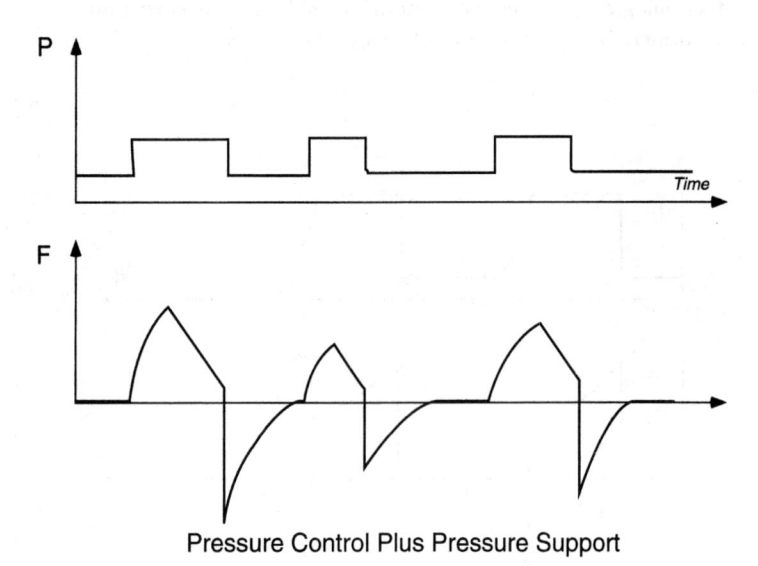

Figure 8.8. Graphic representation of pressure and flow in pressure control plus pressure support mode.

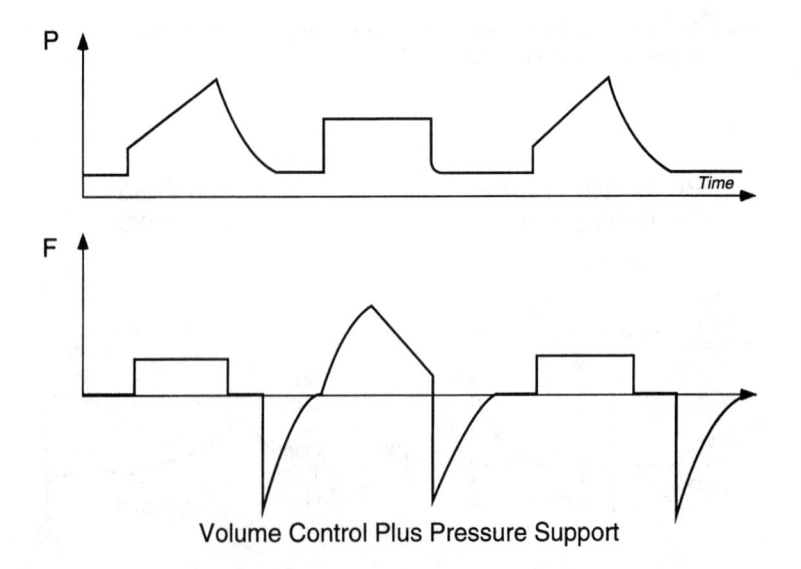

Volume Control Plus Pressure Support

Table 8.4. Advantages and Disadvantages of Commonly Used Ventilators

Pressure Limited
Advantages
  Preset peak inspiratory pressure prevents excessive inflating pressures
  Decreased risk of barotrauma
  Provides static inspiratory pressure plateau, which helps $\dot{V}/\dot{Q}$ matching and intrapulmonary shunting in diseases of decreased compliance and low functional residual capacity (neonatal respiratory distress syndrome)
Disadvantages
  Delivered tidal volume is variable, depending on inspiratory flow, inspiratory time, circuit, and patient compliance
  Changes in lung compliance and airway resistance are difficult to detect because the peak inflating pressure is constant

Volume Limited
Advantages
  A constant preset tidal volume is delivered to the circuit
  Changes in the patient's pulmonary mechanics (compliance, airway resistance) are suggested by changes in inflating pressures
  Better suited to ventilating patients with variable pulmonary pathology
Disadvantages
  Delivered tidal volume to the patient can vary with extremes of circuit compliance and peak inspiratory pressure ("lost" compressible volume)
  High peak inflating pressures may be reached to deliver preset Vt
  Increased risk of barotrauma
  Delivered tidal volumes less than 100 mL are difficult to ensure

Pressure Support
Advantages
  Patient triggered
  Favorable pattern of ventilation for patient who is spontaneously breathing
  Improved patient-ventilator synchrony
  Exercises the diaphragm
Disadvantages
  Adequate tidal volume is difficult to ensure as delivered volume is variable

Reprinted with permission from Savarese A, Zucker H. The pediatric pulmonary system. In: Bell C, Hughes C, Oh T, eds. The pediatric anesthesia handbook. St. Louis: Mosby-Year Book.

1–3 mL/kg. Beneficial effects, as evidenced by improved Pao_2/PAo_2 and decreased oxygenation index, have been noted when compared with conventional mechanical ventilation (31).

Liquid Ventilation

Attempts at improving lung compliance have led to ventilation with oxygenated perfluorocarbons. Successful reduction in airway pressures and improved compliance have been seen with total liquid ventilation (TLV). Improved $\dot{V}/\dot{Q}$ matching and more effective gas exchange have been seen with this therapy. Partial liquid ventilation (PLV) requires less perfluorocarbons, and it allows for gas exchange through in vivo bubble oxygenation. With fewer adverse cardiovascular side effects (32) and reports of improved cardiorespiratory function in animal models (33), the use of PLV may be advantageous to the patient who has undergone a Fontan procedure and has respiratory failure.

EXTUBATION

Extubation of the cardiac patient should be considered when adequate hemostasis, optimal cardiac output, favorable hemodynamics, normothermia, and appropriate mental status exists. Gradual diminution in the settings on the mechanical ventilator should parallel improvements in the clinical status and arterial blood gases. Development of hypoxemia or hypercarbia may warrant a further period of support. Fio_2 requirements of less than 0.40 in the presence of a satisfactory Pao_2 should be achieved and documented. A PEEP of less than or equal to 5 cm H_2O is encouraged as is a negative inspiratory force of -20 to -30 cm H_2O pressure. Vital capacities of greater than 15 mL/kg are ideal. After an adequate level of consciousness is noted and complete resolution or reversal of neuromuscular blockade is attained, the cardiac intensivist considers removal of the tracheal tube. Prior to extubation of any patient it is advisable to have all necessary equipment, including bag-valve-mask, laryngoscopes, endotracheal tubes, suction, and pharmacologic agents, at the bedside in preparation for an emergent and unanticipated reintubation. Adherence to extubation criteria avoids the adverse hemodynamic effects caused by excessive catecholamine release seen with an unsuccessful extubation of the congenital heart disease patient (Table 8.5).

Although early extubation (less than 12 hours) is acceptable in the stable postoperative cardiac patient more than 1 year of age, it is highly recommended that neonates and infants with complex lesions who have undergone palliative or reparative surgery remain intubated and sedated for the first few hours postoperatively. Data from Anand and Hickey (12) show that the use of fentanyl and neuromuscular blockade in the postoperative period have decreased morbidity in the neonate undergoing complex congenital heart disease surgery. Untoward hemodynamic events in neonates not anesthetized in the early postoperative period may be secondary to elevations in pulmonary vascular resistance on stimulation of the airway (e.g., suctioning, tracheal tube repositioning).

A child who presumably met criteria for extubation and then fails to breath spontaneously or maintain adequate gas exchange must be evaluated for a residual anatomic

Table 8.5. Extubation Criteria

Pulmonary
 Vital capacity > 15 cc/kg
 Alveolar to arterial (Aa) difference for oxygen < 350 mm Hg (F_{IO_2} = 1.0)
 Arterial/alveolar partial pressure of oxygen > 0.75
 pH > 7.35
 Pa_{CO_2} < 45 unless pH > 7.35
 Vd/Vt < 0.6
 No pneumothoraces
 No pleural effusions
 Negative inspiratory force of −20 to −30 cm H_2O
Cardiac
 Sinus rhythm or stable pacemaker rhythm
 Adequate stroke volume
 Adequate capillary refill (< 3 seconds)
 Optimal filling pressures
 Adequate stroke volume as assessed by arterial waveforms
 Minimal inotropic support
Neurologic
 Conscious
 No residual neuromuscular blockade
 Minimal sedative agents administered within 2–4 hours of extubation
Other
 Favorable nutritional status
 Normal white blood cell count
 Optimal hematocrit for palliated or repaired patients
 Normothermia

lesion through the use of echocardiography and/or cardiac catheterization. Further evaluation of pulmonary causes of respiratory failure should be sought, including pleural effusions, pneumothoraces, pneumonia, atelectasis, paralyzed hemidiaphragm, airway obstruction (proximally or distally), vocal cord paralysis (secondary to recurrent laryngeal nerve injury), and reactive airway disease. Other factors that should be addressed are neurologic causes, including pharmacologic (oversedation, residual neuromuscular blockade); and physiologic causes (hypoxic ischemic events, intracranial hemorrhage, choreoathetosis).

SUMMARY

Successful postoperative recovery of the pediatric cardiac patient is dependent on many factors. Intubation and mechanical ventilation comprise but one key component in the myriad of issues facing the cardiac intensivist. An impairment in oxygen delivery or carbon dioxide removal can prolong ICU stay. Ventilatory strategies, which result in dys-synchrony between patient effort and mode of support, result in excessive work of breathing, agitation, increased oxygen consumption, and potential development of pneumothoraces, atelectasis, and negative inspiratory force pulmonary edema. These detrimental side effects of poorly chosen and inadequately adjusted ventilatory modes can also impair the ability to wean the infant or child from mechanical ventilation. A thorough understanding of the cardiac diagnosis, preoperative evaluation (ECG, ECHO, catheterizations, electrophysiologic studies, pulmonary function tests, lung scans), surgical and medical options, operative procedures, intraoperative management, anesthetic agents used, and potential postoperative complications must be understood by the cardiac intensivist caring for the critically ill pediatric cardiology patient. Perturbations in normal respiratory physiology affects cardiac hemodynamics, which indirectly alters length of stay, morbidity, mortality, and outcome (24). Similarly, although respiratory failure requiring intubation and mechanical ventilation may be secondary to intrinsic pulmonary pathology, interdependence of the cardiac and respiratory systems makes evaluation of possible cardiac causes paramount when faced with a child who is not recuperating in the expected fashion.

REFERENCES

1. Cote C, Todres ID. The pediatric airway. In: Cote C, Ryan J, Todres ID, et al. A practice of anesthesia for infants and children. 2nd ed. Philadelphia: WB Saunders, 1993:55–83.
2. Miller RA. A new laryngoscope. Anesthesiology 1941;2:317.
3. MacIntosh PR. New laryngoscope. Lancet 1943;1:205.
4. Fearon B, Whalen J. Tracheal dimensions in the living infant. Ann Otol Rhinol Laryngol 1967;76:965–974.
5. Cole F. Pediatric formulas for the anesthesiologist. American Journal of Diseases of Children 1957;94:672–673.
6. Morgan G, Stewart D. Linear airway dimensions in children—Including those with cleft palate. Can Anaesth Soc J 1982;1–8.
7. Linko K, Paloheimo M, Tammish T. Capnography for detection of accidental oesphageal intubation. Acta Anaesthesiol Scand 1983;27:199–202.
8. Quartararo C, Bishop M. Complications of tracheal intubation: prevention and treatment. Semin Anesthes 1990;11:119.
9. Sellick B. Cricoid pressure to control regurgitation of stomach contents during induction of anesthesia. Lancet 1961;2:404.
10. Segan J, Merrill D, Chapleau M, et al. Hemodynamic changes during endotracheal suctioning are mediated by increased autonomic activity. Pediatr Res 1993;33:649–652.
11. Anand K, Hickey PP. Pain and its effects in the human neonate and fetus. N Engl J Med 1987;317:1321–1329.
12. Anand K, Hickey P. Halothane-morphine compared with high-dose sufentanil for anesthesia and postoperative analgesia in neonatal cardiac surgery. N Engl J Med 1992;326:1–9.
13. Anand K, Brown M, Bloom S. Studies on the hormonal regulation of fuel metabolism in the human newborn infant undergoing anaesthesia and surgery. Horm Res 1985;22:115–128.
14. Hickey P, Hansen D. Fentanyl and sufentanil-oxygen-pancuronium anesthesia for cardiac surgery in infants. Anesth Analg 1983;63:117–124.

15. Wessel DL. Perioperative care: management of the infant and neonate with congenital heart disease. In: Castaneda A, Jonas R, Mayer J, et al. Cardiac surgery of the neonate and infant. Philadelphia: WB Saunders, 1994:65–87.
16. Downes J. The historical evolution, current status, and prospective development of pediatric critical care. Progress in pediatric critical care. Crit Care Clin North Am 1992;8(1):1–13.
17. Ibsen B. The anaesthetist's viewpoint on treatment of respiratory complications in poliomyelitis during the epidemic in Copenhagen. Proc R Soc Lond B Biol Sci 1954;47:72.
18. Thurlbeck WM. Postnatal human lung growth. Thorax 1982;37:564–571.
19. Gerhardt T, Bancalau E. Chest wall compliance in full-term and premature infants. Acta Paediatr Scand 1980;69:359–364.
20. Savarese A, Zucker H. The pediatric pulmonary system. In: Bell C, Hughes C, Oh T, eds. The pediatric anesthesia handbook. St. Louis: Mosby-Year Book, 1991.
21. Wilson B, Cheifetz I, Meliones J. Optimizing mechanical ventilation in infants and children. Bird Products Corporation, Palm Springs, CA, 1995.
22. Wernovsky G, Chang A, Wessel D. Intensive care. In: Emmanouilides G, Allen H, Riemenschneider T, Gutgesell H, eds. Moss & Adams heart disease in infants, children, and adolescents (including the fetus and young adult). 5th ed. Baltimore: Williams & Wilkins, 1995.
23. Fields A. Mechanical ventilation II. In: Pediatric Critical Care Clinical Review Series. Part 3. Society of Critical Care Medicine, Anaheim, CA, 1991.
24. Meliones J, Kern F, Schulman S, et al. Pathophysiological approach to respiratory support for patients with congenital heart disease. Progress in Pediatric Cardiology. Special issue: pediatric cardiovascular intensive care 1995;4:3.
25. Life support systems in system SV 300: ventilatory modes. How they work–how they are used? Siemens-Elema AB, Danvers, MA, 1994.
26. Abrahams E, Yoshihara G. Cardiorespiratory effects of pressure controlled ventilation in severe respiratory failure. Chest 1990;98:1445–1449.
27. Wessel D, Wernovsky G, Chang A. Perioperative care of the critically ill child with congenital heart disease. In: Current Concepts in Pediatric Critical Care 1995;113–114.
28. Fisher D. Anesthesia equipment for pediatrics. In: Gregory G, ed. Pediatric anesthesia. 3rd ed. New York: Churchill Livingstone, 1994.
29. Carlton GC, Howland WS, Ray C, et al. High-frequency jet ventilation. A prospective, randomized evaluation. Chest 1983;84:551.
30. Meliones JN, Bove EL, Dekeon MK, et al. High-frequency jet ventilation improves cardiac function after the Fontan procedure. Circulation 1991;84:III–364.
31. Arnold JH, Hanson JH, Toro-Figuero LO, et al. Prospective, randomized comparison of high-frequency oscillatory ventilation and conventional mechanical ventilation in pediatric respiratory failure. Crit Care Med 1994;22:1530–1539.
32. Herman LJ, Fuhrman BP, Papo MC, et al. Cardiorespiratory effects of perfluorocarbon-associated gas exchange at reduced oxygen concentrations. Crit Care Med 1995;23:553.
33. Leach CL, Fuhrman BP, Morin FC III, et al. Perfluorocarbon-associated gas exchange (partial liquid ventilation) in respiratory distress syndrome: a prospective, randomized, controlled study. Crit Care Med 1993;21:1270.

Cardiopulmonary Interactions

Desmond Bohn, MB FRCPC

Our knowledge and understanding of cardiovascular and respiratory physiology has tended to develop along parallel lines. The great physiologists of the late 19th and early 20th centuries who defined for us the laws that govern our understanding of cardiovascular physiology were largely unaware of the major hemodynamic changes that we now know occur during the passage of blood from the venous to the arterial side of the circulation. Starling's classic observations on the effect of the changes in filling pressure on cardiac output presumed that the right heart pumped blood to the left side of the heart without any there being hemodynamic change associated with respiration. For years pulmonary circulation was referred to as the "minor circulation," and it was considered that pulmonary disease was important only so far as it limited full oxygenation of the blood. Both the heart and lungs subserve the same vital function, namely the delivery of oxygenated blood to the tissues. With the development of intensive care and in particular positive pressure ventilation, we now appreciate that the heart and lungs are more than two independent but connected circulations, and that they share the same body cavity means that disease processes affecting either organ will impact on the other. With the development of our ability to measure hemodynamic changes in the critically ill, has come the realization that the passage of venous return through the thoracic cavity is associated with major hemodynamic changes during the respiratory cycle, whether during spontaneous or positive pressure ventilation. These important interactions between the heart and lungs can be influenced by either a primary cardiorespiratory disease process or the therapies used in intensive care treatment; it is important, therefore, to have a fundamental understanding of the normal physiology of cardiopulmonary interactions as a prelude to an explanation of how these can change with therapeutic interventions in the critically ill patient.

CARDIOPULMONARY CIRCULATION

Perhaps the easiest way to begin to understand the fundamentals of the complex interaction between the systemic and pulmonary circulations is to use a model of two pumps connected in series enclosed within a chamber where the pressure is constantly changing. The reservoir for the filling of the right heart (venous return) lies entirely outside the thorax; it is consequently subject to atmospheric pressure, whereas the large venous connections are mostly intrathoracic and subject to negative pressure, at least for part of the respiratory cycle. On the other hand the reservoir for left heart filling (the pulmonary circulation) and the pumping chamber lie entirely within the thorax, although the pump ejects against a high impedance circulation that is largely extrathoracic (systemic vascular resistance). Because intrapleural pressure is constantly changing during the respiratory cycle it follows that the resulting fluctuations in intrathoracic pressure will affect the output from the pump by altering preload or filling on the right side and afterload on the left side. Two further factors influence the performance of the left and right ventricles; in the first place we now know that they do not function as merely two separate pumping chambers connected in series, but because muscle fibers interconnect both ventricles and share a common septum, changes in the contractile state of one ventricle will be reflected in the other, a phenomenon known as "ventricular interdependence" (1). Both pumping chambers are also constrained within a viscoelastic membrane (the pericardium) which, although it does not normally have a significant influence on function, can inhibit contraction in situations where intrapericardial pressure increases. Finally, changes in lung volume, independent of any change in intrathoracic pressure, alter the caliber of the pulmonary vascular bed and thereby influence right ventricular afterload. These various changes and their point of impact are summarized in Figure 9.1.

To simplify this complex series of interactions, the best approach is to follow the sequence of events in the cardiac cycle and then examine the effect of changes in intrathoracic pressure and lung volume on each phase of the cardiac cycle from the venous to the arterial side of the circulation, namely (*a*) venous return and right atrial filling, (*b*) right ventricular output, (*c*) pulmonary vascular resistance, and (*d*) left ventricular output.

VENOUS RETURN (PRELOAD)

In the spontaneously breathing healthy human a fundamental principle of normal cardiovascular physiology is the ability to balance the outputs of the left and right ventricles, and that in the event of a sudden change in either venous return or cardiac output, the balance is restored within a few heartbeats. Although the normal heart pumps

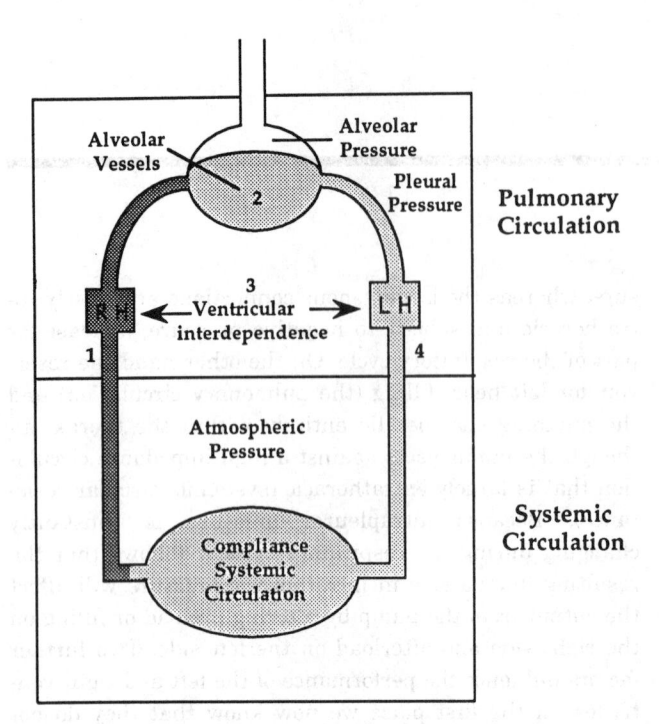

Figure 9.1. A summary of cardiopulmonary interactions represented in a two compartment model of the circulation. Both the right heart (*RH*) and left heart (*LH*) are subjected to pleural (intrathoracic) pressure, whereas the systemic vasculature is subjected to atmospheric pressure. The respiratory cycle alters cardiac output through the effect of intrathoracic pressure preload at (*1*) and afterload at (*4*) and by changing intra-alveolar pressure at (*2*). In addition, a direct interaction occurs between the right and left heart at (*3*) through ventricular interdependence.

all the blood returned to it from the venous side of the circulation, differing changes in venous return to the right atrium occur during the inspiratory and expiratory phases of respiration. Forces governing venous return and how these are influenced by respiration have been defined in Guyton's classic experiments (2). Pressure generated for return of blood flow to the heart is the driving pressure (mean systemic pressure) minus the back pressure to venous return, which in this instance is the right atrial pressure. Acute elevations in right atrial pressure result in a fall in cardiac output until compensated for by a change in compliance in the venous capacitance system. Pressure within the venous system is determined by compliance and volume of the vascular bed. With total circulatory arrest, the mean systemic pressure is 7 mm Hg on both sides of the heart (2). Negative pleural pressure occurring during a normal spontaneous inspiration produces a decrease in right atrial pressure, resulting in increased right atrial filling (Fig. 9.2). The filling pressure gradient for venous return to the right atrium is usually about 5 mm Hg, and it is determined by the difference between the extrathoracic and intrathoracic venous pressures. As negative intrathoracic pressure increases the caliber of intrathoracic veins one might suppose that a dramatic increase in venous return might occur during a rapid reduction in right atrial pressure produced by a deep inspiration. In the normal human there is flow limitation, as this augmentation of venous return by negative intrathoracic pressures is limited by the fact that venae cavae collapse at the thoracic inlet while the intrathoracic cavae are maintained patent by a series of valves. In these conditions, maximal venous return occurs at right atrial pressures of zero and that decreasing the right atrial pressure to less than zero relative to the periphery will not result in any further increase in right heart filling. Although negative pressures in relation to atmosphere can be measured in the right atrium during inspiration, transmural pressure, which is the difference between the intracavity right atrial pressure and pleural pressure, is always positive (Fig. 9.2). Similarly, the rise in intra-abdominal pressure that occurs during inspiration will result in collapse of the abdominal portion of the inferior vena cava (IVC). Where conditions of flow limitation do not exist, a rise in intra-abdominal pressure will cause an increase in venous return to the right atrium, but this rise in pressure on the IVC will result in an increase in impedance for venous return from the peripheral veins. Although these concepts are relatively straightforward, the total effect of spontaneous respiration on the right heart is somewhat more complicated. The increase in venous return to the right atrium that occurs during inspiration increases preload to the right heart but at the same time the rise in right atrial pressure decreases this gradient, so in effect differing and opposite effects occur during a single inspiratory cycle. Different rules govern venous return and right heart filling when intrathoracic pressure becomes positive. These changes will be described in the section on positive pressure respiration.

RIGHT VENTRICULAR OUTPUT

The function of the right ventricle is to pump desaturated venous blood with a high CO_2 content through what is normally a low resistance pulmonary vascular bed. Blood flow through the lung to the left atrium is sustained by the pressure differential between the pulmonary artery, the downstream pressure in the pulmonary resistance vessels, and the intracavity pressure in the left atrium. To accomplish this requires only 20 to 30 mm Hg at rest, although this can rise to 50 mm Hg with severe exercise when venous return can increase by three to four times normal (3). The morphometry of the right ventricle shows that its structure is well adapted to this function in that it

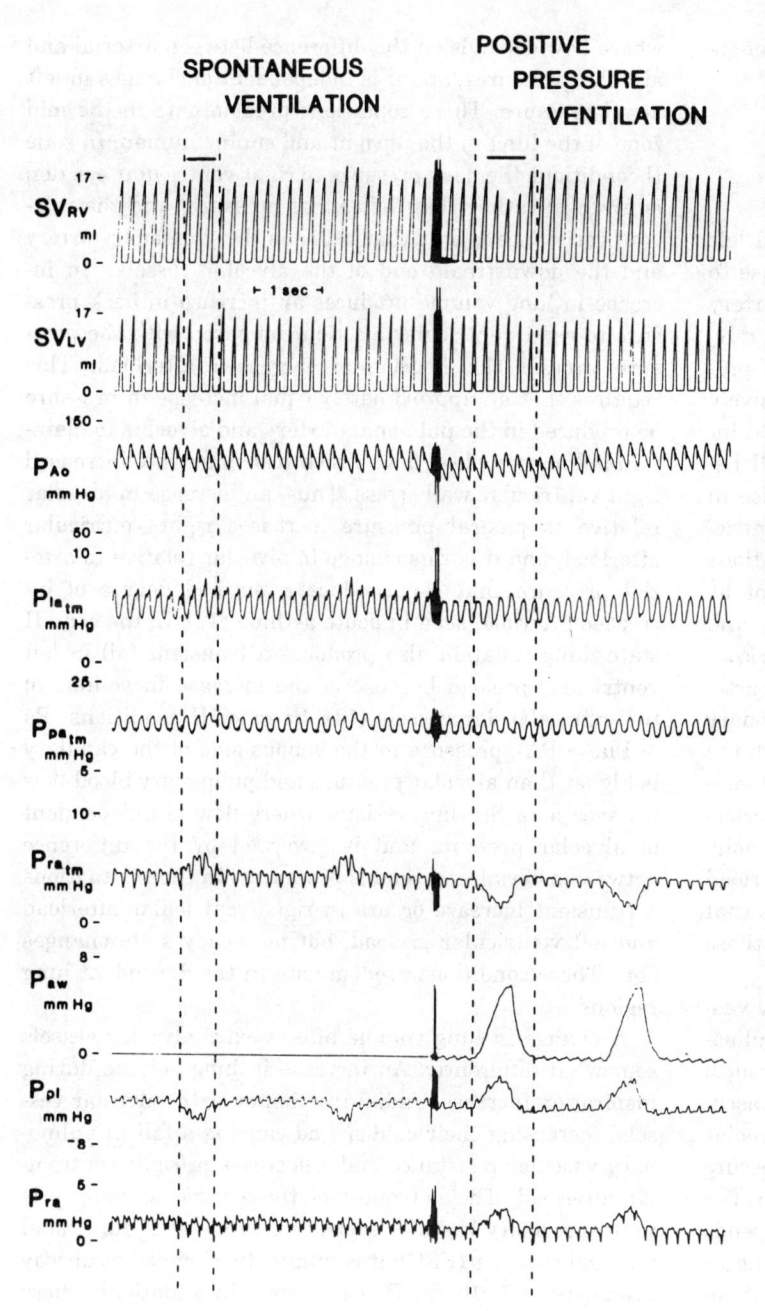

Figure 9.2. The changes in hemodynamics during the respiratory cycle associated with spontaneous and positive pressure ventilation in the normal heart. The *dashed line* indicates inspiration. The reduction in pleural pressure during inspiration in spontaneous respiration increases right atrial filling and the transmural pressure rises together with right ventricular stroke volume. A slight fall occurs in left ventricular stroke volume, which then rises at the beginning of expiration. The transmural left atrial pressure rises probably because of increased left ventricular afterload. During the inspiratory phase of positive pressure respiration venous return, transmural right atrial pressure and right ventricular stroke volume fall, but this is not reflected in the left side until late in inspiration. SVrv, right ventricular stroke volume; Svlv, left ventricular stroke volume; Pao, aortic pressure; Pla$_{tm}$, transmural left atrial pressure; Ppa$_{tm}$, transmural pulmonary artery pressure; Pra$_{tm}$, transmural right atrial pressure; Paw, alveolar pressure; Ppl, pleural pressure; Pra, right atrial pressure. (From Pinsky MR. Cardiopulmonary interactions: the effects of negative and positive changes in pleural pressure on cardiac output. In: Dantzer DR, ed. Cardiopulmonary critical care. 2nd ed. Philadelphia: WB Saunders, 1991:87–120.)

is a relatively flat, crescent-shaped, heavily trabeculated, thin-walled chamber that serves as a low pressure, high volume displacement pump. That the right ventricle and pulmonary circulation are essentially a low pressure system with the generation of modest systolic pressures has led some investigators to question the right ventricle's importance in maintaining normal circulatory homeostasis. Several studies have shown that experimental destruction of myocardium in the right ventricular free wall or its replacement (4–8) or removal of intraventricular septum (9) does not result in alteration in cardiac output or a rise in right atrial pressure. The introduction of the Fontan procedure for the surgical correction of obstructive lesions of the right heart has also shown that effective pulmonary blood flow can be sustained in the absence of a right ventricle when the pulmonary vascular resistance is not elevated. However, in diseases associated with sustained elevations in pulmonary vascular resistance, which demand an increase in driving pressure to sustain pulmonary blood flow, the right ventricle hypertrophies and undergoes an adaptation to a thick-walled pressure chamber capable of generating pressures up to and above systemic levels.

PULMONARY VASCULAR BED

The pulmonary vasculature bridges the right and left heart, and it has a great capacity to dilate in response to increased pulmonary blood flow. That pulmonary artery pressure rarely rises no higher than 50 mm Hg even during severe exercise is attributable to recruitment of previously nonperfused vessels. In situations with excessively high pulmonary blood flow associated with left to right intracardiac shunting, the pulmonary vasculature will become abnormally muscularized, which results in a rise in pulmonary vascular resistance and increased right ventricular afterload. These will be increased further in situations in which either a fixed arteriolar obstruction is present, as in primary pulmonary hypertension, or in acute and chronic hypoxemia exists, although whether this vasoconstriction occurs at the level of the capillary, venule, or arteriole remains a matter of some dispute. As the pulmonary vascular resistance is both the afterload against which the right ventricle contracts as well as the preload for left ventricle filling, changes in its caliber influence the performance of both ventricles. Pulmonary circulation is wholly intrathoracic; therefore, both right ventricular afterload and left ventricular preload are modulated by forces that change intrathoracic pressure, more particularly those pressures produced by changing lung volume.

To examine the effect of respiration on pulmonary vascular resistance it has been convenient to think of pulmonary vessels as being divided into two functional groups: those that behave as if they were exposed to an extravascular pressure that reflects pleural pressure (extra-alveolar vessels) and those exposed to an extravascular pressure that reflects alveolar pressure (intra-alveolar vessels). The change in blood flow in the intra-alveolar vessels depends on their position within the different zones of the lung as outlined by West and Dollery (10) who defined the relationship between pressures in the alveolus (PA) and pulmonary artery (Pa) and left atrium (Pla). Where zone I (lung apex) conditions apply pressure within the arterial end of the vessel is less than alveolar pressure (PA > Pa > Pla) and is therefore insufficient to open the vessels, which remain collapsed. Behavior of these vessels can be described in terms of a Starling resistor where no flow occurs regardless of left atrial pressure (11). These conditions exist in the uppermost parts of the lung in the upright human or in the superior part of the lung when supine. Where zone II conditions apply (Pa > PA > Pla), arterial pressure is higher than alveolar and the intra-alveolar vessels behave as Starling resistors surrounded by alveolar pressure where flow depends on the difference between arterial and alveolar pressures, and it is independent of changes in left atrial pressure. These conditions predominate in the mid zone of the lung in the upright and supine human. In zone II conditions the back pressure to right ventricular ejection is alveolar rather than left atrial pressure, and the relevant resistance is only that between the pulmonary artery and the downstream end of the alveolar vessels. An increase in lung volume produces an increase in back pressure to right ventricular ejection compared with the pressure around the heart and increased afterload. This requires that an approximately equal increase in pressure be produced in the pulmonary artery and alveolus to maintain pulmonary blood flow, which translates into increased right ventricular wall stress. Thus, an increase in alveolar relative to pleural pressure increases right ventricular afterload, and it is this change in alveolar relative to arterial pressure that can produce a marked degree of increased afterload seen in acute asthma (12). In the zone II state, lung inflation also produces a transient fall in left ventricular preload because of the increase in volume of the extra-alveolar vessels (13). In zone III conditions (Pa > Pla > PA), pressure in the venous side of the capillary is higher than alveolar pressure and pulmonary blood flow behaves as a Starling resistor where flow is independent of alveolar pressure and is governed by the difference between arterial and venous pressures. In these situations a transient increase occurs in right ventricular afterload and left ventricular preload, but no steady state changes (14). These conditions predominate in the dependent lung regions.

A change in lung volume affects extra-alveolar vessels somewhat differently. An increase in lung volume during inspiration increases radial traction on extra-alveolar vessels, increasing their caliber and causing a fall in pulmonary vascular resistance and a decrease in right ventricular afterload. The net effect of these various changes is that pulmonary vascular resistance is lowest at functional residual capacity (FRC); it is minimally changed at airway pressures of 5–10 cm H_2O and rises in situations where vessels are compressed during lung collapse or lung overdistention (15). Loss of FRC, for instance, as seen with pulmonary edema or atelectasis, results in a rise in pulmonary vascular resistance, as will lung overdistention due to airway obstruction or high peak airway pressure ventilation that puts the lung on the flat portion of the pressure volume curve. In this situation zone I conditions would predominate throughout the lung (PA > Pa > Pla), and pulmonary vascular resistance would be increased. Changes in transpulmonary pressure will have the same effect on pulmonary vascular resistance, whether they are produced by positive or negative changes in pleural pressure.

THE RIGHT VENTRICLE

Although the right and left ventricles function as circulations in series, structure and function of one intimately affects the other. The two chambers differ in terms of their morphometry, but the function of one ventricle is related to the other by muscle fibers that encircle both chambers, a common deformable septum, and the pericardium that surrounds them both. This symbiotic relationship has been termed "ventricular interdependence" and it affects both systolic and diastolic functions.

The right ventricle can be considered to be made up of four anatomically distinct components: 1) right ventricle free wall, 2) septal wall, anchored to the left ventricle, 3) inflow portion of the cavity, and 4) outflow portion. Contraction of the right ventricle is anything but homogeneous, and it functions like two different chambers connected in series. The heavily trabeculated inflow portion at the apex is electrically activated, and it contracts before the outflow tract giving rise to an almost peristaltic action when visualized angiographically. It is integrated with the left ventricle by being directly attached to the septal wall and by an anatomic attachment of muscle fibers between the free walls of both chambers. The close anatomic arrangement of the right ventricle with the left in fact enhances the efficiency of its contraction. Continuity of muscle fibers between the two free walls means that they are pulling together toward a common center of gravity, thereby enhancing contraction (16). Right ventricular ejection is also enhanced by left ventricular contraction. Isolated heart studies have shown that increasing left ventricular volume increases the pressure generated by the right ventricle (17–19). In addition, angiographic studies have shown rightward displacement of either a normal muscular or artificial septum associated with left ventricular contraction (9, 20–23). The geometry of the right ventricle is entirely different from that of the left ventricle as can be seen when comparing the two chambers in cross section. The right ventricle is crescent shaped, whereas the left has an entirely different configuration with a structure that conforms well with its function. It is thick walled and ellipsoid in shape, which allows for an efficient and homogeneous contraction capable of generating high pressures. Although the intraventricular septum forms a common boundary between the two chambers, functionally it can be considered an extension of the left ventricular free wall because the muscle fiber alignment closely resembles that part of the heart (22) and makes an important contribution to left ventricular systolic ejection. A common septum may further influence the function of one ventricle in conjunction with the other. The septum acts as a fixation point for the right ventricular free wall, and, as it contracts, it shifts in relation to the different diastolic pressures in either chamber. Depending on its radius of curvature, this can either help or hinder right ventricular ejection. Septum conformation also aids systolic ejection of the right ventricle by anchoring the free wall and thereby creating a radial force that draws it toward the septum. The position and curvature of the septum is determined by the balance of forces between the two chambers. Normally, high pressures within the left ventricular chamber create an axial force that results in bowing of the septum toward the right ventricle during systole, whereas the radial forces produced by the alignment of muscle fibers within the septum predominate in the direction of the left ventricular free wall. Any acute change in either the volume or pressure of the right ventricle can result in shift in septal position, which alters the distensibility of the left ventricle, thereby decreasing it's compliance. In extreme situations it can have an adverse effect on left ventricular function, leading to the erroneous assumption that the left ventricle is also abnormal. This can be particularly pronounced in advanced pulmonary vascular disease where it is not uncommon for pressures in the right ventricle to approach or even exceed systemic pressures. In this situation, the septal muscle hypertrophies and its motion is altered (24). Leftward deviation of the septum, especially at the base of the right ventricle, can result in encroachment on the left ventricular outflow tract and compromise its function. This may be part of the explanation for the acute falls in cardiac output and development of pulmonary edema occasionally seen with the use of vasodilator therapy in pulmonary hypertension. Similar distortions in ventricular geometry are seen in patients with cor pulmonale and right ventricular enlargement.

In addition to ventricular interdependence produced by a shared septum, common myocardial muscle, and the intact pericardium, direct mechanical compression of the chambers from inflation and deflation of the lung (mechanical heart-lung interactions) also affect left ventricular function. Santamore et al. (25) have shown a decrease in left ventricular diastolic volume and an increase in right ventricular volume during a spontaneous inspiration. In the isolated heart Janicki et al. (26) demonstrated that if left ventricular end-diastolic volume is held constant while right ventricular end-diastolic volume is increased then left ventricular end-diastolic pressure will rise. Therefore, if left ventricular filling pressure remains constant during an acute distention of the right ventricle, then the stroke volume of the left ventricle will decrease. This diastolic interdependence is thought to be responsible for the decrease in left ventricular stroke volume seen during spontaneous respiration. Studies in intact humans and experimental animals, on the other hand, have shown that, although diastolic compliance of the left ventricle is altered by septal wall shift during right ventricular filling, this does not affect systolic function in the absence of cardiopulmonary disease (27). Robotham (28) has suggested that the change in right ventricular volume that is seen to occur as a consequence of diastolic interdependence during negative intrathoracic pressure, as well as an acute change in left ventricular afterload, contribute to the decrease in left ventricular stroke volume and the increase in end-diastolic pressure seen with inspiration. The corollary of this is the finding of systolic interdependence. As the right ventricular volume rises the end-systolic volume of the left ventricle decreases (29), indicating that the left ventricular stroke volume is maintained. Thus, systolic interdependence is a compensatory mechanism for the reduction in left ventricular output due to diastolic interdependence (30).

The pericardium can also limit acute changes in chamber size and influence cardiac function both directly and indirectly through the mechanism of ventricular interdependence. In the normal situation, the pericardium has some minor influence on both diastolic and systolic function of the ventricles in that ventricular interaction is enhanced during diastole by transmission of pressures throughout the myocardium. Any influence that the pericardium may have on function of either ventricle is related to a change in transmural pressure across the wall of the myocardium, which in this instance is the difference between intracavity and intrapleural pressure. Therefore, changes in intrapericardial pressure cannot be examined in isolation without making reference to pressure changes in the thorax produced by respiration. In situations wherein intrapericardial pressure increases, as in the dilated failing heart or with the development of pericardial fluid accumulation, major alterations can occur in systolic and diastolic performance of both ventricles. However, constraint on ventricular function because of changes in intrapericardial pressure will always be more pronounced in diastole compared with systole. Development of pericardial effusion will interfere with diastolic filling, and the greater the effusion and the more rapidly it develops, the greater will be the compromise to ventricular function (31). Intrapericardial pressure also contributes to ventricular interdependence, being increased in situations of cardiac tamponade (32) and reduced following pericardectomy (33). As most coronary blood flow occurs during diastole, pericardial constraint on the right ventricular free wall can limit coronary perfusion in situations where the ventricle has hypertrophied (34, 35). This seems to be particularly important in situations of right ventricular failure where the dilated failing heart is constrained within the pericardial cavity, resulting in a rise in intrapericardial pressure and interference with diastolic filling. Goldstein et al. (36) have shown that following right ventricular failure produced by infarction, intrapericardial pressure rises and left ventricular filling decreases. This impairment of diastolic function was confirmed to be caused by an alteration in the diastolic pressure-volume relationship of the ventricle, which could be relieved by pericardiotomy (37). The effect of pericardial constraint on cardiac function has also been demonstrated after open heart surgery, particularly in situations where right ventricular failure is compromised by the development of pulmonary hypertension (38). The mechanical constraint on diastolic function produced by intrathoracic pressure provides the rational basis for the practice of either delaying sternal closure or reopening the sternum in the postoperative period in situations of increased myocardial edema following cardiopulmonary bypass (39).

LEFT VENTRICLE

The left ventricle differs from the right in its anatomic configuration, being a thick-walled, spherical chamber capable of supporting high systemic pressures. Systolic function of the left ventricle is governed by contractility, heart rate, and afterload forces against which it contracts, defined as the "systolic wall stress." This consists of aortic pressure and the forces acting across the chamber wall. In the normal situation, wherein no gradient exists between left ventricle and aortic pressure, wall stress is the major component of left ventricular afterload, and it correlates well with left ventricular end-systolic volume (40, 41). Preload for filling of the left ventricle comes from pulmonary venous return and left atrial filling, and because this reservoir and the chamber itself lie within the thorax, both preload and afterload for the left ventricle can be said to be influenced by changes in intrathoracic pressure.

Changes in intrathoracic pressure produced by respiration have important and hitherto underemphasized effects on left ventricular function, which become significant in the failing heart. To evaluate the significance of these various forces and the effect of positive or negative intrathoracic pressure on left ventricular preload and afterload it is important to understand the changes in cardiac output and heart function secondary to respiration.

The most commonly observed change in left heart function that occurs with spontaneous respiration is an initial a fall in arterial pressure during inspiration caused by a decrease in left ventricular stroke volume (28) (Fig. 9.2). Reasons for this have been largely attributed to events occurring on the right side of the circulation and include (a) pooling of blood in the pulmonary circulation because of lung expansion, (b) a phase lag between right and left ventricular output, (c) stimulation of systemic baroreceptors or pulmonary stretch receptors, and (d) right ventricle filling causing a change in left ventricular diastolic compliance or ejection mediated through ventricular interdependence. If left atrial and ventricular diastolic pressures were measured relative to atmosphere then a fall in these pressures could be demonstrated during inspiration, which would support the concept that the principal cause of the decrease in left sided output during inspiration was pooling of blood in the lungs secondary to lung expansion. However, it has been shown that during inspiration in both the intact animal and the isolated lung preparation, pulmonary venous return actually increases at the same time that left ventricular stroke volume is falling (42, 43). This apparent paradox is explained when these pressures are related to intrapleural pressure where it can be shown that transmural (intracavity minus intrapleural) filling pressures on the left side actually increase during inspiration (44, 45) (Fig. 9.2). Thus it is more valid to define the afterload as being the left ventricular transmural pressure, which in this instance is the intracavity pressure minus the intrapleural pressure (Fig. 9.3). Although studies of pulmonary transit time have shown that it takes one to two cardiac cycles for a change in right-sided output to be reflected in the left side (46, 47), the phase lag theory is unlikely to fully explain the decrease in left ventricular ejection associated with a reduction in intrathoracic pressure. In experiments where preload through the pulmonary circulation was maintained constant by replacing the right ventricle with roller pump in close chested, spontaneously breathing dogs, stroke volume still declined during inspiration (48). This finding does not mean that changes in output of the right side of the heart must not at some stage affect the left side as the two circulations are connected in series, which accounts for the observation that blood pressure and left ventricular stroke volume may rise after an initial fall (49). In this situation the increase in venous return eventually overrides the other factors that tend to impede left ventricular output. Neural receptors that have been suggested to influence left ventricular function include stretch receptors in the lung mediated via the vagus nerve and intra and extrathoracic baroreceptors that are mediated by the autonomic system. Reliable experimental data suggest that neither of these is likely to be a major mechanism in the fall of left-sided output. Robotham et al. (48) found significant falls in left ventricular stroke volume still occurring in vagotomized animals during a Müller maneuver (inspiratory effort against a closed glottis), where intrapleural pressure falls but lung volume remains unchanged. A decrease in left ventricular stroke volume during inspiration is still seen even after autonomic blockade of vagal and sympathetic efferent nerves. Diastolic ventricular interdependence does influence left ventricular preload but any reduction is offset by the increased left ventricular output because of systolic interdependence (50).

Abundant experimental and clinical evidence indicates that negative intrathoracic pressure has a significant inhibitory effect on left ventricular ejection by increasing afterload, and that this is particularly important in the failing heart. This increase in afterload can become even more pronounced in situations of decreased lung compliance such as pulmonary edema or lung disease where increasingly negative swings in intrathoracic pressure occur. The observation afterload increases with negative intrathoracic pressure has been confirmed by studies of left ventricular function during spontaneous breathing with increased inspiratory loads, which demonstrated that both left ventricular end-diastolic and end-systolic volumes are increased (49, 51). However this occurs independently of changes in lung volume as has been demonstrated in experiments showing that afterload was found to increase during a Müller maneuver where negative swings in intrathoracic pressure are associated with no change in lung volume (45). Brinker et al. (52) and Guzman et al. (53) have confirmed septal wall displacement during the Müller

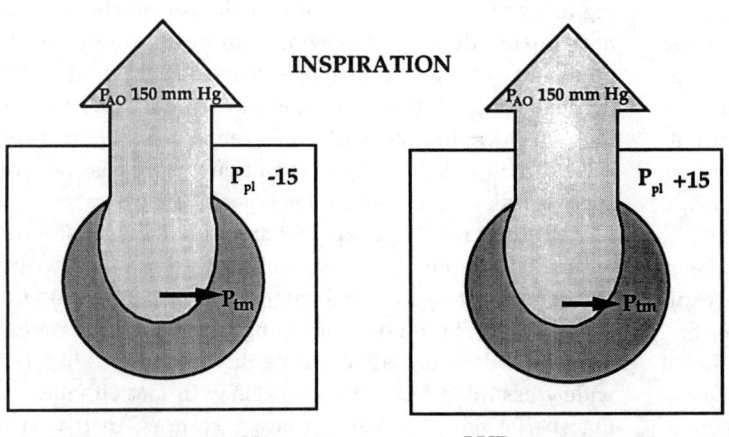

Figure 9.3. The change in left ventricular afterload as represented by the systolic transmural pressure ($LVtmsyst$) with the same systemic pressure during spontaneous inspiration at -15 mm Hg pleural pressure (P_{pl}) and positive pressure inspiration at $+15$ mm Hg. The increase in intrathoracic pressure associated with positive pressure ventilation results in a reduction in left ventricular afterload. Pao, aortic pressure.

maneuver that was associated with decreased diastolic compliance and volume of the left ventricle. Sustained decreases in intrathoracic pressure have also been shown clinically to result in mild degrees of left ventricular dysfunction when associated with ischemic heart disease (54). Because the generation of large negative intrathoracic pressures can impede both diastolic and systolic performance of the left ventricle it is not surprising that this occasionally results in acute left ventricular failure and pulmonary edema. This has been well documented during acute upper airway obstruction occurring with laryngospasm during anesthesia (55–57) and with croup and epiglottitis (58–60). It can also occur following the relief of upper airway obstruction (61) and during status asthmaticus where at the peak of inspiration negative intrathoracic pressures of up to −40 cm H_2O can be produced (62).

Changes in lung volume also affect left ventricular function independent of the change in intrathoracic pressure. Lung expansion changes pulmonary venous system capacitance, thereby altering pulmonary blood flow depending on the underlying pulmonary blood volume and vascular tone (13, 63). Increasing lung volume also restricts cardiac filling in a similar fashion to cardiac tamponade by encroachment of the lung on the cardiac fossa (64). This can have important implications in positive pressure ventilation in status asthmaticus where overinflation of the lung caused by rapid respiratory rates and inadequate expiratory time can result in low output and cardiac arrest. The overall effect of a negative intrathoracic pressure on left ventricular function is therefore a balance between its effect on the preload and left ventricular systolic ejection (afterload) (65, 66).

SPONTANEOUS RESPIRATION AND ABNORMAL HEART FUNCTION

Left Ventricular Failure

In the normal individual a decrease in intrathoracic pressure tends to both augment cardiac output by increased systemic venous return and diminish it by increasing left ventricular afterload, the net result being a balance between these opposite effects. Whether the increase in afterload on the left ventricle becomes hemodynamically significant depends on the underlying pump function. If ventricular function is normal, the negative intrathoracic pressure associated with spontaneous breathing will result in little or no significant hemodynamic change (67, 68). Some of the studies that have examined the magnitude of the afterload effect produced by increased negative or positive intrathoracic pressure have tended to underestimate its significance because of different methods of measuring afterload. Considering the left ventricle in isolation, in situations wherein a major change in intrathoracic pressure is associated with increasing negative intrapleural pressures secondary to lung disease or positive intrapleural pressures secondary to mechanical ventilation, aortic pressure does not reflect left ventricular afterload. This was confirmed in a study by Buda et al. of patients (69) in whom ventricular volumes were measured and plotted against aortic pressure and transmural aortic pressure (aortic pressure minus intrapleural pressure). Physiologically more consistent function curves for the left ventricular ejection were obtained when transmural pressure was used for the pressure load for left ventricular ejection. If the left ventricular filling pressure is unchanged, similar changes in left ventricular afterload can result from either reducing aortic pressure by vasodilator therapy or increasing intrathoracic pressure if the net result is no change in transmural pressure. Although acute impairment of left ventricular ejection associated with the generation of large negative intrathoracic pressures can be demonstrated when ventricular function is normal (49, 51, 69), only comparatively recently has it been shown in the presence of left ventricular failure. Rasanen et al. (70) showed that changing from spontaneous to positive pressure breathing in patients with myocardial infarction resulted in a decrease in the pattern of injury seen on the electrocardiogram (ECG), and they subsequently confirmed that the myocardial sparing only occurred when the negative swings in intrathoracic pressure were abolished (71, 72). Similarly Beach et al. (73) described a series of patients with left ventricular failure supported with positive pressure ventilation who could not tolerate weaning to spontaneous ventilation until left ventricular function was improved with inotropic support. Based on these findings, we can conclude that in patients with overt cardiac failure or borderline left ventricular function, the increased afterload associated with the negative intrathoracic pressure generated during spontaneous respiration will result in worsening heart failure. Furthermore, in situations where pulmonary edema develops following myocardial infarction, the pulmonary venous congestion and alveolar flooding that occur leads to a fall in lung compliance, which translates into increased respiratory work and greater negative intrathoracic pressure. Under these conditions using positive pressure ventilation or continuous positive airway pressure (CPAP) may result in rapid improvement in the situation with interruption of the cycle of increasingly negative intrathoracic pressure producing an ever-decreasing lung compliance. Therefore, increasing intrathoracic pressure, far from adversely affecting cardiac output as has been widely assumed for many years, may in fact enhance cardiac performance in certain circumstances. Increased intrathoracic pressure, therefore, has differing effects on left ventricular ejection depending on whether function is normal or compromised.

Congenital Heart Disease

Congenital heart disease in children frequently produces changes within the lung and results in respiratory symptoms that sometimes make it difficult to distinguish whether the primary disease process is within the lung or heart. Lesions that produce abnormal patterns of pulmonary blood flow through the lungs can produce changes in mechanics that can both mimic lung disease and, by increasing respiratory work and oxygen consumption, aggravate heart failure. The extent of these changes depend on whether pulmonary blood flow is increased, as in the situation of a left-to-right intracardiac shunt, or decreased in right-to-left shunts. The combination of increased pulmonary blood flow and pulmonary hypertension is well recognized to produce severe respiratory symptoms (74). Respiratory distress and atelectasis in the spontaneously breathing child can result from compression of the large bronchi by an enlarged left atrium or pulmonary artery dilation. The left atrium lies immediately inferior to both main stem bronchi, and the left main stem bronchus, left upper lobe bronchus, and right middle lobe bronchus are the most common sites of obstruction (75). Infantile lobar emphysema has also been described in association with pulmonary stenosis (74). Rabinovitch et al. (76) described compression of large bronchi by dilated main pulmonary arteries and compression of intrapulmonary bronchi by tufts of abnormal pulmonary vessels in the tetralogy with absent pulmonary valve syndrome. Any of these abnormalities can result in lobar atelectasis, emphysema, intermittent attacks of wheezing, and blood gas abnormalities. These respiratory symptoms are more likely to occur after the first 2 months of life, when the pulmonary vascular resistance drops and left-to-right shunting increases and before the end of the first year, when the airways become more cartilaginous and less liable to compression (75). In addition to compression of large airways, children with left-to-right shunts can be susceptible to bronchiolar narrowing because of the high flows and pulmonary venous pressure producing interstitial and alveolar edema. Hordof et al. (77) described clinical and radiologic manifestations of peripheral airways obstruction in infants with ventricular septal defect (VSD) associated with increased pulmonary to systemic flow ratios, which regressed with closure of the defect. Motoyama et al. (78) demonstrated an increased airways resistance measured by expiratory flow volumes in patients with large right-to-left shunts prior to corrective cardiac surgery. These changes were reversed following closure of the defect (78).

The importance of the association between increases in pulmonary vascular reactivity and increased airways resistance has been demonstrated in children undergoing corrective surgery for congenital heart disease. Motoyama et al. (79) measured forced expiratory flows (FEF) in children under general anesthesia at the time of corrective cardiac surgery. They found that increased pulmonary blood flow (PBF), secondary to left-to-right shunts, was associated with a decrease in FEF75. Furthermore, when they performed a morphometric analysis on lung biopsy material taken at the time of surgery they observed that patients with grade B morphometric changes (Rabinovitch) showed prominent smooth muscle hypertrophy and narrowing of the lumen of alveolar ducts and respiratory bronchioles. Schindler et al. (80) demonstrated that rises in pulmonary artery pressure in the postoperative period are associated with marked increases in measured airways resistance and that smooth muscle is increased in the airways of these children. Those observations may explain the finding of a sudden episodes of bronchospasm commonly seen in patients who develop rapid rises in pulmonary artery pressure following corrective cardiac surgery for lesions such as VSD and arteroventricular (AV) septal defect. It is likely that some of the bronchoconstrictor responses seen in pulmonary hypertension may be mediated, at least in part, by the leukotriene products of arachidonic metabolism. Leukotrienes C4 and D4, mediators of bronchoconstriction in asthma, have recently been shown to be present in large quantities in the lung lavage fluid of infants with persistent pulmonary hypertension (PPH) (81).

Changes in lung compliance are also seen in congenital cardiac disease (82–84). Bancalari et al. (82) found that both total and specific lung compliance were significantly lower in children with congenital heart disease, in whom increased pulmonary blood flow was seen, compared with lesions with a normal or decreased pulmonary blood flow. When pulmonary blood flow was increased but pulmonary artery pressure was normal, compliance was unchanged, suggesting that it was the pressure level rather than the increased flow within the lung that actually caused the alteration in compliance. Decreased pulmonary compliance has also been described in newborn infants with persistent pulmonary hypertension (85). It is these changes in compliance that are responsible for the increased respiratory rate and decreased tidal volume seen during spontaneous respiration in children with left-to-right intracardiac shunts (86). In the infant and small child with a highly compliant chest wall this is frequently associated with chest wall retraction and intercostal recession. With increasing age these become less prominent as pulmonary vascular resistance rises secondary to increased flow and left-to-right shunting diminishes.

POSITIVE INTRATHORACIC PRESSURE AND CARDIAC FUNCTION

Normal Heart

With the introduction of positive pressure ventilation it was recognized from the very outset that major effects on hemodynamics were associated with its use. Cournaud (87) first showed the association between decreased cardiac output and increased airway pressure in normal humans more than 40 years ago. The explanation for this finding was that increased intrathoracic pressure is transmitted to the systemic venous system, which reduced caval blood flow and the gradient for right atrial filling. This finding has been confirmed since then in numerous studies showing that in the absence of cardiopulmonary disease positive intrathoracic pressure reduces cardiac output in the normovolemic and more especially in the hypovolemic state through the mechanism of decreased venous return (2, 88–92). However, the effects of positive pressure ventilation on cardiac function in disease states are much more complex when applied in the setting of cardiopulmonary disease, where changes in lung mechanics, pulmonary vascular resistance, or ventricular function can modify hemodynamic responses. To understand these differences it is important to examine the complex cardiopulmonary interactions that occur in the normal state with positive intrathoracic pressure.

With a rise in intrathoracic pressure, at the same time that systemic venous return decreases, the increase in pleural pressure causes the right ventricle volume to decrease because of the decreased transmural right atrial pressure, which in turn leads to a fall in right ventricular stroke volume (Fig. 9.2). In the normovolemic, and to a greater extent hypovolemic state, the pulmonary venous blood flow to the left atrium falls significantly, whereas in the hypervolemic state pulmonary venous return would be increased because of augmented antegrade flow. These same principles have also been shown to apply when the increase in pleural pressure occurs without a change in lung volume as in Valsalva's maneuver (93–95). What has been less widely appreciated is that in the normal situation an initial increase occurs in both aortic pressure and left ventricular output early in the inspiratory phase of positive pressure ventilation before falling toward the end of inspiration (91, 96, 97) and that this increase in aortic pressure is more pronounced at faster respiratory rates (91) (Fig. 9.4). In contrast, changes in respiratory rate have little effect on pulmonary artery flow, which declines during inspiration and rises during expiration (91). It therefore appears that increased pleural pressure will have different effects on both the right and left ventricle output at different phases of the respiratory cycle where a fall in pulmonary artery flow and rise in pulmonary artery pressure are seen at the same time as a rise occurs in both

pressure and flow in the aorta early in the inspiratory phase of positive pressure ventilation. These differing effects require more detailed analysis. Among the theories that have been advanced to account for these differences are a phase lag due to pulmonary transit time, reduction in left ventricular afterload associated with positive pleural pressure, increased left ventricular preload because of forward flow of pulmonary venous blood caused by lung expansion, and increased left ventricular compliance due to ventricular interdependence. That pulmonary transit time has little or no bearing on the asynchrony between right and left ventricles has been demonstrated in the intact animal by Robotham et al. (98). In these experiments in which right ventricle output was replaced by a roller pump to maintain a constant left-sided preload, aortic flow still increased during the early phase of inspiration despite the elimination of the variation in right ventricular output. In a further series of experiments in open chest animals, where pleural pressure is no longer a factor, and with the right ventricle decompressed, eliminating the ventricular interdependence factor, Robotham and Mitzner also showed that the application of positive pressure to the lung still resulted in increased left ventricular output (99). They were also able to demonstrate that following a sustained inspiration with a constant flow into the pulmonary artery,

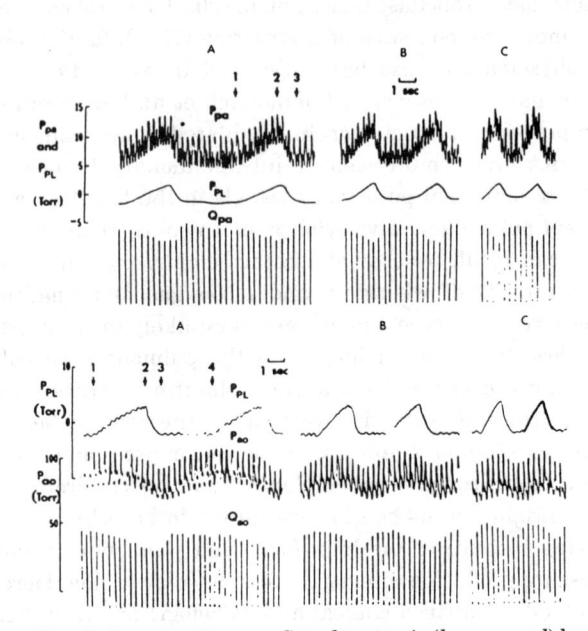

Figure 9.4. Pulmonary (*top panel*) and systemic (*lower panel*) hemodynamic changes associated with positive pressure ventilation in the anesthetized dog at (**A**) slow, (**B**) medium, and (**C**) fast respiratory rates. Pulmonary artery pressure and flow increase with the rise in pleural pressure associated with inspiration. At the same time aortic pressure and flow fall, reaching a minimum early in expiration (**A**). With increasing respiratory rates aortic pressure and flow increase during inspiration, reaching a minimum late in expiration. P_{pa}, pulmonary artery pressure; P_{pl}, pleural pressure; Q_{pa}, pulmonary arterial flow; Q_{ao}, aortic flow. (From Scharf SM, Brown R, Saunders N, et al. Hemodynamic effects of positive pressure inflation. J Appl Physiol 1980;49:124.)

aortic flow drops abruptly with the following inspiration and rises again with the first lung inflation following an expiratory apneic pause. The conclusion that could be drawn from these studies is that changes in lung volume and pulmonary vascular resistance are the major influences on the variation in left ventricular output.

Additional factors have been suggested to play a part in the reduced cardiac output seen with the application of positive end expiratory pressure (PEEP) in the absence of cardiopulmonary disease. These include diminished ventricular contractility and ventricular compression by lung distention (64). Rankin et al. (27) found that application of PEEP in the normal human and animal heart resulted in a fall in cardiac output because of decreased preload (venous return) and increased afterload (pulmonary vascular resistance). The net result was a decrease in left ventricular end-diastolic volume caused by decreased preload but no change in systolic right ventricular function. Several studies (48, 100, 101) have shown that left ventricular dimensions are altered by both intermittent positive pressure ventilation and PEEP in that the septal-to-free-wall and anterior-to-posterior minor axis dimensions diminish, which is consistent with an overall decrease in left ventricular end-diastolic volume. These changes tend to be more pronounced with intermittent positive pressure ventilation than with PEEP (100), and the effect is greater in the septal-to-free-wall dimension, which suggests that ventricular interdependence is the important mechanism that contributes to the decreased left ventricular preload seen with the application of PEEP. Septal-to-free-wall changes are more likely to represent laterally acting forces produced by mechanical heart-lung interactions than by actual septal wall shift per se (64, 102). PEEP, in addition to increasing pleural pressure, increases lung volume and FRC, depending on lung and chest wall compliance. If it overdistends the lung and increases pulmonary vascular resistance, an increase in right ventricular volume will occur, which will adversely affect left ventricular compliance through interventricular dependence. However, in the situation where the appropriate amount of PEEP is being used, lung volume will be recruited and the end expiratory volume will be at FRC and pulmonary vascular resistance will fall. In this situation right ventricular volume will diminish and, therefore, any decrease in left ventricular size cannot be attributed to ventricular interdependence. Clear evidence shows that the pressure within and size of the ventricular chambers can be directly affected by lung inflation. This observation has been confirmed in a study where intraventricular pressures were directly measured during intermittent positive pressure ventilation with PEEP. It was shown in this study that the intracavity pressures rose slightly at the end expiratory point and this was even more exaggerated at end inspiration, a phenomenon referred to as "heart-lung interdependence" (103). It has also been suggested that PEEP may reduce cardiac output and left ventricular stroke volume by depressing the contractile state of the left ventricle (104–107), perhaps through the release of a circulating myocardial depressant factor. The introduction of more sophisticated measurement techniques of left ventricular function has added further clarification, and no evidence supports the notion that the contractile state of the left ventricle is decreased with increased intrathoracic pressure, either in the setting of a normal lung or in acute pulmonary edema (108, 109). However, raised intrathoracic pressure does have the potential to adversely affect contractility in the setting of marginal coronary blood flow. PEEP has been reported to cause a decrease in myocardial blood flow in experimental animals (110, 111), and Tittley et al. (112) have shown that the application of 15 cm H_2O after coronary artery bypass surgery resulted in small but measurable amounts of markers of marginal coronary perfusion in half the patients without a change in ventricular function.

POSITIVE PRESSURE VENTILATION AND PEEP IN CARDIOPULMONARY DISEASE

Right Ventricle

Positive pressure ventilation and PEEP have differing effects on right ventricular function depending on the presence or absence of underlying cardiac or pulmonary disease and on the level of end expiratory pressure used. PEEP is frequently used in pulmonary failure associated with pulmonary edema and low lung compliance as a method of increasing FRC and improving oxygenation. If this were the only consideration then it would simply be a case of increasing PEEP until the best PaO_2 was achieved. However, the potential adverse effects of PEEP on right ventricular preload means that the most important therapeutic goal is the level of PEEP that gives the best combination of oxygenation and cardiac output, thereby achieving maximal oxygen delivery (oxygen content–cardiac output). This has been termed best or optimal PEEP by Suter et al. (113). In a study of patients with acute respiratory distress syndrome (ARDS) they found that the optimal PEEP level in each individual patient was that which produced the highest static lung compliance, but that this level varied between 0 and 15 cm H_2O. It is a simple exercise to apply increasing amounts of PEEP in the setting of ARDS, but to define the changes in hemodynamics produced by this therapy has proved more difficult. The magnitude of these changes depends partly on factors that influence the underlying cardiovascular status (circulating volume, ventricular dysfunction, increased pulmonary vascular resistance) and on factors within the lung that may modulate the transmission of airway (alveolar) pressure to the pleural space and therefore to heart and vascular structures. Decreased lung compliance will reduce pressure transmission (114), whereas increased thoracic compliance will enhance it (115). This is illustrated by studies showing the application of increasing increments of PEEP up to 25 cm H_2O in the setting of severe pulmonary failure with low lung compliance has not been associated with any change in right ventricular ejection even at the highest PEEP levels, although stroke volume did decrease because of reduced preload (116, 117). However in the setting of severely depressed baseline right ventricular ejection in humans, the application of PEEP has been shown to result in the depression of contractile function (118). The reason for this difference may lie in underlying right ventricular ischemia. Schulman et al. (119) have shown differing effects of PEEP before and after coronary ligation in the intact animal. In the normal heart no change occurred in right ventricular volume or systolic performance, but following right coronary artery ligation right ventricular ejection fraction declined associated with an increase in end-systolic volume. PEEP can further compromise flow in a marginal right coronary circulation because of decrease in flow associated with the rise in right ventricular systolic pressure (120, 121) and intrapericardial pressure (122). Similar observations on the differing effect of PEEP on right ventricular ejection fraction have been made in adults with ischemic heart disease after cardiopulmonary bypass (123). Patients with pronounced right coronary artery stenosis had diminished right ventricular ejection fraction and increased right ventricular end-diastolic volume, whereas no effect was seen in patients with minor coronary artery stenosis. Paradoxically, in situations where severe right ventricular failure results in profoundly low cardiac output, ventilation with high peak inflation pressures at rapid rates can result in a rapid improvement in hemodynamics. Serra et al. (124) reported a dramatic improvement in four children with profound right ventricular failure after corrective cardiac surgery when switching from conventional ventilator settings to higher frequency (50/min) high volume (tidal volume [TV] 30 mL/kg) ventilation. Increased intrathoracic pressure in this situation probably acts as a right ventricular assist device in increasing forward flow from a dilated and noncontractile right ventricle in much the same way that it produces forward flow in simultaneous ventilation compression cardiopulmonary resuscitation (CPR).

Taking all these factors into consideration, it is not unusual to see a fall in cardiac output and stroke volume with high levels of positive pressure ventilation with PEEP in ARDS. The mechanisms that have been invoked as a cause for this decrease include decreased venous return, increased right ventricular afterload, decreased left ventricular compliance, and decreased ventricular contractility. Conflicting data exist regarding the most important factors, and the interpretation depends on how various measurements were made. As is seen with positive pressure ventilation in the normal lung, the increase in pleural pressure with PEEP reduces venous return to the right atrium in ARDS (116, 117, 125). None dispute that this is a major factor in reducing right ventricular preload, which is frequently compensated for by increasing filling pressures. In patients with severe acute respiratory failure, levels of PEEP above 10 cm H_2O have been associated with a slight increase in right ventricular afterload (109, 117, 125, 126). One explanation for this is that positive pressure applied to the lung is also known to alter pulmonary vascular resistance by compressing the intra-alveolar vessels while increasing the cross-sectional diameter of extra-alveolar vessels by radial traction. The former effect will increase pulmonary vascular resistance, whereas the latter will cause a decrease. Which effect predominates depends on the underlying condition of the lung. Jardin et al. (127) have shown that pulmonary vascular resistance increases with positive intrathoracic pressure in humans with normal lungs, thereby increasing right ventricular afterload. However, in the setting of acute respiratory failure, underlying pulmonary vascular resistance is increased (128) and compliance is reduced. These changes will modify the effect of positive pressure ventilation as only part of the increased airway pressure will be transmitted to the pleural space (115). This was confirmed in a subsequent study by Jardin et al. that examined the effect on right ventricular function of changes in intrathoracic pressure at different phases of the respiratory cycle produced by positive pressure ventilation in patients with ARDS. Right ventricular ejection fraction decreased while diastolic volume increased during inspiration because of increased right ventricular wall stress or afterload (129).

Positive pressure ventilation with high PEEP also affects left ventricular output through the mechanism of ventricular interdependence. At very high PEEP levels (over 25 cm H_2O) lung inflation will significantly increase right ventricular afterload. This flattens and leftward shifts the intraventricular septum, which in turn encroaches on left ventricular filling and reduces left ventricular preload (69, 126, 130). These changes are frequently compensated for by expansion of circulating volume, which by increasing right ventricular preload, can compensate for right ventricular overloading by increasing myocardial segment length (109, 117, 125, 126, 131, 132). Decreased ventricular compliance caused by direct mechanical heart-lung interaction from lung inflation has also been advanced as an explanation of the decrease in left ventricular preload in ARDS (110, 133), which would reduce diastolic compliance and impede filling. However, more sophisticated techniques using direct measurements of pressure at the surface of the heart has shown little change in compliance (134). Finally, although data in experimental animals would suggest that PEEP reduces myocardial contractility (106, 111), human studies of patients with ARDS do not support this finding

(125, 135). On the contrary, Jardin et al. (126) have shown an increase in contractility with PEEP in ARDS. The situation can be different, e.g., with underlying coronary ischemia, where contractility can be adversely affected by the addition of PEEP. The effect of PEEP in left ventricular afterload in ARDS is similar to that in normal lungs in that a reduction occurs in left ventricular transmural pressure. In summary, with positive pressure ventilation at moderate levels of PEEP (5–15 cm H_2O) in ARDS, decreased venous return is the most important mechanism leading to a decreased cardiac output.

Depending on the underlying lung compliance, patients who can maintain adequate spontaneous ventilation in ARDS with continuous positive airways pressure (CPAP) may achieve better oxygenation for the same level of PEEP with less adverse hemodynamic effect and, therefore, better oxygen delivery because of the lower mean airway pressures (136–139). Dhainaut et al. (139) have observed that when patients were changed from spontaneous respiration to CPAP in ARDS a decrease was seen in right ventricular end-systolic and end-diastolic volumes, suggesting a fall in right ventricular afterload. Jardin et al. (127) observed the opposite effects in normal subjects without lung disease. The explanation for this discrepancy lies in when FRC is normal, pulmonary vascular resistance is at its lowest and right ventricular afterload is minimal. CPAP application in normal individuals increases lung volume above FRC and compresses the extra-alveolar vessels, thereby increasing right ventricular afterload. In ARDS, FRC is considerably reduced and pulmonary vascular resistance is increased at these low lung volumes, a situation that can be reversed by the application of CPAP. Dhainaut et al. (139) also demonstrated during CPAP both cardiac output and oxygen consumption decrease but that with volume expansion cardiac output increases while oxygen consumption remains low, suggesting decreased oxygen demand. They suggested that the explanation for the reduced demand is the reduction in oxygen consumed by the work of breathing following CPAP application.

As with the well known effect of pH on pulmonary vascular resistance, additional evidence exists of a beneficial effect of positive pressure on lung mechanics that helps in controlling pulmonary artery pressure. Mechanical ventilation by stretching the lung releases prostaglandins (140, 141), which cause pulmonary vasodilation and help explain the rapid reductions in pulmonary artery pressure that are seen immediately after the onset of hyperventilation before there has been any time for a change in $PaCO_2$. In addition, in patients with abnormal right ventricle function and normal lungs a reduction of the transmitted airway pressure from mechanical ventilation may cause a decrease in pulmonary vascular resistance and reduce the afterload on the right ventricle. Kocis et al. (142) have shown that switching from conventional to jet ventilation in patients following the Fontan procedure, at matched $PaCO_2$ levels a substantial decrease occurred in mean airway pressure associated with a 59% reduction pulmonary vascular resistance and a 25% increase in cardiac output. Changes in lung volume may also account for the abrupt rises in pulmonary artery pressure when weaning from mechanical ventilation to CPAP. Jenkins et al. (143) have shown that when weaning from low intermittent mandatory ventilation (IMV) setting to CPAP in a group of children following cardiac surgery FRC falls and pulmonary artery pressure and pulmonary vascular resistance rise, especially in children with underlying pulmonary hypertension. Studies in newborn infants following corrective surgery for congenital heart disease show that compliance is low in the postoperative period and the application of CPAP frequently results in improvements in FRC and PaO_2 (144, 145).

Left Ventricle

Although substantial experimental and human evidence shows that in the setting of normal cardiac function preload factors are the predominant forces responsible for respiratory variation in left ventricular function during positive pressure ventilation, with or without PEEP, and that these can be compensated for by volume infusion (87, 125, 131, 146), the situation is clearly different with a failing left ventricle. Abundant clinical data show that increased pleural pressure in the setting of left ventricular failure can result in improved cardiac output by decreasing afterload (147, 148). The extreme example of this would be the discovery that during ventricular fibrillation wherein no left ventricular function output occurs, raising pleural pressure by coughing results in forward blood flow out of the thorax by a combination of the direct effect on the heart and great vessels as well as decreased afterload. This phenomenon is commonly referred to as "cough CPR" (149). Some of the most interesting insights into the effects of intrathoracic pressure elevation in the setting of left ventricular failure come from the work of Pinsky et al. (150). In their animal model left ventricular failure was induced with large doses of beta blockade while adequate venous return was maintained by volume infusion. To study the effects of large increases in intrathoracic pressure on cardiac function without overdistending the lung and causing increased pulmonary vascular resistance and pulmonary barotrauma, they reduced thoracic cage compliance by applying a thoracoabdominal binder (150). Tidal volumes of 35 mL/kg were used to produce a "phasic high intrathoracic pressure support" ventilation (PHIPS). The study showed an improvement in both left and right ventricular function curves with increased intrathoracic pressure, a finding they attributed to a decrease in left ventricular wall stress analogous to the use of vasodilator therapy in congestive heart failure. The same technique was applied to a group of patients with cardiogenic shock, and when conventional ventilator settings were changed to a PHIPS technique cardiac output and mean arterial pressure improved (151). Although it is clear that these large changes in intrathoracic pressure augment cardiac output in the failing heart, the mechanism responsible for this action is a balance between the effect on left ventricular preload and afterload. Large changes in lung volume will affect intra and extra-alveolar blood volume (13) and result in increased forward flow in a manner analogous to cough CPR. At the same time increased intrathoracic pressure will reduce left ventricular afterload. These differing mechanisms were studied in a further series of experiments by Pinsky et al. (88) where they varied respiratory frequency, percent inspiratory time, mean, and swings in intrathoracic pressure using a jet ventilator under normal conditions and during acute left ventricular failure. They found that despite a decrease in transmural left atrial pressure a rise in intrathoracic pressure resulted in an increase in left ventricular stroke volume. Furthermore, this increase in stroke volume continued until a lower limit of left atrial pressure was reached after which there was no further augmentation of left ventricular stroke volume. This demonstrates that when cardiac function is reduced and filling pressures are elevated an increase in intrathoracic pressure can result in an increase in cardiac output despite a fall in filling pressures. However this augmentation becomes limited once a critical value is reached when cardiac output becomes again dependent on filling pressures. A similar effect has been described when intrathoracic pressure is increased by the addition of PEEP in the setting of left ventricular dysfunction in humans. Application of PEEP in this situation did not result in a decrease in cardiac output until the filling pressure fell below 15 mm Hg (147). These data and data from human studies showing enhanced cardiac performance with increased intrathoracic pressure in the setting of cardiogenic shock (70, 71) would suggest that this aspect of the beneficial effect of increased intrathoracic pressure on left ventricular performance was preload dependent, being least beneficial when left ventricular filling was reduced and most beneficial where left ventricular filling pressures were elevated. The predominant hemodynamic effect of increased intrathoracic pressure will be caused by changes in preload if contractility and circulating volume are normal, whereas in situations of reduced left ventricular function where filling pressures are frequently elevated, the principal hemodynamic change will be alterations in left ventricular wall stress (afterload). This has been confirmed in human studies where nasal CPAP has been used to treat adult patients with congestive heart failure. The application of 5 cm H_2O in patients with congestive cardiac failure and a pulmonary capillary wedge pressure (PCWP) greater than 12 mm Hg resulted an increase in the measured cardiac output, whereas it remained unchanged or fell in patients where cardiac failure was associated with a normal filling pressure (152) (Fig. 9.5). A further study, in which 5, 7.5, and 10 cm H_2O were applied, showed a similar beneficial effect in that left ventricular systolic transmural pressure (afterload) fell (153). The same group demonstrated improved left ventricular function and symptomology in a randomized controlled trial of nocturnal nasal CPAP in patients with heart failure associated with Cheyne-Stokes respiration and central sleep apnea (154).

It has also become evident that hemodynamic changes that occur with increased intrathoracic pressure vary according to different phases in the cardiac cycle. This has been demonstrated in the recent studies by Pinsky et al. (155) where positive pressure ventilation was linked to the cardiac cycle by the use of a jet ventilator in animals with left ventricular failure. When positive pressure was timed to occur early in diastole in normal animals, left ventricular stroke volume was decreased, whereas when it was timed to coincide with early systole no effect was seen. In addition it was noted that positive pressure was phased with early diastole, the reduction in stroke volume of the right ventricle preceded that of the left ventricle by one to two heartbeats, suggesting that the reduction was caused by reduced venous return. In the animals with left ventricular failure, increased intrathoracic pressure in phase with systole increased left ventricular stroke volume compared with diastole, although the increased intrathoracic pressure in either phase was associated with increased stroke volume when compared with apnea. These investigators then compared the hemodynamic effects of increases in intrathoracic pressure synchronized to early and late systole. They found that although increased intrathoracic pressure in both phases of the systolic cycle was associated with an increase in stroke volume when compared with apnea, early systolic phase ventilation resulted in an increase in stroke volume without a change in aortic pressure, whereas late systolic ventilation increased both stroke volume and pressure. These findings would suggest that positive pressure ventilation synchronized with early cardiac systole allows for left ventricular ejection into a volume-depleted thoracic aorta. These principles have recently been applied in the clinical arena for the ventilatory management of patients with severe congestive cardiomyopathy who are undergoing heart transplantation (156). Pinsky compared the effects of high frequency jet ventilation (HFJV) synchronized with cardiac systole and found HFJV asynchronous with the cardiac cycle and conventional ventilation at similar levels of intrathoracic pressure. They found that the change to synchronous HFJV was associated with an increase in cardiac output compared with the other modes of ventilation. Similar improvements in cardiac output with synchronized HFJV have been reported by MacIntyre in patients being ventilated for heart failure (157).

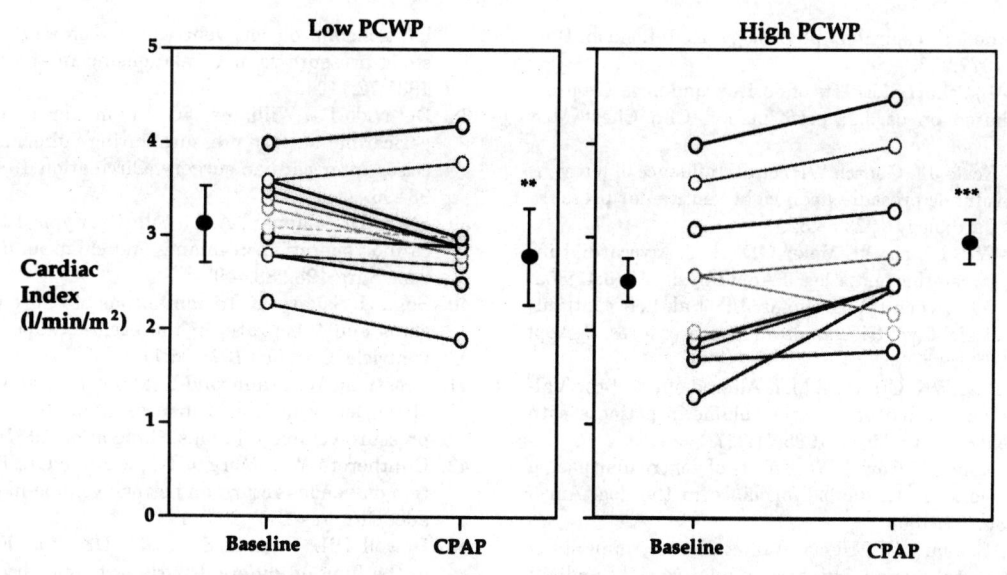

Figure 9.5. The effect of nasal continuous positive airway pressure (*CPAP*) on cardiac output in 22 patients with congestive heart failure. Individual data for patients with high and low pulmonary capillary wedge pressures (*PCWP*) are shown together with the mean standard error of the mean (SEM) for the grouped data. With the application of CPAP cardiac index rose in 10 of the 11 patients in the high PCWP group, whereas it decreased in 9 of 11 in the low PCWP group. ** $P < .025$, *** $P < .001$ compared with baseline. (Reprinted with permission from Bradley TD, Holloway RM, McLaughlin PR, et al. Cardiac output response to continuous positive airway pressure in congestive heart failure. Am Rev Respir Dis 1992;145:377–382.)

SUMMARY

Interaction between the cardiac and respiratory systems as the blood flows through the thorax are complex and become increasingly important in the presence of cardiorespiratory disease. Spontaneous and positive pressure ventilation have differing and often opposite effects on cardiac function. Alteration in cardiac output that occurs with respiration is caused by changes in both pleural pressure and lung volume, the former affecting right heart filling and left heart afterload, whereas changes in lung volume affect pulmonary vascular resistance and right ventricular afterload. Changes in preload and afterload in either ventricle can affect the opposite chamber by the mechanism of ventricular interdependence. In left ventricular failure the positive intrathoracic pressure generated by mechanical ventilation can cause a reduction in stroke volume because of inhibition of right ventricle filling, but this is frequently more than compensated for by the decrease in left ventricular afterload.

REFERENCES

1. Bove AA, Santamore WP. Ventricular independence. Prog Cardiovasc Dis 1981;23:365.
2. Guyton AC. Effect of cardiac output by respiration, opening the chest, and cardiac tamponade. In: Guyton AC, Jones CE, Coleman CE, eds. Circulatory physiology: cardiac output and its regulation. Philadelphia: WB Saunders, 1991:378–386.
3. Ekelund LG, Holmgren A. Central hemodynamics during exercise. Circ Res 1967;20 & 21:33.
4. Bakos ACP. The question of the function of the right ventricular myocardium: an experimental study. Circulation 1950;1:724.
5. Donald DE, Essex HE. Pressure studies after inactivation of the major portion of the canine right ventricle. Am J Physiol 1954;176:155.
6. Kagan A. Dynamic responses of the right ventricle following extensive damage by cauterization. Circulation 1952;5:816.
7. Starr I, Jeffers WA, Meade RH Jr. The absence of conspicuous increments of venous pressure after severe damage to the right ventricle of the dog, with a discussion of the relation between clinical congestive failure and heart disease. Am Heart J 1943;26:291.
8. Sawatani S, Mandell G, Kusaba E, et al. Ventricular performance following ablation and prosthetic replacement of right ventricular myocardium. Trans Am Soc Artif Intern Organs 1974;20:629.
9. Shimazaki Y, Kawashima Y, Mori T, et al. Ventricular function of single ventricle after ventricular septation. Circulation 1980;61:653.
10. West JB, Dollery CT. Distribution of blood flow and the pressure-flow relations of the whole lung. J Appl Physiol 1965;20:175.
11. Hughes JMB, Glazier JB, Maloney JE, et al. Effect of lung volume on the distribution of pulmonary blood flow in man. Respir Physiol 1968;4:58.
12. Permutt S. Relation between pulmonary artery pressure and pleural pressure during the acute asthmatic attack. Chest 1973;63(Suppl):25.
13. Brower R, Wise RA, Hassapoyannes C, et al. Effect of lung inflation on lung blood volume and pulmonary venous flow. J Appl Physiol 1985;58:954.
14. Permutt S, Wise RA, Brower RG. How changes in pleural and alveolar pressure cause changes in afterload and preload. In: Scharf SM, Cassidy SS, eds. Heart-lung interactions in health and disease. New York: Marcel Dekker, 1989:243.

15. Nunn JF. Applied respiratory physiology. 2 ed. London: Butterworths, 1977:213.
16. Robotham JL, Scharf S. Effects of positive and negative pressure ventilation on cardiac performance. Clin Chest Med 1983;4:161.
17. Oboler AA, Keefe JF, Gaasch WH, et al. Influence of left ventricular isovolumic pressure upon right ventricular pressure transients. Cardiology 1973;58:32.
18. Santamore WP, Lynch PR, Meier GD, et al. Myocardial interaction between the ventricles. J Appl Physiol 1976;41:362.
19. Santamore WP, Lynch PR, Heckman JL, et al. Left ventricular effects of right ventricular developed pressures. J Appl Physiol 1976;41:925.
20. Little WC, Barr WK, Crawford MH. Altered effect of the Valsalva maneuver on left ventricular volume in patients with cardiomyopathy. Circulation 1985;71:227.
21. Badke FR, Boinay P, Covell JW. Effects of ventricular pacing on regional left ventricular performance in the dog. Am J Physiol 1980;238:H858.
22. Pearlman AS, Clark CE, Henry WL, et al. Determinants of ventricular septal motion: influence of relative right and left ventricular size. Circulation 1976;54:83.
23. Weymann AE, Wann S, Feigenbaum H, et al. Mechanism of abnormal septal motion in patients with right ventricular volume overload: a cross sectional echocardiographic study. Circulation 1976;54:179.
24. Likoff MJ, Sutton MGSJ, Weber KT, et al. The effect of chronic pulmonary hypertension on left ventricular size and dynamics. Circulation 1978;66:327.
25. Santamore WP, Bove AA, Heckman JL. Right and left ventricular pressure volume response to positive end expiratory pressure. Am J Physiol 1984;246:H114.
26. Janicki JS, Reeves RC, Weber KT, et al. Application of a pressure servo system developed to study ventricular dynamics. J Appl Physiol 1974;37:376.
27. Rankin JS, Olsen CO, Arentzen CE, et al. The effects of airway pressure on cardiac function in intact dogs and man. Circulation 1982;66:108.
28. Robotham JL. Cardiovascular disturbances in chronic respiratory insufficiency. Am J Cardiol 1981;47:941.
29. Weber KT, Janicki JS, Shroff S, et al. Contractile mechanisms and interaction of the right and left ventricles. Am J Cardiol 1981;47:686.
30. Slinker BK, Glantz SA. End systolic and end diastolic ventricular interdependence. Am J Physiol 1986;251:H1062.
31. Janicki JS, Weber KT. The pericardium and ventricular interaction, distensibility and function. Am J Physiol 1980;238:H494.
32. Reddy PS, Curtis EL, O'Toole JD, et al. Cardiac tamponade: hemodynamic observations in man. Circulation 1971;58:265.
33. Taylor RR, Covell JW, Sonnenblick EH, et al. Dependence of ventricular distensibility on filling of the opposite ventricle. Am J Physiol 1967;213:711.
34. Jarmakani JMM, McHole PA, Greenfield JCJ. The effect of the cardiac tamponade on coronary hemodynamics in the awake dog. Cardiol Res 1973;9:112.
35. O'Rourke RA, Fischer DP, Escobar EE, et al. Effect of acute pericardial tamponade on coronary blood flow. Am J Physiol 1967;212:549.
36. Goldstein JA, Vlahakes GH, Verrier ED, et al. The role of right ventricular systolic dysfunction and elevated intrapericardial pressure in the genesis of low output in experimental right ventricular infarction. Circulation 1982;65:513.
37. Goto Y, Yamamoto J, Saito M, et al. Effects of right ventricular ischemia on left ventricular geometry and the end-diastolic pressure-volume relationship in the dog. Circulation 1985;72:1104.
38. Del Nido PJ, Williams WG, Villamater J, et al. Changes in pericardial surface pressure during pulmonary hypertensive crises after cardiac surgery. Circulation 1987;76(Suppl III):93–96.
39. Shore DF, Capuani A, Lincoln C. Atypical tamponade after cardiac operation in infants and children. J Thorac Cardiovasc Surg 1982;83:449.
40. Suga H, Sagawa K. Instantaneous pressure volume relationships and their ratio in the excised, supported canine left ventricle. Circ Res 1974;35:117.
41. Grossman W, Braunwald E, Mann T, et al. Contractile state of the left ventricle in man as evaluated from end-systolic pressure-volume relations. Circulation 1977;56:845.
42. Guntheroth WG, Morgan BC, Mullins GL. Effect of respiration on venous return and stroke volume in cardiac tamponade. Circ Res 1967;20:381.
43. Howell JBL, Permutt S, Proctor DF, et al. Effect of inflation of the lung on different parts of pulmonary vascular bed. J Appl Physiol 1961;16:71.
44. Robotham JL, Lixfield W, Holland L, et al. The effects of positive end expiratory pressure on right and left ventricular performance. Am Rev Respir Dis 1980;121:667.
45. Summer WR, Permutt S, Sagawa K, et al. Effects of spontaneous respiration on canine left ventricular function. Circ Res 1979;45:719–728.
46. Franklin DL, Van Citters RL, Rushmer RF. Balances between right and left ventricular output. Circ Res 1962;10:17.
47. Maloney JE, Bergel DH, Glazier JB, et al. Transmission of pulsatile blood pressure and flow through the isolated lung. Circ Res 1968;23:11.
48. Robotham JL, Rabson J, Permutt S, et al. Left ventricular hemodynamics during respiration. J Appl Physiol 1979;47:1295–1303.
49. Scharf SM, Brown R, Tow DE, et al. Cardiac effects of increased lung volume and decreased pleural pressure in man. J Appl Physiol 1979;47:257.
50. Janicki JS, Shroff SG, Weber KT. Ventricular interdependence. In: Scharf SS, ed. Heart-lung Interactions in health and disease. New York: Marcel Dekker, 1989.
51. Scharf SM, Brown R, Saunders N, et al. Effects of normal and loaded spontaneous inspiration on cardiovascular function. J Appl Physiol 1979;47:582.
52. Brinker JA, Weiss JL, Lappe DL, et al. Leftward septal displacement during right ventricular loading in man. Circulation 1980;61:623.
53. Guzman PA, Maughan WL, Lin FCP, et al. Trans-septal pressure gradient with leftward septal displacement during the Mueller maneuver in man. Br Heart J 1981;46:657.
54. Scharf SM, Bianco JA, Tow DE, et al. The effects of large negative intrathoracic pressure on left ventricular function in patients with coronary artery disease. Circulation 1981;63:871–875.
55. Conzanitis DA, Leijala M, Pesoner E, et al. Acute pulmonary edema due to laryngeal spasm. Anesthesiology 1982;37:1198.
56. Lee KWT, Downes JJ. Pulmonary edema secondary to laryngospasm in children. Anesthesiology 1983;59:347.
57. Jackson FN, Rowland V, Corssen G. Laryngospasm induced pulmonary edema. Chest 1980;78:819.
58. Travis KW, Todrea ID, Shannon DC. Pulmonary edema associated with croup and epiglottitis. Pediatrics 1977;59:695.

59. Stradling JR, Bolton P. Upper airways obstruction as cause of pulmonary edema. Lancet 1982;1:1353.
60. Oswalt CE, Gates GA, Holstrom FMG. Pulmonary edema as a complication of acute upper airway obstruction. JAMA 1977;238:1833.
61. Sofer S, Bar-Ziv J, Scharf SM. Pulmonary edema following relief of upper airway obstruction. Chest 1984;86:401.
62. Stalcup SA, Mellins RB. Mechanical forces producing pulmonary edema in acute asthma. N Engl J Med 1977;297:592.
63. Sylvester JT, Mitzner W, Ngeow Y, et al. Hypoxic constriction of alveolar and extra-alveolar vessels in isolated pig lungs. J Appl Physiol 1983;54:1660.
64. Lloyd TCJ. Mechanical cardiopulmonary interdependence. J Appl Physiol 1982;52:333.
65. Peters J, Kindred MK, Robotham JL. Transient analysis of cardiopulmonary interactions. I. Diastolic events. J Appl Physiol 1988;64:1506.
66. Peters J, Kindred MK, Robotham JL. Transient analysis of cardiopulmonary interactions. II. Systolic events. J Appl Physiol 1988;64:1518.
67. Polianski JM, Huchon GJ, Gaudebout CC, et al. Pulmonary and systemic effects of increased negative inspiratory intrathoracic pressure in dogs. Am Rev Respir Dis 1986;133:49.
68. Rebuck AS, Read J. Assessment and management of severe asthma. Am J Med 1971;51:788.
69. Buda AJ, Pinsky MR, Ingels NB, et al. Effect of intrathoracic pressure on left ventricular performance. N Engl J Med 1979;301:453–459.
70. Rasanen J, Nikki P, Heikkila J. Acute myocardial infarction complicated by respiratory failure: the effects of mechanical ventilation. Chest 1984;85:21.
71. Rasanen J, Heikkila J, Downs J, et al. Continuous positive airway pressure by face mask in acute cardiogenic pulmonary edema. Am J Cardiol 1985;55:296.
72. Rasanen J, Vaisanen IT, Heikkila J, et al. Acute myocardial infarction complicated by left ventricular dysfunction and respiratory failure. Chest 1985;87:158.
73. Beach T, Millen E, Grenvik A. Hemodynamic response to discontinuance of mechanical ventilation. Crit Care Med 1973;1:85.
74. Stanger P, Lucas RVJ, Edwards JE. Anatomic factors causing respiratory distress in acyanotic congenital cardiac disease. Special reference to bronchial obstruction. Pediatrics 1969;43:760.
75. Lister G, Pitt BR. Cardiopulmonary interactions in the infant with congenital heart disease. Clin Chest Med 1983;4:219.
76. Rabinovitch M, Grody S, David I, et al. Compression intrapulmonary bronchi by abnormally branching pulmonary arteries associated with absent pulmonary valves. Am J Cardiol 1982;50:804.
77. Hordof AJ, Mellins RB, Gersony WM, et al. Reversibility of chronic obstructive lung disease in infants following repair of ventricular septal defect. J Pediatr 1977;90:187.
78. Motoyama EK, Laks H, Oh T, et al. Deflation flow-volume (DFV) curves in infants with congenital heart disease (CDH): evidence for lower airway obstruction. Circulation 1978;58:107.
79. Motoyama EK, Tanaka T, Fricker FJ, et al. Peripheral airway obstruction in children with congenital heart disease and pulmonary hypertension (PAH). Am Rev Respir Dis 1986;133:A10.
80. Schindler MB, Bohn DJ, Bryan AC, et al. Increased respiratory system resistance and bronchial smooth muscle hypertrophy in children with acute postoperative pulmonary hypertension. Am J Respir Crit Care Med; 1995;152:1347.
81. Stenmark KR, James SL, Voelkel NF, et al. Leukotriene C4 and D4 in neonates with hypoxemia and pulmonary hypertension. N Engl J Med 1983;309:77.
82. Bancalari E, Jesse MJ, Gelband H, et al. Lung mechanics in congenital heart disease with increased and decreased pulmonary blood flow. J Pediatr 1977;90:192.
83. Wallgren G, Geubelle F, Koch G. Studies of the mechanics of breathing in children with congenital heart lesions. Acta Paediatr 1960;49:415.
84. Howlett G. Lung mechanics in normal infants and infants with congenital heart disease. Arch Dis Child 1972;47:707.
85. Yeh TF, Lilien LD. Altered lung mechanics in neonates with persistent fetal circulation syndrome. Crit Care Med 1981;9:83.
86. Lees MH, Burnell RH, Morgan CL, et al. Ventilation perfusion relationships in children with heart disease and diminished pulmonary blood flow. Pediatrics 1968;42:778.
87. Courand A, Motley HL, Werko L, et al. Physiological studies of the effects of intermittent positive pressure breathing on cardiac output in man. Am J Physiol 1948;152:162.
88. Pinsky MR, Matuschak GM, Klain M. Determinants of cardiac augmentation by elevations in intrathoracic pressure. J Appl Physiol 1985;58:1189–1198.
89. Brecker GA, Hubay CA. Pulmonary blood flow and venous return during spontaneous respiration. Circ Res 1955;3:210.
90. Scharf SM, Caldini P, Ingram RHJ. Cardiovascular effects of increasing airway pressure in the dog. Am J Physiol 1977;232:H35.
91. Scharf SM, Brown R, Saunders N, et al. Hemodynamic effects of positive pressure inflation. J Appl Physiol 1980;49:124.
92. Charlier AA, Jaumin PM, Pouleur H. Circulatory effects of deep inspirations, blocked expirations and positive pressure inflations at equal transpulmonary pressure in conscious dogs. J Physiol 1974;241:589.
93. Parisi AF, Harrington JJ, Askenazi J, et al. Echocardiographic evaluation of the Valsalva maneuver in healthy subjects and patients with and without heart failure. Circulation 1976;54:921.
94. Brooker JZ, Alderman EL, Harrison DC. Alterations in left ventricular volumes induced by Valsalva manoeuver. Br Heart J 1974;36:713.
95. Korner PI, Tonkin AM, Uther JB. Reflex and mechanical circulatory effects of graded Valsalva maneuvers in normal man. J Appl Physiol 1976;40:434.
96. Morgan BC, Martin WE, Hornberger JF. Intermittent positive pressure respiration. Anesthesiology 1966;27:584.
97. Morgan BC, Crawford EW, Guntheroth WG. The hemodynamic effects of changes in blood volume during intermittent positive pressure ventilation. Anesthesiology 1969;30:297.
98. Robotham JL, Cherry D, Mitzner W, et al. A re-evaluation of the hemodynamic consequences of positive pressure ventilation. Crit Care Med 1983;11:783.
99. Robotham JL, Mitzner W. A model of the effects of the left ventricle. J Appl Physiol 1979;46:41.
100. Robotham JL, Bell RC, Badke FR, et al. Left ventricular geometry during positive end expiratory pressure in dogs. Crit Care Med 1985;13:617.
101. Visner MS, Arentzen CE, O'Connor MJ, et al. Alterations in left ventricular three dimensional dynamic geometry and systolic function during acute right ventricular hypertension in the conscious dog. Circulation 1983;67:353.

102. Wallis TW, Robotham JL, Compean R, et al. Mechanical heart-lung interactions with positive end expiratory pressure. J Appl Physiol 1983;54:1039.
103. Robotham JL, Badke FR, Kindred MK, et al. Regional left ventricular performance during normal and obstructed spontaneous respiration. J Appl Physiol 1983;55:569.
104. Ashton JH, Cassidy SS. Reflex depression of cardiovascular function during lung inflation. J Appl Physiol 1985;58:137.
105. Grindlinger GA, Manny J, Justice R, et al. Presence of negative inotropic agents in canine plasma during positive end-expiratory pressure. Circ Res 1979;45:460.
106. Liebman PR, Patten MT, Manny J, et al. The mechanism of depressed cardiac output on positive end expiratory pressure (PEEP). Surgery 1978;83:594.
107. Manny J, Grindlinger G, Mathe AA, et al. Positive end expiratory pressure, lung stretch, and decreased myocardial contractility. Surgery 1978;84:127.
108. Johnston WE, Vinten-Johansen J, Santamore WP, et al. Mechanism of reduced cardiac output during positive end expiratory pressure in the dog. Am Rev Respir Dis 1989;140(5):1257–1264.
109. Calvin JE, Driedger AA, Sibbald WJ. Positive end-expiratory pressure (PEEP) does not depress left ventricular function in patients with pulmonary edema. Am Rev Respir Dis 1981;124:121.
110. Cassidy SS, Mitchell JH, Johnson RLJ. Dimensional analysis of right and left ventricles during positive-pressure ventilation in dogs. Am J Physiol 1982;242:H549.
111. Manny J, Patten MT, Liebman PR, et al. The association of lung distention, PEEP and biventricular failure. Ann Surg 1978;187:151.
112. Tittley JG, Fremes SE, Weisel RD, et al. Hemodynamic and myocardial metabolic consequences of PEEP. Chest 1985;88:496.
113. Suter PM, Fairley HB, Isenberg MD. Optimum end expiratory airway pressure in patients with acute pulmonary failure. N Engl J Med 1975;292:284.
114. Pontoppidian H, Wilson RS, Rie MA, et al. Respiratory intensive care. Anesthesiology 1977;47:96.
115. Jardin F, Genevray B, Brun-Ney D, et al. Influence of lung and chest wall compliances on transmission of airway pressure to the pleural space in critically ill patients. Chest 1985;88:653.
116. Potkin R, Hudson L, Weaver J, et al. Effect of positive end expiratory pressure on right and left ventricular function in patients with the adult respiratory distress syndrome. Am Rev Respir Dis 1987;135:307.
117. Viquerat C, Righetti A, Suter P. Biventricular volumes and function in patients with ARDS ventilated with PEEP. Chest 1983;83:509.
118. Schulman DS, Biondi JW, Matthay RA, et al. Effect of positive end expiratory pressure on right ventricular performance: importance of baseline right ventricular function. Am J Med 1988;84:57.
119. Schulman DS, Biondi JW, Zohgbi S, et al. Coronary flow limits right ventricular performance during positive end-expiratory pressure. Am Rev Respir Dis 1990;141(6):1531–1537.
120. Brooks H, Kirk E, Vokonas P, et al. Performance of the right ventricle under stress: relation to right coronary flow. J Clin Invest 1971;50:2176.
121. Bishop S, White F, Bloor C. Regional myocardial blood low during acute myocardial infarction in the conscious dog. Circ Res 1976;38:429.
122. Fessler J, Braver R, Wise R, et al. Effect of positive pleural pressure on myocardial perfusion [Abstract]. Am Rev Respir Dis 1988;37:293.
123. Boldt J, Kling D, Bormann B, et al. Influence of PEEP ventilation immediately after cardiopulmonary bypass on right ventricular function. Chest 1988;94(3):566–571.
124. Serra J, McNicholas KW, Moore R, et al. High frequency, high volume ventilation for right ventricular assist. Chest 1988;93(5):1035–1037.
125. Dhainaut JF, Devaux JY, Monsallier JF, et al. Mechanisms of decreased left ventricular preload during continuous positive pressure ventilation in ARDS. Chest 1986;90:74.
126. Jardin F, Farcot JC, Boisante L, et al. Influence of positive end expiratory pressure on left ventricular performance. N Engl J Med 1981;304:387.
127. Jardin F, Farcot JC, Gueret P, et al. Echocardiographic evaluation of ventricles during continuous positive airway pressure breathing. J Appl Physiol 1984;56:619.
128. Zapol WM, Snider MT. Pulmonary hypertension in severe acute respiratory failure. N Engl J Med 1977;296:476.
129. Jardin F, Delorme G, Hardy A, et al. Reevaluation of hemodynamic consequences of positive pressure ventilation: emphasis on cyclic right ventricular afterloading by mechanical lung inflation. Anesthesiology 1990;72:966.
130. Olsen CO, Tyson GS, Maier GW, et al. Dynamic ventricular interaction in the conscious dog. Circ Res 1983;52:85.
131. Qvist J, Pontoppidan H, Wilson RS, et al. Hemodynamic responses to mechanical ventilation with PEEP. Anesthesiology 1975;42:45.
132. Prewitt RM, Oppenheimer L, Sutherland JB, et al. Effect of positive end expiratory pressure on left ventricular mechanics in patients with hypoxic respiratory failure. Anesthesiology 1981;55:409.
133. Scharf SM, Brown R, Saunders N, et al. Changes in canine left ventricular size and configuration with positive end expiratory pressure. Circ Res 1979;44:672.
134. Fewell JE, Abendschein DR, Carlson J, et al. Continuous positive pressure ventilation does not alter ventricular pressure volume relationship. Am J Physiol 1981;240:H821.
135. Van Trigh P, Spray TL, Pasque MK, et al. The effect of PEEP on left ventricular diastolic dimensions and systolic performance following myocardial revascularization. Ann Thorac Surg 1982;33:585.
136. Shah DM, Newell JC, Dutton RE, et al. Continuous positive airway pressure versus positive end expiratory pressure in respiratory distress syndrome. J Thorac Cardiovasc Surg 1977;14:557.
137. Simmoneau G, Lemaire F, Harf A, et al. A comparative study of the cardiorespiratory effects of continuous positive airway pressure breathing and continuous positive pressure ventilation in acute respiratory failure. Int Care Med 1982;8:61.
138. Schlobohm RM, Falltrick RT, Quan SF, et al. Lung volumes, mechanisms and oxygenation during spontaneous positive pressure ventilation: the advantage of CPAP over EPAP. Anesthesiology 1981;55:416.
139. Dhainaut JF, Aoute P, Monsallier JF, et al. Improvement of RV performance by continuous positive airway pressure in ARDS. J Crit Care 1987;2:15.
140. Berend N, Christopher KL, Voelkel NF. The effect of positive end-expiratory pressure on functional residual capacity: role of prostaglandin production. Am Rev Respir Dis 1982;126:646.
141. Berry EM, Edmonds JF, Wyllie JH. Release of prostaglandin E2 and unidentified factors from ventilated lungs. Br J Surg 1971;58:189.

142. Kocis KC, Meliones JN, Dekeon MK, et al. High frequency jet ventilation for respiratory failure after congenital heart surgery. Circulation 1992;86(Suppl II):127–132.
143. Jenkins J, Lynn A, Edmonds J, et al. Effects of mechanical ventilation on cardiopulmonary function in children after open heart surgery. Crit Care Med 1985;13:77.
144. Hatch DJ, Taylor BW, Glover WJ, et al. Continuous positive airway pressure after open heart operations in infancy. Lancet 1973;9:469.
145. Gregory GA, Edmunds LHJ, Kitterman JA, et al. Continuous positive airway pressure and pulmonary and circulatory function after cardiac surgery in infants less than three months of age. Anesthesiology 1975;43:426.
146. Braunwald E, Binion JT, Morgan WL, et al. Alterations in central blood volume and cardiac output induced by positive-pressure breathing and counteracted by metaraminol (Aramine). Circ Res 1957;5:670.
147. Grace MP, Greenbaum DM. Cardiac performance in response to PEEP in patients with cardiac dysfunction. Crit Care Med 1982;10:358–360.
148. Mathru M, Rao TLK, El-etr AA, et al. Hemodynamic response to changes in ventilatory pattern in patients with normal and poor left ventricular reserve. Crit Care Med 1982;10:423.
149. Criley JM, Balfuss AH, Vissel GL. Cough-induced cardiac compression: self-administered form of cardiopulmonary resuscitation. JAMA 1976;236:1246.
150. Pinsky MR, Summer WR, Wise RA, et al. Augmentation of cardiac function by elevation of intrathoracic pressure. J Appl Physiol 1983;54:950–955.
151. Pinsky MR, Summer WR. Cardiac augmentation by phasic high intrathoracic pressure support in man. Chest 1983;84:370.
152. Bradley TD, Holloway RM, McLaughlin PR, et al. Cardiac output response to continuous positive airway pressure in congestive heart failure. Am Rev Respir Dis 1992;145:377–382.
153. Naughton MT, Rahman A, Hara K, et al. Effect of continuous positive airway pressure on intrathoracic and left ventricular transmural pressures in patients with congestive heart failure. Circulation 1995;91(6):1725–1731.
154. Naughton MT, Liu PP, Benard DC, et al. Treatment of congestive heart failure and Cheyne-Stokes respiration during sleep by continuous positive airway pressure. Am J Respir Crit Care Med 1995;151(1):92–97.
155. Pinsky MR, Matuschak GM, Bernardi L, et al. Hemodynamic effects of cardiac cycle-specific increases in intrathoracic pressure. J Appl Physiol 1986;60:604.
156. Pinsky MR, Marquez J, Martin D, et al. Ventricular assist by cardiac cycle-specific increases in intrathoracic pressure. Chest 1987;91:709–715.
157. MacIntyre NR. The effects of jet ventilation synchronized to cardiac systole in MICU patients. Chest 1987;92:665.

Cardiopulmonary Resuscitation

10

Duncan J. Macrae, MB, FRCA

Cardiopulmonary resuscitation (CPR) is the application of therapy aimed at preserving the integrity of vital organs during cardiorespiratory arrest with the ultimate aim of restoring spontaneous circulation. Cardiorespiratory arrest, characterized by apnea and pulselessness, can occur instantly as in ventricular fibrillation, over minutes as with asphyxiation, or over hours as with shock or hypoxemia. In contrast to adult cardiac patients with ischemic heart disease, cardiac arrest in children in the cardiac intensive care setting is usually not a consequence of primary ventricular fibrillation but rather a result of a gradual deterioration of cardiac or respiratory function (Table 10.1).

Only a few children who sustain cardiac arrest in the hospital survive to discharge (1–3). These studies report an incidence of survival to hospital discharge after inhospital arrest as 9 to 15.5%, with the additional sequelae of major neurologic impairment in up to one third of these surviving children. The series reported by Zaritsky et al. (1) illustrates a better outcome in children who had an isolated respiratory arrest, with a 40% survival in this population at hospital discharge. No reports have been made of outcome following cardiorespiratory arrest in the context of a pediatric cardiac intensive care unit (CICU).

In view of the dismal outcome of cardiorespiratory arrest in children, the best strategy is to make strong efforts to prevent this event through *anticipatory* care as well as early detection and treatment of problems in the CICU setting. An example of this strategy would be vigilance to maintain an adequate diastolic pressure (above 25 mm Hg) in a patient with single ventricle physiology in order to avoid myocardial ischemia and cardiovascular collapse.

This chapter reviews management during cardiopulmonary resuscitation and the reader is encouraged to refer to the appropriate chapter for arrhythmia management (Chapter 30, *Diagnosis and Management of Cardiac Arrhythmias*), specific pharmacologic agents (Chapter 5, *Cardiovascular Pharmacology*), and mechanical ventilation (Chapter 8, *The Airway and Mechanical Ventilation*).

MANAGEMENT OF IMPENDING CARDIORESPIRATORY ARREST

Early recognition of cardiorespiratory arrest is essential if resuscitation is to be effective. Although monitoring modalities such as the electrocardiogram, invasive and noninvasive blood pressure measurements, transcutaneous oximetry, and blood gas analysis are particularly helpful when assessing patients in the intensive care setting, no substitute exists for astute clinical observation and physical examination in diagnosing impending respiratory or cardiovascular collapse.

Cardiorespiratory arrest is diagnosed clinically by the sudden onset of pallor, loss of consciousness, apnea, and pulselessness. In a sedated, critically ill child monitored in an intensive care setting, loss of a transducible arterial waveform and a dramatic fall in end-tidal carbon dioxide concentration reliably herald the onset of cardiac arrest even if the electrocardiogram is still detectable. Loss of pressure trace from a previously reliable intra-arterial catheter must be assumed to indicate cardiorespiratory arrest; the inclination to favor a diagnosis of monitor malfunction over a true cardiac arrest must be avoided.

It is also essential to establish absence of a detectable cardiac output before initiating cardiopulmonary resuscitation (CPR). Absence of peripheral pulses does not always equate with absence of cardiac output; in situations such as extreme vasoconstriction or hypovolemia, central circulation may be preserved and, therefore, a pulse waveform may be detectable on an arterial pressure tracing while undetectable by palpation. In situations with severe bradycardia in which cardiac output can be compromised, appropriate management includes securing the airway to assure adequate oxygenation and then, depending on blood pressure, instituting appropriate use of intravenous agents such as atropine or epinephrine.

Resuscitation protocols and routines are necessary to enable efficient treatment to be performed in stressful situations in the CICU setting. It is vital to remember in any given situation, particularly with patients with distracting complex intracardiac physiology, the basic airway-breathing-circulation (ABC) algorithm (4, 5). Basic protocols used by resuscitation teams in the CICU setting should follow published recommendations from the European Resuscitation Council (ERC) (4) and the American Heart Association (AHA) (5), but the special circumstances pertaining to children's cardiac intensive care should also take into account.

Caution must be taken when resuscitating children judged to be in a state of impending cardiorespiratory arrest as injudicious delivery of sedative drugs can suppress endogenous catecholamine production and sympathetic

Table 10.1. Common Causes of Pediatric Inhospital Cardiac Arrest

Airway—ventilatory causes
Airway obstruction
Endotracheal tube obstruction
Hypoxia
Failure of a mechanical ventilator
Cardiac causes
Primary pulseless arrhythmia
    Ventricular fibrillation
    Pulseless ventricular tachycardia
Impaired myocardial performance
    Other arrhythmias
    Electrolyte disturbances
    Severe acidosis
    Pacemaker malfunction
    Drug toxicity (e.g., digitalis)
    Sepsis
Mechanical—surgical causes
Tension pneumothorax
Pericardial tamponade
Hypovolemia

tone, and positive pressure ventilation can reduce venous return. Both of these interventional maneuvers have the potential to further impair cardiac output and precipitate full cardiorespiratory arrest. Unless the airway is acutely compromised, consideration should be given to administration of oxygen followed by intravenous fluids and inotropic drugs before securing the airway through intubation and ventilation. Resuscitation of children in impending cardiorespiratory arrest requires a constant cycle of assessment, action, and reassessment.

MANAGEMENT OF CARDIORESPIRATORY ARREST

Airway and Breathing

The first step in treating any child with cardiac arrest is to ensure that a clear airway exists and that ventilation is adequate. In the CICU, many patients are intubated and ventilated, but the resuscitation team must not be misled by the apparently secure airway under these circumstances. The endotracheal tube must be carefully checked to exclude obstruction or displacement and the respiratory equipment should be examined to exclude mechanical malfunction. If endotracheal tube displacement or blockage is suspected, the tube should be removed and bag and mask ventilation undertaken until reintubation can be safely accomplished. If a mechanical malfunction is suspected, the child should be separated from the potentially defective equipment and ventilation to the lungs provided manually or with an alternative system. It is also essential to examine the child for signs of a tension pneumothorax. If in doubt, the chest should be drained percutaneously without waiting for radiologic confirmation.

Circulatory Support

Cardiac massage aims to produce blood flow from the heart into the aorta and thus maintain a cardiac output. Blood flow to vital organs is provided by cardiac massage, which can be performed by external chest compression (closed chest massage) or direct manual compression of the heart (open chest massage). Absolute vital organ blood flow (heart and brain) during properly conducted CPR is severely reduced compared with prearrest values; blood flows to other organs (gastrointestinal tract, liver, and kidneys) can be even further reduced, especially with the administration of vasocontricting agents. In a study conducted in dogs, conventional CPR with epinephrine resulted in cerebral and myocardial blood flows of 15 and 5% of the prearrest values, respectively (6).

Blood flow to the myocardium during CPR is dependent on the pressure gradient between the aorta and right atrium during the relaxation (diastolic) phase of the CPR cycle. Coronary perfusion pressure, an indirect assessment of myocardial blood flow, is a reliable predictor of return of spontaneous circulation during adult CPR; however, little data are available on children (7). Treatment algorithms have recently been modified with a recommendation on the use of high dose epinephrine, emphasizing the importance of maximizing coronary perfusion pressure during CPR. Goetting (7) studied coronary perfusion pressure in 17 children in during CPR, and noted coronary perfusion pressure deteriorated without epinephrine.

Cerebral blood flow is dependent on aortic pressure and intracranial or right atrial pressure during the chest compression phase of the CPR cycle. It is clear that CPR does not halt progression of cerebral ischemic injury in adults (8). Few data exist on the adequacy of cerebral blood flow during CPR in children; however, as in adults, CPR duration is a determinant of the quality of neurologic survival (3, 9). Recently it has become possible to study cerebral oxygen saturation noninvasively using infrared spectroscopy. With this technique, McCormick et al. demonstrated a rapid fall in cerebral oxygen saturation with the onset of cardiac arrest treated with CPR; saturation did not rise until spontaneous circulation returned (10).

Closed Chest Cardiac Massage

The mechanism of blood flow during CPR is controversial. Two principal models, the thoracic pump model (in which the mechanism is thought to be increase in intrathoracic pressure) and the cardiac pump model (in which the mechanism involves compression of the heart between the spine and the sternum) are reviewed in detail elsewhere

(11). It is, however, generally accepted that the heart is directly compressed during closed chest compression in neonates and children because of the compliant nature of their chest wall.

Chest compression should be performed by depressing the lower third of the sternum to a depth related to the child's age, of approximately one third to one half of the thoracic depth (5). Recent work using a pediatric animal model suggests that a technique of "circumferential compression," that is, surrounding the chest with both hands and depressing the sternum with both thumbs, improves perfusion pressure during CPR (12). This confirms earlier reports of its efficacy in neonates (13). When using this technique, care must be taken to allow the chest to re-expand fully during the decompression phase of the CPR cycle.

Open Chest Cardiac Massage

Open chest CPR can be physiologically superior to closed chest massage. During open massage, intrathoracic pressure is not raised, resulting in lower right atrial and intracranial pressures and thus improved coronary and cerebral perfusion pressures (14, 15). Open chest CPR has been shown to improve outcome after failure of conventional closed chest techniques in an animal model (16). No adequate studies, however, compare outcome of open and closed chest cardiac massage in children sustaining cardiac arrest while in the hospital.

Open chest cardiac massage is frequently employed in the postoperative cardiac intensive care unit where skilled personnel are immediately available to perform manual compressions when the chest is already open or to gain access to the heart via the recently closed sternotomy incision. Open cardiac massage is the only effective method of cardiac compression in patients with an open sternal wound following cardiac surgery, as splints (employed to separate the sternal wound edges) lift the sternum away from the heart and make closed compressions ineffective. Open massage may also be preferred in patients with large conduits lying under the sternum, as closed cardiac massage, which compresses the heart, probably compresses the conduit as well. There is also the added advantage of direct visualization of the heart so that cardiac tamponade and tension pneumothorax as potential causative factors can be excluded.

Open cardiac massage can be seriously considered especially if return of spontaneous circulation has not occurred within 15 minutes of commencing CPR. During open cardiac massage, the aorta may be partially occluded by a clamp or digital pressure, thereby enhancing coronary and brain perfusion. In a study comparing outcome of CPR with and without occlusion of the descending aorta, all 10 dogs in the occlusion group were successfully resuscitated and survived 48 hours compared with only one 48-hour survivor in the nonocclusion group (17).

Vascular Access

Rapid access to the circulation is obviously vital for drug and fluid administration during pediatric CPR. Venous access should be sought through cannulation of any accessible vein, and it should be achieved without interrupting cardiac massage. Central vein drug administration has been shown to lead to more rapid onset of drug action in adult CPR (18), and central lines should certainly be used during pediatric CPR if they are in place at the time of the arrest. Because neck and subclavian vein cannulations are difficult to achieve during cardiac massage, femoral vein cannulation is preferred. Both the ERC (4) and AHA (5) recommend alternative routes to vascular access if venous access is not achieved rapidly (e.g., within three attempts or 90 seconds).

For drug administration, any form of vascular access is preferred to the endotracheal route, which has previously been recommended for emergency administration of lipid-soluble drugs (including epinephrine, atropine, lidocaine, and naloxone). Epinephrine delivery by the tracheal route requires a ten times higher dose than the regular intravenous dose to achieve similar blood levels (19, 20). Required doses of the other drugs via this route are unknown and doubt exists regarding the reliability of this route during CPR.

Intraosseous access, used since the 1940s (21), provides rapid and reliable access to the circulation in children if venous access cannot be achieved readily. Complications of the technique include osteomyelitis and bony fractures. A specially designed intraosseous needle or a Jamshidi bone marrow needle is inserted into the bone marrow cavity following which all resuscitation drugs and fluids can be safely administered. The site usually recommended for intraosseous infusion in children is the tibia 2 cm below the tibial tuberosity, but other sites (including distal femur, sternum, or iliac crest) can be employed in older children.

Blind intracardiac administration of drugs is usually not recommended because of considerable risks associated with the technique, including coronary artery damage, laceration, pericardial tamponade, and failure to deliver drug into the blood stream.

Adrenergic Agonists

Use of adrenergic agonists during CPR was first described in the classic paper by Redding and Pearson in 1963 (22). They subsequently demonstrated that the successful use of epineprine in CPR was a result of increased aortic diastolic pressure, probably because of the effects of epinephrine in raising peripheral vascular tone (23). A similar outcome was observed in adult CPR when pure α

agonist drugs such as methoxamine (24) and norepinephrine (25) were used. The relative efficacy of epinephrine and α agonist drugs is debatable. In a laboratory study (24), only 27% of dogs receiving an α agonist and a β agonist were resuscitated successfully; it appears that β-adrenergic stimulation on the hypoxic myocardium increases oxygen demand, which may not be met during CPR.

High dose epinephrine use is somewhat controversial. The importance of epinephrine in raising peripheral vascular tone and thereby decreasing flow to nonvital organs while increasing coronary blood flow during CPR is universally recognized, and it is the basis on which recent high dose epinephrine strategy was devised (26, 27). Both the AHA and ERC recently included a higher dose of epinephrine (0.1 mg/kg) in their resuscitation guidelines (4, 5). High dose epinephrine has been shown to improve both myocardial and cerebral blood flows in animals with cardiac arrest (28) and to improve neurologic outcome in pediatric CPR (26). Evidence from three recent multicenter trials of high dose epinephrine in adult CPR, however, showed that, although spontaneous circulation occurred more frequently in the high dose patient group, outcome did not improve (27, 29, 30). Higher doses of epinephrine may have disadvantages such as increase in myocardial oxygen consumption, increase in subendocardial ischemia, and higher likelihood of precipitating tachyarrhythmias. Further studies of the use of high-dose epinephrine in children are needed.

Isoproterenol is a synthetic catecholamine with β_1 and β_2 receptor stimulating properties. Its routine administration during CPR is not recommended because the β_1 effects of the drug increases myocardial oxygen demand, and the β_2 effects of the drug induces vasodilation, lowering aortic diastolic pressure and, therefore, coronary perfusion pressure. The combination of these effects results in worsening of myocardial oxygen balance. Isoproterenol, however, can be used with extreme caution in resuscitation for some forms of bradycardia (e.g., children with high degree atrioventricular [AV] block who are not pulseless or significantly hypotensive).

Calcium

Calcium has long been accepted as a useful drug in cardiac resuscitation (31). Recent CPR guidelines have limited indications for calcium administration because evidence suggests that calcium administration can lead to cell death. In cases of ionized hypocalcemia, however, cardiac contractility is impaired and an attenuated myocardial response to catecholamines is evident. Experimental studies have demonstrated that, whereas raising calcium to normal values in subjects with ionized hypocalcemia improves cardiac contractility, induced hypercalcemia causes vasoconstriction without any further increase in cardiac output.

Calcium may not be indicated in cardiac arrest except in cases of electromechanical dissociation, hypocalcemia, hyperkalemia, hypermagnesemia, or calcium channel blocker overdose. Choice of calcium salt between gluconate and choride has been long debated. Several studies have shown that similar elevations of ionized calcium occur when equimolar amounts of chloride and gluconate are administered. One recent study, however, concludes that chloride salt produced greater elevations in ionized calcium (32). Rapid administration of calcium can cause severe bradycardia and extravasation can lead to tissue necrosis.

Acidosis

Sodium Bicarbonate

Management of acidosis, and in particular, sodium bicarbonate use during CPR, is controversial. Metabolic acidosis occurs from inadequate tissue oxygen delivery, anaerobic metabolism, and production of lactic acid. Acidosis has the potential to cause systemic vasodilation, pulmonary vasoconstriction, depression of the inotropic state of the myocardium, and attenuation of cardiac responsiveness to catecholamines (33–35). Intubation and ventilation correct hypoxemia, but they do not improve tissue blood flow, which remains severely compromised even with effective chest compressions.

During CPR, poor tissue flow results in substantial gradients of P_{CO_2} and pH developing between arterial and venous blood. Occurrence of a marked arteriovenous CO_2 gradient is caused by impaired CO_2 elimination from tissues in the low flow circulation. Carbon dioxide content relationship to tissue blood flow is illustrated by applying the Fick equation to CO_2 content:

$$Cv_{CO_2} - Ca_{CO_2} = V_{CO_2}/Q$$

(Cv_{CO_2} mixed venous content CO_2, Ca_{CO_2} arterial content CO_2, V_{CO_2} carbon dioxide production, Q cardiac output)

Thus, a large arteriovenous CO_2 gradient exists when cardiac output is low as in cardiac arrest. In this context, bicarbonate administration is unlikely to improve the situation as hydrogen ions are buffered in a reaction that results in production of carbon dioxide in tissues.

$$HCO_3^- + H + \leftrightarrow H2CO_3 \leftrightarrow H_2O + CO_2$$

This is disadvantageous to myocardial cells during CPR, as it is clear that tissue CO_2 levels remain high until tissue blood flow increases. Furthermore, bicarbonate ion is readily available to extracellular fluid, but the ion diffuses across cell membranes slowly. In contrast, CO_2 diffuses rapidly across cell membranes and has the potential to temporarily worsen intracellular acidosis. Effects of excess CO_2 during CPR cannot be overcome by hyperventilation as the small amount of blood flowing through the pulmonary circulation during CPR is usually well oxygenated and efficiently rid of CO_2. It is low pulmonary blood flow, not failure to remove of CO_2 from pulmonary capillary blood, that impairs tissue CO_2 removal and pulmonary CO_2 excretion during CPR.

Although no clear evidence is found that treatment of acidosis improves outcome of cardiopulmonary resuscitation (36, 37), less controversial indications exist for its use in the CICU. Relevance is seen of the influence of even modest acidemia on pulmonary vascular resistance. Rudolph and Yuan noted that the pulmonary vascular resistance doubled as the pH fell from 7.40 to 7.20 in a normoxic animal model (38). Rapid onset of metabolic or respiratory acidosis can severely compromise patients susceptible to pulmonary hypertensive crises and those with critically balanced pulmonary and systemic circulations (e.g., pre and postoperative babies with 'Norwood' physiology). In addition, sodium bicarbonate is advocated in the therapy for hyperkalemia.

THAM

Tris(hydroxymethyl) aminomethane, or tromethamine (THAM), is an organic amine that combines with hydrogen ions. In contrast to bicarbonate, THAM combines with carbonic acid and lowers CO_2 levels; it does not impose an obligatory sodium load. THAM, however, can induce systemic vasodilation which can adversely affect outcome of CPR. Other side effects include hyperkalemia, hypoglycemia, and apnea. Hydrogenated THAM is excreted by the kidney, and therefore it should not be used in children with renal failure.

Sodium Carbonate

Sodium carbonate also buffers with reduction in P_{CO_2}. It is a highly alkaline solution that can be hazardous to administer. Carbicarb is an experimental preparation composed of equimolar amounts of sodium bicarbonate and sodium carbonate. Sodium carbonate consumes the CO_2 generated by sodium bicarbonate. Only limited animal and clinical data are available on the use of Carbicarb in CPR, and therefore its role is not yet established (39).

Based on the findings outlined above, any known preexisting metabolic acidosis should be corrected once lung ventilation is established. If no pre-existing acidosis is present and the arrest is brief (1 to 2 minutes), sodium bicarbonate administration may be unnecessary. If, however, arrest is prolonged, particularly when CPR duration exceeds 10 minutes, sodium bicarbonate should probably be administered. Bicarbonate administration can be guided by arterial acid-base estimations, aiming for pH 7.2–7.4.

Atropine

Atropine, a parasympatholytic drug, is the drug of choice for bradyarrhythmias, asystole, and electromechanical dissociation. Side effects include tachycardia and paradoxic bradycardia (if a dose of less than 0.1 mg is administered) (40).

Glucose

Hypoglycemia can induce a shocklike state with hypotension, tachycardia, and poor perfusion and, therefore, glucose status must be rapidly ascertained in pediatric cardiac arrest. Hyperglycemia, on the other hand, is undesirable during CPR because laboratory studies suggest that hyperglycemia worsens neurologic outcome following cardiac arrest by supporting the development of intracellular lactic acidosis (41). Clinical studies in children also support the adverse influence of hyperglycemia on outcome (42). It seems rational to avoid hyperglycemia during and immediately after CPR and only to administer glucose solutions with guidance from blood glucose monitoring.

MONITORING DURING CPR

Hemodynamic Monitoring

Hemodynamic monitoring is essential for the effective mechanical and pharmacologic management of cardiopulmonary arrest so that myocardial and cerebral blood flows could be maximized. The electrocardiogram should be recorded continuously during all cardiac arrests as a guide to heart rhythm and its treatment. Cardiopulmonary arrest can occur with maintenance of a normal rhythm (especially in some cases when a paced rhythm is maintained); these states are termed "pulseless electrical activity" or "electromechanical dissociation" (EMD). Primary ventricular fibrillation occurs rarely in children, and it is managed as in adults by defibrillation, followed if necessary by drug therapy (43). In addition, adequacy of compressions should be assessed by palpation of a peripheral pulse or detection of a pulsatile waveform of relevant magnitude transduced from an indwelling arterial catheter. This is important as a minimal diastolic pressure is needed to maintain myocardial perfusion and maximize chance for return of spontaneous circulation. Pulmonary arterial (PA) catheter data may document prodromal elevations in pulmonary artery pressure in a child at risk of life-threatening pulmonary hypertension. PA catheters also provide a ready means of sampling mixed venous blood, which provides an indirect indication of adequacy of oxygen delivery to tissues.

Transthoracic and transesophageal echocardiography are invaluable in the assessment of cardiac function, both in patients at risk of cardiopulmonary arrest and in assessment of cardiac function after a successful resuscitation. Echocardiographic assessment in the CICU during the performance of CPR can also be made for the rapid exclusion of pericardial tamponade.

Respiratory Monitoring

Adequate air entry should be assessed by auscultation of breath sounds, best assessed bilaterally in both axillae. Pulse oximetry can be used to detect peripheral pulsation and transcutaneous oxygen saturation during CPR, but frequently it proves unreliable because of movement artifact or severe vasoconstriction. Arterial oxygenation is best assessed during CPR by direct arterial gas analysis.

Blood gas abnormalities during CPR are complex. Severely lowered cardiac output and tissue perfusion promote anaerobic metabolism and lactic acidosis. Venous acidosis develops as tissue beds drain carbon dioxide and lactate in high concentrations, reflecting reduced tissue blood flow. Pco_2 in pulmonary venous blood increases because of the markedly lowered pulmonary blood flow and consequent reduced CO_2 excretion.

End-tidal carbon dioxide ($ETco_2$) measurements can first be used to confirm endotracheal tube placement. Menegazzi and Heller showed that in adult CPR tracheal placement of the tube was confirmed provided the $ETco_2$ was accurate after seven or more ventilations (44). In addition, $ETco_2$ measurement is reflective of blood flow to the lungs, and it may be of benefit during CPR, reflecting resuscitation efficacy and indicating return of spontaneous circulation (45). During periods of normal cardiac output, the balance of lung ventilation and perfusion ensures that $ETco_2$ concentrations reflect arterial CO_2 tension. At low levels of cardiac output, however, the dramatic reduction in pulmonary blood flow distorts this relationship, and it is the predominant influence on $ETco_2$. $ETco_2$ concentrations increase with more effective CPR (31), and normalize when spontaneous circulation is restored. A dramatic change in $ETco_2$ from a low to a high value, because of improved CO_2 delivery to the lung, is an early indication of return of spontaneous circulation. It is known that bicarbonate administration causes a temporary increase in $ETco_2$ without any increase in cardiac output. It should be noted that $ETco_2$ measurement during CPR has not yet been shown to improve the outcome, and its routine use must await the outcome of clinical trials (46).

Neurologic Monitoring

Neurologic examination, although frequently performed during CPR, should not be relied on to predict outcome (47). The electroencephalogram recorded *during* CPR is a poor predictor of outcome, but it can be useful to predict outcome *after* resuscitation. Persistence of a pupillary light response during CPR is encouraging, but the converse, large dilated and apparently fixed pupils, may not indicate irreversible brain injury but may simply be a reflection of epinephrine administration during CPR. Some children who survive a cardiac arrest managed with closed-chest CPR (15 minutes or more in duration) are neurologically handicapped; good outcomes are rare after 25 minutes (48).

POSTRESUSCITATION STABILIZATION

Following resuscitation, normal cardiac output and tissue oxygen delivery must be restored as rapidly as possible. Inotropic drugs or mechanical support devices may be required to support the heart. Mechanical ventilation of the lungs is usually continued in the immediate postresuscitation period as a means of best ensuring optimal blood gases. The aim should be to achieve normal arterial oxygen saturations together with control of arterial carbon dioxide levels such that hypercarbic cerebral vasodilation is avoided. Deliberate hyperventilation (e.g., to $Paco_2$ less than 30 mm Hg) may not be necessary after a global cerebral ischemic injury, and it can worsen outcome by contributing to cerebral vasoconstriction.

A chest radiograph should be obtained and examined carefully for features including rib fractures, pneumothoraces, atelectases, pulmonary edema, and device positions, including endotracheal tube and monitoring lines. A complete postarrest echocardiographic examination will provide evidence of ventricular function and assist in maximizing cardiac performance through adjustments to cardiotonic drugs; important postoperative residua can also be detected. Pericardial tamponade must be excluded, particularly in patients resuscitated with external cardiac massage.

BRAIN RESUSCITATION

Cerebral blood flow during CPR is affected by CPR duration, central venous pressure, and age. With sudden circulatory arrest at normothermia, brain oxygen stores are rapidly depleted, resulting in loss of consciousness in 10 to 20 seconds. It is widely recognized that the maximal period of no flow that is consistent with complete functional and structural brain recovery is 4 to 5 minutes. This correlates well with the time course of glucose and adenosine triphosphate depletion in various models of brain ischemia. During complete ischemia, calcium shifts occur, lactic acidosis develops, and levels of free fatty acids and excitatory amino acids increase. In no-reflow situations (i.e., death), histologic integrity of the brain is observed; after periods of ischemia in excess of 1 hour, however, early reperfusion triggers processes that lead to neuronal damage. These damaging processes are thought to be brought about by substances including free radicals and excitatory amino acids formed during the ischemic period, which are only able to induce damage after the onset of reperfusion, so-called reperfusion injury.

General Measures

Basic brain resuscitation focuses on achieving a robust postresuscitation circulation capable of delivering a sufficient quantity of well oxygenated blood to the brain at adequate pressure. Hypoglycemia and hyperglycemia should be controlled, and factors increasing cerebral oxygen requirement such as hyperthermia, inadequate analgesia, and seizures must be effectively managed.

Patients who have suffered a brain injury should be fluid restricted. Fluid restriction is intended to maintain a relatively high plasma osmolality aimed at reducing severity of postinjury cerebral edema. In recommending fluid restriction, the assumption is that the patient has an adequate circulating volume. Steroids are of little benefit after global cerebral injury and osmotic diuretics such as mannitol have not been shown to improve cerebral outcome after cardiac arrest.

Hypertension often occurs spontaneously following resuscitation as epinephrine administered during CPR is washed out. A brief period (1 to 5 minutes) of relative hypertension followed by controlled normotension abolished evidence of a "no-reflow" area in a dog model (49). In addition, Safar recommends attempting to generate systolic pressures of 200 mm Hg for 1 to 5 minutes following resuscitation in adults (50). No data are available, however, to support the use of this strategy in children.

Cerebral hyperthermia raises oxygen consumption and compromises the delicate oxygen supply-demand balance of the injured brain, and it should be avoided. Mild hypothermia (34°C) has been shown to be beneficial after global or focal brain ischemia (51, 52). The protective effect of mild hypothermia is presumably multifactorial, as it cannot be fully explained by the modest reduction in oxygen consumption of about 7% at 34°C.

In patients who have doubtful neurologic recovery or even suspected global coma, neurologic consultation as well as appropriate neurologic testing should be carried out without delay (see Chapter 24 *Neurologic Disorders* for discussion of brain death).

Specific Therapies

Various therapies have been proposed to modify reperfusion injury of the brain after sudden cardiac arrest, and these have been reviewed recently. Large-scale clinical trials of postarrest therapy with thiopentone (BRCTI study) (53), and the calcium channel blocker lidoflazin (BRCTII study) (54) have failed to show improved brain recovery in the adult population. Although the BRCTII study failed to demonstrate a clear benefit for lidoflazin treatment postarrest, theoretic benefits of calcium channel blockade in preventing cerebral vasospasm and modifying calcium loading of neurons have encouraged others to investigate newer calcium channel blocking agents such as nimodipine. Until the results of further studies are available, routine use of calcium channel blockers for cerebral protection following cardiac arrest cannot be recommended in either adults or children.

Activation of excitatory amino acid receptors causes a large influx of calcium into neurones, leading to cell death (55). The importance this potential mechanism of brain injury and others such as free radical-induced reperfusion injury remains to be determined in humans, and thus the place of anti-free-radical therapy and receptor blockers in human brain resuscitation is uncertain (50).

NEW TECHNIQUES IN CPR

A number of mechanical techniques have been investigated aimed at improving blood flow to vital organs and hence outcome of CPR.

Simultaneous Compression-Ventilation

By delivering ventilation to coincide with each compression, simultaneous compression-ventilation (SCV-CPR) aims to augment intrathoracic pressure and blood flow during closed chest CPR. Some hemodynamic studies in animals demonstrated improved carotid blood flow compared with conventional CPR, but studies in small animals (in which direct cardiac compression was thought to be the predominant blood flow mechanism) did not show any advantage for SCV-CPR over conventional CPR. Human studies have been disappointing (56), and no study has demonstrated increased survival with SCV-CPR.

Pneumatic Vest CPR

Pneumatic vest CPR employs an inflatable vest resembling a large blood pressure cuff that wraps around the chest. The cuff is inflated phasically by an air pump to deliver chest compressions; because of the circumferential nature of the device, these inflations are unlikely to produce direct cardiac compressions. In an adult human study, vest CPR increased aortic pressure and coronary perfusion pressure and significantly improved initial resuscitation rate (57). The influence of vest CPR on survival in adults has yet to be determined, and pediatric studies are not yet available. In addition, the technique is less traumatic than conventional CPR, but it is unlikely to be useful in the cardiac surgical patient owing to presence of devices (dressings, wires, drains) that would interfere with fit of the vest.

Active Compression-Decompression

Active compression-decompression (ACD-CPR) involves the use of a handheld suction device to assist the decompression phase of closed-chest CPR with the theory that more blood will then be drawn back into the thorax. Animal studies have shown that cerebral perfusion pressure and coronary diastolic perfusion pressure are augmented when the technique is used (58). In addition, a randomized study of the technique in adult human in-hospital cardiac arrest demonstrated a much improved initial resuscitation rate with ACD-CPR (62%) than with standard CPR (30%) (59). Despite the higher initial resuscitation rate, however, only 2 of the 62 patients studied survived to hospital discharge. It is interesting to speculate that the technique may be particularly helpful in patients with a Fontan circulation, in whom augmentation of prepulmonary blood volume is important.

Extra-Corporeal Circulation

Extra-corporeal mechanical support techniques can be used to support children with severe circulatory dysfunction, suffering from reversible pathologies, who are in imminent danger of cardiorespiratory arrest (60). Extra-corporeal circuits take time to prepare, and most pediatric CICUs cannot offer immediate mechanical support if cardiac arrest occurs. In view of the severely reduced cerebral blood flow during CPR, mechanical support cannot be recommended after cardiac arrest unless cannulation is immediate, or return of spontaneous circulation (ROSC) to a "low output" state occurs.

REFERENCES

1. Zaritsky A, Nadkarni V, Getson P, et al. CPR in children. Ann Emerg Med 1987;16:1107–1111.
2. Lewis JK, Minter MG, Eshelman SF, et al. Outcome of pediatric resuscitation. Ann Emerg Med 1983;12:297–299.
3. Gillis J, Dickson D, Rieder M, et al. Results of inpatient pediatric resuscitation. Crit Care Med 1986;14:469–471.
4. Paediatric Life Support Working Party of the European Resuscitation Council. Guidelines for Paediatric Life Support. BMJ 1994;308:1349–1355.
5. Guidelines for cardiopulmonary resuscitation and emergency care. JAMA 1992;268:2171–2302.
6. Paradis NA, Martin GB, Rivers EP, et al. Coronary perfusion pressure and return of spontaneous circulation in human cardiopulmonary resuscitation. JAMA 1990;263:1106–1113.
7. Goetting MG. Effect of basic life support and epinephrine on coronary perfusion pressure in pediatric cardiac arrest. Crit Care Med 1994;22:A153.
8. Brain Resuscitation Clinical Trial I Study Group. Abramson NS, Safar P, Detre KM. Neurologic recovery after cardiac arrest: effect of duration of ischemia. Crit Care Med 1985;13:930.
9. Nichols DG, Kettrick RG, Swerdlow DB. Factors influencing outcome of cardiopulmonary resuscitation in children. Pediatr Emerg Care 1986;2:1.
10. McCormick PW, Stewart M, Goetting MG, et al. Regional cerbrovascular oxygen saturation measured by optical spectroscopy in humans. Stroke 1991;22:596–602.
11. Schleien CL, Kulux JW, Schaffner H, et al. Cardiopulmonary resuscitation. In: Rogers MC, ed. Textbook of pediatric intensive care. Vol. 1. Baltimore: Williams & Wilkins, 1992:3–51.
12. Menegazzi JJ, Auble TE, Nicklas KA, et al. Two thumb versus two finger chest compression during CPR in a swine model of cardiac arrest. Ann Emerg Med 1993;22:240–243.
13. David R. Closed chest cardiac massage in the newborn infant. Pediatrics 1988;81:552–554.
14. Del Guercio LRM, Feins NR, Cohn JD, et al. Comparison of blood flow during external and internal cardiac massage in man. Circulation 1965;3(Suppl 1):1-171–1-180.
15. Sanders AB, Kern KB, Ewy GA, et al. Improved resuscitation from cardiac arrest with open-chest massage. Ann Emerg Med 1984;13:672–675.
16. Kern KB, Sanders AB, Ewy GA. Open chest cardiac massage after closed chest compression in a canine model: when to intervene. Resuscitation 1987;15:51–57.
17. Tang W, Weil H, Noc M, et al. Augmented efficacy of external CPR by intermittent occlusion of the ascending aorta. Circulation 1993;88:1916–1921.
18. Hedges JR, Barson WB, Doan LA, et al. Central versus peripheral intravenous routes in cardiopulmonary resuscitation. Am J Emerg Med 1984;2:385–390.
19. Ralston SH, Tacker WA, Showen L, et al. Endotracheal versus intravenous epinephrine during electromechanical dissociation with CPR in dogs. Ann Emerg Med 1985;14:1044–1048.
20. Quinton DN, O'Byrne G, Aitkenhead AR. Comparison of endotracheal and peripheral intravenous adrenaline in cardiac arrest. Is the tracheal route reliable? Lancet 1987;I:828–829.
21. Heinild S, Sodergaard T, Tudvad F. Bone marrow infusion in childhood: experience from a thousand infusions. J Pediatr 1947;30:400–412.
22. Redding JS, Pearson JW. Evaluation of drugs for cardiac resuscitation. Anesthesiology 1963;24:203–207.
23. Pearson JW, Redding JS. Influence of peripheral vascular tone on cardiac resuscitation. Anesth Analg 1965;44:746–752.
24. Olson DW, Thakur R, Stueven HA, et al. Randomized study of epinephrine versus methoxamine in prehospital ventricular fibrillation. Ann Emerg Med 1989;18:250–253.
25. Brown CG, Robinson L, Jenkins J, et al. The effect of norepinephrine versus epinephrine on regional cerebral blood flow during cardiopulmonary resuscitation. Am J Emerg Med 1989;7:278–282.
26. Goetting MG, Paradis NA. High-dose epinephrine improves outcome from pediatric cardiac arrest. Ann Emerg Med 1991;20:22–26.
27. Brown CG, Martin DR, Pepe PE, et al. A comparison of standard-dose and high-dose epinephrine in cardiac arrest outside the hospital. N Engl J Med 1992;327:1051–1055.
28. Brown CG, Werman HA. Adrenergic agonist during cardiopulmonary resuscitation. Resuscitation 1990;19:1–16.
29. Steill IG, Hebert PC, Weitzman BN, et al. High-dose epinephrine in adult cardiac arrest. N Engl J Med 1992;327:1045–1050.
30. Callaham ML, Madsen CD, Barton CW, et al. A randomized clinical trial of high-dose epinephrine and norepinephrine vs

standard-dose epinephrine in prehospital cardiac arrest. JAMA 1992;268:2667–2672.
31. Kay J, Blalock A. The use of calcium chloride in the treatment of cardiac arrest in patients. Surg Gynecol Obstet 1951;93:97–102.
32. Broner CW, Stidham GL, Westen-Kirchner DF, et al. A prospective randomized double-bind comparison of calcium chloride and calcium gluconate therapies for hypocalcemia. J Pediatr 1990;117:986–989.
33. Steinhart CR, Permutt S, Gurtner GH, et al. B-adrenergic activity and cardiovascular response to severe respiratory acidosis. Am J Physiol 1983;1983:H46–H54.
34. Steenbergen C, Deleeuw G, Rick T, et al. Effects of acidosis and ischemia on contractility and intracellular pH of rat heart. Circ Res 1977;41:849–858.
35. Wood WB, Manley ES, Woodbury RA. The effects of CO_2 induced respiratory acidosis on the depressor and pressor components of the dogs blood pressure response to epinephrine. J Pharmacol Exp Ther 1963;139:238–247.
36. Guerci A, Chandra N, Johnson E, et al. Failure of sodium bicarbonate to improve resuscitation from ventricular fibrillation in dogs. Circulation 1986;74:IV75–IV79.
37. Federiuk CS, Sanders AB, Kern KB, et al. The effect of bicarbonate on resuscitation from cardiac arrest. Ann Emerg Med 1991;20:1173–1177.
38. Rudolph AM, Yuan S. Response of the pulmonary vasculature to hypoxia and H+ ion changes. J Clin Invest 1966;45:399.
39. Grazmuri RJ, Planta MV, Weil MH, et al. Cardiac effects of carbon dioxide-consuming and carbon dioxide-generating buffers during cardiopulmonary resuscitation. J Am Coll Cardiol 1990;15:482–490.
40. Myers R. Lactic acid accumulation as a cause of brain edema and cerebral necrosis resulting from oxygen derivation. In: Korbin RGC, ed. Advances in perinatal neurology. New York: Spectrum, 1979:84–114.
41. Aswal S, Schneider S, Tomasi L, et al. Prognostic implications of hyperglycemia and reduced cerebral blood flow in childhood near drowning. Neurology 1990;40:820–823.
42. Gutgesell HP, Tacker WA, Geddes LA, et al. Energy dose for ventricular defibrillation of children. Pediatrics 1976;58:898–901.
43. Kottmeier CA, Gravenstein JS. The parasympathomimetic activity of atropine and atropine methylbromide. Anesthesiology 1968;29:1125–1133.
44. Menegazzi JJ, Heller MB. Endotracheal tube confirmation with colorimetric CO_2 detectors. Anesth Analg 1990;71:441–442.
45. Gudipati CV, Weil MH, Bisera J, et al. End-expired carbon dioxide: a noninvasive monitor of cardiopulmonary resuscitation. Circulation 1988;77:234–239.
46. Gasman JD, Fishman RS, Raffin TA. Monitoring cardiopulmonary resuscitation: role of blood and end-tidal carbon dioxide tension. Crit Care Med 1995;23:797–798.
47. Jorgensen EO, Malchow-Moller A. Cerebral prognostic signs during cardiopulmonary resuscitation. Resuscitation 1979;6:217.
48. Orlowski JP. How much resuscitation is enough resuscitation? Pediatrics 1992;90:997–998.
49. Sterz F, Leonov Y, Safer P, et al. Hypertension with or without hemodilution after cardiac arrest in dogs. Stroke 1990;21:1178–1184.
50. Safar P. Cerebral resuscitation after cardiac arrest: research initiatives and future directions. Ann Emerg Med 1993;22:324–349.
51. Sterz F, Safar P, Johnson DW, et al. Mild hypothermic cardiopulmonary resuscitation improves outcome after prolonged cardiac arrest in dogs. Resuscitation 1991;24:27–47.
52. Kuboyama K, Safar P, Radovsky A, et al. Delay in cooling negates the beneficial effect of mild resuscitative cerebral hypothermia after cardiac arrest in dogs: a prospective randomized study. Crit Care Med 1993;21:1348–1358.
53. Brain Resuscitation Clinical Trial I study group. Abramson NS, Safar P. Randomized clinical study of thiopental loading in comatose survivors of cardiac arrest. N Engl J Med 1986;314:397–403.
54. Brain Resuscitation Clinical Trial 2 study group. Abramson NS, Sutton-Tyrell KA. Randomized clinical study of a calcium-entry blocker (lidoflazine) in the treatment of comatose survivors of cardiac arrest. N Engl J Med 1991;324:1225–1331.
55. Benveniste H, Jorgensen MB, Diemer NH, et al. Calcium accumulation by glutamate receptor activation is involved in hippocampal cell damage after ischemia. Acta Neurol Scand 1988;78:529–536.
56. Krischer JP, Fine EG, Weisfeldt ML, et al. Comparison of prehospital conventional and simultaneous compression-ventilation cardiopulmonary resuscitation. Crit Care Med 1989;17:1263–1269.
57. Halperin HR, Sitlik JE, Gelfand M, et al. A preliminary study of cardiopulmonary resuscitation by circumferential compression of the chest with use of a pneumatic vest. N Engl J Med 1993;329:762–768.
58. Lindner KH, Pfenninger EG, Lurie KG, et al. Effects of active compression-decompression resuscitation on myocardial and cerebral blood flow in pigs. Circulation 1993;88:1254–1263.
59. Cohen TJ, Goldner BG, Maccaro PC, et al. A comparison of active compression-decompression cardiopulmonary resuscitation with standard cardiopulmonary resuscitation for cardiac arrests occurring in the hospital. N Engl J Med 1993;329:1918–1921.
60. ECMO registry report. Ann Arbor: Extracorporeal Life Support Organization, 1995.

Invasive and Noninvasive Monitoring

Ian Adatia, MBChB, FRCP(C), and Peter N. Cox, MBChB, FRCP(c)

Repeated careful clinical observation and documentation of the observed changes in a patient's condition are fundamental to all bedside monitoring. If the results of sophisticated monitoring devices yield ambiguous results, a moment's reflection and clinical examination of the patient often resolves the apparent conundrum. However, continuous monitoring devices offer real advantages in the management of patients to whom access is limited or rapid hemodynamic changes are occurring.

NONINVASIVE MONITORING

Blood Pressure Monitoring

The first measurements of intravascular pressure, cardiac output, and ventricular volume were invasive (Fig. 11.1) and carried out by Stephen Hale, who published his experiments in 1733. Frederick Akhbar Mahomed was the first person to systematically estimate arterial pressure. His sphygmograph (Fig. 11.2) is an ingenious method for the quantitative, noninvasive measurement of arterial pressure. It was a modification of instruments designed earlier by Vierodt and Marey. Pressure on the button overlying the radial artery was adjusted by a thumbscrew, the pressure itself being recorded in ounces troy weight on the adjacent dial. The first sphygmomanometer was designed by von Basch, but modern instruments are based on Riva-Rocci's method described in 1896. Von Recklinghausen introduced the wide cuff in 1901, and the auscultatory method was described by Korotkoff in 1905 (1). The traditional auscultatory method of blood pressure measurement with cuff and pressure gauge is fraught with difficulties if access to the patient is limited, the patient is a small uncooperative infant, and when frequent recordings are required. Thus two techniques—Doppler and oscillometric—will be discussed briefly before direct intravascular measurements.

Doppler Measurement of Blood Pressure

A Doppler ultrasound probe is taped to the radial or brachial artery. The Doppler signal can be transmitted audibly or via an oscilloscope. A cuff wrapped around the upper arm is inflated until the Doppler signal is obliterated and then deflated until the signal first becomes audible again. This is the systolic blood pressure. This method has been validated in low flow states and in small children (2). However, diastolic pressure and mean pressure are less easily determined.

Oscillometric Measurement of Blood Pressure

The oscillometric method has the advantage of being readily automated. The Dinamap machine acronym for Device for Indirect Non Invasive Mean Arterial Pressure is an example. This instrument is based on the oscillometric principle that blood flow through a vessel produces oscillation of the arterial wall that is transmitted to an inflatable cuff encircling the extremity. As cuff pressure decreases, a characteristic change occurs in the magnitude of oscillation at the levels at which systolic, diastolic, and mean pressures are registered. Thus, systolic pressure is recorded when a rapid increase in oscillation amplitude occurs. This coincides with the point at which arterial pressure just exceeds pressure created by the cuff. As pressure in the cuff continues to decline, amplitude of oscillation reaches a maximum; this point is taken as mean pressure. The point at which a sudden decrease in oscillation occurs is taken as diastolic pressure. Accuracy of Dinamap blood pressures has been validated in children, and it correlates well with direct intravascular radial artery pressures (3).

Accuracy and complications of these two techniques are related to the cuff. If the cuff is too narrow the pressure recorded will be erroneously high and if too wide may be too low. The American Heart Association recommends that the width of the inflatable bladder should be 40% of the midcircumference of the limb and the length should be twice this width (4). Complications result from prolonged or frequent inflations leading to petechiae or ulnar nerve palsy, the latter particularly if the cuff edge is not placed well above the elbow.

Both techniques are unreliable and inadequate in patients with low cardiac output, hypotension, dysrhythmia with frequent beat to beat changes in blood pressure, and in whom diastolic pressure measurement is important. The technique can also be limited in cases of significant corporal edema after cardiopulmonary bypass, especially in the vasoconstricted state. In such circumstances direct intravascular pressure measurement with on-line display of beat to beat variation is required.

Pulse Oximetry

Apparently, Stadie in 1919 first demonstrated a relationship between cyanosis and arterial hypoxemia (5). Cyanosis can be detected by clinical inspection of the lips and buccal mucosa, but pitfalls in the clinical estimation of arterial hypoxemia are manifold. The well-oxygenated plethoric newborn may appear cyanosed. Poor skin circulation and ambient lighting can affect the ability to reliably estimate desaturation clinically, especially if assessing the ear lobe or nail bed color (5). A number of studies have demonstrated the value of pulse oximetry monitoring in both detection and avoidance of hypoxemic episodes in children, especially those under 2 years of age. Of course monitoring of arterial oxygen saturation on the cardiac intensive care unit (CICU) is as important in the detection of untoward hypoxemia as it is for detecting unacceptably high arterial saturations in the management, for instance, of the patient with the hypoplastic left heart syndrome or other common mixing lesion. It has become an indispensable monitor for rapid evaluation of airway adequacy, gas exchange, and cardiovascular status including heart rate. It can be used to facilitate rapid weaning of FIO_2 in the early postoperative period, and it can substantially assist airway evaluation after extubation.

Principle of Pulse Oximetry

Pulse oximeter measures quantity of hemoglobin saturated with oxygen in arterial blood. It depends on two principles (6). First, oxygenated and reduced hemoglobin have different absorption spectra. Second, at a constant light intensity and hemoglobin concentration, oxygen saturation of hemoglobin is a logarithmic function of the intensity of the transmitted light (Beer Lambert Law). The oximeter probe, consists of at least two light-emitting diodes (light source) and a light detector. Most of the light emitted is absorbed by connective tissue, skin, bone, and venous blood. However, this fraction remains constant throughout the cardiac cycle, but with each systole an influx of arterialized blood is seen, which is accompanied by a small increase in light absorption. Two wave lengths of light, which have different absorption spectra for reduced hemoglobin and oxyhemoglobin, are transmitted from the light-emitting diodes through the arterial bed (either finger, toe,

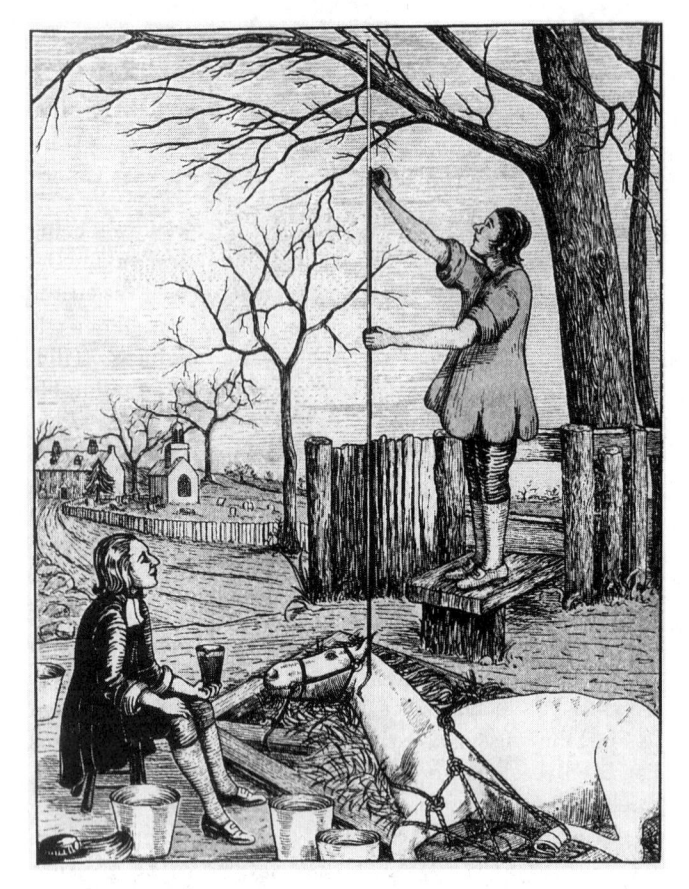

Figure 11.1. Stephen Hales and assistant measuring blood pressure in the horse. (Reprinted with permission from Fishman AP, Richards DW, eds. Circulation of the blood—men and ideas. New York: Oxford University Press, 1964.)

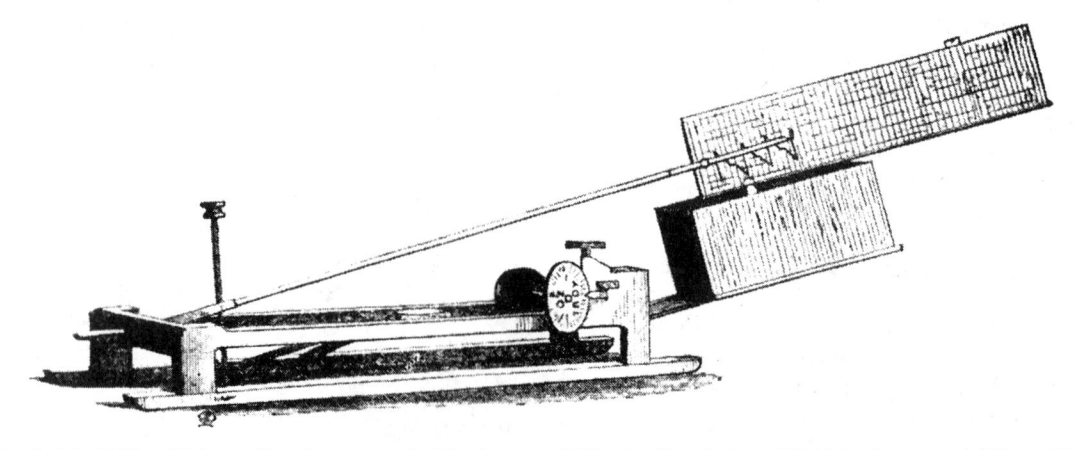

Figure 11.2. Frederick Akhbar Mahomed's sphygmograph. The first device used to systematically estimate arterial pressure noninvasively. (Reprinted with permission from Fishman AP, Richards DW, eds. Circulation of the blood—men and ideas. New York: Oxford University Press, 1964.)

earlobe, or hypothenar eminence in neonates). Light absorption at the two wavelengths is compared. A microprocessor compares the ratio of pulsatile and baseline absorption. This ratio represents the ratio of oxyhemoglobin:reduced hemoglobin. Oxygen saturation is calculated based on experimental data. No mathematic relationship is found between oxygen saturation and the oxyhemoglobin:reduced hemoglobin ratio (7). Attenuated light intensity is measured by a detector and converted to an electrical signal that is analyzed by a microprocessor to give pulse rate and oxygen saturation.

At 660 nm oxyhemoglobin transmits up to ten times more light than reduced hemoglobin. Whereas at 940 nm, reduced hemoglobin transmits more light than oxyhemoglobin. Pulse oximeters, which employ two light wavelengths, measure "functional saturation," which is the percentage of oxyhemoglobin compared with the sum of oxyhemoglobin and reduced hemoglobin. By comparison, oximeters with four to six light-emitting diodes can measure additional hemoglobin species and "fractional saturation," which represents the percentage of oxyhemoglobin compared with the sum of oxyhemoglobin and reduced hemoglobin and, in addition, carboxyhemoglobin and methemoglobin.

Limitations and Pitfalls in Pulse Oximetry Use

Hypoxemia Pulse oximeters have repeatedly demonstrated the high prevalence of unexpected hypoxemia (8). However, pulse oximeters have a high potential for error at saturations below 80% as calibration is carried out in healthy volunteers without producing severe hypoxemia. Errors are further apparent below values of 60%. In the range of 56 to 99.5% correlation coefficients of 0.82–0.99 have been reported (6). Nevertheless, in a review of 244 values of oxygen saturations less than 80%, 30% of values were in error by more than 5% (9). As it is not uncommon for children with congenital heart disease to have saturations between 60 and 88% it is prudent to establish the error with co-oximetry and to regard the values as a useful indicator of trends.

Hyperoxia The oxygen dissociation curve flattens out at the high range so that at saturations above 90 to 95% large changes in Pao$_2$ will accompany small changes in saturation. This is important in the avoidance of hyperoxia in the premature infant (10).

Dyes and Pigment

Indocyanine green dye used for dye dilution curves causes apparently low oxygen saturations as displayed by the pulse oximeter. Injections of methylene blue cause similar problems. Effects are usually transitory, lasting until the dye is diluted and cleared from the circulation. The cause of low oxygen saturation readings in this instance is usually obvious (11–13).

Nail polish will cause up to 6% lower saturation readings. This is most marked with blue nail polish, least with red (14). A similar effect has been noted in burn victims whose fingers are stained with silver nitrate (14). The problem can be circumvented by applying the probe sideways on the finger (15).

Skin color and pulse oximeter readings have been investigated with variable results. Small but clinically insignificant errors occur in the darkest skin colors (16).

Ambient Lighting

Surgical, fluorescent, or heating lamps can lead to falsely high displayed saturations. These problems are easily remedied by shielding the probe with an opaque cover (11, 17).

Motion

Heavy shaking such as occurs during external cardiac massage can introduce error in the pulse oximeter reading. However, under most clinical conditions such as during transport these errors are minimal. Susceptibility of a pulse oximeter to motion error can be reduced by increasing the signal averaging time, but this obviously delays the response when the saturations are changing rapidly. Motion artifact is more readily apparent if the pulse oximeter is correlated with an electrocardiographic waveform (11).

Methemoglobinemia

As stated, pulse oximeters are empirically calibrated using healthy volunteers with methemoglobin and carboxyhemoglobin levels usually less than 2%. Thus high levels of either hemoglobin species will affect pulse oximetry reading (11). Abnormal carboxyhemoglobin levels are unlikely to be a major problem in the child with congenital heart disease. However, with the emergence of inhaled nitric oxide therapy monitoring, methemoglobin levels have assumed new importance as prolonged and high doses of nitric oxide can produce significant methemoglobinemia (18–20). Methemoglobin has the same absorption coefficient at both 660 nm and 940 nm, and it will tend to produce absorption of 1:1 at both wavelengths. This corresponds with an oxygen saturation of 85% in normal volunteers. Therefore, if sufficient methemoglobin is present the pulse oximeter will be biased to read 85%. A high methemoglobin level may mask profound desaturation (21, 22).

INVASIVE MONITORING

Insertion of Intravascular Monitoring Lines

Insertion of intravascular lines is often essential in the management of the patient with congenital heart disease. However, their necessity always should be considered carefully and they should be removed as soon as the clinical condition permits. Risk of subtle or severe systemic thromboembolic events is a constant hazard in patients with centrally placed catheters in this patient population. Relatively large cannulas left in small veins for prolonged periods are much more likely to end in vessel thrombosis. This complication can be devastating if vascular access is required repeatedly for future diagnostic or therapeutic cardiac catheterization. It is essential that the major upper body veins remain patent in patients likely to require palliation with cavopulmonary anastomoses or those who may undergo cardiac transplantation and repeated myocardial biopsies.

Certain points are germane to insertion of any intravascular line.

1. Position the patient carefully before beginning the procedure with gentle but secure restraints. Adequate sedation and judicious use of local anesthesia are important in the fragile neonate.
2. Be certain that heart rate monitor, pulse oximeter, and blood pressure cuff are attached and functioning and that someone is present to watch the patient, monitors, and airway. The patient will be hidden by drapes and the operator will be concentrating on the technicalities of line insertion.
3. A few moments reflection about how the cardiac anatomy and physiology will dictate where the line is placed and affect the information derived from pressure transduction and blood sampling is worthwhile. Thus, a left radial arterial line is inappropriate in a child who has or will undergo repair of coarctation of the aorta with a left subclavian flap. A right radial line will provide different information from a posterior tibial line before coarctation repair and in the neonate with a right-to-left ductal shunt, unless the origin of the right subclavian artery is aberrant. Most neonates undergoing a modified Blalock-Taussig shunt will receive it on the right side. Therefore, right radial artery and right subclavian vein lines should be avoided prior to and after surgery. In contrast, a child with an aberrant right subclavian vein, a right aortic arch, or a dominant left superior vena cava can receive a left-sided modified Blalock-Taussig shunt. Before placing a left internal jugular or subclavian vein catheter, review the echocardiography report to ascertain the presence or absence of a left superior vena cava to coronary sinus (Fig. 11.3). If the tip of the venous line is in the atrium and the child has an obligate left-to-right atrial shunt (hypoplastic left heart, mitral outrace) or total anomalous pulmonary venous connection to the systemic veins or coronary sinus, oxygen saturations cannot be used reliably to estimate arteriovenous oxygen differences or cardiac output.

   Alternatively, early cannulation of the umbilical artery of a neonate with critical aortic stenosis or the umbilical vein in transposition of the great arteries may be prudent to facilitate later therapeutic aortic valve dilation or balloon atrial septostomy, thus preserving the femoral artery and vein, respectively, for later use.
4. Finally, it is prudent to transduce the waveform from the catheter before infusing potent or corrosive drugs. In a cyanosed and hypotensive patient it may not be apparent by color and force of ejection of the blood alone whether the artery or vein has been entered.

Arterial Access

Intra-arterial lines offer the opportunity to monitor beat to beat changes in arterial pressure and intermittent blood gas analysis. Commonly the radial, femoral, dorsalis pedis,

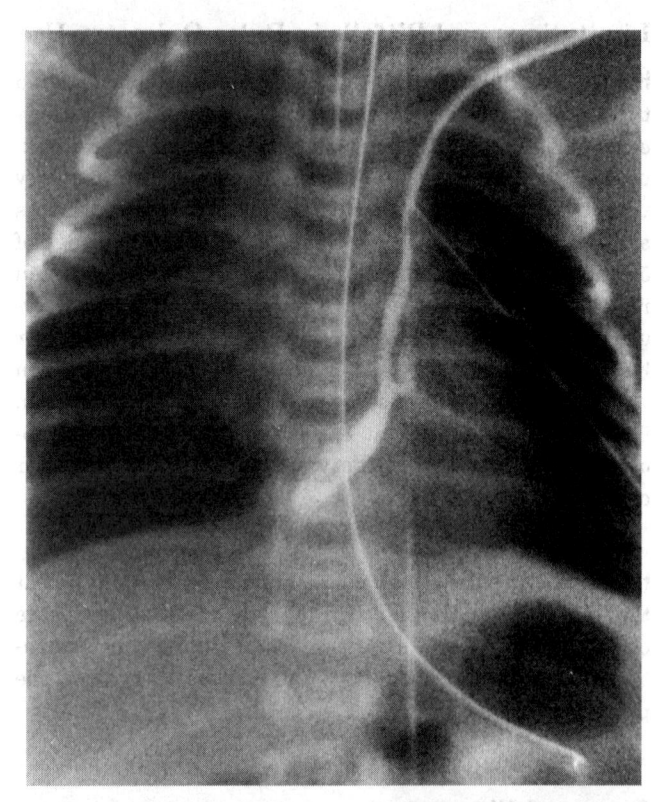

Figure 11.3. Venogram demonstrating a left superior vena cava to coronary sinus in a patient with pulmonary atresia with intact septum. A monitoring line left low in the coronary sinus may result in dysrhythmias or thrombosis of the coronary sinus.

and posterior tibial arteries are used. Less often, the axillary or in the newborn the umbilical artery can be used. Percutaneous entry is usually possible but on occasion a cut-down may be required to expedite vascular access.

Radial Artery Cannulation

Percutaneous radial artery cannulation can be performed in most infants and children. Complications are minor and without major sequelae (23–25). Serious limb ischemia is rare except in cases of pre-existing vascular injury. Transient radial artery occlusion is common after removal of the line, although most can be recannulated (23, 25). Complication rate increases after 4 days in situ (23). A modified Allen's test can be used to test ulnar and palmar arcade adequacy prior to insertion of a radial line. Allen's original test described in 1929 was used to evaluate palmar collaterals in thromboangitis obliterans (26). Value of the modified Allen's test is questionable in the absence of peripheral vascular disease, and it is not predictive of ischemic damage after cannulation (24). Vigorous flushing of an occluded line can result in retrograde cerebral emboli (27).

Procedure

Patient's hand is gently secured to a board. A small roll under the dorsal aspect of the wrist produces extension of the wrist. Skin is cleaned with antiseptic solution and infiltrated with lidocaine. Radial pulse is palpated and the artery pierced with a No. 24 or No. 22 angiocatheter. Once the vessel is entered the cannula is advanced over the stylet into the artery. Alternatively, the vessel is transfixed, the stylet withdrawn, and the cannula gently withdrawn until free flow of arterial blood is seen. A small intravascular guidewire is advanced into the artery and the cannula advanced over the wire. The cannula is attached to the transducer and then fixed in place securely.

Umbilical Artery Cannulation

The umbilical artery can be cannulated in the newborn during the first 72 hours of life. However, we prefer use of radial, posterior tibial, or femoral artery lines except in circumstances as indicated above. Umbilical lines have an uncertain link with necrotizing enterocolitis and the neonate with duct-dependent congenital heart disease, low diastolic pressures, and subsequent systemic steal can be at increased risk. Serious complications are more frequent than seen with radial lines and include infection, lower limb or mesenteric ischemia, and aortic thrombosis.

Procedure for Umbilical Artery Cannulation

The umbilical stump is prepared in a sterile fashion. It is transected with a scalpel. Usually two small muscular walled arteries and a larger thin walled vein are present. The umbilical stump is stabilized with two pairs of forceps and the artery orifice probed and dilated with a pair of iris forceps. The catheter is advanced gently into the vessel and blood withdrawn to confirm the intravascular location. The catheter tip is left either at the level of the diaphragm or low in the descending aorta; its position is confirmed by x-ray. The catheter is secured in place and connected to the transducer to monitor pressure.

Central Venous Access

Central venous access offers the opportunity to measure central venous pressure, deliver potent drugs or high osmolarity nutritional solutions centrally, and repeatedly sample blood to monitor venous oxygen saturations and other metabolic parameters. Multilumen catheters are useful.

In the patient with single ventricle physiology who has undergone palliation with a cavopulmonary anastomosis a line inserted via the upper limb or neck veins will measure pulmonary artery pressure. This can be an important parameter to follow. However, if access is required only to infuse inotropes, it is prudent to insert the line elsewhere as thrombosis or occlusion of the superior vena cava will limit pulmonary blood flow. Catheters inserted from below should reach the inferior cava-atrial junction for accurate assessment of atrial pressures. In the patient with single ventricle physiology and an adequate atrial septectomy, monitored pressures will reflect systemic ventricle filling pressures. If complete atrial or ventricular mixing is seen care should be taken with line flushing or bolus administration of drugs as inadvertent infusion of air or clot has the potential to result in paradoxic systemic embolism.

The optimal site for monitoring mixed venous saturation in a patient with an intracardiac shunt is usually the superior vena cava. Venous oxygen saturations drawn from the inferior vena cava or right atrium can be misleading. An erroneously high or low saturation can be drawn if streaming comes from the renal veins or coronary sinus, respectively.

Additional and often neglected uses of atrial pressure monitoring is in elucidating atrial dysrhythmias (Fig. 11.4) and assessing atrioventricular synchrony during pacing.

Percutaneous Femoral Vein Catheterization

Femoral venous catheter insertion offers several advantages over internal jugular or subclavian vein cannulation. The anatomy is readily appreciated by palpation, potential for pneumothorax is avoided, and hemorrhagic complications from inadvertent arterial entry or venous laceration are easily controlled by compression. Relative disadvantages are proximity to the perineum and a potential for infection, although when care is taken the incidence of infection is probably no greater (28) than at other sites. It is,

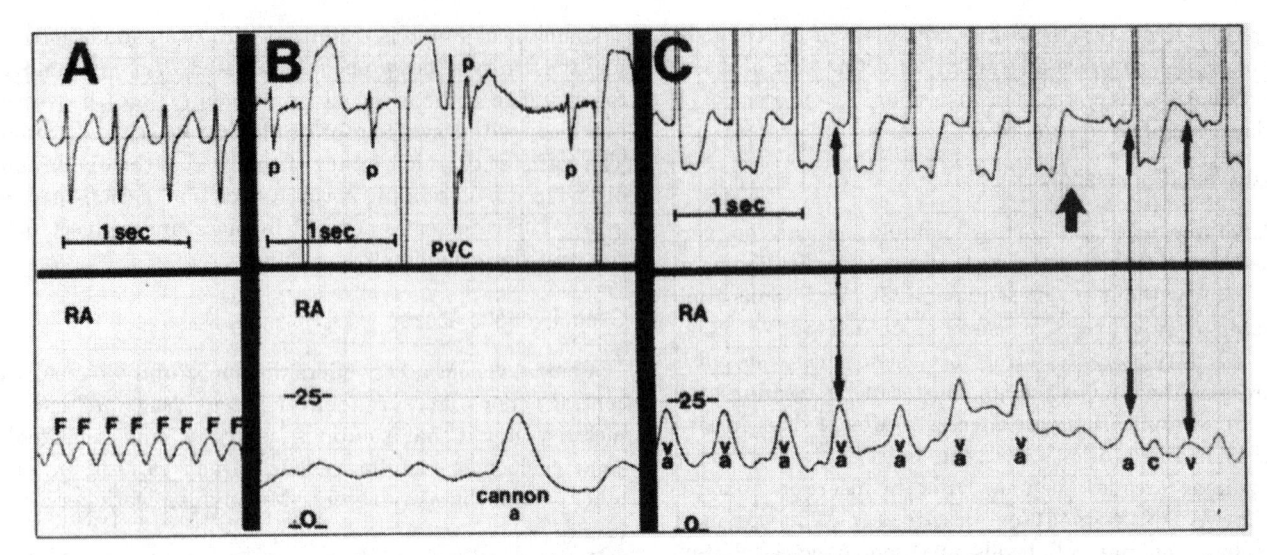

Figure 11.4. **A.** Right atrial (*RA*) pressure waveform demonstrates mechanical flutter waves (*F*) at 300/minute. **B.** Right atrial pressure waveform demonstrates a cannon wave, which is caused by atrial systole (*P*) at a time when the tricuspid valve has been closed by a premature ventricular contraction (*PVC*). **C.** Right atrial pressure waveform during paroxysmal supraventricular tachycardia demonstrates regular cannon waves. The sequence of atrial and ventricular contraction is reversed, but the two events remain associated, which causes the cannon waves to be regular. When tachycardia ceases (*large arrow*), normal A, C, and V waves appear with sinus rhythm. Note that the right atrial pressure is higher during tachycardia because of the cannon waves. (Reprinted with permission from Sharkey S. Beyond the wedge: clinical physiology and the Swan-Ganz Catheter. Am J Med 1987;83:111–122.)

however, worth remembering that cardiac catheterization in young children is most easily accomplished from the leg, and some procedures (e.g., balloon atrial septostomy) cannot be performed from the neck. Thus, a large groin hematoma will be viewed poorly by colleagues in the cardiac catheterization laboratory, and it may delay an important therapeutic or diagnostic procedure in an unstable child. Equally, successful femoral vein cannulation may require alternative venous access if essential drugs are to be infused during cardiac catheterization.

Procedure

The patient's hips are elevated with a rolled towel to facilitate femoral artery palpation. Legs are secured gently. Skin is prepared and draped using a sterile technique. The inguinal ligament, which runs between the superior anterior iliac spine and the symphysis pubis, is located. The femoral arterial pulse is palpated as it passes beneath the inguinal ligament. The femoral vein runs medially to this vessel under the inguinal ligament toward the umbilicus. Overlying tissue is infiltrated with lidocaine. With fingers on the femoral pulse, the needle is inserted medially below the inguinal crease. A characteristic give is present as the needle enters the vein, and gentle aspiration results in a free flow of blood. A guidewire is inserted through the needle and if well placed will pass without resistance up the vessel. The needle is removed over the wire, the skin nicked with a scalpel blade, and the dilator passed over the wire to free the subcutaneous tissue. The dilator is removed and the catheter guided over the wire into the vein. Free flow of blood with aspiration confirms an intravascular position, and the waveform on connection to the transducer confirms it is in the venous circulation. An x-ray will demonstrate exactly the final position.

Internal Jugular and Subclavian Vein Catheterization

Vascular catheterization via the internal jugular or subclavian vein offers the advantages of easier access to the line than the femoral vein, during cardiac surgery, sternal reopening, or cardiac catheterization. However, complications do arise as a result of internal jugular and subclavian lines insertion, especially in the immediate postoperative period. Reported complications (Table 11.1) include bleeding; hemothorax, pneumothorax, and chylothorax; inadvertent arterial entry; pericardial tamponade; dysrhythmias; sepsis; and thrombosis (29–36). Complications of indwelling lines occur in approximately 5% of children, most in those aged less than 5 years. Line sepsis is reported as 1.4 septic episodes per 100 catheterizations (37). Line patency can be prolonged with continuous infusion of a solution containing 0.25–1.0 U/mL of heparin.

Procedure: Internal Jugular Vein

The patient is positioned with the head turned to the contralateral side with a roll under the neck to allow the

Table 11.1. Complications of Pulmonary Artery Catheterization

Central venous access
   Arterial puncture
   Bleeding
   Neuropathy
   Pneumothorax
   Air embolism
Catheter manipulation
   Ventricular tachycardia[a]
   Ventricular fibrillation[a]
   Right bundle branch block[a]
   Complete heart block (in patients with prior left bundle branch block)[a]
Catheter position
   Pulmonary artery rupture[a]
   Positive catheter-tip cultures
   Sepsis
   Thrombophlebitis
   Venous thrombosis
   Pulmonary infarction[a]
   Mural thrombus[a]
   Endocarditis[a]

[a] Complications more frequently (or exclusively) associated with pulmonary artery than with central venous catheterization.
Modified from Roizen M, Berger D, Gabel R, et al. Practice guidelines for pulmonary artery catheterization. Anesthesiology 1993;78:380–394.

head to fall back. The Trendelenburg position, not always feasible, increases venous distension and reduce the chance of air embolism. Alternatively, gentle pressure over the liver increases jugular venous distension. Sternal and clavicular heads of the sternocleidomastoid are identified with the apex of the triangle above the clavicle (Fig. 11.5) (36). The area is prepared and draped in a sterile manner and lidocaine infiltrated. Carotid pulse is palpated medially. The needle is attached to a syringe and inserted at the apex of the triangle at 45° angle, and it is directed caudally and toward the ipsilateral nipple with continuous gentle suction. On venous entry blood is aspirated, the wire is threaded into the vein, needle removed, subcutaneous tissue dilated, and catheter advanced over the wire as described above. If blood is not aspirated within 1–2 cm of needle insertion it may have passed through the vein. If this is the case blood will be aspirated during gentle withdrawal of the needle. The technique can be modified in the newborn to use the palpable carotic artery as the primary medial landmark. The needle enters the skin above the lateral edge of the carotid artery, and it is aimed laterally toward the ipsilateral nipple.

Procedure: Subclavian Vein

The patient is positioned with the head in the midline and a rolled towel placed longitudinally between the shoulder blades. The Trendelenburg position can be used. The area is prepared as above. The subclavian vein runs under the medial part of the clavicle toward the sternal notch (Fig. 11.6). The skin is punctured with the needle at the midclavicular point or just laterally. It is "walked" under the clavicle and then directed medially toward the sternal notch, but remaining parallel to the coronal plane with continuous gentle aspiration until the vessel is entered. The wire is inserted, needle removed, and catheter introduced over a wire using the Seldinger technique.

Percutaneous venous entry is successful in most cases, but it is clearly more difficult in the smaller patient. Nevertheless, variations and anomalies in venous anatomy can thwart attempts at percutaneous placement in up to 16% of cases (38). Subclavian vein position may be altered by previous surgical dissection during placement of a modified Blalock-Taussig shunt. The shunt itself may be inadvertently punctured if the needle approach is directed too posteriorly. Recent availability of direct visualization of the vessel during cannulation with small handheld ultrasound imagers promises to increase successful placement with fewer complications.

Pulmonary Artery Swan-Ganz

Bedside insertion of pulmonary artery catheters was first described by Bradley in 1964 (39). Swan et al (40) refined the technique by the addition of an inflatable balloon at the tip that renders the catheter buoyant, flow directable, easier to wedge, and less likely to cause perforation of the heart or vessels. The concept of a balloon-tipped catheter was communicated first by Lategola and Rahn to whom credit is given by Swan et al. (40). With pressure monitoring, such catheters can be directed into the pulmonary artery without recourse to fluoroscopy (Fig. 11.7). Modern catheters incorporate a proximal side hole to monitor right atrial pressure, a thermistor to estimate cardiac output by thermodilution, as well as an end hole to measure pulmonary artery pressure. When the balloon is inflated the pulmonary artery wedge pressure, or more appropriately the pulmonary artery occlusion pressure, which is a reflection of left atrial pressure, can be recorded. The catheter can be left in situ to monitor changes in response to treatment and volume administration. In addition, cardiac output can be measured and pulmonary and systemic vascular resistance calculated.

Indications

Pulmonary artery catheters are a useful means of measuring and repeatedly monitoring pulmonary artery pressure as well as cardiac output and pulmonary capillary wedge pressure or left atrial pressure. Intrapulmonary shunt fraction can also be estimated. Pulmonary artery catheter insertion may be indicated in patients with myo-

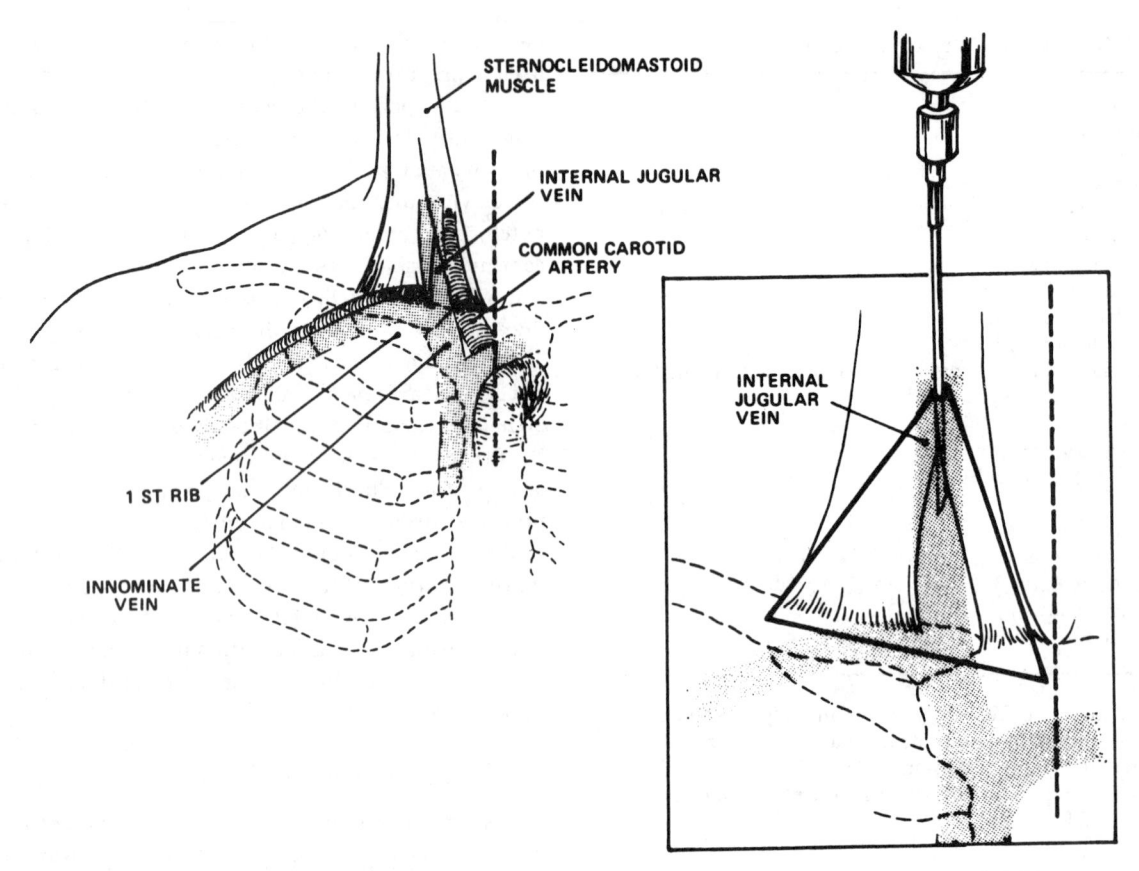

Figure 11.5. Diagram of the landmarks used during percutaneous internal jugular vein entry. (Reprinted with permission from Prince S, Sullivan R, Hackel A. Percutaneous catheterization of the internal jugular vein in infants and children. Anesthesiology 1976;44:170–174.)

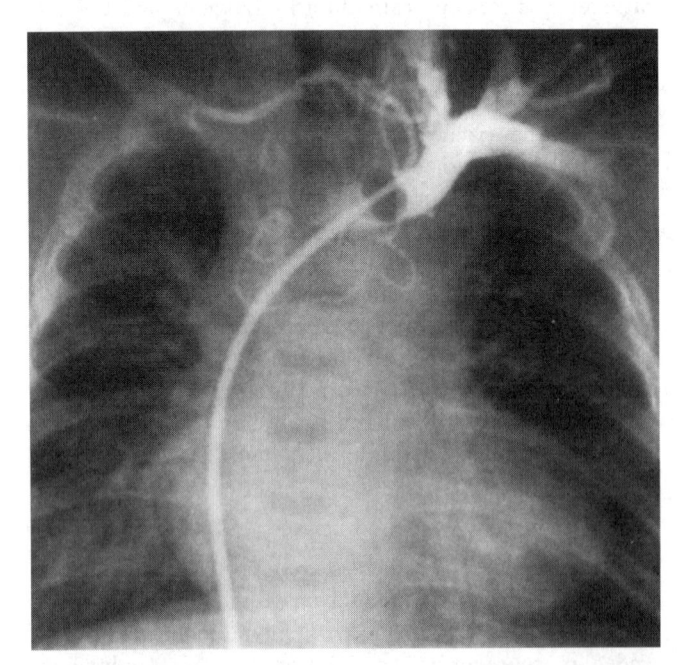

Figure 11.6. Venogram demonstrating the relationship of the axillary, subclavian and internal jugular vein as they drain into the superior caval vein.

carditis, cardiomyopathy, pulmonary hypertension, or acute respiratory distress syndrome (ARDS) complicating congenital heart disease.

Procedure: Pulmonary Artery Catheters

Percutaneous insertion of such catheters is best from either the left subclavian or right internal jugular veins, but it can be accomplished from the femoral vein. Using a modified Seldinger technique following guidelines described above for percutaneous catheter insertion catheters, a sheath is inserted into a central vein. A side arm adapter equipped with a one-way valve offers additional vascular access and prevents bleeding and air emboli. A flexible sleeve protects the catheter outside the body and allows sterile repositioning later. The catheter is advanced as far as the right atrium; the balloon inflated with carbon dioxide and manipulated into the pulmonary artery. In general catheters can be manipulated into the pulmonary artery by watching the pressure tracing (Fig. 11.7) (41, 42). In difficult cases catheter positioning can be aided greatly by bedside fluoroscopy or echocardiography. Catheters can be inserted in children with few complications (43). Final

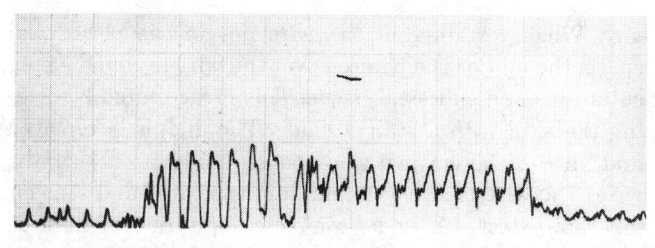

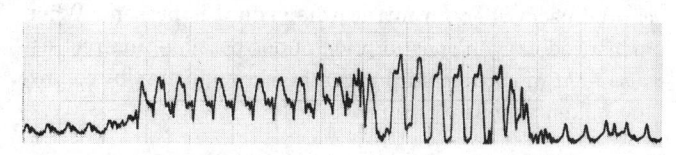

Figure 11.7. Pressure tracings during placement of a pulmonary artery catheter. From left to right: right atrium, right ventricle, pulmonary artery, pulmonary artery wedge pressure. Catheter withdrawn from wedge position in right panel.

Table 11.2. Situations When Pulmonary Artery Capillary Wedge Pressure and Left Ventricle End-Diastolic Pressure May Not Correlate

Mitral valve disease
Pulmonary vascular disease
Pulmonary venous disease
Positive end-expiratory pressure above 10 cm H_2O
Noncompliant LV dependent on atrial systole

Cardiac Output Determination

Determination of cardiac output is usually accomplished by an indicator technique (45–49). The principle of indicator techniques is that a fluid's rate of flow can be calculated by adding a known quantity of indicator, which is then added or removed, at a known rate. The indicators used in clinical practice are oxygen, cold saline, or green dye (see Chapter 13).

Fick's Principle

In 1870 Adolf Fick published in the brief proceedings of the Würzburg Physikalische-Medizinische gesellschaft for July 9, 1870 his principle to measure cardiac output using oxygen as the indicator (50). The beguilingly simple Fick principle states that the total oxygen absorbed per minute, divided by the uptake of oxygen into the blood per unit of blood flowing (i.e., arteriovenous oxygen difference), gives the total blood flow through the lungs. Thus, the faster the blood flow, the less oxygen taken up per unit of flowing blood. Hence the higher the mixed venous oxygen content. Thus

Cardiac Output
= Oxygen consumption/arteriovenous oxygen content

Or

Cardiac Output
= Oxygen consumption/(Systemic Arterial O_2 saturation − SVC O_2 saturation) * Hb * 10 * 1.36

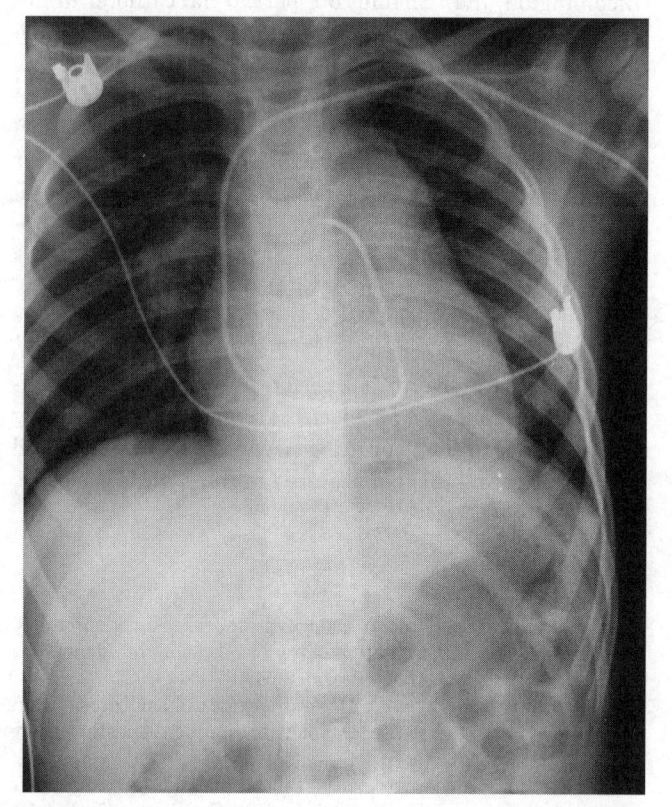

Figure 11.8. Catheter tip positioned in the origin of the right pulmonary artery in a patient with pulmonary hypertension. On inflation of the balloon the catheter will float distally down the right pulmonary artery until wedged.

catheter position should not be too distal to avoid erosion of a small pulmonary artery or rupture during balloon inflation (43, 44) (Fig. 11.8).

Pulmonary Artery Capillary Wedge Pressure

Pulmonary artery capillary wedge pressure has been shown to be an accurate reflection of left atrial and left ventricular end-diastolic pressure. However, in certain circumstances this relationship may not hold (Table 11.2).

Limitations of this technique are the difficulty measuring oxygen consumption in the intubated and ventilated patient. However, this can be accomplished if the F_{IO_2} is 0.3 or less. The advantage of the Fick technique is that it can be used when an intracardiac shunt is present. When measured oxygen consumption is not possible, indirect assessment of cardiac output can be accomplished by following mixed venous oxygen saturation.

Pericardiocentesis

Pericardiocentesis is indicated to relieve acute tamponade, to drain an effusion that is rapidly increasing in size, especially in a child who is deteriorating clinically, and to obtain bacteriologic or immunologic specimens in suspected infectious or immune-mediated pericarditis.

Uncomplicated anterior and inferior collections of pericardial fluid can be safely aspirated and drained on the intensive care unit with echocardiographic guidance using a modified Seldinger technique and 8 F modified pigtail catheters with enlarged side holes as described by Lock et al. (49, 51). Posterior effusions are more safely dealt with in the cardiac catheterization laboratory when fluoroscopy can be used to aid better needle placement.

Procedure

Careful preparation is essential. Reliable venous access should be ensured and a volume expander such as 5% albumen should be available at the bedside. Blood should have been cross matched and quickly available. Although a bleeding diathesis is not an absolute contraindication (49), coagulation studies should be checked and corrected when possible. Gentle but secure restraints should be placed around the child's legs and arms. Blood pressure, pulse rate, electrocardiogram, and pulse oximeter should be monitored throughout. The child may be adequately sedated with ketamine and midazolam and the airway supervised continuously.

The patient is positioned sitting with 30 to 45° degree elevation to encourage anterior and inferior pooling of fluid. Pericardial space and amount of fluid are imaged by subxyphoid echocardiography. If the rim of fluid is less than 4–5 mm it is probably unsuitable for percutaneous drainage.

Subxyphoid and subcostal areas are prepared in a sterile fashion and draped with sterile towels. Skin and subcutaneous tissue down to the xiphoid is infiltrated with lidocaine. A 6 cm long thin-wall 18 gauge needle attached to a syringe is advanced posteriorly under the subcostal prominence and toward the fluid, which will be posteriorly, and toward the left scapular tip. Gentle aspiration is maintained. As soon as fluid is aspirated, the needle is held steady and a 0.038 J-tipped guidewire is advanced well into the pericardial space and the needle withdrawn. If any doubt to the position of the wire is present, especially when the fluid is bloody, it should be confirmed by echocardiography. When certain that the wire lies in the pericardial space, the dilator is advanced over the wire to free the subcutaneous and subcostal tissue. This is facilitated by nicking the skin with a scalpel blade. The dilator is removed and an 8 F, 50 cm pigtail catheter is advanced over the wire. The wire is removed and fluid aspirated and sent for laboratory tests. After as complete aspiration of fluid as possible the pigtail is sutured in position and hooked up to closed gentle suction drainage (10–20 cm H_2O) or allowed to drain by gravity.

Pericardial drainage sets are available from Cook (Bloomington, Ind). Smaller 5 F pericardial catheter drainage setups for the child less than 6 kg are also available. Confirmation of adequate drainage by echocardiography is useful; regularly scheduled chest radiographs while the drain is in place may detect inadvertent pneumopericardium or malposition. Drains can be safely left in place for several days (52), but the risk of infection must be continually assessed.

Success rate is high and complications few with this technique. Inadvertent entry of the pleural space or abdominal cavity has been described (51). The smaller (less than 6 kg) child can be at an increased risk of complications, especially myocardial perforation (52). Although often described, use of an electrocardiographic monitoring lead attached to the aspirating needle is unnecessary and cumbersome, and it is not required in the routine case (53).

REFERENCES

1. Pickering G. Systemic arterial hypertension. In: Fishman A, Richards D, eds. Circulation of the blood—men and ideas. New York: Oxford University Press, 1964:487–541.
2. Waltemath C, Preuss D. Determination of blood pressure in low-flow states by the Doppler technique. Anesthesiology 1971;34:77–79.
3. Park M, Menard S. Accuracy of blood pressure measurement by the Dinamap monitor in infants and children. Pediatrics 1987;79:907–914.
4. Kirkendall W, Feinleib M, Freis E, et al. Recommendations for human blood pressure determination by sphygmomanometer. Circulation 1980;62:1146A–1155A.
5. Kelman G, Nunn J. Clinical recognition of hypoxaemia under fluorescent lamps. Lancet 1966;II:1400–1403.
6. Taylor M, Whitwam J. The current status of pulse oximetry. Anaesthesia 1986;41:943–949.
7. Schnapp L, Cohen N. Pulse oximetry uses and abuses. Chest 1990;98:1244–1250.
8. Severinghaus JW, Kelleher JF. Recent developments in pulse oximetry. Anesthesiology 1992;76:1018–1038.
9. Webb R, Ralston A, Runciman W. Potential errors in pulse oximetry. II. Effects of changes in saturation and signal quality. Anaesthesia 1991;46:207–212.
10. Fanconi S, Doherty P, Edmonds J, et al. Pulse oximetry in pediatric intensive care: comparison with measured saturations and transcutaneous oxygen tension. J Pediatr 1985;107:362–366.
11. Ralston A, Webb R, Runciman W. Potential errors in pulse

oximetry. III. Effects of interference, dyes, dyshaemoglobins and other pigments. Anaesthesia 1991;46:291–295.
12. Eisenkraft J. Methylene blue and pulse oximetry readings: spuriouser and spuriouser! Anesthesiology 1988;68:171.
13. Scheller M, Unger R, Kelner M. Effects of intravenously administered dyes on pulse oximetry readings. Anesthesiology 1986;65:550–552.
14. Coté C, Goldstein E, Fuchsman W, et al. The effect of nail polish on pulse oximetry. Anesth Analg 1988;67:683–686.
15. White P, Boyle W. Nail polish and oximetry. Anesth Analg 1989;68:545–547.
16. Ries A, Prewitt L, Johnson J. Skin color and ear oximetry. Chest 1989;96:287–290.
17. Costarino A, Davis D, Keon T. Falsely normal saturation reading with pulse oximeter. Anesthesiology 1987;67:830–831.
18. Wessel DL, Adatia I, Giglia TM, et al. Use of inhaled nitric oxide and acetylcholine in the evaluation of pulmonary hypertension and endothelial function after cardiopulmonary bypass. Circulation 1993;88(Part 1):2128–2138.
19. Wessel DL, Adatia I, Thompson JE, et al. Delivery and monitoring of inhaled nitric oxide in patients with pulmonary hypertension. Crit Care Med 1994;22:930–938.
20. Adatia I, Lillehei C, Arnold JH, et al. Inhaled nitric oxide in the treatment of postoperative graft dysfunction after lung transplantation. Ann Thorac Surg 1994;57:1311–1318.
21. Rieder H, Frei F, Zbinden A, et al. Pulse oximetry in methaemoglobinaemia. Anaesthesia 1989;44:326–327.
22. Barker SJ, Tremper KK, Hyatt J. Effects of methemoglobinemia on pulse oximetry and mixed venous oximetry. Anesthesiology 1989;70:112–117.
23. Miyasaka K, Edmonds J, Conn A. Complications of radial artery lines in the paediatric patient. Canad Anaesth Soc J 1976;23:9–14.
24. Slogoff S, Keats A, Arlund C. On the safety of radial artery cannulation. Anesthesiology 1983;59:42–47.
25. Bedford R, Wollman H. Complications of percutaneous radial-artery cannulation. Anesthesiology 1973;38:228–235.
26. Allen E. Thromboangitis obliterans: methods of diagnosis of occlusive arterial lesions distal to the wrist with illustrative cases. Am J Med Sci 1929;178:237–244.
27. Lowenstein E, Little J, Lo H. Prevention of cerebral embolization from flushing radial-artery cannulas. N Engl J Med 1971;25:1414–1415.
28. Stenzel J, Green T, Fuhrman B, et al. Percutaneous femoral venous catheterizations: a prospective study of complications. J Pediatr 1989;114:411–415.
29. Poole J. Subclavian vein catheterization for cardiac surgery in children. Anaesth Intensive Care 1980;8:81–83.
30. Groff D, Ahmed N. Subclavian vein catheterization in the infant. J Pediatr Surg 1974;9:171–174.
31. Filston H, Grant J. A safer system for percutaneous subclavian venous catheterization in newborn infants. J Pediatr Surg 1979;14:564–570.
32. Venkataraman S, Orr R, Thompson A. Percutaneous infraclavicular subclavian vein catheterization in critically ill infants and children. J Pediatr 1988;113:480–485.
33. Eichelberger M, Rous P, Hoelzer D, et al. Percutaneous subclavian venous catheters in neonates and children. J Pediatr Surg 1981;16:547–553.
34. Hüttel M, Christensen P, Olesen A. Subclavian venous catheterization in children. Acta Anaesthesiol Scand 1985;29:733–735.
35. Hayashi Y, Uchida O, Takaki O, et al. Internal jugular vein catheterization in infants undergoing cardiovascular surgery: an analysis of the factors influencing successful catheterization. Anesth Analg 1992;74:688–693.
36. Prince S, Sullivan R, Hackel A. Percutaneous catheterization of the internal jugular vein in infants and children. Anesthesiology 1976;44:170–174.
37. Smith-Wright D, Green T, Lock J, et al. Complications of vascular catheterization in critically ill children. Crit Care Med 1984;12:1015–1017.
38. Alderson P, Burrows F, Stemp L, et al. Use of ultrasound to evaluate internal jugular vein anatomy and to facilitate central venous cannulation in paediatric patients. Br J Anaesth 1993;70:145–148.
39. Bradley R. Diagnostic right-heart catheterisation with miniature catheters in severely ill patients. Lancet 1964;2:941–942.
40. Swan H, Ganz W, Forrester J, et al. Catheterization of the heart in man with use of a flow-directed balloon-tipped catheter. N Engl J Med 1970;283:447–451.
41. Roizen M, Berger D, Gabel R, et al. Practice guidelines for pulmonary artery catheterization, a report by the American Society of Anesthesiologists task force on pulmonary artery catheterization. Anesthesiology 1993;78:380–394.
42. Sharkey S. Beyond the wedge: clinical physiology and the Swan-Ganz Catheter. Am J Med 1987;83:111–122.
43. Introna R, Martin D, Pruett J, et al. Percutaneous pulmonary artery catheterization in pediatric cardiovascular anesthesia; insertion techniques and use. Anesth Analg 1990;70:562–566.
44. Kelly T, Morris G, Crawford E, et al. Perforation of the pulmonary artery with Swan-Ganz catheters. Ann Surg 1981;6:686–692.
45. Fegler G. Measurement of cardiac output in anaesthetized animals by a thermo-dilution method. Q J Exp Physiol 1954;39:153.
46. Freed M, Keane J. Cardiac output measurement by thermodilution in infants and children. J Pediatr 1978;92:39–42.
47. Levett J, Replogle R. Thermodilution cardiac output: a critical analysis and review of the literature. J Surg Res 1979;27:392–404.
48. Wessel H, Paul M, James G, et al. Limitations of thermal dilution curves for cardiac output determinations. J Appl Physiol 1971;30(5):643–652.
49. Lock J, Bass J, Kulik T, et al. Chronic percutaneous pericardial drainage with modified pigtail catheters in children. Am J Cardiol 1984;53:1179–1182.
50. Hamilton W, Richards D. The output of the heart. In: Fishman A, Richards D, eds. Circulation of the blood—men and ideas. New York: Oxford University Press, 1964.
51. Lock J, Keane J, Fellows K. Diagnostic and interventional catheterization in congenital heart disease. Boston: Martinus Nijhoff, 1987:141–143.
52. Zahn E, Houde C, Benson L, et al. Percutaneous pericardial catheter drainage in childhood. Am J Cardiol 1992;70:678–680.
53. Spodick D. Drainage of pericardial fluid. Am J Cardiol 1993;71:502.

Section III:

Perioperative Care of Congenital Heart Disease

Part A: General Principles
Preoperative Care

12

Bradley S. Marino, MD, and Gil Wernovsky, MD

SPECIAL CONSIDERATIONS FOR THE NEONATE

Although most pediatric patients who undergo cardiac surgery are diagnosed and treated preoperatively as outpatients, the neonate with significant, unrepaired congenital heart disease (CHD) frequently requires preoperative assessment and management in an intensive care unit setting. Approximately one third of all children born with congenital heart defects become critically ill during the first year of life and either die or receive surgical treatment (1). Critical congenital heart defects that are palliated or not corrected can cause progressive and irreversible secondary organ damage, principally to the heart, lungs, and central nervous system, and they can interfere with normal postnatal changes, such as myocardial hyperplasia, coronary angiogenesis, and pulmonary vascular and alveolar development (2, 3). In addition to these anatomic and functional sequelae, psychomotor and cognitive abnormalities may be present and limit the development of the child with palliated or uncorrected critical congenital heart disease (4). Over the past decade it has become apparent that the cumulative morbidity and mortality of palliative operations, followed by later repair, is greater than that of early corrective procedures. *Primary reparative surgery in the neonate offers the opportunity to decrease mortality caused by the primary defect and also to prevent secondary damage to other organ systems* (5).

Expanding the scope of reparative operations to the neonate has altered the demographic makeup of cardiac patients scheduled for surgery in the intensive care unit. Of the ~2500 annual admissions to the Cardiac Intensive Care Units of Children's Hospital of Philadelphia, Boston Children's Hospital, and CS Mott Children's Hospital, 25% are neonates and more than 50% are aged less than 1 year (Kulik T and Wessel DL, personal communication). Optimal management requires a multidisciplinary team approach, combining the disciplines of cardiology, cardiac surgery, cardiac anesthesia, neonatology, intensive care, and nursing (6, 7).

Care of the critically ill neonate requires an appreciation of the special structural and functional features of neonatal organ systems, the "transitional" neonatal circulation, and the secondary effects of congenital heart lesions on other organ systems. The neonate appears to respond to physiologically stressful circumstances rapidly and profoundly with drastic changes in pH, serum lactate and glucose concentrations, and temperature (8). Neonates have diminished fat and carbohydrate reserves relative to older infants and children. The higher metabolic rate and oxygen consumption of the neonate account for the rapid appearance of hypoxemia when these infants become apneic. Liver and kidney immaturity can be associated with reduced protein synthesis and glomerular filtration such that drug metabolism is altered and hepatic synthetic function is reduced. These issues can be further compounded by the fact that the neonate's total body water is greater than that of the older child, and that the capillary system of the neonate has the propensity to leak fluid from the intravascular space (9). This is especially prominent in the lung of the neonate where the pulmonary vascular bed is nearly fully recruited at rest and the lymphatic recruitment required to handle increases in pulmonary blood flow may be unavailable (10).

The neonate may be more likely to maintain blood pressure when a state of impending shock exists, lulling the practitioner into a false sense of security immediately prior to circulatory collapse. Systemic blood pressure is not always a reliable indicator of the adequacy of preload or satisfactory oxygen delivery. The neonatal myocardium is less compliant than that of the older child, is less tolerant of increases in afterload, and is less responsive to increases in preload (11–14). The potential for sustained or labile changes in pulmonary vascular resistance is common in neonates and concern over inciting pulmonary hypertensive events has deterred some from pursuing a reparative approach in neonates. Finally, the extreme stress responses to cardiopulmonary bypass must be considered in the overall approach to the management of these patients (15, 16).

These factors do not preclude intervention in the neonate but simply dictate that extraordinary vigilance must be applied to the care of these children, and that management plans emerge to account for their immature physiology. Whereas the neonate may be more labile than the older child, ample evidence indicates that this age group is more resilient to metabolic or ischemic injury. In fact, the neonate may be particularly capable of coping with some forms of stress. Hypoxia tolerance in the neonate is characteristic of many species and the "plasticity" of the neurologic system in the newborn is well described (17–19). For example, neonates with obstructive left heart lesions frequently present with profound metabolic acidosis and shock, but they can frequently be effectively resuscitated without persistent organ system impairment or sequelae as the rule rather than the exception. Elasticity and mobility of vascular structures in the neonate improve the technical aspects of surgery. Reparative operations in the neonate take advantage of normal postnatal changes, allowing more normal growth and development in crucial areas such as myocardial muscle, pulmonary parenchyma, and coronary and pulmonary capillary beds. Increasing evidence indicates that postoperative, pulmonary hypertension is more common in the slightly older infant, who has been exposed to weeks or months of high pulmonary pressure and flow (20, 21). This observation seems especially true in such lesions as truncus arteriosus, complete atrioventricular canal defects, and transposition of the great arteries with ventricular septal defect. Finally, cognitive and psychomotor abnormalities associated with months of hypoxemia or abnormal hemodynamics can be diminished or eliminated by early repair (4).

A regionalized approach to perinatal medical care, with organized transport systems and outreach education programs, has both optimized resuscitation and stabilization of newborns with congenital heart disease and expedited the transfer of these infants to critical care units.

In critical congenital heart lesions ultimate outcome depends on timely and accurate assessment of the structural anomaly and evaluation and resuscitation of secondary organ damage. It is therefore critical that pediatricians, pediatric cardiologists, and neonatologists are able to rapidly evaluate and participate in the initial medical management of neonates with congenital heart disease. Because up to 20% of patients with severe congenital heart disease are premature neonates weighing less than 2500 g at birth, a multidisciplinary preoperative approach involving several subspecialty services is frequently required (22). Crucial in this process is the continued communication among medical, surgical, and nursing disciplines. Optimal perioperative management involves:

1. Initial stabilization, airway management, establishment of vascular access, and in most newborns, maintenance of a patent ductus arteriosus.
2. Complete and thorough noninvasive delineation of anatomic defect(s).
3. Evaluation and treatment of secondary organ dysfunction, particularly of the brain, kidneys, and liver.
4. Cardiac catheterization, if necessary.
5. Surgical management, if necessary, when cardiac, pulmonary, renal, and central nervous system functions are optimized.

This chapter delineates the general principles of perioperative care, and it is divided into discussions on the clinical presentations of congenital heart disease in the neonate, fetal echocardiography, evaluation of the neonate with suspected congenital heart disease, evaluation and management of the cyanotic neonate, stabilization and transport, confirmation of the diagnosis, evaluation of other pertinent organ systems, and finally, palliative versus corrective surgery.

CLINICAL PRESENTATIONS OF CONGENITAL HEART DISEASE IN THE NEONATE

Timing of presentation and accompanying symptomatology depends on the nature and severity of the anatomic defect, in utero effects (if any) of the structural lesion, and, following birth, alterations in cardiovascular physiology secondary to the effects of ductus arteriosus closure and fall in pulmonary vascular resistance.

In the first few weeks of life, the many heterogeneous forms of heart disease present in a suprisingly limited number of ways. Signs and symptoms include (a) cyanosis, (b) congestive heart failure or shock, (c) asymptomatic heart murmur, and (d) arrhythmia. (See Section I, Chapter 4, *Cardiac Diagnostic Evaluation*, for additional discussions on these four presentations of congenital heart disease.) Although an increasing number of neonates with congenital heart disease are diagnosed prior to delivery by fetal echocardiography (23) (see below), most congenital heart anomalies are not discovered until after birth. Not infrequently the clinician is diverted away from a diagnosis of congenital heart disease because of the report of a "normal" prenatal ultrasound performed for screening purposes. Conversely, the diagnosis of "heart disease" should not deter the clinician from performing a complete noncardiac evaluation searching for additional medical problems (e.g., sepsis). Table 12.1 delineates the most common congenital heart defects presenting at different points during the neonatal period (24).

FETAL ECHOCARDIOGRAPHY

It is increasingly common for infants to be born with a diagnosis of probable congenital heart disease because of the increasing use of obstetric ultrasound and fetal echocardiography. Recommended timing for fetal echocardiography is 18 to 22 weeks gestation, although reasonable images can be obtained as early as 12 to 16 weeks gestation. Transvaginal ultrasound is being investigated for diagnostic purposes in fetuses in the first trimester. Indications for fetal echocardiography are summarized in Table 12.2 (25, 26). Referral for the indications delineated has resulted in finding significant structural and or functional heart disease with approximate frequency as follows: family history 1%; maternal diabetes 5%; fetal arrhythmia 10%; obstetrician's suspicion of congenital heart disease

Table 12.1. Frequency Distribution of Congenital Heart Defects Based on Age at Diagnosis

Diagnosis	Patients (%)
Age on Admission: 0–6 Days (n = 537)	
D-Transposition of the great arteries	19
Hypoplastic left heart syndrome	14
Tetralogy of Fallot	8
Coarctation of the aorta	7
Ventricular septal defect	3
Others	49
Age on Admission: 7–13 Days (n = 195)	
Coarctation of the aorta	16
Ventricular septal defect	14
Hypoplastic left heart syndrome	8
D-Transposition of the great arteries	7
Tetralogy of Fallot	7
Others	48
Age on Admission: 14–28 Days (n = 177)	
Ventricular septal defect	16
Coarctation of the aorta	12
Tetralogy of Fallot	7
D-Transposition of the great arteries	7
Patent ductus arteriosus	5
Others	53

Adapted from Flanagan MF, Fyler DC. Cardiac disease. In: Avery GB, Fletcher MA, MacDonald M, eds. Neonatology: pathophysiology and management of the newborn. Philadelphia: JB Lippincott, 1994:524.

Table 12.2. Indications for Fetal Echocardiography

Fetal Risk Factors Associated with Congenital Heart Disease
  Extracardiac anomalies
    Abnormal karyotype
      Trisomies (13, 18, 21)
      Partial trisomy 22
      Turner's syndrome (XO)
    Congenital malformations: duodenal atresia, esophageal atresia or tracheoesophageal fistula, omphalocele, diaphragmatic hernia, renal dysgenesis, hydrocephalus
  Arrhythmias
    Unsustained irregular rhythm
    Sustained tachycardia
    Sustained bradycardia
  Suspected cardiac anomaly on level I scan
  Small for gestational age
  Nonimmune hydrops fetalis
  Two-vessel umbilicus
Maternal Risk Factors Associated with Congenital Heart Disease
  Congenital heart disease
  Cardiac teratogen exposure
    Lithium carbonate
    Amphetamines
    Alcohol
    Anticonvulsants: phenytoin, valproic acid, carbamazepine, trimethadione
    Isotretinoin
  Maternal metabolic disorders
    Diabetes mellitus
    Phenylketonuria
  Infection
    Rubella
    Cytomegalovirus
    Coxsackie virus
  Collagen vascular disease
  Polyhydramnios
  Oligohydramnios
Familial Risk Factors Associated with Congenital Heart Disease
  Congenital heart disease
  Genetic syndromes
    Noonan
    Tuberous sclerosis
    Marfan
    Holt-Oram
    DiGeorge
    Hypertrophic cardiomyopathy

Adapted from Friedman AH, Copel HA, Kleinman CS. Fetal echocardiography and fetal cardiology: indications, diagnosis, and management. Sem Perinatol 1993;17(2):76.

from screening four chamber view 40%; other major organ system defect, involving abnormal karyotype, 25%; maternal drug ingestion or abuse 0 to 1% (26).

Although the most severe forms of congenital heart anomalies can be accurately diagnosed by fetal echocardiography, some lesions such as coarctation of the aorta, small ventricular and atrial septal defects, total anomalous pulmonary venous return, and mild aortic or pulmonary stenosis can be missed by fetal echocardiography (23, 27). Although, the main anomaly in complex congenital heart disease is generally identified by fetal echocardiography, complete definition of the exact anatomy of the cardiac malformation often requires postnatal echocardiography.

Sustained or intermittent fetal tachyarrhythmias or bradyarrhythmias can be detected on routine obstetric screening ultrasound examinations. If a fetal arrhythmia is found a more complete fetal echocardiogram should be performed to rule out associated structural heart disease and to further delineate the arrhythmia.

Therapeutic interventions of prenatally diagnosed congenital heart disease remain limited and primarily involve redirecting delivery to a tertiary care center and drug therapy for tachyarrhythmias. Pregnancy termination may be considered in some circumstances. Lesions that may warrant delivery of the neonate with known congenital heart disease at or near a tertiary care center, are those that are ductal dependent for systemic blood flow (hypoplastic left heart syndrome, interrupted aortic arch, coarctation of the aorta, severe aortic stenosis); ductal dependent for pulmonary blood flow (critical pulmonic stenosis, pulmonic atresia with intact ventricular septum, tetralogy of Fallot with pulmonary atresia, tricuspid atresia, and Ebstein's anomaly); those that may require intervention to improve intracardiac mixing after birth (transposition of the great arteries); or those that may require emergency surgery (obstructed total anomalous pulmonary venous return). Spontaneous delivery at term is usually preferable to elective induction, unless nonimmune hydrops fetalis is present. The full-term infant is easier to manage from a cardiorespiratory and hemodynamic standpoint, and has a nutritional reserve accumulated during the third trimester that the premature neonate does not possess. The full-term neonate is also less likely to suffer from electrolyte abnormalities, respiratory distress syndrome, necrotizing enterocolitis, and intraventricular hemorrhage.

EVALUATION OF THE NEONATE WITH SUSPECTED CONGENITAL HEART DISEASE

Initial evaluation of the neonate with suspected congenital heart disease includes a thorough history, physical examination with four extremity blood pressure measurements, chest radiograph, electrocardiogram, hyperoxia test, and echocardiogram, if indicated. A complete discussion of this evaluation can be found in Chapter 4. Interpretation of the chest radiograph is described in Chapter 27, *Perioperative Radiographic Studies*.

Blood pressure measurement, manually or with an automated Dynamapp (Johnson and Johnson Criticare, Piscataway, NJ), should be performed on all four extremities when congenital heart disease is suspected. A systolic pressure more than 10 mm Hg higher in the upper body relative to the lower body is abnormal and suggests coarctation of the aorta, aortic arch hypoplasia, or interrupted aortic arch. It should be noted that testing for a systolic blood pressure gradient is specific for an arch abnormality, but it is not very sensitive; a systolic blood pressure gradient will not be present in the neonate with an arch abnormality in whom the ductus arteriosus is patent and nonrestrictive. *Therefore, lack of a systolic blood pressure gradient in the newborn does not conclusively rule out coarctation or other arch abnormalities, but the presence of a systolic pressure gradient is diagnostic of an aortic arch abnormality.*

Hyperoxia Test

In all neonates with suspected critical congenital heart disease, a properly performed hyperoxia test is most likely to be the most sensitive and specific tool in the initial evaluation. A hyperoxia test should be performed in neonates with resting pulse oximetry less than 95%, cyanosis, or circulatory collapse. The hyperoxia test consists of obtaining a baseline right radial (preductal) arterial blood gas measurement when the child is breathing room air, $F_{IO_2} = 0.21$, and then repeating the measurement with the child inspiring 100% oxygen, $F_{IO_2} = 1.00$. Arterial partial pressure of oxygen (P_{O_2}) should be measured directly via arterial puncture, although properly acquired transcutaneous oxygen monitor (TCOM) values for P_{O_2} are also acceptable. Pulse oximetry cannot be used for documentation, as a neonate given 100% inspired oxygen who has an oxygen saturation of 100% may have an arterial P_{O_2} of 80 mm Hg, which is abnormal, or greater than 500 mm Hg, which is normal. Measurements of P_{O_2} should be made at both preductal and postductal sites, as a difference in saturations is helpful diagnostically. If preductal saturation is different than postductal saturation, "differential cyanosis" exists. Differential cyanosis is discussed fully in Chapter 4. Interpretation of the hyperoxia test is delineated in Table 12.3 (28):

The neonate who "fails" a hyperoxia test is likely to have congenital heart disease with ductal-dependent systemic or pulmonary blood flow, and should receive prostaglandin E_1 until anatomic definition can be accomplished.

When the hyperoxia test suggests that cardiac disease is responsible for the hypoxia, chest radiograph and electrocardiogram may be used to help delineate which of the cardiac structural defects is most likely until definitive echocardiography can be carried out.

EVALUATION OF THE CYANOTIC NEONATE

Cyanosis is the physical sign characterized by blue mucous membranes, nail beds, and skin. Cyanosis can be perceived when an absolute concentration of deoxygenated hemoglobin of at least 3 g/dL is present. It is the absolute concentration of desaturated hemoglobin, not the ratio of oxygenated to deoxygenated hemoglobin (% saturation), that determines the presence of cyanosis.

Cyanosis indicates arterial oxygen desaturation (hypoxemia), except when polycythemia or methhemoglobinemia are present. Factors that influence whether cyanosis will appear include the hematocrit, which reflects the absolute concentration of hemoglobin, and the factors that affect the O_2 dissociation curve, which have an impact on oxygen saturation. Parameters that affect the O_2 dissociation curve include pH, P_{CO_2}, temperature, level of 2,3-diphosphoglycerate, and the ratio of adult to fetal hemoglobin. For example, consider two infants with an oxygen saturation of 85%. The polycythemic newborn, with a hemoglobin of 22 g/dL, will have 3.3 g/dL (15% of 22 g/dL) of desaturated hemoglobin, and will appear cyanotic, whereas the anemic in-

Table 12.3. Interpretation of the Hyperoxia Test

	$FiO_2 = 0.21$ PaO_2 (% saturation)		$FiO_2 = 1.00$ PaO_2 (% saturation)	$PaCO_2$
Normal	70 (95)		> 200 (100)	40
Pulmonary disease	50 (85)		> 150 (100)	50
Neurologic disease	50 (85)		> 150 (100)	50
Methemoglobinemia	70 (95)		> 200 (100)	35
Cardiac disease				
Parallel circulation[a]	< 40 (< 75)		< 50 (< 85)	35
Restricted PBF[b]	< 40 (< 75)		< 50 (< 85)	35
Complete mixing without restricted PBF[c]	50–60 (85–93)		< 150 (< 100)	35
PPHN	Preductal	Postductal		
PFO (no right-to-left shunt)	70 (95)	< 40 (< 75)	Variable	35–50
PFO (with right-to-left shunt)	< 40 (< 75)	< 40 (< 75)	Variable	35–50

PBF, pulmonary blood flow; PFO, patent foramen ovale; PPHN, persistent pulmonary hypertension of the newborn.
[a] e.g., D-transposition of the great arteries.
[b] e.g., Tricuspid atresia with pulmonary stenosis or atresia, pulmonary atresia or critical pulmonary stenosis with intact ventricular septum, or tetralogy of Fallot.
[c] e.g., Truncus arteriosus, total anomalous pulmonary venous return, single ventricle, hypoplastic left heart syndrome, tricuspid atresia without pulmonary stenosis or atresia.
Adapted from Barone, MA. The Harriet Lane Handbook. 14th ed. St. Louis: Mosby-Yearbook, 1996.

fant with 10 g/dL of hemoglobin and only 1.5 g/dL (15% of 10 g/dL) of deoxygenated hemoglobin may not.

Cyanosis caused by hypoxemia should not be confused with acrocyanosis, which is blueness of the extremities due to peripheral vasoconstriction noted in the first 24 to 48 hours of life. Neonates with acrocyanosis have pink mucosal membranes.

Differential diagnosis of cyanosis in the newborn is delineated in Table 12.4, and it is subdivided into (a) cardiac, (b) neurologic, (c) pulmonary, and (d) hematologic causes. Differentiating cardiac and respiratory causes of cyanosis in the neonate is a common clinical problem. Pulmonary causes of hypoxemia and cyanosis result from intrapulmonary right-to-left shunting. Hypoxemia and cyanosis in the neonate from neurologic causes is typically due to hypoventilation. Clinical cyanosis without hypoxemia can be present in infants with polycythemia or methemoglobinemia. Polycythemic infants are plethoric from venous congestion in the distal extremities.

A full discussion on the evaluation and management of the cyanotic neonate is delineated in Section I, Chapter 4.

STABILIZATION AND TRANSPORT

Once a diagnosis of congenital heart disease is suspected, the infant must be stabilized and arrangements made to make a definitive anatomic diagnosis. This may involve transport of the neonate to another medical center where a pediatric cardiologist is available.

Initial Resuscitation

For the neonate who presents with cyanosis, congestive heart failure, or shock, simultaneous attention is devoted to the basics of advanced life support and maintenance of a patent ductus arteriosus. A stable airway must be maintained to allow for adequate ventilation. Reliable venous access is essential; the umbilical vein should be used if patent. An arterial line assists in monitoring blood pressure, acid-base status, and oxygenation of the patient. In the neonate this can be most reliably obtained through the umbilical artery. Volume resuscitation, inotropic support, and correction of metabolic acidosis are required to maximize cardiac output and tissue perfusion.

A blood glucose level should be checked to determine if hypoglycemia is present. In the initial evaluation of a newborn with cyanosis or circulatory collapse, a sepsis workup is usually performed, and the patient is started on appropriate antibiotics.

Airway Management and Supplemental Oxygen

If respiratory distress or profound cyanosis is present, the infant should be intubated, sedated, and mechanically ventilated. If possible, intubation should be performed

Table 12.4. Differential Diagnosis of Cyanosis in the Neonate

Cardiac
  Ductal Independent Mixing Lesions
    Truncus arteriosus
    Total anomalous pulmonary venous return without obstruction
    D-transposition of the great arteries[a]
  Lesions with Ductal Dependent Pulmonary Blood Flow
    Tetralogy of Fallot
    Ebstein's anomaly
    Tetralogy of Fallot with pulmonary atresia[b]
    Critical pulmonic stenosis
    Tricuspid valve atresia with normally related great arteries[b]
    Pulmonic valve atresia with intact ventricular septum
    Heterotaxy[b]
  Lesions with Ductal Dependent Systemic Blood Flow
    Hypoplastic left heart syndrome
    Interrupted aortic arch
    Critical coarctation of the aorta
    Critical aortic stenosis
Neurological
  Central Nervous System Dysfunction
    Drug-induced depression of respiratory drive
    Postasphyxial cerebral dysfunction
    Intraventricular hemorrhage
    Subarachnoid hemorrhage
    Subdural hematoma
    Meningitis
    Encephalitis
    Sepsis
    Shock
    Seizures
    Hypoglycemia
  Respiratory Neuromuscular Dysfunction
    Cardiac
    Neurological
      Central nervous system dysfunction
      Respiratory neuromuscular dysfunction
    Neonatal myasthenia gravis
    Botulism
    Werdnig-Hoffman disease
    Phrenic nerve paralysis
Pulmonary
  Primary Lung Disease
    Respiratory distress syndrome
    Persistent pulmonary hypertension of the newborn (PPHN)
    Transient tachypnea of the newborn
    Meconium aspiration
    Pneumonia
    Pulmonary hemorrhage
    Cystic adenomatoid malformation
    Pulmonary hypoplasia
    Pulmonary arteriovenous malformation
  Airway Obstruction
    Choanal stenosis or atresia
    Macroglossia
    Thyroid goiter
    Cystic hygroma
    Vocal cord paralysis
    Laryngotracheomalacia
    Laryngeal web
    Vascular ring or pulmonary sling
    Tracheoesophageal fistula
    Tracheal or bronchial stenosis
    Mediastinal mass (teratoma, thymoma)
    Absent pulmonary valve syndrome
    Pierre-Robin syndrome
  Extrinsic Compression of the Lungs
    Pneumothorax, chylothorax, hemothorax
    Pleural effusion
    Pulmonary interstitial emphysema,
    Congenital diaphragmatic hernia
    Thoracic dystrophies or dysplasias
Hematologic
  Methemoglobinemia
  Polycythemia

[a] A patent ductus arteriosus may improve mixing, especially with an intact ventricular septum (see Chapter 19.1).
[b] Most forms.

with neuromuscular blockade and sedation (see Chapter 7, *Principles of Sedation and Analgesia* and Chapter 8, *The Airway and Mechanical Ventilation*). Rather than "rules" dictating the concentration of supplemental O_2, the child with suspected congenital heart disease should receive supplemental oxygen to titrate oxygen saturation to 80 to 85%. (See also Chapter 18, *Single Ventricle Lesions*.)

Prostaglandin E_1

The neonate who "fails" the hyperoxia test or has an equivocal result in addition to other signs or symptoms of congenital heart disease, or the neonate who presents in shock within the first 3 weeks of life is highly likely to have congenital heart disease. These neonates are likely to have congenital lesions that depend on blood flow through a patent ductus arteriosus for either pulmonary or systemic blood flow, or need the patent ductus arteriosus to promote intercirculatory mixing. Administration of prostaglandin E_1 has been shown to open the ductus arteriosus (29), and, depending on the lesion, increase pulmonary blood flow, systemic blood flow, or intercirculatory mixing. As the ductus becomes patent hypoxemia is minimized and the metabolic acidosis that results from persistent hypoxemia or low systemic blood flow corrects (29). In the severely hypoxemic neonate with ductal-dependent pulmonary blood flow, oxygen saturation will increase as pulmonary blood flow increases. Neonates who present in shock or congestive heart failure in the first few weeks of life have ductal-dependent systemic flow until proved otherwise, and resuscitation will not be successful until the ductus is opened. In neonates with transposition of the great arteries, maintenance of a patent ductus arteriosus improves intercirculatory mixing.

Administered as a continuous intravenous infusion PGE_1 has adverse reactions that must be anticipated. Common side effects include fever (14%), apnea (12%), and peripheral vasodilation (10%). Other deleterious reactions include bradycardia (7%), seizures (4%), tachycardia (3%), edema (1%), and in extremely rare cases cardiac arrest (1%) (30).

Apnea resulting from PGE_1 therapy typically occurs within the first 24 hours of administration, but it can occur at any time during administration. Infants who are begun on PGE_1 require continuous cardiorespiratory monitoring. For those neonates in whom transport to another facility is planned, consideration should be made for control of the airway and mechanical ventilation before transport. Factors influencing the decision toward intubation are severity of cyanosis and hemodynamic instability, gestational age of the patient, transport distance, and skill of the transport team in emergent intubation.

The usual starting dose is 0.025–0.1 µg/kg/min. Once a therapeutic effect has been achieved, the dose may be decreased to as low as 0.025 µg/kg/min without loss of therapeutic effect. Response to PGE_1 is often immediate if patency of the ductus is important for the hemodynamic state of the infant. Failure to respond to PGE_1 can mean an incorrect initial diagnosis, the ductus is unresponsive to PGE_1, which occurs in the older infant, or an absent ductus.

Rarely, the patient may become progressively unstable after the institution of PGE_1 therapy. Clinical deterioration after institution of PGE_1 is an important diagnostic finding that identifies the congenital heart defect as one that has obstructed blood flow out of the pulmonary veins or left atrium. Lesions that have impaired blood flow out of the left atrium include hypoplastic left heart syndrome with restrictive patent foramen ovale, mitral atresia with restrictive foramen ovale, transposition of the great arteries with intact ventricular septum and a restrictive foramen ovale, and total anomalous pulmonary venous connection with obstruction. If clinical deterioration occurs with PGE_1, then urgent plans for echocardiography and interventional catheterization or cardiac surgery should be made.

Typically, PGE_1 causes peripheral vasodilation that manifests itself as cutaneous flushing and, in many cases, hypotension. Because of this phenomenon, a separate intravenous line should be secured for volume administration in any infant receiving PGE_1, especially those who require transport. If hypotension is noted a 10–20 mL/kg bolus of normal saline, lactated Ringer's, 5% albumin, or plasmanate will generally normalize the infant's blood pressure. It is prudent to remeasure an arterial blood gas, and reassess the infant's capillary refill and vital signs within 15–30 minutes of starting the PGE_1 infusion.

Inotropic Agents

For the neonate or infant in cardiogenic shock, continuous infusion of an inotropic agent may improve myocardial contractility and thereby enhance tissue perfusion of the vital organs and periphery. Care should be taken to replete the intravascular volume before instituting vasoactive agents.

Sympathomimetic amines are the inotropic agents most commonly used for hemodynamic stabilization (see Chapter 5, *Cardiovascular Pharmacology*). Sympathomimetic amines may be endogenous (dopamine and epinephrine) or synthetic (dobutamine and isoproterenol). Dopamine and dobutamine are recommended for the neonate with hypotension and tachycardia, as these agents have less chronotropic properties. Dopamine is a precursor of norepinephrine, and it stimulates dopaminergic, β_1, and α-adrenergic receptors in a dose-dependent manner. Dopamine improves myocardial contractility, thereby increasing stroke volume, cardiac output, and mean arterial pressure, as well as urine output with a low incidence of side effects at doses less than 10 µg/kg/min. Dobutamine, an analogue of dopamine, stimulates β_1 receptors predominantly, with relatively weak β_2 and α-receptor stimulating activity. In comparison with dopamine, dobutamine lacks renal vasodilating properties and does not depend on norepinephrine release from peripheral nerves for its effect. Few data are available concerning the use of dobutamine in neonates, although clinical experience has been favorable. A combination of low dose dopamine, up to 5 µg/kg/min, and dobutamine, 5–10 µg/kg/min, can be used to minimize the potential peripheral vasoconstriction induced by high doses of dopamine while maximizing the dopaminergic effects on renal perfusion.

Isoproterenol and epinephrine are recommended for the neonate with hypotension and a normal or low heart rate, as these agents have both inotropic and chronotropic effects. Isoproterenol stimulates both β_1 and β_2 receptors. In comparison to dobutamine it has a greater chronotropic effect and a stronger vasodilatory effect via its β_2 mechanism. Because of its strong chronotropic effect it should be started at a low dose and increased slowly to titrate effect. Chronotropic effects appear before inotropic effects in responsive hearts, and isoproterenol can produce tachyarrhythmias. The heart usually accommodates quickly to the chronotropic properties to allow the dose to be raised further for inotropic needs. The recommended starting dose is 0.05–0.10 µg/kg/min. Epinephrine, has α_1, α_2, β_1, and β_2 effects. It is most commonly used when the previously listed inotropic infusions at high doses and in combination fail to produce the desired cardiac response. Recommended starting dose is 0.05–0.10 µg/kg/min. Adverse reactions to the sympathomimetic amines include tachycardia, atrial and ventricular arrhythmias, and increased afterload caused by peripheral vasoconstriction. Tachycardia increases myocardial oxygen consumption, whereas atrial and ventricular arrhythmias and peripheral vasoconstriction may decrease cardiac output.

Transport

After resuscitation and stabilization is complete, the neonate with suspected congenital heart disease often needs to be transferred to an institution that provides subspecialty care in pediatric cardiology and cardiac surgery. A successful transport involves two transitions of care for the neonate: from the referring hospital staff to the transport team, and from the transport staff to the accepting hospital staff. The need for accurate, detailed, and complete communication of information between the respective teams cannot be overemphasized. If possible, the pediatric cardiologist accepting the patient should be included in formulating a management plan for the neonate while the neonate is still at the referring hospital.

Reliable vascular access should be secured for the neonate receiving continuous infusions of PGE_1 or inotropic agents during transport. Many neonates receiving a PGE_1 infusion will be intubated for transport. All intubated patients should have gastric decompression by nasogastric tube or orogastric tube and should not receive nutrition by mouth or nasogastric tube.

Acid-base status and oxygen delivery should be evaluated prior to transport with an arterial blood gas measurement. Although most noncardiac patients are transported receiving supplemental oxygen at or near 100%, this is often not the inspired oxygen concentration of choice for the neonate with congenital heart disease (see above). This management decision for transport is particularly important for those infants with ductal-dependent systemic or pulmonary blood flow and complete intracardiac mixing with single ventricle physiology, and it emphasizes the need to consult with a pediatric cardiologist prior to transport to achieve optimal transport care (see Chapter 18).

In neonates, *hypotension is a late finding in shock*. More sensitive signs of impending decompensation include persistent tachycardia, poor tissue perfusion, and metabolic acidosis. Treatment of shock should occur prior to transport during the stabilization phase of management. Before leaving the referring hospital, the patient's most current hemodynamic status (capillary refill, heart rate, systemic blood pressure, acid-base status) should be reassessed and relayed to the receiving hospital.

CONFIRMING THE DIAGNOSIS

Echocardiography

Two-dimensional echocardiology, supplemented with Doppler and color Doppler, has become the primary diagnostic modality for anatomic definition in pediatric cardiology. Echocardiography quickly provides information about the structure and function of the heart and great vessels. The echocardiogram in the neonate is not "noninvasive"; a complete echocardiogram on a newborn suspected of having congenital heart disease may take an hour or more to perform, and it may not be well tolerated by a sick and/or premature neonate. Temperature instability from exposure during this extended period may be detrimental to the newborn infant. Extension of the neck for suprasternal notch views of the aortic arch may be problematic, particularly in the neonate with respiratory distress or a tenuous airway. Therefore, in sick neonates a medical staff person other than the individual performing the echocardiogram should observe the patient's vital signs and respiratory status. A thorough description of echocardiography and its use in diagnosis can be found in Chapter 28, *Echocardiography*.

Cardiac Catheterization

The role of pediatric cardiac catheterization has changed dramatically over the last decade. Prior to the era of Doppler echocardiography, it was the primary means of defining cardiac anatomy and for assessing hemodynamics. Catheterization is presently used to obtain hemodynamic information that cannot be obtained by echocardiography, to look at anatomy not identified echocardiographically, and for therapeutic interventions. Congenital cardiac lesions that still require catheterization for anatomic definition include distal pulmonary artery stenoses, aorticopulmonary collaterals, and certain types of coronary artery anomalies. Usual indications for neonatal catheterization are shown in Table 12.5. Cardiac catheterization is described fully in Chapter 29, *Cardiac Catheterization in the Critically Ill Cardiac Patient*.

EVALUATION OF ADDITIONAL ORGAN SYSTEMS

Genetics

A careful search for other congenital anomalies is essential, as congenital heart disease is accompanied by at least one extracardiac malformation 25% of the time (31). The spectrum of associated defects in children with congenital

Table 12.5. Indications for Neonatal Catheterization[a]

Interventions
  Therapeutic
    Balloon atrial septostomy
    Balloon pulmonary valvuloplasty
    Balloon aortic valvuloplasty
    Balloon angioplasty of native coarctation of the aorta
    Coil embolization of abnormal vascular communications
  Diagnostic
    Endomyocardial biopsy
Anatomic Definition
  Coronary arteries
    Pulmonary atresia with intact ventricular septum
    Transposition of the great arteries
    Tetralogy of Fallot
  Aortic to pulmonary artery collateral vessels
    Tetralogy of Fallot with pulmonary atresia
  Distal pulmonary artery anatomy
Hemodynamic Measurements

[a] All the therapeutic interventions listed above have alternate surgical options and their use depends on institutional experience.

heart disease is broad and likely reflects the complexity of the developmental process during cardiogenesis.

Congenital heart disease and extracardiac malformations occur with chromosomal abnormalities, single gene defects, and syndromes and associations of unknown cause. Chromosomal anomalies causing both cardiac and noncardiac defects include trisomy 13, trisomy 18, trisomy 21, and monosomy X (Turner syndrome). Noonan syndrome, Holt-Oram syndrome, and Ellis-van Creveld syndrome are single gene defects that can result in both cardiac and extracardiac congenital dysmorphisms. Examples of syndromes of unknown cause that result in cardiac and noncardiac anomalies include Alagille's syndrome, thrombocytopenia absent radius (TAR) syndrome, and Williams syndrome. Associations of unknown cause that contain multiple congenital defects include VACTERL and CHARGE. Table 12.6 summarizes common chromosomal anomalies, single gene defects, and syndromes and associations of unknown cause in which congenital heart disease is present.

The association of cardiovascular defects and other midline defects has been studied using the population-based registry of the Metropolitan Atlanta Congenital Defects Program (32). This group reviewed associations among neural tube defects (anencephaly, spina bifida, encephalocele), oral clefts, omphalocele, tracheoesophageal fistula, imperforate anus, conotruncal heart defects, and diaphragmatic hernia. Oral clefts, omphalocele, tracheoesophageal fistula, and imperforate anus were found to be in association with conotruncal defects more commonly than expected by chance alone. No cases of neural tube defects or diaphragmatic hernia were identified in babies with conotruncal congenital heart defects. Chromosome 22 alterations, first noted in velocardiofacial syndrome, are linked with conotruncal malformations (tetralogy of Fallot, truncus arteriosus, interrupted aortic arch, aortic arch abnormalities and conoventricular septal defects). Therefore, children with conotruncal congenital heart lesions should be evaluated for karyotypic evaluation (33).

If the child's congenital heart disease is thought to be part of a syndrome, a genetics consultation should be obtained to assist in diagnosis and long-term management. Any defects noted that may affect the child's intraoperative or postoperative course should be evaluated by the appropriate specialist to minimize any untoward effects the defect may have on the surgical procedure or catheterization. Airway anomalies should be evaluated by otolaryngology or pediatric pulmonology. If gastrointestinal anomalies are present, such as diaphragmatic hernia, Hirschsprung's disease, malrotation (heterotaxy), tracheoesophageal fistula, omphalocele, gastroschisis, intestinal atresia, or imperforate anus, a pediatric gastroenterology or pediatric surgery specialist should be consulted.

Central Nervous System

Imaging studies are often needed to complete the preoperative evaluation. If the child is thought to have a chromosomal anomaly, syndrome, or association that has both cardiac and central nervous system defects then the brain should be imaged. Magnetic resonance imaging (MRI) assists in imaging of the cerebral cortex, ventricular size, posterior fossa, and brainstem, whereas computed tomography (CT) scan of the head defines cortical gray and white matter and ventricular size. If the neonate with suspected congenital heart disease is premature, a screening head ultrasound is recommended to rule out intraventricular hemorrhage prior to surgery, interventional catheterization, or placement onto extracorporeal membrane oxygenation or cardiopulmonary bypass. The infant or child with congenital heart disease who has seizures may need a neurology consultation and an electroencephalogram. See Chapter 24, *Neurologic Disorders* for a full discussion on the interaction between the central nervous system and heart disease.

Renal

Children who have ductal-dependent systemic flow are at risk for prerenal renal failure, unless arterial flow to the kidneys through the patent ductus arteriosus can be guaranteed. If arterial flow to the kidneys is inadequate, dopamine can be started to cause dilation of the renal arterioles and the splanchnic circulation.

Because a higher incidence of urinary tract anomalies is found in children with congenital heart disease (3 to 6%

Table 12.6. Common Chromosomal Anomalies, Syndromes, and Associations Including Congenital Heart Disease

Chromosomal Anomalies

Chromosome	Incidence	Extracardiac Features	Cardiac Features
Trisomy 13 (Patau's Syndrome)	1/7000–8000	Facies (midfacial hypoplasia, cleft lip, microphthalmia coloboma, low set ears); brain anomalies (microcephaly, holoprosencephaly)	≥ 80% have cardiac defects; VSD most common; secundum ASD; PDA; BAV; BPV
Trisomy 18 (Edward's Syndrome)	1/7000 female/male = 3:1	SGA; facies (dolichocephaly, prominent occiput, short palpebral fissures, low set posteriorly rotated ears, small mandible); short sternum; "rocker bottom feet"; crossing fifth and index fingers with "clenched fists"	≥ 95% have cardiac defects; VSD most common (60% malalignment, 35% conoventricular); 95% CPVND with regurgitation; 25% TOF or DORV
Trisomy 21 (Down Syndrome)	1/650	Facies (brachycephaly, flattened occiput, midfacial hypoplasia, mandibular prognathism, upslanting palpebral fissures, epicanthal folds, Brushfield spots, large tongue); simian creases, clinodactyly with short 5th finger; pronounced hypotonia	40% have cardiac defects (50% CAVC, ASD primum, inlet VSD; 20 to 30% conoventricular VSD, secundum ASD, PDA, or CoA; 10–15% TOF);
Monosomy X (Turner's Syndrome)	1/2500	Lymphedema of hands, feet; short stature; short webbed neck; facies (triangular with downslanting palpebral fissures; low set ears); shield chest	35% have cardiac defects (40% BAV, aortic stenosis, CoA; 20% VSD, secundum ASD, PDA; 5 to 10% aortic dilatation)

Single Gene Defects

Syndrome	Incidence and Inheritance	Extracardiac Features	Cardiac Features
Noonan	1/2000 Autosomal Dominant	Facies (hypertelorism, epicanthal folds, broad forehead, downslanting palpebral fissures, ptosis); low set ears; short webbed neck with low hairline; shield chest; short stature; cryptorchidism in males	50% have cardiac defect; usually valvar pulmonary stenosis caused by valve dysplasia; peripheral pulmonary artery stenosis; hypertrophic cardiomyopathy with or without pulmonary stenosis
Holt-Oram	Autosomal Dominant	Spectrum of upper limb and shoulder girdle anomalies; radial hypoplasia; phocomelia; small stature; small chest	50% have cardiac defect; usually secundum ASD or VSD
Alagille	Autosomal Dominant	Direct hyperbilirubinemia; facies (micrognathia, broad forehead, deep set eyes); vertebral anomalies	Peripheral pulmonary artery stenosis most common
Ellis-van Creveld	Autosomal Recessive	Short distal extremities; polydactyly; hypoplastic nails; dental anomalies	50% have cardiac defect, usually endocardial cushion defect or common atrium
Thrombocytopenia-Absent Radius (TAR)	Autosomal Recessive	Thrombocytopenia; absent or hypoplastic radii; leukemoid granulocytosis in the first year of life	33% have cardiac defect, usually TOF; VSD; ASD; dextrocardia
Williams	Mostly sporadic, some familial inheritance noted	SGA, FTT; short stature; facies ("elfin" with short palpebral fissures, flat nasal bridge, blue eyes with stellate iris, long philtrum, anteverted nares, prominent lips); friendly personality; characteristic mental deficiency (motor more reduced than verbal performance)	50% have cardiac defect most commonly supravalvar aortic stenosis; valvular aortic stenosis; peripheral pulmonary artery stenosis

Associations (Name)	Incidence	Extracardiac Features	Cardiac Features
VACTERL	0.16/1000	Vertebral defects; anal atresia; tracheoesophageal fistula; radial and renal anomalies; limb defects	50% have cardiac defects; most commonly VSD and TOF
CHARGE		Coloboma; choanal atresia; growth and mental deficiency; genital hypoplasia (in males); ear anomalies and/or deafness	85% have cardiac defect; most commonly conotruncal anomalies (TOF, truncus arteriosus, aortic arch anomalies)

VSD, ventricular septal defect; ASD, atrial septal defect; PDA, patent ductus arteriosus; BAV, bicuspid aortic valve; BPV, bicuspid pulmonic valve; SGA, small for gestational age; CPVND, congenital polyvalvar nodular dysplasia; DORV, double outlet right; TOF, tetralogy of Fallot; CAVC, complete atrioventricular canal; CoA coarctation of the aorta; FTT, failure to thrive; VSD, ventricular septal defect.

of the infants with congenital heart disease compared with 1.4% of the general population), a renal ultrasound should be considered to delineate any abnormal urinary anatomy (34). Urinary anomalies seen with congenital heart anomalies include hydronephrosis, ureteral duplication, unilateral renal agenesis, position abnormalities, and renal dysplasia (35). Children who have both urinary tract and cardiac defects often have multiple congenital defects, and it is in this group that a screening renal ultrasound should be mandatory. See Chapter 25, *Renal Issues* for a detailed discussion of renal issues pertinent to congenital heart disease.

Gastrointestinal

When ductal-dependent systemic blood flow is present, there may be inadequate intestinal arterial blood flow; if ductal-dependent pulmonary blood flow is present, there may be hypoxemic intestinal blood flow. In both cases there may be inadequate oxygen delivery to the intestine and an increased risk of necrotizing enterocolitis (NEC). The premature neonate is much more at risk for NEC than the full-term neonate.

Because infants with ductal-dependent systemic or pulmonary blood flow are at risk for NEC, they should be fed enterally with care. Advantages of enteral feeding include higher caloric intake than what can be provided through a peripheral intravenous line, avoidance of cholestasis and chronic liver disease from parenteral nutrition, and maintenance of a vital intestinal mucosa. The main disadvantage of enteral feeding to the child with critical congenital heart disease is that if bowel ischemia or hypoxemia are present, feeding the child might result in bacterial invasion into the intestinal mucosa and NEC.

Full-term infants with critical congenital heart disease should be given intravenous fluid during stabilization and transport, and they are usually kept on intravenous fluid until their surgical procedure is performed. If the child's definitive procedure will not occur within the first few days of life the newborn can be fed orally, if tolerated, or by nasogastric tube. Premature infants less than 34 weeks gestation may not be able to feed orally because of central nervous system immaturity; they should be fed by nasogastric tube until reaching a suitable size for surgical intervention, which is approximately 1600–1800 g. Chapter 26, elaborates on topics in gastroenterology that pertain to congenital heart disease.

TIMING AND TYPE OF SURGERY

For the neonate with congenital heart disease requiring surgical intervention, the cardiology and cardiac surgery teams responsible must decide on timing and type of surgery. In the neonate who has sustained end-organ damage secondary to hypoxia-ischemia, medical management should continue, if possible, until evidence is seen of recovery of secondary organ function, to minimize surgical morbidity and risk. In addition, sepsis should be evaluated for and ruled out. Delaying surgery a few days also allows adequate time for the family to understand the complexity of the heart defect and the proposed intervention.

REFERENCES

1. Fyler DC, Rothman KJ, Parisi-Buckley L, et al. The determinants of five year survival of infants with critical congenital heart disease. Cardiovascular Clinics 1981;11:393–405.
2. Rabinovitch M, Herrera-Deleon V, Castaneda AR, et al. Growth and development of the pulmonary vascular bed in patients with tetralogy of Fallot, with or without pulmonary atresia. Circulation 1981;64:1234–1249.
3. Flanagan MF, Fujii AM, Colan SD, et al. Myocardial angiogenesis and coronary perfusion in left ventricular pressure-overload hypertrophy in the young lamb. Evidence for inhibition with chronic protamine administration. Circ Res 1991;68:1458–1470.
4. Newburger JW, Silbert AR, Buckley LP, et al. Cognitive function and age at repair of transposition of the great arteries in children. N Engl J Med 1984;310:1495–1499.
5. Castaneda AR, Mayer JE Jr, Jonas RA, et al. The neonate with critical congenital heart disease: repair—a surgical challenge. J Thorac Cardiovasc Surg 1989;98:869–875.
6. Hazinski MF. Physician-nurse interaction in the intensive care unit. In: Holbrook PR, ed. Textbook of pediatric critical care. Philadelphia: WB Saunders, 1993;1166–1179.
7. Moynihan PJ, Wernovsky G, Hickey PA, et al. Complication rates of transthoracic intracardiac lines removed by critical care nurses [Abstract]. Circulation 1992;86(Suppl I):702A.
8. Anand KJS, Sippell WG, Aynsley-Green A. Randomized trials of fentanyl anesthesia in pre-term babies undergoing surgery: effects on the stress response. Lancet 1987;1:62–66.
9. Mills AN, Haworth SG. Greater permeability of the neonatal lung: postnatal changes in surface charge and biochemistry of porcine pulmonary capillary endothelium. J Thorac Cardiovasc Surg 1991;101:909.
10. Feltes TF, Hansen TN. Effects of an aorticopulmonary shunt on lung fluid balance in the young lamb. Pediatr Res 1989;26:94–97.
11. Reller MD, Morton MJ, Giraud GD. Severe right ventricular pressure loading in fetal sheep augments global myocardial blood flow to submaximal levels. Circulation 1992;86:581–588.
12. Romero TE, Friedman WF. Limited left ventricular response to volume overload in the neonatal period: a comparative study with the adult animal. Pediatr Res 1979;13:910–915.
13. Thornburg KL, Morton MJ. Filling and arterial pressure as determinants of RV stroke volume in the sheep fetus. Am J Physiol 1983;244:H656.
14. Friedman WF. The intrinsic physiologic properties of the developing heart. Prog Cardiovasc Dis 1972;15:87–111.
15. Anand KJS, Phil D, Hansen DD, et al. Hormonal metabolic stress response in neonates undergoing cardiac surgery. Anesthesiology 1990;73:661–670.
16. Anand KJS, Hickey PR. Halothane-morphine compared with high-dose sufentanil for anesthesia and postoperative analgesia in neonatal cardiac surgery. N Engl J Med 1992;326:1–9.

17. Fisher DJ, Heymann MA, Rudolph AM. Fetal myocardial oxygen and carbohydrate consumption during acutely induced hypoxemia. Am J Physiol 1982;242:H657.
18. Brooks-Gunn J, Liaw FR, Klebanov PK. Effects of early intervention on cognitive function of low birth weight preterm infants. J Pediatr 1992;120:350–359.
19. Lenn NJ. Plasticity and responses of the immature nervous system to injury. Semin Perinatol 1987;11:117–131.
20. Clapp S, Perry BL, Farooki ZQ, et al. Down's syndrome, complete atrioventricular canal, and pulmonary vascular obstructive disease. J Thorac Cardiovasc Surg 1990;100:115–121.
21. Hanley FL, Heinemann MK, Jonas RA, et al. Repair of truncus arteriosus in the neonate. J Thorac Cardiovasc Surg 1993;105:1047–1056.
22. Fyler DC. Report of the New England Regional Infant Cardiac Program. Pediatrics 1980;65(Suppl):377.
23. Benacerraf BR, Sanders SP. Fetal echocardiography. Radiol Clin North Am 1990;28:131–147.
24. Flanagan MF, Fyler DC. Cardiac disease. In: Avery GB, Fletcher MA, MacDonald M, eds. Neonatology: pathophysiology and management of the newborn. Philadelphia: JB Lippincott, 1994;524.
25. Friedman AH, Copel JA, Kleinman CS. Fetal echocardiography and fetal cardiology: indications, diagnosis, and management. Semin Perinatol 1993;17:76.
26. Emmanouilides GC, Allen HA, Riemenschneider TA, et al. Moss and Adams' heart disease in infants, children, adolescents, including the fetus and the young adult. 5th ed. Baltimore, Williams & Wilkins, 1995:555.
27. Allan LD, Sharland GK, Milburn A, et al. Prospective diagnosis of 1,006 consecutive cases of congenital heart disease in the fetus. J Am Coll Cardiol 1994;23:1452–1458.
28. Barone, MA. The Harriet Lane handbook. 14th ed. St. Louis: Mosby-Year Book, 1996;155.
29. Heymann MA. Pharmacologic use of prostaglandin E1 in infants with congenital heart disease. Am Heart J 1981;101:837–843.
30. Physicians' Desk Reference. 50th ed. Montvale, NJ: Medical Economics, 1996;2636.
31. Fyler DC. Nadas' pediatric cardiology. Philadelphia: Hanley & Belfus, 1992;37.
32. Khoury MJ, Cordero JF, Mulinare J, et al. Selected midline defect associations: a population study. Pediatrics 1989;84:266–272.
33. Emmanouilides GC, Allen HA, Riemenschneider TA, et al. Moss and Adams' heart disease in infants, children, adolescents, including the fetus and the young adult. 5th ed. Baltimore, Williams & Wilkins, 1995:619–620.
34. Greenwood RD, Rosenthal A, Parisi L, et al. Extracardiac abnormalities in infants with congenital heart disease. Pediatrics 1975;55:485–492.
35. Murugasu B, Yip WCL, Tay JSH, et al. Sonographic screening for renal tract anomalies associated with congenital anomalies of the urinary system. J Clin Ultrasound 1990;18:79–83.

Postoperative Care

13

Stephen J. Roth, MD, MPH

Improved techniques in pediatric cardiac surgery, pediatric anesthesia, echocardiography, diagnostic and interventional cardiac catheterization, and pediatric intensive care since the 1970s have dramatically increased the treatment options for children with significant congenital heart disease (CHD). Because of the complexity and heterogeneity of structural defects in patients with CHD, and the physiologic derangements which derive from them, the critical care of these children has shifted from the adult cardiac intensive care unit (ICU) into units dedicated to pediatric general or pediatric cardiac intensive care. This shift has paralleled the change in philosophy and surgical practice at many institutions of performing reparative operations on neonates and infants instead of an initial palliative procedure followed by definitive repair during childhood (1). Although the ICU team requires the knowledge and technical skills to manage postoperative pediatric cardiac patients of all ages and some young adults with CHD, expertise in the care of neonates and infants is thus of growing importance (2).

Successful postoperative management of patients with CHD who undergo either reparative or palliative operations depends on a thorough knowledge of the following:

1. Precise anatomic diagnosis of the patient's cardiac defect(s).
2. Pathophysiologic effects of the defect(s) on the cardiovascular system and other organs prior to surgery.
3. Patient's noncardiac medical and surgical history plus the preoperative medication regimen.
4. Anesthetic agents used in the operating room.
5. Details of the operation including intraoperative support times (e.g., duration of cardiopulmonary bypass and circulatory arrest) and technical features, plus the potential for residual defects and adverse occurrences that are most commonly encountered following that specific operation.
6. Intraoperative complications, such as dysrhythmias, air embolism, or bleeding, and their management.
7. Evaluation of data obtained from physical examination, hemodynamic monitoring, echocardiography, and cardiac catheterization (if necessary).
8. General ICU management including the use of mechanical ventilators, anesthetic and sedation medications, antimicrobial agents, and parenteral nutrition.
9. Pharmacology of drugs that affect the cardiovascular system, including inotropes, vasodilators, diuretics, and antiarrhythmics.
10. Indications for selected procedures, including pacing, pericardiocentesis, and mechanical support of the failing myocardium with extracorporeal membrane oxygenation (ECMO) or a ventricular assist device (VAD).

This chapter focuses on the specialized equipment required to manage postoperative cardiac patients, initial postoperative assessment following transition from the operating room, interpretation of bedside monitoring data, management of fluid and electrolyte balance, and evaluation and support of cardiac output.

CARDIAC ICU: ENVIRONMENT AND SPECIALIZED EQUIPMENT

Successful postoperative care requires that the ICU possess specific physical features and specialized equipment, as well as a coordinated, multidisciplinary team with expertise in cardiac surgery, cardiology, cardiac anesthesia, intensive care, cardiac nursing, and respiratory therapy. Because the ICU functions in many centers as a recovery room, it is essential that patients can be transported safely from the operating room within 5 minutes. Bed space designs that incorporate both open architecture and isolation rooms are useful. It is preferable for the unit performing post-ICU care to be located adjacent to the ICU, so patients requiring readmission can be transferred quickly.

Pediatric cardiac intensive care requires the standard equipment and laboratory services present in a general pediatric medical or surgical ICU or neonatal ICU plus additional specialized equipment (Table 13.1). Electronic physiologic monitors in each bed space should have the capacity for continuous display of heart rate, electrocardiogram (ECG), arterial blood pressure and arterial pressure tracing; and additional pressure tracings from the pulmonary artery (PA), right atrium (RA), or another central venous site; and left atrium (LA) respiratory rate and body temperature. Monitors must have alarms to alert staff when a monitored variable deviates from its set limits so a response can be initiated immediately. A display of variables such as heart rate and arterial blood pressure in graphic format is a special monitor function that is useful in detecting trends and reconstructing the events surrounding

Table 13.1. Specialized Equipment in the Pediatric Cardiac Intensive Care Unit

Cardiac output computer
Access to cooximeter
External pacemaker equipment
    Bedside single- and dual-chamber external pacemakers
    Transthoracic pacemaker
    Skin leads for temporary transthoracic pacing
    Portable pulse stimulator
    Electrical cables for synchronized cardioversion
Access to echocardiography machine
Mediastinal cart for sternotomy and sternal closure
Access to ECMO and VAD circuits
Delivery and monitoring system for inhaled nitric oxide

ECMO, extracorporeal membrane oxygenation; VAD, ventricular assist device.

changes in hemodynamic status. For example, when evaluating the mechanism of an episode of supraventricular tachycardia, a graphic trend analysis of the ECG can reveal whether the heart rate changed suddenly, suggesting a re-entrant mechanism, or gradually, suggesting an automatic focus or sinus tachycardia. Each monitor should be connected to a printer so that a copy of the ECG, pressure tracings, or graphic trend profiles can be prepared. A cardiac output computer, either as a portable unit or a module used with the bedside monitor, should be accessible to determine thermodilution cardiac outputs. A pulse oximeter for continuous arterial oxygen saturation monitoring at each bed space, and a cooximeter for measurement of blood oxygen saturation should be available. Ideally, all monitors would be components of a clinical information system to allow on-line data display, storage, and analysis.

Because dysrhythmias and conduction abnormalities are common in postoperative cardiac patients (3), the ICU must be equipped to provide cardiac pacing using either temporary epicardial wires placed during surgery, transvenous or transesophageal pacing catheters, or transthoracic leads. Portable, battery-operated, external single- and dual-chamber pacemakers are used for cardiac pacing with either temporary epicardial wires (atrial, ventricular, or both) or transvenous pacing catheters. In patients who require emergent pacing (e.g., sudden complete heart block) but lack a pacing catheter or wire(s), external transthoracic pacing with skin leads may be necessary for a limited time (less than 1 hour) until either a pacing catheter or wire(s) can be inserted. A portable pulse stimulator for use with either epicardial wires or an esophageal pacing catheter is also necessary. The pulse stimulator can be programmed to provide consistent pacing at greater outputs than bedside external pacemakers in patients whose wire thresholds are high (e.g., greater than 18–20 mA). It can also be used to generate single or multiple atrial beats at preset pulse widths and amplitudes for interrupting supraventricular tachycardias. Electrical cables for linking a defibrillator to the bedside ECG monitor should be available for synchronized direct-current cardioversions.

An echocardiography machine must be immediately available to the ICU at all times for imaging patients during emergency situations such as cardiopulmonary resuscitation or suspected acute tamponade.

Occasionally, postoperative patients require a sternotomy in the ICU because of severely compromised cardiac output (e.g., tamponade from chest bleeding or constrictive chest wall forces from edema) or profound cyanosis (e.g., shunt thrombosis with shunt-dependent pulmonary blood flow). A mediastinal cart with the sterile surgical equipment to open and explore the chest should be available for emergent or planned sternotomy procedures. For patients with profound myocardial failure, the capability of initiating mechanical support with either ECMO or VAD within 30 to 45 minutes should exist.

Inhaled nitric oxide, although classified in the United States in 1997 as an investigational drug by the Food and Drug Administration (FDA), has important applications in the treatment of pulmonary artery hypertension in patients with CHD (4). When this potent, selective pulmonary vasodilator gains FDA approval, a system for effective and safe inhaled nitric oxide administration and monitoring will become standard equipment in the cardiac ICU.

TRANSITION FROM THE OPERATING ROOM TO THE ICU AND INITIAL POSTOPERATIVE ASSESSMENT

Transition from operating room to ICU is a time of increased risk for patients, because they must be transported with fewer monitoring capabilities and are converted to new monitoring and support equipment before a thorough postoperative assessment can be performed. Guidelines discussed below provide a general strategy for the initial assessment and management of postoperative cardiac patients.

The ICU team should be familiar with the salient historical details of each patient scheduled for cardiac surgery plus the surgical plan before the patient is taken to the operating room. This is best accomplished by attending regularly scheduled, multidisciplinary preoperative conferences. As surgery is concluding and approximately 30 minutes before transfer, the ICU is called with a concise report of the procedure, current hemodynamic and respiratory status of the patient, medication regimen, and any important complications. Between report and the patient's arrival, appropriate equipment and medications (e.g., a dopamine infusion) are prepared in the ICU. When a patient's surgery is particularly difficult or significant alterations in the surgical plan occur, it can be beneficial for the

ICU physician or cardiologist to visit the operating room to discuss technical or management issues with the surgical team. Patients are transported by the anesthesiologist and at least one member of the surgical team and operating room nursing team.

On the patient's arrival in the ICU, the initial goals of care are to convert efficiently from transport to bedside monitoring equipment and to communicate clearly the details of the operating room course. Maintenance of adequate gas exchange and oxygenation, and uninterrupted delivery of any vasoactive drugs are critical to achieving an uncomplicated transfer. A complete description of the operation is presented to the ICU team while the patient is being connected to bedside monitoring equipment and infusion pumps, and other necessary equipment (e.g., mechanical ventilator and suction for gastric or chest tube evacuation). The description should include details of anesthetic use, airway and ventilator management, and the surgery. Significant details of surgery would include the duration of cardiopulmonary bypass (CPB) and circulatory arrest (if utilized), any concerns about myocardial protection, observations about the recovery of myocardial function, typical systemic arterial and intracardiac pressures after CPB, any dysrhythmias or bleeding problems, and ongoing medication requirements. Postoperative orders should also be reviewed and a decision reached about the use of analgesic, sedative, and neuromuscular blockade agents during the first few hours.

A comprehensive postoperative assessment should be performed by the ICU team soon after arrival (Table 13.2).

Table 13.2. Components of the Initial Postoperative Assessment in the Intensive Care Unit

Laboratory Evaluation
Chest radiograph
Electrocardiogram
Blood gas analysis, preferably from an arterial sample
Serum Na^+, K^+, and Cl^-, glucose levels
Ionized Ca^{2+} level
Hemoglobin or hematocrit, white blood cell count, and platelet count

Postoperative Evaluation by the ICU Physician
Review of patient's underlying cardiac defect(s), history of prior interventions, and preoperative pathophysiology and clinical status
Review of anesthesia record and operative note
Verification of current medication dosages, ventilator settings (if mechanically ventilated), and intravenous fluid rates
Physical examination focusing on the cardiovascular and respiratory systems
Interpretation of data from bedside monitoring and initial laboratory testing
Documentation in the medical record of physical examination and laboratory findings, evaluation of the adequacy of the procedure, and plans for the first postoperative night

Vital signs should document core temperature, heart rate and rhythm (e.g., spontaneous or paced), respiratory rate, arterial blood pressure, pressures from additional intravascular catheters (e.g., RA or other central venous pressure [CVP], LA, and PA), and arterial oxygen saturation by pulse oximetry. The core temperature of patients who have undergone procedures using hypothermia can be 33° to 35°C; low heart rates in these patients often reflect low body temperature. Arterial oxygen desaturation in cardiac patients can be secondary either to right-to-left shunting at intracardiac or other vascular levels (e.g., a patent ductus arteriosus [PDA] or systemic venous to pulmonary venous collaterals) or to pulmonary venous desaturation. Physical examination should focus primarily on cardiovascular and respiratory function, but it should be as complete as possible based on the patient's condition. The examination is performed with the patient's diagnosis and described surgery in mind, so that procedure adequacy can be evaluated. For example, in the patient who has undergone complete repair of tetralogy of Fallot (TOF), the examiner should specifically assess for evidence of a residual ventricular septal defect, right ventricular dysfunction, and residual right ventricular outflow tract obstruction.

A determination of the appropriateness of intravenous (IV) fluid composition and rate should be made (see *Postoperative Management of Fluid Balance and Electrolytes*), and rates of both urine and chest tube output should be noted and interpreted based on the patient's weight. CPB can induce hemolysis, which may cause transient hemoglobinuria (5, 6). Excessive chest tube output (defined as the need for reoperation) (7) from ongoing bleeding should prompt a discussion of possible bleeding sites with the surgeon and a laboratory evaluation of coagulation status. Patients with extensive aortic suture lines require special attention to blood pressure control, because hypertension can exacerbate bleeding from the aorta. An acute, significant decrease in chest tube output is also concerning, especially when associated with increased RA or LA pressure and hypotension. If the chest tubes become obstructed but bleeding continues, cardiac tamponade may follow.

Based on the patient's ventilatory requirements in the operating room, the anesthesiologist will recommend the mode of mechanical ventilatory support and initial settings in ventilator-dependent patients. The ICU team must know the ventilatory mode and settings in order to evaluate the adequacy of gas exchange and oxygenation during the early postoperative period. Details of past problems with the upper airway (e.g., subglottic stenosis) or lower airway (e.g., reactive airway disease) should also be reviewed. Close monitoring of patients undergoing early extubation (e.g., in the operating room or within the first few hours of recovery), an increasingly popular strategy driven by cost concerns to reduce ICU stay, is also important (8, 9).

Initial laboratory evaluation should include the tests listed in Table 13.2. A comparison of pre- and postoperative frontal chest radiographs is used to evaluate changes in heart size and shape, changes in the appearance of lung parenchyma, pleural spaces, and lung volumes, and to determine the position of new hardware. Precise location must be established of all tubes (endotracheal, gastric, and chest), intracardiac or other central catheters (RA, CVP, LA, PA), wires (sternal, temporary atrial and ventricular epicardial pacing, permanent pacing), devices placed at catheterization (coils, stents, or occluders), and clips (Fig. 13.1). Tubes and catheters that are inappropriately positioned, such as an endotracheal tube with its tip in the right main stem bronchus, should be adjusted and a follow-up radiograph obtained to assess the result.

A 12- or 15-lead ECG is obtained to document the rhythm and to compare with the preoperative ECG. It is important to determine if the patient is in a regular sinus rhythm with appropriate atrioventricular (AV) node function. The atrial contribution to ventricular filling, which occurs in AV synchrony from atrial systole, significantly increases cardiac output (10, 11) (Fig. 13.2). Because decreased cardiac function occurs frequently as a result of surgery and CPB, it is important to maintain AV synchrony for recovery, especially in patients with a palliated circulation. The ECG should be assessed for new abnormalities, including bundle branch block (e.g., complete right bundle branch block is typical following repair of TOF) and ST-T wave changes suggestive of myocardial ischemia.

Accurate interpretation of the initial arterial blood gas (ABG) analysis requires an understanding of the patient's postoperative cardiac anatomy and physiology, plus findings from the physical examination and other laboratory tests. Most intubated patients, except those with palliated single-ventricle physiology (e.g., hypoplastic left heart syndrome [HLHS] following the Norwood procedure) (12), receive a high fraction of inspired oxygen (F_{IO_2}) until an adequate P_{O_2} on the the first ICU ABG is confirmed. This practice reduces the likelihood of arterial desaturation from inadequate alveolar P_{O_2} levels during transfer from the operating room. Ventilator changes can then be made based on the adequacy of ventilation and oxygenation and knowledge of the patient's clinical status.

The cause of unexpected abnormalities of either pH, P_{CO_2}, or P_{O_2} must be evaluated promptly, and interventions instituted to correct them. In the patient with a physiologically corrected circulation who has no right-to-left

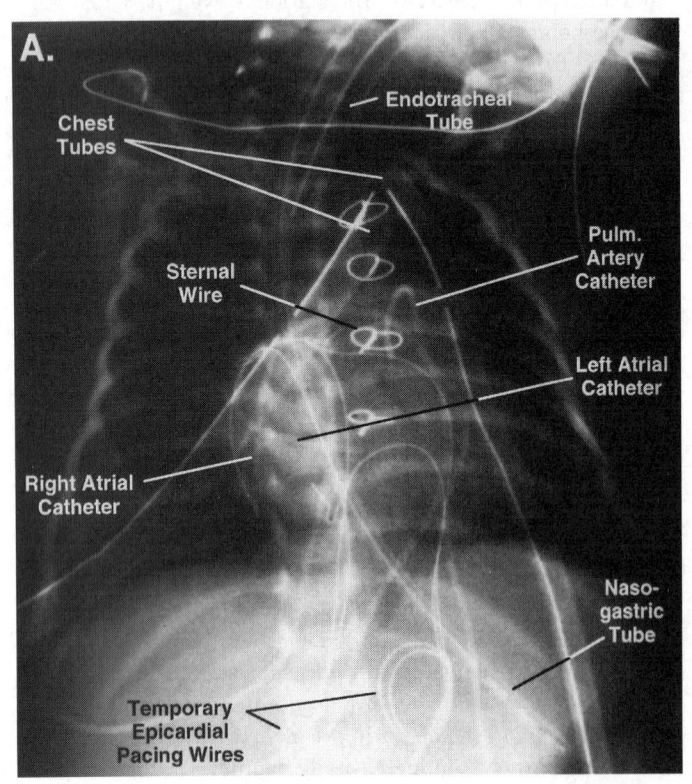

Figure 13.1. Postoperative frontal chest radiograph (**A**) and schematic drawing (**B**) showing the position of tubes, wires, and transthoracic intracardiac catheters in an infant following reparative cardiac surgery. *Ao*, aorta, *PA*, pulmonary artery.

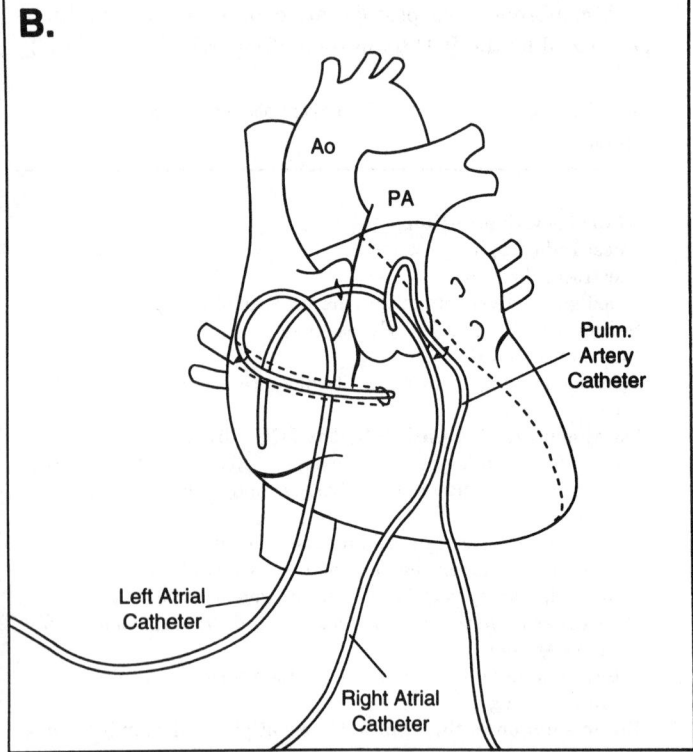

**BASELINE RHYTHM
(COMPLETE HEART BLOCK)**

CI = 2.2 liters/min/m²

**EPICARDIAL PACING:
VVI PACING**

CI = 2.5 liters/min/m²

**EPICARDIAL PACING:
A-V SEQUENTIAL PACING**

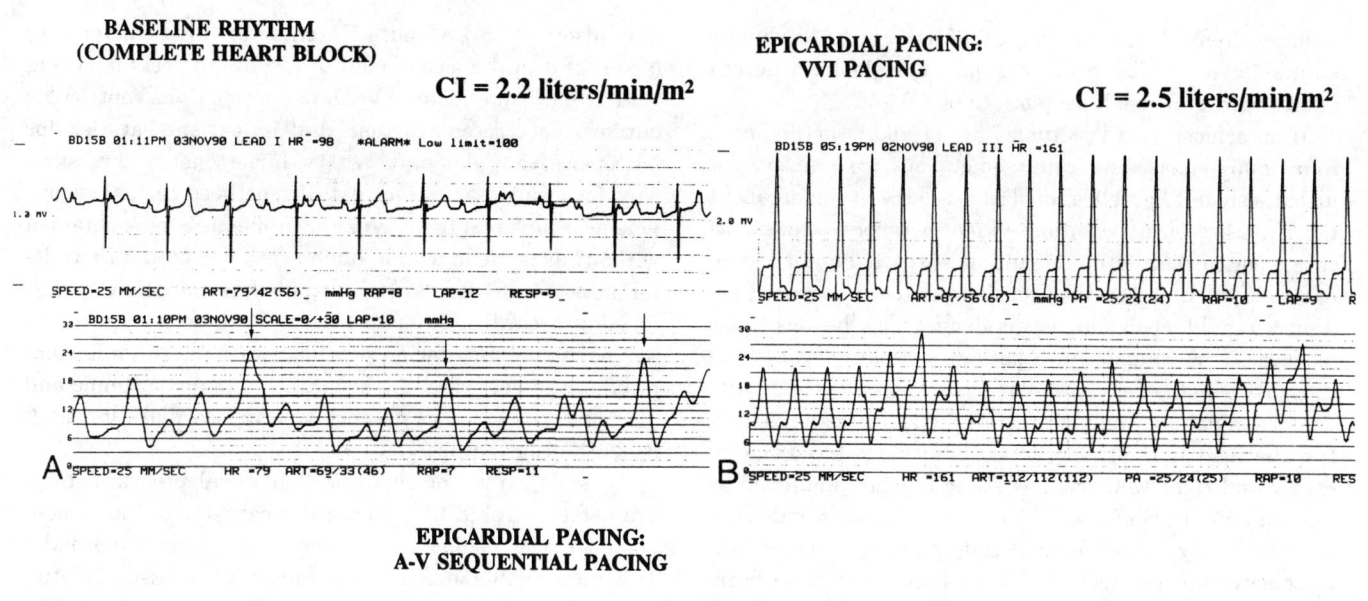

CI = 3.4 liters/min/m²

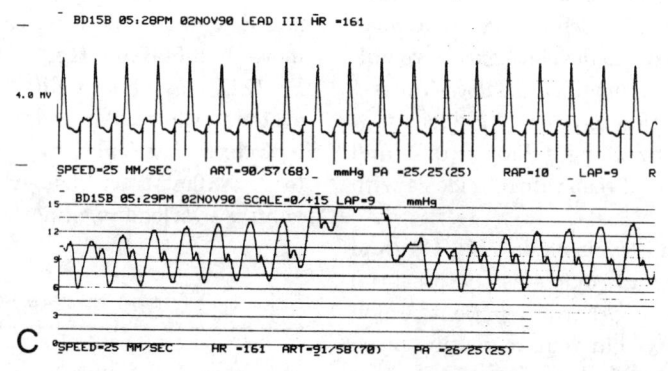

Figure 13.2. Hemodynamic response to epicardial pacing in a 1-year-old with complete heart block (*CHB*) 24 hours after inlet ventricular septal defect repair. Bedside monitor tracing of the ECG (*upper panel*) and left atrial (*LA*) pressure (*lower panel*) are shown. **A.** CHB with atrioventricular (*AV*) dissociation and ventricular escape rate = 98 beats per minute. Blood pressure = 69/33 mm Hg (mean 46) with thermodilution cardiac index (CI) = 2.2 L/min/M². Mean LA pressure = 10 mm Hg with "cannon" waves (arrows) on LA tracing. **B.** With ventricular pacing at 161 beats per minute, blood pressure increased to 87/56 mm Hg (mean 67), CI increased to 2.5 L/min/M², and mean LA pressure = 12 mm Hg. **C.** On re-establishing AV synchrony with dual-chamber pacing at 161 beats per minute, blood pressure = 91/58 mm Hg (mean 70), CI improved further to 3.4 L/min/M², and mean LA pressure = 9 mm Hg with a more normal wave form. (Reproduced with permission from Wernovsky G, Chang A, Wessel D. Intensive care. In: Emmanoulides G, Riemenschneider T, Allen H, et al, eds. Heart disease in infants, children, and adolescents. 5th ed. Baltimore: Williams & Wilkens, 1995.)

shunting and no significant parenchymal lung abnormalities on chest radiograph, an appropriate ABG would have a normal pH (7.34–7.45), normal P_{CO_2} (35–45 mm Hg), and an elevated P_{O_2} (often greater than 300 mm Hg) because of the high F_{IO_2} (typically 1.0). In contrast, a patient with single-ventricle physiology and clear lungs who has mixing of pulmonary and systemic venous blood should have a normal pH and P_{CO_2}, but a P_{O_2} less than 55 mm Hg (13, 14). In any patient with complete mixing of pulmonary and systemic venous blood, a high F_{IO_2} will not produce a normal or elevated P_{O_2} because of intracardiac right-to-left shunting. Causes of reduced arterial P_{O_2} other than intracardiac right-to-left shunting include alterations in gas exchange producing pulmonary venous desaturation such as intrapulmonary shunt, ventilation/perfusion (V/Q) mismatch, diffusion impairment, or alveolar hypoventilation (15). Patients who have a normal P_{O_2} and arterial oxygen saturation can appear cyanotic, however (16). Their cyanosis occurs in the distal extremities (acrocyanosis) and derives from either low cardiac output with an elevated arteriovenous (A-V) O_2 difference or from polycythemia. In both situations cyanosis is caused by an increased quantity of reduced hemoglobin in the capillaries (e.g., acyanotic adults have ≈ 2.25 g of reduced hemoglobin, whereas adults with cyanosis have more than 3.0 g).

If an acidosis (pH less than 7.34) or alkalosis (pH more than 7.45) exists, the cause—metabolic, respiratory, or mixed—should be determined and a decision made about the necessity of intervention. When metabolic acidosis occurs, poor cardiac output should be suspected and an evaluation of the cause of the acidosis initiated. In selected patients a mild acidemia or alkalemia may be desirable, however. For example, in a patient with an elevated but responsive pulmonary vascular resistance (PVR) who undergoes repair of complete atrioventricular canal defect, the afterload on the right ventricle may be reduced significantly and right ventricular systolic function improved by maintaining a pH of 7.45–7.5 (17, 18). Patients with Fontan physiology, whose nonpulsatile pulmonary blood flow is sensitive to changes in PVR, often respond with increased O_2 saturations and decreased right-sided filling pressures when a mild alkalosis is induced to decrease PVR. In contrast, a patient with HLHS who has undergone a palliative Norwood procedure and develops excessive pulmonary blood flow through a modified Blalock-Taussig shunt may experience a reduction in pulmonary blood flow when the PVR is increased by using a $F_{IO_2} = 0.21$ and hypoventilating to achieve a mild respiratory acidosis with a pH of 7.30–7.33 (19).

Determination of the serum levels of Na^+, K^+, Cl^-, and ionized Ca^{2+}, and the hemogram completes the essential initial postoperative blood testing. For any patient receiving medications preoperatively that require routine blood level monitoring (e.g., phenobarbital), a determination in the early postoperative period is appropriate.

Laboratory and physical examination data are combined to form an impression of the patient's status and to develop a plan for initial management. These data and the impression and plan should be documented thoroughly in the medical record within a few hours of admission to the ICU.

INTERPRETATION OF PRESSURE DATA FROM INTRAVASCULAR CATHETERS

Postoperative patients are admitted to the ICU with one or more intravascular catheters, depending on their cardiac diagnosis, type of surgery, and anticipated requirements for hemodynamic monitoring. All patients have an arterial catheter in place, with a distal extremity location such as a radial artery preferred. Patients undergoing intracardiac surgery for defects more complex than a secundum atrial septal defect typically have one or two RA catheters. Neonates and infants, especially those with complex disease (e.g., transposition of the great arteries or truncus arteriosus) who require major reconstructive procedures, may also have a LA and a PA catheter. PA catheters are also useful in the assessment of residual defects following ventricular septal defect (VSD) closure or right ventricular outflow tract reconstruction, and in patients at risk for postoperative pulmonary artery hypertension. Pressure, waveform, and saturation data from these catheters provide as complete a hemodynamic profile as can be obtained without inserting a double-lumen catheter with a thermistor into the PA for cardiac output determination or performing a cardiac catheterization. Data from continuous hemodynamic monitoring provide a rational basis for manipulating heart rate, intravascular volume, systemic and pulmonary vascular resistance, and myocardial contractility with drug therapy.

Possible causes of abnormal left atrial pressure (LAp) are listed in Table 13.3. At cardiac catheterization in nonpostoperative pediatric patients, mean LAp is normally 1–2 mm Hg higher than the mean RA pressure (RAp), which ranges between 1 and 6 mm Hg (average 3 mm Hg) and varies significantly with respiration (20). Mean LAp and RAp in postoperative cardiac patients are higher, often more than 6–8 mm Hg, but should be less than 12–14 mm Hg (21). Any abnormality that causes an elevation of the systemic ventricular end diastolic pressure can raise LAp, including ventricular hypertrophy from pressure overload (e.g., outflow tract obstruction), ventricular dilation from volume overload (e.g., aortic regurgitation), and poor ven-

Table 13.3. Causes of Elevated or Reduced Left Atrial Pressure

Elevated
Elevated systemic ventricular end diastolic pressure
    Decreased systemic ventricular systolic or diastolic function
    Systemic ventricular hypertrophy
    Systemic ventricular volume overload
Mitral valve disease
    Stenosis with absent or restrictive interatrial communication
    Regurgitation
    Obstructive mass (e.g., thrombus)
Large left-to-right shunt
Chamber hypoplasia
Intravascular volume overload
Cardiac tamponade
Tachyarrhythmia
Artifactual
    Catheter tip not in body of left atrium (e.g., in a ventricle or wedged)
    Pressure transducer below level of heart
    Pressure transducer improperly calibrated or zeroed

Reduced
Low intravascular fluid status
Inadequate preload
Artifactual
    Catheter malfunction (e.g., cracked or clotted)
    Pressure transducer above level of heart
    Pressure transducer improperly calibrated or zeroed

tricular systolic function (20). Mitral valve disease can elevate LAp. However, a patient can have severe mitral valve stenosis or actual atresia and normal LAp if an unrestrictive interatrial communication (e.g., a congenital secundum atrial septal defect [ASD] or a defect created by surgical atrial septectomy) also exists. Volume overload, either from excessive fluid administration or from a large left-to-right shunt defect, such as an unrestrictive VSD or PDA, which increases pulmonary blood flow and LA return, also can elevate LAp. Cardiac tamponade, which raises diastolic pressures throughout the heart and impairs cardiac filling, is another cause. Hypoplasia of the LA (e.g., in Shone's syndrome or total anomalous pulmonary venous connection) can limit LA compliance following surgical repair (22, 23). Elevated LAp can be anticipated in these patients, and the upper limit of acceptable pressure may be somewhat higher. Certain dysrhythmias, including AV dissociation and rhythms of junctional or ventricular origin with retrograde AV node conduction, increase LAp by causing the atria to contract when the atrioventricular valves are closed. This phenomenon generates "cannon waves" on the LA pressure waveform (Fig. 13.2A). Both supraventricular and ventricular tachycardias can elevate LAp by impairing atrial emptying.

When evaluating a patient whose LAp is abnormally high, it is also important to exclude artifactual causes. These include improper positioning of the catheter tip (e.g., tip in the ventricle or "reverse" wedged in a pulmonary vein), placement of the pressure transducer below heart level, or improperly calibrating or zeroing the transducer.

Reduced LAp, if accurate, suggests either that the patient has low intravascular volume or inadequate preload. The difference in these conditions is illustrated by the following scenarios: (a) the patient in negative fluid balance from excessive chest bleeding who develops hypotension with a LAp = 3 mm Hg has low intravascular volume, and (b) the failing Fontan patient with high PVR, RAp more than 20 mm Hg, LAp = 3 mm Hg, and hypotension despite 40 mL/kg IV fluid has inadequate preload. Typically, low arterial and central venous pressures together with reduced LAp suggest low intravascular volume. A bolus of IV crystalloid or colloid at 5–10 mL/kg would be expected to raise LAp, CVP, and arterial blood pressure in this situation.

Possible causes of abnormalities in RAp are shown in Table 13.4. Elevations in RAp are usually not as pronounced as those in LAp because RA compliance is greater (24). Therefore, when significant RAp elevation occurs (e.g., more than 15 mm Hg), especially in neonates, it suggests significant disease, and it typically is poorly tolerated. Ascites and tissue edema are common manifestations of high RAp, as is pleural effusion in the newborn, in part because of increased resistance to lymphatic drainage into systemic veins with elevated central venous pressure (25).

Table 13.4. Causes of Elevated or Reduced Right Atrial Pressure

Elevated
Decreased right (or single) ventricular compliance
    Abnormal ventricular systolic or diastolic function
    Right ventricular hypertrophy
    Right ventricular volume overload
Tricuspid valve disease
    Stenosis with absent or restrictive interatrial communication
    Regurgitation
    Obstructive mass (e.g., thrombus)
Left ventricular-to-right atrial shunt
Intravascular volume overload
Cardiac tamponade
Tachyarrhythmia
Artifactual
    Catheter tip not in body of right atrium (e.g., in a ventricle or wedged)
    Pressure transducer below level of heart
    Pressure transducer improperly calibrated or zeroed
Reduced
Low intravascular volume status
Inadequate preload
Artifactual
    Catheter malfunction (e.g., cracked or clotted)
    Pressure transducer above level of heart
    Pressure transducer improperly calibrated or zeroed

Reductions in RAp usually result from low intravascular volume status. Patients with normal or elevated RAp can develop low RAp when beginning therapy with intravenous afterload-reducing agents such as nitroprusside, amrinone, and milrinone (26–28). Vasodilation of systemic and venous capacitance vessels causes this lowering of RAp, and may necessitate the administration of IV fluids.

Causes of elevations and reductions in pulmonary artery pressure (PAp) are outlined in Table 13.5. Normal mean PAp in non-postoperative pediatric patients varies between 10 and 20 mm Hg (average 13 mm Hg) (29). Mean PAp in postoperative cardiac patients is often more than 13 mm Hg, but it should be less than 25 mm Hg (30). Pulmonary artery hypertension is an important cause of right ventricular dysfunction in postoperative patients that can be precipitated or exacerbated by CPB (31). Patients at increased risk of postoperative pulmonary artery hypertension include the following:

1. Documented preoperative pulmonary artery hypertension, especially in those patients with reduced pulmonary vasoreactivity in response to 100% oxygen or nitric oxide.
2. Neonates, especially within the first days of life when PVR can intermittently be increased.
3. Specific cardiac lesions such as the pulmonary venous hypertensive diseases (e.g., obstructed total anomalous

Table 13.5. Causes of Elevated or Reduced Pulmonary Artery Pressure

Elevated
Mechanical obstruction of the pulmonary circulation
  Anatomic defects (e.g., pulmonary vein or branch pulmonary artery stenosis)
  Pulmonary embolus
Pulmonary arteriolar smooth muscle hypertrophy (e.g., primary pulmonary hypertension, pulmonary vascular obstructive disease)
Inflammatory response to cardiopulmonary bypass
Mechanical obstruction of the airways
  Atelectasis
  Excessive airway pressure (mechanically ventilated patients)
  Pleural effusion
  Tension pneumothorax
  Chest wall disease
Airway hyper-reactivity (e.g., asthma)
Lung hypoplasia
Alveolar hypoxia
Low serum pH
Hyperviscosity (from polycythemia)
Elevated LAp (e.g., elevated systemic ventricular end-diastolic pressure, mitral stenosis)
High pressure left-to-right shunt lesion (e.g., unrestrictive VSD or large PDA)
Persistent pulmonary hypertension of the newborn
Artifactual
  Catheter tip in incorrect position (e.g., in aorta across a PDA or in ventricle)
  Pressure transducer below level of heart
  Pressure transducer improperly calibrated or zeroed
Reduced
Low intravascular volume
Severe obstruction to pulmonary blood flow
Low cardiac output
Artifactual
  Catheter malfunction (e.g., cracked or clotted)
  Pressure transducer above level of heart
  Pressure transducer improperly calibrated or zeroed

LAp, left atrial pressure; PDA, patent ductus arteriosus; VSD, ventricular septal defect.

pulmonary venous connection, mitral stenosis, or pulmonary vein stenosis) and long-term left-to-right shunts with unrestricted pulmonary blood flow (e.g., unrepaired transposition of the great arteries with VSD, complete atrioventricular canal defect, truncus arteriosus, or large VSD).
4. Severely impaired systemic ventricular function with high end diastolic pressure.
5. Reactive (e.g., asthma) or fixed (e.g., scoliosis with restrictive chest wall anatomy) lung disease.

In these patients and others whose pulmonary blood flow is more sensitive to elevations in PVR than normal (e.g., Fontan patients), it is particularly important to detect rapidly and treat aggressively low serum pH and alveolar hypoxia, because pH and oxygen are both potent regulators of PVR (32, 33). PAp should be compared with the simultaneous arterial blood pressure when evaluating the degree of pulmonary artery hypertension. Although elevated, a PAp = 50/25 mm Hg in a patient following VSD closure whose arterial blood pressure = 120/70 mm Hg is less concerning for a significant residual VSD than a second VSD patient with identical PAp whose simultaneous arterial blood pressure = 70/40 mm Hg. In the former patient, systolic PAp is less than one half the systemic blood pressure, but in the latter patient, it is five sevenths the systemic blood pressure. Artifactual elevations in PAp are produced by problems similar to those described for LA and RA catheters. Decreased PAp can be caused by either low intravascular volume, severe proximal obstruction to pulmonary blood flow (e.g., pulmonary valve stenosis), or low cardiac output. As noted, in the first instance, LAp and RAp should also be low, whereas in the third scenario, either can be abnormally high.

INTERPRETATION OF OXYGEN SATURATION DATA FROM INTRAVASCULAR CATHETERS

Oxygen saturation data, and at times Po_2 determination, complement pressure data available from LA, RA, and PA catheters and are also important for optimal postoperative management. Table 13.6 provides a list of the causes of elevated and decreased oxygen saturations in the RA, LA, and PA. Correct interpretation of saturation data from catheters in these locations depends on accurate knowledge of the patient's cardiac anatomy and respiratory status, and the position of each catheter tip, which is obtained by inspecting both the patient's chest radiograph and pressure waveform tracings. As an example, the tip of a surgically placed RA catheter may lie in the body of the RA, but it may also be located in the inferior vena cava (IVC), superior vena cava, or coronary sinus.

Right atrial oxygen saturation values measured at cardiac catheterization in children with normal cardiac outputs and no intracardiac shunts who are breathing room air (Fio_2 = 0.21) vary between 69 and 87% (mean 78%) (34). Expected values in repaired postoperative patients with adequate cardiac output and no significant residual defects are somewhat lower, but they vary widely depending on the patient's metabolic and hemodynamic state. An abnormally high RA oxygen saturation raises the possibility of a left-to-right shunt through an ASD or anomalous pulmonary venous return. In patients who have undergone repair of common atrioventricular canal defects, left ventricular-to-right atrial shunts can occur as a residual defect. Pathologic conditions that significantly increase cardiac output and oxygen delivery such as "warm" septic

Table 13.6. Causes of Elevated or Reduced Right Atrium, Left Atrium, or Pulmonary Artery Oxygen Saturation

Location	Elevated	Reduced
Right Atrium	Atrial level left-to-right shunt Anomalous pulmonary venous return Left ventricular-to-right atrial shunt Increased oxygen delivery Decreased oxygen extraction Increased dissolved oxygen content Catheter tip position (e.g., near renal veins)	Increased oxygen extraction (e.g., low cardiac output) Decreased arterial oxygen saturation with a normal A-V O_2 difference Anemia Catheter tip position (e.g., near the coronary sinus)
Left Atrium	Normally fully saturated	Atrial level right-to-left shunt Pulmonary venous desaturation (e.g., ventilation-perfusion mismatch) Improper catheter position
Pulmonary Artery	Significant residual left-to-right shunt Small left-to-right shunt with incomplete mixing of blood Erroneous catheter tip position (e.g., "wedged" in the distal pulmonary artery)	Increased oxygen extraction (e.g., low cardiac output, fever) Decreased arterial oxygen saturation with a normal A-V O_2 difference Anemia

A-V, arteriovenous.

shock can result in elevated systemic venous oxygen saturation; however, this state is rarely encountered in young children. Use of an elevated F_{IO_2} (e.g., 0.4–1.0) will increase the dissolved O_2 content of blood, which may elevate the oxygen saturation. Catheter tip location in the IVC near the renal veins, where blood has a relatively elevated oxygen saturation because of high renal blood flow, can also produce high oxygen saturations.

An abnormally low RA oxygen saturation can occur in several situations, the most important of which is decreased cardiac output (fever, lung disease, and anemia are other causes). To help determine if a low RA saturation is caused by decreased cardiac output, the A-V O_2 difference should be calculated or estimated. Normally, the A-V O_2 difference is less than 30% (35). Therefore, a patient with a RA saturation of 50% and a normal systemic arterial saturation of 98% could have decreased cardiac output, because the A-V O_2 difference is increased at 48%. However, a patient with single-ventricle physiology and intracardiac right-to-left shunting, which produces a systemic saturation of 75%, has a normal A-V O_2 difference with a RA saturation of 50%, and cardiac output may be normal. In the latter patient, reduced RA saturation is caused by low systemic oxygen saturation from the mixing of deoxygenated and oxygenated blood, not increased oxygen extraction. Knowledge of the catheter tip position is also important in interpreting reduced RA saturations, because locations with lower saturations, such as the coronary sinus and hepatic veins, can yield samples with saturations that are lower than the "true" mixed venous O_2 saturation (obtained from thoroughly mixed venous blood in the pulmonary artery) (36, 37).

Because blood returning to the LA from the pulmonary veins is normally fully saturated with oxygen, abnormal elevations in LA saturation do not occur. Unless the LA catheter is not positioned properly (e.g., the tip is in the RA through an ASD), reductions in oxygen saturation will be caused by either right-to-left shunting at the atrial level or desaturation of pulmonary venous blood. Abnormalities generating higher RAp than LAp in the presence of an atrial communication can lead to right-to-left shunting, including tricuspid valve stenosis or regurgitation, right ventricular systolic or diastolic dysfunction, and AV dissociation. Significant right-to-left atrial shunting causes systemic arterial desaturation, and frequently explains the desaturation observed in neonates and young infants following complete repair of TOF and truncus arteriosus. In these patients the patent foramen ovale is not closed surgically so that the RA, which develops elevated pressure from early postoperative right ventricular dysfunction, can decompress (38). Echocardiography, especially when combined with color Doppler flow mapping or saline contrast injection into the RA catheter, is useful for proving the existence of an interatrial communication.

Pulmonary venous desaturation from altered gas exchange is the other important cause of LA oxygen desaturation. The chest radiograph should be inspected for abnormalities that could cause V/Q mismatch such as consolidation, atelectasis or lobar collapse, pulmonary edema, pleural effusion, or pneumothorax. Patients with no apparent lung disease who have reduced RA saturations because of low cardiac output (as in cardiomyopathy) or a decreased ratio of pulmonary blood flow (Q_p) to systemic blood flow (Q_s) (i.e., Q_p/Q_s less than 1) from ventricular level right-to-left shunting (as in TOF) should have a normal LA saturation.

Oxygen saturation data from PA catheters are especially useful in identifying residual left-to-right shunts following surgery to repair VSD(s). The absolute value of the PA saturation has been demonstrated to be a better predictor of a significant postoperative left-to-right shunt than the difference or "step-up" (with PA more than RA) in RA and PA saturations (30, 39). Specifically, a PA saturation greater than 80% in patients receiving O_2 at a F_{IO_2} less than 0.5 within 48 hours of VSD or TOF repair was a sensitive indicator of a significant left-to-right shunt (Q_p/Q_s more than 1.5) 1 year following surgery (30, 39). Occasionally, however, the left-to-right shunt will be overestimated because the PA catheter samples a stream of LV blood from a small residual defect (Q_p/Q_s = 1.1–1.5 if the PA catheter were repositioned to sample true mixed venous blood). It is also possible for a patient to have a PA oxygen saturation less than 80%, but still have a large left-to-right shunt. Abnormalities that cause this scenario include low cardiac output with increased O_2 extraction, severe anemia, and excessive O_2 consumption (e.g., high fever). Differences in saturation of 5 to 10% between RA and PA can occur without shunting because of variability in the venous saturation at specific locations around the RA (e.g., hepatic versus renal veins, as noted above) (34). This normal difference in O_2 saturation, which has been documented primarily in catheterization laboratory studies, is likely to be exaggerated in postoperative patients because of greater variability in catheter positioning.

The LA, RA, and PA catheters placed in the operating room for monitoring intracardiac pressures and oxygen saturations are typically single lumen catheters. In addition to these monitoring functions, they can also be used for the infusion of IV fluids, blood products, medications, and parenteral nutrition solutions. If it is important to obtain accurate measurements of cardiac output and calculate other hemodynamic variables for either diagnostic or therapeutic purposes, a double-lumen PA catheter containing a thermistor can be inserted into the PA. Use of these catheters and interpretation of cardiac output data collected from them are discussed in the section, *Cardiac Output: Determination of Cardiac Output Status and Support of the Postoperative Myocardium*. As less invasive techniques such as transesophageal echocardiography gain in utility and popularity (40), the need for PA catheter placement may diminish.

The decision to remove an intracardiac catheter is based on the patient's postoperative course and the possible complications of continued catheter use. Unless a patient is hemodynamically unstable and LAp data are required for optimal management, the LA catheter is usually removed on the first postoperative day. The PA catheter is also usually taken out within a day of surgery, except in patients who remain critically ill or who require continued monitoring of pulmonary artery hypertension. Coagulation indices, including the prothrombin and partial thromboplastin times and platelet count, should be measured and corrected, if significantly abnormal, before discontinuing these catheters. Appropriately crossmatched blood should be available in case significant bleeding occurs. Typically, at least one chest tube is still in place when the LA and PA catheters are removed; if bleeding occurs, the risk of cardiac tamponade is lowered because the blood can be evacuated by the indwelling chest tube(s). Because these catheters are discontinued early in the postoperative period, most patients are still mechanically ventilated. Catheter removal during the period of intubation provides an additional factor of safety should a bleeding complication occur, and it allows for optimal sedation and analgesia without compromising respiratory status. RA catheters can remain in place for up to 2 weeks, but they should be removed as soon as they are no longer necessary.

Reported complication rates associated with intracardiac catheter usage are approximately 1 to 2% (41, 42). The most common complication is bleeding at the time of catheter removal. Bleeding accompanies the discontinuance of PA and LA catheters more often than RA catheters. Additional complications at removal include catheter breakage and entrapment. Catheter retrieval, either in the operating room or cardiac catheterization laboratory, may be required in these instances. Complications that can occur with the use of any intravascular catheter, such as infection and embolus, must also be considered when contemplating how long to maintain a catheter. Since many patients are at increased risk of embolic stroke because of intracardiac communications, interventions such as a low-dose heparin infusion or use of heparin-bonded catheters should be considered to reduce the likelihood of thrombus formation, especially in neonates and infants (43–45).

POSTOPERATIVE MANAGEMENT OF FLUID BALANCE AND ELECTROLYTES

Postoperative cardiac patients experience derangements in normal fluid balance, electrolyte balance, calcium (Ca^{2+}) and magnesium (Mg^{2+}) homeostasis, and renal function because of interventions required both to accomplish surgery and to manage recovery in the ICU. These derangements are typically more pronounced in patients who have undergone procedures using CPB, but all postoperative patients are at risk because of the requirement for general anesthesia and IV fluid administration.

Patients who return to the ICU following surgery with CPB typically have significant total body water and salt overload from dilution of blood with crystalloid in the bypass circuit (e.g., to a hematocrit of 20%) (46–48). Neonates and young infants appear to acquire a relatively greater excess of fluid than older children, at times experiencing intraoperative weight gains of 600–1000 g (i.e., 20 to 25% of preoperative weight) (21, 49). The additional fluid distributes diffusely throughout the body, including into the soft tissues, lungs, kidneys, brain, and myocardium. The mechanism for this process appears to be generalized capillary leak from endothelial damage caused by exposure to CPB and/or ischemia-reperfusion injury (50, 51). In anticipation of this extracellular fluid overload, some institutions employ strategies such as ultrafiltration during the final period of CPB (52) or routine placement of a peritoneal dialysis catheter at the inferior aspect of the sternotomy incision for either simple drainage or dialysis in the ICU (53). Other strategies in development focus on prophylactic interventions to prevent or mitigate reperfusion injury, such as selective inhibition of adhesion molecule interactions between leukocytes and endothelium (54, 55). A urinary catheter is routinely placed in the bladder prior to surgery for continuous monitoring of urine production during and after surgery.

In the first 2 to 4 hours following admission to the ICU, most patients who have undergone CPB produce more than 1 mL/kg/h of urine. After this initial period of adequate urine output, the rate often decreases to less than 1 mL/kg/h and may continue at lower rates for up to 48 hours. The brief initial period of increased output occurs because of intraoperative volume administration followed by an osmotic diuresis. This osmotic diuresis is caused by either hyperglycemia from the elevated glucose concentration of the CPB priming solution and the stress response to surgery or to intraoperative mannitol administration (56–58). During the 12 to 18 hours after the hyperglycemia and glycosuria resolve, the kidneys often respond poorly to diuretic agents, in part because of inappropriate secretion of antidiuretic hormone (SIADH). Therefore, diuretic therapy is typically initiated on postoperative day 1, because it is seldom effective before that time. Neonates may require more time to excrete excess fluid compared with infants and children because of a lower glomerular filtration rate (GFR) (59). Reduced GFR in neonates also leads to decreased metabolism of drugs excreted by the kidneys (e.g., the muscle relaxants metocurine iodide and vecuronium), requiring dosing adjustments to prevent excessive drug levels, particularly in the early postoperative period.

Initial management of postoperative patients should account for excessive fluid and salt administered during CPB. Sodium overload results from the electrolyte composition of crystalloid solutions used to fill ("prime") the bypass circuit. For example, Plasmalyte A (Baxter, Deerfiled, IL), a commonly employed crystalloid priming solution, contains 140 mEq/L of Na^+. In the first 24 hours, the total rate of IV fluid administration is typically set at one half to two thirds of the maintenance fluid rate. The maintenance fluid rate can be calculated using either the surface area method (maintenance = 1500–1700 $mL/m^2/d$) or the caloric expense method (maintenance = 100 mL/kg/d [less than 10 kg] + 50 mL/kg/d [10–20 kg] + 20 mL/kg/d [more than 20 kg]) (60). At weights between 5 and 30 kg, these two methods provide similar volumes. Neonates and young infants, who have a decreased ability to maintain normal blood glucose levels, receive an IV solution with a greater glucose concentration (e.g., 10% dextrose with one fourth normal saline [$D_{10}1/4NS$]), whereas older infants and children receive a solution containing less glucose (e.g., 5% dextrose with one fourth normal saline [$D_51/4NS$]). Blood glucose and serum electrolyte measurements should be made within 1 hour of admission to the ICU and then every 4 to 6 hours during the initial 24 hours after surgery in higher risk patients. Fluid restriction is discontinued as urine output improves, usually on postoperative day 1 or 2. Potassium, primarily in the form of potassium chloride (KCl), is added to the IV fluid solution to treat low serum K^+ only after adequate urine output has been established.

Although sodium intake restriction may be appropriate initially, the need for fluid administration is ultimately dictated by interpreting the patient's hemodynamic state in light of the measured filling pressures and requirement for blood products or colloid. Examples of situations in which a maintenance or greater IV fluid rate is appropriate would be the following:

1. Modified Blalock-Taussig shunt in the polycythemic patient, to decrease the risks of both inadequate shunt flow from low intravascular volume and shunt thrombosis.
2. Cavopulmonary anastomosis or Fontan procedure, to provide adequate preload for nonpulsatile pulmonary blood flow.
3. The patient with normal blood pressure after aortic coarctation repair, a procedure performed without CPB and typically not accompanied by fluid overload.

A thorough assessment of the postoperative patient's fluid balance and electrolyte status should be made at least once a day in the ICU. Sources of data for this assessment include physical examination, monitored variables such as systemic blood pressure, CVP or RAp, LAp (if available), heart rate, and fluid input and output volumes, and laboratory determinations of serum electrolytes, blood urea nitrogen, creatinine, hematocrit, and urinalysis. Daily weight measurement can be useful, but it is often difficult to perform with accuracy because of equipment attached to the patient (e.g., tubes, catheters, and leads), especially in the early postoperative period.

Although patients are often total body fluid overloaded following surgery, they can become depleted of intravascular volume from ongoing chest tube drainage or capillary leak. Significant intravascular volume depletion presents as reduced systemic blood pressure, decreased filling pressures (CVP or RAp, and LAp), and sinus tachycardia. In the patient whose pulmonary blood flow is dependent on systemic blood pressure (e.g., tricuspid atresia with a modified Blalock-Taussig shunt), systemic oxygen desaturation can subsequently occur. Treatment consists of an IV infusion of 5–10 mL/kg of fluid at an infusion rate that is determined by the degree of hemodynamic compromise, and the effects on systemic blood pressure, filling pressures, and heart rate evaluated. The type of fluid to infuse depends on knowledge of the patient's postoperative physiology, hematocrit, coagulation status, and type of ongoing fluid losses. If the hematocrit is adequate and bleeding is well controlled, either a crystalloid (e.g., lactated Ringer's or normal saline ± dextrose) or colloid (e.g., 5% human serum albumin) solution is administered. If the patient is anemic but not bleeding, packed red blood cells should be considered, especially in palliated patients with systemic oxygen desaturation from right-to-left shunting. If significant bleeding is present, packed red blood cells plus additional blood products (e.g., fresh frozen plasma, platelets, or cryoprecipitate) should be infused, depending on the patient's coagulation profile.

Treatment of fluid overload with diuretics following CPB is usually not initiated until 12 to 24 hours after surgery. Patients with a stable blood pressure, including those receiving vasoactive drugs, are candidates for diuretic therapy. Diuretic agent choice varies between institutions, but the loop diuretic furosemide is a common choice. Patients either receive intermittent furosemide dosing (e.g., 1–2 mg/kg dose IV two or three times daily) or a constant infusion at a rate of 0.1–0.4 mg/kg/h. Treatment with a constant infusion has the possible advantage of precipitating smaller short-term fluctuations in intravascular volume, and may be preferable in patients at risk of hemodynamic lability (61, 62). If diuresis is not adequate with one agent, a second agent with a different site of action in the kidney tubules can be added. The thiazide diuretic chlorothiazide 10 mg/kg per dose IV twice a day, the thiazide-like agent metolazone 0.5 mg per dose once a day in infants, and 1.0 mg/kg dose once a day in children (available only in enteral formulations), or the osmotic agent mannitol at 0.25–1.0 g/kg per dose IV as needed are possible choices. Mannitol should be used with caution in patients who have low cardiac output and poor renal perfusion. If mannitol is not excreted, it can cause a prolonged increase in oncotic pressure, leading to a shift of extravascular fluid into the intravascular space that raises filling pressures and exacerbates congestive heart failure.

Another strategy commonly employed to accentuate urine output is a constant, low-dose infusion of the catecholamine dopamine. In the kidney the two other endogenous catecholamines, norepinephrine and epinephrine, bind to α_1 adrenergic receptors in the afferent and efferent arterioles of the glomeruli (63). Receptor binding and activation increases arteriolar resistance, which decreases glomerular blood flow causing lower GFR. Dopamine binds to specific dopaminergic receptors (designated DA_1) in the renal arterioles, and at lower doses (5 µg/kg/min or less via a continuous IV infusion) can counteract the α-receptor–mediated effects of norepinephrine and epinephrine by lowering resistance (64, 65). Although used routinely in many institutions, the value of "renal dose" dopamine (3 µg/kg/min or less) has not been evaluated in a prospective, randomized study. In adults higher dopamine doses (e.g., more than 10–15 µg/kg/min) reduce renal blood flow and urine output (66). The effect of higher-dose dopamine on kidney function can be different in adults and infants; no significant reduction in urine output was observed in one study of 15 critically ill infants who received more than 20 µg/kg/min of dopamine (67).

Diuretic therapy accelerates excretion of excess water and Na^+, which may reduce the duration of mechanical ventilation and ICU stay. However, diuretics can also cause electrolyte imbalances, which require careful monitoring and management. Treatment with either loop or thiazide diuretics, and especially combined diuretic therapy, is a common cause of hyponatremia, hypokalemia, and hypochloremia. In addition to mild hyponatremia (serum Na^+ = 128–135 mEq/L) and variable degrees of hypokalemia, the usual outcome of continued diuretic therapy is development of a hypochloremic metabolic alkalosis from accentuated losses of K^+, hydrogen ion, and Cl^- from the renal tubules (68). Total body K^+ and Cl^- are diminished, and serum levels of each are abnormally low. Serum bicarbonate levels are typically elevated to 30–40 mEq/L. The compensatory response to metabolic alkalosis is reduced respiratory drive, causing decreased minute ventilation and CO_2 retention. Additional common causes of hypokalemia in postoperative cardiac patients are listed in Table 13.7.

In myocardial cells the electrophysiologic effects of hypokalemia include increased duration of the action potential and the effective refractory period, and accentuated automaticity. Electrocardiographic manifestations of hypokalemia begin with T wave flattening or inversion and the appearance of prominent U waves, and can progress to atrial or ventricular dysrhythmias if the patient is receiving digoxin (69). Younger patients usually tolerate hypokalemia well, whereas adults have a significant incidence of atrial and ventricular arrhythmias (70). KCl supplementa-

Table 13.7. Common Causes of Abnormal Serum Potassium, Calcium, and Magnesium Levels in Postoperative Cardiac Patients

Potassium

Hypokalemia

Total body K$^+$ deficit
  Diuretic therapy
  Nondiuretic kidney losses
    Osmotic diuresis (e.g., hyperglycemia)
    Elevated aldosterone
    Medications
      Amphotericin B
      Gentamicin
  Recovery from acute renal failure
  Losses from the gastrointestinal tract
    Nasogastric suctioning
    Persistent vomiting or diarrhea
K$^+$ Redistribution
  Alkalemia

Hyperkalemia

Total body K$^+$ excess
  Excessive administration
  Blood transfusion
  Cell death
  Acute renal failure
  Medications
    K$^+$-sparing diuretics
    Angiotensin-converting enzyme inhibitors
K$^+$ redistribution
  Acidemia
  Hypertonicity
  Medications
    Digoxin
    Succinylcholine
Artifact
  Prolonged tourniquet use
  Hemolysis

Calcium

Hypocalcemia

Citrate-anticoagulated blood transfusion
Diuretic therapy (loop diuretics)
Acute respiratory alkalosis
Low serum parathyroid hormone level
  DiGeorge syndrome
Hyperphosphatemia
Vitamin D deficiency
  Renal insufficiency
  Inadequate intake or absorption

Hypercalcemia

Excessive Ca^{2+} dosing

Magnesium

Hypomagnesemia

Excessive renal excretion
  Medications
    Diurectics (especially furosemide)
    Gentamicin
    Amphotericin B
    Cyclosporin A
Citrate-anticoagulated blood transfusion
Cardiopulmonary bypass
Inadequate Mg^{2+} intake
  Malabsorption
  Insufficient Mg^{2+} in diet or parenteral nutrition solution

Hypermagnesemia

Increased Mg^{2+} intake
  Excessive supplementation
  Mg^{2+}-containing antacids
Decreased Mg^{2+} excretion
  Renal insufficiency

---

tion to achieve normal serum K$^+$ levels (3.5–5.5 mEq/L) can be administered either enterally or parenterally. However, treatment of dysrhythmias presumed to be secondary to hypokalemia should generally be performed with IV supplementation, because gastrointestinal absorption is unreliable, especially in the early postoperative period. Because the transmembrane distribution of K$^+$ contributes to the resting membrane potential of cells, acute, dramatic fluctuations in the serum concentration of K$^+$ can precipitate life-threatening arrhythmias (70). Therefore, the following guidelines should be followed when administering KCl IV: (*a*) infuse 0.5 mEq/kg/dose or less, (*b*) infusion dose over 1 hour or more, (*c*) continuous ECG monitoring throughout dosing. Concentrated KCl (e.g., more than 80–100 mEq/L) should be infused through a central venous line (CVL) because of pain at peripheral infusion sites and the risk of tissue necrosis from extravasation.

Although hyperkalemia is not encountered as frequently as hypokalemia, it can also precipitate life-threatening electrophysiologic problems. Table 13.7 lists common causes of hyperkalemia. Normal K+ balance depends on the rates of urinary, and to a lesser extent, gastrointestinal excretion, so that higher urine flow rates through the distal tubules in the kidney lead to greater K+ excretion (71). Excessive total body K+ results from either increased loading (e.g., KCl supplementation in IV fluid or total parenteral nutrition solutions, large or rapid blood transfusions, or cell death with release of intracellular K+) or decreased excretion (e.g., acute renal failure with low GFR or medications that inhibit normal renal tubular K+ excretion, such as spironolactone or the angiotensin-converting enzyme [ACE] inhibitors). Redistributions of K+ into extracellular spaces can be caused by acidemia (metabolic more than respiratory acidosis), hypertonicity, or specific medications including digoxin and the depolarizing muscle relaxant succinylcholine (72).

When a serum K+ result shows hyperkalemia (K+ more than 5.5 mEq/L), appropriate initial responses include reviewing the method used to obtain the sample plus the patient's status for causative clues, repeating the test to confirm the value, and obtaining an ECG. Artifactual causes include sampling from a catheter through which a K+-containing solution is running or measuring K+ in a sample from an ischemic extremity (e.g., prolonged tourniquet application) or from hemolyzed blood. However, if a repeat determination from a properly obtained sample shows an elevated K+, further evaluation is indicated. The ECG should be inspected for evidence of the following abnormalities (these appear in the order listed as the severity of hyperkalemia increases): (*a*) tall, peaked T waves, (*b*) diminished R wave amplitude, (*c*) widening of the QRS interval, (*d*) prolongation of the PR interval, (*e*) flattening or disappearance of the P wave, and (*f*) "sine wave" QRS morphology from blending of P and QRS waves (Fig. 13.3) (69). Cardiac rhythm can degenerate to ventricular fibrillation or asystole, especially if the serum K+ level is greater than 8.0 mEq/L.

If the serum K+ level is 5.5–6.5 mEq/L and no ECG abnormalities exist, interventions should consist of discontinuing exogenous K+ supplementation and any medications that inhibit renal excretion, and close monitoring. If the serum K+ level is greater than 6.5 mEq/L and ECG changes suggestive of hyperkalemia are observed, the interventions described above plus one or more of the following maneuvers, based on severity, should be performed:

1. Administer Ca^{2+} IV over several minutes, either as calcium chloride (10%, 10–25 mg/kg) or calcium gluconate (10%, 50–100 mg/kg) through a CVL. (Note: avoid rapid Ca^{2+} infusions in patients with digoxin toxicity, because this could precipitate ventricular fibrillation) (73).
2. Administer sodium bicarbonate IV 1–2 mEq/kg over several minutes to generate an alkalemia and redistribute K+ into cells.
3. Administer regular insulin (0.1–0.3 U/kg) with glucose (1g/kg) IV over 15–30 minutes and then as continuous infusions to promote cotransport of K+ into cells with glucose. Note: Interventions 1 and 2 produce only brief (minutes) reductions in serum K+, whereas combined insulin and glucose infusions can produce a more sustained reduction. All three maneuvers, however, only shift extracellular K+ into cells. They do not promote K+ elimination from the body. To eliminate excess K+, intervention 4, 5, or 6 is necessary.
4. Administer a diuretic (e.g., furosemide 1–2 mg/kg IV) if the patient can respond with an increase in urine output.
5. Administer the K+-binding resin sodium polystyrene sulfonate 1–2 g/kg in 1 mL 70% sorbitol per gram resin either orally, by nasogastric tube, or per rectum (use early in patients with renal insufficiency).
6. Prepare to initiate either hemodialysis or peritoneal dialysis in patients with renal failure while temporizing the hyperkalemia with maneuvers 1, 2, 3, and 5 above.

Adequate levels of ionized Ca^{2+}, the physiologically active form of Ca^{2+} in the body, are essential for normal contractile function of cardiac muscle, vascular smooth muscle, and skeletal muscle (74). Routine monitoring of ionized Ca^{2+} levels instead of total serum Ca^{2+} has become standard practice in most ICUs. Normal serum ionized Ca^{2+} levels are 1.14–1.30 mmol/L, with slightly higher values for newborns in the first hours of life (75, 76). Avoidance of significant hypocalcemia is important, because postoperative cardiac patients commonly have some degree of systolic dysfunction, and Ca^{2+} is a potent positive inotrope (77). Common causes of abnormal serum Ca^{2+} levels are listed in Table 13.7. Patients with conotruncal defects and

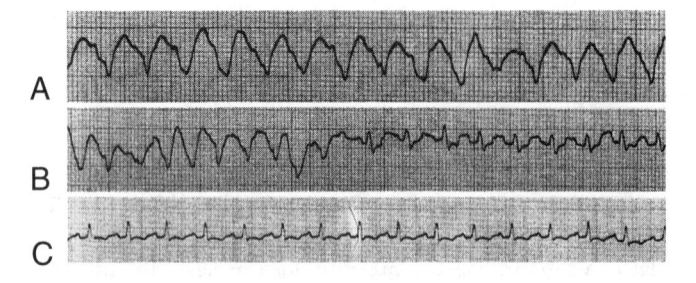

Figure 13.3. ECG (lead II) in a patient with hyperkalemia (serum K+ = 9.0 mEq/L) during acute renal failure showing "sine wave" QRS morphology (**A**), conversion to a more normal QRS morphology with a bolus of IV calcium gluconate (**B**), and maintenance of the normalized QRS morphology during a continuous calcium infusion (**C**). (Reproduced with permission from Campieri C, Fatone F, Mignani R, et al. Nephron 1987;47:312.)

aortic arch anomalies such as truncus arteriosus, TOF, and interrupted aortic arch type B who have DiGeorge syndrome (now termed CATCH 22 syndrome because of microdeletions in chromosome 22) are at increased risk of hypocalcemia from hypoparathyroidism (78, 79). Transfusion of large volumes of citrate-anticoagulated blood, which occurs during the treatment of excessive chest tube bleeding, reduces ionized Ca^{2+} because citrate chelates Ca^{2+} (80). Loop diuretics promote increased renal tubular excretion of Ca^{2+} (in contrast, thiazide diuretics spare Ca^{2+} relative to Na^+ and K^+) and increase urinary losses. An acute respiratory alkalosis from hyperventilation reduces ionized Ca^{2+} levels because more Ca^{2+} binds to serum proteins (more than 50% of total serum Ca^{2+} is normally protein bound) when pH is elevated.

Urgency in treating hypocalcemia depends primarily on the patient's hemodynamic status. Because the ionized Ca^{2+} should be monitored as frequently as serum electrolyte levels for 24 to 48 hours following surgery, patients should not progress to develop the skeletal muscle signs of hypocalcemia such as fasiculations or tetany. Any patient who is hemodynamically unstable or who requires significant inotropic support to maintain an adequate systemic blood pressure should receive Ca^{2+} if the ionized Ca^{2+} level is low (i.e., less than 1.0 mmol/L). If multiple, intermittent bolus doses of calcium chloride (10%, 25 mg/kg IV) or calcium gluconate (10%, 100 mg/kg IV) are needed to achieve a normal level, a continuous infusion of Ca^{2+} can be used. Patients with stable and normal systemic blood pressure probably do not require supplementation until their ionized Ca^{2+} is less than 0.8 mmol/L (81). Bolus and infusion Ca^{2+} ideally should be administered through a CVL, because extravasation can cause tissue necrosis. Ca^{2+} and sodium bicarbonate should not be given together through the same IV catheter, because precipitates can form.

Abnormalities of serum Mg^{2+}, particularly hypomagnesemia, have recently become better recognized as important contributors to morbidity in postoperative adult and pediatric cardiac patients (82, 83). A study by Weise et al. revealed that 81% of children developed hypomagnesemia within 5 days of cardiac surgery (84). The physiologically active form of Mg^{2+}, as with Ca^{2+}, is ionized. Routine measurement of ionized Mg^{2+} is not yet available in most diagnostic laboratories, so either serum total Mg^{2+} or ultrafilterable (free of serum proteins) Mg^{2+} is determined. Normal levels of serum total Mg^{2+} vary based on multiple factors including age (e.g., lower values in neonates) and diet, so reference values differ between laboratories (85, 86). For older children and adults, serum total Mg^{2+} less than 0.7–0.8 mmol/L, and for neonates, serum total Mg^{2+} less than 0.6 mmol/L, are recommended to diagnose hypomagnesemia.

Magnesium has multiple cardiovascular and noncardiovascular functions. Its important cardiovascular functions include energy metabolism in adenosine triphosphate-dependent processes (e.g., myocardial contraction), maintenance of cell membrane electrical potential, and regulation of vascular tone (87). Common causes of abnormal serum Mg^{2+} levels are listed in Table 13.7. The primary risk to patients with significant hypomagnesemia is ventricular dysrhythmias; ventricular tachycardia and fibrillation plus torsade de pointes can all occur with hypomagnesemia (88, 89). Total Mg^{2+} should be measured along with ionized Ca^{2+} when evaluating the cause of ventricular ectopic activity. Supplementation with magnesium sulfate ($MgSO_4$) 15–30 mg/kg IV is an appropriate component of the treatment of hypomagnesemic patients with ventricular ectopy. $MgSO_4$ should be infused over 15 to 30 minutes to avoid the most common side effects of IV administration—flushing, weakness, and hypotension—and hemodynamic status should be closely monitored. Hypermagnesemia is an unusual problem in the ICU that predominantly manifests with peripheral and central nervous system signs and symptoms.

CARDIAC OUTPUT: DETERMINATION OF CARDIAC OUTPUT STATUS AND SUPPORT OF THE POSTOPERATIVE MYOCARDIUM

Maintaining adequate cardiac output is a critical determinant of success in managing the recovery of postoperative cardiac patients. Qualitative and quantitative determination of cardiac output in the ICU is accomplished by physical examination, evaluation of bedside monitoring data, noninvasive imaging (radiography and echocardiography), and bedside cardiac output measurements. When sufficient data are not available from these sources to diagnose or optimize the patient's cardiovascular status, cardiac catheterization may be required. It is important to note that the possibility of residual or undiagnosed structural defects should be investigated aggressively before attributing low cardiac output to the effects of intraoperative support techniques (e.g., CPB) (90).

Assessing Cardiac Output

Cardiac output (CO) is the quantity of blood delivered to the systemic circulation per unit time, and it is mathematically defined as the product of ventricular stroke volume (units = liters/beat) multiplied by heart rate (units = beats/minute) (91). Because CO is a function of body mass, and patients vary significantly in size, CO is usually indexed to body surface area (BSA, units = $meter^2$). Therefore, CO is expressed as cardiac index (CI), where CI = CO/BSA (units = liters/minute/$meter^2$ or $L/min/M^2$). Cardiac output varies inversely with age, so that normal values for CI in children at rest are 4.0–5.0 $L/min/M^2$, whereas normal, resting CI at age 70 is 2.5 $L/min/M^2$ (92).

Factors determining ventricular stroke volume include afterload (impedance to ventricular emptying), preload (atrial filling pressures), and myocardial contractility.

Physical examination always provides useful clinical information about the patient's CO status, but it can be limited by ongoing supportive measures (e.g., sedation or anesthesia, neuromuscular blockade, and mechanical ventilation). The patient's mental status (difficult to assess in the early postoperative period), vital signs, cardiac impulse, peripheral perfusion, and liver size provide the best information. Inadequate CO can be manifested by one or more of the following physical examination features:

Mental status: lethargy or decreased responsiveness or irritability

Vital signs: core hyperthermia (extremity skin temperature may be cool from vasoconstriction), tachycardia, bradycardia (can immediately precede cardiac arrest), tachypnea, hypotension (for age and weight), narrow pulse pressure

Cardiac impulse: abnormally increased (e.g., outflow tract obstruction, shunt lesion) or decreased (e.g., poor systolic function)

Peripheral perfusion: cool temperature or pale color of skin in the extremities, prolonged distal extremity capillary refill (more than 3 seconds), poorly palpable pulses

Liver size: enlarged (more than 2–3 cm below the costal margin) or normal/small (e.g., from hypovolemia)

Bedside monitoring and laboratory data should be combined with physical examination findings to determine the degree and cause (abnormality of heart rate, afterload, preload, or contractility) of the deficit in CO. Abnormalities of the routine parameters monitored in the ICU and tested in the diagnostic laboratory that can occur when CO is inadequate include the following:

ECG tracing: rhythm other than normal sinus

Arterial wave form: blunted upstroke, narrow pulse pressure

RAp or CVP, LAp: low in hypovolemia (usually accompanied by tachycardia) and high with ventricular dysfunction, decreased ventricular compliance, or cardiac tamponade

Urine output: less than 1.0 mL/kg/h in neonates, infants, and children and less than 25 mL/h in older patients

Mixed venous O_2 saturation: decreased (less than 65 to 70%) because of reduced tissue blood flow and greater O_2 extraction (increased A-V O_2 difference)

Acid-base balance: increased arterial lactate concentration (more than 2.2 mM) from tissue hypoxia; metabolic acidosis on blood gas analysis

Electrolytes, blood urea nitrogen (BUN), and creatinine (Cr): hyperkalemia, elevated BUN (e.g., from hypovolemia), and elevated Cr (e.g., from decreased renal blood flow and low GFR)

Chest radiography: cardiac enlargement (e.g., dilation from decreased systolic function or a large volume load, pericardial effusion), abnormal pulmonary blood flow (increased in a large left-to-right shunt or decreased with severe pulmonary stenosis), or pulmonary edema (elevated pulmonary venous pressure)

For some patients an adequate evaluation of low CO cannot be achieved with the data from physical examination, routine bedside monitoring, and routine laboratory testing. In these situations it is appropriate to perform an echocardiogram to assess the overall adequacy of the operation. Goals of echocardiographic examination in these patients are the following:

1. Thoroughly image all areas of the heart manipulated during the operation.
2. Confirm the anatomic details of the operation.
3. Scan for any possible residual defects (e.g., shunts, valve stenosis or regurgitation, obstructed anastomosis).
4. Rate ventricular systolic function, either qualitatively or quantitatively (using M-mode echocardiography to measure left ventricular shortening fraction).
5. Image for potential complications of the operation (e.g., pericardial effusion from bleeding).

Because transthoracic imaging can be technically limited by postoperative changes in the chest wall or equipment (e.g., an open sternum or chest tubes), it may be necessary to perform a transesophageal echocardiogram (40, 93, 94). The capacity to perform two-dimensional and Doppler imaging via either transthoracic or transesophageal approaches at any time in the ICU is essential for optimal postoperative care.

If quantification of CO or other hemodynamic parameters (e.g., systemic vascular resistance [SVR] and PVR) is necessary to diagnose or optimally manage a patient, then either bedside CO measurements or cardiac catheterization must be performed. Echocardiographic techniques that use quantitative Doppler flow measurements are available for noninvasive estimates of CO, but these techniques are prone to greater inaccuracies than invasive measurements (95, 96). The two most commonly used non-echocardiographic techniques are the Fick method and thermodilution method. Both methods are based on the

Fick principle (97), and they are indicator dilution techniques. The Fick principle allows for determination of flow using an indicator (oxygen in the Fick method and temperature in thermodilution) when flow cannot be directly measured. In quantitative terms, if both the concentration (mg/mL) of indicator in a fluid and the rate (mg/min) of indicator removal or addition can be measured, then the flow (mL/min) can be calculated as follows:

$$\frac{\text{Rate of removal or addition}}{\text{Change in concentration}} = \frac{\text{mg/min}}{\text{mg/mL}} = \text{mL/min}$$

For the Fick method, total pulmonary blood flow is calculated by dividing the total quantity of oxygen absorbed per minute by the oxygen uptake from blood per unit of blood flowing (i.e., the A-V O_2 difference). Therefore, CO (i.e., pulmonary blood flow) = oxygen consumption/A-V O_2 difference. Although more difficult to perform in mechanically ventilated patients breathing supplemental oxygen, the Fick method has the important advantage of continued accuracy in the presence of an intracardiac shunt.

The bedside technique used most commonly in the ICU is the thermodilution method (98, 99). In thermodilution the indicator (temperature) is added to the circulation by injecting an IV bolus of cold, sterile fluid, which can either be saline, dextrose solution, or water. Thermodilution requires a double-lumen PA balloon catheter equipped with a thermistor that allows for cold indicator injection into the RA and measurement of the change in blood temperature in the PA. Percutaneous placement of this catheter via a femoral, subclavian, or internal jugular vein can be performed in the ICU. After insertion and attachment to a pressure transducer, catheter tip position is deduced by analysis of both pressures and pressure waveforms (See Fig. 11.7 in Chapter 11, *Invasive and Noninvasive Monitoring*) (100). Ideally, the distal port of the catheter will be positioned in the main or a central branch PA and the proximal port in the RA. A chest radiograph should be obtained to verify catheter position.

If the bedside monitor does not contain the computer software for performing CO determinations, a portable CO unit can be employed. A bucket with ice containing several sterile syringes and a bottle of sterile normal saline is prepared 30 minutes before the measurements to allow for complete temperature equilibration. The patient's height, weight, and a calibration factor, which corrects for the type of catheter and injectate characteristics, are entered into the computer. Injectate volume is based on the patient's weight; typical volumes are 1–3 mL (less than 10 kg), 3–5 mL (10–30 kg), and 10 mL (more than 30 kg). A temperature probe is placed into the ice and the thermistor is connected to the computer. The first syringe of cold saline is rapidly injected into the proximal port, and it is used only to cool the catheter, not for a measurement. Three rapid (less than 2 seconds), consecutive injections of identical volume are made during the same portion of the respiratory cycle (e.g., after exhalation) and as close together in time as possible for the measurement. The computer will generate output curves, which should be inspected, and calculate CI based on weight and height data (Fig. 13.4). The three CI readings should vary by less than 15%.

If performed carefully, thermodilution CO determinations achieve 90 to 95% accuracy when compared with val-

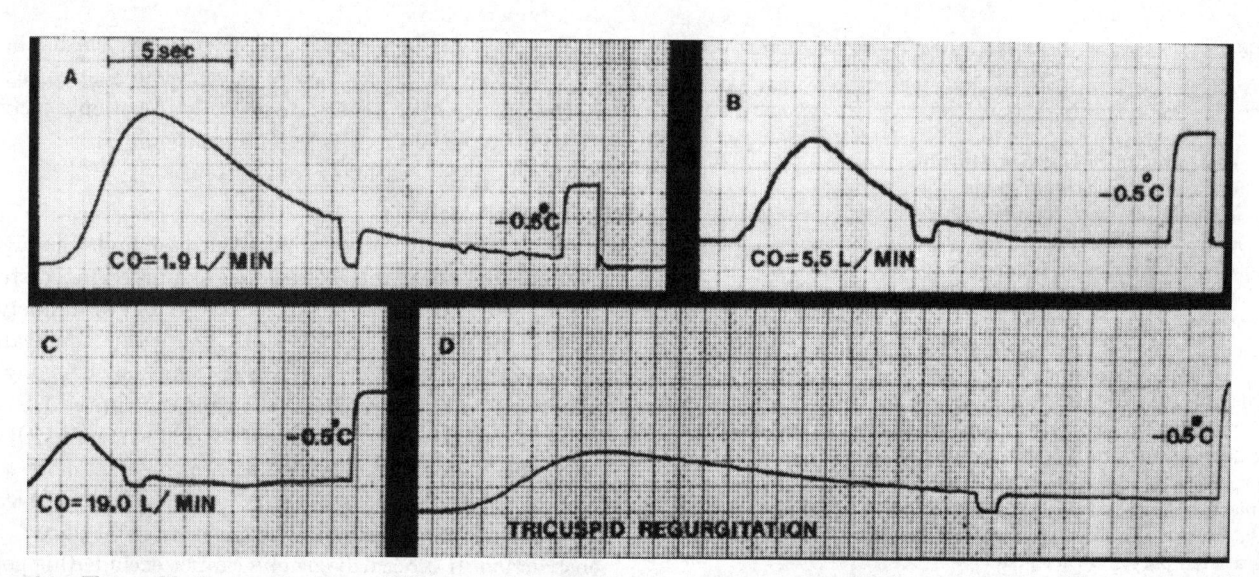

Figure 13.4. Thermodilution cardiac output (CO) curves. Time (sec) is represented by the ordinate and temperature (°C) by the abscissa. **A**, Low cardiac output. **B**, Normal cardiac output. **C**, High cardiac output. **D**, In significant tricuspid regurgitation or pulmonary regurgitation (not shown), an inadequate curve is generated for CO calculation by the computer. Notches on the descending portion of each curve are artifacts produced by the computer. (Reproduced with permission from Sharkey S. Amer J Med 1987; 83:111–122.)

ues obtained by the classic Fick oxygen consumption method (91). Multiple sources of error are possible when using the thermodilution method, however (101, 102). These errors and their effects on measurement values are provided in Table 13.8. Changes in temperature in the PA are used to calculate pulmonary blood flow. In the absence of intracardiac shunting, pulmonary blood flow is equal to systemic blood flow and therefore systemic CO. Shunting produces errors in measurement. A left-to-right shunt will increase pulmonary blood flow, reduce the temperature change between RA and PA, and thus overestimate CO (see Fig. 13.4C). The amount of indicator "lost" in a right-to-left shunt (i.e., included in shunted blood) is difficult to predict. Other errors that decrease the temperature difference between RA and PA (e.g., an inadequate injectate volume, elevated injectate temperature, insufficiently cooled catheter, and prolonged injection time) generate overestimates. Specific errors of catheter positioning, such as placing the thermistor on or near the PA wall (which will not cool as efficiently as blood), can falsely elevate the CO. The magnitude of overestimation can be greater in patients with lower CO, because blood moving at reduced velocity through the right ventricle can acquire more heat from the heart (103). Errors that exaggerate the temperature difference in the PA, such as an excessive injectate volume, low injectate temperature (lower than the temperature of the probe in the bucket of ice), and narrow distance between injectate site and thermistor, produce an underestimation (see Fig. 13.4A). Normal fluctuations in PA temperature, which occur as a result of respiratory and cardiac cycle variations, can generate unpredictable errors in measurement. Respiratory variation can be reduced by always injecting after exhalation. Significant tricuspid and pulmonary regurgitation can affect the electronic analysis of CO curves such that the computer will be unable to compute a value (see Fig. 13.4D).

If invasive bedside CO measurements in combination with echocardiographic data do not provide a sufficient explanation for the patient's low CO state, then cardiac catheterization should be considered. Specific indications for catheterization of critically ill postoperative patients are discussed in Chapter 29, *Cardiac Catheterization in the Critically Ill Cardiac Patient.*

Support of the Postoperative Myocardium

Low CO in the postoperative patient can result from one or a combination of factors including the following:

1. Residual (e.g., aortic arch obstruction) or unrecognized (e.g., additional muscular VSD after complete common atrioventricular canal or TOF repair) structural defects.
2. Continuation of preoperative ventricular dysfunction.
3. Myocardial dysfunction related to intraoperative support techniques (e.g., ischemia-reperfusion injury, effects of CPB and hypothermia, inadequate myocardial protection).
4. Type of surgical procedure (e.g., right ventricular [RV] dysfunction after right ventriculotomy in repair of TOF).
5. Complication of surgery (e.g., compromised coronary artery perfusion).
6. Dysrhythmia (e.g., junctional ectopic tachycardia) or loss of normal conduction (e.g., complete heart block).
7. Pulmonary hypertension (especially in patients lacking an atrial or ventricular communication).
8. Infection (e.g., catheter-related sepsis).

It is especially important to consider and thoroughly evaluate the possibility of residual or unrecognized structural defects, because medical management is unlikely to reverse the patient's low CO state, and it can significantly increase the risks of a corrective procedure by delaying reintervention. For example, in the neonate with HLHS who has undergone a Norwood procedure, low systemic CO coupled with high arterial oxygen saturation (e.g., more than 85% in room air) and a chest radiograph showing cardiomegaly and congested lungs suggest residual aortic arch obstruction. If echocardiography cannot exclude this possibility, cardiac catheterization should be performed to evaluate the adequacy of arch augmentation. In some situations, however, low CO after CPB can be anticipated, even when the repair is excellent. Neonates with transposition

---

Table 13.8. Factors Affecting the Accuracy of Thermodilution Cardiac Output Measurements

Overestimation of Cardiac Output
Left-to-right intracardiac shunt
Inadequate injectate volume
Insufficient volume placed into syringe
Loss of volume during injection (e.g., catheter leak)
Elevated injectate temperature
Inadequate catheter cooling with initial (premeasurement) injection
Prolonged injection time (> 4–5 s)
Catheter malposition
Thermistor tip on or near pulmonary artery wall

Underestimation of Cardiac Output
Excessive injectate volume
Injectate temperature lower than temperature probe value
Catheter malposition with narrow distance between right atrium port and thermistor

Variable Effects on Measured Cardiac Output
Right-to-left intracardiac shunt
Physiologic fluctuations in pulmonary artery blood temperature
Use of incorrect calibration factor, height, or weight

of the great arteries (TGA) develop a predictable decline in CI (average decrease = 32%), with the lowest CI occurring 9 to 12 hours after repair with the arterial switch operation (21). Inotropic support, afterload reduction, and continued use of neuromuscular blockade and anesthesia during the first postoperative night in these patients can attenuate the decline in CO and mitigate the adverse effects of postoperative stimuli (e.g., endotracheal tube suctioning).

One or more of the factors contributing to CO—heart rate, preload, afterload, and contractility—can be manipulated when treating the patient with low CO. Following surgery, patients in sinus rhythm may have either abnormally high (sinus tachycardia) or low (sinus bradycardia) resting heart rates. Elevated sinus rates, which are more common, can be caused by medications (e.g., catecholamines, pancuronium), fever, pain and anxiety, and depressed ventricular function. Tachyarrhythmias, whether of sinus node origin or generated from an abnormal supraventricular, junctional, or ventricular focus, can decrease CO by compromising ventricular filling or depressing ventricular function (104, 105). Bradycardia can be secondary to hypothermia (e.g., incomplete rewarming after CPB with hypothermia), sinus node dysfunction (e.g., edema from atrial surgery), severely depressed ventricular function, or medications (e.g., digoxin). Neonates and young infants, whose CO is more heart-rate dependent than that of children and adults, are particularly affected by low heart rates (106). Because the normal range of heart rate varies with age, knowledge of age-adjusted normal values is important (107).

Preload effects on ventricular stroke volume are demonstrated by the Frank-Starling mechanism, where increased ventricular filling during diastole produces enhanced myofibril shortening in systole, resulting in a greater volume of blood pumped per heart beat (108, 109). Characteristics of patients with decreased preload on physical examination and from bedside monitoring and laboratory data have been discussed in previous sections. Patients who have undergone specific procedures typically require additional preload, especially in the early postoperative period. Procedures in this group include: (a) a right ventriculotomy (e.g., complete repair of TOF or placement of a right ventricle-to-PA homograft in the Rastelli procedure), (b) a cavopulmonary anastomosis (e.g., bidirectional Glenn shunt or modified Fontan procedure), (c) a systemic-to-pulmonary artery shunt (e.g., modified Blalock-Taussig shunt), and (d) operations complicated by pulmonary hypertension (e.g., repair of obstructed total anomalous pulmonary venous connection or mitral stenosis). Filling pressures of 12–15 mm Hg may be necessary in these patients to provide the preload necessary to generate an adequate CO.

Increased afterload is frequently encountered in the ICU, and it often complicates operations, which also cause decreased myocardial contractility (110). Both pulmonary and systemic vascular beds can develop elevated resistance that will lower CO. When PVR is elevated, right ventricular output can be compromised, leading to extravascular fluid accumulation (e.g., pleural effusion, ascites, persistent tissue edema), cyanosis (via right-to-left shunting when an intracardiac communication exists), and systemic hypotension (severe reduction in pulmonary blood flow in patients without shunts). When SVR is increased, either because of excessive catecholamine levels or loss of normal vasodilatory function from inflammation, patients will initially develop poor peripheral perfusion and low urine output. Treatment of excessive afterload includes recognizing and ameliorating conditions that exacerbate vasoconstriction (e.g., hypoxia, acidosis, hypothermia, and pain) and administering vasodilating agents. A phosphodiesterase inhibitor (amrinone or milrinone) is frequently combined as a second-line agent with an inotrope (e.g., dopamine), because these agents act synergistically to increase CO without significantly elevating the heart rate (27, 28). The neonatal myocardium in particular benefits from afterload reduction therapy.

Decreased myocardial contractility is commonly encountered in postoperative patients, especially following procedures with CPB. Pharmacologic augmentation of contractility with inotropic medications and reduction of afterload with vasodilators are essential in the treatment of low CO. A detailed discussion of the mechanism of action and pharmacokinetics of vasoactive drugs is presented in Chapter 5, *Cardiovascular Pharmacology*. The algorithms in Figure 13.5 provide guidelines for the use of these agents, either individually or in combination, in commonly encountered postoperative situations.

When assessing the value of pharmacologic support of a postoperative patient with low CO, it is important to consider first the patient's intravascular volume status, serum Ca^{2+} level, cardiac rhythm, and level of sedation. If low intravascular volume or inadequate preload exists, an infusion of IV crystalloid or colloid should be administered. For example, in the initial 12 hours following fenestrated Fontan repair, patients often require additional IV fluid to generate adequate right-sided venous pressures to overcome elevated PVR and maintain CO (111). In the hypocalcemic patient, IV Ca^{2+} should be given, because a positive inotropic effect may be achieved by normalizing serum ionized Ca^{2+}. If the patient is not in normal sinus rhythm, an attempt should be made to correct the dysrhythmia with cardiac pacing, drug therapy, or electrical cardioversion. Depth of sedation should also be considered, because mild-to-moderate hypotension in the deeply sedated or paralyzed and anesthetized patient who is vasodilated but maintains adequate distal perfusion and urine output may not require treatment with an inotrope. Inotropic treatment of hypotension that is either mild (10 to 20% de-

A. Mild-to-Moderate Hypotension

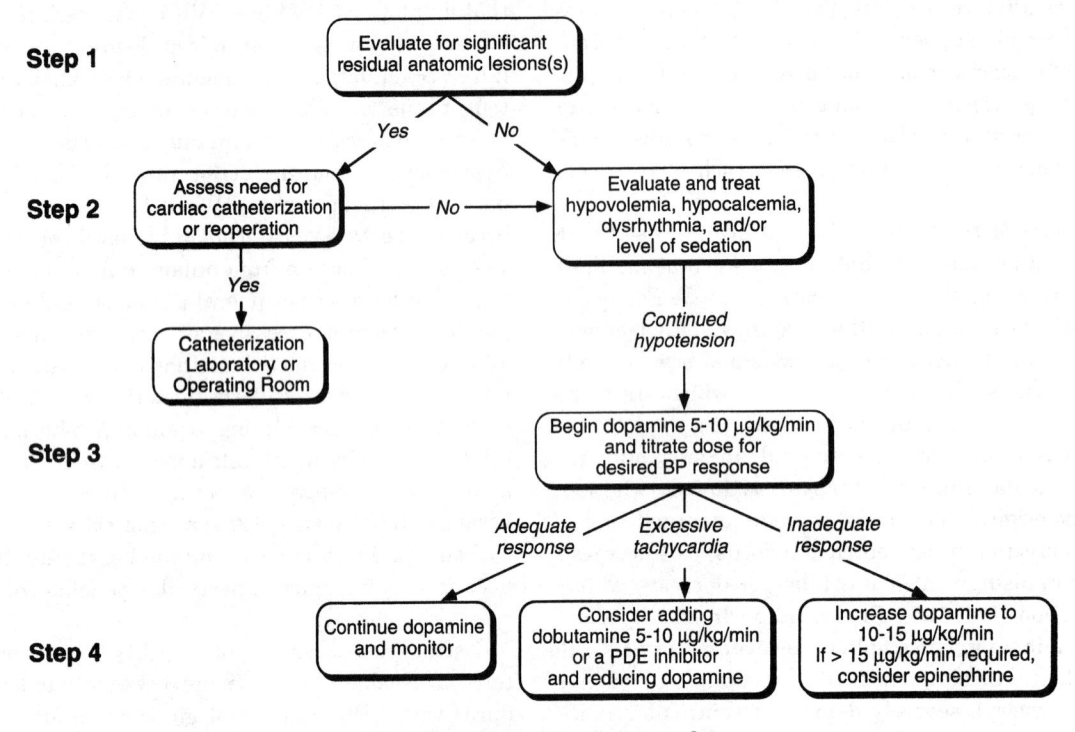

Step 1: Evaluate for significant residual anatomic lesions(s)

- Yes → **Step 2:** Assess need for cardiac catheterization or reoperation
  - Yes → Catheterization Laboratory or Operating Room
  - No → Evaluate and treat hypovolemia, hypocalcemia, dysrhythmia, and/or level of sedation
- No → Evaluate and treat hypovolemia, hypocalcemia, dysrhythmia, and/or level of sedation

Continued hypotension ↓

Step 3: Begin dopamine 5-10 μg/kg/min and titrate dose for desired BP response

Step 4:
- Adequate response → Continue dopamine and monitor
- Excessive tachycardia → Consider adding dobutamine 5-10 μg/kg/min or a PDE inhibitor and reducing dopamine
- Inadequate response → Increase dopamine to 10-15 μg/kg/min. If > 15 μg/kg/min required, consider epinephrine

B. Severe Hypotension

Part A Steps 1-4 with inadequate BP response to dopamine > 15 μg/kg/min

↓

Begin epinephrine at 0.05-0.1 μg/kg/min and titrate dose for desired BP response to ≤ 0.3 μg/kg/min

- Adequate response → Continue epinephrine and monitor
- Inadequate response, low SVR → Consider adding norepinephrine 0.01-0.2 μg/kg/min
  - Adequate response → Continue norepinephrine and epinephrine and monitor
  - Inadequate response → Evaluate need for mechanical support with VAD or ECMO
- Inadequate response, normal or high SVR → Evaluate need for mechanical support with VAD or ECMO

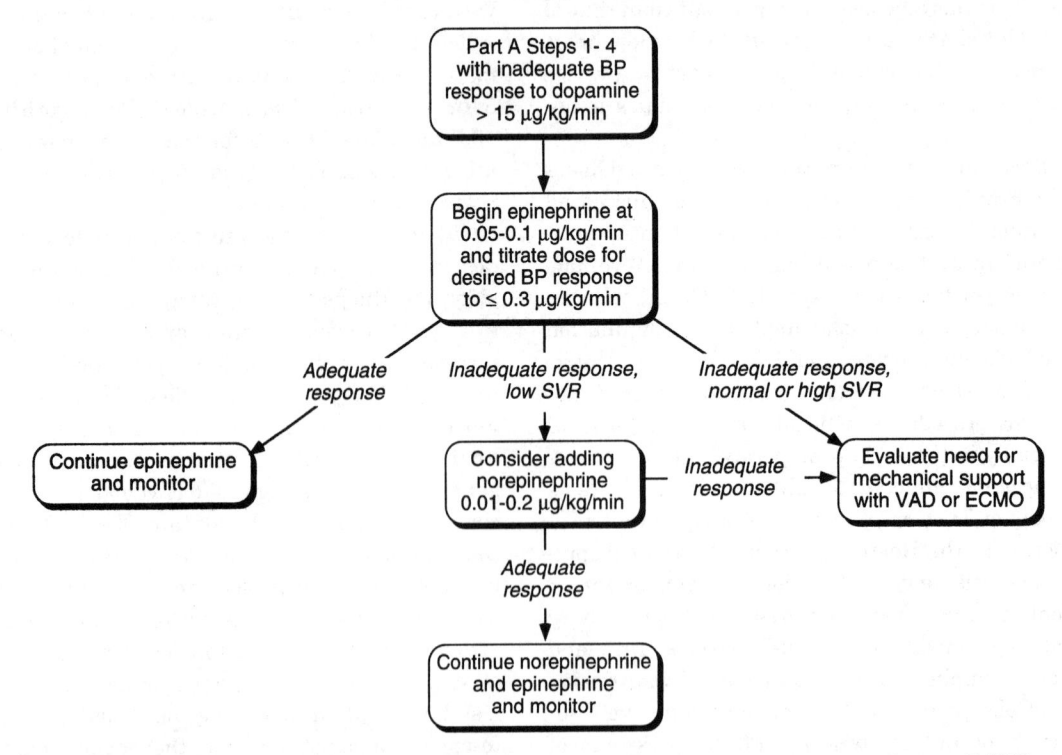

Figure 13.5. Algorithms for the use of inotropic and afterload-reducing medications in postoperative patients. *BP*, blood pressure; *PDE*, phosphodiesterase inhibitor; *SVR*, systemic vascular resistance; *VAD*, ventricular assist device; *ECMO*, extracorporeal membrane oxygenation; *CO*, cardiac output.

C. Normal or Mildly Decreased BP with Low CO and Elevated SVR

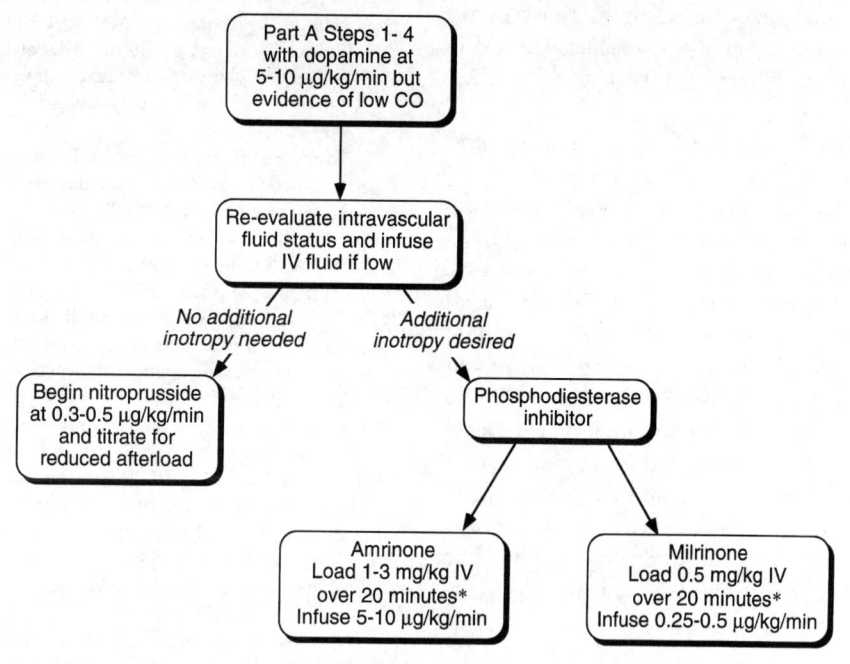

```
Part A Steps 1-4
with dopamine at
5-10 µg/kg/min but
evidence of low CO
        │
        ▼
Re-evaluate intravascular
fluid status and infuse
IV fluid if low
   │              │
No additional    Additional
inotropy needed  inotropy desired
   │              │
   ▼              ▼
Begin nitroprusside   Phosphodiesterase
at 0.3-0.5 µg/kg/min  inhibitor
and titrate for        │          │
reduced afterload      ▼          ▼
                   Amrinone    Milrinone
                   Load 1-3    Load 0.5
                   mg/kg IV    mg/kg IV
                   over 20     over 20
                   minutes*    minutes*
                   Infuse      Infuse
                   5-10        0.25-0.5
                   µg/kg/min   µg/kg/min
```

*Vasodilation during the loading dose of either PDE inhibitor can cause hypotension; IV fluid should be available during administration of loading dose.

Figure 13.5. (continued).

crease in normal mean arterial blood pressure for age) or moderate (20 to 30% decrease in normal mean arterial blood pressure for age) usually begins with dopamine. An infusion at a dose of 5–10 µg/kg/min is initiated, and the infusion rate titrated to produce the desired systemic blood pressure. If dose-dependent tachycardia develops, dobutamine at 5–10 µg/kg/min can be added and dopamine reduced. Dobutamine produces less tachycardia in adults (112), so that a combination of the two drugs may adequately increase blood pressure with only mild tachycardia. For treatment of mild-to-moderate hypotension, dobutamine as a single agent may be less effective than dopamine because it causes a reduction in SVR (113). When dopamine at 15–20 µg/kg/min is required to achieve adequate blood pressure, addition of a more potent inotrope such as epinephrine (see below) should be considered. Dopamine at low doses (3 µg/kg/min or less) has a minimal effect on CO, but it stimulates dopaminergic receptors in the kidney and may lead to increased renal perfusion and greater urine production.

Patients with severe hypotension (more than 30% decrease in normal mean arterial blood pressure for age) or an inadequate response to high doses of dopamine (e.g., 15–20 µg/kg/min) are candidates for treatment with epinephrine. Epinephrine is a more potent inotrope than dopamine because of its greater myocardial α_1- and β_1-adrenoceptor—mediated effects, and it is preferred for treatment of severe ventricular dysfunction. Epinephrine is infused at rates of 0.01–1.0 µg/kg/min and should be administered by CVL. At high doses (i.e., 0.5 µg/kg/min or more) both renal and peripheral extremity perfusion can be significantly compromised, and tachycardia is common. Lower-dose epinephrine (e.g., less than 0.1 µg/kg/min) or dopamine is useful in combination therapy with an IV afterload-reducing agent such as amrinone, milrinone, or sodium nitroprusside for treatment of significant ventricular dysfunction and elevated SVR. Examples of scenarios in which combination therapy with an inotrope and afterload-reducing agent are effective include (a) complicated reparative surgery with anticipated postoperative reduction in CO in the neonate (e.g., arterial switch operation and VSD closure for TGA/VSD or repair of TOF with pulmonary atresia) or young infant (e.g., repair of truncus arteriosus), (b) complicated palliative surgery with longer intraoperative support times (e.g., Norwood procedure for HLHS) and (c) modified Fontan repair (the single ventricle must overcome both SVR and PVR in series). Norepinephrine is used infrequently in postoperative pediatric patients because of its marked vasoconstrictive effects. However, two situations for which IV doses of 0.01–0.5 µg/kg/min by CVL can be considered include (a) severe hypotension and low SVR (e.g., "warm" shock from sepsis), and (b) temporary support of profoundly decreased CO while preparing to initiate mechanical support with a VAD or ECMO.

In patients with mild or borderline hypotension and bradycardia from either sinus node dysfunction or AV block, isoproterenol can be used in place of atrial pacing for chronotropy. Doses in the range of 0.01–0.05 µg/kg/min by infusion typically elevate the heart rate. Because of its β_2-adrenoceptor–mediated effects on the peripheral vasculature, isoproterenol can lower SVR and exacerbate hypotension, especially in the patient with low intravascular volume. In some institutions isoproterenol is preferred to atrial pacing for bradycardia in the denervated heart following orthotopic cardiac transplantation, because it provides inotropic as well as chronotropic support.

If postoperative patients require continued therapy with oral inotropic and afterload-reducing agents, the choices are limited. Digoxin is the only oral inotrope currently in widespread use in the United States. It is started at 8–10 µg/kg/d divided twice a day when inotropes administered by IV infusion, such as dopamine, are being reduced or discontinued. If the child is unable to ingest digoxin, it can be administered at the same dose IV until enteral feeding is tolerated. Digoxin is commonly used in children in the following situations: (a) persistent volume load (e.g., shunted single-ventricle patients), (b) right ventriculotomy with decreased CO postoperatively (e.g., complete repair of TOF), and (c) persistence of poor ventricular systolic function after surgery. The ACE inhibitors, captopril and enalapril, are used to replace the IV afterload-reducing agents. A test dose of captopril 0.1 mg/kg should be administered initially, followed by close blood pressure monitoring for 4 to 6 hours. Therapeutic captopril doses range between 0.1–2 mg/kg/d (neonates), 0.5–6 mg/kg/d (children), and 12.5–25 mg/dose (adolescents), and are given in three doses a day. Enalapril has the advantage of dosing only twice a day.

REFERENCES

1. Castaneda A, Jonas R, Mayer JJ, et al, eds. Cardiac surgery of the neonate and infant. Philadelphia: WB Saunders, 1994:65–66.
2. Wernovsky G, Chang A, Wessel D. Intensive care. In: Emmanoulides G, Riemenschneider T, Allen H, et al, eds. Heart disease in infants, children, and adolescents. Baltimore: Williams & Wilkins, 1995:398.
3. Krongrad E. Postoperative arrhythmias in patients with congenital heart disease. Chest 1984;85:107–113.
4. Adatia I, Wessel D. The use of inhaled nitric oxide in congenital heart disease. In: Weir E, Archer S, Reeves J, eds. Nitric oxide and radicals in the pulmonary vasculature. Armonk, NY: Futura, 1996:463–491.
5. Kirklin J, Blackstone E, Kirklin J. Cardiopulmonary bypass: studies on its damaging effects. Blood Purif 1987;5:168–187.
6. Salama A, Hugo F, Heinrich D, et al. Deposition of terminal C5b-9 complement complexes on erythrocytes and leukocytes during cardiopulmonary bypass. N Engl J Med 1988;318:408–414.
7. Kirklin J, Barratt-Boyes B. Postoperative care. In: Kirklin J, Barratt-Boyes B, eds. Cardiac surgery. New York: Churchill Livingstone, 1993:222–224.
8. Barash P, Lescovich F, Katz J, et al. Early extubation following pediatric cardiothoracic operation: a viable alternative. Ann Thorac Surg 1980;29:228–233.
9. Laussen P, Reid R, Stene R, et al. Tracheal extubation of children in the operating room after atrial septal defect repair as part of a clinical practice guideline. Anesth Analg 1996;82:988–993.
10. Braunwald E. Hemodynamic significance of atrial systole. Am J Med 1964;37:778–779.
11. Mitchell J, Gupta D, Payne R. Influence of atrial systole on effective ventricular stroke volume. Circ Res 1965;17:11–18.
12. Norwood W. Hypoplastic left heart syndrome. Ann Thorac Surg 1991;52:688–695.
13. Wernovsky G, Chang A, Wessel D. Intensive care. In Emmanoulides G, Riemenschneider T, Allen H, et al, eds. Heart disease in infants, children, and adolescents. Baltimore: Williams & Wilkins, 1995:404–405; 422–423.
14. Chang A, Farrell P, Murdison K, et al. Hypoplastic left heart syndrome: hemodynamic and angiographic assessment after initial reconstructive surgery and relevance to modified Fontan procedure. J Am Coll Cardiol 1991;17:1143–1149.
15. West J, ed. Pulmonary pathophysiology. Baltimore: Williams & Wilkins, 1982:19–41.
16. Nadas A. Hypoxemia. In: Fyler D, ed. Nadas' pediatric cardiology. Philadelphia: Hanley & Belfus, 1992:73.
17. Wessel D, Hickey P, Hansen D. Pulmonary and systemic hemodynamic effects of hyperventilation in infants after repair of congenital heart disease. Anesthesiology 1987;67:A526.
18. Morray J, Lynn A, Kahana M. The effect of pH and Pco_2 on pulmonary and systemic hemodynamics following surgery in children with congenital heart disease and pulmonary hypertension. Anesthesiology 1986;65:A451.
19. Jonas R, Lang P, Hansen D, et al. First-stage palliation of hypoplastic left heart syndrome. J Thorac Cardiovasc Surg 1986;92:6–13.
20. Lock J. Hemodynamic evaluation of congenital heart disease. In: Lock J, Keane J, Fellows K, eds. Diagnostic and interventional catheterization in congenital heart disease. Norwell: Martinus Nijhoff, 1987:35.
21. Wernovsky G, Wypij D, Jonas R, et al. Postoperative course and hemodynamic profile after the arterial switch operation in neonates and infants. A comparison of low-flow cardiopulmonary bypass and circulatory arrest. Circulation 1995;92:2226–2235.
22. Shone J, Sellers R, Anderson R, et al. The developmental complex of "parachute mitral valve," supravalvular ring of left atrium, subaortic stenosis, and coarctation of aorta. Am J Cardiol 1963;11:714–725.
23. Mathew R, Thilenius O, Replogle R, et al. Cardiac function in total anomalous pulmonary venous return before and after surgery. Circulation 1977;55:361–370.

24. Suga H. Importance of atrial compliance in cardiac performance. Circ Res 1974;35:39–43.
25. Laine G, Allen S, Katz J, et al. Effect of systemic venous pressure on lymph flow and lung edema formation. J App Physiol 1986;61:1634–1638.
26. Applebaum A, Blackstone E, Kouchoukos N. Afterload reduction and cardiac output in infants early after intracardiac surgery. Am J Cardiol 1977;39:445–452.
27. Lawless S, Zaritsky A, Miles M. The acute pharmacokinetics and pharmacodynamics of amrinone in pediatric patients. J Clin Pharmacol 1991;31:800–803.
28. Chang A, Atz A, Wernovsky G, et al. Milrinone: systemic and pulmonary hemodynamic effects in neonates after cardiac surgery. Crit Care Med 1995;23:1907–1914.
29. Krovetz L, McLoughlin T, Mitchell M, et al. Hemodynamic findings in normal children. Pediatr Res 1967;1:122–130.
30. Lang P, Chipman C, Siden H, et al. Early assessment of hemodynamic status after repair of tetralogy of Fallot: a comparison of 24 hour (intensive care unit) and 1 year postoperative data in 98 patients. Am J Cardiol 1982;50:795–799.
31. Hickey P, Hansen D. Pulmonary hypertension in infants; postoperative management. In: Yacoub M, ed. Annual of cardiac surgery. London: Current Science, 1989:16–22.
32. Chang A, Zucker H, Hickey P, et al. Pulmonary vascular resistance in infants after cardiac surgery: the role of carbon dioxide and hydrogen ion. Crit Care Med 1995;23:568–574.
33. Rudolph A, Yuan S. Response of the pulmonary vasculature to hypoxia and H^+ ion concentration changes. J Clin Invest 1966;45:399–411.
34. Freed M, Miettinen O, Nadas A. Oximetric detection of intracardiac left-to-right shunts. Br Heart J 1979;42:690–694.
35. Little W, Braunwald E. Assessment of cardiac function. In: Braunwald E, ed. Heart disease. Philadelphia: WB Saunders, 1997:439.
36. Dexter L, Haynes F, Burwell C, et al. Studies of congenital heart disease. II. The pressure and oxygen content of blood in the right auricle, right ventricle, and pulmonary artery in control patients with observations on the oxygen saturation and source of pulmonary "capillary" blood. J Clin Invest 1947;26:554–560.
37. Barratt-Boyes B, Wood E. The oxygen saturation of blood in the venae cavae, right-heart chambers, and pulmonary vessels of healthy subjects. J Lab Clin Med 1957;93–106.
38. Hanley F, Heinemann M, Jonas R, et al. Repair of truncus arteriosus in the neonate. J Thorac Cardiovasc Surg 1993;105:1047–1056.
39. Vincent R, Lang P, Chipman C, et al. Assessment of hemodynamic status in the intensive care unit immediately after closure of ventricular septal defect. Am J Cardiol 1985;55:526–529.
40. Wolfe L, Rossi A, Ritter S. Transesophageal echocardiography in infants and children: use and importance in the cardiac intensive care unit. J Am Soc Echocardiogr 1993;3:286–289.
41. Moynihan P, Wernovsky G, Hickey P, et al. Complication rates of transthoracic lines removed by critical care nurses [Abstract]. Circulation 1992;86 (Suppl 1):702A.
42. Gold J, Jonas R, Lang P, et al. Transthoracic monitoring lines in pediatric surgical patients: a ten year experience. Ann Thorac Surg 1986;42:185–191.
43. Petaja J, Lundstrom U, Sairanen H, et al. Central venous thrombosis after cardiac operations in children. J Thorac Cardiovasc Surg 1996;112:883–889.
44. Krafte-Jacobs B, Sivit CJ, Mejia R, et al. Catheter-related thrombosis in critically ill children; comparison of catheters with and without heparin bonding. J Pediatr 1995;126:50–54.
45. David M, Andrew M. Venous thromboembolic complications in children. J Pediatr 1993;123:337–346.
46. Kirklin J, Westaby S, Blackstone E, et al. Complement and the damaging effects of cardiopulmonary bypass. J Thorac Cardiovasc Surg 1983;86:845–857.
47. Smith E, Naftel D, Blackstone E, et al. Microvascular permeability after cardiopulmonary bypass. J Thorac Cardiovasc Surg 1987;94:225–233.
48. Maehara T, Novak I, Elliot M. Peri-operative changes in total body water in children undergoing open heart surgery. Eur J Cardiothorac Surg 1991;5:258–265.
49. Rosenthal S, LaJohn L. Effect of age on transvascular fluid movement. Am J Physiol 1975;228:134–140.
50. Quillen J, Sellke F, Brooks L, et al. Ischemia-reperfusion impairs endothelium-dependent relaxation of coronary microvessels but does not affect large arteries. Circulation 1990;82:586–594.
51. Kirklin J, Barratt-Boyes B. Hypothermia, circulatory arrest, and cardiopulmonary bypass. In: Kirklin J, Barratt-Boyes B, eds. Cardiac surgery. New York: Churchill Livingstone, 1993:83–97.
52. Naik S, Knight A, Elliot M. A prospective randomized study of a modified technique of ultrafiltration during pediatric open-heart surgery. Circulation 1991;84 (Suppl III):III-422–III-431.
53. Mee R. Dialysis after cardiopulmonary bypass in neonates and infants. J Thorac Cardiovasc Surg 1992;103:1021–1022.
54. Lefer DJ, Shadelya SM, Serrano Jr, et al. Cardioprotective actions of a monoclonal antibody against CD-18 in myocardial ischemia-reperfusion injury. Circulation 1993;88:1779–1787.
55. Lefer DJ, Flynn DM, Phillips LM, et al. A novel sialyl Lewis^x analog attenuates neutrophil accumulation and myocardial necrosis after ischemia and reperfusion. Circulation 1994;90:2390–2401.
56. Anand K, Hansen D, Hickey P. Hormonal-metabolic stress responses in neonates undergoing cardiac surgery. Anesthesiology 1990;73:661–670.
57. Anand K, Hickey P. Halothane-morphine compared with high-dose sufentanil for anesthesia and postoperative analgesia in neonatal cardiac surgery. N Engl J Med 1992;326:1–9.
58. Benzing G, Francis P, Kaplan S, et al. Glucose and insulin changes in infants and children undergoing hypothermic open-heart surgery. Am J Cardiol 1983;52:133–136.
59. Guignard J, Torrado A, Da Cunha O, et al. Glomerular filtration rate in the first three weeks of life. J Pediatr 1975;87:268–272.
60. Wood E, Lynch R. Fluid and electrolyte balance. In: Fuhrman B, Zimmerman J, eds. Pediatric critical care. St. Louis: Mosby-Year Book, 1992:672.
61. Singh N, Kissoon N, Al Mofada S, et al. Comparison of continuous versus intermittent furosemide administration in postoperative pediatric cardiac patients. Crit Care Med 1992;20:17–21.
62. Yetman A, Singh N, Parbtani A, et al. Acute hemodynamic and neurohormonal effects of furosemide in critically ill pediatric patients. Crit Care Med 1996;24:398–402.

63. DiBona G. Neural control of renal tubular solute and water transport. Miner Electrolyte Metab 1989;15:44–50.
64. Schmidt M, Imbs J. Pharmacological characterization of renal vascular dopamine receptors. J Cardiovasc Pharmacol 1980;2:595–605.
65. Girardin E, Berner M, Rouge J, et al. Effect of low dose dopamine on hemodynamic and renal function in children. Pediatr Res 1989;26:200–203.
66. Goldberg L. Cardiovascular and renal actions of dopamine: potential clinical applications. Pharmacol Rev 1972;24:1–29.
67. Perez C, Reimer J, Schreiber M. Effect of high dose dopamine on urine output in newborn infants. Crit Care Med 1986;14:1045–1049.
68. Wong H, Chundu K. Metabolic alkalosis in children undergoing cardiac surgery. Crit Care Med 1993;21:884–887.
69. Garson A. Electrocardiography. In: Garson A, Bricker J, McNamara D, eds. The science and practice of pediatric cardiology. Philadelphia: Lea & Febiger, 1990:747.
70. Moore S, Wilkoff B. Rhythm disturbances after cardiac surgery. Semin Thorac Cardiovasc Surg 1991;3:24–29.
71. Wright F. Flow dependent transport processes: filtration, absorption, secretion. Am J Physiol 1982;243:F1–F11.
72. Ponce S, Jennings A, Madias N, et al. Drug-induced hyperkalemia. Medicine 1985;64:357–370.
73. Hastreiter AR, Vander Horst, Chow-Ting E. Digitalis toxicity in infants and children. Pediatr Cardiol 1984;5:131–148.
74. Morgan JP, Perreault CL, Morgan KG. The cellular basis of contraction and relaxation in cardiac and vascular smooth muscle. Am Heart J 1991;121:961–968.
75. Lougheed JL, Mimouni F, Tsang RC. Serum ionized calcium concentrations in normal neonates. Am J Dis Child 1988;142:516–518.
76. Jordan CD, Flood JG, Laposata M, et al. Normal reference laboratory values. N Engl J Med 1992;327:718–724.
77. Opie L. Regulation of myocardial contractility. J Cardiovasc Pharmacol 1995;26 (Suppl 1):S1–S9.
78. Wilson D, Burn J, Scambler P, et al. DiGeorge syndrome; part of CATCH 22. J Med Genet 1993;30:852–856.
79. Cuneo BF, Langman CB, Ilbawi MN, et al. Latent hypothyroidism in children with conotruncal cardiac defects. Circulation 1996;93:1702–1708.
80. Delinger J, Nahrwold M, Gibbs P, et al. Hypocalcemia during rapid blood transfusion in anesthetized man. Br J Anaesth 1976;48:995–1000.
81. Zaloga G. Hypocalcemia in critically ill patients. Crit Care Med 1992;20:251–262.
82. Aglio L, Stanford G, Maddi R, et al. Hypomagnesemia is common following cardiac surgery. J Cardiothorac Vasc Anesth 1991;5:201–208.
83. Satur C, Stubington S, Jennings A, et al. Magnesium flux during and after open heart operations in children. Ann Thorac Surg 1995;59:921–927.
84. Weise K, Thompson S, Besunder J. Hypomagnesemia after cardiac surgery in children: patterns and complications of treatment [Abstract]. Third Pediatric Critical Care Colloquim, Santa Monica, CA 1989;October 26–28.
85. Salem M, Munoz R, Chernow B. Hypomagnesemia in critical illness. Crit Care Clin 1991;7:225–252.
86. Munoz R, Khilnani P, Ziegler J, et al. Ultrafilterable hypomagnesemia in neonates admitted to the neonatal intensive care unit. Crit Care Med 1994;22:815–820.
87. Arsenian M. Magnesium and cardiovascular disease. Prog Cardiovasc Dis 1993;35:271–310.
88. Boriss M, Papa L. Magnesium: a discussion of its role in the treatment of ventricular dysrhythmia. Crit Care Med 1988;16:292–293.
89. Ramee S, White C, Svinarich J, et al. Torsades de pointes and magnesium deficiency. Am Heart J 1985;109:164–167.
90. Jonas R, Krasna M, Sell J, et al. Myocardial failure is a rare cause of death after pediatric cardiac surgery [Abstract]. J Am Coll Cardiol 1991;17:110a.
91. Grossman W. Blood flow measurement: the cardiac output. In: Grossman W, Baim D, eds. Cardiac catheterization, angiography, and intervention. Baltimore: Williams & Wilkins, 1996:109–124.
92. Guyton A, Jones C, Coleman, eds. Circulatory physiology: cardiac output and its regulation. Philadelphia: WB Saunders, 1973:4–80.
93. Marcus B, Wong P, Wells W, et al. Transesophageal echocardiography in the postoperative child with an open sternum. Ann Thorac Surg 1994;58:235–236.
94. Chin A, Vetter J, Seliem M, et al. Role of early postoperative surface echocardiography in the pediatric cardiac intensive care unit. Chest 1994;105:10–16.
95. Mellander M, Sabel K, Caidahl K, et al. Doppler determination of cardiac output in infants and children: comparison with simultaneous thermodilution. Pediatr Cardiol 1987;8:241–246.
96. Sanders S, Yeager S, Williams R. Measurement of systemic and pulmonary blood flow and Qp/Qs ratio using doppler and two-dimensional echocardiography. Am J Cardiol 1983;51:952–956.
97. Fick A. Uber die messung des blutquantums in den herzventriken. Sits der Physik-Med ges Wurtzberg 1870;16.
98. Ganz W, Donoso R, Marcus HS, et al. A new technique for measurement of cardiac output by thermodilution in man. Am J Cardiol 1971;27:392–396.
99. Forrester JS, Ganz W, Diamond G, et al. Thermodilution cardiac output determination with a single flow-directed catheter. Am Heart J 1972;83:306–311.
100. Bridges NB, Freed MD. Cardiac catheterization. In: Emmanouilides GC, Riemenschneider TA, Allen HD, et al, eds. Heart disease in infants, children, and adolescents. Baltimore: Williams & Wilkins, 1995:318–322.
101. Wessel H, Paul M, James G, et al. Limitations of thermal dilution curves for cardiac output determinations. J Appl Physiol 1971;30:643–652.
102. Freed M, Keane J. Cardiac output measured by thermodilution in infants and children. J Pediatr 1978;92:39–42.
103. Van Grondelle A, Ditchey R, Groves B, et al. Thermodilution method overestimates low cardiac output in humans. Am J Physiol 1983;245:H690–II692.
104. Mukharji J, Rehr R, Hastillo A, et al. Comparison of atrial contribution to cardiac hemodynamics in patients with normal and severely compromised cardiac function. Clin Cardiol 1990;13:639–643.
105. Leinbach R, Chamberlain D, Kastor J, et al. A comparison of the hemodynamic effects of ventricular and sequential A-V pacing in patients with heart block. Am Heart J 1969;78:502–508.
106. Anderson PAW. Physiology of the fetal, neonatal, and adult heart. In: Polin RA, Fox WW, eds. Fetal and neonatal physiology. Philadelphia: WB Saunders, 1992:740–753.
107. Davignon A, Rautaharju P, Boiselle E, et al. Normal ECG standards for infants and children. Pediatr Cardiol 1979;1:123–152.
108. Starling EH. The Linacre lecture on the law of the heart. London: Logmans, Green & Co. 1918.

109. Frank O. Zur dynamik des herzumuskels. Z Biol 1895;32:370–447.
110. Wessel D. Hemodynamic responses to perioperative pain and stress in infants. Crit Care Med 1993;21(Suppl 9):s361–362.
111. Castaneda A, Jonas R, Mayer JJ, et al. Cardiac surgery of the neonate and infant. Philadelphia: WB Saunders, 1994:263–268.
112. Sakamoto T, Yamada T. Hemodynamic effects of dobutamine in patients following open heart surgery. Circulation 1977;55:525–533.
113. Leier CV, Heban PT, Huss P, et al. Comparative systemic and regional hemodynamic effects of dopamine and dobutamine in patients with cardiomyopathic heart failure. Circulation 1978;58:466–475.

Cardiopulmonary Bypass

14

John E. Mayer, Jr, MD

"Cardiopulmonary bypass" is a term generally used to describe the techniques by which some of the major functions of the heart and lungs are temporarily replaced with a mechanical system to support the patient while surgical interventions on the cardiovascular or pulmonary systems are carried out. In simplest terms, this apparatus consists of a pumping device to deliver blood to the patient and an oxygenator in which gas exchange occurs. Virtually all current systems also incorporate a heat exchanger by which the temperature of the blood in the oxygenator can be altered, thereby allowing control of the patient's temperature.

Bypass systems for cardiac operations, initially employed clinically in the early 1950s, were associated with significant mortality and morbidity, but with improvements in materials and bypass techniques, cardiac operations using cardiopulmonary bypass are now safely carried out on a daily basis throughout the world. However, cardiopulmonary bypass remains an "unphysiologic" state, and despite recent improvements it is still associated with morbidity and mortality. In this chapter the ways in which various techniques of cardiopulmonary bypass can be utilized to carry out intracardiac operations in infants and children are discussed, including problems and limits of current techniques in this patient population. Because repair of most defects requires that the heart and sometimes the entire circulation be arrested, techniques of cardioplegia and deep hypothermic circulatory arrest are also discussed.

PRINCIPLES AND MECHANICS OF CARDIOPULMONARY BYPASS

The primary function of cardiopulmonary bypass is to circulate blood of appropriate composition to the body to maintain viability of the patient during surgery. Maintaining viability obviously involves provision of oxygen and removal of carbon dioxide, but constraints imposed by the need to provide suitable operating conditions and by the damaging effects of unmodified cardiopulmonary bypass itself require that a number of other variables including pH, temperature, hematocrit, oncotic pressure, electrolyte and glucose composition, and the pharmacologic milieu be manipulated as well. These various manipulations are directed at minimizing the damaging effects of cardiopulmonary bypass, and offsetting the deleterious effects of cardiac or whole body ischemia required to provide suitable conditions to conduct the repair.

BASICS OF CARDIOPULMONARY BYPASS

Basic components of a cardiopulmonary bypass (Fig. 14.1) circuit are a pump (generally a roller pump), an oxygenator (to provide for gas exchange), a reservoir (to temporarily store blood collected from the operative field and from the venous cannulas), and a system of tubing and cannulas to carry blood between the patient and the pump oxygenator.

Cannulation

To establish cardiopulmonary bypass, the surgeon must introduce cannulas into the systemic arterial and systemic venous systems (Fig. 14.1). In most cases, the arterial cannula is inserted into the ascending aorta, but any medium to large size systemic artery can be used for access to the arterial system. A venous cannula(s) is generally inserted into the right atrium and/or directly into the superior and inferior vena cavae. Arterial blood is returned to the patient from the oxygenator via the arterial cannula, and venous blood is drained from the patient to the bypass system via the venous cannulas. In most systems, the venous blood is *siphoned* from the patient into a reservoir by the force of gravity. Therefore, venous cannulas must be of relatively large caliber to minimize resistance to blood flow. Active suction can be used to drain blood from the patient to the pump oxygenator, but this is much more traumatic to the blood and results in hemolysis and protein denaturation. Return of venous blood to the oxygenator by siphonage requires that the column of venous return blood not be broken by air entering the venous cannulas. If air does enter the venous cannulas, then an "air lock" can result, which interrupts the siphon effect and will therefore stop venous return to the oxygenator. For this reason *tourniquets* are generally placed around the superior and inferior vena caval cannulas to prevent air from being "sucked" into the venous cannulas if the right side of the heart is to be opened.

Once the blood reaches the reservoir of the oxygenator, it then passes through the oxygenator itself where gas exchange occurs. Blood is also brought from the operating field to the reservoir by means of *cardiotomy suction devices*. These cardiotomy suction devices are simply suction

Figure 14.1. Basic components of cardiopulmonary bypass. Venous blood is drained from the heart via a cannula in the right atrium (shown here), or alternatively, bicaval cannulation in the superior vena cava (*SVC*) and inferior vena cava (*IVC*). Blood drains by gravity to a venous reservoir, and mixes with blood drained from the operative field by cardiotomy suction catheters. After passing through a heat exchanger, the blood is passed through an oxygenator—where oxygen and carbon dioxide are titrated—through a roller pump, micropore filter, and back to the body via an aortic cannula (see text).

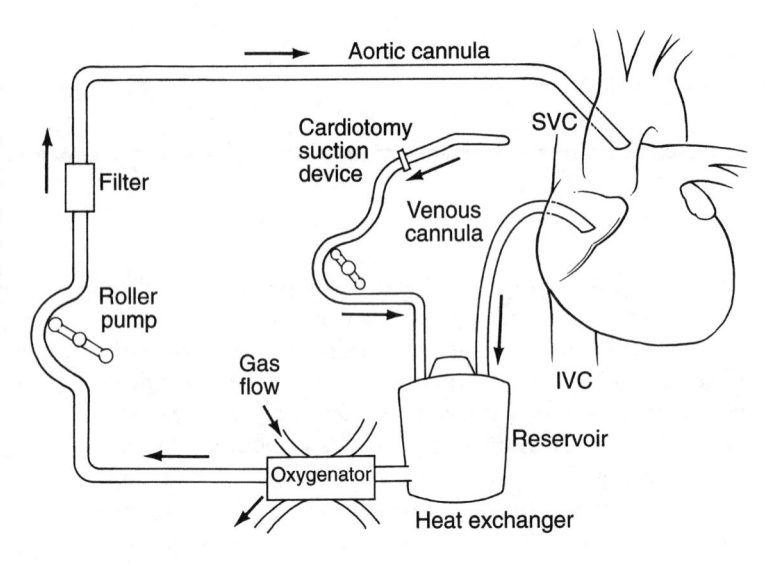

catheters connected to auxiliary roller pump heads, which create the suction. Blood aspirated from the operative field into the cardiotomy suction is returned to the venous reservoir. Blood that has passed through the oxygenator is pumped back into the patient through the arterial cannula that has been introduced into the systemic arterial system (usually the ascending aorta). This pumping of the blood is generally carried out with a roller pump, which compresses the tubing containing the blood in a rotary fashion within the pump housing and thereby forces the blood in the tubing back toward the patient. In some membrane oxygenator systems, the pump is proximal to the membrane.

Although all operations involving cardiopulmonary bypass are conducted using the basic cannulas, tubing, pump, and oxygenator outlined, a number of variations can be used depending on the anatomic defect to be repaired and the size of the patient. The typical sequence of events in most open-heart operations involves several basic steps. Once the patient is anesthetized, prepared, and draped, a midline sternotomy incision is carried out, and the pericardial sac is entered. Purse string sutures are placed in the sites where placement of arterial (ascending aorta) and venous (right atrium and/or vena cavae) cannulas is planned. Heparin is given to prevent thrombosis from occurring in the cannulas, tubing, or the pump oxygenator. After ensuring that the patient is heparinized (usually by checking activated clotting time [ACT]), the arterial and venous cannulas are inserted, cleared of air, and connected to the corresponding tubing of the pump oxygenator.

Extracorporeal Circulation and Circulatory Arrest

Cardiopulmonary bypass is then instituted by removing the clamp(s) occluding the venous cannula(s) and starting the roller pump to force fluid out of the oxygenator and into the patient. Initially, this fluid is the "priming" solution contained within the oxygenator, but within the first minute on bypass, the priming fluid is completely mixed with the patient's own blood. Once it is determined that no problems exist with the function of the cardiopulmonary bypass apparatus and circuit, the heat exchanger in the oxygenator is cooled, resulting in a lowering of the patient's body temperature. (In neonatal operations, cooling is begun immediately at the start of bypass.) Some degree of hypothermia is used in most cardiopulmonary bypass operations in infants and children for reasons addressed in the discussion of hypothermia. After bypass is established, tourniquets are generally placed around the superior and inferior vena cavae. When the tourniquets are tightened to compress the walls of the vena cavae against the outside of the cannulas, air cannot enter into the venous cannulas and air lock formation is prevented. Caval tourniquets also force all systemic venous return (except coronary sinus return) to drain to the oxygenator rather than load the heart, and this situation is termed "*total* cardiopulmonary bypass." At this point (or shortly before) mechanical ventilation is stopped because the lungs are not contributing to gas exchange.

For most intracardiac repairs, surgeons induce myocardial ischemia by "cross clamping" the aorta between the site where the arterial cannula has been inserted and the root of the aorta where the coronary arteries arise from the sinuses of Valsalva (Fig. 14.2). To protect the heart during this period of induced ischemia, it is chemically arrested to eliminate any mechanical work by infusing "cardioplegia" solution via a small catheter inserted into the proximal ascending aorta. The important components of the cardioplegia solution are outlined in the section on Myocardial Protection. In most pediatric centers, the cardioplegia solution is made quite cold (6 to 8°C), and as the cold solution is administered into the aortic root (and thus into the coronary circulation), the heart is cooled as well. By eliminating coronary blood flow, no coronary sinus blood enters the right atrium, thereby improving exposure within the heart. Intracardiac repair is then completed in the cold, arrested heart.

Some blood flow will return to the left side of the heart during "total cardiopulmonary bypass" because the blood that reaches the lungs via the bronchial arteries will drain out of the lungs via the pulmonary veins. Therefore, it is frequently necessary to "vent" the left side of the heart to prevent both the operative field from being obscured and the left ventricle from being distended by this pulmonary venous return. Vent catheters are frequently inserted into the left atrium and directed across the mitral valve. In some situations, particularly in neonates, size constraints may make it awkward to insert two venous cannulas plus a vent catheter, and the entire circulation can be arrested by simply turning off the bypass pump. Use of "deep hypothermia" (less than 18°C) improves the safety of this period of total body ischemia (see discussion on hypothermia). This technique is appropriately termed "deep hypothermia with circulatory arrest" (DHCA) (Fig. 14.3).

Whenever the left side of the heart is entered, either during the repair or with a vent catheter, air will enter the left-sided chambers. At the completion of the operation, this air can be ejected into the systemic arterial circulation once the heart begins to beat. Therefore, the left side of the heart must be "de-aired" prior to the time when the heart might begin to beat. Typically, this de-airing is accomplished by filling the left heart with either blood or saline solution via the left heart vent catheter or by allowing the left heart to fill with the bronchial artery return. Air contained in the chambers in the left side of the heart is vented out through a hole in the ascending aorta proximal to the aortic clamp (usually at the cardioplegia catheter insertion site). Once the left side of the heart is de-aired, the intracardiac portion of the repair is completed, and the aortic clamp is removed to restore coronary blood flow. This coronary blood flow washes the cardioplegia solution out of the coronary vascular bed, and frequently the heart will begin beating spontaneously. If the heart rhythm returns as ventricular fibrillation, then the heart can be electrically defibrillated. "Partial bypass" is established by loosening the caval tourniquets. Blood passing through the oxygenator is usually partially rewarmed during the time just before the coronary blood flow is re-established, and the body temperature is brought up toward normothermic levels.

Weaning from Cardiopulmonary Bypass

Once systemic temperature reaches 35 to 36°C and the heart appears to be contracting well, the patient is "weaned" from bypass. This weaning process involves reducing the rate at which the bypass pump is turning while partially occluding the venous drainage tubing. This forces some of the blood returning from the body through the vena cavae to load the heart. As the heart begins to eject, mechanical ventilation of the lungs is initiated. Once the heart is adequately filled, as judged by inspection and by measurement of atrial filling pressures, the mechanical pump is stopped. At this point all of the systemic and pulmonary blood flow is provided by the patient's heart, and

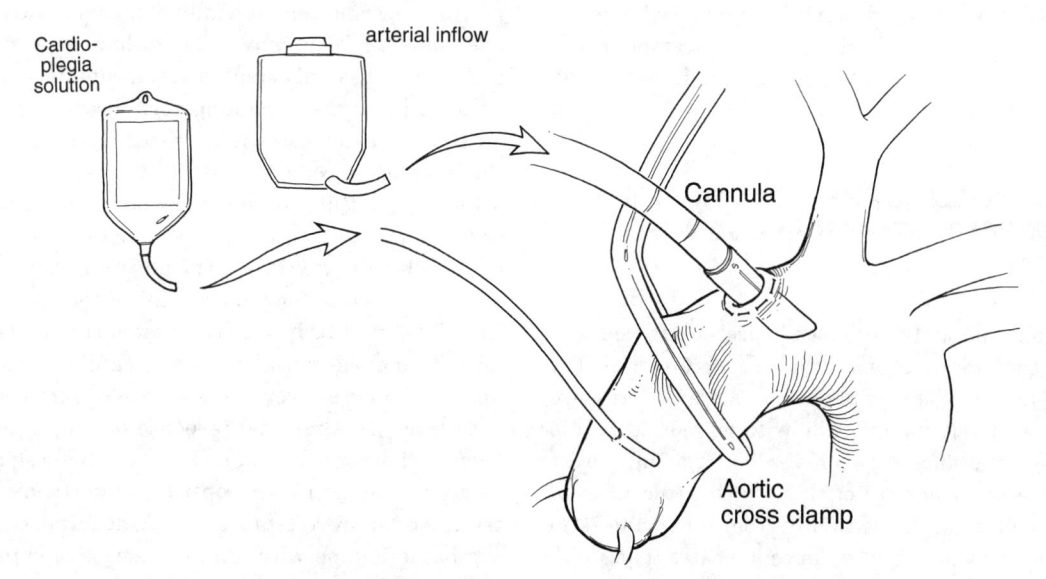

Figure 14.2. The cardioplegia solution is placed proximal to the aortic cross clamp to enter the coronary arteries. Oxygenated blood from cardiopulmonary bypass is inserted distal to the aortic cross clamp (see text).

Figure 14.3. A. Whole body temperature (*y-axis*) changes during cardiopulmonary bypass (*CPB*) using profound hypothermia (see text). **B.** For operations not requiring profound hypothermia and circulatory arrest, cardiopulmonary bypass is typically carried out at 25 to 28°C (see text).

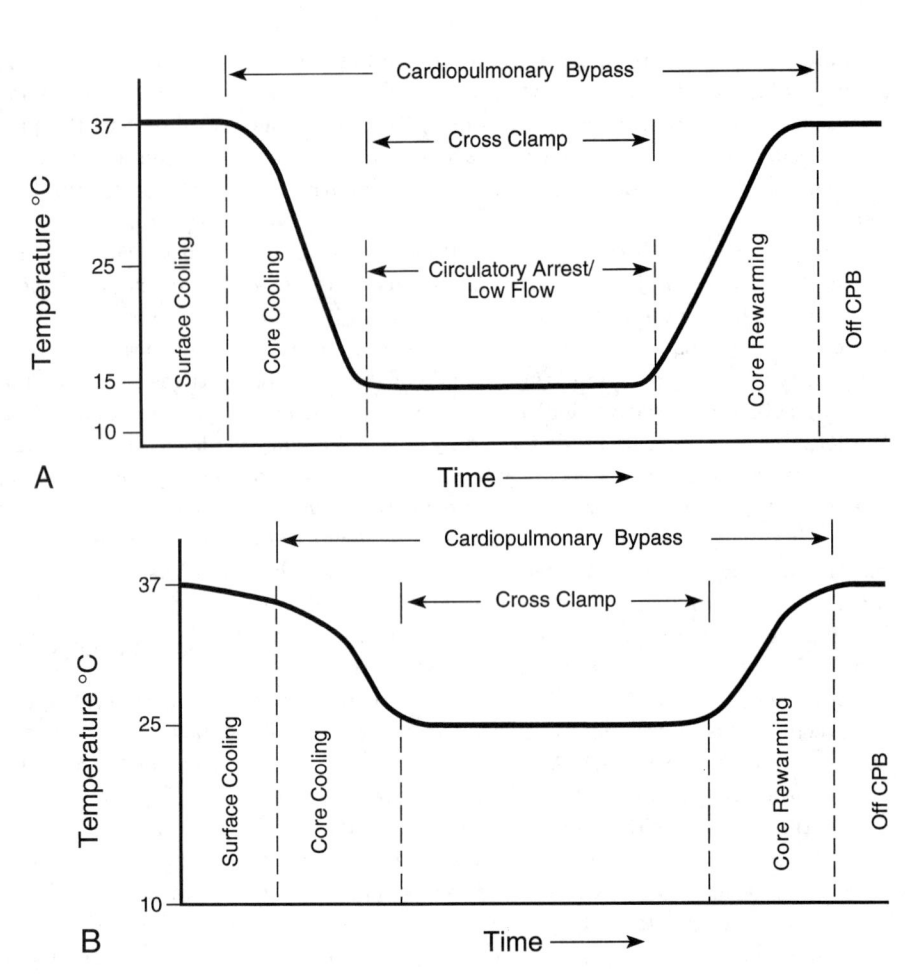

oxygenation depends on the patient's respiratory system. After assuring that the patient's hemodynamics and ventilation are satisfactory, the cannulae are removed and the cannulation sites are secured. Heparin is reversed with intravenous administration of protamine. The completeness of this reversal can be assessed by rechecking the activated clotting time after protamine is completed.

PROBLEMS RESULTING FROM CARDIOPULMONARY BYPASS AND INTERVENTIONS TO MINIMIZE MORBIDITY

Circulation

Use of a roller pump to force blood back into the patient from the oxygenator is a significant departure from the normal physiology of the circulation. Arterial pressure waveform is relatively nonpulsatile with no more than a 5 to 10 mm Hg difference between the highest and lowest pressures. The consequences of this nonpulsatile arterial flow are difficult to separate totally from other effects of cardiopulmonary bypass, but evidence indicates that a pulsatile waveform may be associated with better tissue perfusion, lower systemic arterial resistance, and less accumulation of extracellular fluid, particularly following a period of reduced perfusion (1, 2). It is only relatively recently, however, that a reliable system to provide pulsatile flow has become commercially available. The ability to deliver pulsatile flow may be more limited in neonates and infants because only small arterial cannulas (10–12 F) can be placed into the ascending aorta because of its small diameter, and these cannulas generally dampen the pulsatile waveform considerably. Newer model roller pumps achieve pulsatility by causing wide variations in the speed of the roller pump, and they seem more effective at producing a pulsatile waveform. The advantages of pulsatile flow over nonpulsatile flow in the clinical setting remain a subject of debate (3). In general, systemic vascular resistance falls during the initial phases of cardiopulmonary bypass and then progressively rises to levels higher than baseline with time (3). The renal response to nonpulsatile flow has been well described, and includes an increase in renin production, which, in turn, contributes to the increase in systemic vascular resistance (4). A generalized increase in sympathetic tone with adrenal release of epinephrine has also been documented in adults (5) and to an even greater degree in neonates (6). Total bypass flow rates nearly equal to the cardiac output of an anesthetized patient are generally attainable, but pump output must not exceed the venous return to the pump, as this would result in the pump "running dry," with air being pumped into the patient.

One of the functions of the perfusionist, therefore, is to regulate arterial output of the pump (by altering pump head speed) to match the rate at which venous blood is returning to the pump oxygenator system. This regulation is accomplished by maintaining a constant level of blood in the reservoir portion of the system, but close communication between the perfusionist and the surgeon is necessary to maintain smooth control of the system. Minor changes in venous cannula position can significantly alter venous return, which is detected by the perfusionist as a fall in the reservoir level. To compensate for fluid losses, including urine output and fluid sequestration in the tissues, during bypass the perfusionist may also need to add volume in the form of crystalloid or blood to maintain an adequate level of perfusate in the reservoir. In most clinical systems, blood loss in the operative field is returned to the bypass circuit using "cardiotomy" suction catheters, which are connected to separate roller pump heads (see above).

As a general approach, perfusion flow rate rather than perfusion pressure is the criterion for setting bypass parameters. In infants initial flow rates of approximately 150–200 mL/kg/min are used, and only rarely are attempts made to intervene pharmacologically to elevate perfusion pressures. In fact, α-adrenergic blockade with phentolamine (0.1 mg/kg) is frequently used in an attempt to improve tissue perfusion and to enhance the evenness of cooling prior to the onset of circulatory arrest (as described below).

Respiration

Oxygen introduction and carbon dioxide removal occurs in the oxygenator portion of the cardiopulmonary bypass apparatus. This gas exchange must occur across an interface between the gas(es) introduced into the oxygenator and the plasma and erythrocytes that are in the oxygenator at that moment. In the early oxygenator systems, this interface was created by direct contact between the blood and the gas source, either by spreading the blood into thin films that were then exposed to oxygen (disk oxygenator) or by introducing "bubbles" of oxygen into the blood so that gas exchange would occur across the blood-gas bubble interface (bubble oxygenator). Amounts of oxygen transferred into the blood and carbon dioxide removed are controlled both with the composition of the "ventilating" gas supplied to the oxygenator and by the flow rate. Higher gas flow rates tend to remove more CO_2, but higher gas flow rates were frequently necessary to achieve adequate oxygen transfer. Carbon dioxide was added to the ventilating gas to control arterial CO_2 concentration. In more recently designed oxygenators, thin-walled "membranes" are interposed between the gas and blood (membrane oxygenators) in an attempt to reduce the deleterious effects of the direct gas-blood interface on the plasma proteins and the formed elements of the blood. Similar relationships between the flow rates and composition of the "ventilating" gas for the oxygenator and the arterial blood gas composition exist as for the bubble oxygenators. The gas exchange characteristics of these various oxygenators vary, and therefore familiarity with a particular system is important for the perfusionist to anticipate the flow rate and gas composition of the particular oxygenator to achieve the appropriate blood gas concentrations in the arterial outflow to the patient. In general, all systems can achieve normal to supernormal levels of oxygen and normal to hypocapnic levels of CO_2 in the blood leaving the oxygenator.

Respiration at the cellular level is dependent on several variables during bypass. On bypass at normothermic temperatures, total body oxygen consumption is related to blood flow, and bypass flows of at least 2 L/min/m^2 are required to achieve typical oxygen consumption for anesthetized patients (110–130 mL/min/m^2). If bypass flow rates are lower than these values, then total body O_2 delivery falls and metabolic acidosis can result (3). However, as temperatures are reduced, O_2 consumption falls and bypass flow requirements are likewise reduced with less dependence of total body O_2 consumption on bypass flow rate (7). To improve both operating conditions and overall tolerance to cardiopulmonary bypass, most surgeons now use at least moderate levels of hypothermia, allowing reduced flow rates during cardiac operations on bypass (25°C). Deep hypothermia (less than 20°C) with circulatory arrest is used in many repairs in neonates and infants (see below).

Optimal management of respiration, particularly pH and P_{CO_2}, under hypothermic conditions remains unsettled. In general, two strategies, termed "pH stat" and "alpha stat," have been used. In the pH stat approach, P_{CO_2} and pH are maintained at 40 torr and 7.40, respectively, during hypothermia. These values are the "corrected" values that account for the patient's temperature and they are not the values obtained when the sample is introduced into a blood gas analyzer (which brings the temperature of the blood to 37°C prior to analysis). Therefore, the actual P_{CO_2} result from the blood gas analyzer (at 37°C) of a sample collected at a patient temperature of 20°C would be approximately 65 torr to yield a "corrected" value of 40 torr. Similarly, to achieve a "corrected" pH value of 7.40 for the patient at 20°C, the blood gas analyzer would yield a reading of 7.16. Functionally, these blood gas targets can be achieved by adding CO_2 to the gases entering the oxygenator as cooling was carried out. With the alpha stat strategy, P_{CO_2} is reduced, and consequently pH rises during hypothermia. Target values as measured in the blood gas analyzer are approximately P_{CO_2} = 40 torr and pH = 7.40. At 20°C, actual P_{CO_2} is considerably lower (17.6 torr) with an actual pH of almost 7.7.

Interestingly, in "natural" situations of hypothermia, both strategies are used in different species. Hibernating mammals use a pH stat strategy whereas poikilothermic species (e.g., reptiles, frogs) generally use an alpha stat strategy (8) and reduce P_{CO_2} by relative hyperventilation in response to lower temperatures. In humans and in many other "homeotherms" temperature variations are found in various parts of the arterial system (and body) under normal conditions, but these variations occur at a relatively constant total CO_2 content (9).

Actual sampling of the arterial blood shows that lower temperatures are associated with lower P_{CO_2} and higher pH in accordance with values obtained with the alpha stat strategy (9). Change in blood pH per degree Centigrade is approximately −0.0147. It appears from studies in a variety of mammalian and other species that the goal of P_{CO_2} (and consequent pH) regulation is to maintain a constant state of ionization of the intracellular proteins (9). The two ionizing species with a pK in the physiological pH range (6–8) are the imidazole moiety of histidine and the alpha NH_3^+ terminal group of peptide chains, with the histidine groups being much more numerous. The ratio of nonprotonated (nonionized) imidazole groups to the total of protonated (NH_3^+) and protonated imidazole groups is denoted by the symbol $alpha_{Im}$. This ratio is physiologically important because the tertiary and quartenery structures of proteins are optimized at a narrow ratio. In addition, the pK of $alpha_{Im}$ varies inversely with temperature. The result is that the ionization state of the imidazole moieties change appreciably with temperature. However, this change can be offset if the P_{CO_2} also falls and the pH rises (9). The implication is that because the ionization state of the intracellular proteins does not change with temperature changes (if these pH and P_{CO_2} conditions are met), then the enzymatic functions of these proteins will not be impaired by temperature change. It is noteworthy that ionization of water also varies inversely with temperature, so that the pH of water rises with a fall in temperature, and the change in pH of water per degree Centigrade is also −0.0147. It therefore seems that the alpha stat strategy for the regulation of P_{CO_2} on bypass during hypothermic conditions most closely mimics the strategy employed by the organism in response to changes in temperature conditions, and it has been adopted by many units as the method by which to regulate blood gas tensions and pH.

Studies comparing the alpha-stat and pH stat strategies on oxygen consumption during bypass procedures in adults have yielded conflicting results (10, 11), but Ekroth et al. (12) noted an inverse correlation between creatine phosphokinase BB levels and pH in infants having operations using circulatory arrest. Other data from Jonas et al. (13) suggest that alkaline pH during the cooling phase of bypass (alpha-stat) prior to circulatory arrest is associated with a worse cognitive outcome. The question of whether the alpha-stat or the pH-stat strategy is optimal if the tissue is to be made ischemic remains to be more definitively answered, although some evidence favors the alpha-stat strategy when myocardial preservation during ischemia is considered (14).

Temperature

As indicated, some degree of hypothermia is used in most cardiac operations. The rationales for the use of hypothermia are multiple, but they are centered around safely providing optimal operating conditions to conduct the operation. The protective effects of hypothermia for tissues exposed to periods of reduced or absent blood flow during experimental cardiac surgery were investigated by Bigelow et al. (15) in 1950, and the principle of hypothermic protection was used by Lewis and Tauffic (16) in 1953 for a clinical "open heart" operation in which an atrial septal defect was closed during a short period of circulatory arrest at a moderate level of hypothermia without any cardiopulmonary bypass.

The mechanism by which hypothermia is protective during ischemia is not completely defined, but it must involve the reduced metabolic demands of the tissues as a result of the lower temperatures. The effect of temperature on metabolic rate (as reflected by oxygen consumption) is described by the term Q_{10}, which is the ratio of oxygen consumption at two different temperatures (10 degrees apart). For humans, this value has been estimated to be approximately 1.9, and therefore oxygen consumption at 20°C is reduced to about 20% of that at 37°C (17). It seems likely, however, that hypothermia has other protective effects beside reducing metabolic rate. If the central nervous system has a safe ischemic period of 5 minutes at normothermia, then a fivefold reduction in metabolic demand would only be expected to increase the "safe" interval of ischemia to 25 minutes. Clinically, it had seemed that total circulatory arrest times of up to 45 to 50 minutes are well tolerated neurologically in most cases, suggesting that hypothermia probably has other protective effects besides that of reducing metabolism.

The technique of DHCA provides ideal operating conditions for most intracardiac repairs in neonates and infants (Fig. 14.3A). With this technique, bypass is established with single aortic and single right atrial cannulas with the perfusate (pump prime) precooled to approximately 25°C. Cooling is carried out predominantly with perfusion on cardiopulmonary bypass (core-cooling), although some *surface cooling* is achieved after anesthesia induction by using a cooling blanket and exposing the child to ambient temperature. Cooling on bypass is generally carried out for at least 10 to 15 minutes, and the tympanic and rectal temperatures are brought to less than 20°C. Ice in a plastic bag is generally placed around the head, and the cooling blanket remains cold during the period of circulatory arrest. The ductus (or ligamentum) arteriosus (and/or any systemic to pulmonary artery shunt) is ligated to prevent runoff of systemic blood flow into the pulmonary circulation, and to prevent air entry into the aortic arch during the period of circulatory arrest. After clamping the aorta and administering cardioplegia, blood is drained to the oxygenator by leaving the venous line open and stopping the arterial inflow to the patient. Before the heart is opened, the venous line is occluded to prevent air from entering the venous line tubing and causing an air lock. Cardiac repair is then carried out, and after completion of those parts of the repair in which circulatory arrest is necessary for visualization, the right atrium is closed and the venous cannula is reinserted.

To shorten the circulatory arrest time, *low flow bypass* (approximately 50 mL/kg/min) can also be restarted using cardiotomy suction for venous return while the atrium is closed. With increasing experience and use of metal-tipped right-angled venous cannulas directly inserted into the superior and inferior vena cavae, and when necessary for visualization inside the heart, bypass flow can be reduced to "low flow" levels or ceased altogether. Using these techniques, circulatory arrest duration can be significantly reduced and in many cases completely eliminated. The one type of operation demanding a period of complete circulatory arrest involves reconstruction of the aortic arch. All other operations can be performed without circulatory arrest. Some surgeons avoid circulatory arrest unless absolutely necessary, whereas others use it in a variety of circumstances because it provides ideal operative conditions—a bloodless operative field in a still, nonbeating heart.

Once the atrium is closed, circulation can be resumed, and generally rewarming is begun, keeping the temperature of the heat exchanger no more than 10°C above the temperature of the blood returning from the patient to prevent gases from coming out of the solution. Careful attention to the rates of cooling and rewarming of the rectal, esophageal, and tympanic probes may uncover residual anatomic problems particularly in the aortic arch.

The safe period of circulatory arrest in human neonates and infants has not been established with certainty (3), but periods of 45 to 60 minutes appear to be well tolerated in most patients. However, more recent data from a prospective trial in patients undergoing arterial switch operations for transposition of the great arteries shows that the incidence of postoperative seizures is related to the length of DHCA (18). Early postoperative seizure activity also seems to correlate with worse scores on certain developmental tests at 1 year postoperatively as well (19). In contrast, O'Connor et al. (20) have shown that 1 hour of circulatory arrest at 13°C in dogs was associated with neither functional or anatomic evidence of injury, and Tharion et al. (21) reported a low incidence of neurologic problems after circulatory arrest in children. Transient seizure activity has been noted in approximately 5 to 15% of patients (3, 18), and an occasional patient will develop choreoathetoid movements (see Chapter 24, *Neurologic Disorders*).

Despite these favorable clinical results with DHCA, Greeley et al. (22) have shown that recovery of cerebral blood flow after a period of DHCA is remarkably lower than if hypothermic bypass without DHCA was used. Interaction of preoperative, intraoperative, and postoperative events on ultimate neurologic outcome makes evaluation of the impact of DHCA alone difficult, but Blackwood et al. (23) reported that developmental outcome was not different between a group of patients undergoing operations using circulatory arrest and a group having repairs on bypass without arrest. Evidence indicates that continuous hypothermic bypass without circulatory arrest can result in severe neurologic injury, particularly if hemodilution is not used (24, 25).

One side effect of hypothermia of unknown significance is fluid sequestration in the tissues. This effect occurs even without bypass, and it was reported in both animals and humans undergoing surface cooling to 25°C by Chen et al. (26). No explanation has been made for this effect, but it may involve changes in capillary permeability or sequestration of whole blood and plasma in certain portions of the circulatory bed with hypothermia. From a postoperative management perspective, it is difficult to wean patients from mechanical ventilation when a significant amount of chest wall and total body edema are present. Diuretic use and resolution of the inflammatory response to cardiopulmonary bypass with the passage of time after surgery (usually 1 to 3 days) typically allows the mobilization of this fluid and weaning from mechanical ventilation.

Hematocrit and Oncotic Pressure

Reduction of the hematocrit during the period of cardiopulmonary bypass (hemodilution) appears to be desirable, and it is widely used for a number of reasons. First, with hypothermia blood viscosity increases, which contributes to a rise in the resistance to blood flow, particularly in the microcirculation (3). When this factor is added to the nonpulsatile nature of bypass flow, significant underperfusion of the microcirculation can occur during bypass with resulting tissue ischemia. The importance of hemodilution during hypothermia was suggested by early experiences reported by Bjork et al. (24) and Egerton et al. (25) using deep hypothermia with normal hematocrit, where a high incidence of significant neurologic deficits was seen when deep hypothermia (even without circulatory arrest) was used. It is also of interest that hibernating (hypothermic) mammals are observed to become naturally hemodiluted during their period of hibernation (27). A second advantage to hemodilution is reducing blood products use to "prime" the cardiopulmonary bypass circuit with its attendant reduction in risk of transfusion-associated diseases. Current "target" hematocrit while on bypass is 20 to 25%, and this is achieved by using a balanced crystalloid priming solution (pH = 7.4) and adding citrated whole blood to the prime (when necessary) to account for the patient's prebypass hematocrit and calculated blood volume. The amount of crystalloid and blood added to the prime is calculated so that the mixed final hematocrit of the patient plus oxygenator circuit will be in the desired range. Hemodilution with nonblood priming solutions also results in a fall in the protein concentration of the blood, and concerns have been expressed regarding the development of tissue edema as a result of the decreased oncotic pressure (3). However, Marelli et al. were unable to show any significant advantages in adding albumin to the priming solution (28). Most infants undergoing operations on bypass do seem to accumulate a considerable amount of extravascular fluid, and some evidence suggests that the capillary beds of immature animals are more "leaky" than those of the mature animal (29). However, the impact of this fluid accumulation on ultimate outcome after cardiac surgery is unclear.

Electrolyte and Glucose Composition

Logic would seem to dictate that concentrations of serum electrolytes and glucose should be maintained within normal ranges to maintain the normal milieu for the cells of the body. Such a strategy has been used, in general, for most of these constituents, but at least two exceptions are worth noting. Glucose concentrations during cardiopulmonary bypass have frequently been raised by use of glucose containing priming solutions with the goal of inducing an osmotic diuresis during bypass and thereby attempting to minimize the risk of renal failure in the post-bypass period (3). However, evidence suggests that elevated glucose levels can have a deleterious effect on the outcome of central nervous system tissue subjected to ischemia (30). Ekroth et al. (12) have shown that levels of creatine kinase BB, which is thought to be specific for central nervous system injury, were highly correlated with elevations of glucose prior to circulatory arrest (12). Therefore, it is typical to use a priming solution for bypass that does not contain glucose, particularly when circulatory arrest is anticipated.

Calcium is generally thought to be involved in the ischemia-reperfusion process, and massive increases in intracellular calcium have been noted during reperfusion after lethal periods of ischemia (31). Rebeyka et al. (32, 33) have suggested that hypothermia induces intracellular accumulation of calcium, and therefore have recommended that cardioplegic arrest of the heart should be effected prior to reaching deep hypothermic levels to prevent this hypothermia-induced rise in intracellular calcium, which will increase the metabolic demands during ischemia. When applied to the whole organism, it might infer that reduced levels of calcium, prior to or immediately following ischemia, may reduce ischemic injury, but the advantages of such an approach at this point are hypothetical. One approach is to induce hypocalcemia during preischemic cooling, particularly in neonatal patients, as a result of using a calcium-free crystalloid priming solution and citrated bank blood in the pump prime. Bank blood that is added to the pump prior to bypass is not supplemented with calcium once heparin is added. Ionized calcium concentrations generally are in the range of 0.2 to 0.3 mM/L during the preischemic cooling phase, and they are not raised to normocalcemic levels until midway through the postischemic rewarming period near the end of bypass. Advantages of this strategy of calcium management remain unproved in the clinical arena, but studies in neonatal lambs suggest that myocardial preservation is improved when preischemic cooling is carried out under hypocalcemic conditions (34). All other electrolytes are maintained within the normal ranges.

Pharmacologic Manipulations

As discussed, cardiopulmonary bypass remains an unphysiologic state, and it results in a number of deleterious effects on the patient as reviewed recently by Kirklin and Kirklin (35). As these effects have become known (and sometimes before the mechanisms of the effects were precisely characterized), a variety of pharmacologic manipulations have been introduced to offset the ill effects of bypass. The most obvious effect of bypass is on the circulating blood, and the contact of the blood with the inner surfaces of the bypass tubing and oxygenator results in prompt thrombus formation unless the coagulation system is inhibited. Therefore, heparin must be given to the patient before the blood makes contact with any of these surfaces. Heparin acts by enhancing the activity of antithrombin III (heparin cofactor), which inhibits the serine active sites of many of the factors in the coagulation cascade including thrombin (36). A low incidence of deficiency of this heparin cofactor is found in the general population (36), but the recommendation has been made that a prolonged clotting time be confirmed after heparin administration, but before initiation of bypass. Clinically significant deficiencies of this cofactor have generally been reported only in adults (36), and they can be reversed by administering normal (fresh frozen) plasma. Platelet function and numbers are also impaired by cardiopulmonary bypass (35, 37), and a variety of platelet inhibiting agents have been employed experimentally to reduce these effects

(35, 38, 39). However, agents such as prostacyclin (38, 39), dipyridamole, and iloprost have potent vasodilator effects that can significantly lower perfusion pressure on bypass. Concern has been expressed that the platelets activated in the bypass circuit may then aggregate and lodge in the microcirculation, leading to organ dysfunction (39); preventing this effect could theoretically reduce bypass morbidity. The anticoagulant effect of heparin is reversed with protamine once the patient is separated from bypass. However, a number of problems with the hemostatic system frequently remain. In infants and children, generally it is necessary to replace clotting factors and platelets with fresh whole blood and component therapy.

Bypass also elicits a generalized inflammatory response from the contact of the blood and plasma with the nonendothelial surfaces of the pump oxygenator (35), which involves the kallikrein-bradykinin system and complement activation (35, 40). C3a is released in the early phases of bypass and continues to be produced throughout the duration of bypass (35, 40, 41). More recently, elevated levels of other inflammatory cytokines have been demonstrated, including interleukin-8, which may contribute to the inflammatory effects of bypass (42). Granulocytes are also activated during bypass with rises in plasma levels of granulocyte myeloperoxidase, lactoferrin, and elastase (40). Levels of lactoferrin and elastase could be reduced with infusion of nifedipine during bypass, but this agent did not affect the levels of C3a (40). Oxygen-free radicals and hydrogen peroxide are also produced by neutrophils during bypass (41). Experimentally, it has been shown that inhibition of leukocyte function with a platelet activating factor antagonist or leukocyte depletion improves recovery of the isolated heart after a period of extracorporeal circulation and hypothermic ischemia (43). It has recently been demonstrated that bypass induces cardiac and skeletal muscle to produce the mRNA for adhesion molecules, which interact with neutrophils to promote leukocyte adhesion and transmigration (44). Experimentally, bypass has been shown to increase microvascular permeability, which appears to result from an increase in the size of large pores in the microvascular bed (45). Corticosteroids have been used as an additive to the bypass priming solution at many institutions, and they were initially added based on observations of beneficial effects in patients in low cardiac output following cardiac operations (46). The multiple anti-inflammatory effects of steroids, including reduction of complement activation during bypass (47), can be a more rational justification for steroid use prior to bypass.

Mannitol, which was originally used to induce an osmotic diuresis, has now been shown to be a free radical scavenger, and therefore it may have significant benefit in reducing free radical injury, which occurs during reperfusion after a period of ischemia (48). To offset the remarkable increases in catecholamines induced by cardiopulmonary bypass and hypothermia with the consequent effects on systemic vascular resistance, phentolamine is also added to the bypass priming solution in many institutions, based initially on the favorable effects noted in postoperative patients (46).

Myocardial Protection

Myocardial preservation during surgically induced myocardial ischemia has been the subject of hundreds of publications in recent years. Most surgeons now employ hypothermic cardioplegia during periods of myocardial ischemia, although clinical and experimental evidence has not conclusively proved its value particularly in the immature myocardium (49, 50). However, the consequences of incomplete myocardial protection during surgically induced myocardial ischemia can have a dominant effect on the postoperative course, including low cardiac output, elevated atrial filling pressures, and requirements for increased intotropic support. It should be emphasized, however, that low cardiac output following repair of a congenital heart defect should prompt a rapid search for residual anatomic problems *before* poor myocardial function caused by ischemia or reperfusion injury is invoked as an explanation for the low cardiac output (see Chapter 13, *Postoperative Care*).

Despite numerous experimental studies, multiple problems are associated with extrapolating experimental animal data to the human infant. Furthermore, significant variations are found among species (51). Finally, remarkably few clinical studies compare various methods of myocardial protection, due at least in part to the difficulties in measuring load and geometry-independent indices of ventricular function in patients. Despite these problems, cardioplegic solutions are used by most surgeons, and their basic components are potassium (to achieve diastolic arrest) and cold temperature to reduce the metabolic demands of the heart during ischemia. Magnesium, which is an important component in the St. Thomas solution, probably has a beneficial effect through an antagonism of calcium entry into the myocardial cells during ischemia (52, 53). Oxygenation of the cardioplegic solution has been shown to have benefit experimentally (54). Adding free radical scavengers to the cardioplegia solution has been reported to be of benefit experimentally (48). Substrate modification, particularly by the addition of amino acids such as aspartate and glutamate, has also been shown to be of benefit experimentally (55–57).

Control of reperfusion conditions, particularly with regard to perfusion pressure, seems to have an important impact on recovery of function in the experimental setting (58). It is not uncommon for surgeons to employ a low initial reperfusion pressure strategy (59, 60). Single dose cardioplegia, rather than multiple doses, seems to provide better myocardial protection in immature rabbits (61), but it has not been proved clinically. Using current "state of the art" approaches to myocardial protection, most patients with an anatomically complete repair do not require high dose inotropic support if the myocardial ischemic times are less than 120 minutes. It should be noted however that current techniques do not provide complete protection of the myocardium, and some myocardial dysfunction should be anticipated during the first 24 hours after many operations (see Chapter 13).

A number of more recent laboratory studies have emphasized the importance of vascular events occurring during ischemia and reperfusion in the recovery of ventricular function (43, 58, 62, 63), and several of these studies point to a particularly important role for the endothelium (58, 63) and endothelial-leukocyte interactions (43). Clinical studies will be necessary before the applicability of these concepts to the clinical situation can be proved.

SUMMARY

Reparative cardiac surgery of all types requires cardiopulmonary bypass and periods of myocardial and total body ischemia to provide satisfactory surgical conditions for the repair. Despite improved materials and better understanding of the pathophysiology of this form of support, its application remains limited by the mechanical and biochemical effects of bypass and tissue ischemia. Continued efforts are necessary to further reduce the morbidity of tissue ischemia and cardiopulmonary bypass to allow safer conduct of reparative operations for congenital heart defects.

REFERENCES

1. Mori F, Ivey TD, Itoh T, et al. Effects of pulsatile reperfusion on postischemic recovery of myocardial function after global hypothermic cardiac arrest. J Thorac Cardiovasc Surg 1987;93:719–727.
2. Bregman D, Marrin CAS, Spotnitz HM. Pulsatile flow in extracorporeal circulation. In: Ionescu MI, ed. Techniques in extracorporeal circulation. 2nd ed. London: Butterworths, 1981:601–626.
3. Kirklin JW, Barratt-Boyes B. Hypothermia, circulatory arrest, and cardiopulmonary bypass. In: Kirklin JW, Barratt-Boyes B, eds. Cardiac surgery. 1st ed. New York: John Wiley and Sons, 1986:29–82.
4. Bartlett RH, Gazzaniga AB. Physiology and pathophysiology of extracorporeal circulation. In: Ionescu MI, ed. Techniques in extracorporeal circulation. 2nd ed. London: Butterworths, 1981:1–3.
5. Tan CK, Glisson SN, El-Etr AA, et al. Levels of circulating norepinephrine and epinephrine before, during, and after cardiopulmonary bypass operation in man. J Thorac Cardiovasc Surg 1976;71:928–931.
6. Anand KJS, Phil D, Hansen DD, et al. Hormonal-metabolic stress responses in neonates undergoing cardiac surgery: survivors and non-survivors. Anesthesiology 1990;73:661–670.
7. Hickey RF, Hoar PF. Whole body oxygen consumption during low-flow hypothermic cardiopulmonary bypass. J Thorac Cardiovasc Surg 1983;86:903–906.
8. White FN. A comparative physiological approach to hypothermia. J Thorac Cardiovasc Surg 1981;82:821–831.
9. Reeves RB, Rahn H. Patterns in vertebrate acid-base regulation. In: Wood SC, Lenfant C, eds. Evolution of respiratory processes: a comparative approach. 1st ed. New York: Marcel Dekker, 1979:225–252.
10. Alston RP, Singh M, McLaren AD. Systemic oxygen uptake during hypothermic cardiopulmonary bypass: effects of flow rate, flow character, and arterial pH. J Thorac Cardiovasc Surg 1989;98:757–768.
11. Tuppurainen T, Settergren G, Stensved P. The effect of arterial pH on whole body oxygen uptake during hypothermic cardiopulmonary bypass in man. J Thorac Cardiovasc Surg 1989;98:769–773.
12. Ekroth R, Thompson RJ, Lincoln C, et al. Elective deep hypothermia with total circulatory arrest. Changes in plasma creatinine kinase BB, blood glucose, and clinical variables. J Thorac Cardiovasc Surg 1989;97:30–35.
13. Jonas RA, Bellinger DC, Rappaport LA, et al. Relation of pH strategy and developmental outcome after hypothermic circulatory arrest. J Thorac Cardiovasc Surg 1993;106:362–368.
14. Becker H, Vinten-Johansen J, Buckberg GD, et al. Myocardial damage caused by keeping pH 7.40 during systemic deep hypothermia. J Thorac Cardiovasc Surg 1981;82:810–820.
15. Bigelow WG, Callaghan JC, Hopps JA. General hypothermia for experimental intracardiac surgery. Ann Surg 1950;132:531–539.
16. Lewis FJ, Tauffic M. Closure of atrial septal defects with the aid of hypothermia: experimental accomplishments and the report of one successful case. Surgery 1953;33:52–58.
17. Harris EA, Seelye ER, Barratt-Boyes B. Respiratory and metabolic acid-base changes during cardiopulmonary bypass in man. Br J Anaesth 1970;42:912.
18. Newburger JW, Jonas RA, Wernovsky G, et al. A comparison of the perioperative neurologic effects of hypothermic circulatory arrest versus low flow cardiopulmonary bypass in infant heart surgery. N Engl J Med 1993;329:1057–1064.
19. Bellinger DC, Jonas RA, Rappaport LA, et al. Developmental and neurologic status of children after heart surgery with hypothermic circulatory arrest or low flow cardiopulmonary bypass. N Engl J Med 1995;332:549–555.
20. O'Connor JV, Wilding T, Farmer P, et al. The protective effect of profound hypothermia on the canine central nervous system during one hour of circulatory arrest. Ann Thorac Surg 1986;41:255–259.
21. Tharion J, Johnson DC, Celermajer JM, et al. Profound hypothermia with circulatory arrest: nine years' clinical experience. J Thorac Cardiovasc Surg 1982;84:66–72.
22. Greeley WJ, Ungerleider RM, Smith LR, et al. The effects of deep hypothermic cardiopulmonary bypass and total circulatory arrest on cerebral blood flow in infants and children. J Thorac Cardiovasc Surg 1989;97:737–745.
23. Blackwood MJA, Haka-Ikse K, Steward DJ. Developmental outcome in children undergoing surgery with profound hypothermia. Anesthesiology 1986;65:437–440.
24. Bjork VO, Hultquist G. Contraindications to profound hypothermia in open heart surgery. J Thorac Cardiovasc Surg 1962;44:1.
25. Egerton N, Egerton WS, Kay JH. Neurologic changes following profound hypothermia. Ann Surg 1963;157:366–382.
26. Schubert T, Vetter H, Owen P, et al. Adenosine cardioplegia:

adenosine versus potassium cardioplegia: effects on cardiac arrest and postischemic recovery in the isolated rat heart. J Thorac Cardiovasc Surg 1989;98:1057–1065.
27. Kent KM, Popovic V. Cardiovascular responses in hypothermia and hibernation. Physiologist 1965;8:318.
28. Marelli D, Paul A, Samson R, et al. Does the addition of albumin to the prime solution in cardiopulmonary bypass affect clinical outcome? J Thorac Cardiovasc Surg 1989;98:751–756.
29. Harake B, Power GC. Thoracic duct lymph flow: a comparative study in newborn and adult sheep. J Dev Physiol 1986;8:87–95.
30. Siemkowicz I, Gjedde A. Postischemic coma in rat: effect of different preishcemia blood glucose levels on cerebral metabolic recovery after ischemia. Acta Physiol Scand 1980;110:225–232.
31. Fitzpatrick D, Karmazyn M. Comparative effects of calcium channel blocking agents and varying extracellular calcium concentration on hypoxia/reoxygenation and ischemia/reperfusion-induced cardiac injury. J Pharmacol Exp Ther 1984;84:761–768.
32. Williams WG, Rebeyka IM, Tibshirani RJ, et al. Warm induction blood cardioplegia in the infant. J Thorac Cardiovasc Surg 1990;100:896–901.
33. Rebeyka IM, Diaz RJ, Augustine JM, et al. Effect of rapid cooling contracture on ischemic tolerance in immature myocardium. Circulation 1991;84(Suppl III):III-389–III-393.
34. Aoki M, Nomura F, Kawata H, et al. Effect of calcium and preischemic hypothermia on recovery of myocardial function after cardioplegic ischemia in neonatal lambs. J Thorac Cardiovasc Surg 1993;105:207–213.
35. Kirklin JK, Kirklin JW. Cardiopulmonary bypass for cardiac surgery. In: Sabiston DC, Spencer FC, eds. Surgery of the chest. 5th ed. Philadelphia: WB Saunders, 1990:1107–1125.
36. Rosenberg JS, Rosenberg RD. Advances in the understanding of the anticoagulant function of heparin. In: Silverglade A, ed. A heparin symposium. 1st ed. Tenafly, NJ: Therapeutic Research Press, 1975:66–78.
37. Addonizio VP, Fisher CA, Jenkin BK, et al. Iloprost (ZK36374), a stable analogue of prostacyclin, preserves platelets during simulated extracorporeal circulation. J Thorac Cardiovasc Surg 1985;89:926–933.
38. DeSesa VJ, Huval W, Leluk S, et al. Disadvantages of prostacyclin infusion during cardiopulmonary bypass: a double-blind study of 50 patients having coronary revascularization. Ann Thorac Surg 1984;38:514–519.
39. Fish KJ, Sarnquist FH, van Steenis C, et al. A prospective, randomized study of the effects of prostacyclin on platelets and blood loss during coronary bypass operations. J Thorac Cardiovasc Surg 1986;91:436–442.
40. Riegel W, Spillner G, Schlosser V, et al. Plasma levels of main granulocyte components during cardiopulmonary bypass. J Thorac Cardiovasc Surg 1988;95:1014–1019.
41. Cavarocchi NC, England MD, Schaff HV, et al. Oxygen free radical generation during cardiopulmonary bypass: correlation with complement activation. Circulation 1986;74(Suppl III):III-130–III-133.
42. Kalfin RE, Engelman RM, Rousou JA, et al. Induction of interleukin-8 expression during cardiopulmonary bypass. Circulation 1993;88(Part 2):401–406.
43. Kawata H, Sawatari K, Mayer JE. Evidence for the role of neutrophils in reperfusion injury after cold cardioplegic ischemia in neonatal lambs. J Thorac Cardiovasc Surg 1992;103:908–918.
44. Kilbridge PM, Mayer JE, Newburger JW, et al. Induction of intercellular adhesion molecule-1 and E-selectin mRNA in heart and skeletal muscle of pediatric patients undergoing cardiopulmonary bypass. J Thorac Cardiovasc Surg 1994;107:1183–1192.
45. Smith EJ, Naftel DC, Blackstone EH, et al. Microvascular permeability after cardiopulmonary bypass. J Thorac Cardiovasc Surg 1987;94:225–233.
46. Dietzman RH, Ersek RA, Lillehei CW. Low output syndrome, recognition and treatment. J Thorac Cardiovasc Surg 1969;57:138–150.
47. Cavarocchi NC, Pluth JR, Schaff HV, et al. Complement activation during cardiopulmonary bypass. J Thorac Cardiovasc Surg 1986;91:252–258.
48. Gardner TJ, Stewart JR, Casale AS, et al. Reduction of myocardial ischemic injury with oxygen-derived free radical scavengers. Surgery 1983;94:423–427.
49. Fujiwara T, Heinle J, Britton L, et al. Myocardial preservation in neonatal lambs: comparison of hypothermia with crystalloid and blood cardioplegia. J Thorac Cardiovasc Surg 1991;101:703–712.
50. Bull CM, Cooper J, Stark J. Cardioplegic protection of the child's heart. J Thorac Cardiovasc Surg 1984;88:287–293.
51. Baker JE, Boerboom LE, Olinger GN. Is protection of ischemic neonatal myocardium by cardioplegia species dependent? J Thorac Cardiovasc Surg 1990;99:280–287.
52. Reynolds TR, Geffin GA, Titus JS, et al. Myocardial preservation related to magnesium content of hyperkalemic cardioplegic solutions at 8°C. Ann Thor Surg 1989;47:907–913.
53. Geffin GA, Love TR, Hendren WG, et al. The effects of calcium and magnesium in hyperkalemic cardioplegic solutions on myocardial preservation. J Thorac Cardiovasc Surg 1989;98:239–250.
54. Bodenhamer RM, DeBoer WV, Geffin GA, et al. Enhanced myocardial protection during ischemic arrest. J Thorac Cardiovasc Surg 1983;85:769–780.
55. Rosenkranz ER, Okamoto F, Buckberg GD, et al. Safety of prolonged aortic clamping with blood cardioplegia. III. Aspartate enrichment of glutamate-blood cardioplegia in energy-depleted hearts after ischemic and reperfusion injury. J Thorac Cardiovasc Surg 1986;91:428–435.
56. Rosenkranz ER, Okamoto F, Buckberg GD, et al. Safety of prolonged aortic clamping with blood cardioplegia. II. Glutamate enrichment in energy-depleted hearts. J Thorac Cardiovasc Surg 1984;88:402–410.
57. Robertson JM, Vinten-Johansen J, Buckberg GD, et al. Safety of prolonged aortic clamping with blood cardioplegia. J Thorac Cardiovasc Surg 1984;88:395–401.
58. Sawatari K, Kadoba K, Bergner KA, et al. Influence of initial reperfusion pressure after hypothermic cardioplegia on endothelial modulation of coronary tone in neonatal lambs. Impaired coronary vasodilator response to acetycholine. J Thorac Cardiovasc Surg 1991;101:777–782.
59. Fujiwara T, Kurtts T, Silvera M, et al. Physical and pharmacological manipulation of reperfusion conditions in neonatal myocardial preservation. Circulation 1988;78(Suppl II):II-444.
60. Lazar HL, Wei J, Dirbas FM, et al. Controlled reperfusion following regional ischemia. Ann Thor Surg 1987;44:350–355.
61. Kempsford RD, Hearse DJ. Protection of the immature heart. J Thorac Cardiovasc Surg 1990;99:269–279.
62. Kawata H, Aoki M, Mayer JE Jr. Nitroglycerine improves functional recovery of neonatal lamb hearts after 2 hours of cold ischemia. Circulation 1993;88(Suppl II):II-366–II-371.
63. Hiramatsu T, Forbess JM, Miura T, et al. Effects of L-arginine and L-nitro-arginine methyl ester on recovery of neonatal lamb hearts after cold ischemia: evidence for an important role of endothelial production of nitric oxide. J Thorac Cardiovasc Surg 1995;109:81–87.

Part B: Perioperative Care by Lesion

Shunt Lesions

15.1: Aorticopulmonary Window

Anthony C. Chang, MD, and Winfield Wells, MD

Aorticopulmonary window, a rare lesion, also known as aortopulmonary septal defect, is a vascular communication between the ascending aorta and the main pulmonary artery (1). As with other conotruncal cardiac malformations, 22q11 chromosomal deletion can be associated with this defect (2).

ANATOMY

This lesion results from a failure of the aortopulmonary septum to form, thus placing this defect in the spectrum from hemitruncus to truncus arteriosus, the latter lacking two distinct semilunar valves (3) (Fig. 15.1.1).

Communication between the ascending aorta and the main pulmonary artery can be variable both in size and in location (either close to the semilunar valves or closer to the right pulmonary artery). Aortic origin of the right pulmonary artery can also be associated with this defect. Occasionally, one or both coronary arteries can arise anomalously from either the aorticopulmonary window or the pulmonary artery.

Associated Lesions

This defect can be associated with ventricular septal defect, coarctation of the aorta, or interrupted aortic arch (4).

PATHOPHYSIOLOGY

Left-to-right shunting leads to increased pulmonary blood flow and pulmonary hypertension with left ventricular volume overload (similar to a patent ductus arteriosus).

Clinical Course

Patients usually have symptoms and signs of congestive heart failure after pulmonary vascular resistance falls in the first weeks of life. Because of the usual large size of the defect, pulmonary hypertension can be irreversible as early as 1 year of life (5).

SURGERY

Preoperative Evaluation

For preoperative evaluation, see Section 15.2, on patent ductus arteriosus.

Echocardiography

Usually echocardiography alone is sufficient for the diagnosis, although this defect can be missed or be confused with patent ductus arteriosus even by the experienced echocardiographer. The aorticopulmonary defect is visualized with the aid of color Doppler (6). Indirect evidence includes diastolic flow reversal in the abdominal aorta secondary to runoff to the pulmonary arteries.

Cardiac Catheterization

Cardiac catheterization is usually not indicated unless clinical evidence indicates measurement of pulmonary vascular resistance is necessary.

Transcatheter device closure of this defect with a double umbrella device has been reported (7).

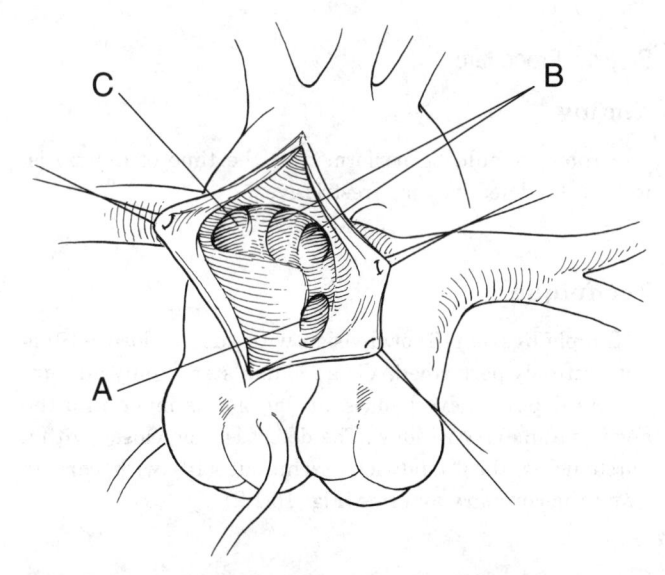

Figure 15.1.1. A composite of the various types of aorticopulmonary window. **A.** The simplest form of this lesion, consisting of a communication between the ascending aorta and the main pulmonary artery. **B.** The more complex form of this lesion, which involves both the main pulmonary artery and the origin of the right branch pulmonary artery. **C.** The variation in which the right pulmonary artery appears to originate separately from the ascending aorta.

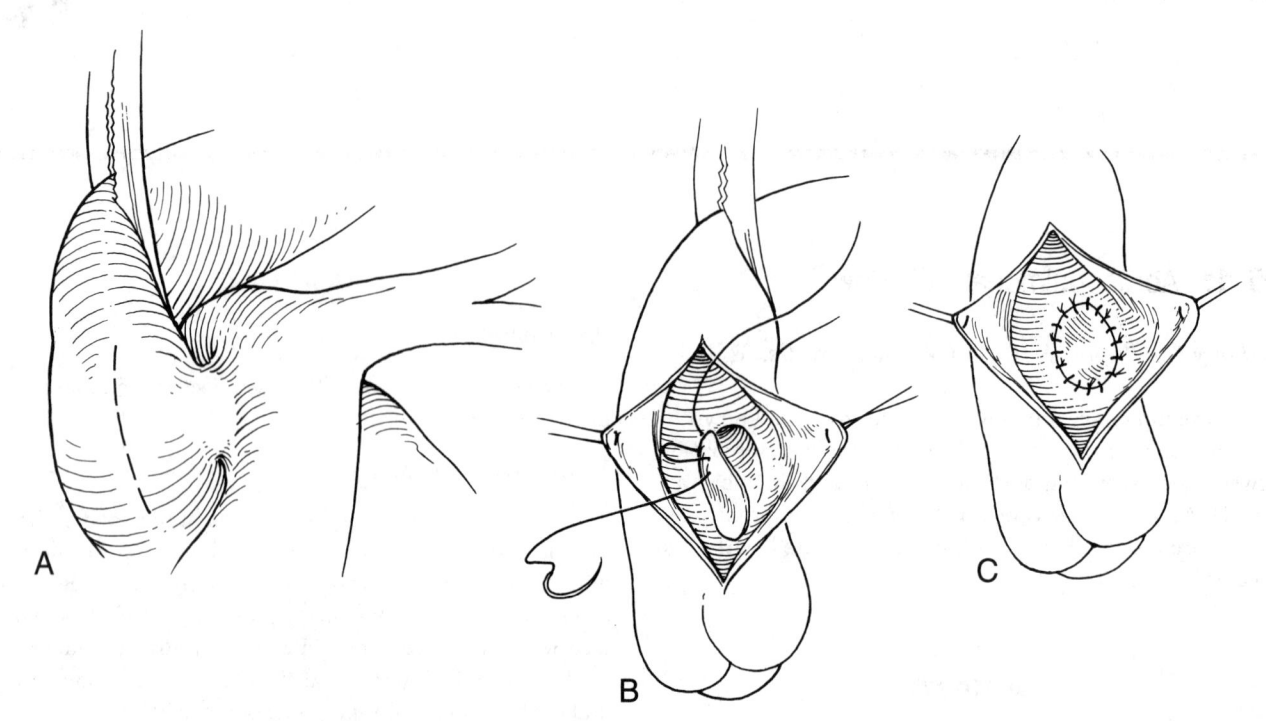

Figure 15.1.2. Repair of simple aorticopulmonary window. Cardiopulmonary bypass with moderate hypothermia and cardioplegic arrest is typically used. **A.** The external appearance of an aorticopulmonary window between the ascending aorta and main pulmonary artery is shown. The *broken line* indicates the position of the incision when the window is approached through an anterior ascending aortotomy. **B.** The aortotomy has been opened, and the window is visualized between the posterior aspect of the ascending aorta and main pulmonary artery. Patch closure of the defect has been initiated. **C.** Patch closure of the defect has been completed. Subsequent to this, the ascending aortotomy is closed, completing the repair. Some surgeons prefer an incision directly into the external wall of the window itself rather than into the aorta. The repair is essentially the same as described.

Surgical Procedure

Timing

Surgery should be performed at the time of diagnosis, unless the defect is very "restrictive."

Technique

Simple ligation (8) or division with suture closure (9) is not routinely performed. Via a median sternotomy and under cardiopulmonary bypass, an incision is made into the aorticopulmonary window. The defect is then closed with a patch using the "sandwich" technique (10) with care to avoid the coronary arteries (Fig. 15.1.2).

Mortality

In most centers, mortality for uncomplicated aortopulmonary window should approach 0%, unless interrupted aortic arch is associated (11). Long-term sequelae include pulmonary artery distortion.

Postoperative Management

Postoperative care of patients after repair is usually uneventful. Ideal monitoring consists of arterial line and central venous pressure line; pulmonary artery line may be indicated if pulmonary hypertension is present.

Specific Postoperative Problems

Pulmonary Hypertension

Preoperative pulmonary vascular resistance of more than $7.3 \text{ U} \cdot \text{m}^2$ has been reported to increase postoperative pulmonary hypertension and mortality (12). Residual shunt after repair is rarely significant, but it should be ruled out if pulmonary artery hypertension is present. Management should be carefully directed using measures to avoid pulmonary hypertensive crises. See Chapter 32, *Pulmonary Hypertension* for more details.

REFERENCES

1. Kutsche LM, Van Mierop LHS. Anatomy and pathogenesis of aorticopulmonary septal defect: analysis of 286 reported cases. Am J Cardiol 1987;59:443–447.

2. Takahashi K, Kido S, Hoshino K, et al. Frequency of a 22q11 deletion in patients with conotruncal cardiac malformations: a prospective study. Eur J Pediatr 1995;154:878–881.
3. Richardson JV, Doty DB, Rossi NP, et al. The spectrum of anomalies of aortopulmonary septation. J Thorac Cardiovasc Surg 1979;78:21–29.
4. Davies MJ, Dyamenahalli U, Leanage RR, et al. Total one stage repair of aortopulmonary window and interrupted aortic arch in a neonate. Pediatr Cardiol 1996;17:122–124.
5. Blieden LC, Moller JH. Aorticopulmonary septal defect: an experience with 17 patients. Br Heart J 1974;36:630–635.
6. Balaji S, Burch M, Sullivan ID. Accuracy of cross-sectional echocardiography in diagnosis of aortopulmonary window. Am J Cardiol 1991;67:650–658.
7. Stamato T, Benson LN, Smallhorn JF, et al. Transcatheter closure of an aortopulmonary window with a modified double umbrella occluder system. Cathet Cardiovasc Diagn 1995;35:165–167.
8. Doty DB, Richardson JV, Falkovsky GE, et al. Aortopulmonary septal defect: hemodynamics, angiography, and operation. Ann Thorac Surg 1981;32:244–250.
9. Richardson JV, Doty DB, Rossi NP, et al. The spectrum of anomalies of aortopulmonary septation. J Thorac Cardiovasc Surg 1979;78:21–27.
10. Ravikumar E, Wright CM, Hawker RE, et al. The surgical management of aortopulmonary window using the anterior sandwich patch closure technique. J Cardiovasc Surg 1988;29:629.
11. Tkebuchava T, von Segesser LK, Vogt PR, et al. Congenital aortopulmonary window: diagnosis, surgical technique and long term results. Eur J Cardiothorac Surg 1997;11:293–297.
12. van Son JA, Puga FJ, Danielson GK, et al. Aortopulmonary window: factors associated with early and late success after surgical treatment. Mayo Clin Proc 1993;68:128–133.

15.2 Patent Ductus Arteriosus

Anthony C. Chang, MD, and Winfield Wells, MD

As an isolated defect, patent ductus arteriosus is common. Evidence of a higher incidence of patent ductus arteriosus is found in children living at high altitude (1). Maternal rubella is also an associated condition. Patent ductus arteriosus has a higher incidence among premature neonates, estimated to be at about 20% in neonates weighing 1750 g or less (2). Since the introduction of indomethacin and now ibuprofen as pharmacologic therapy for closure of the ductus arteriosus (3, 4), the need for surgical ligation has decreased.

ANATOMY

A patent ductus arteriosus is a vascular communication between the junction of the main and left pulmonary arteries and the lesser curvature of the descending aorta just distal to the left subclavian artery. Several variations are seen in the anatomy of the ductus arteriosus. Also significant differences are found between the ductus arteriosus tissue and the pulmonary artery tissue in both intima and media (5). The left recurrent laryngeal nerve is located near the ductus arteriosus (Fig. 15.2.1).

Associated Lesions

Atrial septal defect, ventricular septal defect, common atrioventricular canal, and ductal-dependent lesions are associated lesions (see specific sections in text for additional information).

PATHOPHYSIOLOGY

Pathophysiology includes left-to-right shunting leading to increased pulmonary blood flow, left atrial dilation, and left ventricular volume overload (similar to ventricular septal defect [VSD]).

As in VSD, the degree of shunting is determined by the size of the communication, unless the defect is unrestrictive, in which case the shunting is then determined by the relative resistances between the systemic and pulmonary circulations. The increase in left atrial pressure as a result of the left-to-right shunt and increase in pulmonary blood flow can lead to an additional left-to-right shunt via a stretched foramen ovale.

After birth, with the removal of the placenta (the major source of prostaglandin in utero) as well as increase in metabolism of the lungs (where prostaglandins are metabolized), the ductus starts to constrict (starting at the pulmonary end) and reaches functional closure. Closure of the ductus arteriosus is also dependent on arterial P_{AO_2}, prostaglandins, thromboxanes, and so forth (6). Ductal closure may be delayed in premature neonates because metabolism of prostaglandin is altered (owing to immature lung tissue) and sensitivity to prostaglandin is increased. In addition, the response to oxygen by vasoconstriction is altered in the premature neonate (7). Finally, as pulmonary vascular resistance falls with age or with improving lung function with surfactant therapy, the left-to-right shunt via the ductus arteriosus can increase and contribute to symptomatology (8).

At about 2 weeks of age, anatomic closure occurs because the ductus undergoes degenerative changes and becomes fibrotic, and thus becomes the ligamentum arteriosum.

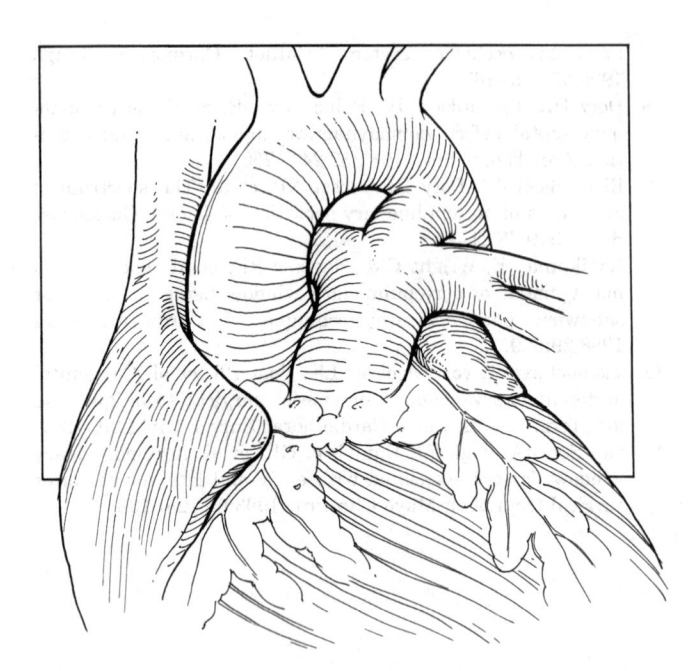

Figure 15.2.1. Typical appearance of ductus arteriosus from an anterior perspective. Note that the structure arises from the main pulmonary artery, has a definable length, and enters the descending aorta well beyond the left subclavian artery on the internal curvature of the aorta. The segment of aorta between the subclavian artery and the ductus insertion is the aortic isthmus. In otherwise normal hearts, the insertion sites of the ductus arteriosus are constant; however, the ductus length and diameter can vary substantially. When a patent ductus arteriosus exists in association with other complex congenital heart disease such as tetralogy of Fallot, pulmonary atresia, interrupted aortic arch, or other arch anomalies, the anatomy of patent ductus arteriosus, including its site of origin on the pulmonary and systemic arteries, can vary significantly.

Clinical Course

Premature neonates have less compensatory mechanisms to cope with the left-to-right shunt observed with a patent ductus arteriosus (9). Congestive heart failure, apnea, or respiratory compromise can occur if the ductus is large, and it is associated with high morbidity in the premature neonate (10). In addition, multisystem organ failure (renal failure, necrotizing enterocolitis, and central nervous system problems) can ensue. If the ductus is small, usually just a systolic murmur is present.

In the full-term neonate, spontaneous closure after the first few months of life is relatively uncommon. Recurrent pulmonary infections and congestive heart failure occur. Pulmonary vascular obstructive disease can occur within the first year of life if untreated. Other potential problems in older children include infective endocarditis or aneurysm formation that may rupture.

SURGERY

Preoperative Evaluation

Physical Examination

A systolic murmur in the left sternal border is usually auscultated in neonates and a continuous murmur in the second left intercostal space is often heard in older children. Absence of any murmur can also be a finding. Bounding peripheral pulses can be present and a wide pulse pressure with a low diastolic pressure can be seen especially in neonates with a large ductus arteriosus. Hyperactive precordium is also seen in these patients.

Chest Roentgenogram

Cardiomegaly with a prominent main pulmonary artery segment and increased pulmonary vascularity is the usual finding.

Electrocardiography

Left atrial enlargement and biventricular hypertrophy can be present.

Echocardiography

Usually echocardiography alone is sufficient for the diagnosis, especially with the advent of color Doppler (Fig. 15.2.2; see color plate 15.2.2). Usually seen is left atrial and left ventricular dilatation. Pulmonary artery pressure can be estimated by continuous wave Doppler interrogation of the ductus arteriosus. Noninvasive studies are useful in serial examination of the ductus arteriosus, especially with indomethacin treatment (11).

Cardiac Catheterization

Cardiac catheterization is usually unnecessary unless evidence is found for pulmonary hypertension or associated lesions that are readily delineated by echocardiography.

Transcutaneous catheter occlusion of the ductus arteriosus can be performed with minimal complications with an occluder device, coils, or the new Gianturco-Grifka vascular occlusion device (12–15). Certain patients, such as those with very large patent ductus arteriosus or patients who are very small (because relatively large catheters are introduced via the femoral vein), may not be suitable candidates for this intervention. Complications with transcatheter closure include embolization and residual shunt.

Surgical Procedure

Timing

In premature neonates, a national collaborative study showed that ductal closure can be as high as 79% with use of indomethacin but surgical closure should be considered after medical failure (defined as three doses of indometha-

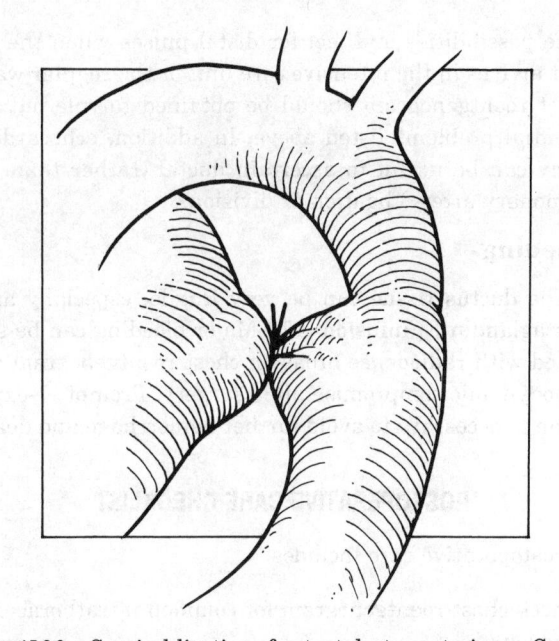

Shunt Lesions 205

Figure 15.2.3. Surgical ligation of patent ductus arteriosus. Cardiopulmonary bypass is not used. The surgical perspective via a left thoracotomy is shown. A suture ligature has been placed in the midportion of the ductus arteriosus to achieve closure. In children beyond the newborn period, typically three separate suture ligatures are placed to minimize the chance of recanalization of the ductus. In premature infants, a single ligature is typically placed using either suture material or metal clips.

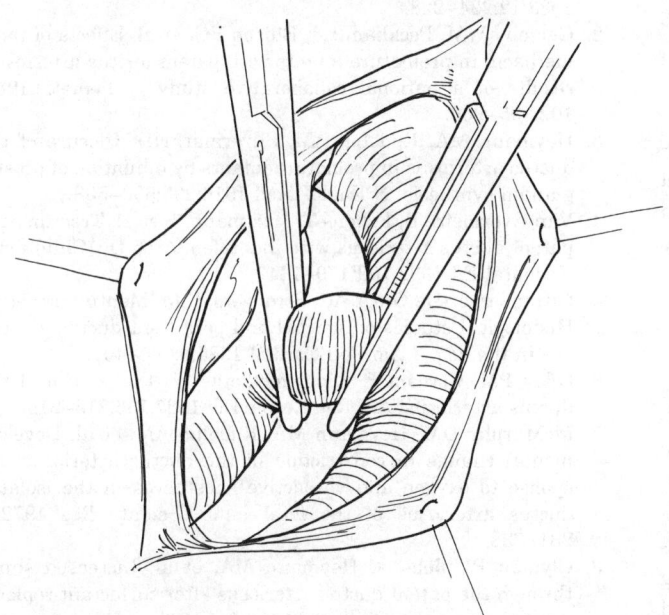

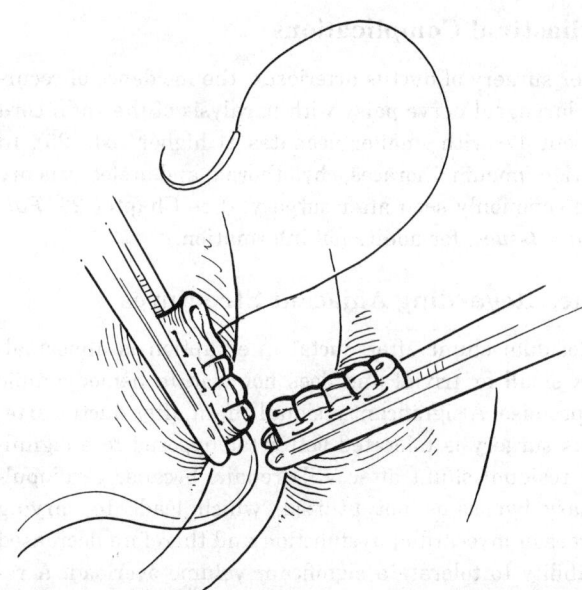

cin). In addition, furosemide use has been associated with ductal patency, probably through a prostaglandin-mediated process (16). Contraindications to indomethacin therapy include renal dysfunction, necrotizing enterocolitis, bleeding, shock, or myocardial ischemia. Indomethacin should *not* be used without echocardiographic confirmation of patent ductus arteriosus as certain congenital heart lesions can coexist and indomethacin use to close the ductus may be disastrous in certain diagnoses (e.g., coarctation of the aorta) (17).

In older children, surgical or catheter closure of a large ductus arteriosus should be considered in the first 6 months of life. If the ductus arteriosus is small, intervention is controversial.

Technique

Ligation Via a left thoracotomy and with the left lung displaced, the recurrent laryngeal nerve is identified as it curves around the inferior part of the ductus arteriosus. The ductus arteriosus is ligated doubly or triply with circumferential sutures. Recanalization and hemorrhage has occurred with simple suture ligation (17) (Fig. 15.2.3).

Division With a large ductus arteriosus, division may be the preferred technique. Via a left thoracotomy and with

Figure 15.2.4. Surgical division of patent ductus arteriosus. The surgical perspective via a left thoracotomy is shown. The adventitia overlying the aortic isthmus and ductus arteriosus has been opened and is retracted with sutures. Clamps have been placed across the aortic and pulmonary ends of the ductus arteriosus. The ductus is then divided between the clamps and each of the ends is oversewn with a running suture technique. Following this, the clamps are carefully removed and the overlying adventitia is closed. This technique is typically performed in older patients, especially those with anatomic variants that have a large diameter and short length, or in older patients who have acquired degenerative changes within the ductus arteriosus.

the left lung displaced, the ductus is identified. With vascular clamps on either side and with sutures in place at both ends, the ductus is partially and then completely divided after initial stitches are placed on the aortic end. The aortic end is oversewn, followed by the pulmonary end (Fig. 15.2.4).

Recently, the video-assisted thorascopic surgery (VATS) technique has been successfully applied to closure of the ductus arteriosus (19, 20).

Mortality

In most centers, mortality for uncomplicated patent ductus ligation should approach 0%. In premature neonates, mortality may be slightly higher (21). Results with surgical ligation is comparable to use of indomethacin (22). Complications can include recurrence of patency after surgical ligation (23).

Postoperative Management

In premature neonates, surgery is at times performed in the neonatal intensive care unit to avoid increased morbidity with transfer to the operating room (24). In older patients, postoperative care of patients after patent ductus ligation is usually uneventful and early extubation in the operating room is performed. In the absence of intraoperative complications, intensive care monitoring is not routine.

Specific Postoperative Problems

Mediastinal Complications

For surgery of ductus arteriosus, the incidence of recurrent laryngeal nerve palsy with paralysis of the vocal cord is about 4% with smaller neonates at higher risk (25). In addition, pneumothoraces, chylothorax, and atelectasis are more commonly seen after surgery. (See Chapter 23, *Pulmonary Issues*, for additional information.)

Issues Regarding Adjacent Structures

Residual shunt after ductal interruption is almost always small or trivial and does not lead to hemodynamic compromise. A significant residual shunt after ductus arteriosus surgery is tolerated better (as opposed to a significant residual shunt after VSD repair) because cardiopulmonary bypass is not utilized, which leads to varying degrees of myocardial dysfunction and therefore decreased capability to tolerate a significant volume overload. A residual shunt detectable by color Doppler echocardiography is comparable between surgical ligation and catheter device closure to be as high as 20 to 25% (26).

Aorta, left pulmonary artery, and left main stem bronchus, however, can all be mistaken for the ductus arteriosus and ligated. The caretaker should have vigilance to these possibilities and feel for distal pulses when the patient arrives in the intensive care unit or the regular ward. Chest roentgenogram should be obtained to rule out the potential problems listed above. In addition, echocardiography can be useful to ascertain ductal (rather than left pulmonary artery) ligation or division.

Bleeding

The ductus tissue can be very fragile, especially after prostaglandin E_1 infusion (27). Major bleeding can be suspected with radiodense areas on chest roentgenogram and hemodynamic compromise after surgery. Prompt re-exploration is necessary to avoid further hemorrhage and death.

POSTOPERATIVE CARE CHECKLIST

Postoperative care includes:

- Check chest roentgenogram for common intrathoracic problems.
- Feel pulses to rule out ligation of nonductus vascular structures (e.g., aorta or left pulmonary artery).
- Pay attention to possibility of hemorrhage.

REFERENCES

1. Miao C, Zuberbuhler JA, Zuberbuhler JR. Prevalence of congenital cardiac anomalies at high altitude. J Am Coll Cardiol 1988;12:224–228.
2. Gersony WM, Peckham GJ, Ellison RC, et al. Effects of indomethacin in premature infants with patent ductus arteriosus: results of a national collaborative study. J Pediatr 1983; 102:895–906.
3. Heymann MA, Rudolph AM, Silverman NH. Closure of the ductus arteriosus in premature infants by inhibition of prostaglandin synthesis. N Engl J Med 1976;295:530–538.
4. Van Overmeire B, Follens T, Hartmann S, et al. Treatment of patent ductus arteriosus with ibuprofen. Arch Dis Child Fetal Neonatal Ed 1997;76:F179–184.
5. Gittenberger-De Groot AC, Strengers JLM, Mentink M, et al. Histological studies on normal and persistent ductus arteriosus in the dog. J Am Coll Cardiol 1985;6:394–401.
6. Olley PM, Coceani F. Lipid mediators in the control of the ductus arteriosus. Am Rev Respir Dis 1987;136:218–219.
7. McMurphy DM, Heymann MA, Rudolph AM, et al. Developmental change in constriction of the ductus arteriosus: response to oxygen and vasoactive substances in the isolated ductus arteriosus of the fetal lamb. Pediatr Res 1972;6: 231–238.
8. Clyman RI, Jobe A, Heymann MA, et al. Increased shunt through the patent ductus arteriosus after surfactant replacement therapy. J Pediatr 1982;100:101–108.
9. Lebowitz EA, Novick JS, Rudolph AM. Development of myocardial sympathetic innervation in the fetal lamb. Pediatr Res 1972;6:887–893.
10. Jones RWA, Pickering D. Persistent ductus arteriosus complicating the respiratory distress syndrome. Arch Dis Child 1977;52:274–281.
11. Smallhorn JP, Gow R, Olley PM, et al. Combined noninvasive assessment of the patent ductus arteriosus in the preterm in-

fant before and after indomethacin treatment. Am J Cardiol 1984;54:1300–1304.
12. Khan MAA, Yousef SA, Mullins CE, et al. Experience with 205 procedures of transcatheter closure of ductus arteriosus in 182 patients, with special reference to residual shunts and long-term followup. J Thorac Cardiovasc Surg 1992;104:1721–1727.
13. Rashkind WJ, Mullins CE, Hellenbrand WE, et al. Nonsurgical closure of patent ductus arteriosus: clinical application of the Rashkind PDA occluder system. Circulation 1987;75:583–592.
14. Alwi M, Kang LM, Samion H, et al. Transcatheter occlusion of native persistent ductus arteriosus using conventional Gianturco coils. Am J Cardiol 1997;79:1430–1432.
15. Grifka RG, Miller MW, Frischmeyer KJ, et al. Transcatheter occlusion of a patent ductus arteriosus in a Newfoundland puppy using the Gianturco-Grifka vascular occlusion device. J Vet Intern Med 1996;10:42–44.
16. Green TP, Thompson TR, Johnson DE, et al. Furosemide promotes patent ductus arteriosus in premature infants with respiratory distress syndrome. N Engl J Med 1983;308:743–748.
17. Chang AC, Hanley FL, Lock JE, et al. Management and outcome of low birth weight neonates with congenital heart disease. J Pediatr 1994;124:461–466.
18. Daniels SR, Reller MD, Kaplan S. Recurrence of patency of the ductus arteriosus after surgical ligation in premature infants. Pediatrics 1984;73:56–58.
19. Laborde F, Noirhomme P, Karam J, et al. A new video-assisted thoracoscopic surgical technique for interruption of patent ductus arteriosus in infants and children. J Thorac Cardiovasc Surg 1993;105:278–280.
20. Burke RP, Wernovsky GW, van der Velde M, et al. Video assisted thorascopic surgery for congenital heart disease. J Thorac Cardiovasc Surg 1995;109:499–507.
21. Wagner HR, Ellison RC, Zierler S, et al. Surgical closure of patent ductus arteriosus in 268 preterm infants. J Thorac Cardiovasc Surg 1984;87:870–875.
22. Zerella JT, Spies RJ, Deaver DC, et al. Indomethacin versus immediate ligation in the treatment of 82 newborns with patent ductus arteriosus. J Pediatr Surg 1983;18:835.
23. Daniels SR, Reller MD, Kaplan S. Recurrence of patency of the ductus arteriosus after surgical ligation in premature infants. Pediatrics 1984;73:56–58.
24. Mortier E. Ongenae M, Vermassen F, et al. Operative closure of patent ductus arteriosus in the neonatal intensive care unit. Acta Chir Belg 1996;96:266–268.
25. Fan LL, Campbell DN, Clarke DR, et al. Paralyzed left vocal cord associated with ligation of patent ductus arteriosus. J Thorac Cardiovasc Surg 1989;98:611–613.
26. Sorensen KE, Kristensen BO, Hansen OK. Frequency of occurrence of residual ductal flow after surgical ligation by color-flow mapping. Am J Cardiol 1991;67:653–654.
27. Calder AL, Kirker JA, Neutze JM, et al. Pathology of the ductus arteriosus treated with prostaglandins: comparison with untreated. Pediatr Cardiol 1984;5:85–92.

15.3 Atrial Septal Defect

Anthony C. Chang, MD, and Jeffrey Jacobs, MD

An isolated atrial septal defect is one of the most common congenital heart defects accounting for 5 to 10% of all congenital heart disease. These defects are also often seen in conjunction with many other congenital heart defects. It is more common in females than in males (2:1).

ANATOMY

The true atrial septum is composed of the septum primum and the septum secundum. It merges with the two vena cavae at the superior and inferior cavoatrial junctions, and with the atrioventricular canal septum as the tricuspid valve is approached.

Types of Atrial Septal Defect

Ostium Secundum Type

Ostium secundum atrial septal defect is the most common type and the only true atrial septal defect (Fig. 15.3.1). It is centrally located in the region of the fossa ovalis (and therefore also called "fossa ovalis" type defect), and it occurs as a result of septum primum deficiency. This deficiency may take various forms from attenuation to complete absence to multiple perforations.

Ostium Primum Type

See Chapter 15.5, *Common Atrioventricular Canal,* for information on this type of defect.

Sinus Venosus Type

Sinus venosus type defects are not true defects in the atrial septum, but rather defects where the atrial septum merges with the vena cavae. Two subtypes are found: First, the superior vena caval type, which is located high, immediately below the superior vena cava orifice. This type of defect is commonly associated with partial anomalous pulmonary venous drainage of the right upper and middle pulmonary veins. Second, the inferior vena caval type, which is located low, at the right atrial-inferior vena cava junction. As in the superior vena cava type of atrial septal defect, this type can also be associated with partial anomalous pulmonary venous drainage.

Coronary Sinus Type

A rare defect, the coronary sinus type is located in the roof of the coronary sinus (also termed "unroofed coronary sinus"). It is formed as a result of full or partial absence of the wall between the coronary sinus and left atrium. This defect leads to drainage of left atrial blood into the coro-

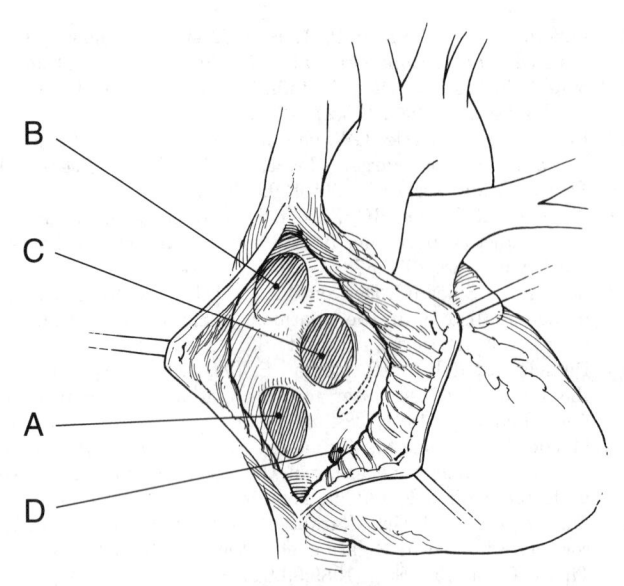

Figure 15.3.1. Anatomy of atrial septal defects. The four types of intra-atrial communications are shown. **A.** The ostium secundum atrial septal defect, the only true atrial septal defect. The lesion results from a defect in the development of the septum primum. Complete absence of the septum primum results in a large defect that extends down to the inferior vena cava. Multiple perforations in an otherwise well-developed septum primum can result in a "fenestrated" atrial septal defect. If the septum primum is normally developed, but does not fuse to the limbus (septum secundum), the defect is termed a "foramen ovale." **B.** The superior vena caval type of sinus venosus defect is shown. In this defect, the atrial septum itself is intact, however, malalignment is seen between the atrial septum and the entrance of the superior vena cava into the atrium. Partial anomalous pulmonary venous return from the upper portion of the right lung is commonly found in association with this defect. **C.** The ostium primum defect is shown. This defect, which is more extensively described in Chapter 15.5, *Common Atrioventricular Canal Defects,* is caused by a defect in the development of the atrioventricular canal septum. **D.** The position of the coronary sinus is shown. A defect in the common wall between the coronary sinus and the left atrium results in a communication between the two atria. In essence, the coronary sinus defect is a sinus venosus defect of the left side.

nary sinus, and then into the right atrium. It can also be associated with a persistent left superior vena cava.

Other Anatomic Notes

A patent foramen ovale is closely related to the ostium secundum atrial septal defect, occurring in the same position. The distinction between the two is that in patent foramen ovale, there is no deficiency of the septum primum. A patent foramen ovale is present in up to 34% of pediatric patients (1). The patent foramen ovale is a normal interatrial communication in the fetus that functionally closes postnatally as the left atrial pressure supercedes the right atrial pressure, allowing the mobile septum primum to drift against the rigid limbus of the septum secundum.

Right-to-left shunting will occur through the foramen ovale if right atrial pressure exceeds left atrial pressure and if the septum primum has not physically sealed itself against the limbus.

An aneurysm of the atrial septum is a bulging of the septum primum that can be associated with structural heart disease or supraventricular dysrhythmias, but it usually resolves with age and maturational changes in the atrial septum (2).

A common atrium denotes a large defect that is essentially absence of both the septum primum and secundum. It is rare and usually associated with the heterotaxy syndromes or other complex lesions.

Associated Lesions

Partial anomalous pulmonary venous drainage, pulmonary stenosis, mitral valve anomalies (including prolapse) are associated lesions.

PATHOPHYSIOLOGY

Left-to-right shunting at the atrial level leading to right atrial dilation, right ventricular volume overload, and increased pulmonary blood flow are pathophysiologic findings.

The degree of left-to-right shunting depends not only on the size of the atrial defect but also on the relative compliance of the ventricles during diastole. Left-to-right shunting progressively increases with age (as right ventricular compliance improves). Blood flow across the defect occurs predominantly in diastole, when the mitral and tricuspid valves open and filling occurs in the ventricles. Another important factor that can influence the quantity of shunting is the size of the defect itself. A defect is described as nonrestrictive when equal pressures occur in both atria and the quantity of shunting is solely determined by the left and right ventricular compliances. A defect is considered restrictive if its size is small enough to provide resistance to flow across it.

Clinical Course

Infants and children are usually asymptomatic despite the volume overload on the right ventricle. Congestive heart failure usually occurs after the second or third decade of life as a result of chronic right ventricular volume overload; however, congestive heart failure can occur in up to 5% of children before the first year of life (3). In older patients (more than 15 years of age), chronic right ventricular dilation can lead to decreased left ventricular distensibility and congestive heart failure (4). Pulmonary hypertension is rare in childhood (5), but it can occur in up to 13% of unoperated patients younger than 10 years of age (6, 7). Surgical closure of the atrial septal defect once pulmonary vascular obstructive disease occurs is debatable and may not be recommended for pulmonary vascular resistance much greater than 8 U.m² (8). Atrial fibrillation and flutter may be related to degree of left to right shunt (9) or age (10), and it can be present in up to 13% of unoperated patients over age 40 years (11). Sinoatrial node dysfunction can occur in 65% of older patients before surgical correction (12), but conduction abnormalities are less frequent in children (13). Paradoxic emboli via an atrial septal defect can lead to cerebrovascular accidents (14). Cyanosis can occur as a result of right-to-left shunt at the atrial level in the presence of elevated pulmonary vascular resistance. Rarely, in superior vena cava-type of sinus venosus atrial septal defect, the degree of superior vena cava override can be severe and lead to significant venous drainage into the left atrium and cause cyanosis. Bacterial endocarditis is unusual in patients with atrial septal defects without associated lesions.

SURGERY

Preoperative Evaluation

Physical Examination

A systolic ejection murmur in the pulmonic area (second left interspace) is heard as a result of increased pulmonary blood flow. A widely split S_2 is found (as a result of delay in the right ventricle emptying). In addition, an early to mid-diastolic rumble at the left sternal border can also be present.

Chest Roentgenogram

Cardiomegaly with an enlarged right atrium and ventricle is seen with a prominent main pulmonary artery segment and increased pulmonary vascularity.

Electrocardiography

Right axis deviation and right ventricular hypertrophy with an incomplete right bundle branch block pattern (rsR′) in the right precordial leads are seen. Right atrial enlargement (tall p wave in lead II) can also be present.

Echocardiography

The defect is visualized in the atrial septum with right ventricular volume overload (Fig. 15.3.2; see color plate 15.3.2). Usually echocardiography alone is sufficient for the diagnosis, although an associated partial anomalous drainage of the right upper or middle pulmonary vein can be occasionally missed. "Paradoxic" interventricular septal motion is seen. Color Doppler echocardiography can demonstrate flow across the defect (15). In older patients, transesophageal echocardiography may be necessary to confirm the diagnosis (16).

Cardiac Catheterization

Cardiac catheterization is usually not indicated unless a coexisting lesion or presence of pulmonary hypertension are suspected. When performed, findings include (*a*) an oxygen saturation step-up from the superior vena cava to the right atrium of more than 10% and (*b*) a pressure gradient across the pulmonary valve (as much as 40 mm Hg) secondary to increased pulmonary blood flow.

For some secundum type defects that are not excessive in size (less than 22 mm in size) and are centrally located, catheter closure of defect can be done in the cardiac catheterization laboratory with umbrella-like or buttoned devices (17, 18).

Surgical Procedure

Timing

Repair is traditionally recommended between 3 to 5 years of life; however, this is partly due to historical reasons as a holdover from the time when cardiopulmonary bypass in younger children carried a definable risk. Spontaneous closure of some small secundum type defects can occur in up to 87% of infants in the first year of life (19–21). Closure electively at 1 year of age or earlier if symptoms are present may minimize overall morbidity (22). Surgical closure of small defects, however, is controversial (23).

Technique

For secundum type atrial defects, a median sternotomy, or right anterior submammary thoracotomy for cosmetic purposes (24), is made for exposure. Cardiopulmonary bypass is used either with aortic cross clamping and cardioplegia, or with electrical fibrillation. Through an oblique right atrial incision, suture or patch (pericardial or Dacron) closure of the defect is performed. Patch closure is preferred for large secundum defects (to minimize tension). One potential hazard during repair is air embolism because the left side of the heart is open to air.

For sinus venosus type defect, a median sternotomy is used along with cardiopulmonary bypass and aortic cross clamp and cardioplegia. Various surgical techniques are used, but the general principle is to use a patch to close the defect and at the same time baffle the anamolous pulmonary veins to the left atrium. Repair is close to the sinoatrial node (Fig. 15.3.3).

Mortality

In most centers, mortality for uncomplicated atrial septal defects should approach 0%.

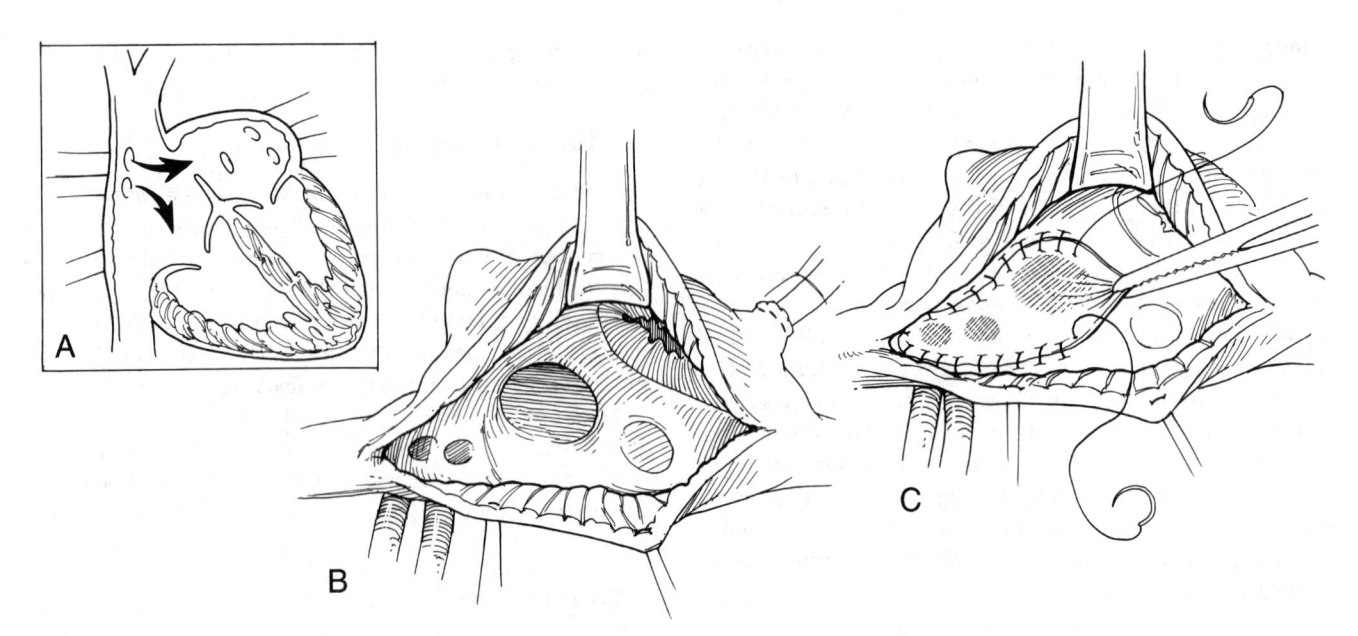

Figure 15.3.3. Repair of sinus venous defect with partial anomalous pulmonary venous return. **A.** A cross-sectional schematic shows the intra-atrial communication and the abnormal drainage of the veins from the right upper lung field into the right atrium. **B.** The surgical perspective is shown. The patient has been placed on cardiopulmonary bypass using moderate hypothermia and aortic cross-clamping. A right atriotomy incision has been performed, and the edges of the right atrial incision have been retracted to show the internal anatomy of the atrial septum. The superior vena cava enters the right atrium from the left side of the figure and the inferior vena cava enters the right atrium from the right side. The large opening in the atrial septum represents the sinus venosus defect, and the two smaller openings represent the orifices of two right upper lung field pulmonary veins that are draining anomalously into the right atrium. The intact fossa ovalis is seen to the right-hand side of the sinus venous defect. **C.** Patch repair of the sinus venous defect with concomitant baffling of the anomalously draining pulmonary veins is accomplished using a single patch. In this technique, a somewhat redundant patch is placed as a hood over the sinus venosus defect and around the orifices of the anomalously draining pulmonary veins. The patch eliminates communication between the left and right atria and also allows the anomalous veins to drain under the patch across the sinus venosus defect into the left atrium. Following placement of the patch, the right atrial incision is closed and the patient is weaned from cardiopulmonary bypass.

Postoperative Management

Postoperative care of patients after atrial septal defect repair is usually uneventful and early extubation in the operating room is sometimes performed.

Ideal monitoring consists of arterial line and central venous pressure line. Monitoring of left atrial pressure in older patients and of pulmonary arterial pressure in patients with preoperative pulmonary hypertension may be indicated.

Specific Postoperative Problems

Sinoatrial Node Dysfunction

Injury to the sinoatrial node can occur as a result of either direct trauma or as a consequence of interruption of its blood supply. This can be manifested in a subtle fashion by inappropriate chronotropic response to anemia, stress, or inotropic agents, and also by the presence of atrial arrhythmias or junctional rhythm. Postoperative dysrhythmias can occur in 23% of patients after repair (25), and up to 2% of patients may even need a pacemaker after surgery (26). The risk for sinoatrial node dysfunction has been noted to be higher with sinus venosus type atrial septal defect repair (27).

Close monitoring of heart rhythm is warranted during the immediate postoperative period as manifestations of this rhythm disturbance may be subtle.

Postpericardiotomy Syndrome

Postpericardiotomy syndrome manifests sometimes with fever, malaise, lymphocytosis, nausea, vomiting, or abdominal pain in the first few days or weeks after surgery; a friction rub may not be present on physical examination. Cardiomegaly on chest roentgenogram can correlate with echocardiographic examination of a sizable pericardial effusion. In addition, tachycardia and even hemodynamic compromise can occur. Patients can, however, be asymptomatic.

The postpericardiotomy syndrome can be initially treated with either aspirin, nonsteroidal anti-inflammatory agents, or even steroids. With any suggestion of hemodynamic compromise, intravenous fluids should be given and a pericardiocentesis performed without delay. (For details, please refer to Chapter 33, *Miscellaneous Topics*).

Left Ventricular Dysfunction

Although uncommon, left ventricular dysfunction is a potential problem in older patients (more than 15 years of age) who have had chronic right ventricular dilation. The left ventricular failure is a reflection of chronic right ventricular volume overload and decreased left ventricular compliance, rather than irreversible myocardial dysfunction. Closure of the atrial septal defect may lead to transient elevated left atrial pressure and pulmonary edema (28).

Inotropic support and/or afterload reduction may be indicated in selected patients with left ventricular dysfunction. Digoxin may also be indicated. If indicated, positive pressure ventilation can also be useful to overcome decompensation secondary to pulmonary edema.

Pulmonary Hypertension

Postoperative mortality is considerably higher in patients with atrial septal defects who had preoperative pulmonary vascular resistance of more than $8\ U \cdot m^2$ (29). Fortunately, this phenomenon is uncommon in the pediatric patient population. (For treatment, please refer to Chapter 32, *Pulmonary Hypertension*.)

Residual Atrial Septal Defect

The incidence of residual atrial shunt after surgery is typically low, but it has been reported to be as high as 15% (30). These residual shunts are usually of no hemodynamic consequence and do not require reoperation. Rarely, patch or suture line dehiscence can occur, causing a large residual defect which requires reoperation.

Venous Obstruction

After repair of superior vena cava type of sinus venosus atrial septal defect, obstruction to superior vena cava and pulmonary veins may occur (31). Superior vena caval obstruction is manifested by facial edema whereas right pulmonary venous obstruction can be demonstrated on chest roentgenogram as a focal right lung field pulmonary interstitial edema.

Cyanosis

In the repair of large atrial septal defects, the eustachian valve may be mistaken for the lower rim of the atrial septal defect. This may lead to the patch placed in such a way that the blood from the inferior vena cava is directed to the left atrium.

Atrioventricular Block

After repair of coronary sinus type of atrial septal defect, atrioventricular block can occur because of the proximity of the atrioventricular node to the defect. Temporary pacing or even permanent pacemaker placement may be indicated.

POSTOPERATIVE CARE CHECKLIST

Postoperative care checklist includes:

- Be aware of clinical signs for pericardial effusion.
- Monitor heart rate for sinoatrial node dysfunction.
- Maintain vigilance for signs of noncompliant left ventricle in older patients.

REFERENCES

1. Hagen PT, Scholz DG, Edwards WD. Incidence and size of patent foramen ovale during the first 10 decades of life: an autopsy of 965 normal hearts. Mayo Clin Proc 1984;59:17–20.
2. Wolf WJ, Casta A, Sapire DW. Atrial septal aneurysms in infants and children. Am Heart J 1987;113:1149–1153.
3. Hunt CE, Lucas RV. Symptomatic atrial septal defect in infancy. Circulation 1973;47:1042–1048.
4. Booth DC, Wisenbaugh T, Smith M, et al. Left ventricular distensibility and passive elastic stiffness in atrial septal defect. J Am Coll Cardiol 1988;12:1231–1236.
5. Haworth SG. Pulmonary vascular disease in secundum atrial defect in childhood. Am J Cardiol 1982;51:265–272.
6. Cherian G, Uthaman CB, Durairaj M, et al. Pulmonary hypertension in isolated secundum atrial septal defect: high frequency in young patients. Am Heart J 1983;105:952–957.
7. Steele PM, Fuster V, Cohen M, et al. Isolated atrial septal defect with pulmonary vascular obstructive disease: long-term follow-up and prediction of outcome after surgical correction. Circulation 1987;76:1037–1042.
8. Dalen JE, Haynes FW, Dexter L. Life expectancy with atrial septal defect: influence of complicating pulmonary vascular disease. JAMA 1967;200:442–446.
9. Sealy WC, Farmer JC, Young WG, et al. Atrial dysrhythmias and atrial secundum defects. J Cardiovasc Thorac Surg 1968;57:245–250.
10. Ruschhaupt DG, Khoury L, Thilenius OG, et al. Electrophysiologic abnormalities of children with secundum atrial septal defect. Am J Cardiol 1984;53:1643–1647.
11. Gault JH, Morrow AG, Gay WA, et al. Atrial septal defect in patients over the age of forty years: clinical and hemodynamic studies and the effects of operation. Circulation 1968;37:261–272.
12. Benedini G, Affatato A, Bellandi M, et al. Preoperative sinus node function in adult patients with atrial septal defect. Eur Heart J 1985;6:261.
13. Karpawich PP, Antillon JR, Cappola PR, et al. Pre and postoperative electrophysiologic assessment of children with secundum atrial septal defect. Am J Cardiol 1985;55:519–521.
14. Lechat P, Mas JL, Lascault G, et al. Prevalence of patent foramen ovale in patients with stroke. N Engl J Med 1988;318:1148–1152.
15. Suzuki Y, Kambara H, Kadota K, et al. Detection of intracardiac shunt flow in atrial septal defect using a real-time two-dimensional color-coded Doppler flow imaging system and comparison with contrast two-dimensional echocardiography. Am J Cardiol 1985;56:347–350.

16. Hanrath P, Schluter M, Langenstein BA, et al. Detection of ostium secundum atrial septal defects by transesophageal cross-sectional echocardiography. Br Heart J 1983;49: 350–358.
17. Rome JJ, Keane JF, Perry SB, et al. Double umbrella closure of atrial defects: initial clinical applications. Circulation 1990;82:751–758.
18. Rao PS, Wilson AD, Levy JM, et al. Role of buttoned double-disk device in the management of atrial septal defects. Am Heart J 1992;123:191–200.
19. Cockerham JT, Martin TC, Guitierrez FR, et al. Spontaneous closure of secundum atrial septal defect in infants and young children. Am J Cardiol 1983;52:1267–1271.
20. Mahoney LT, Truesdell SC, Krzmarzick TR, et al. Atrial septal defects that present in infancy. Am J Dis Child 1986;140:1115–1118.
21. Radzik D, Davignon A, van Doesburg N, et al. Predictive factors for spontaneous closure of atrial septal defects diagnosed in the first 3 months of life. J Am Coll Cardiol 1993;22: 851–853.
22. Murphy JG, Gersh BJ, McGoon MD, et al. Long-term outcome after surgical repair of isolated atrial septal defect. N Engl J Med 1990;323:1645–1650.
23. Moss AJ, Siassi B. The small atrial septal defect—operate or procrastinate? Am J Cardiol 1973;32:978–981.
24. Lancaster LL, Mavroudis C, Rees AH, et al. Surgical approach to atrial septal defect in the female: right thoracotomy versus sternotomy. Am Surg 1990;56:218–221.
25. Bink-Boelkens M, Meuzelaar KJ, Eygelaar A. Dysrhythmias after atrial surgery in children. Am Heart J 1983;106: 125–130.
26. Bolens M, Friedli B. Sinus node function and conduction system before and after surgery for secundum atrial septal defect: an electrophysiologic study. Am J Cardiol 1984;53:1415–1420.
27. Bink-Boelkens ME, Velvis H, Homan van der Heide JJ. Dysrhythmias after atrial surgery in children. Am Heart J 1983;106:125–130.
28. Sondergard T, Paulsen PK. Some immediate consequences of closure of atrial septal defects of the secundum type. Circulation 1984;69:905–913.
29. Rahimtoola SH, Kirklin JW, Burchell HB. Atrial septal defect. Circulation 1968;67:2–12.
30. Pastorek JS, Allen HD, Davis JT. Current outcomes of surgical closure of secundum atrial septal defect. Am J Cardiol 1994;74:75–77.
31. Friedli B, Guerin R, Davignon A, et al. Surgical treatment of partial anomalous pulmonary venous drainage. A long-term followup study. Circulation 1972;45:159–170.

15.4 Ventricular Septal Defect

Anthony C. Chang and Jeffrey Jacobs, M.D.

A communication between the ventricles is the most common congenital heart defect. It can be an isolated defect, in association with other simple defects (atrial septal defect [ASD], patent ductus arteriosus [PDA]), or part of more complex heart defects (tetralogy of Fallot, common atrioventricular canal, double outlet right ventricle).

ANATOMY

The ventricular septum is divided into four parts: the membranous septum, and the inlet, trabecular, and outlet parts of the muscular septum.

Types of Ventricular Septal Defect

A composite of various types of ventricular septal defect (VSD) is shown in Figure 15.4.1.

Perimembranous Type

Also termed conoventricular, subaortic, infracristal, or membranous type, the perimembranous type defect is the one most commonly found. The defining characteristic is that the defect occurs directly adjacent to the membranous septum and the fibrous trigone of the heart where the aortic, mitral, and tricuspid valves are in fibrous continuity. Tricuspid valve tissue sometimes forms an aneurysm of the membranous septum, which is a mechanism of defect closure in these cases (1).

Subpulmonary Type

Also termed supracristal, infundibular, intracristal, outlet, conoseptal, conal, or doubly committed subarterial type, subpulmonary defects are located above the crista supraventricularis within the outlet septum, and they border on the semilunar valves. These defects, more common in Asians, are associated with aortic insufficiency because the aortic cusps (right or noncoronary) can prolapse into the defect itself because of loss of annular support for the aortic valve (2).

Muscular Type

Muscular types of defects can be located anywhere in the muscular septum, including apical, anterior, posterior, or midseptum inlet and outlet. The defining characteristic is that the entire rim of the defect is muscular. When multiple muscular defects are present, the term "Swiss cheese" septum is used.

Malalignment Type

Malignment type is a large defect created by "malalignment" between the infundibular septum and the

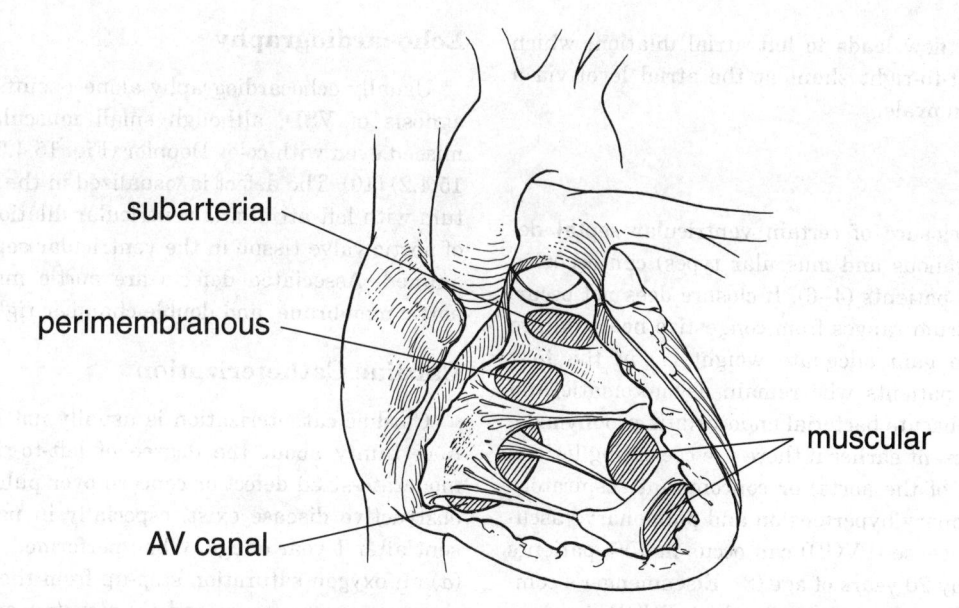

Figure 15.4.1. This composite figure shows the various types of ventricular septal defect. The perimembranous defect is adjacent to the membranous septum and can vary greatly in size. The defect may extend into the inlet, into the outlet or into the anterior muscular ventricular septum. The conduction system of the heart runs along the inferior posterior border of perimembranous defect. The tricuspid valve anulus defines the posterior border of the perimembranous defect.

The subarterial defect lies completely within the conal septum with the superior border of the defect defined by the semilunar valves. Leaflet tissue from the aortic valve can prolapse into the defect.

Muscular defects are defined by the fact that the entire rim of the defect is made up of ventricular septal muscle. The position and size of the defects may vary widely. These defects are typically defined by their position, such as apical muscular defect, anterior muscular defect, or midmuscular defect.

Malalignment defects occur in a position very similar to perimembranous defects; however, they are characterized less by an absence of ventricular septal tissue and more by the malalignment of the conal septum and trebecular muscular septum. Malalignment defects typically occur as one component of a more complex cardiac defect.

AV Canal defects or inlet type defects occur adjacent to the tricuspid and mitral valve anuli under the septal leaflet of the tricuspid valve. These defects are typically associated with the spectrum of arterioventricular canal defects. However, similar defects may occur in isolation.

trabecular muscular septum. The malalignment can be anterior displacement of the infundibular septum, which occurs in lesions such as tetralogy of Fallot, or posterior displacement in lesions such as interrupted aortic arch.

Canal Type

(Also termed "inlet" type), these defects are located posteriorly within the area confined by the tricuspid valve septal leaflet papillary muscles. The defect borders the tricuspid valve anulus.

Associated Lesions

Patent ductus arteriosus, atrial septal defect, pulmonary stenosis (valvar and subvalvar, the so-called "double chamber right ventricle"), subaortic stenosis (usually discrete membranous type), and coarctation of the aorta are associated lesions.

PATHOPHYSIOLOGY

Left-to-right shunting at the ventricular level leading left atrial dilation, left ventricular volume overload, and increased pulmonary blood flow, are pathophysiologic findings in VSD.

The degree of left-to-right shunt via the ventricular septal defect is determined by both the size of the defect and the pulmonary vascular resistance. If the VSD is *restrictive* (smaller than the aortic root diameter), the degree of shunting is determined by the size of the defect. If, however, the VSD is *unrestrictive* (no pressure gradient between right and left ventricles), then the degree of left-to-right shunting is determined by the pulmonary vascular resistance. The fall in pulmonary vascular resistance in neonates with large defects is abnormally delayed (3).

In contrast to atrial level shunting in an ASD, ventricular level shunting occurs predominantly in systole, when the atrioventricular (AV) valves are closed and the semilunar valves (aortic and pulmonary) are open. The increased pulmonary blood flow leads to left atrial dilation, which can lead to a left-to-right shunt at the atrial level via a stretched foramen ovale.

Clinical Course

Spontaneous closure of certain ventricular septal defects (perimembranous and muscular types) can occur in up to 50% of the patients (4–6). If closure does not occur, the clinical spectrum ranges from congestive heart failure and/or failure to gain adequate weight (7) in the first weeks of life to patients who remain asymptomatic and who only take subacute bacterial endocarditis prophylaxis. Patients may present earlier if there are coexisting lesions (e.g., coarctation of the aorta) or concomitant respiratory infections. Pulmonary hypertension and pulmonary vascular obstructive disease (PVOD) can occur in 15% patients with large VSD by 20 years of age (8). Eisenmenger's complex denotes a clinical condition in which PVOD develops and causes pulmonary vascular resistance to rise above systemic vascular resistance. At this point, the pulmonary artery pressures become suprasystemic causing shunting to occur from right to left, leading to cyanosis. Bacterial endocarditis in patients with VSD can occur (9).

SURGERY

Preoperative Evaluation

Physical Examination

On physical examination a systolic murmur is present that is harsh in nature and holosystolic in duration, located at the left sternal border, and it can be associated with a thrill. In addition, an early to mid-disatolic rumble at the apex signifies increased flow across the mitral valve secondary to a large left-to-right shunt. A diastolic murmur (early descrecendo type) of aortic insufficiency can also be present.

Chest Roentgenogram

On roentgenogram, cardiomegaly with an enlarged left atrium and ventricle is seen with a prominent main pulmonary artery segment and increased pulmonary vascularity.

Electrocardiography

Biventricular or left ventricular hypertrophy is usually present for large defects. Left atrial enlargement can also occur. If right ventricular hypertrophy is present, the diagnosis of subpulmonary stenosis (secondary to double chamber right ventricle) or pulmonary hypertension should be considered.

Echocardiography

Usually echocardiography alone is sufficient for the diagnosis of VSD, although small muscular type can be missed even with color Doppler (Fig. 15.4.2; see color plate 15.4.2) (10). The defect is visualized in the ventricular septum with left atrial and ventricular dilation. The presence of aortic valve tissue in the ventricular septal defect is examined. Associated defects are aortic insufficiency, subaortic membrane, and double chamber right ventricle.

Cardiac Catheterization

Cardiac catheterization is usually not indicated unless uncertainty about the degree of left-to-right shunt in a moderate-sized defect or concern over pulmonary vascular obstructive disease exist, especially in patients who present after 1 year of age. When performed, findings include (a) an oxygen saturation step-up from the right atrium to the pulmonary artery and (b) elevated pulmonary artery pressure.

Surgical Procedure

Timing

Correction is usually recommended early if the ventricular septal defect is large and symptoms and signs are found for congestive heart failure or failure to gain weight. With perimembranous and muscular defects, if the patient is compensating well, surgery can be delayed up to a year of life because spontaneous closure is possible. Because spontaneous closure does not occur with malalignment or AV canal type defects, surgery should not be delayed with these defects. Surgery in the first year of life has also been demonstrated to lead to better recovery of left ventricular mechanics (11) as well as better weight gain (12).

If the defect is not closed at the end of first year of life and pulmonary artery pressures are suspected to be half or greater than those of systemic, cardiac catheterization is performed and the VSD should be surgically closed if the shunt is more than 2:1. In patients with a small or moderate VSD who were managed medically, almost 95% remain in New York State Heart Association class I at 15 year follow-up (13). If a patient is older than 2 years of age and has evidence of elevated pulmonary vascular resistance of greater than 8 U.m^2 without response to pulmonary vasodilators, surgical correction is controversial (14). If aortic insufficiency is associated with the defect of any size, surgical closure is recommended to halt the progression of valve insufficiency (15).

Technique

Perimembranous Ventricular Septal Defect The defect is exposed via a right atriotomy and with the tricuspid valve retracted (Fig. 15.4.3). The VSD is visualized by looking

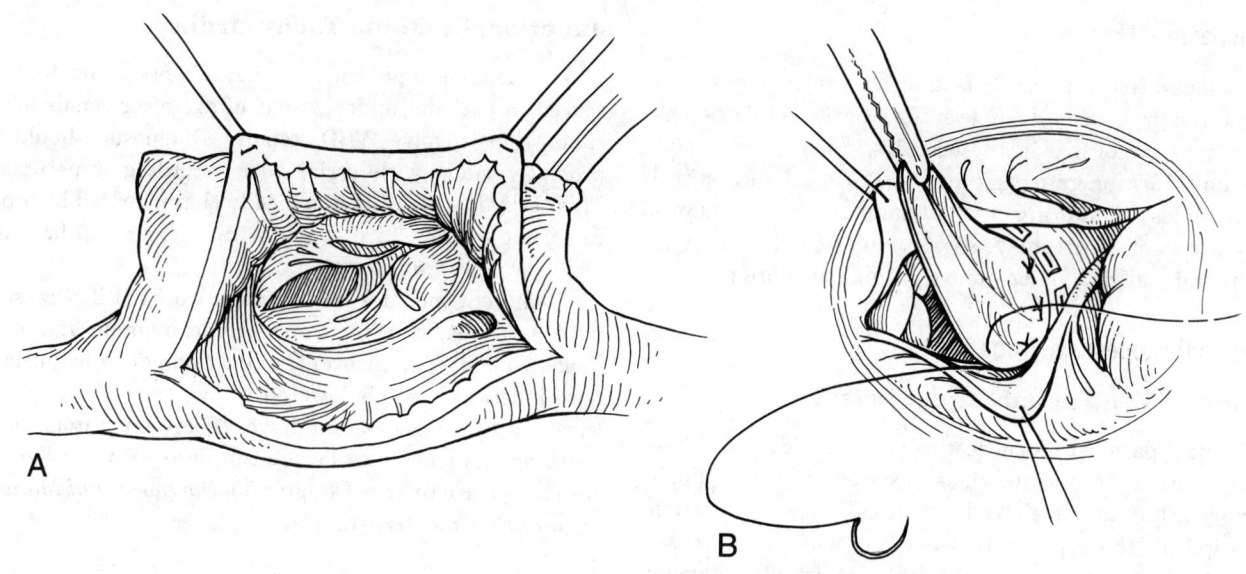

Figure 15.4.3. Repair of Perimembranous VSD. Cardiopulmonary bypass with moderate hypothermia and cardioplegic arrest are utilized. The typical perimembranous VSD is approached surgically through a right atrial incision. The surgeon then visualizes the defect by looking through the tricuspid valve onto the right ventricular aspect of the ventricular septum, which is adjacent to the commissure formed by the anterior and septal leaflets of the tricuspid valve. The tricuspid leaflets are retracted to expose the rim of the defect which is partially made up of the anulus of the tricuspid valve itself. The remainder of the rim of the defect is ventricular muscle. The superior rim of the perimembranous defect is very close to the aortic valve anulus and injury to the aortic valve must be avoided. The posterior and inferior rim of the defect is very close the conduction system and deep sutures in this area must be avoided in order to prevent surgically induced heart block. Various patch materials can be used to close the defect using either interrupted sutures or a running suture technique.

through the tricuspid valve orifice to the right ventricular aspect of the interventricular septum. The septal leaflet of the tricuspid valve is partially detached if necessary. The defect is closed with a patch using interrupted pledgeted sutures or a running suture. Care must be taken to avoid the conduction system which is situated close to the defect. The tricuspid valve is then repaired if necessary.

Subpulmonary Ventricular Septal Defect The defect is closed via an approach from the pulmonary artery via a pulmonary arteriotomy or from the infundibulum of the right ventricle via a small horizontal infundibulotomy. Sutures are placed in the fibrous tissue between the great arteries or within the sinuses of the pulmonary artery to secure the patch (16).

Muscular Ventricular Septal Defect The midmuscular defect (17) is exposed via a right atriotomy and the defect is closed using a patch with interrupted pledgeted sutures. Care must be taken to avoid the conduction system. Left ventriculotomy for closure of apical VSDs is controversial because it may be associated with left ventricular aneurysms and late dysfunction. Catheter device closure with an umbrella is an alternative approach to these defects (18). With anterior or apical muscular VSD, an approach via a right ventriculotomy may sometimes be preferred to exposure through a right atriotomy and tricuspid valve orifice.

Malalignment Type For information, see under other lesions.

AV Canal Type The defect is closed via an approach from the right atrium, looking through the tricuspid valve orifice.

Other Surgical Procedures

Pulmonary Artery Banding For multiple muscular type VSD, surgical correction is more difficult because of exposure. An alternative intervention is pulmonary artery banding. Pulmonary artery banding may also be preferable in the patient with active infectious pneumonitis (to avoid cardiopulmonary bypass and further lung parenchymal insult).

Mortality

Mortality is less than 5% (19, 20), and it was 8% in an earlier series with repair during the first year of life (21). The morbidity and mortality may be higher for children with multiple muscular VSD and associated lesions.

Postoperative Management

Postoperative care of patients after ventricular septal defect repair is usually uneventful. Early extubation is sometimes performed in the operating room or intensive care unit. Ideal monitoring consists of arterial and central venous lines. Monitoring of left atrial pressure and pulmonary artery pressure may also be indicated. In addition, atrial and ventricular temporary pacing wires are placed.

Specific Postoperative Problems

Residual Ventricular Septal Defect

Clinical parameters suggestive of a significant residual VSD after surgery include sinus tachycardia, elevated pulmonary artery and left atrial pressures, oxygen saturation step-up from the superior vena cava or right atrium to the pulmonary artery of more than 10%, persistent metabolic acidosis, oliguria, cardiomegaly, pulmonary edema, and a heart murmur (22). A residual defect may not be well tolerated postoperatively because of the myocardial dysfunction usually observed after cardiopulmonary bypass (23).

Inotropic and mechanical ventilatory support may need to be escalated to maintain adequate systemic cardiac output. If the residual VSD is deemed significant, however, reoperation should be pursued without delay.

Pulmonary Hypertension

Pulmonary hypertension found postoperatively may be caused by residual VSD, postoperative changes in pulmonary vascular resistance, or undiagnosed branch pulmonary artery stenosis. Episodic elevation of pulmonary artery pressures suggests postoperative pulmonary hypertension. Assessment for residual or previously undiagnosed defects must be done prior to or simultaneously with institution of specific therapy for pulmonary hypertension. (For treatment, please refer to Chapter 32, *Pulmonary Hypertension*.)

Heart Block

A postoperative complication, heart block can occur in up to 10% of patients after VSD closure. The bundle of His courses posterior-inferiorly to the perimembranous defect. It is more common after perimembranous type VSD closure (but uncommon after muscular or subpulmonary type defect closures) (24). Heart block is also particularly common after repair of a canal type VSD with straddling of the tricuspid valve. The conduction problem may be transient and mainly caused by edema near sutured areas.

Treatment involves atrioventricular synchronous temporary pacing, but it is usually prudent to wait at least 7 days before implantation of a permanent pacemaker.

Junctional Ectopic Tachycardia

Junctional ectopic tachycardia is more commonly observed in patients under 1 year of age after repair for lesions that involve VSD repair. Diagnosis should be promptly made with atrial wire recording if necessary. This tachydysrhythmia is typically characterized by a narrow complex tachycardia with a rate above 150 bpm and atrioventricular dissociation.

Treatment includes hypothermia (to 34°C if necessary) with paralysis, and intravenous procainamide and/or esmolol. In addition, atrioventricular pacing can be initiated once junctional rate is lowered to less than 150 bpm. Because catecholamines can have effects on automaticity, these agents should be lowered in dose. (For further discussion, please refer to Chapter 30, *Diagnosis and Management of Cardiac Arrhythmias*).

POSTOPERATIVE CARE CHECKLIST

Postoperative care checklist includes:

- Monitor pulmonary artery pressures for pulmonary hypertension and rule out residual VSD in a timely fashion.
- If patient shows signs of low cardiac output, assessment for a residual or previously undiagnosed defect must be aggressively pursued.

REFERENCES

1. Freedom RM, White RD, Pieroni DR et al. The natural history of the so-called aneurysm of the membranous ventricular septum in childhood. Circulation 1974;49:375–384.
2. Rhodes L, Keane JF, Fellows KE et al. Long followup (up to 43 years) of ventricular septal defect with audible aortic regurgitation. Am J Cardiol 1990;66:340–345.
3. Rudolph AM. The effects of postnatal circulatory adjustments in congenital heart disease. Pediatrics 1965;36:763–772.
4. Moe DG, Guntheroth WG. Spontaneous closure of uncomplicated ventricular septal defect. Am J Cardiol 1987;60:674–678.
5. Ramaciotti C, Keren A, Silverman NH. Importance of perimembranous ventricular septal aneurysm in the natural history of isolated perimembranous ventricular septal defect. Am J Cardiol 1986;57:268–272.
6. Ramaciotti C, Vetter JM, Bornemeier RA, Chin AJ. Prevalence, relation to spontaneous closure, and association of muscular ventricular septal defects with other cardiac defects. Am J Cardiol 1995;75:61–65.
7. Levy RJ, Rosenthal A, Miettinen OS et al. Determinants of growth in patients with ventricular septal defects. Circulation 1978;57:793–797.
8. Hoffman JIE, Rudolph AM, Heymann MA. Pulmonary vascular disease with congenital heart lesions: pathologic features and causes. Circulation 1981;64:873–877.
9. Ellis JH, Moodie DS, Sterba R et al. Ventricular septal defect in the adult: natural and unnatural history. Am Heart J 1987;114:115–120.

10. Helmcke F, Souza A, Nanda NC et al. Two-dimensional and color Doppler assessment of ventricular septal defect of congenital origin. Am J Cardiol 1989;63:1112–1116.
11. Cordell D, Graham TP, Atwood GF, Boerth RC, Boucek RJ, Bender HW. Left heart volume characteristics following ventricular septal defect closure in infancy. Circulation 1976;54:294–298.
12. Weintraub RG, Menahem S. Early surgical closure of a large ventricular septal defect: influence on long term growth. J Am Coll Cardiol 1991;18:552–558.
13. Kidd L, Driscoll DJ, Gersony WM et al. Second natural history study of congenital heart defects: results of treatment of patients with ventricular septal defects. Circulation 1993;87(suppl I):138–151.
14. Neutze JM, Ishikawa T, Clarkson PM, Calder AI, Barratt-Boyes BG, Kerr AR. Assessment and followup of patients with ventricular septal defect and elevated pulmonary vascular resistance. Am J Cardiol 1989;63:327–331.
15. Karpawich PP, Duff DF, Mullins CE, Cooley DA, McNamara DG. Ventricular septal defect with associated aortic valve insufficiency. J Thorac Cardiovasc Surg 1981;82:182–189.
16. Backer CL, Idriss FS, Zales VR et al. Surgical management of the conal (supracristal) ventricular septal defect. J Thorac Cardiovasc Surg 1991;102:288–296.
17. Serraf A, Lacour Gayet F, Bruniaux J et al. Surgical management of isolated multiple ventricular septal defects. J Thorac Cardiovasc Surg 1992;103:437–443.
18. Lock JE, Block PC, McKay RG et al. Transcatheter closure of ventricular septal defects. Circulation 1988;78:361–368.
19. Okita Y, Miki S, Kusuhara K et al. Long term results of aortic valvuloplasty for aortic regurgitation associated with ventricular septal defect. J Thorac Cardiovasc Surg 1988;96:769–774.
20. Hardin JT, Muskett AD, Canter CE, Martin TC, Spray TL. Primary surgical closure of large ventricular septal defects in small infants. Ann Thorac Surg 1992;53:397–401.
21. Yeager SB, Freed MD, Keane JF et al. Primary surgical closure of ventricular septal defect in the first year of life: results in 128 infants. J Am Coll Cardiol 1984;3:1269–1276.
22. Vincent RN, Lang P, Dhipman CW et al. Assessment of hemodynamic status in the intensive care unit immediately after closure of ventricular septal defect. Am J Cardiol 1985;55:526–529.
23. Cyran SE, Hannon DW, Daniels SR et al. Predictors of postoperative ventricular dysfunction in infants who have undergone primary repair of ventricular septal defect. Am Heart J 1987;113:1144–1148.
24. Blake RS, Chung EE, Wesley H et al. Conduction defects, ventricular arrhythmias, and late death after surgical closure of ventricular septal defects. Br Heart J 1982;47:305–315.

15.5 Common Atrioventricular Canal

Anthony C. Chang, MD, and
Redmond P. Burke, MD

Also called an "endocardial cushion defect" or "atrioventricular septal defect," common atrioventricular canal involves a single atrioventricular annulus that drains both atria, and it is common in children with Down's syndrome.

ANATOMY

The endocardial cushions, derived from mesenchymal tissue, form the atrioventricular valves and the septum of the atrioventricular canal. The normally formed atrioventricular canal septum merges with the lower part of the atrial septum and the upper part of the ventricular septum, thereby partitioning the two atria and the two ventricles and also separating tricuspid and mitral valves. When these cushions fail to fuse, common atrioventricular canal results.

Three basic potential components are found in this defect: (*a*) an ostium primum defect creating an interatrial communication, (*b*) an interventricular communication in the inlet portion of the ventricles, and (*c*) abnormal formation of the atrioventricular valves.

Types of Common Atrioventricular Canal Defect

Partial Atrioventricular Canal Defect, or Ostium Primum Defect

Also termed "incomplete" atrioventricular canal, partial atrioventricular canal defect is an interatrial communication associated with a cleft in the anterior leaflet of the left atrioventricular valve and usually some degree of left atrioventricular valve insufficiency. No interventricular communication exists; two separate atrioventricular valves are present (Fig. 15.5.1).

"Transitional" Atrioventricular Canal Defect

In the transitional atrioventricular canal defect variant, an ostium primum defect is present and the atrioventricular valves may only be partially separated into two valves. Dense attachments of the chordae to the crest of the muscular septum are such that the interventricular communication may be small or moderate, often with multiple individual communications.

Complete Atrioventricular Canal Defect

Present in the complete atrioventricular canal defect variant are an ostium primum defect, a large (nonrestrictive) interventricular communication, and a large common

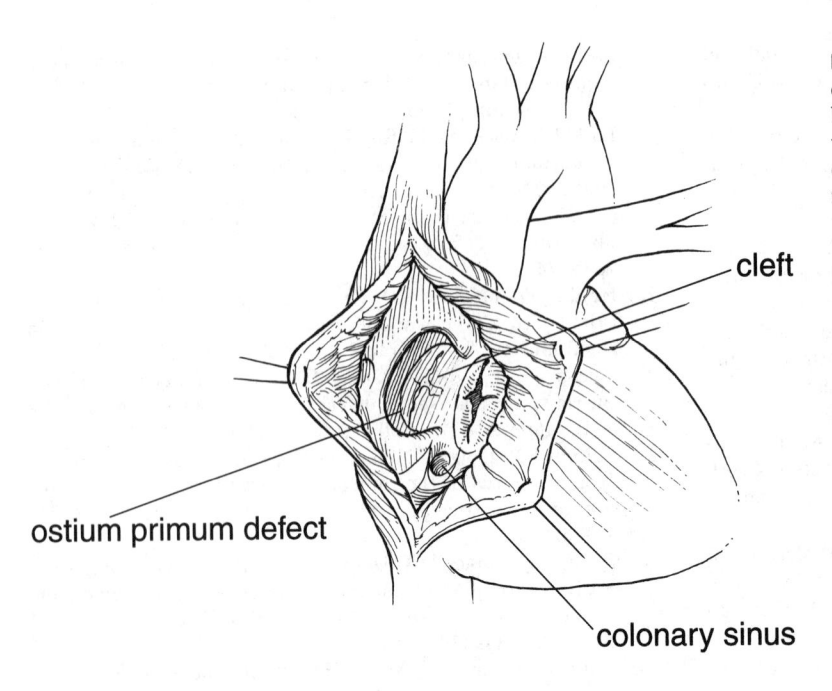

Figure 15.5.1. Anatomy of partial atrioventricular (AV) canal defect. A longitudinal right atrial incision has been made with retraction of the atrial tissue to reveal the intra-atrial and atrioventricular canal anatomy. The most common form of partial AV canal is illustrated. Note the large ostium primum defect that provides unrestricted communication between the left and right atria. The anterior margin of this defect is made up by the adjacent portions of the left and right AV valve anuli. The septal leaflets of both the left and right AV valves are abnormally formed. Most typically, a deep cleft is found in the anterior (septal) leaflet of the left-sided AV valve. The coronary sinus is displaced inferiorly. The conduction bundle, which is not shown in the illustration, is also displaced inferiorly. The "gooseneck" deformity of the left ventricular outflow tract is usually present in partial AV canal defects; however, it is typically less severe than in more complete forms of AV canal defect.

(single) atrioventricular valve. Rastelli A, B, and C forms of atrioventricular canal defect are recognized (Fig. 15.5.2). This anatomic classification scheme relates the superior atrioventricular valve leaflet cordal attachments to the crest of the ventricular septum (1). In type A, the superior leaflet cords are attached to the crest of the interventricular septum. In type B, the superior leaflet cords are inserted into the papillary muscle in the right ventricle. In type C, the superior leaflet is described as "free-floating" and therefore the cords do not attach to the ventricular septum at all.

Other Anatomic Notes

Just as an ostium primum defect does not have a ventricular component, an interventricular defect of the endocardial cushion type without an ostium primum defect can also exist. In addition, ventricular hypoplasia of either the right or left ventricle may exist and preclude a biventricular repair (2). An isolated cleft in the left atrioventricular valve without atrial or ventricular communications may also exist.

The term "override" denotes anatomic arrangement with the atrioventricular valve annulus presiding over the ventricular septum, and the term "straddling" denotes having chordae attach to the "other" ventricular side of the septum.

Associated Lesions

Patent ductus arteriosus, tetralogy of Fallot, coarctation of the aorta, subaortic stenosis, left superior vena cava, and asplenia or polysplenia are associated lesions.

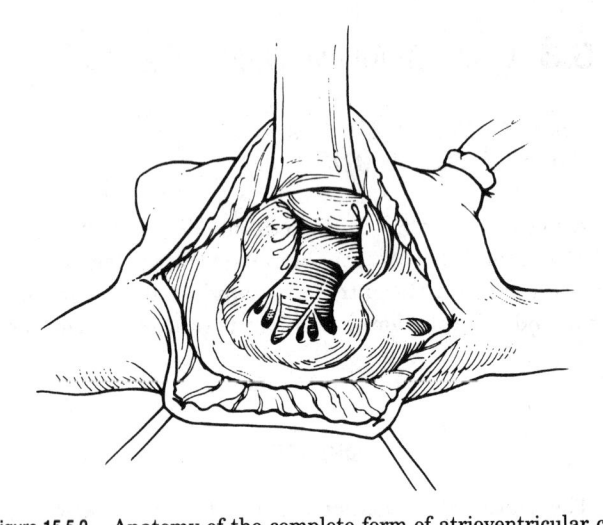

Figure 15.5.2. Anatomy of the complete form of atrioventricular canal defect. A longitudinal right atriotomy has been performed and the atrial free wall edges have been retracted. Note that there is one large atrioventricular valve ring. On the atrial side of the valve is seen a large ostium primum defect. On the ventricular side of the valve is seen a large interventricular communication as well. The coronary sinus is displaced inferiorly along with the conduction bundle. Note that the valve leaflets on the inferior and superior side of the anulus straddle the ventricular septum, with components of the leaflets in both the left and right ventricles. These are the superior and inferior bridging leaflets. The Rastelli classification of complete atrioventricular canal defects is based on the position of the cordal attachments of the superior bridging leaflet. A, B, and C forms are recognized. A "gooseneck" deformity of the left ventricular outflow tract is also present in essentially all cases of complete atrioventricular canal defect.

PATHOPHYSIOLOGY

In the partial form of atrioventricular canal (ostium primum defect), the pathophysiology resembles that of secundum atrial septal defect, unless significant left atrioventricular valve regurgitation is present. In the complete form of atrioventricular canal, the pathophysiology resembles that of a ventricular septal defect with an associated atrial septal defect, with left-to-right shunting at both atrial and ventricular levels leading to biatrial and biventricular volume overload. If atrioventricular valve regurgitation is present, it could worsen the ventricular volume overload.

Clinical Course

In ostium primum defect, congestive heart failure and failure to gain weight usually occur after infancy unless mitral regurgitation or left-sided hypoplasia is severe. In addition, frequent pulmonary infections can occur. In complete atrioventricular canal, congestive heart failure is common by 2 months of age. Other symptoms include failure to gain weight and recurrent respiratory infections. Pulmonary hypertension and irreversible pulmonary vascular obstructive disease can occur by 1 year of age (3). Down's syndrome children may have upper airway obstruction and pulmonary hypoplasia as contributing factors for elevated pulmonary vascular resistance (4), but it is uncertain whether these children have a higher likelihood of developing pulmonary vascular obstructive disease at an earlier age compared with those children with normal chromosomes (5).

SURGERY

Preoperative Evaluation

Physical Examination

A systolic regurgitant murmur of atrioventricular valve regurgitation can be heard in the lower left sternal border or at the apical area. A hyperactive precordium may be present. P_2 can be loud.

Chest Roentgenogram

Cardiomegaly with enlarged atria and ventricles is seen with a prominent main pulmonary artery segment and increased pulmonary vascularity.

Electrocardiography

The QRS axis is leftward and superior at −30 to −150 (with Q waves in leads I and aVL and deep S wave in aVF). Biatrial and biventricular hypertrophy can be present.

Echocardiography

Atrioventricular canal has a cleft in the anterior leaflet of the left atrioventricular valve, characterized by a break in continuity of the atrioventricular valve. In ostium primum defect, the lower atrial septum is absent. In complete atrioventricular canal, attention is given to the atrioventricular valve morphology and degree of regurgitation (Fig. 15.5.3). Particular issues such as the morphology of the papillary muscles, valve attachments to the crest of the ventricular septum, and presence of ventricular hypoplasia and subaortic narrowing can be delineated by echocardiography.

Cardiac Catheterization

Cardiac catheterization is usually not indicated for ostium primum defects. For complete common atrioventricular canal, cardiac catheterization is usually not indicated in patients younger than 4 months of age if echocardiographic findings are thought to be definitive. However, if morphologic questions remain, the patients's clinical course is atypical, or the patient is older than 6 months, catheterization may be necessary.

When performed, cardiac catheterization findings include (a) 75 to 85% oxygen saturation in the atria and ventricles and (b) systemic pressure in both the right ventricle and the pulmonary arteries. On left ventriculography, the gooseneck deformity of the elongated and narrowed left ventricular outflow tract is classically seen.

Surgical Procedure

Timing

For ostium primum defects, surgery has been traditionally recommended when the patient is 3 to 5 years of age; however, many groups now perform elective repair in infants 1 to 2 years of age. Postponement of surgery in patients with left atrioventricular valve regurgitation, however, has been associated with valve damage and less satisfactory postoperative left atrioventricular valve function.

For complete atrioventricular canal defect, the ideal age for surgery remains controversial. Because a potential need exists for left atrioventricular valve valvuloplasty and, rarely, valve replacement, early elective repair in patients less than 3 months of age may be less advisable. Otherwise, surgery should probably be performed between 3 and 6 months of life, particularly in children with Down's syndrome (6).

With these defects, if left atrioventricular valve insufficiency is moderate to severe and left ventricular function is suboptimal, preoperative inotropic support may be indicated.

Figure 15.5.3. Apical four-chamber view from an infant with common atrioventricular canal. Both a primum type atrial septal defect (*ASD I*) and a canal type ventricular septal defect (*VSD*) are depicted with *arrows*. RA, right atrium; LA, left atrium; RV, right ventricle; LV, left ventricle.

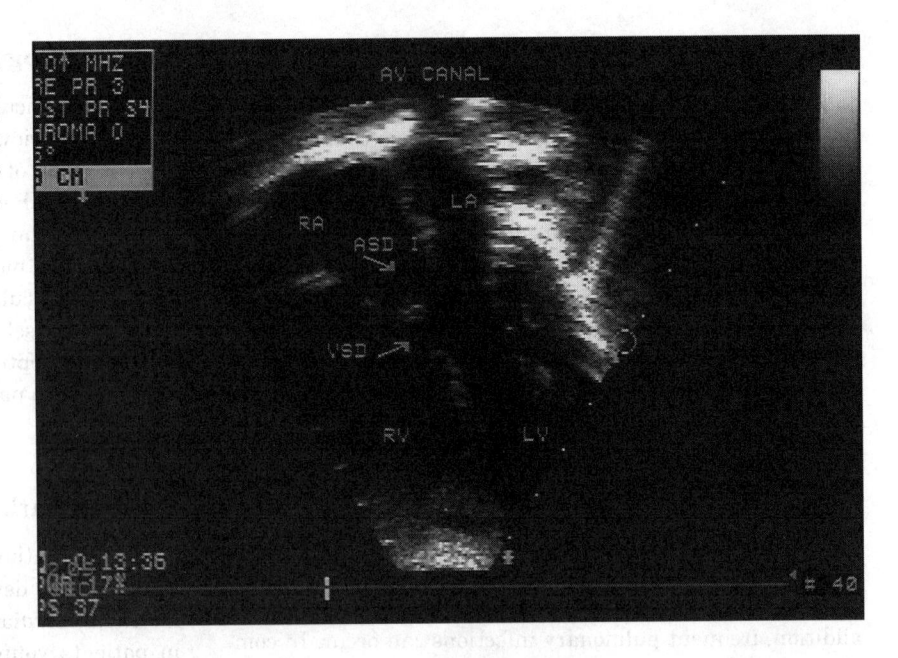

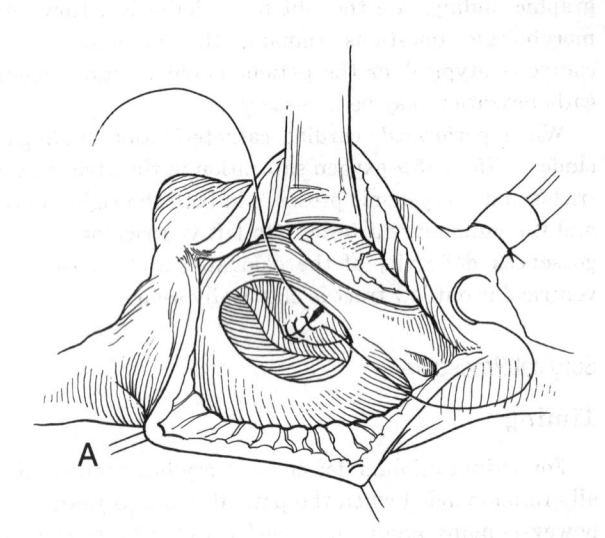

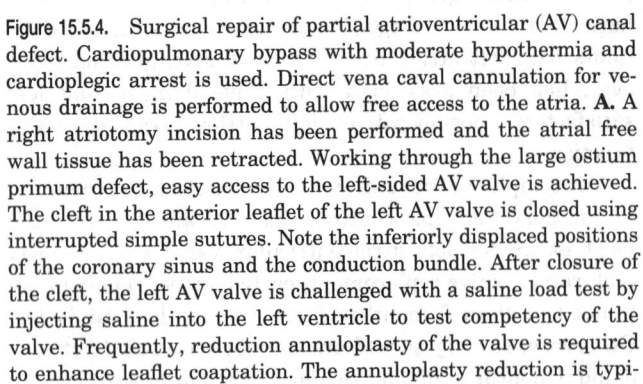

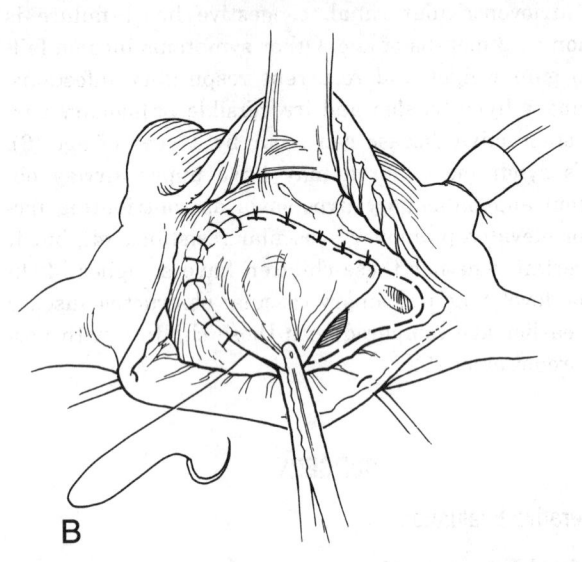

Figure 15.5.4. Surgical repair of partial atrioventricular (AV) canal defect. Cardiopulmonary bypass with moderate hypothermia and cardioplegic arrest is used. Direct vena caval cannulation for venous drainage is performed to allow free access to the atria. **A.** A right atriotomy incision has been performed and the atrial free wall tissue has been retracted. Working through the large ostium primum defect, easy access to the left-sided AV valve is achieved. The cleft in the anterior leaflet of the left AV valve is closed using interrupted simple sutures. Note the inferiorly displaced positions of the coronary sinus and the conduction bundle. After closure of the cleft, the left AV valve is challenged with a saline load test by injecting saline into the left ventricle to test competency of the valve. Frequently, reduction annuloplasty of the valve is required to enhance leaflet coaptation. The annuloplasty reduction is typically performed where the base of the commissures meets the anulus. After satisfactory reconstruction of the left AV valve, the ostium primum defect is closed with a patch. Various materials can be used. However, Dacron and other materials with a relatively rough surface are avoided because such materials have been associated with severe hemolysis caused by a jet of left AV valve regurgitation impacting on the patch, leading to red cell trauma. Depending on surgeon preference, the patch can be placed around the defect alone or it may encompass the coronary sinus as well, allowing the coronary sinus to drain into the left atrium. In some cases this latter technique can avoid injury to the conduction system with more certainty. In the illustration shown in **B**, the patch is placed directly around the rim of the defect, allowing the coronary sinus to drain physiologically into the right atrium.

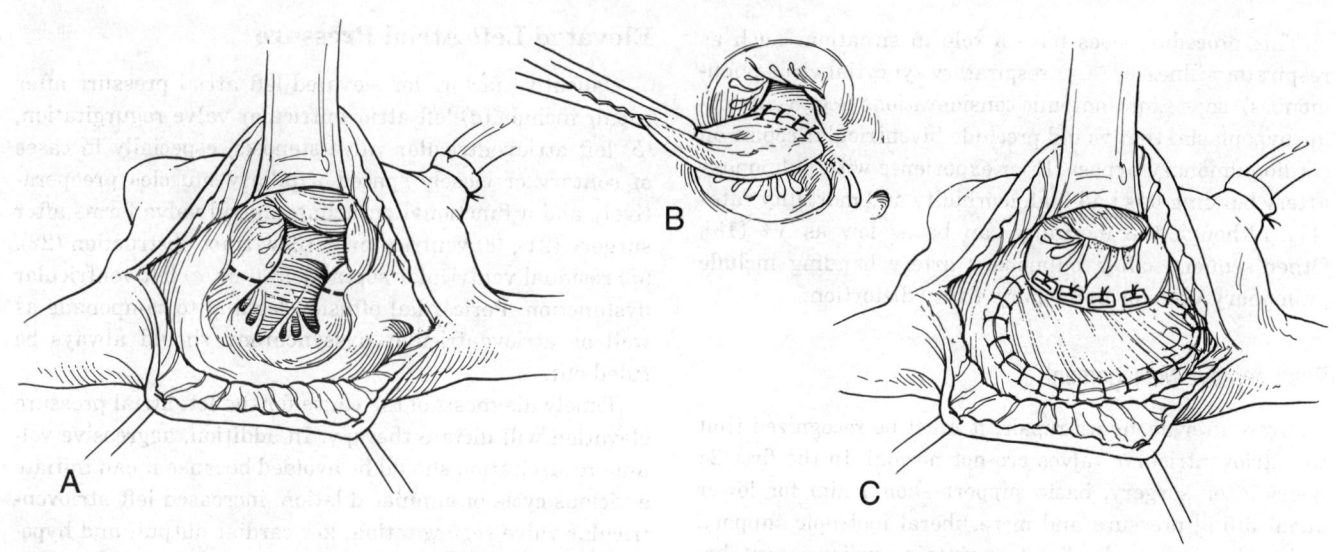

Figure 15.5.5. Surgical repair of complete atrioventricular (AV) canal defect. The "single patch" and "double patch" repair techniques have been described. The "single patch" technique is shown here. The repair proceeds using cardiopulmonary bypass and either moderate or deep hypothermia with cardioplegic arrest. Deep hypothermic circulatory arrest use depends on surgeon preference. Exposure of the AV canal is achieved through a longitudinal right atriotomy as shown in **A**. The *broken lines* show the incisions in the superior and inferior bridging leaflets. These incisions parallel the crest of the ventricular septum and divide the bridging leaflets into left ventricular and right ventricular components. Following this a patch, typically of pericardium, is placed along the crest of the interventricular septum to obliterate the interventricular communication. As this suture line proceeds it approaches the AV valve ring on both the superior and inferior aspects as shown in **B**. The cut edges of the superior and inferior bridging leaflets on both the left and right ventricular sides are then attached to the patch with interrupted pledgeted sutures as shown in **C**. Finally, the patch is sewn to the edge of the ostium primum defect to obliterate the interatrial communication created by the ostium primum defect. As shown in **C**, the atrial component of the patch passes around the coronary sinus allowing the coronary sinus to drain to the left atrium. Following completion of the reconstruction the atrial incision is closed and the patient is weaned from cardiopulmonary bypass.

Technique

In ostium primum defect, repair is always performed via median sternotomy with cardiopulmonary bypass; a right atriotomy incision is used (Fig. 15.5.4). The edges of the cleft in the left atrioventricular valve are approximated with interrupted sutures and tested for valve competency.

The interatrial communication is sometimes closed with autologous pericardial patch to avoid the possibility of synthetic material-induced hemolysis in the event of significant mitral regurgitation. Carpentier has suggested an alternative approach to repair of the mitral valve without closing the cleft (7); however, this is not widely accepted, especially in infants.

In complete atrioventricular canal, a right atriotomy is performed. One or two patches (8) are used to repair the defect (Fig. 15.5.5). The common atrioventricular valve is separated into right and left valves, and the left-sided cleft is closed. The patch is sutured to the top of the interventricular septum to close the interventricular communication and the valve leaflets are then attached to the patch. The ostium primum defect is then patch closed as well. A valve annuloplasty (or a left atrioventricular valve prosthesis) or pericardial patch augmentation may be necessary to achieve valve competence (9, 10).

If common atrioventricular canal is associated with a lesion such as tetralogy of Fallot, the surgical technique combines features of both lesions (11).

Mortality

For primum atrial septal defect, mortality is considered to be less than 5% with late postoperative residua of residual left atrioventricular valve regurgitation in about 10% of patients (12). Mortality rate may be higher if left ventricular hypoplasia is present. For complete atrioventricular canal correction, mortality in the first year of life has been reported to be about 10% (13, 14), although the hospital mortality in the first 6 months of life has recently decreased to less than 2% (15).

Other Surgical Procedures

Pulmonary Artery Banding Pulmonary artery banding can serve as an adequate palliative surgery for common atrioventricular canal (16); however, it is recommended in only a few specific situations. Pulmonary artery banding is performed without cardiopulmonary bypass via a lateral thoracotomy.

This procedure does have a role in situations such as respiratory illnesses (e.g., respiratory syncytial virus pneumonitis), sepsis, or anatomic considerations (e.g., ventricular hypoplasia) that would preclude biventricular repair on cardiopulmonary bypass. Prior experience with pulmonary artery banding has had high morbidity and mortality rates (17), although the mortality can be as low as 5% (18). Other sequelae after pulmonary artery banding include pulmonary valve or pulmonary artery distortion.

Postoperative Management

Even after adequate repair, it must be recognized that the atrioventricular valves are not normal. In the first 24 hours after surgery, basic support should aim for lower atrial filling pressure and more liberal inotropic support, rather than volume loading to maintain cardiac output, because volume loading can encourage atrioventricular valve regurgitation.

Ideal monitoring consists of arterial, central venous pressure, left atrial pressure, and pulmonary artery pressure lines. In addition, atrial and ventricular temporary pacing wires are placed.

Specific Postoperative Problems

Pulmonary Hypertension

The incidence of postoperative pulmonary hypertension is high, and it is correlated with older patient age at operation. These episodes are related to immediate postoperative mortality (19). It is important to rule out anatomic causes of elevated pulmonary artery pressure that mimic pulmonary hypertension, such as severe left atrioventricular valve regurgitation or stenosis and residual ventricular septal defect. Evidence also indicates that postoperative pulmonary vascular resistance is higher in children with Down's syndrome than those without (20). (For treatment, please refer to Chapter 32, *Pulmonary Hypertension*.)

Low Cardiac Output

The single most important concern is dehiscence of the repair of the left atrioventricular valve. Other possibilities include residual ventricular septal defect (see Chapter 15.4, *Ventricular Septal Defect*). The incidence of reoperation for residual left atrioventricular valve regurgitation can be as high as 5 to 10%, and it is associated as a risk factor for death.

Because severe left atrioventricular valve regurgitation can lead to annular dilation and more atrioventricular valve regurgitation, aggressive afterload reduction is mandatory. If the patient is hemodynamically unstable, the strategy should involve reoperation without delay.

Elevated Left Atrial Pressure

Causative factors for elevated left atrial pressure after repair include (*a*) left atrioventricular valve regurgitation, (*b*) left atrioventricular valve stenosis, especially in cases of solitary or closely spaced papillary muscles preoperatively and a functional parachute mitral valve forms after surgery (21), (*c*) ventricular outflow tract obstruction (22), (*d*) residual ventricular septal defect, or (*e*) left ventricular dysfunction. Pericardial effusion leading to tamponade as well as atrioventricular dyssynchrony should always be ruled out.

Timely diagnosis of the cause for the left atrial pressure elevation will dictate therapy. In addition, aggressive volume resuscitation should be avoided because it can initiate a vicious cycle of annular dilation, increased left atrioventricular valve regurgitation, low cardiac output, and hypotension. Reoperation may be necessary in selected cases.

Heart Block

The atrioventricular node is in a different position in a patient with atrioventricular canal (23). In addition, sinoatral node dysfunction is common in atrioventricular canal defects, and complete heart block can occur after surgery (24).

Atrial pacing can improve cardiac output if sinoatrial node dysfunction is present. In addition, atrioventricular sequential pacing is necessary with heart block, and it is preferable to ventricular pacing alone because left atrioventricular valve regurgitation may worsen with sole ventricular pacing.

Residual Ventricular Septal Defect

See Chapter 15.4, *Ventricular Septal Defect*.

Junctional Ectopic Tachycardia

See Chapter 13, *Ventricular Septal Defect*, and Chapter 30, *Diagnosis and Management of Cardiac Arrhythmias*.

POSTOPERATIVE CARE CHECKLIST

Postoperative care checklist includes:

- Avoid overaggressive volume resuscitation.
- Monitor pulmonary artery pressures for pulmonary hypertension and rule out significant left atrioventricular valve regurgitation.
- Hemodynamic deterioration anytime after repair if severe left atrioventricular valve regurgitation until proved otherwise.

REFERENCES

1. Rastelli GC, Kirklin JW, Titus JL. Anatomic observations on the complete form of persistent common atrioventricular canal with special reference to atrioventricular valves. Mayo Clin Proc 1966;41:296–308.
2. Cohen MS, Jacobs ML, Weinberg PM, et al. Morphometric analysis of unbalanced common atrioventricular canal using two dimensional echocardiography. J Am Coll Cardiol 1996;28:1017–1023.
3. Newfeld EA, Sher M, Paul MH, et al. Pulmonary vascular disease in complete atrioventricular canal defect. Am J Cardiol 1977;39:721–726.
4. Cooney TP, Thurlbeck WM. Pulmonary hypoplasia in Down's syndrome. N Engl J Med 1982;307:1170–1173.
5. Clapp S, Perry BL, Farooki ZQ, et al. Down syndrome, complete atrioventricular canal, and pulmonary vascular obstructive disease. J Thorac Cardiovasc Surg 1990;100:115–121.
6. Yamaki S, Yasui H, Kado H, et al. Pulmonary vascular disease and operative indications in complete atrioventricular canal defect in early infancy. J Thorac Cardiovasc Surg 1993;106:398–405.
7. Carpentier A. Surgical anatomy and management of the mitral component of atrioventricular canal defects. In: Anderson RH, Shinebourne EA, eds. Pediatric cardiology. Edinburgh: Churchill Livingstone 1978:477–490.
8. Weintraub RG, Brawn WJ, Venables AW, et al. Two-patch repair of complete atrioventricular septal defect in the first year of life: results and sequential assessment of atrioventricular valve function. J Thorac Cardiovasc Surg 1990;99:320–326.
9. Capouya ER, Laks H, Drinkwater DC, et al. Management of the left atrioventricular valve in the repair of complete atrioventricular septal defects. J Thorac Cardiovasc Surg 1992;104:196–203.
10. van Son JA, Van Praagh R, Falk V, et al. Pericardial patch augmentation of the tissue deficient mitral valve in common atrioventricular canal. J Thorac Cardiovas Surg 1996;112:1117–1119.
11. Vargas FJ, Coto ED, Mayer JE, et al. Complete atrioventricular canal and tetralogy of Fallot: surgical considerations. Ann Thorac Surg 1986;42:258–265.
12. King RM, Puga FJ, Danielson GK, et al. Prognostic factors and surgical treatment of partial atrioventricular canal. Circulation 1986;74(Suppl 1):142–146.
13. Bender HW Jr, Hammon JW, Hubbard SG, et al. Repair of atrioventricular canal malformation in the first year of life. J Thorac Cardiovasc Surg 1982;84:515–522.
14. Chin AJ, Keane JF, Norwood WI, et al. Repair of complete common atrioventricular canal in infancy. J Thorac Cardiovasc Surg 1982;84:437–445.
15. Hanley FL, Fenton K, Mayer JE, et al. Repair of atrioventricular canal defects in infancy: twenty year trends. J Thorac Cardiovasc Surg 1993;106:387–397.
16. Epstein ML, Moller JH, Amplatz KK, et al. Pulmonary artery banding in infants with complete atrioventricular canal. J Thorac Cardiovasc Surg 1979;78:28–31.
17. Bender HW, Hammon JW, Hubbard SC, et al. Repair of atrioventricular canal malformation in the first year of life. J Thorac Cardiovasc Surg 1982;84:515–522.
18. Silverman NH, Levitsky S, Fisher E, et al. Efficacy of pulmonary artery banding in infants with complete atrioventricular canal. Circulation 1983;68(Suppl 2):II-148–II-1153.
19. Pozzi M, Remig J, Fimmers R, et al. Atrioventricular septal defects: analysis of short and medium term results. J Thorac Cardiovasc Surg 1991;101:138–142.
20. Morris CD, Magilke D, Reller M. Down's syndrome affects results of surgical correction of complete atrioventricular canal. Pediatr Cardiol 1992;13:80–84.
21. Tandon R, Moller JH, Edwards JE. Single papillary muscle of the left ventricle associated with persistent common atrioventricular canal: variant of parachute mitral valve. Pediatr Cardiol 1986; 7:111–114.
22. Chang CI, Becker AE. Surgical anatomy of left ventricular outflow tract obstruction in complete atrioventricular septal defect: a concept for operative repair. J Thorac Cardiovasc Surg 1987;94:897–903.
23. Bharati S, Lev M, McAllister HA, et al. Surgical anatomy of the atrioventricular valve in the intermediate type of common atrioventricular orifice. J Thorac Cardiovasc Surg 1980;79:884–892.
24. Portman MA, Beder SD, Ankeney JL, et al. A 20-year review of ostium primum defect repair in children. Am Heart J 1985;110:1054–1062.

15.6 Anomalous Pulmonary Venous Connection

Anthony C. Chang, MD, and
Redmond P. Burke, MD

Total anomalous pulmonary venous connection is a congenital defect in which all of the pulmonary veins drain anomalously into a systemic venous structure rather than directly into the left atrium. This chapter focuses primarily on total anomalous pulmonary venous connection.

ANATOMY

Embryologically, the pulmonary veins misconnect with a venous compartment rather than with the left atrium. A common collecting reservoir called "the pulmonary venous confluence" is usually found.

Types of Total Anomalous Pulmonary Venous Connection

Supracardiac

In the supracardiac type of venous connection the common pulmonary venous confluence drains into the innominate vein via a vertical vein (and then into the right atrium), or it drains directly into the superior vena cava (Fig. 15.6.1).

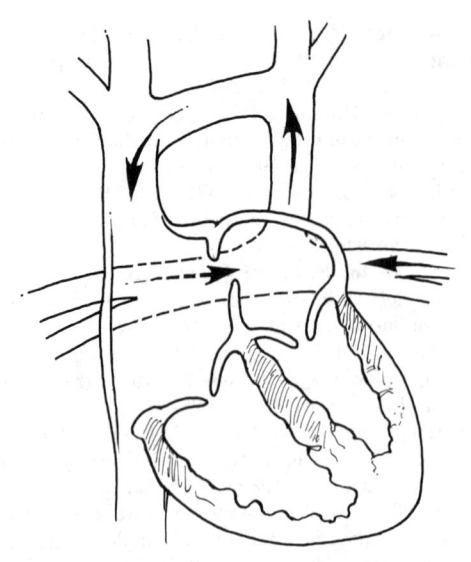

FIGURE 15.6.1. The cross-sectional anatomy of the supracardiac type of total anomalous pulmonary venous return is shown. The *arrows* indicate blood flow returning from the left and right lungs. The veins fail to connect to the back of the left atrium, but instead drain via an ascending vein to the innominate vein and finally to the superior cava and back to the right atrium. Typically, the left atrium and left ventricle are mildly hypoplastic. An atrial septal defect is always present in this lesion, providing the only access of blood to the left atrium and systemic circulation.

Intracardiac

The common pulmonary venous confluence drains into a dilated coronary sinus or directly into the right atrium in the intracardiac type of venous connection.

Infracardiac

In the infracardiac type of venous connection the left and right pulmonary veins drain downward via a common pulmonary vein that is vertically oriented and which then drain into the portal system by passing through the diaphragm. From there, the blood drains into the inferior vena cava via the ductus venosus.

Other Anatomic Notes

In "mixed" drainage patterns, the four pulmonary veins can anomalously drain into more than one venous structure (e.g., the right pulmonary veins draining into the right atrium while the left pulmonary veins draining into the vertical vein).

In partial anomalous pulmonary venous connection, the most common types are (*a*) right pulmonary veins to the superior vena cava (often associated with a sinus venosus type atrial septal defect); (*b*) left pulmonary veins to the left innominate vein via a vertical vein; and (*c*) scimitar syndrome, in which is found partial or complete anomalous drainage of the right pulmonary veins to the inferior vena cava at the level of the diaphragm. This syndrome is often associated with right lung and right pulmonary arterial hypoplasia, bronchial anomalies, dextrocardia, and anomalous arterial supply from the descending aorta to the right lung (1).

Associated Lesions

Anomalous pulmonary venous connection is associated with atrial septal defect, asplenia, or polysplenia.

PATHOPHYSIOLOGY

Two basic pathophysiologic states are seen in total anomalous pulmonary venous connection: obstructed and unobstructed.

In the *obstructed* pulmonary venous pathophysiology, pulmonary venous hypertension is seen with resultant pulmonary edema. In addition, reflex pulmonary arteriolar vasoconstriction and pulmonary hypertension are seen with resultant right heart failure.

In the unobstructed pulmonary venous pathophysiology, pulmonary venous return is to the systemic venous circulation and blood from both venous systems is mixed. Right atrial and ventricular dilation are present. Systemic cardiac output is maintained by a right-to-left shunt at the atrial level.

Obstruction to pulmonary venous return in this lesion can be caused by a number of mechanisms. In the supracardiac type, the vertical vein can be compressed between the pulmonary artery and the main stem bronchus (the so-called "hemodynamic vise"). Anatomic narrowing of the venous structures can also exist. Although the intracardiac type is rarely obstructed, it can become so from a narrowed pulmonary venous confluence as it enters the coronary sinus (2, 3). Lastly, the infracardiac type, which obstructs most commonly, can be occluded at the diaphragm from a closing ductus venosus or from resistance in the liver parenchyma (hepatic sinusoids). These obstructions create a pathologic anatomic substrate of intimal fibrosis of the pulmonary veins and muscular changes in the pulmonary arterioles (4) as well as lymphangiectasia (5).

In the *unobstructed* forms, right ventricular failure results from the volume load to that side. As a result of right side dilation, the left atrium and ventricle can be relatively small and less compliant.

The pathophysiology of partial anomalous pulmonary venous connection is similar to that of an atrial septal defect: left-to-right shunting at the atrial level leading to right atrial dilation, increased pulmonary blood flow, and right ventricular volume overload.

Clinical Course

In obstructed total anomalous pulmonary venous connection (TAPVC), cyanosis with respiratory compromise occurs early in the postnatal period, and it can often be severe, requiring immediate resuscitation (see below) and surgical correction. In unobstructed TAPVC, the clinical presentation is usually later and consists of congestive heart failure. Pulmonary hypertension can occur late.

SURGERY

Preoperative Evaluation

Physical Examination

In the obstructed form of TAPVC, severe cyanosis is present and a systolic murmur of tricuspid regurgitation can sometimes be present. Hepatomegaly may be present from right ventricular failure.

In the unobstructed form of TAPVC (as well as partial anomalous pulmonary venous connection), the physical examination can resemble that of secundum atrial septal defect (fixed split of S_2, systolic ejection murmur in the pulmonic area, and so forth).

Chest Roentgenogram

In obstructed TAPVC, gross pulmonary interstitial edema is present without cardiomegaly. In the unobstructed form, cardiomegaly and increased pulmonary vascularity are seen. In some older children, the vertical vein can be seen, and thus it is termed "the snowman configuration" (with the left vertical vein being the left half of the snowman).

In partial anomalous pulmonary venous connection, cardiomegaly with an enlarged right atrium and ventricle is seen with a prominent main pulmonary artery segment and increased pulmonary vascularity. A distended vertical vein can be seen. In patients with scimitar syndrome, often a distinctive crescent-shaped shadow is seen in the right lower lung field.

Electrocardiography

Right atrial enlargement and right ventricular hypertrophy are usually seen with total anomalous pulmonary venous connection.

Echocardiography

Color Doppler has greatly improved the sensitivity of making the diagnosis of anomalous pulmonary venous connection. Each of the four pulmonary veins is carefully sought and identified. The entire length of the pulmonary venous drainage is carefully studied to rule out any potential area of narrowing (Fig. 15.6.2; see color plate 15.6.2).

Indirect evidence for this lesion includes dilated innominate vein and superior vena cava, dilated right ventricle, right-to-left atrial shunting at the foramen ovale, and small-appearing left atrium and ventricle. In addition, evidence may be found of pulmonary hypertension.

The diagnosis of partial anomalous pulmonary venous connection can be difficult, but it is improved with the use of both color Doppler and transesophageal echocardiography (6).

Cardiac Catheterization

Cardiac catheterization is usually not indicated unless there is ambiguity concerning site(s) of pulmonary venous drainage. Cardiac catheterization is risky particularly in neonates with obstructed pulmonary veins, and it should be avoided if at all possible.

Surgical Procedures

Timing

If the patient has obstructed pathophysiology, surgical correction should be emergently performed. Without surgery, mortality is almost 100% in the first year of life (7).

Because of severe pulmonary venous obstruction, mechanical ventilation should be instituted quickly with positive end-expiratory pressure. In infracardiac type TAPVC, one may prefer to avoid placing an umbilical venous catheter. Prostaglandin E_1 should not be instituted because a potential exists for worsening of oxygenation if severe obstruction of pulmonary venous drainage is present (increase in pulmonary blood flow can aggravate the severity of obstruction). However, there is a potential for ductus venosus to relax with prostaglandin E_1 in infracardiac TAPVC.

In patients with partial anomalous pulmonary venous connection, as with secundum atrial septal defect, surgery is usually recommended between 3 and 5 years of life to minimize the likelihood of developing pulmonary vascular disease.

Technique

In surgery for total anomalous pulmonary venous connection, the basic aspect of surgical repair involves anastomosing the pulmonary venous confluence to the left atrium to achieve proper drainage.

Supracardiac Type Repair Via a median sternotomy and under cardiopulmonary bypass, the heart is gently lifted anteriorly. An incision is then made in the transverse pulmonary venous trunk located posterior to the heart, and an anastomosis is fashioned between the pulmonary venous trunk and the left atrium in a side-to-side manner. The vertical vein is then ligated (Fig. 15.6.3).

FIGURE 15.6.3. Surgical repair of supracardiac total anomalous pulmonary venous return. Following median sternotomy and institution of cardiopulmonary bypass with moderate or deep hypothermia and cardioplegia arrest access to the posterior pericardial space is required. The pulmonary veins are situated just beneath the parietal pericardium. The posterior parietal pericardium can be approached either by lifting ventricular mass out of the pericardial sack or as shown in **A** by lifting the right atrial appendage anteriorly. Counter incisions in the back of the left atrium and in the transverse pulmonary veins are made as shown in **B** and the left atrium and pulmonary veins are anastomosed with a running suture technique. The completed anastomosis is shown in **C**. The procedure also entails closure of the atrial septal defect, ligation of a patent ductus arteriosus, if present, and ligation of the abnormal ascending vein.

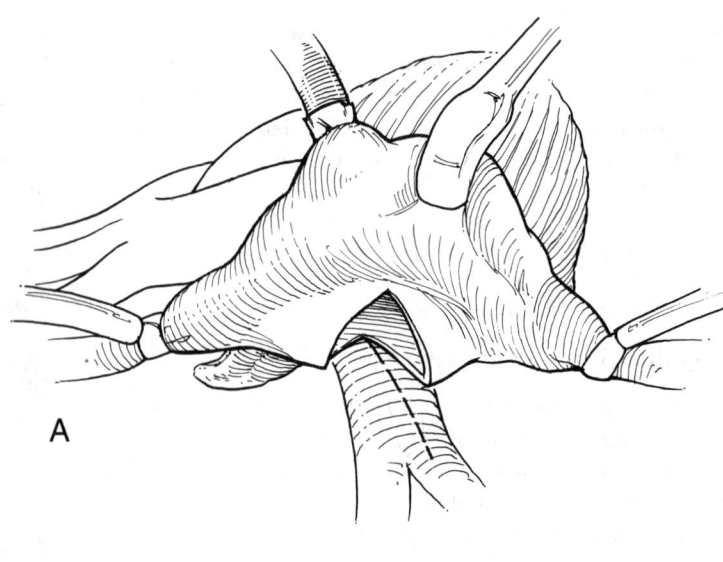

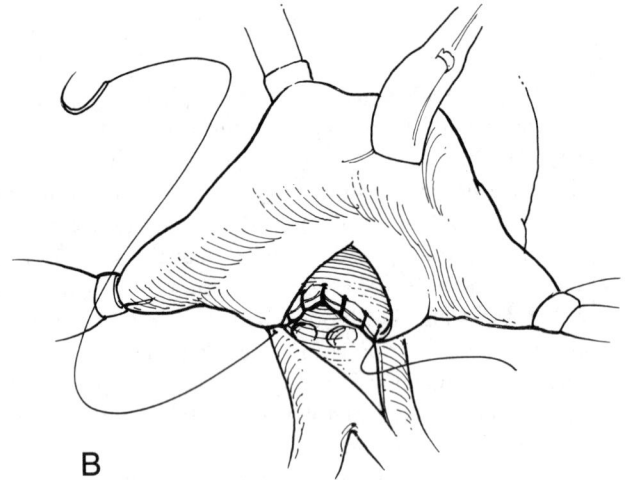

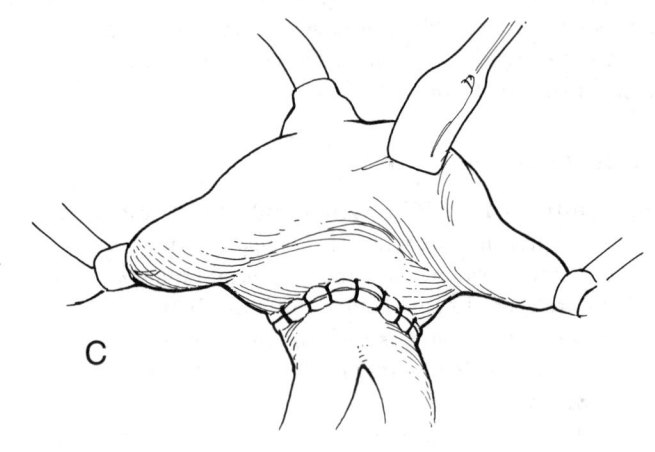

Intracardiac Type Repair Via a median sternotomy and under cardiopulmonary bypass, the coronary sinus is unroofed by cutting the wall between the coronary sinus and the left atrium via a right atriotomy. A patch is then placed around the margins of the foramen ovale and the coronary sinus ostium to allow both pulmonary venous blood and coronary sinus blood to drain into the left atrium.

Infracardiac Type Repair Via a median sternotomy and under cardiopulmonary bypass, the vertically oriented pulmonary vein confluence and the left atrium are anastomosed in a side-to-side fashion. The descending vein is then ligated.

In patients with partial anomalous pulmonary venous connection, surgery is dictated by the type of anomalous connection.

Right Pulmonary Veins to the Superior Vena Cava A patch is sewn along the wall of the superior vena cava so that the anomalous pulmonary veins drain into the left atrium via a tunnel. The superior vena cava is augmented to avoid obstruction (8).

Left Pulmonary Veins to the Left Innominate Vein via a Vertical Vein Via a sternotomy or left thoracotomy, the pulmonary vein is anastomosed to the left atrial appendage (9, 10).

Scimitar Syndrome In scimitar syndrome, a partial or complete anomalous drainage occurs in the right pulmonary veins to the inferior vena cava. If the pulmonary veins are low on the inferior vena cava, the pulmonary veins are detached from their inferior vena cava connection and anastomosed to the wall of the right atrium. If the pulmonary veins are not low, they are left alone. A portion of the interatrial septum is then excised to create an atrial septal defect. These pulmonary veins then drain into the left atrium via an interatrial baffle that is created.

Mortality

Mortality, which is presently as low as 5%, correlates with preoperative morbidity (11, 12). Pulmonary venous obstruction can occur in 5 to 10% of patients, and it often occurs not at the site of the original anastomosis; it is associated with considerable mortality (13–15). Late postoperative dysrhythmias can also occur.

In patients with partial anomalous pulmonary venous connection, mortality is less than 5% with postoperative sequelae consisting of systemic venous obstruction and sinoatrial node dysfunction (16).

Postoperative Management

Postoperative care of patients after TAPVC repair can be challenging mainly because of preoperative morbidity, especially respiratory insufficiency.

Ideal monitoring consists of arterial, central venous pressure, left atrial, and pulmonary artery lines. In addition, atrial and ventricular temporary pacing wires are particularly useful after surgery.

Specific Postoperative Problems

Low Cardiac Output

Previously dilated right-sided structures have influenced sizes of the left atrium and ventricle (17) as well as compliances of these structures (18). Low cardiac output can therefore occur as a result of the left ventricle being relatively noncompliant, with less effective stroke volume per heart beat (19).

Postoperative therapy consists of maintenance of optimal heart rate with either sequential pacing or with isoproterenol because cardiac output in this lesion may be more heart-rate dependent compared with others. Filling pressure to the left ventricle may need to be maintained at 15 mm Hg or so because of the poorly compliant nature of the left ventricle. This underfilling of the left side can also be exacerbated in the presence of pulmonary hypertension and right ventricular dilation. Overaggressive volume replacement should be avoided because this may lead to excessive and rapid left atrial pressure elevation, which can then lead to pulmonary hypertension and worsening of left atrial hypertension.

Respiratory Insufficiency

Severe respiratory compromise results from fulminant pulmonary edema prior to surgery, and therefore it is exacerbated by cardiopulmonary bypass. Therapy includes paralysis and sedation to maximize ventilatory efficiency and positive end-expiratory pressure to improve alveolar oxygenation. In the most severe cases, extracorporeal membrane oxygenation may be necessary to support oxygen delivery.

Pulmonary Hypertension

As a result of medial hypertrophy of the pulmonary arterioles, pulmonary hypertension can occur in as much as 50% of patients, particularly neonates (20). This problem remains a significant risk factor for death in the immediate postoperative period (21). Monitoring with a pulmonary artery line has been instrumental in lowering postoperative mortality (22).

If pulmonary artery pressures are elevated, residual pulmonary venous obstruction must be first ruled out, either with echocardiogram (transesophageal echocardiogram can be particularly useful) or cardiac catheterization, before measures are instituted to treat pulmonary hypertension. Even intravenous magnesium sulfate has been reported to treat this postoperative problem in total anomalous pulmonary venous connection (23).

It is important to appreciate the physiology that may ensue following lowering of pulmonary artery pressure and increase in pulmonary blood flow. Occasionally, the increase in preload in this situation to the left side of the circulation may precipitate a vicious cycle of (a) increased left atrial pressure, (b) increased pulmonary artery pressure, (c) decreased compliance of the left ventricle, and (d) increased left atrial pressure. (See Chapter 32, *Pulmonary Hypertension,* for additional information.)

Perioperative Dysrhythmias

Dysrhythmias, which can occur in up to 20% of patients, consist mainly of supraventricular tachydysrhythmias (24). (See Chapter 30, *Diagnosis and Management of Cardiac Arrhythmias,* for additional information.)

POSTOPERATIVE CARE CHECKLIST

The postoperative checklist includes:

- Monitor pulmonary artery pressures closely and suspect pulmonary venous obstruction.
- Be aware of decreased left-sided compliance and avoid aggressive volume resuscitation.

REFERENCES

1. Canter CE, Martin TC, Spray TL, et al. Scimitar syndrome: a report of nine cases. Am J Cardiol 1986;58:652–654.
2. DeLeon MM, DeLeon SY, Roughneen PT, et al. Recognition and management of obstructed pulmonary veins draining to the coronary sinus. Ann Thorac Surg 1997;63:741–744.
3. Jonas RA, Smolinsky A, Mayer JE, et al. Obstructed pulmonary venous drainage with total anomalous pulmonary venous connection to the coronary sinus. Am J Cardiol 1987;59:431–435.
4. Haworth SG, Reid L. Structural study of pulmonary circulation and of the heart in total anomalous pulmonary venous return in early infancy. Br Heart J 1977;39:80–87.

5. Yamaki S, Tsunemoto M, Shimada M, et al. Quantitative analysis of pulmonary vascular disease in total anomalous pulmonary venous connection in sixty infants. J Thorac Cardiovasc Surg 1992;104:728–735.
6. Ammash NM, Seward JB, Warnes C, et al. Partial anomalous pulmonary venous connection: diagnosis by transesophageal echocardiography. J Am Coll Cardiol 1997;29:1351–1358.
7. Burroughs JT, Edwards JE. Total anomalous pulmonary venous connection. Am Heart J 1960;59:913–931.
8. Okabe H, Matsunaga H, Kawauchi M, et al. Rotation advancement flap method for correction of partial anomalous pulmonary venous drainage into the superior vena cava. J Thorac Cardiovasc Surg 1990;99:308–311.
9. Kalmansohn RB, Maloney JV, Kalmansohn RW. Partial anomalous pulmonary venous connection with unusual variations. N Engl J Med 1961;264:1233–1235.
10. Van Meter C, LeBlanc JG, Culpepper WS, et al. Partial anomalous pulmonary venous return. Circulation 1990;82(Suppl IV):195–198.
11. Serraf A, Bruniaux J, Lacour-Gayet F, et al. Obstructed total anomalous pulmonary venous return. J Thorac Cardiovasc Surg 1991;101:601–606.
12. Lupinetti FM, Kulik TJ, Beekman RH, et al. Correction of total anomalous pulmonary venous connection in infancy. J Thorac Cardiovasc Surg 1993;106:880–885.
13. van der Velde M, Parness IA, Colan SD, et al. Two dimensional echocardiography in the pre- and post-operative management of total anomalous pulmonary venous connection. J Am Coll Cardiol 1991;18:1746–1753.
14. Lamb RK, Qureshi SA, Wilkinson JL, et al. Total anomalous pulmonary venous drainage: seventeen year surgical experience. *J Thorac Cardiovasc Surg* 1988;96:368–375.
15. Kelley LM, Cheatham JP, Kugler JD, et al. Postnatal atresia of extraparenchymal pulmonary veins, fulminant necrotizing pulmonary arteritis and elevated circulating immune complexes. J Am Coll Cardiol 1987;9:1043–1048.
16. Gustafson RA, Warden HE, Murray GF, et al. Partial anomalous pulmonary venous connection to the right side of the heart. J Thorac Cardiovasc Surg 1989;98:861–868.
17. Rosenquist GC, Kelly JL, Chandra R, et al. Small left atrium and change in contour of the ventricular septum in total anomalous pulmonary venous connection: a morphometric analysis of 22 infant hearts. Am J Cardiol 1985;55:777–782.
18. Hammon JW, Bender HW, Graham TP, et al. Total anomalous pulmonary venous connection in infancy: ten years' experience including studies of postoperative ventricular function. J Thorac Cardiovasc Surg 1980;80:544–551.
19. Parr GV, Kirklin JW, Pacifico AD, et al. Cardiac performance in infancy after repair of total anomalous pulmonary venous connection. Ann Thorac Surg 1974;17:561–569.
20. Sano S, Brawn WJ, Mee RBB. Total anomalous pulmonary venous drainage. J Thorac Cardiovasc Surg 1989;97:886–892.
21. Lincoln CR, Rigby ML, Mercanti C, et al. Surgical risk factors in total anomalous pulmonary venous connection. Am J Cardiol 1988;61:608–611.
22. Serraf A, Bruniaux J, Lacour-Gayet F, et al. Obstructed total pulmonary venous return: toward neutralization of a major risk factor. J Thorac Cardiovasc Surg 1991;101:601–606.
23. Lin SC, Teng RJ, Wang JK. Management of severe pulmonary hypertension in an infant with obstructed total anomalous pulmonary venous return using magnesium sulfate. Int J Cardiol 1996;56:131–135.
24. Raisher BD, Grant JW, Martin TC, et al. Complete repair of total anomalous pulmonary venous connection in infancy. J Thorac Cardiovasc Surg 1992;104:443–448.

15.7 Truncus Arteriosus

Anthony C. Chang, MD, and Mohan Reddy, MD

Truncus arteriosus is an uncommon congenital heart lesion representing 1.4% of all congenital cardiac abnormalities. It is the result of failure of the truncus arteriosus to divide into the aorta and pulmonary artery, and it is therefore characterized by a single arterial trunk arising from both ventricles. It is almost always associated with a ventricular septal defect (VSD). This lesion, along with other conotruncal anomalies (e.g., tetralogy of Fallot, double outlet right ventricle, and transposition of the great arteries) and arch obstructive lesions, can be associated with microdeletion of the 22nd chromosome (22q11) (1).

ANATOMY

Truncus arteriosus is defined as a single arterial vessel that originates from the heart, overrides the ventricular septum, and, in the following order, supplies the coronary circulation, the pulmonary arterial circulation, and the systemic circulation. A number of alpha-numeric classification schemes have been derived, particularly by Van Praagh and Collett-Edwards (Fig. 15.7.1). The site of origin of the pulmonary arteries from the truncus is the basis of the more commonly used Collett-Edwards classification: types I–III are characterized by increasing separation of the right and left pulmonary arteries from the truncus, whereas type IV truncus arteriosus is not a true subtype of truncus arteriosus, but it is more accurately considered pulmonary atresia with major aortopulmonary collaterals (Fig. 15.7.2).

The ventricular septal defect in truncus arteriosus has features of both subarterial and tetralogy types of VSD. The VSD results from the absence of the infundibular septum, and the upper border of the VSD is invariably formed by the truncal valve itself. The truncal valve is often dysmorphic, and it can be stenotic and/or regurgitant. It usually has three leaflets, but the number of leaflets can

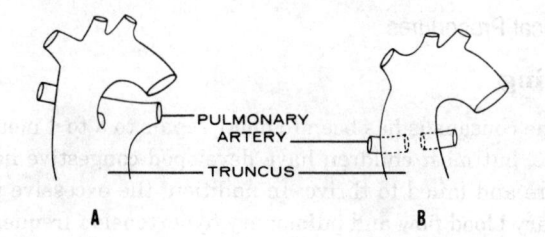

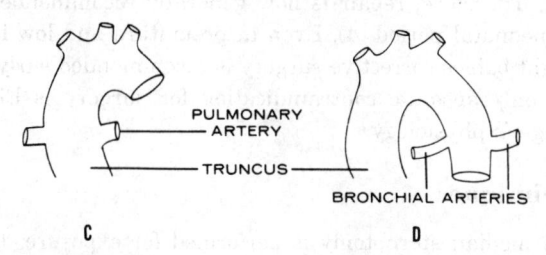

FIGURE 15.7.1. Classification of truncus arteriosus. Type I (**A**); type II (**B**); type III (**C**); type IV (**D**). Reprinted with permission from Fink BW. Congenital heart disease: a deductive approach to its diagnosis. 3rd ed. St. Louis: Mosby-Year Book, 1991.

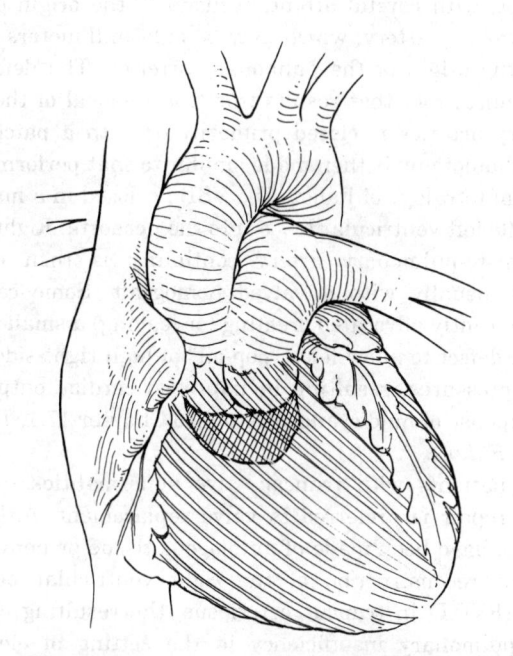

FIGURE 15.7.2. External anatomy of type 1 truncus arteriosus. Note the large truncal valve, which overrides the ventricular septum. The ventricular septal defect is of the subarterial outlet type. It is almost always large and nonrestrictive. The ascending aorta and main pulmonary artery arise from the common trunk. The truncal valve is frequently abnormal with dysmorphic changes and an abnormal number of valve cusps.

vary from two to six. The truncal valve is often balanced equally over the right and left ventricles; however, it can be positioned further over the right ventricle, which may potentially result in subaortic obstruction after repair. In 10 to 15% of cases the aortic arch is either hypoplastic or interrupted. Coronary artery abnormalities are present in nearly half of the cases. Clinically important variations are a high origin of the left coronary artery (making it vulnerable to surgical injury when explanting the pulmonary arteries) and large infundibular or anterior descending artery crossing the right ventricular outflow tract, making it vulnerable at the time of right ventricular outflow tract conduit placement. Lastly, the pulmonary arteries can be either stenotic or hypoplastic.

Associated Lesions

Truncus arteriosus can be associated with aortic arch obstruction, right aortic arch, and atrial septal defect.

PATHOPHYSIOLOGY

Findings include pressure and volume overload to both the right and the left ventricles with the degree of pulmonary blood flow depending on pulmonary vascular resistance; thus this aspect of the pathophysiology resembles single ventricle physiology (See Chapter 18, *Single Ventricle Lesions,* for additional information). The volume and pressure overload can be further increased by truncal valve stenosis or regurgitation. Lastly, coronary ischemia can occur secondary to relatively low diastolic pressure (as a result of the pulmonary circulation runoff).

The amount of pulmonary blood flow is dependent on the presence of stenoses at the origin of the pulmonary arteries as well as the pulmonary vascular resistance. In the absence of pulmonary arterial stenosis, the natural fall in pulmonary vascular resistance results in significant pulmonary overcirculation and symptoms of congestive heart failure within a few weeks of age. This failure may worsen if the patient has truncal valve regurgitation (2).

Clinical Course

If left untreated, this lesion carries a mortality rate of 87% by 6 months of age and 91% by 1 year of age. Because of excessive pulmonary blood flow at high pressure, pulmonary vascular obstructive disease can develop as early as 3 months of age. In addition, pulmonary endothelial dysfunction has been shown to develop as early as a few weeks after birth, which may contribute to postoperative pulmonary hypertension crises if repair is delayed beyond the first few weeks of life.

Truncus arteriosus is usually diagnosed in the neonatal period based on the findings of mild cyanosis, heart murmur, and pulmonary overcirculation. As the pulmonary vascular resistance falls, neonates present with increasing congestive heart failure and failure to thrive in the later weeks of the neonatal period. A small number of patients may be asymptomatic during this time period because of branch pulmonary artery stenosis or persistently elevated pulmonary vascular resistance, both of which can limit pulmonary blood flow. On the other hand, patients with complex truncus arteriosus, such as those with significant truncal stenosis and/or regurgitation or associated interrupted aortic arch, may present earlier with severe congestive heart failure.

SURGERY

Preoperative Evaluation

Physical Examination

Usually signs of congestive heart failure are present. Occasionally, an ejection click may be auscultated. The second heart sound can be single (single S_2) and a harsh systolic murmur is generally heard over the precordium. In addition, an early diastolic murmur may also be heard toward the apex if truncal insufficiency is present.

Chest Roentgenogram

Cardiomegaly with pulmonary edema and increased pulmonary vascularity is evident.

Electrocardiography

Left atrial enlargement may be present. Right, left, or more commonly, biventricular hypertrophy is usually seen.

Echocardiography

Echocardiography alone typically is sufficient to establish the basic diagnosis in uncomplicated truncus arteriosus. In addition to the conotruncal ventricular septal defect, attention must be focused on the number of ventricular septal defects, anatomic abnormalities of the truncal valve, anomalies of the coronary arteries, origins of the pulmonary arteries, and caliber of the aortic arch.

Preoperative quantitative assessment of the truncal valve regurgitation may be underestimated preoperatively because of runoff in the pulmonary circulation. Truncal valve stenosis can be overestimated because of increased flow across the truncal valve from combined ventricular output and truncal valve insufficiency. Lastly, even thymic tissue can be assessed by echocardiography to make the diagnosis of DiGeorge syndrome (3).

Cardiac Catheterization

Cardiac catheterization is generally indicated only in older infants when pulmonary vascular disease is suspected. In addition, children with type IV truncus arteriosus usually require cardiac catheterization for delineation of the aortopulmonary collateral and pulmonary artery anatomy.

Surgical Procedures

Timing

The consensus has been to delay repair to 3 to 4 months of life, but most children have developed congestive heart failure and failed to thrive. In addition, the excessive pulmonary blood flow and pulmonary hypertension frequently resulted in pulmonary hypertension crises following surgery. Therefore, repair is now generally recommended in the neonatal period (4). Even in premature and low birth weight babies corrective surgery is recommended early (5). The only absolute contraindication for surgery is Eisenmenger's physiology.

Technique

A median sternotomy is performed for exposure. Deep hypothermia with low flow (50 mL/kg) technique is routinely employed; circulatory arrest can be avoided except in cases with associated interrupted aortic arch (Fig. 15.7.3). The pulmonary arteries are removed from the aortic root, with careful attention made to the origin of the left coronary artery, which may be only millimeters away from the origin of the pulmonary arteries. The defect in the truncal root that results from the removal of the pulmonary arteries is closed primarily or with a patch. An infundibulotomy is then made similar to that performed in cases of tetralogy of Fallot. The VSD is closed in a manner to baffle left ventricular blood into the neoaorta. Right ventricular-to-pulmonary artery continuity is then established, usually with a valved homograft. Some centers have recently advocated creating (or leaving) a small atrial septal defect to allow for a "pop-off" of high right-sided venous pressures, resulting in improved cardiac output at the expense of mild cyanosis (see also Chapter 17.1, *Tetralogy of Fallot*).

In patients with truncal valve abnormalities truncal valve repair is preferred to valve replacement. Although reports have been made of autologous tissue or nonvalved conduit reconstruction of the right ventricular outflow tract (RVOT) in truncus arteriosus, the resulting obligatory pulmonary insufficiency in the setting of elevated neonatal pulmonary vascular resistance will likely compromise the outcome and is not recommended. In patients with interrupted aortic arch, techniques have been described to reduce the likelihood of bronchial compression (6).

Mortality

Mortality risk for truncus arteriosus is highly dependent on the underlying anatomy. In patients with essentially normal truncal valves and no other significant associated abnormalities, mortality risk is typically less than 10%, but it is higher in patients with arch obstruction, severe truncal valve stenosis or regurgitation, coronary ar-

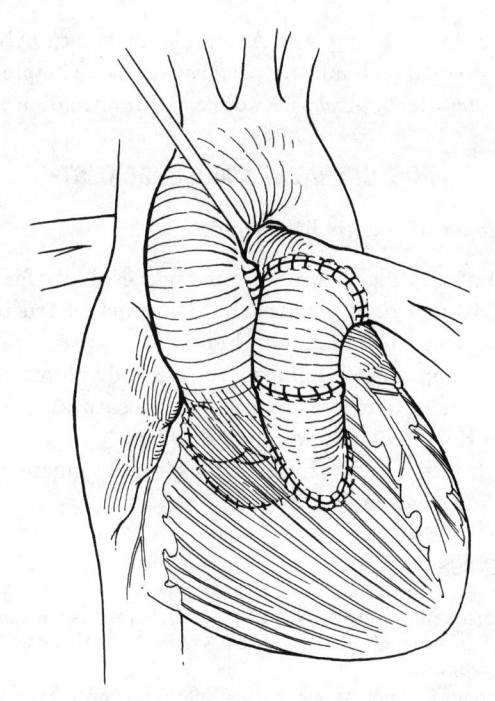

FIGURE 15.7.3. Repair of truncus arteriosus. Cardiopulmonary bypass with moderate or deep hypothermia and cardioplegic arrest are used. The pulmonary arteries are removed from the trunk and this site on the trunk is oversewn with a running suture. The ventricular septal defect is closed, allowing the left ventricle to eject through the truncal valve to the aorta. A valved conduit is placed from the right ventricle into the distal main pulmonary artery. A foraman ovale, if present, is usually left open as in other lesions with major right-sided construction. This practice allows right-to-left atrial shunting if right-sided pump failure develops in the perioperative period. Some surgeons prefer to repair truncus arteriosus without using a right-ventricular-to-pulmonary-artery valved conduit. Various techniques have been described. Increased levels of pulmonary insufficiency and a higher incidence of right heart failure should be anticipated.

tery anomalies, or very low birth weight (7). In addition, conduit obstruction necessitating replacement or revision is common after surgery (8).

Postoperative Management

Postoperative care of patients after truncus arteriosus repair can be challenging mainly because of both pulmonary hypertension and right ventricular dysfunction.

Ideal monitoring consists of arterial, central venous, left atrial, and pulmonary artery lines. In addition, atrial and ventricular temporary pacing wires are particularly useful after surgery.

Specific Postoperative Problems

Pulmonary Hypertensive Crisis

Before medical treatment for pulmonary hypertension is instituted, a large residual VSD should be ruled out. Pulmonary hypertension "crises" are especially prevalent in patients having this repair relatively late in infancy (9); these paroxysmal elevations of pulmonary artery pressure can be life threatening. In these patients an indwelling pulmonary artery catheter is recommended. If the pulmonary artery line is not available, caretakers should use other indirect evidence for pulmonary hypertension (such as elevated central venous pressure, desaturation, tachycardia, hypotension, acidosis, oliguria, and so forth).

Usual ventilatory measures aimed at minimizing pulmonary vascular resistance are routinely instituted in the early postoperative period. Should there be evidence of pulmonary hypertension, it is also helpful to extend the anesthetic period with continuous neuromuscular blockade and high dose fentanyl infusions through the first 24 to 48 hours after surgery. If pulmonary hypertension is not responsive to conventional measures, nitric oxide administration is recommended. Finally, mechanical cardiopulmonary support devices such as extracorporeal membrane oxygenation may be a consideration in refractory cases (10). (See Chapter 32, *Pulmonary Hypertension,* for additional information.)

Low Cardiac Output

In patients after truncus arteriosus repair, poor peripheral perfusion, low mixed venous saturation, metabolic acidosis, and oliguria suggest low cardiac output. Intravascular volume status should be assessed and often preload is insufficient for the degree of right ventricular dysfunction after this surgery; a central venous pressure of 12–15 mm Hg for the immediate postoperative period may be needed to assure an adequate preload to a noncompliant right ventricle.

Mechanical ventilation should be provided with minimal mean airway pressure and the inotropic support/afterload reduction (including phosphodiesterase inhibitors) (11) should be optimized. With no improvement, echocardiography should be promptly performed to assess myocardial function and rule out any residual defects. Regional myocardial dysfunction suggests a coronary ostial problem or an embolic phenomenon. If residual defects (significant VSD, RVOT obstruction, or truncal valve insufficiency) are present, cardiac catheterization and surgery may be necessary. If myocardial edema is significant, chest opening may be necessary to reduce intrathoracic pressure and allow the heart to be less compressed (12). In the absence of residual defects, mechanical ventricular support may be necessary if global myocardial dysfunction appears to be the cause of low cardiac output and pharmacologic support is maximal.

Cyanosis

Right ventricular dysfunction is typically present in the postoperative period. This is usually manifested by elevated right atrial pressure and subsequent right-to-left shunting of blood across the patent foramen ovale. The degree of shunting determines the level of desaturation of arterial blood. As the right ventricular function improves, shunting can potentially reverse and the systemic arterial oxygen saturation improves. Cyanosis caused by lung disease should be distinguished from right ventricular dysfunction by chest roentgenogram and echocardiography (contrast study).

Other than appropriate inotropic support and afterload reduction to ameliorate the degree of right ventricular dysfunction, no other specific therapy is warranted.

Dysrhythmias

Because of the right ventricular incision, complete right bundle branch block is nearly always present on the postoperative 12-lead electrocardiogram. Other commonly seen malignant dysrhythmias following truncus arteriosus repair are junctional ectopic tachycardia, atrial tachycardias, and atrioventricular block. Complete heart block occurs in 3 to 5% of patients. Patients with truncus arteriosus can also be susceptible to isolated ventricular ectopy and seem especially sensitive to changes in electrolytes in the immediate postoperative period, particularly hypokalemia, hypocalcemia, and hypomagnesemia.(See Chapter 30, *Diagnosis and Management of Cardiac Arrhythmias,* for additional information.)

Neoaortic (Truncal) Valve Stenosis/Regurgitation

The truncal valve may have residual stenosis and/or regurgitation following surgery. Afterload reduction should be used judiciously in patients with residual truncal valve stenosis. Truncal valve regurgitation, which can be exacerbated by slower heart rates, may be particularly difficult to manage and when severe, may require valve replacement.

Residual Ventral Septal Defect

Residual VSD following truncus arteriosus repair results in persistent left ventricular volume overload and pulmonary overcirculation. The presence of a loud murmur may not be helpful to exclude VSD as frequently a concomitant turbulence is heard across the right ventricular-to-pulmonary artery homograft. Clinical signs include tachycardia, elevated atrial and pulmonary artery pressures, oliguria, and metabolic acidosis. Hemodynamic instability should prompt caregivers to investigate the presence of an additional or residual VSD; reoperation may be necessary in selected cases. (See Chapter 15.4, *Ventricular Septal Defect,* for additional information.)

Issues Pertaining to Interrupted Aortic Arch

Caretakers should pay special attention to issues relating to DiGeorge syndrome as well as to potential hyperinflation of the left lung (13). A fluorescent in situ hybridization test (FISH) should be performed. (See Chapter 16.4, *Interrupted Aortic Arch,* for additional information.)

POSTOPERATIVE CARE CHECKLIST

Postoperative checklist includes:

- If pulmonary artery pressure is high, evaluate for residual VSD and right ventricle outflow tract obstruction, as well as treat for pulmonary hypertension.
- Institute appropriate pharmacologic and volume support for the right ventricle and allow for desaturation secondary to right-to-left atrial level shunting.
- Pay attention to dysrhythmias, especially junctional ectopic tachycardia.

REFERENCES

1. Johnson MC, Hing A, Wood MK, et al. Chromosome abnormalities in congenital heart disease. Am J Med Genet 1997;70:292–298.
2. Momma K, Ando M, Takao A, et al. Fetal cardiovascular morphology of truncus arteriosus with or without truncal valve insufficiency in the rat. Circulation 1991;83:2094–2100.
3. Yeager SB, Sanders S. Echocardiographic identification of thymic tissue in neonates with congenital heart disease. Am Heart J 1995;129:837–839.
4. Bove EL, Lupinetti FM, Pridjian AK, et al. Results of a policy of primary repair of truncus arteriosus in the neonate. J Thorac Cardiovasc Surg 1993;105:1057–1065.
5. Chang AC, Hanley FL, Lock JE, et al. Management and outcome of low birth weight neonates with congenital heart disease. J Pediatr 1994;124:461–466.
6. Pretre R, Friedli B, Rouge JC, et al. Anterior translocation of the right pulmonary artery to prevent bronchovascular compression in a case of truncus arteriosus and type A interrupted aortic arch. J Thorac Cardiovasc Surg 1996;111:672–674.
7. Oddens JR, Bogers AJ, Witsenburg M, et al. Anatomy of the proximal coronary arteries as a risk factor in primary repair of common arterial trunk. J Cardiovasc Surg (Torino) 1994;35:295–299.
8. Rajashinghe HA, McElhinney DB, Reddy VM, et al. Long term followup of truncus arteriosus repaired in infancy: a twenty year experience. J Thorac Cardiovasc Surg 1997;113:869–878.
9. Bando K, Turretine MW, Sharp TG, et al. Pulmonary hypertension after operations for congenital heart disease: analysis of risk factors and management. J Thorac Cardiovasc Surg 1996;112:1600–1607.
10. Pearson GA, Sosnowski A, Chan KC, et al. Salvage of postoperative pulmonary hypertensive crisis using ECMO via cervical cannulation in a case of truncus arteriosus. Eur J Cardiothorac Surg 1993;7:390–391.
11. Chang AC, Atz AM, Wernovsky G, et al. Milrinone: systemic and pulmonary hemodynamic effects in neonates after cardiac surgery. Crit Care Med 1995;23:1907–1914.
12. Elami A, Permut LC, Laks H, et al. Cardiac decompression after operation for congenital heart disease in infancy. Ann Thorac Surg 1994;58:1392–1396.
13. Sano S, Brawn WJ, Mee RB. Repair of truncus arteriosus and interrupted aortic arch. J Cardiovasc Surg 1990;5:157–162.

Left Ventricular Outflow Tract Obstruction

16.1 Aortic, Subaortic, and Supravalvar Aortic Stenosis

Anthony C. Chang and Redmond P. Burke

AORTIC STENOSIS

Valvar aortic stenosis that presents in infancy represents a spectrum of anatomic variants that range from hypoplastic left heart syndrome to thickened aortic valve. In older children, valvar aortic stenosis can be relatively mild with little sequelae.

ANATOMY

In neonates with aortic stenosis, the valve leaflets are immature and myxomatous and often unicommissural. In addition, the ascending aorta and the left ventricle may be somewhat hypoplastic and endocardial fibroelastosis can be present (1). In older infants, the left ventricle is usually hypertrophied.

In older children, the anatomy of the valve may be bicuspid with fusion of commissures and with the orifice in an eccentric location. The valve leaflets are often thickened. An immature commissure called a "raphe" may also be present. Lastly, the subendocardial layer may be fibrotic (2).

Associated Lesions

Aortic stenosis is associated with other lesions of left ventricular outflow tract obstruction (supravalvar aortic stenosis, bicuspid aortic valve, mitral valve anomalies, and coarctation of the aorta). Aortic insufficiency is often associated. Lastly, some patients have endocardial fibroelastosis.

Pathophysiology

Aortic stenosis that presents in the neonatal period and during infancy leads to pressure overload in the left ventricle and progressive left ventricular concentric hypertrophy and failure, with resultant elevation in end-diastolic pressure and pulmonary edema.

In older children with aortic stenosis, chronic obstruction to systemic blood flow leads to left ventricular pressure overload and concentric hypertrophy.

In neonates with critical aortic stenosis, a patent ductus arteriosus provides an increase in cardiac output by right-to-left shunting. The left ventricle is usually dilated and poorly contractile (rather than hypertrophied as seen in older patients). Inadequate coronary blood flow is found, which is caused by both tachycardia and increased end-diastolic pressure in the left ventricle that are usually associated with heart failure. A gradient may not be accurate under several conditions: (a) presence of a patent ductus arteriosus which provides flow from the right ventricle to the descending aorta; (b) presence of other obstructive lesions, particularly mitral valve stenosis and coarctation of the aorta; and (c) depressed left ventricular function. The elevated left atrial pressure leads to pulmonary edema and pulmonary hypertension with dilation of the right ventricle; in addition, left atrial hypertension leads to stretching of the foramen ovale and to left-to-right shunting at the atrial level. Lastly, end-organ ischemia can result from decreased perfusion and lead to renal failure, necrotizing enterocolitis, and intracerebral bleeds.

In the older child, left ventricular hypertrophy occurs as a compensatory mechanism to maintain optimal wall stress. If the hypertrophy is severe, it leads to subendocardial tissue-blood supply mismatch and subendocardial ischemia. This decrease in coronary blood flow is further exaggerated in situations such as stress or exercise.

Clinical Course

Congestive heart failure or even profound circulatory collapse can occur within the first few weeks of life. Older children can be relatively asymptomatic with aortic stenosis and present with a systolic ejection murmur. In children with more severe obstruction, however, symptoms can include syncopal episodes, exercise intolerance, anginal pain, infective endocarditis, and sudden death.

SURGERY

Preoperative Evaluation

Physical Examination Shock and other signs of circulatory collapse can be present in the critically ill neonate. Some neonates and older infants can also present with signs of congestive heart failure (tachycardia, decreased pulses, gallop rhythm, tachypnea). In these patients, a systolic ejection murmur is usually heard at the apex or the left sternal border but may be absent due to low cardiac output. A systolic ejection click can sometimes be heard.

In the older child, a crescendo-decrescendo systolic murmur at the second right intercostal space (radiating to the jugular notch) with an ejection click can be auscultated. A systolic thrill is sometimes present in the suprasternal notch. Decreased pulse pressure can also be present. Early diastolic murmur secondary to aortic insufficiency is sometimes heard.

Chest Roentgenogram

In neonates and infants, cardiomegaly is usually present with pulmonary edema. In older children, cardiomegaly, if present, is usually mild and it is seen without pulmonary edema. In severe aortic stenosis, left atrial enlargement may be seen.

Electrocardiography

Right ventricular hypertrophy is usually present in infancy. In older children, left ventricular hypertrophy is observed with ST-T segment and T-wave changes that would be consistent with left ventricular strain and/or ischemia. It is controversial whether a direct correlation is seen between symptoms and ST-T segment changes during exercise or rest (3).

Echocardiography

Echocardiographic evaluation alone is usually adequate for surgical or catheter intervention (4). The valve leaflets can be dysplastic and immobile. The stenotic gradient across the aortic valve can be measured using the continuous Doppler principle, and aortic insufficiency is detected using color Doppler. A poststenotic dilation may be present. Some degree of left ventricular hypertrophy and/or dysfunction and even mitral valve regurgitation can be present, especially in neonates. Even if the systolic performance of the heart is preserved, diastolic function can be impaired (5). Importantly, the feasibility for a biventricular repair must be determined by careful assessment of all left-sided structures (including size of the left ventricle and aortic annulus, size and function of the mitral valve, presence of coarctation of the aorta, and so forth).

In older children, the aortic valve more often has a doming appearance. Left ventricular hypertrophy (rather than a dilated left ventricle) is often observed in older patients. The gradient obtained by Doppler echocardiography does not always correlate with the gradient measured by cardiac catheterization (6).

Cardiac Catheterization Diagnostic cardiac catheterization is usually not routine. Findings include narrowed pulse pressure in the ascending aorta, elevated end-diastolic pressure in the left ventricle, and a systolic gradient across the aortic valve.

As an alternative intervention to surgery, percutaneous balloon angioplasty is performed to relieve the aortic stenosis. A balloon dilation catheter is introduced across the aortic valve via a retrograde approach from either the umbilical or femoral arteries. Balloon dilation has also been described using the carotid artery via cutdown (7). The diameter of the balloon is kept less than 100% to minimize chance of postdilation aortic insufficiency. It is not unusual for the gradient across the aortic valve to increase after dilation because the left ventricular function usually improves. Recently, balloon dilation has even been performed in the fetus (8).

Presently, balloon valvotomy offers an alternative given the comparable results to surgical valvotomy (9). Undesirable residua include aortic regurgitation, ileofemoral arterial complications, and bleeding (10, 11).

Preoperative Management in Critically Ill Neonates and Infants

See Chapter 16.5, *Coarctation*, and the section on preoperative management in critically ill neonates and infants for general principles (12).

Surgical Procedure

Timing

When the neonate is metabolically stable, either catheter balloon valvotomy or surgical valvotomy should be performed without delay. In older infants, a gradient measured to be at least 50 mm Hg or presence of symptoms (anginal pain or ST-T segment changes during exercise) even with normal left ventricular function should render the patient a candidate for intervention.

Techniques

A wide range of surgical techniques are available to treat this lesion, but the choice depends on the anatomy of the aortic valve and other structures as well as the age of the patient. It is vital to appreciate that these procedures are usually palliative rather than curative.

Stage I Reconstructive Surgery (Norwood) In selected neonates with severe valvar aortic stenosis who failed attempted aortic valvotomy and in certain neonates with associated left-sided obstructive lesions or hypoplastic structures, a staged approach akin to hypoplastic left heart syndrome may be preferred (13).

Surgical Valvotomy Under cardiopulmonary bypass or under inflow occlusion, the aortic valve is incised via an aortotomy (Fig. 16.1.1).

Bypass Conduit Under cardiopulmonary bypass, placement of a left ventricle-to-thoracic aorta conduit has been described (14).

Aortic Valvuloplasty Aortic valvuloplasty may be the preferred approach with older patients who have an anatomic tricuspid valve. Via a median sternotomy and under car-

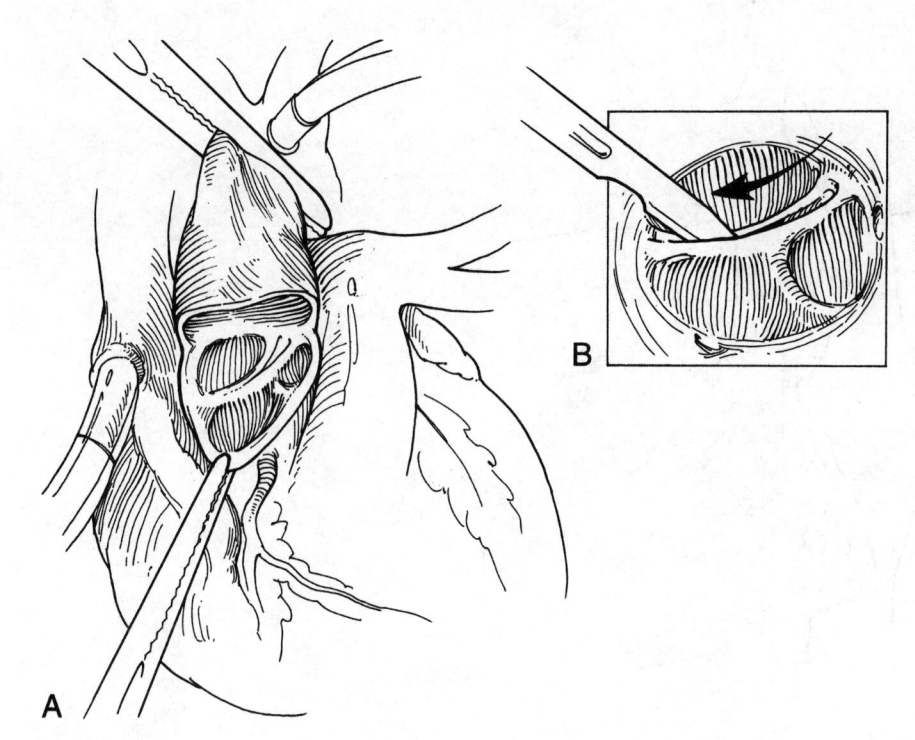

Figure 16.1.1. Repair of aortic stenosis. Cardiopulmonary bypass with moderate hypothermia and cardiologic arrest is typically used, although surgeon preference varies widely. **A.** The aortic cross clamp is in place and the aorta has been surgically opened revealing the deformed aortic valve. **B.** A closeup of the aortic valve. It is bicuspid with a prominent raphe in the anterior valve leaflet, probably representing a vestigial fused commissure. The valve orifice is enlarged using a knife to split the fused commissure between the two leaflets. The incision in the aorta is then closed and the patient weaned from cardiopulmonary bypass.

diopulmonary bypass, the aortic valve is inspected via a longitudinal arteriotomy. Incision of fused commissures is made under direct vision. A recent technique using bovine pericardium to repair the valve has also been reported (15).

Aortic Valve Replacement In certain children who had recurrent aortic stenosis despite surgical or catheter interventions or in those with severe aortic insufficiency, valve replacement may be necessary (16). Bioprosthetic and mechanical valves as well as cryopreserved homografts are used.

Ross Procedure An alternative to prosthetic valve replacement is the Ross operation (17). This operation is also indicated for severe aortic insufficiency. In this operation, the native pulmonary valve (autograft) is excised and used to replace the diseased aortic valve (Fig. 16.1.2). The coronary arteries are translocated to the new aortic valve. The right ventricular outflow tract reconstruction is then completed with homograft.

Problems pertaining to the Ross operation include coronary ischemia, aortic insufficiency, ventricular dysfunction, and right ventricular outflow tract obstruction.

Konno Procedure (Aortoventriculoplasty) Via a median sternotomy and under cardiopulmonary bypass, a longitudinal incision is made in the aorta. A transverse right ventriculotomy is made. The aortic annulus is entered and incision made into the ventricular septum. A prosthetic patch is used to augment the left ventricular outflow tract with the prosthetic aortic valve sutured in place. A pericardial patch is then used to close the right ventriculotomy.

Problems pertaining to the Konno operation include complete heart block, residual ventricular septal defect, right ventricular outflow tract obstruction, and prosthetic valve problems.

A combined Ross-Konno operation recently has been reported for the surgical treatment of critical aortic stenosis (18) (Fig. 16.1.3).

Mortality

Combined mortality for neonates with aortic stenosis has been reported to be as high as 50% (19). Balloon valvotomy has a mortality rate as high as 25% or greater and may be correlated with the underlying anatomy. For surgical valvotomy, mortality is about 2% (20).

Mortality for the Ross or Konno operations can be as low as 4% with normal recovery of left ventricular function (21), but can be considerably higher in neonates and infants (22).

Postoperative Management

Postoperative management is considerably different between the neonate with critical aortic stenosis who presented in shock and the older child with aortic stenosis whose indication for surgery is to lower the chance of sudden death.

Ideal monitoring consists of arterial line, central venous pressure line, and pulmonary artery and left atrial pressure monitoring if ventricular septal defect(s) were present.

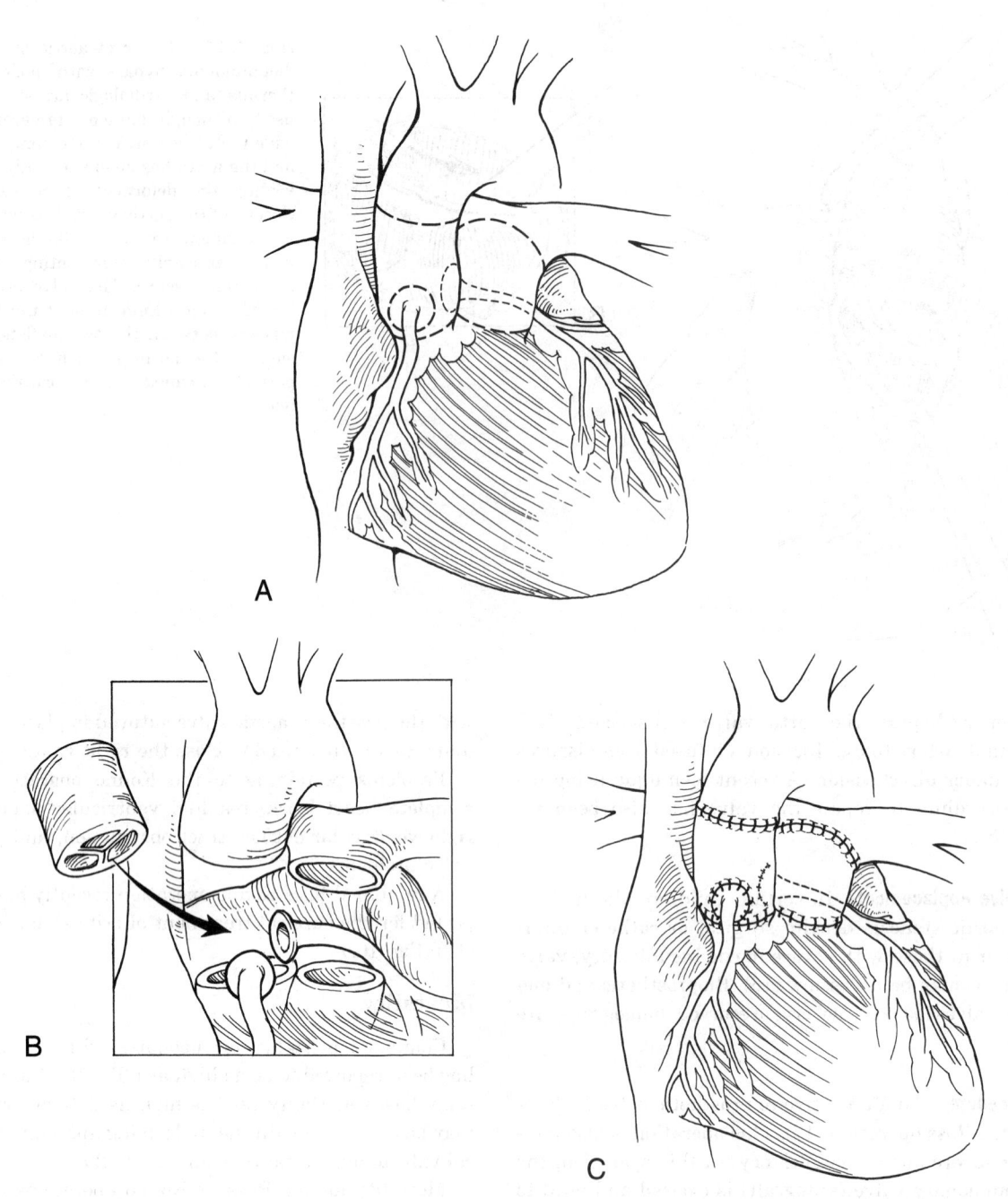

Figure 16.1.2. Aortic valve replacement with the pulmonary autograft (Ross Procedure). Following the institution of cardiopulmonary bypass with moderate hypothermia and cardioplegia arrest, the procedure continues as shown in **A**. The incisions in the native pulmonary valve and in the diseased aorta are shown. First, the pulmonary autograft is harvested by transacting the main pulmonary artery just above the sinotubular junction at the distal end and along the distal infundibulum at the proximal end. The resulting autograft is in a tube of pulmonary artery containing the intact pulmonary valve. The fringe of infundibular muscle harvested with the graft at its proximal margin usually measures approximately 5 mm in thickness. The incision in the ascending aorta proceeds just above the sinutular ridge. The two coronary arteries are removed with a button of sinus of Valsalva tissue. The abnormal valve itself is removed using sharp dissection. The autograft cylinder containing the pulmonary valve is transferred into the left ventricular outflow tract anastomosing the infundibular tissue to the remaining annulus of the left ventricular outflow tract. The coronary buttons are reimplanted into the appropriate sinuses of the autograft and finally the autograft is anastomosed into the end of the ascending aorta. The autograft is shown in **B** being positioned into the left ventricular outflow tract after removal of the abnormal valve. The operation is completed by placing a pulmonary allograft into the right ventricular outflow tract position as shown in **C**.

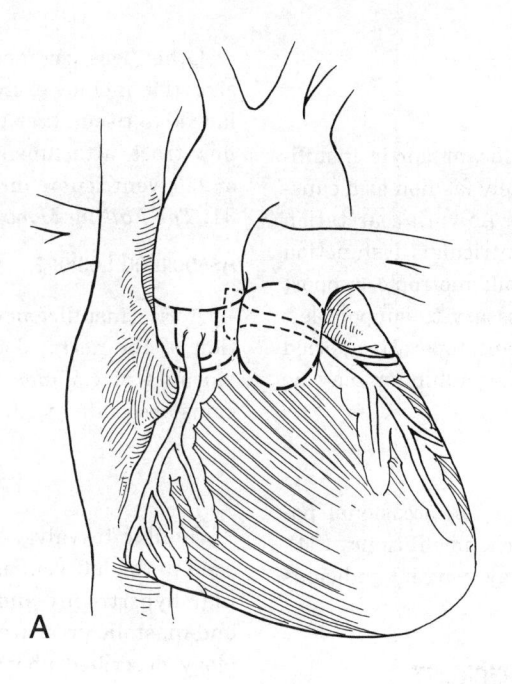

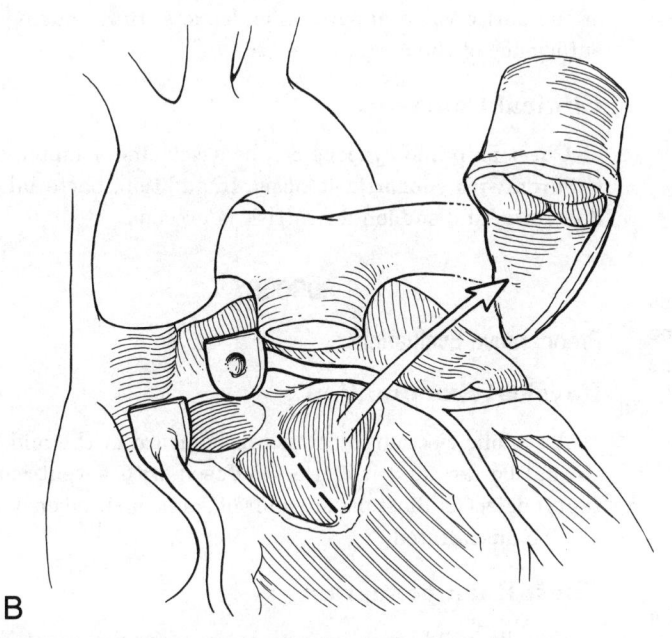

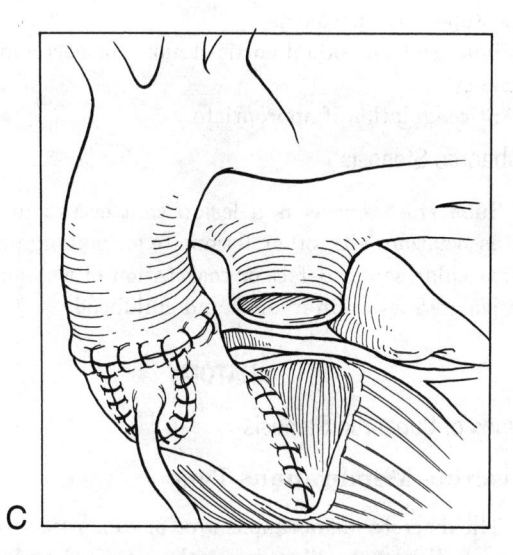

Figure 16.1.3. The Ross-Konno procedure. This procedure is done by use of cardiopulmonary bypass with moderate hypothermia and cardioplegia arrest. With hypoplasia of the subvalvar left ventricular outflow tract, a Konno procedure can be combined with the Ross operation. The incisions on the autograft and on the aorta are shown in **A**. These incisions are similar to the standard Ross procedure; however, the infundibular incision is brought lower onto the free wall of the right ventricle creating a longer "apron" of tissue on the anterior component of the circumference of the autograft. In **B** the autograft has been removed, and it is shown with the accompanying apron of free wall right ventricular infundibulum. The abnormal aortic valve has been removed along with the remainder of the aortic root and the coronary buttons have been mobilized, also shown in **B**. The hypoplastic subvalvar left ventricular tract is shown and the *dotted line* indicates the Konno incision into the ventricular septum. The autograft is then placed into the left ventricular septum and then into the left ventricular outflow tract as in the standard Ross procedure; however, the apron of infundibular tissue is placed into the Konno incision to widen the subvalvar region. This relieves the valvar and subvalvar components of the left ventricular outflow tract disease. The coronary implantations and the remainder of the aortic reconstruction and right ventricular outflow reconstruction are similar to the standard Ross procedure. Shown in **C** is the autograft in place with the Konno addition prior to placement of the right ventricular outflow tract allograft.

Specific Postoperative Problems

Low Cardiac Output

Residual aortic stenosis and significant aortic insufficiency must first be ruled out in a timely fashion as a causative factor(s) for low cardiac output. As with coarctation of the aorta, some degree of left ventricular dysfunction can be present after the intervention; inotropic support and afterload reduction may be necessary to support left ventricular function in the immediate postoperative period (23). An angiotensin-converting enzyme inhibitor may be initiated when enteral feedings begin.

Aortic Insufficiency

After balloon or surgical valvotomy, an occasional patient will have moderate to severe aortic insufficiency (24). This is usually well tolerated but may warrant judicious afterload reduction.

POSTOPERATIVE CARE CHECKLIST

Postoperative care checklist includes:

- Particular attention made to specific procedure-related postoperative problems.
- Vigilance for residual aortic stenosis or aortic insufficiency.
- Anticoagulation if appropriate.

Subaortic Stenosis

Subaortic stenosis is a lesion that occurs in neonates in association with other lesions (e.g., malalignment type ventricular septal defect or coarctation of the aorta) or as an isolated lesion in infancy and childhood.

ANATOMY

Types of Subaortic Stenosis

Discrete Membranous Type

The discrete membranous type of subaortic stenosis is a fibrous diaphragm-like ring with a central orifice that is located below the aortic valve. The aortic valve is sometimes distorted and aortic insufficiency is therefore common. This lesion is almost never seen in neonates.

Fibromuscular Tunnel Type

The fibromuscular tunnel type, which is the less common type of subaortic stenosis, consists of a long segment tunnel-like obstruction below the aortic valve.

Hypertrophic Type

A dynamic outflow tract obstruction, this type of subaortic stenois is a result of hypertrophy of the interventricular septum and the anterior leaflet of the mitral valve.

Other less common anatomic causes for subaortic obstruction include excrescences of right or left atrioventricular valve tissue that protrude into the left ventricular outflow tract, attachments of the mitral valve to the septum, or left ventricular intracavitary obstruction. (See Chapter 31, *The Failing Myocardium*, for additional information.)

Associated Lesions

Aortic insufficiency, ventricular septal defect, coarctation of the aorta, double chambered right ventricle, and variants of common atrioventricular canal are other lesions associated with subaortic stenosis (25).

PATHOPHYSIOLOGY

Similar to valvar aortic stenosis, pressure overload is seen in the left ventricle as well as progressive left ventricular hypertrophy and failure, with resultant elevation in end-diastolic pressure. In addition to the basic pathophysiology described above, the turbulence created below the aortic valve by subvalvar obstruction can lead to distortion of the aortic valve apparatus or leaflets, thus causing insufficiency of the aortic valve (26).

Clinical Course

Chest pain and syncope can be associated symptoms in children with subaortic stenosis. In addition, bacterial endocarditis and sudden death risk is present.

SURGERY

Preoperative Evaluation

Physical Examination

A systolic ejection murmur can be heard at the mid left sternal border, and it can be confused with a ventricular septal defect. A diastolic murmur of aortic insufficiency can also be auscultated.

Chest Roentgenogram

Usually mild cardiomegaly is seen on the roentgenogram. As with aortic stenosis, an occasional patient will have a dilated ascending aorta.

Electrocardiography

Left ventricular hypertrophy can be seen in most patients. Also seen are ST-T segments and T-wave changes consistent with left ventricular strain.

Echocardiography

Echocardiographic assessment is excellent for anatomy and degree of obstruction (27).

Both types of subvalvar obstruction, either discrete or fibromuscular, can be assessed with ultrasound and color

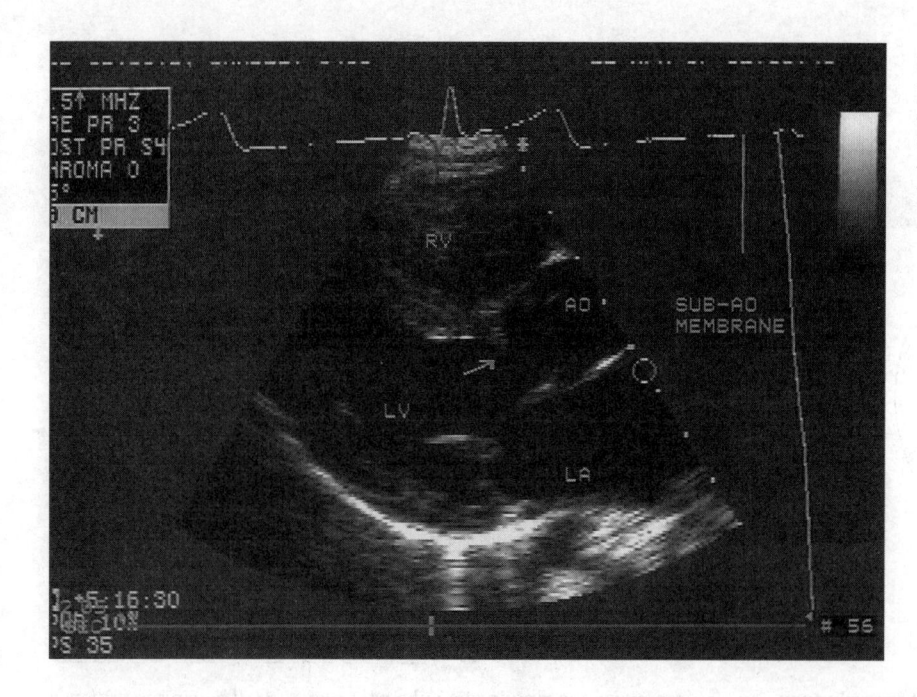

Figure 16.1.4. Parasternal long-axis view from a patient with subvalvular aortic stenosis of the discrete membranous type. The membrane (*arrow*) is seen immediately below the aortic valve (AO). LA, left atrium; LV, left ventricle; RV, right ventricle.

Doppler (Fig. 16.1.4). In addition, the degree of aortic insufficiency can also be estimated. Left ventricular hypertrophy is present at varying degrees. Transesophageal echocardiography has increased the diagnostic sensitivity in assessing this lesion (28).

Cardiac Catheterization

Catheterization is sometimes indicated for exact pressure gradient measurements and angiographic delineation of the left ventricular outflow tract. At times, the pressure gradient is not obtainable if subaortic obstruction is close to the aortic valve. Lastly, the thin membrane of subaortic stenosis may be difficult to delineate on angiography.

Balloon dilation for subaortic stenosis has been performed with acceptable success (29).

Surgical Procedure

Timing

Although somewhat controversial, indications for surgery include a gradient of more than 25 mm Hg, aortic insufficiency, or coexisting lesions (such as ventricular septal defect).

Technique

For discrete membranous type of subaortic stenosis, a median sternotomy is performed (Fig. 16.1.5). Under cardiopulmonary bypass, the membrane is excised via a transverse or longitudinal aortotomy. Resection of excessive muscle in the left ventricular outflow tract may be necessary, and it may lower the incidence of recurrence (30). A recently developed approach via a 4 cm upper sternal incision using cardiac endoscopy to expose and resect the membrane provides good visualization and reduces tissue trauma (personal communication with Redmond Burke).

For tunnel type subaortic stenosis, a median sternotomy is also first performed. Under cardiopulmonary bypass, resection or a Konno (31) procedure, or homograft replacement (32) are performed. In the Konno operation, the aortotomy is into the aortic valve annulus via a surgically created ventricular septal defect. A combined Ross-Konno operation has been described for complex left ventricular outflow tract obstruction with hypoplastic aortic annulus (33). Lastly, a left ventricular to descending aorta conduit can also be placed (34).

Mortality

Mortality is low (less than 5%) with excision of the subaortic membrane (35), but the recurrence for subaortic stenosis can be high (36).

Postoperative Management

Postoperative care of patients after simple subaortic stenosis is usually uneventful and early extubation in the operating room is sometimes performed.

Ideal monitoring consists of arterial line and central venous pressure lines.

Specific Postoperative Problems

As with aortic stenosis, significant residual left ventricular outflow tract stenosis should be assessed. In addition, excision of the subaortic membrane can injure the mitral valve (leading to mitral regurgitation) or create a ventricular septal defect (leading to a left-to-right shunt), and these postoperative residua should be sought. Left bundle

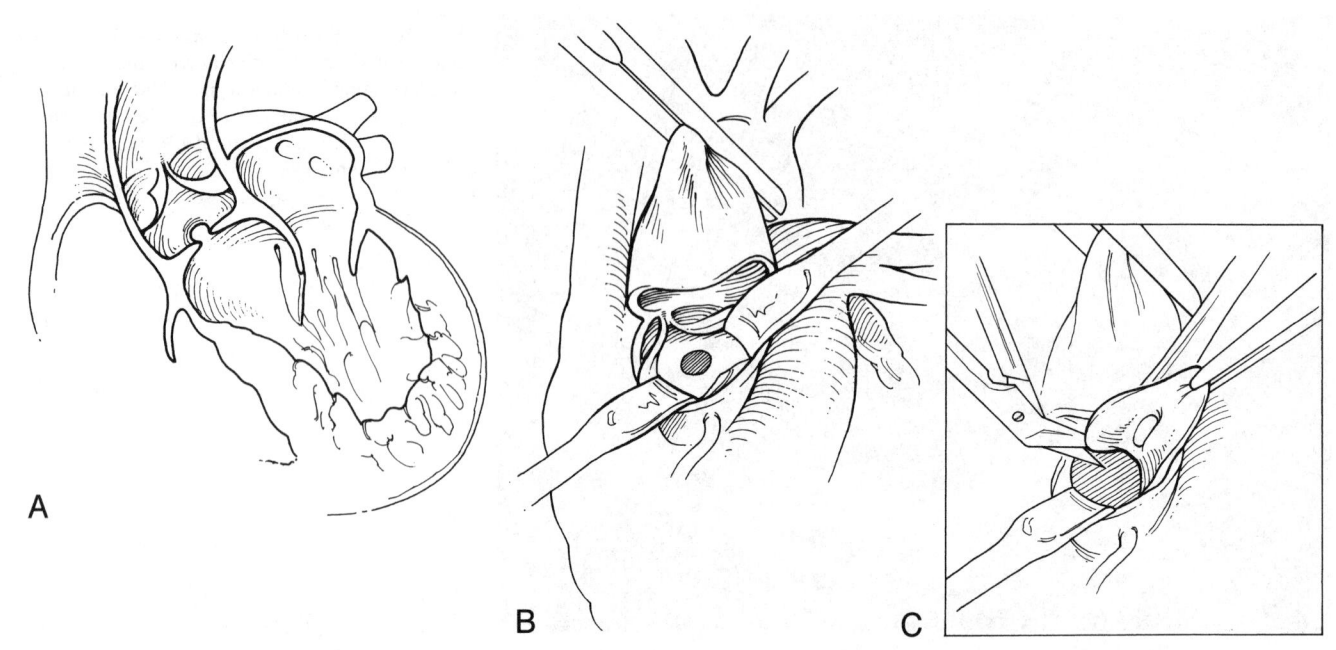

Figure 16.1.5. Cross-sectional anatomy of discrete membranous subaortic stenosis is shown in **A**. This lesion is surgically approached, using cardiopulmonary bypass, with moderate hypothermia and cardioplegia arrest. The aorta is cross-clamped and opened with a transverse incision as shown in **B**. Small instruments are used to retract the aortic valve leaflets revealing the membranous ring in the subaortic region. **C**. The ring is removed completely using sharp dissection. Additionally, a left ventricular outflow tract myectomy is performed to reduce the incidence of recurrence. Following completion of the resection, the aortotomy is closed and the patient weaned from cardiopulmonary bypass.

branch block or even complete heart block can occur secondary to surgical resection in the left ventricular outflow tract.

SUPRAVALVAR AORTIC STENOSIS

Supravalvar aortic stenosis, which is the least common type of aortic stenosis, consists of a localized or diffuse narrowing above the sinotubular junction. It is associated with Williams syndrome (elfin faces, mental retardation, hypercalcemia, abnormal dentition, and auditory hyperacusis) (37) or with a familial autosomal dominant form (38).

ANATOMY

A narrowing is seen above the aortic valve, and its sinuses of Valsalva are associated with a supravalvar ridge and generalized vessel wall thickening. The aortic valve leaflets may also be thickened and abnormal. The coronary arteries at the ostia can be obstructed by the thickened tissue.

Two basic types of supravalvar aortic stenosis occur: (*a*) discrete membranous type (the "hourglass" deformity), which has a discrete narrowing above the sinus of Valsalva, and (*b*) diffuse tubular hypoplasia type. There may be compromise to coronary filling by the narrowing and distortion of the aortic valve leaflets as well as by valve adherence to the supravalvar ridges. Branch vessels of the ascending and descending aorta may also be stenotic at their origin.

In children with Williams syndrome, the tendency is for the supravalvar aortic stenosis to progress with time (39). In addition, patients with Williams syndrome can also have stenoses of the right ventricular outflow tract or of the peripheral pulmonary and renal arteries.

Associated Lesions

Pulmonary stenosis (valvar, subvalvar, or peripheral), aortic stenosis, arch vessel stenosis, coarctation of the aorta, mitral valve anomalies, and renal artery stenosis are lesions associated with supravalvar aortic stenosis.

Pathophysiology

As with valvar and subvalvar aortic stenosis, progressive left ventricular pressure overload and hypertrophy secondary to the obstruction occur. In supravalvar aortic stenosis, the coronary arteries fill under high pressure (which is distinctly different than valvar or subvalvar aortic stenosis) and often become tortuous and dysplastic (40).

Clinical Course

Chest pain and syncope can occur as symptoms with supravalvar stenosis. In addition, similar to aortic stenosis an incidence is seen of bacterial endocarditis and sudden death.

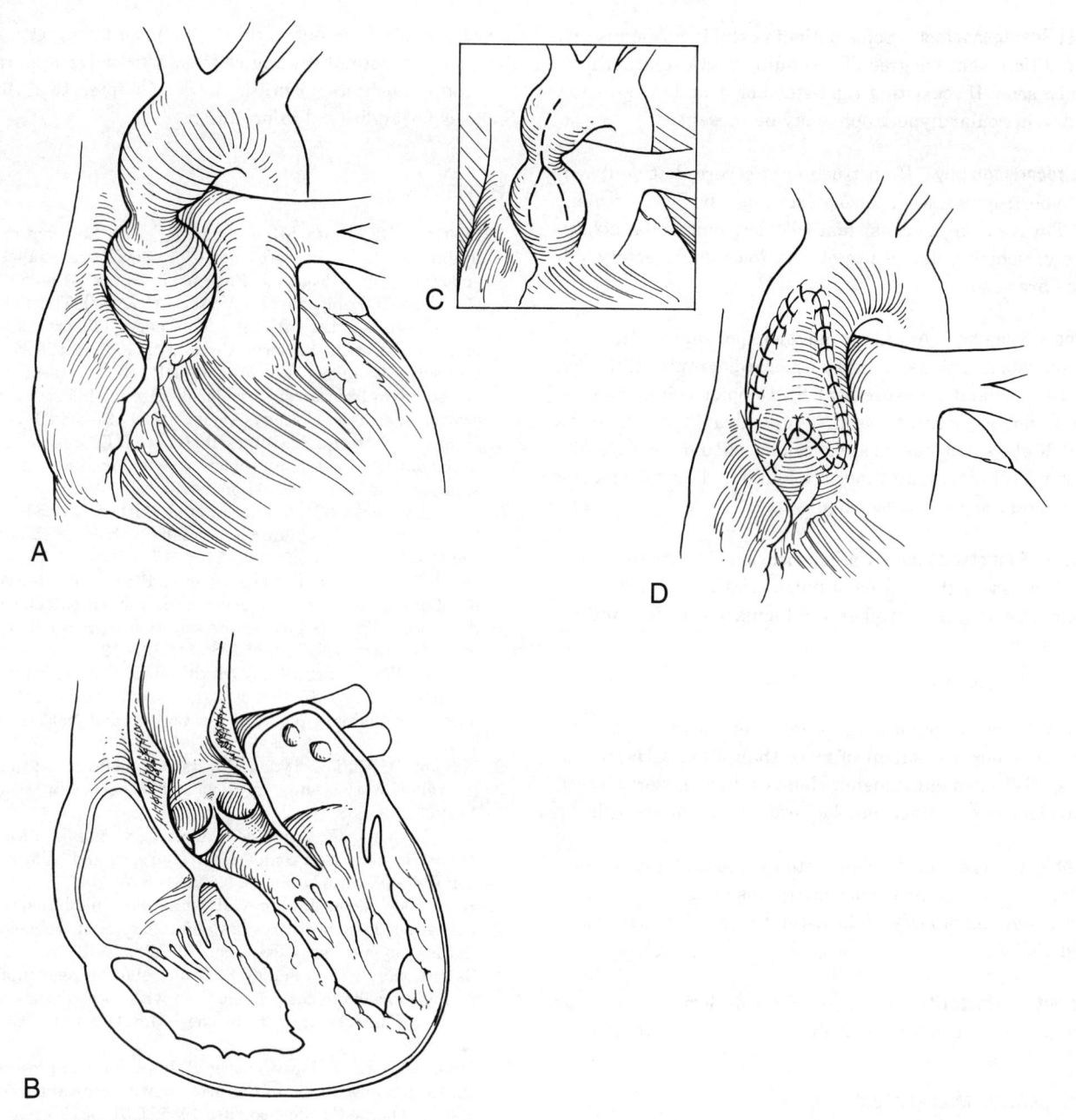

Figure 16.1.6. Repair of discrete supravalvar aortic stenosis. The external appearance of the ascending aorta is shown in **A**. Note the normal diameter of the aortic valve itself, with a discrete hourglass narrowing at the sinotubular junction. A cross-sectional representation is shown in **B**. Note the thickening of the aortic wall at the sinotubular junction. Using cardiopulmonary bypass with moderate hypothermia and aortic cross-clamping, the ascending aorta is incised, as shown in **C**. The incision is begun in the ascending aorta and developed toward the aortic valve. The incision is then bifurcated at the sinotubular ridge into an inverted Y, with one limb entering the right coronary sinus and the other entering the noncoronary sinus. A patch corresponding to this inverted Y incision is then placed in the ascending aorta and sinuses as shown in **D**. In addition, any discrete membranous component of the obstruction can be removed from the sinotubular ridge prior to placement of the patch.

Surgery

Preoperative Evaluation

Physical Examination The physical findings resemble that for valvar aortic stenosis. An interesting physical finding in some patients is differential blood pressures between the right and left upper extremities, due to the Coanda effect (41). This is a physical phenomenon in which a greater proportion of kinetic energy imparted by flow through the obstruction is directed toward the right upper extremity. In addition, pulses in arm and head vessels should be carefully palpated for potential differences as aortic arch vessels can have ostial stenoses.

Chest Roentgenogram Some patients exhibit cardiomegaly. In addition, some degree of ascending aorta dilation may also be seen. If coexisting right-sided obstruction is severe, right ventricular hypertrophy may be present.

Electrocardiography If obstruction is severe, left ventricular hypertrophy is seen. Also present may be ST-T segment and T-wave changes consistent with left ventricular strain. Rarely, ischemic changes secondary to coronary artery stenoses are seen.

Echocardiography Anatomic narrowing of supravalvar aortic stenosis can be assessed by echocardiography, although precise gradient measurement by Doppler echocardiography is not as accurate as that for valvar aortic stenosis (42). Right-sided obstruction lesions should be carefully sought. Technical limitations are found in delineating coronary artery or arch vessel stenoses.

Cardiac Catheterization Catheterization is usually indicated to assess the degree of narrowing of coronary ostia, aortic arch vessels, peripheral pulmonary arteries, and renal arteries.

Surgical Procedure

Timing Indications of surgery for supravalvar aortic stenosis includes a gradient of more than 50 mm Hg, symptoms, ST-T segment ischemic changes during exercise test, or evidence on angiography for coronary ostial stenosis.

Technique Via a median sternotomy and under cardiopulmonary bypass, a inverted Y incision is made and a pantaloon patch angioplasty of the ascending aorta is performed (Fig. 16.1.6).

Mortality Mortality in surgery for this lesion can be as high as 20% but lower for the discrete type of supravalvar aortic stenosis (43).

Postoperative Management

Postoperative care of patients after supravalvar stenosis usually requires more intensive care than that for subaortic membrane resection.

Ideal monitoring consists of arterial line and central venous pressure lines.

Specific Postoperative Problems

As with aortic stenosis, significant residual left ventricular outflow tract stenosis should be assessed. Because of the long suture lines needed for the repair, systemic hypertension should be promptly treated with afterload reduction and/or β-blockade to decrease severity of bleeding. In addition, repair of the supravalvar aortic stenosis can lead to coronary ischemia because of the high incidence of coronary ostial involvement in this lesion prior to surgery. Aortoplasty can potentially injure the aortic valve apparatus (leading to aortic regurgitation). (See Chapter 16.1, *Aortic Stenosis* for additional information.)

REFERENCES

1. Sharland GK, Chita SK, Fagg NLK, et al. Left ventricular dysfunction in the fetus: relation to arotic valve anomalies and endocardial fibroeleastosis. Br Heart J 1991;66:419–424.
2. Cheitlin MD, Rabinowitz M, McAllister H, et al. The distribution of fibrosis in the left ventricle in congenital aortic stenosis and coarctation of the aorta. Circulation 1980;62:823–830.
3. Lambert EC, Menor VA, Wagner HR, et al. Sudden unexpected death from cardiovascular disease in children: a cooperative international study. Am J Cardiol 1974;34:89–96.
4. Huhta JC, Latson LA, Gutgesell HP, et al. Echocardiography in the diagnosis and management of symptomatic aortic valve stenosis in infants. Circulation 1984;70:438–447.
5. Fifer MA, Borow KM, Colan SD, et al. Early diastolic left ventricular function in children and adults with aortic stenosis. J Am Coll Cardiol 1985;5:1147–1154.
6. Oh JK, Taliercio CP, Holmes DR, et al. Prediction of the severity of aortic stenosis by Doppler aortic valve area determination: prospective Doppler-catheterization correlation in 100 patients. J Am Coll Cardiol 1988;11:1227–1234.
7. Fischer DR, Ettedgui JA, Park SC, et al. Carotid artery approach for balloon dilation of aortic valve stenosis in the neonate: a preliminary report. J Am Coll Cardiol 1990;15:1633–1639.
8. Maxwell D, Allan L, Tynan MJ. Balloon dilatation of the aortic valve in the fetus: a report of 2 cases. Br Heart J 1991;65:256–258.
9. Zeevi B, Keane JF, Castaneda AR, et al. Neonatal critical valvar aortic stenosis: a comparison of surgical and balloon dilation therapy. Circulation 1989;80:831–837.
10. Sholler GF, Keane JF, Perry SB, et al. Balloon dilation of congenital aortic stenosis: results and influence of technological features on outcome. Circulation 1988;78:351–360.
11. Galal O, Rao PS, Al-Fadley F, et al. Followup results of balloon aortic valvuloplasty in children with special reference to causes of late aortic insufficiency. Am Heart J 1997;133:418–423.
12. Jonas RA, Lang P, Mayer JE, et al. Importance of prostaglandin E_1 in resuscitation of the neonate with critical aortic stenosis. J Thorac Cardiovasc Surg 1985;89:314–315.
13. Rychik J, Murdison KA, Chin AJ, et al. Surgical management of severe aortic outflow obstruction in lesions other than the hypoplastic left heart syndrome: use of the pulmonary artery to aorta anastomosis. J Am Coll Cardiol 1991;18:809–816.
14. Norwood WI, Lang P, Castaneda AR, et al. Management of infants with left ventricular outflow tract obstruction by conduit interposition between the ventricular apex and thoracic aorta. J Thorac Cardiovasc Surg 1983;86:771–779.
15. Tolan MJ, Daubeney PE, Slavik Z, et al. Aortic valve repair of congenital stenosis with bovine pericardium. Ann Thorac Surg 1997; 63:465–469.
16. Bissett GS III, Meyer RA, Hirschfield SS, et al. Aortic valve replacement in childhood: evaluation of left ventricular function by electrocardiography, echocardiography, and graded exercise testing. Am J Cardiol 1983;52:568–572.
17. Gerosa G, McKay R, Davies J, et al. Comparison of the aortic homograft and the pulmonary autograft for aortic valve root

replacement in children. J Thorac Cardiovasc Surg 1991; 102:51–61.
18. van Son JA, Falk V, Mohr FW, et al. Ross-Konno operation with resection of endocardial fibroelastosis for critical aortic stenosis with borderline sized left ventricle in neonates. Ann Thorac Surg 1997;63:112–116.
19. Gaynor JW, Bull C, Sullivan ID, et al. Late outcome of survivors of intervention for neonatal aortic valve stenosis. Ann Thorac Surg 1995;60:122–125.
20. Deboer DA, Robbins RC, Maron BJ, et al. Late results of aortic valvotomy for congenital valvar aortic stenosis. Ann Thorac Surg 1990;50:69–73.
21. Rubay JE, Shango P, Clement S, et al. Ross procedure in congenital patients: results and left ventricular function. Eur J Cardiothorac Surg 1997;11:92–99.
22. Sudow G, Solymar L, Berggren H, et al. Aortic valve replacement with a pulmonary autograft in infants with aortic stenosis. J Thorac Cardiovasc Surg 1996;112:433–436.
23. Dorn GW, Donner R, Assey ME, et al. Alterations in left ventricular geometry, wall stress, and ejection performance after correction of congenital aortic stenosis. Circulation 1988;78:1358–1365.
24. Justo RN, McCrindle BW, Benson LN, et al. Aortic valve regurgitation after surgical versus percutaneous balloon valvotomy for congenital aortic stenosis. Am J Cardiol 1996;77:1332–1338.
25. Manning P, Mayer J, Sanders S, et al. Unique features and prognosis of primum ASD presenting in the first year of life. Circulation 1994;90:II30–II35.
26. Morrow AG, Fort L III, Roberts WC, et al. Discrete subaortic stenosis complicated by aortic-valvular regurgitation: clinical, hemodynamic, and pathologic studies and the results of operative treatment. Circulation 1965;31:163–171.
27. Wilcox WD, Seward JB, Hagler DJ, et al. DIscrete subaortic stenosis: two-dimensional echocardiographic features with angiographic and surgical correlation. Mayo Clin Proc 1980;55:425–433.
28. Gnanapragasam J, Houston A, Doig W. Transesophageal echocardiography assessment of fixed subaortic obstruction in children. Br Heart J 1991;66:281–284.
29. Labadidi Z, Weinhaus L, Stoeckle H, et al. Transluminal balloon dilation of discrete subaortic stenosis. Am J Cardiol 1987;59:423–425.
30. Lupinetti FM, Pridjian AK, Callow LB, et al. Optimum treatment of discrete subaortic stenosis. Ann Thorac Surg 1992;54:467–471.
31. Konno S, Imai Y, Iida Y, et al. New method for prosthetic valve replacement in congenital arotic stenosis associated with hypoplasia of the aortic valve ring. J Thorac Cardiovasc Surg 1975;10:909–917.
32. Somerville J, Stone S, Ross D. Fate of patients with fixed subaortic stenosis after surgical removal. Br Heart J 1980;43:629–647.
33. Reddy VM, Rajasinghe HA, Teitel DF, et al. Aortoventriculoplasty with the pulmonary autograft: the "Ross-Konno" procedure. J Thorac Cardiovasc Surg 1996;111:158–165.
34. DiDonato RM, Danielson GK, McGoon DC, et al. Left ventricular to aortic conduits in pediatric patients. J Thorac Cardiovasc Surg 1984;88:82–91.
35. Brown J, Stevens L, Lynch L, et al. Surgery for discrete subvalvular aortic stenosis: actuarial survival, hemodynamic results, and acquired aortic regurgitation. Ann Thorac Surg 1985;40:151–155.
36. Jones M, Garnhart GR, Morrow AG. Late results after operations for left ventricular outflow tract obstruction. Am J Cardiol 1982;50:569–578.
37. Williams JCP, Barrett-Boyes BG, Lowe JB. Supravalvar aortic stenosis. Circulation 1961;24:1311–1318.
38. Kahler RL, Braunwald E, Plauth WH, et al. Familial congenital heart disease. Am J Med 1966;40:384–389.
39. Wren C, Oslizlok P, Bull C. Natural history of supravalvular aortic stenosis and pulmonary artery stenosis. J Am Coll Cardiol 1990;15:1625–1630.
40. van Son JAM, Edwards WD, Danielson GK. Pathology of coronary arteries, myocardium, and great arteries in supravalvular aortic stenosis: report of five cases with implications for surgical treatment. J Thorac Cardiovasc Surg 1994;108:21–28.
41. French JW, Guntheroth WG. An explanation of asymmetric upper extremity blood pressure in supravalvular aortic stenosis: the Coanda effect. Circulation 1970;42:31–36.
42. Weyman AE, Caldwell RL, Hurwitz RA, et al. Cross sectional echocardiographic characterization of aortic obstruction. I. Supravalvar aortic stenosis and aortic hypoplasia. Circulation 1978;57:491–497.
43. Keane JF, Fellows KE, LaFarge CG, et al. The surgical management of discrete and diffuse supravalvar aortic stenosis. Circulation 1976;54:112–117.

16.2 Interrupted Aortic Arch

Anthony C. Chang, MD, and Vaughn A. Starnes, MD

Interrupted aortic arch is a relatively uncommon defect in which the aortic arch is either atretic or interrupted, creating either complete disruption in arch continuity or luminal obstruction (without external interruption).

ANATOMY

An interrupted aortic arch can represent the extreme form of coarctation of the aorta or an involution of derivatives of the embryonic aortic arches (Fig. 16.2.1). A causative origin may exist in neural crest migration in type B interrupted aortic arch because it is often associated with DiGeorge syndrome (1).

Types of Interrupted Aortic Arch

The anatomic subtype classification of interrupted aortic arch was introduced by Celoria and Patton (2) (Fig. 16.2.2) as follows:

1. Type A: The interruption is distal to the left subclavian artery. This subtype may be a severe form of coarctation of the aorta. It is associated with transposition of the great arteries.

2. **Type B:** The interruption is between the left subclavian artery and the left carotid artery. This is the most common type; it is associated with DiGeorge syndrome and aberrant origin of the right subclavian artery. Usually present is a posteriorly malaligned ventricular septal defect (VSD). The malalignment of the conal septum with the ventricular septum leads to posterior deviation of the conal septum toward the left ventricular outflow tract (thus creating the subaortic stenosis).
3. **Type C:** The interruption is between the right innominate artery and the left carotid artery. This type is very rare.

Associated Lesions

An interrupted aortic arch can be associated with truncus arteriosus (3), aortopulmonary window, transposition of the great arteries, double outlet right ventricle, or single ventricle. In addition, an aberrant subclavian artery can also be associated with this lesion, and it can manifest as subclavian steal syndrome (4).

PATHOPHYSIOLOGY

See Chapter 16.3, *Coarctation*. Similar to coarctation of the aorta, acute onset of obstruction to systemic blood flow occurs, which results in congestive heart failure with resultant pulmonary edema.

Clinical Course

Most neonates present with varying degrees of congestive heart failure and circulatory shock. Older children and even adults have been diagnosed to have this lesion later on in life.

SURGERY

Preoperative Evaluation

Physical Examination

Congestive heart failure and circulatory shock signs are usually present. Unlike coarctation of the aorta, no sig-

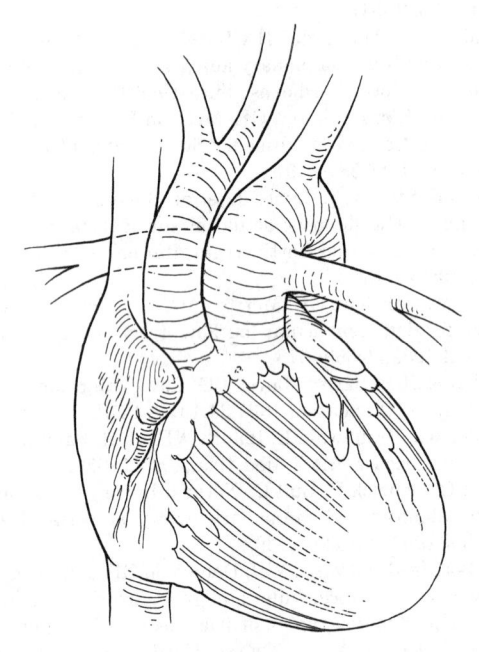

Figure 16.2.1. Anatomy of interrupted aortic arch. Typical external appearance of interrupted aortic arch. Note that the pulmonary artery is substantially larger than the ascending aorta, that the large ductus arteriosus provides a direct connection between the main pulmonary artery and the descending aorta, and that no continuity exists between the ascending aorta and the descending aorta. A ventricular septal defect is almost always present, with posterior malalignment of the conal septum. The conal septal deviation can cause subaortic obstruction. A bicuspid aortic valve is common.

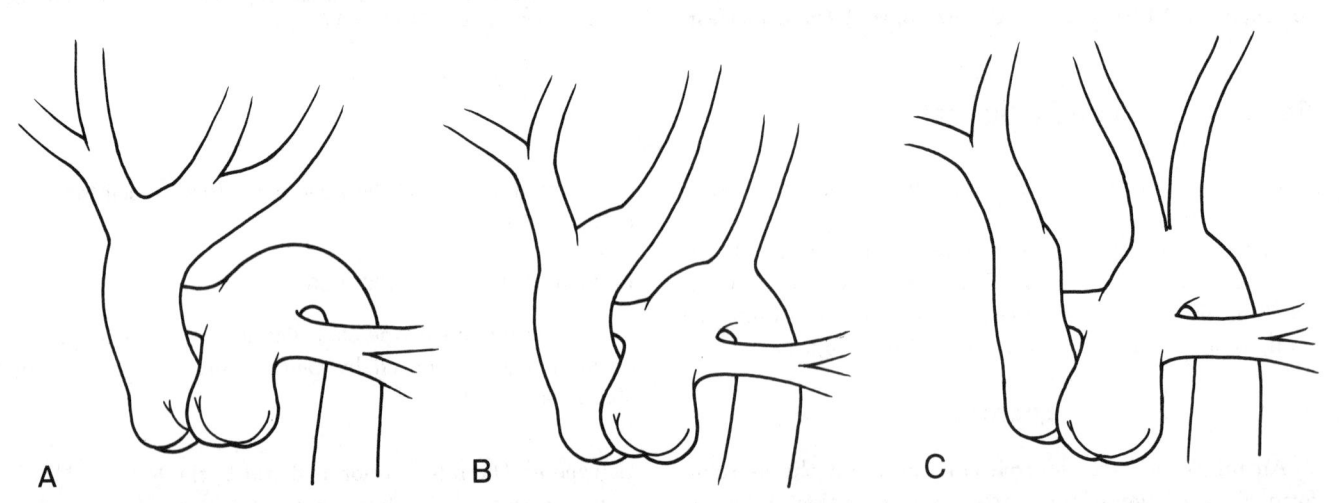

Figure 16.2.2. The three types of interrupted aortic arch. In type **A**, the interruption is at the aortic isthmus between the left subclavian artery and the ductus. In type **B**, the interruption is at the distal aortic arch between the left carotid and left subclavian arteries. In type **C**, the interruption is at the proximal aortic arch between the innominate and left carotid arteries. Type B is the most common form of this lesion. Type C is rare.

nificant differential cyanosis is usually present because a large VSD in this defect creates mixing.

Chest Roentgenogram

Cardiomegaly and increased pulmonary vascularity are seen on the chest roentgenogram.

Electrocardiography

Right ventricular hypertrophy is seen in electrocardiography study.

Echocardiography

Echocardiography alone is usually sufficient for diagnosis (5). In addition to the VSD, other areas of investigation should include subaortic area, aortic valve, and mitral valve (Fig. 16.2.3).

Cardiac Catheterization

Catheterization is usually not indicated for surgery and it would be a higher risk to the patient. Some authors do recommend angiography to delineate the aortic arch anatomy using an upper arm arterial source.

Preoperative Management (see Chapter 16.3)

It is important to balance between systemic and pulmonary blood flow as in neonates with coarctation of the aorta with ventricular septal defect (6).

Surgical Procedure

Timing

As with preoperative care and management for neonates with coarctation of the aorta, surgical correction should be done when renal, pulmonary, and central nervous systems have recovered from any potential initial ischemia. More than 30% of neonates with interruption of the aorta can have renal failure at the time of presentation (7). Unlike coarctation of the aorta, however, cardiopulmonary bypass is needed to repair this lesion.

Technique

Palliative Surgery Technique involves correction of the arch obstruction with a concomitant pulmonary artery band with a plan to close the VSD later in life (8). The results of this strategy has been less than satisfactory (9). One potential disadvantage of a pulmonary artery band in this anatomic substrate is the potential development of subaortic stenosis (10).

In cases of severe subaortic obstruction, a palliative surgery such as reconstructive surgery for hypoplastic left heart syndrome (Norwood operation) is necessary to provide unobstructed flow to the aorta (11).

Corrective Surgery Via a median sternotomy and under cardiopulmonary bypass, the corrective surgery involves arch reconstruction (synthetic bypass graft or reconstruction with or without patch augmentation in an end-to-side fashion) with VSD closure as a single-stage procedure (12) (Fig. 16.2.4). The conal septum may be partially resected to decrease the severity of left ventricular outflow tract obstruction. A recent modification described by Lucianni et al. involves closure of the VSD without resection of the conal septum (13).

Mortality

Recent survival for single-stage or two-stage surgical correction has been as high as 91% or greater (14), but

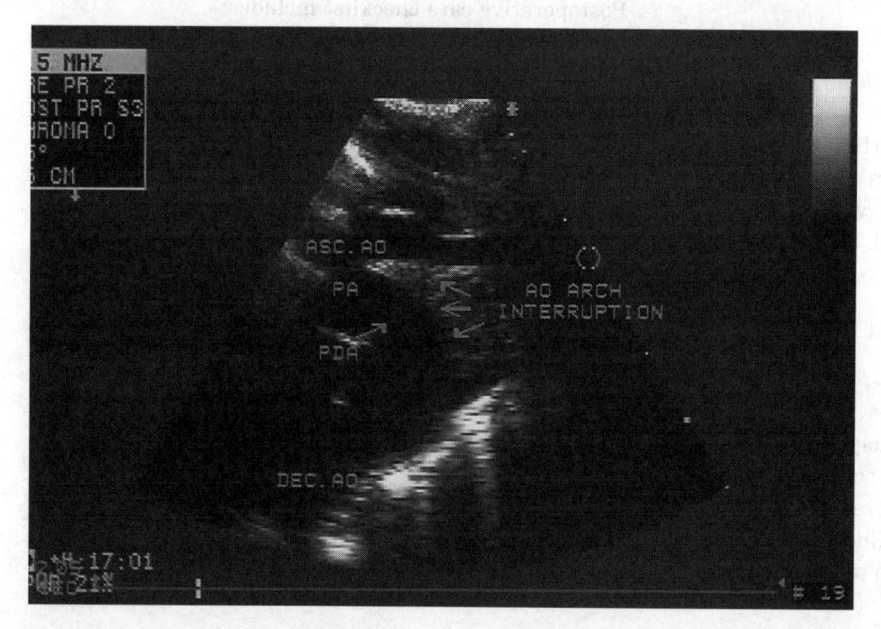

Figure 16.2.3. Suprasternal view from a patient with interrupted aortic arch. The ascending aorta (*ASC.AO*) is interrupted with the patent ductus arteriosus (*PDA*) in continuity with the descending aorta (*DEC.AO*).

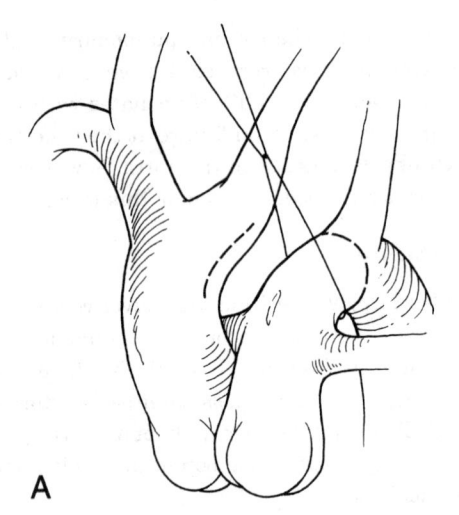

Figure 16.2.4. Repair of type B interrupted aortic arch. The perspective is through a median sternotomy. **A.** The *broken lines* show the anticipated incisions in the ascending aorta and descending aorta, and a suture has been placed around the ductus arteriosus. The procedure is typically performed with the aid of cardiopulmonary bypass and deep hypothermic circulatory arrest. Effective repair requires that all ductal tissue is removed from the descending aorta prior to performing the anastomosis. **B.** The repair has been completed with the anastomosis between the descending aorta and ascending aorta, and ligation of the ductus arteriosus. Ventricular septal defect closure is also performed.

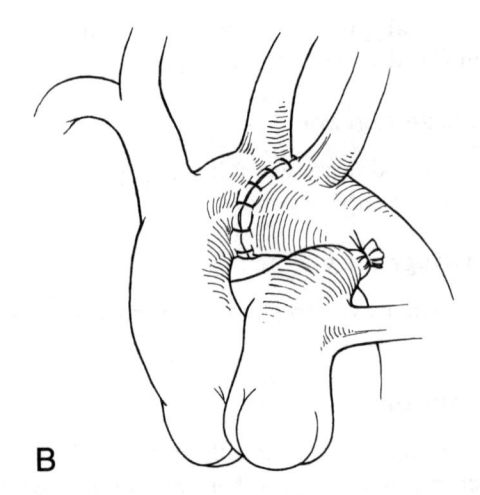

it can be as low as 73% 1 month after repair (15). Late postoperative sequelae include recurrent arch obstruction (25%), which can be balloon dilated (16), and left ventricular outflow tract obstruction (up to 57%), which can be correlated with preoperative subaortic diameter (17).

Postoperative Management (see Chapter 16.3)

Ideal monitoring consists of two arterial lines for blood pressure monitoring (for above and below the arch reconstruction); central venous pressure monitoring; and pulmonary artery and left atrial pressure monitoring.

Specific Postoperative Problems

Pulmonary Hypertension

See Chapter 32, *Pulmonary Hypertension.*

Residual Obstruction After interrupted aortic arch repair, both arch and subaortic areas can remain narrow. If degree of narrowing is severe, surgical reintervention may be necessary when the patient is stabilized after the first surgery.

Residual Ventricular Septal Defect

See Chapter 15.4, *Ventricular Septal Defect.*

Hyperinflation of the Left Lung An uncommon postoperative sequela, hyperinflation of the left lung can occur as a result of the left main stem bronchus being compressed after mobilization and repair of the aortic arch. Chest roentgenogram will show preferential hyperinflation of the left lung. If severe, this postoperative issue may warrant reoperation to ameliorate the anatomic arrangement.

Issues Relating to DiGeorge Syndrome

In addition to hypocalcemia, laboratory investigation should include T cells and chromosomal analysis in cases of DiGeorge syndrome. Hypocalcemia requires vigilance and supplementation. Appropriate genetic counseling should be provided to the family.

POSTOPERATIVE CARE CHECKLIST

Postoperative care checklist includes:

- Vigilance for pulmonary hypertension.
- Check for potential residua after surgery, including left lung inflation status.
- Attention to issues that pertain to DiGeorge syndrome.

REFERENCES

1. Kirby ML, Gale TF, Stewart DE. Neural crest cells contribute to normal aortopulmonary septation. Science 1983;220:1059–1061.
2. Celoria GC, Patton RB. Congenital absence of the aortic arch. Am Heart J 1959;58:407–415.
3. Rajasinghe HA, McElhinney DB, Reddy VM, et al. Long term follow-up of truncus arteriosus repaired in infancy: a twenty-year experience. J Thorac Cardiovasc Surg 1997;113:869–878.
4. Garcia OL, Hernandez FA, Tamer D, et al. Congenital bilateral subclavian steal: ductus dependent symptoms in inter-

rupted aortic arch associated with ventricular septal defect. Am J Cardiol 1979;44:101–104.
5. Riggs TW, Berry TE, Aziz KU, et al. Two-dimensional echocardiographic features of interruption of the aortic arch. Am J Cardiol 1982;55:1385–1390.
6. Lang P, Freed M, Rosenthal A, et al. The use of prostaglandin E_1 in an infant with interruption of the aortic arch. J Pediatr 1977;91:805–807.
7. Serraf A, Lacour-Gayet F, Robotin M, et al. Repair of interrupted aortic arch: a ten-year experience. J Thorac Cardioavsc Surg 1996;112:1150–1160.
8. Irwin ED, Braunlin EA, Foker JE. Staged repair of interrupted aortic arch and ventricular septal defect in infancy. Ann Thorac Surg 1991;52:632–639.
9. Pinho P, Von Oppell UO, Brink J, et al. Pulmonary artery banding: adequacy and long term outcome. Eur J Cardiothorac Surg 1997;11:105–111.
10. Freed MD, Rosenthal A, Plauth WH Jr, et al. Development of subaortic stenosis after pulmonary artery banding. Circulation 1973;47(Suppl 3):7–10.
11. Rychik J, Murdison KA, Chin AJ, et al. Surgical management of severe aortic outflow obstruction in lesions other than hypoplastic left heart syndrome: use of a pulmonary artery to aorta anastomosis. J Am Coll Cardiol 1991;18:809–816.
12. Sell JE, Jonas RA, Mayer JE, et al. The results of a surgical program for interrupted aortic arch. J Thorac Cardiovasc Surg 1988;96:864–877.
13. Luciani GB, Ackerman RJ, Chang AC, et al. One stage repair of interrupted aortic arch, ventricular septal defect, and subaortic obstruction in the neonate: a novel approach. J Thorac Cardiovasc Surg 1996;111:348–358.
14. Karl TR, Sano S, Brawn W, et al. Repair of hypoplastic or interrupted aortic arch via sternotomy. J Thorac Cardiovasc Surg 1992;104:688–695.
15. Jonas RA, Quaegebeur JM, Kirklin JW, et al. Outcomes in patients with interrupted aortic arch and ventricular septal defect: a multiinstitutional study. J Thorac Cardiovasc Surg 1994;107:1099–1113.
16. Sato S, Akiba T, Nakasato M, et al. Percutaneous balloon aortoplasty for restenosis after extended aortic arch anastomosis for type B interrupted aortic arch. Pediatr Cardiol 1996; 17:275–277.
17. Geva T, Hornberger LK, Sanders SP, et al. Echocardiographic predictors of left ventricular outflow tract obstruction after repair of interrupted aortic arch. J Am Coll Cardiol 1993;22: 1953–1960.

16.3 Coarctation of the Aorta

Anthony C. Chang, MD, and Vaughn A. Starnes, MD

Coarctation is a constriction of the thoracic aorta distal to the left subclavian artery. Despite the relatively simple anatomic pathology, the resultant pathophysiology in coarctation can be quite varied. Confusing terms such as "infantile" versus "adult" and "preductal" versus "postductal" coarctation are best avoided. In neonates, coarctation of the aorta is a complex physiologic entity, and it is commonly associated with significant hypoplasia of the aortic arch and ventricular septal defect (1) as well as other complex congenital heart diseases such as truncus arteriosus, double outlet right ventricle, and single ventricle. In older children, coarctation of the aorta is usually an isolated lesion that may be associated with collateral formation. Coarctation is also associated with Turner syndrome.

ANATOMY

Coarctation of the aorta is defined as a narrowing of the upper thoracic aorta caused by posterior infolding or indentation opposite the region of the ductus arteriosus insertion (or "juxtaductal").

One theory postulates that this lesion results from a fetal blood flow pattern of decreased antegrade flow across the ascending aorta (2). Interestingly, coarctation is almost never found in coexistence with lesions with decreased pulmonary blood flow, such as pulmonary stenosis or tetralogy of Fallot (Fig. 16.3.1) (3).

To fully appreciate the complex coarctation syndrome in neonates, the segments of the aortic arch are defined as (*a*) proximal transverse arch: section of the aorta between the innominate vessel and the left carotid artery (usually 60% of the ascending aorta diameter); (*b*) distal transverse arch: section of the aorta between the left carotid and the left subclavian artery (usually 50% of the ascending aorta diameter); and (*c*) the isthmus region: defined as the aorta between the left subclavian artery and the area of the ductus arteriosus (usually 40% of the ascending aorta diameter). The aorta can be hypoplastic at the isthmus or as far proximal as the inominate artery.

Other Anatomic Notes

Coarctation of the aorta can be a part of a developmental complex of left-sided obstructive lesions termed "Shone's complex" that includes parachute-type of mitral stenosis, supravalvar ring of left atrium, subaortic stenosis, and coarctation of the aorta (4). The most severe end of this spectrum merges with hypoplastic left heart syndrome.

Associated Lesions

Coarctation can be associated with bicuspid aortic valve, aortic stenosis, subaortic stenosis, or ventricular

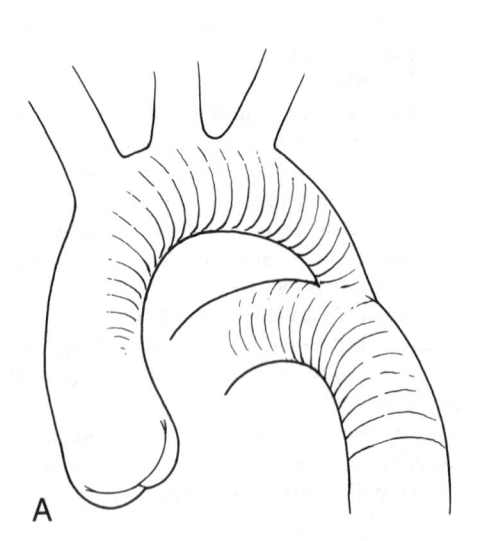

Figure 16.3.1. Types of aortic coarctation. **A.** The typical appearance of aortic coarctation in the newborn infant. The ductus arteriosus is patent. A discrete coarctation is seen in the periductal region with a varying amount of tubular hypoplasia of the aortic isthmus and proximal aortic arch. In some cases, there may also be hypoplasia of the proximal arch and ascending aorta. A bicuspid aortic valve and somewhat hypoplastic aortic annulus may also be present. Of note, major collateral arteries between the upper and lower body are not present. Associated intracardiac defects are common.

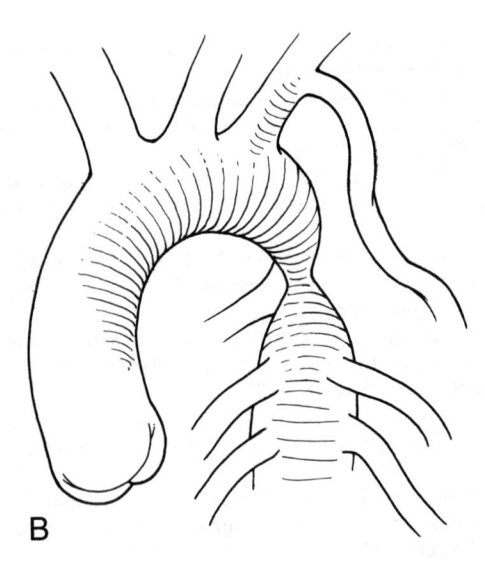

B. The typical appearance of aortic coarctation in a patient presenting beyond infancy. In this lesion a discrete hourglass deformity is present at the level of the ligamentum arteriosum; the aorta proximal to this is usually well developed. There may be poststenotic dilation of the proximal descending aorta and extensive development of arterial collateral vessels between the upper and lower body. The aortic valve may be bicuspid or tricuspid; however, other intracardiac anomalies are unusual.

septal defect. Other less common associated defects include truncus arteriosus, aortopulmonary window, and single ventricle.

PATHOPHYSIOLOGY

Coarctation of the aorta that presents in neonates and infants is a result of a relatively acute onset obstruction to systemic blood flow, thus leading to left ventricular pressure overload and failure with resultant pulmonary edema.

In the older child, the obstruction to systemic blood flow leads to left ventricular pressure overload and concentric hypertrophy. Systemic hypertension occurs and thoracic aortic collaterals commonly develop.

In neonates with coarctation of the aorta, the clinical presentation can be determined by several elements: (a) the rapidity and severity of coarctation narrowing; (b) the patency of the ductus arteriosus; and (c) the presence of associated intracardiac lesions, especially ventricular septal defect.

Because neonates do not tolerate acute rise in afterload, a severe narrowing of the aorta in a relatively short time will bring about left ventricular failure and cardiovascular collapse. In coarctation, a patent ductus arteriosus serves as a conduit to allow passage of blood from the right ventricle to the descending aorta. With closing of the ductus arteriosus, however, cardiovascular collapse will occur. As ventricular function deteriorates and end-diastolic pressure becomes elevated, the left atrial pressure increases, which results in pulmonary edema as well as a left-to-right atrial shunt via a stretched foramen ovale.

In the presence of a coexisting ventricular septal defect, the left ventricle is somewhat protected from the acutely imposed afterload because it can eject into the pulmonary circuit via the defect. Thus, the left ventricle does not have to contend with both an elevated afterload with the coarctation as well as a volume load from the left-to-right ventricular shunt.

Clinical Course

At one extreme of the clinical spectrum, neonates with coarctation of the aorta can present with profound shock, metabolic acidosis, and end-organ ischemia. Organ systems that are often involved include central nervous system (intracranial hemorrhage), renal (acute renal failure), and gastrointestinal (necrotizing enterocolitis). A pulse difference between the upper and lower extremities may not be present in certain situations such as the presence of a ductus arteriosus, coexisting ventricular septal defect, or poor ventricular function. Differential cyanosis may be present from the ductus arteriosus supplying desaturated blood to the lower extremity.

Neonates with coarctation can also present with progressive congestive heart failure, usually before 3 months of age. If the coarctation is more gradual in its development, the patient can even be relatively asymptomatic and instead present with blood pressure differential between the upper and lower extremities. Aortic thrombosis (especially in neonates who have had intra-arterial catheters) and abdominal coarctation should be considered in the differential diagnosis of coarctation of the aorta (5).

A common presentation for coarctation in the older child is the discovery of systolic hypertension or decreased femoral pulses during a routine physical examination in the asymptomatic child. Undesired sequelae in the nonoperated patient include myocardial infarction, cerebral vascular accidents, endocarditis, aortic aneurysms and dissection, congestive heart failure, headaches, lower extremity symptoms such as claudication and coldness, and epistaxis (6, 7). Natural history studies indicate that the average life span is decreased to less than 40 years (8).

SURGERY

Preoperative Evaluation

Physical Examination

Although circulatory shock can be present in the most critically ill neonates, signs of congestive heart failure are present in neonates who are less ill. In some infants, blood pressure differential can exist between upper and lower extremities. In addition, blood pressures in both upper extremities and at least one lower extremity should be taken because the right and/or left subclavian arteries can arise distal to the coarctation and result in a lowered blood pressure from that extremity. Differential cyanosis may be present from the ductus arteriosus supplying desaturated blood to the lower extremity.

In the older child, systolic hypertension, with blood pressure differential between upper and lower extremities, is usually present. With extensive collaterals (intercostal, internal mammary, and spinal) that bypass the obstruction, blood pressure differential may be considerably less or even absent. Absent or delayed femoral pulses may be present. A systolic murmur from the coarctation is heard over the left upper sternal border as well as the left infraclavicular and interscapular area. In addition, a continuous murmur from collateral circulation can be heard anteriorly and posteriorly. A systolic ejection click (from the bicuspid aortic valve) could also be present. Lastly, stigmata for Turner syndrome (webbed neck, widely spaced nipples, and short stature) should be sought.

Chest Roentgenogram

In neonates and infants, cardiomegaly is usually seen with pulmonary edema and pulmonary venous congestion.

Rib notching, representing erosion of the fourth to ninth ribs secondary to enlarged intercostal collateral arteries, can be observed in older children (more than 5 years of age). The "3" sign occurs as a result of the indentation at the site of the coarctation with the poststenotic dilated descending aorta and is best seen in the left paramediastinal area.

Electrocardiography

In neonates and infants, right ventricular hypertrophy (dominant R wave and upright T wave in V_1) is usually seen. Left ventricular hypertrophy, however, is usually seen in older children.

Echocardiography

In neonates and infants, usually echocardiography alone is adequate for definitive diagnosis of coarctation and other coexisting lesions (9) (Fig. 16.3.2; see color plate 16.3.2). A discrete shelf-like membrane is noted posteriorly (opposite the ductal remnant) in the suprasternal notch view. Indirect evidence for coarctation is a delayed upstroke velocity profile with continuous antegrade flow in the abdominal aorta.

Status of the ductus arteriosus is carefully examined. If the ductus arteriosus is widely patent, the shunting pattern is usually right-to-left in systole. If the ductus arteriosus is not patent or restrictive, however, a pressure gradient across the coarctation site can be measured using continuous wave Doppler. It is not always possible to rule out coarctation with 100% certainty when the ductus arteriosus is present.

Left ventricular dysfunction and mitral regurgitation can be present. In addition, left atrial dilation (with bulging of the atrial septum left-to-right) with left-to-right atrial shunt can also be seen. For completeness, the segments of the aortic arch are usually measured. Lastly, coexisting lesions, especially left-sided obstructive lesions and ventricular septal defects, are usually sought.

Echocardiography is sometimes inadequate to confirm the diagnosis in the older child because the area of narrowing may be difficult to image. Magnetic resonance imaging can be used as an alternative imaging tool (10).

Cardiac Catheterization

Cardiac catheterization is usually not indicated in neonates and infants unless uncertainty exists about coexisting lesions or percutaneous balloon angioplasty is being considered to relieve the obstruction.

If performed, findings include a systolic pressure gradient between the left ventricle and the descending aorta. The pressure tracing in the descending aorta can be dampened. Because collaterals may lessen the gradient, the severity of the coarctation is best assessed by the luminal narrowing on aortography.

As an alternative intervention to surgery, percutaneous balloon angioplasty can be performed to relieve the coarctation narrowing. The balloon dilation is achieved by physical disruption of the intimal and medial layers of the aorta. Although the results are good (11–13), gradient relief may be less compared with surgery, and perforation and aneurysmal formation are potential complications (14, 15). This procedure has the advantage that paradoxical hypertension is not observed with the same frequency as surgery (16). In addition, balloon dilation has been effective for recoarctation after surgery (17). Lastly, an advantage of lower cost may be seen with balloon angioplasty (18). Implantation of balloon expandable-stents for coarctation of the aorta has also had good results (19).

Preoperative Management in Critically Ill Neonates and Infants

Preoperative management of critically ill neonates and infants includes the following:

- **Establish Arterial Access**

  Establishment of an arterial line both above (right radial artery) and also below (umbilical, posterior tibial, or dorsalis pedis) the coarctation is useful. Because of potential added risk for necrotizing enterocolitis, one should avoid leaving the umbilical line in place longer than absolutely necessary.

- **Initiate Infusion of Prostaglandin E_1**

  Institution of prostaglandin E_1 before surgical correction for coarctation of the aorta has been demonstrated to improve survival (20). This measure may be indicated for partial or complete opening of the ductus arteriosus or to allow the aortic end of the ductus to relax to allow a wider passage for blood to flow to the descending aorta. It is critically important for the PGE_1 to be administered through a reliable central venous line. Judicious use of a bolus infusion of prostaglandin E_1 may be necessary early in the resuscitation. The response time for PGE_1 to open the ductus arteriosus can range from 15 minutes to as long as 4 hours (21).

  Adequate response to the PGE_1 infusion consists of increased urine output, resolution of metabolic acidosis, and usually a decrease in blood pressure differential between the upper and lower extremities. Only after the ductus arteriosus is established should afterload reduction be aggressively initiated.

- **Appropriate Use of Inotropic Agent**

  Myocardial dysfunction, which may be secondary to metabolic acidosis and/or the acute afterload increase, is usually reversible. One should avoid the use of vasodilating agents in the presence of obstruction in coarctation of the aorta.

- **Institution of Mechanical Ventilation**

  The institution of mechanical ventilation will decrease the work of breathing and contribute to the overall stabilization of the patient. If a large ventricular septal defect is present with the coarctation, it is important to avoid mechanical hyperventilation and high inspired oxygen because these measures can encourage excessive pulmonary blood flow.

- **Correction of Metabolic Acidosis**

  Correction of metabolic acidosis can improve myocardial dysfunction as the myocardium does not contract normally and the inotropic agents may not be effective in an acidic milieu. If the metabolic acidosis persists, necrotizing enterocolitis should be considered and abdominal x-rays obtained.

- **Assessment of End-Organ Ischemia**

  Renal and central nervous system dysfunction should be serially assessed with ultrasound and blood chemistries, especially if cardiopulmonary bypass is considered for the repair.

Surgical Procedure

Timing

In neonates and infants, medical management alone has a high mortality rate (85 to 90%) (22). If cardiopulmonary bypass is needed for extensive arch reconstruction or to correct coexisting lesions, then renal, neurologic, and pulmonary status needs to have had an opportunity to recover. If the coarctation can be adequately repaired without cardiopulmonary bypass (i.e., if the lesion does not have significant tubular hypoplasia), the threshold to achieve full stabilization can be lowered.

Traditional teaching suggests elective repair in the asymptomatic child at 3 to 5 years of age. The rationale for this approach is that by this age the aorta has reached 50% of its adult diameter; an anastomosis made at this time, even if no further growth occurred, would provide an adequate lumen (23). With improved surgical techniques, considerable controversy is seen to operating earlier, even before 1 year of age. Delaying repair beyond late childhood can be associated with higher prevalence of residual hypertension after surgery.

Technique (Fig. 16.3.3)

Resection and End-to-End Anastomosis Via a left posterolateral thoracotomy, the aorta is transected proximal to the coarctation. A coarctectomy is performed to remove ductal tissues as well as the narrowed segment of the aorta. The two ends of the transected aorta are then anastomosed in a way to avoid excessive tension. The anastomosis is performed with a running suture using absorbable suture material (24).

For aortic arch hypoplasia, several modified techniques involving more extensive resection and an end-to-side anastomosis between the descending aorta and the undersurface of the arch may be used.

Among advantages of this technique is that ductal tissue is removed. Disadvantages include tension on the repair and a circumferential scar after surgery. This technique has been reported to have a higher rate of recoarctation (25).

Subclavian Flap Angioplasty Via a left posterolateral thoracotomy and with a clamp placed between the subclavian and carotid arteries, the subclavian artery is divided (26). A longitudinal incision is made from the subclavian artery through the coarctation segment. The intimal shelf of the coarctation segment is excised. The distal end is ligated and the proximal end is fashioned into a vascular flap to patch over the excised coarctation segment.

Although this technique has the advantages of using only native tissue and avoids a circumferential suture line, the blood supply to the left arm is compromised (27). The incidence of reoperation approaches zero with this technique (28).

Patch Aortoplasty Via a left posterolateral thoracotomy, the area of the coarctation is incised longitudinally and the coarctation shelf is trimmed (29). An elliptical-shaped patch (either pericardium or polytetrafluoroethylene) is used to augment the diameter of the aorta. This technique may be necessary in some patients with long coarctation segments or for the neonate who needs an emergent repair.

Advantage of this technique is its technical ease but disadvantages include higher rate of aneurysm formation and recurrence (30). This technique is not commonly used at present.

Bypass Graft Via a left posterolateral thoracotomy, the coarctation is "bypassed" with the use of a graft placed proximal and distal to the coarctation (31). This technique is not commonly used at present.

A coexisting ventricular septal defect can be managed in one of the following ways: (*a*) patch closure (via median sternotomy); (*b*) pulmonary artery banding placed at the time of coarctation repair (32); or (*c*) no surgical intervention at the time of coarctation repair with careful postoperative monitoring for signs of congestive heart failure (33).

Mortality

Mortality for coarctation repair in neonates and infants can be 13% (34), but it can be higher with associated ventricular septal defects (35) or other left-sided obstructive lesions (36). Recurrent coarctation is a late complication. In the older child, mortality is reported to be less than 1%.

Postoperative Management

Ideal monitoring consists of arterial line, central venous pressure line, and pulmonary artery; left atrial pressure monitoring may be necessary if ventricular septal defect(s) were present.

Specific Postoperative Problems

Paradoxical Hypertension

Systemic hypertension, which can persist after repair, appears to be bimodal. The cause for this hypertension is thought to be multiple, including increased catecholamines (37), derangement of the renin-angiotensin axis (38), or a disrupted baroreceptor response (39). The sympathetic nervous system may be responsible for the initial hypertension, which is primarily systolic in nature, and the renin-angiotensin system for the later hypertension, which has a diastolic component. This postoperative problem is less common in patients younger than 5 years of age (40, 41).

Hypertension needs to be treated appropriately because it can increase the degree of postoperative bleeding from either the anastomotic site or the intercostal arteries; it is also correlated with postcoarctectomy syndrome (see below). Sedation and/or analgesia should be adequate to address any pain-induced elevation in blood pressure. Use of vasodilators such as hydralazine or nitroprusside (42) in conjunction with a β-blocker such as propranolol (43) or esmolol (44) can be efficacious. The β-blocker is usually effective in attenuating the reflex tachycardia often observed with hydralazine. Prophylactic β-blockade has been found to be effective in ameliorating paradoxical hypertension and lowering plasma renin activity (45). Lobetalol, a combined α- and β-blocker, has the advantage of preventing unopposed receptor-mediated vasoconstriction, and it has been used with good results.

Systolic hypertension can persist after the immediate postoperative period, so an angiotensin converting enzyme inhibitor (captopril or enalapril), which can block the renin-angiotensin system can be used when enteral medications are administered (46).

Postcoarctectomy Syndrome

Postcoarctectomy syndrome is a postoperative problem that is most likely caused by mesenteric arteritis secondary to the introduction of pulsatile flow and subsequent vessel injury or reflex vasoconstriction after surgery. This is manifested by abdominal pain and/or distension, and can be even accompanied by ascites, fever, and leucocytosis. Infarction of bowel can occur. Lastly, long-term sequelae of the gastrointestinal tract can be serious; it can include ulceration, stenosis, fibrosis, and malabsorption (47). This postoperative state is most common in older pa-

A

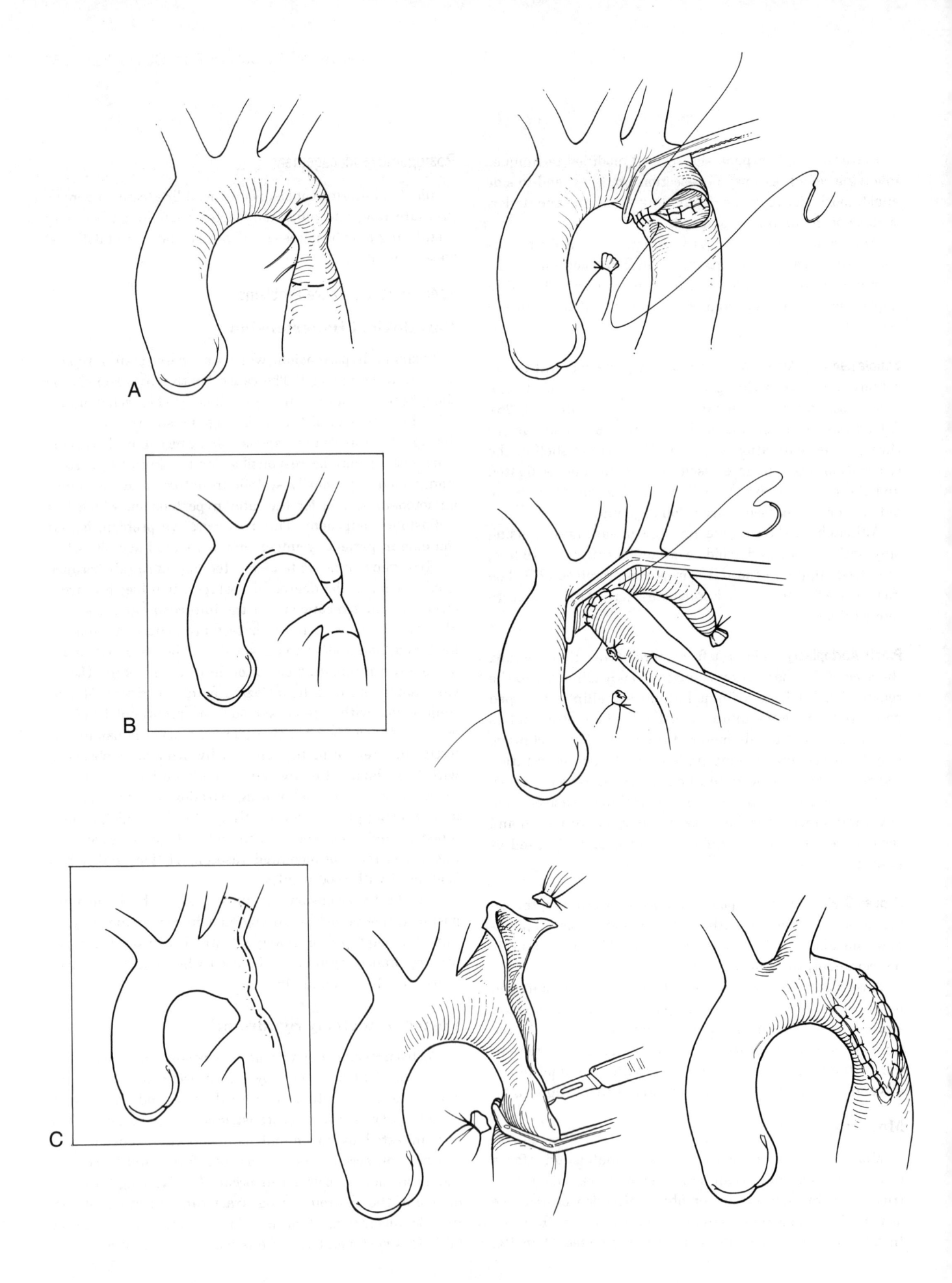

B

C

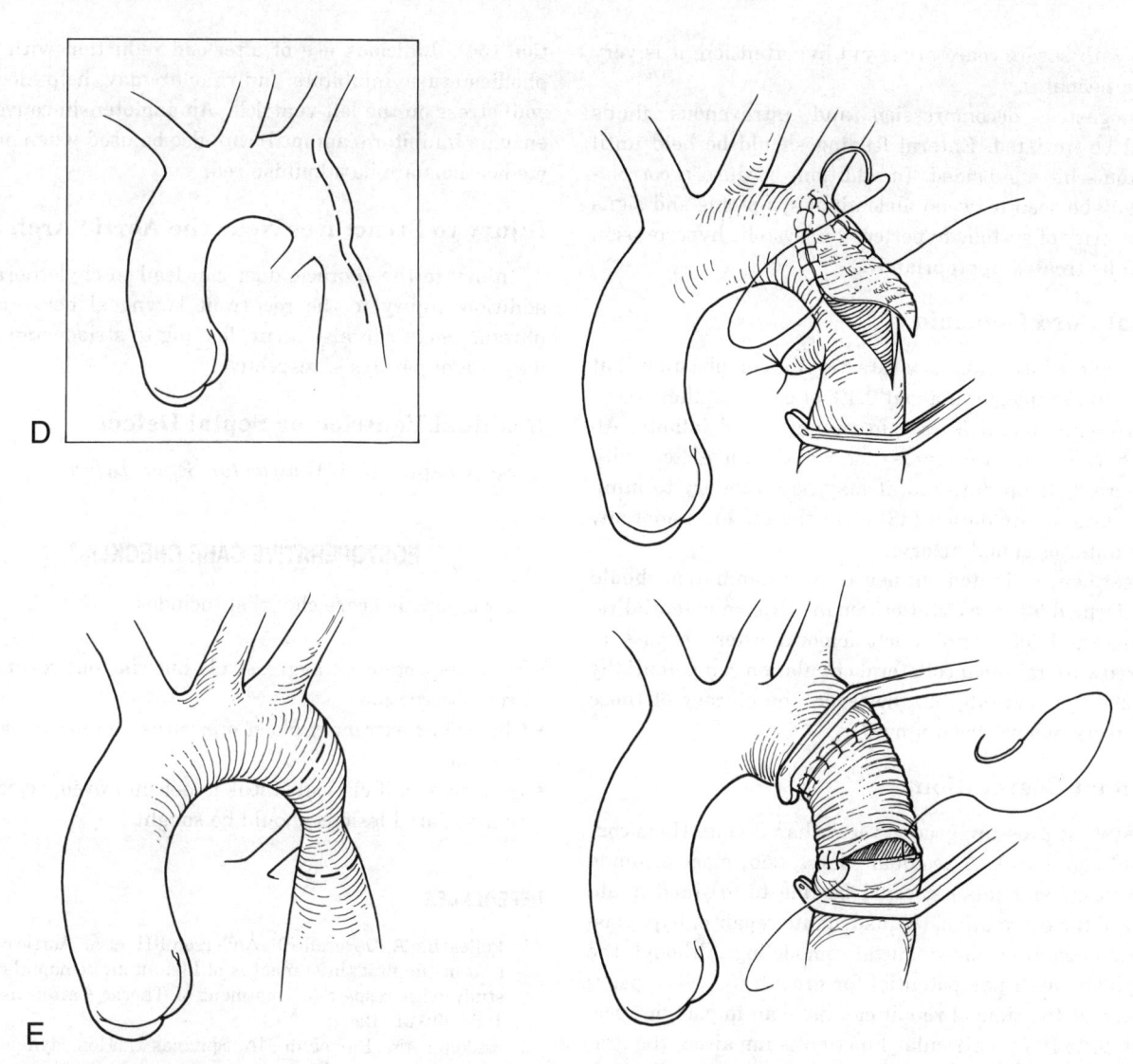

Figure 16.3.3. Repair of aortic coarctation. Aortic coarctation is approached surgically through a left posterolateral thoracotomy incision. Cardiopulmonary bypass is not necessary in the great majority of cases. **A.** End-to-end repair technique is shown. The sites of transsection of the aorta are shown by the *broken lines*. The proximal aortic cross clamp is shown in position on the aortic isthmus. The ductus arteriosus or ligamentum arteriosum has been ligated and divided. An end-to-end anastomosis of the descending aorta and aortic isthmus is performed using a running suture technique. **B.** The more aggressive aortic end-to-side anastomosis is shown. The *dotted lines* represent the points of incision. This technique is used when arch hypoplasia is present, typically in the newborn. The ductus arteriosus is divided and ligated, and the hypoplastic aortic isthmus is divided and ligated. The coarctation and all ductal tissue are resected from the descending aorta. The proximal side-biting clamp is placed opposite the origins of the left carotid and innominate arteries and a longitudinal incision is made in the under surface of the aortic arch between the left carotid and innominate arteries. The descending aorta is then mobilized and anastomosed end-to-side to the ascending aorta, leaving the hypoplastic distal arch as an end vessel to the left carotid and left subclavian arteries. **C.** The subclavian flap aortoplasty is shown. The *dotted lines* represent the surgical incisions. The subclavian artery is ligated distally as it exits from the thorax. The proximal stump of the subclavian artery is then opened longitudinally onto the aorta beyond the isthmus and aortic coarctation. The flap created by the opened subclavian artery is then turned down onto the aorta to augment the hypoplastic area. The ductus arteriosus is ligated and divided. This is a commonly performed procedure in the neonatal period, especially when proximal arch hypoplasia is not severe. **D.** Patch aortoplasty. The *dotted line* indicates the line of incision. Following this, a synthetic patch or pericardial patch is used to augment the hypoplastic area and coarctation site. The ductus arteriosus in this illustration is ligated. It should be noted that this procedure can be performed expeditiously with minimal dissection and the ductus arteriosus can remain patent. These features occasionally make the patch aortoplasty the procedure of choice; however, it is currently only rarely used as a primary procedure. **E.** The prosthetic interposition graft. The *dotted lines* indicate the lines of resection. Following this, an appropriate diameter synthetic graft of Dacron or Gortex is interposed between the aortic arch and the descending aorta. Use of this procedure is also limited to unusual circumstances when the coarctation is long-segment, or in other circumstances when mobilization of the aorta is limited, such as reoperation for coarctation.

tients with severe coarctation and hypertension; it is very rare in neonates.

Nasogastric decompression and intravenous fluids should be initiated. Enteral feeding should be held until symptoms have subsided. In addition, because a correlation may be seen between abdominal symptoms and signs and severity of systolic hypertension, systolic hypertension should be treated appropriately.

Spinal Cord Ischemia

Spinal cord ischemia is a catastrophic complication that results in paraplegia in about 0.4% of patients after coarctation repair, but it is rare in neonates and infants. Although this complication is not clearly correlated with aorta cross clamp duration, it may be secondary to minimal collateral circulation (48) or to the intrinsic anatomy of the anterior spinal artery.

Treatment is limited but neurologic examination should be performed after coarctation repair. Evoked potential recordings and left atrial-to-left femoral artery bypass in children with minimal collateral circulation can potentially decrease the risk (49, 50); however, the efficacy of these maneuvers has not been proved.

Residual Coarctation

A systolic pressure gradient less than 20 mm Hg is considered significant. A residual coarctation, more common in neonates and infants, could be due to (a) inadequate repair of the coarctation, (b) inadequate repair of hypoplastic arch or isthmus, or (c) ductal remodeling. Although the hypoplastic arch has potential for growth (51), it appears that age at the time of repair can have an impact on recoarctation (52). If ventricular function is impaired, the gradient may not be present. "Recurrent coarctation," which refers to a gradient after initial success of repair, may be due to inadequate growth of the repair.

If the patient is hemodynamically and clinically stable, this postoperative residuum can be remedied by balloon dilation about 2 months after surgery. If the patient fails to wean from the ventilator, surgical revision is recommended.

Low Cardiac Output

In neonates and some infants low cardiac output can persist after coarctation repair due to preoperative left ventricular dysfunction (53). It is imperative to seek any residual or undiagnosed lesions (such as residual coarctation or ventricular septal defect) if the patient is not improved.

The left ventricular dysfunction is usually reversible with appropriate inotropic support, although some long-term studies have shown persistent myocardial dysfunction (54). Judicious use of afterload reduction with phosphodiesterase inhibitors (milrinone) may help decrease wall stress on the left ventricle. An angiotensin-converting enzyme inhibitor (captopril) can also be used when enteral medications are be administered.

Injury to Structures Near the Aortic Arch

Injury to the thoracic duct can lead to chylothorax. In addition, injury to the recurrent laryngeal nerve or the phrenic nerve can also occur, leading to stridor and hemidiaphragm paralysis, respectively.

Residual Ventricular Septal Defect

See Chapter 15.4, *Ventricular Septal Defect*.

POSTOPERATIVE CARE CHECKLIST

Postoperative care checklist includes:

- Treat hypertension aggressively but rule out residual arch obstruction.
- Check four extremity blood pressures and neurologic function.
- In neonates, if clinical status is not improved, residual or associated lesions should be sought.

REFERENCES

1. Pellegrino A, Deverall PB, Anderson RH, et al. Aortic coarctation in the first three months of life: an anatomopathological study with respect to treatment. J Thorac Cardiovasc Surg 1985;89:121–126.
2. Rudolph AM, Heymann MA, Spitznas U. Hemodynamic considerations in the development of narrowing of the aorta. Am J Cardiol 1972;30:514–521.
3. Shinebourne EA, Elseed AM. Relation between fetal flow patterns, coarctation of the aorta, and pulmonary blood flow. Br Heart J 1094;36:498–507.
4. Shone JD, Sellers RD, Anderson RC, et al. The developmental complex of parachute mitral valve, supravalvar ring of left atrium, subaortic stenosis, and coarctation of the aorta. Am J Cardiol 1963;11:714–725.
5. McFaul RC, Keane JT, Nowicki ER, et al. Aortic thrombosis in the neonate. J Thorac Cardiovasc Surg 1981;81:334–339.
6. Liberthson RR, Pennington G, Jacobs ML, et al. Coarctation of the aorta: review of 234 patients and clarification of management problems. Am J Cardiol 1979;43:835–840.
7. Strauss RG, McAdams AJ. Dissecting aneurysm in childhood. J Pediatr 1970;76:578–584.
8. Reifenstein GH, Levine SA, Gross RE. Coarctation of the aorta: a review of 104 autopsied cases of the adult type, 2 years of age or older. Am Heart J 1947;33:146–153.
9. Huhta JC, Gutgesell HP, Latson LA, et al. Two-dimensional echocardiographic assessment of the aorta in infants and children with congenital heart disease. Circulation 1984;70:417–424.

10. Boxer RA, LaCorte MA, Singh S, et al. Nuclear magnetic resonance imaging in evaluation and follow-up of children treated for coarctation of the aorta. J Am Coll Cardiol 1986;7:1095–1098.
11. Beekman RH, Rocchini AP, Dick M, et al. Percutaneous balloon angioplasty for native coarctation of the aorta. J Am Coll Cardiol 1987;10:1078–1084.
12. Rao PS, Thapar MK, Galal O, et al. Follow-up results of balloon angioplasty of native coarctation in neonates and infants. Am Heart J 1990;120:1310–1314.
13. McCrindle BW, Jones TK, Morrow WR, et al. Acute results of balloon angioplasty of native coarctation versus recurrent aortic obstruction are equivalent. J Am Coll Cardiol 1996;28:1810–1817.
14. deLezo JS, Fernandez R, Sancho M, et al. Percutaneous transluminal angioplasty for aortic isthmus coarctation in infancy. Am J Cardiol 1984;54:1147–1149.
15. Brandt B, Marvin WJ, Rose EF, et al. Surgical treatment of coarctation of the aorta after balloon angioplasty. J Thorac Cardiovasc Surg 1987;94:715–719.
16. Choy M, Rochinni AP, Beekman RH, et al. Paradoxical hypertension after repair of coarctation of the aorta in children: balloon angioplasty versus surgical repair. Circulation 1987;75:1186–1194.
17. Lock JE, Bass JL, Amplatz K, et al. Balloon dilation angioplasty of coarctation in infants and children. Circulation 1983;68:109–116.
18. Shim D, Lloyd TR, Moorehead CP, et al. Comparison of hospital charges for balloon angioplasty and surgical repair in children with native coarctation of the aorta. Am J Cardiol 1997;79:1143–1146.
19. Bulbul ZR, Bruckheimer E, Love JC, et al. Implantation of balloon expandable stents for coarctation of the aorta. Cathet Cardiovasc Diagn 1996;39:36–42.
20. Leoni F, Huhta JC, Douglas J, et al. Effect of prostaglandin on early surgical mortality in obstructive lesions of the systemic circulation. Br Heart J 1984;52:654–659.
21. Freed MD, Heymann MA, Lewis AB, et al. Prostaglandin E_1 in infants with ductus arteriosus-dependent congenital heart disease. Circulation 1981;64:899–905.
22. Shinebourne EA, Tam ASY, Elseed AM, et al. Coarctation of the aorta in infancy and childhood. Br Heart J 1976;38:375–380.
23. Moss AJ, Adams FH, O'Loughlin BJ, et al. The growth of the normal aorta and of the anastomotic site in infants following surgical resection of coarctation of the aorta. Circulation 1959;19:338–349.
24. Cobanoglu A, Teply TF, Grunkemeier GL, et al. Coarctation of the aorta in patients younger than 3 months. J Thorac Cardiovasc Surg 1985;89:128–135.
25. Penkoske PA, Williams WG, Olley PM, et al. Subclavian arterioplasty: repair of coarctation of the aorta in the first year of life. J Thorac Cardiovasc Surg 1984;87:894–900.
26. Campbell DB, Waldhausen JA, Pierce WS, et al. Should elective repair of coarctation of the aorta be done in infancy? J Thorac Cardiovasc Surg 1984;88:929–938.
27. van Son JA, van Asten WN, van Lier HJ, et al. Detrimental sequelae on the hemodynamics of the upper left limb after subclavian flap angioplasty in infancy. Circulation 1990;81:996–1004.
28. Moulton AL, Brenner JI, Roberts G, et al. Subclavian flap repair of coarctation of the aorta in neonates. J Thorac Cardiovasc Surg 1984;87:220–235.
29. Clarkson PM, Brandt PWT, Barratt-Boyes BG, et al. Prosthetic repair of coarctation of the aorta with particular reference to Dacron onlay patch grafts and late aneurysm formation. Am J Cardiol 1985;56:342–346.
30. Rheuban KS, Gutgesell HP, Carpenter MA, et al. Aortic aneurysm after patch angioplasty for aortic ischemic coarctation in childhood. Am J Cardiol 1986;58:178–185.
31. Jacob T, Cobanoglu A, Starr A. Late results of ascending aorta-descending aorta bypass graft for recurrent coarctation of the aorta. J Thorac Cardiovasc Surg 1988;95:782–787.
32. Neches WH, Park SC, Lenox CC, et al. Coarctation of the aorta with ventricular septal defect. Circulation 1977;55:189–194.
33. Graham TP, Burger J, Boucek RJ, et al. Absence of left ventricular volume loading in infants with coarctation of the aorta and a large ventricular septal defect. J Am Coll Cardiol 1989;14:1545–1552.
34. Quaegebeur JM, Jonas RA, Weinberg AD, et al. Outcomes in seriously ill neonates with coarctation of the aorta. J Thorac Cardiovasc Surg 1994;108:841–854.
35. Hammon JW, Graham TP, Boucek RJ, et al. Operative repair of coarctation of the aorta in infancy: results with and without ventricular septal defect. Am J Cardiol 1985;55:1555–1559.
36. Vogel M, Freedom RM, Smallhorn JF, et al. Complete transposition of the great arteries and coarctation of the aorta. Am J Cardiol 1984;53:1627–1632.
37. Benedict CR, Grahame-Smith DG, Fisher A. Changes in plasma catecholamines and dopamine beta-hydroxylase after corrective surgery for coarctation of the aorta. Circulation 1978;57:598–602.
38. Rocchini AP, Rosenthal A, Barger AC, et al. Pathogenesis of paradoxical hypertension after coarctation resection. Circulation 1976;54:382–387.
39. Beekman RH, Katz BP, Moorehead-Steffens C, et al. Altered baroreceptor function in children with systolic hypertension after coarctation repair. Am J Cardiol 1983:52:112–116.
40. Will RJ, Walker OM, Traugott RC, et al. Sodium nitroprusside and propranolol therapy for management of postcoarctectomy hypertension. J Thorac Cardiovasc Surg 1978;75:722–729.
41. Anyanwu E, Klemm C, Achatzy R, et al. Surgery of coarctation of the aorta: a nine-year review of 253 patients. Thorac Cardiovasc Surg 1984;32:350–357.
42. Will RJ, Walker OM, Traugott RC, et al. Sodium nitroprusside and propranolol therapy for management of postcoarctectomy hypertension. J Thorac Cardiovasc Surg 1978;5:722–729.
43. Gidding SS, Rocchini AP, Beekman R, et al. Therapeutic effect of propranolol on paradoxical hypertension after repair of coarctation of the aorta. N Engl J Med 1985;312:1224–1228.
44. Smerling A, Gersony WM. Esmolol for severe hypertension following repair of aortic coarctation. Crit Care Med 1990;18:1288–1290.
45. Leenen FH, Balfe JA, Pelech AN, et al. Postoperative hypertension after repair of coarctation of the aorta in children: a protective effect of propranolol? Am Heart J 1987;113:1164–1173.
46. Casta A, Conti VR, Talaki A, et al. Effective use of captopril on postoperative paradoxical hypertension of coarctation of the aorta. Clin Cardiol 1982;5:551–558.
47. Mays ET, Sergenat CK. postcoarctectomy syndrome. Arch Surg 1965;91:58–65.
48. Brewer LA, Fosburg RG, Mulder GA, et al. Spinal cord complications following surgery for coarctation of the aorta: a study of 66 cases. J Thorac Cardiovasc Surg 1972;64:368–381.

49. Krieger KH, Spencer FC. Is paraplegia after repair of coarctation of the aorta due principally to distal hypotension during aortic cross clamping? Surgery 1985;97:2–6.
50. Luosto R, Kyllonen KEJ, Merikallio E. Surgical treatment of coarctation of the aorta with minimal collateral circulation. Scand J Thorac Cardiovasc Surg 1980;14:217–220.
51. Sade RM, Crawford FA, Hohn AR, et al. Growth of the aorta after prosthetic patch aortoplasty for coarctation in infants. Ann Thorac Surg 1984;38:21–25.
52. Bergdahl L, Bjork VO, Jonasson R. Surgical correction of coarctation of the aorta: influence of age on late results. J Thorac Cardiovasc Surg 1983;85:532–536.
53. Graham TP, Atwood GF, Boerth RC, et al. Right and left heart size and function in infants with symptomatic coarctation. Circulation 1977;56:641–647.
54. Sigurdardottir LY, Helgason H. Echocardiographic evaluation of systolic and diastolic function in postoperative coarctation patients. Pediatr Cardiol 1997;18:96–110.

Right Ventricular Outflow Tract Obstruction 17

17.1 Tetralogy of Fallot

Thomas L. Spray, MD, and Gil Wernovsky, MD

ANATOMY

Tetralogy of Fallot (TOF), described initially in the early 19th century, includes the association of four anatomic findings: ventricular septal defect (VSD), subpulmonary stenosis, aortic "override" of the ventricular septum, and right ventricular hypertrophy. The "tetralogy" that Fallot described is actually the result of a single anatomic abnormality: anterior malalignment of the infundibular septum with the muscular septum (Fig. 17.1.1).

Associated Anatomic Abnormalities

Associated anatomic abnormalities include:

- Anomalous origin of the left anterior descending (LAD) from the right coronary artery crossing the right ventricular outflow tract
- Dual LAD supply
- Right aortic arch
- Multiple VSDs
- Persistent left superior vena cava

In addition to "straight-forward" tetralogy of Fallot, additional constellations of anatomic defects occur with relatively high frequency (discussed below). These include TOF with (*a*) pulmonary atresia, (*b*) absent pulmonary valve, and (*c*) complete atrioventricular (AV) canal.

PATHOPHYSIOLOGY

Preoperative physiology is mainly dependent on the degree of subpulmonary stenosis. In patients with minimal obstruction to pulmonary blood flow, the physiology is similar to that in patients with a left-to-right shunt through a VSD; these patients will have pulmonary overcirculation, a large pulmonary to systemic flow ratio, and symptoms of congestive heart failure (CHF). These patients have little to no right-to-left shunting and are occasionally labeled "pink tets." Alternatively, severe obstruction to pulmonary blood flow may be present with a significant right-to-left shunt at the VSD level. These patients are hypoxemic and may have oxygen saturations in the 70 to 80% range. Despite the hypoxemia, they tend to grow and develop fairly normally. In between these two extremes are patients who are "balanced" with enough pulmonary stenosis to "protect" the pulmonary arteries from overcirculation and pulmonary hypertension. These patients may have minimal to mild hypoxemia (oxygen saturations ≈ 90%) and are typically asymptomatic.

Hypercyanotic "Spells"

The classic TOF spell involves (*a*) agitation or irritability, (*b*) hyperpnea, (*c*) profound cyanosis, and (*d*) syncope. Auscultation during the spell frequently reveals an absent murmur, caused by minimal flow across the obstructive right ventricular outflow tract. If frequent or inadequately managed, these spells can lead to severe disability or even death. Initial treatment typically consists of (*a*) supplemental oxygen, (*b*) sedation (subcutaneous or intravenous [IV] morphine 0.1 mg/kg), and (*c*) volume expansion. The "knee-chest position" has been advocated for these children to increase both systemic venous return and systemic vascular resistance. In some very agitated and hypoxemic children, this positioning tends to worsen the situation as it can be very upsetting and increase the irritability.

It is particularly important for the physicians and nurses at the bedside to keep the situation (and patient) calm. Frequently, the most effective position for these children is to be held by a parent over the shoulder, with knees bent and with supplemental oxygen being given by an additional person. In the case of persistent cyanosis despite these maneuvers, agents to increase systemic afterload (e.g., phenylephrine, 5 to 20 µg/kg/dose IV) can reverse the spell in some cases. Emergency surgery or even extracorporeal circulation (ECMO) is occasionally, but rarely indicated.

PREOPERATIVE EVALUATION

Physical Examination/Electrocardiography/Chest Radiography

A harsh systolic ejection murmur is typically audible at the mid to upper left sternal border; the intensity of the murmur is related to the degree of obstruction to pulmonary blood flow. Patients who are hypoxemic and unrepaired into childhood—rare in the current era—may have signs of polycythemia and clubbing. The electrocardiogram (ECG) typically shows right axis deviation and right ventricular hypertrophy, with upright T waves in the right precordial leads. The chest radiograph may show in-

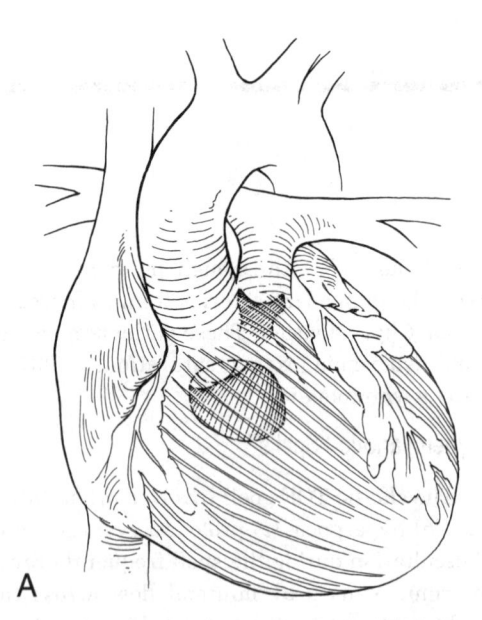

Figure 17.1.1. Anatomy of tetralogy of Fallot. **A.** The external cardiac anatomy of tetralogy of Fallot is shown. Note the hypoplastic pulmonary annulus and the somewhat enlarged and anteriorly displaced aorta. **B.** A cutaway of the right ventricular infundibulum reveals the hypertrophied right ventricular muscle, the increased musculature at the level of the infundibulum, the narrowed subpulmonary region and hypoplastic pulmonary anulus, and the malalignment of the ventricular septal defect with aortic override.

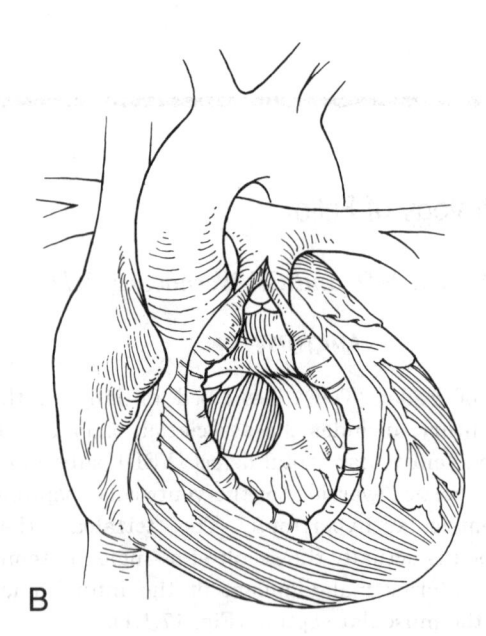

Figure 17.1.2. Subcostal sagittal view from an infant with tetralogy of Fallot. A large malalignment ventricular septal defect (VSD) is seen with anterior malalignment of the infundibular septum (arrow). IVS, intraventricular septum; LA, left atrium; RV, right ventricle.

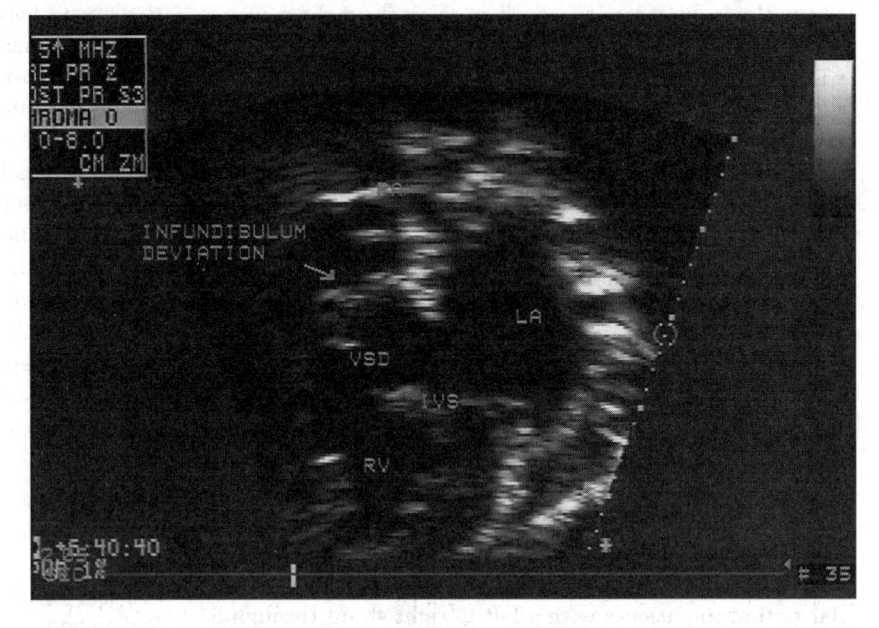

creased, normal, or decreased pulmonary blood flow depending on the severity of the subpulmonary obstruction. The heart may appear "boot-shaped." One should look for the presence of a right aortic arch. The thymus may be absent in patients with microdeletion of the 22nd chromosome.

Echocardiography/Catheterization

Echocardiography is generally sufficient to establish the basic diagnosis. In addition to the anterior malalignment VSD, additional anatomic abnormalities as listed above must be ruled out (Fig. 17.1.2). Cardiac catheterization is typically not indicated for physiologic measurements; in fact, crossing the right ventricular outflow tract with a catheter can induce tetralogy spells. However, some institutions recommend cardiac catheterization to exclude multiple VSDs and coronary abnormalities in particular. Cardiac catheterization is always indicated prior to repair of TOF with pulmonary atresia and diminutive pulmonary arteries, due to the high prevalence of aorticopulmonary collaterals and abnormalities of pulmonary arterial branching (see Chapter 29, *Cardiac Catheterization in the Critically Ill Cardiac Patient*).

SURGERY

Timing

Controversy exists regarding management of both asymptomatic and symptomatic children with TOF. In asymptomatic patients, repair has been advocated anywhere from the time of diagnosis (even in the neonatal period) to 1 year or so of age. For symptomatic and/or cyanotic patients, depending on institutional preference, complete repair can be performed as a single stage procedure or an intermediate aortopulmonary shunt can be performed, followed by complete repair at a later date. Although a shunt can be performed with low risk, an intermediate shunt is associated with a higher incidence of distal pulmonary artery stenoses at the shunt insertion site. In addition, the patient continues to have abnormal physiology until complete repair is undertaken. For these reasons, most centers now favor complete repair in nearly all patients with uncomplicated tetralogy of Fallot, and we currently recommend elective repair between 2 and 4 months of age in the asymptomatic patient.

Technique

A median sternotomy is made for exposure. Cardiopulmonary bypass with aortic cross clamping and cardioplegia is instituted. The operation can be performed with bicaval cannulation while the patient is on cardiopulmonary bypass or, alternatively, utilizing deep hypothermic circulatory arrest. In a transventricular repair, a right ventricular incision is made in the infundibulum; the excision is extended through the pulmonary annulus if it is hypoplastic. This allows exposure of the VSD, which is closed with a patch. A patch is then used to close the infundibulotomy, extending the patch through the annulus if the incision was extended superiorly (Fig. 17.1.3). Transannular patches result in pulmonary regurgitation, which can have significant hemodynamic consequences on right-sided heart function as the right ventricle is typically hypertrophied and noncompliant (1, 2). Alternatively, the VSD and subpulmonary stenosis can be approached using a combined transatrial, transpulmonary approach.

The pulmonary artery should also be inspected for areas of branch stenosis; constriction of ductal tissue at the origin of the left pulmonary artery (LPA) may result in its "coarctation" (3), which should be dealt with at the time of the complete repair. Finally, many centers have recently advocated creating (or leaving) a small atrial septal defect to allow for a "pop off" of high right-sided venous pressures, resulting in improved cardiac output at the expense of mild cyanosis (4).

Mortality

Mortality risk for uncomplicated TOF should be less than 3 to 5% (2, 5–7).

POSTOPERATIVE ISSUES

The repair should be evaluated in the operating room using a combination of transesophageal echocardiography, measurements of right ventricular pressure, and pulmonary artery oxygen saturations. Once the surgeon is comfortable that no hemodynamically significant residual VSD or residual right ventricular outflow tract obstruction exists, the patient is separated from cardiopulmonary bypass and brought to the intensive care unit.

Monitoring will include an arterial line, continuous ECG, central venous monitoring line, temporary pacing wires, and typically a left atrial line. Pulmonary artery catheters may be placed if residual VSD, right ventricular outflow tract obstruction, or pulmonary hypertension are suspected (8). Postoperative care of patients with TOF is typically uneventful with most patients being extubated within 24 hours of surgery.

Specific Postoperative Problems

Residual (or Previously Undiagnosed) VSD

Residual VSD in patients with TOF may be poorly tolerated. In particular, small (3 to 4 mm) VSDs that might be well tolerated by other patients with large left-to-right shunt lesions (VSD, truncus arteriosus, complete atrioventricular canal, and so forth) seem to have a greater hemodynamic impact postoperatively in patients with TOF. This may be due to the coexisting pulmonary regurgitation, noncompliance of the ventricles, a left ventricle not previously volume loaded, or a combination of all of these factors. Patients with hemodynamically important residual VSDs typically have inappropriately elevated heart rates and atrial pressures. In particular, the left atrial pressure (LAP) may be significantly higher than the right atrial pressure, which is the reverse of the normal postoperative course in TOF. An oxygen saturation in the pulmonary artery of more than 80% has been correlated with late catheterization findings of a hemodynamically important residual VSD (8). In patients with hemodynamic instability following TOF repair, the presence of an additional or residual VSD should be promptly and thoroughly investigated.

Residual Right Ventricular Outflow Tract Obstruction

Patients with residual right ventricular outflow tract obstruction may have residual murmurs on auscultation, but they typically tolerate the obstruction fairly well in the immediate perioperative period. However, residual ob-

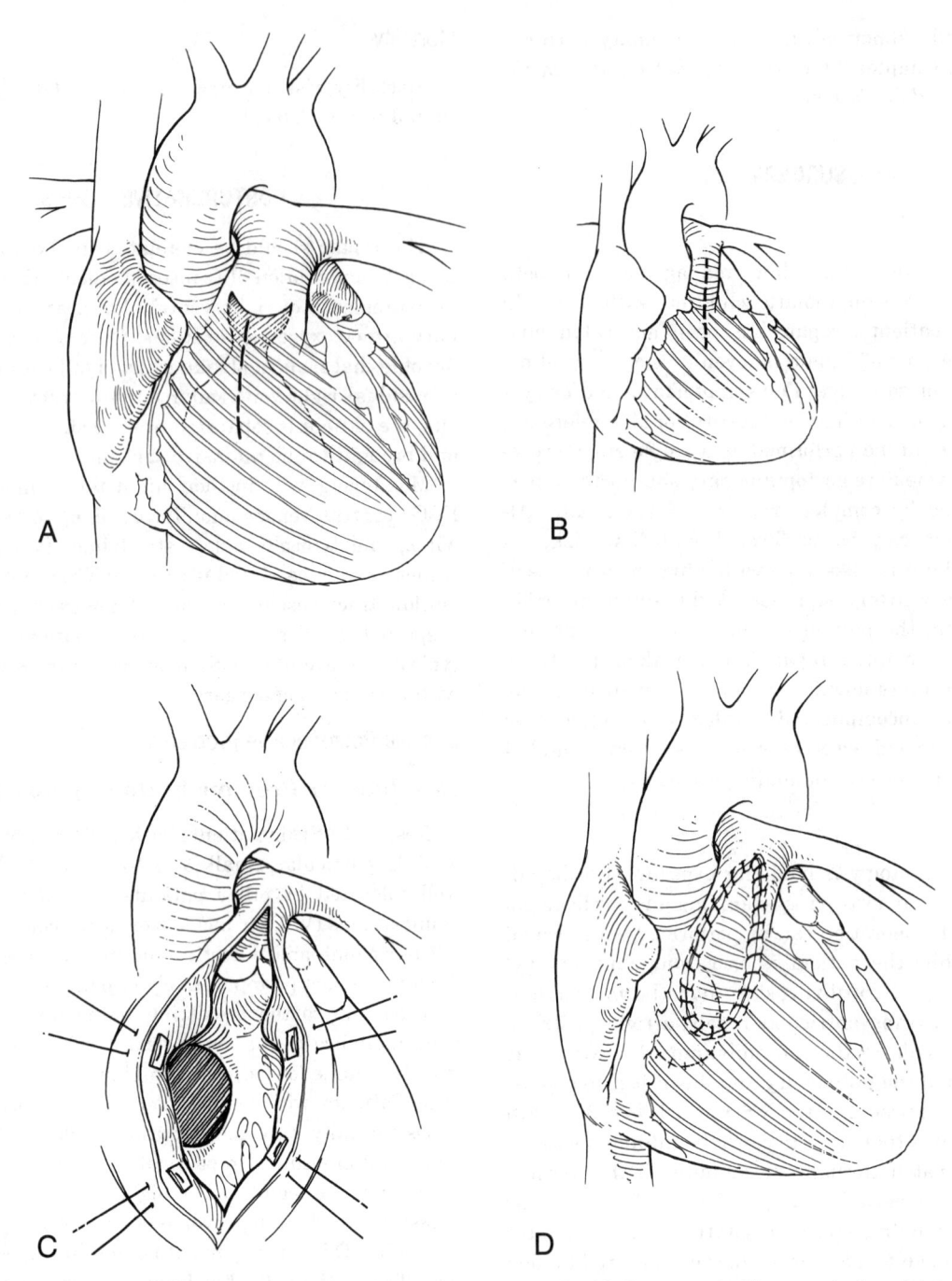

Figure 17.1.3. Repair of tetralogy of Fallot. The position of the subvalvar infundibular incision is shown in **A**. This incision is used when the pulmonary anulus is adequate and a transannular patch is not necessary. When the pulmonary valve anulus is inadequate, a transannular incision is required as shown in **B**. A transannular incision has been performed in **C**, and the edges of the infundibular muscle have been retracted laterally. The hypoplastic bicuspid pulmonary valve is revealed along with malalignment of the ventricular septal defect. The repair proceeds by resecting the hypertrophied septal and parietal bands of the infundibulum to relieve the infundibular stenosis. The ventricular septal defect is patched taking care not to injure the overriding aorta beneath the superior aspect of the defect. A transannular patch is placed to augment the right ventricular outflow tract at the levels of the infundibulum, valve anulus, and main pulmonary artery, as shown in **D**. When a transannular patch is used, postoperative pulmonary insufficiency is a certainty. Some surgeons prefer to add a "monocusp" to the transannular patch to reduce the amount of pulmonary insufficiency in the postoperative period.

struction across the right ventricular outflow tract has been associated with increased problems late after repair, including ventricular arrhythmias and an increased likelihood of late reoperation.

Right Ventricular Dysfunction

Low cardiac output may also be attributable to right ventricular dysfunction. This is typically related to the combination of the right ventricular incision and pulmonary regurgitation, but as mentioned, a residual VSD or right ventricular outflow tract obstruction must be ruled out. The patient with right ventricular dysfunction typically has signs of low systemic cardiac output coupled with signs of elevated central venous pressure (hepatomegaly, edema, and so forth). Pleural effusions are not uncommon in this setting. The time course for recovery is typically 3 to 5 days. In the interim, inotropic support, digoxin, and diuretics are the mainstays of therapy. In addition, right ventricular afterload can be reduced with ventilatory maneuvers to decrease the pulmonary vascular resistance. These patients with transient, postoperative right-sided heart failure are those who benefit the most from the maneuver to leave the foramen ovale patent (4). Patients with signs of severely compromised systemic output from right-sided heart failure who do not have an atrial communication may have one created using trans-septal techniques in the cardiac catheterization laboratory.

Electrophysiologic Abnormalities

Complete heart block (CHB) can occur in 3 to 5% of patients. Although in many cases CHB is transient, brief periods of CHB in the operating room should prompt the caregivers in the intensive care unit to test the temporary pacemaker wires and have a pacemaker ready at the bedside. Bifascicular block occurs in 8 to 12% of patients with TOF. Essentially all patients with a right ventricular incision have a right bundle branch block pattern on the 12-lead ECG. In many cases, this is due to slowing of the peripheral conduction across the infundibulum; intracardiac electrophysiologic studies have shown that only a fraction of patients with right bundle branch block on the scalar ECG have "central" block (i.e., from injury to the His-Purkinje system). Junctional ectopic tachycardia (JET) occurs in a surprisingly high frequency of patients undergoing TOF repair, typically during the first postoperative night, and characterized by AV dissociation with rapid junctional rates as high as 200 to 230 beats per minute. We have observed a surprisingly high number of patients who have transient CHB in the operating room, followed by JET 12 to 24 hours later in the cardiac intensive care unit. Hemodynamic instability with JET warrants treatment. A combination of core cooling (34°C to 35°C) and antiarrhythmic agents (procainamide, amiodarone) can typically slow the junctional rate to below 150 to 160 beats per minute. Should the hemodynamics still be suboptimal, atrial pacing can then be used to re-establish AV synchrony (see Chapter 30, *Diagnosis and Management of Cardiac Arrhythmias*).

POSTOPERATIVE CARE CHECKLIST

Postoperative care checklist includes:

- Evaluate for residual VSD and right ventricular outflow obstruction and dysfunction.
- Continuous monitoring of heart rate with evaluation for arrhythmia (JET, ventricular ectopy, CHB).
- Temporary pacemaker available at bedside in some cases.

Tetralogy of Fallot with Pulmonary Atresia

Also referred to as "pulmonary atresia with ventricular septal defect" (PA/VSD), the intracardiac anatomy of TOF with pulmonary atresia (TOF/PA) is identical to that of TOF—an anterior malalignment-type of VSD with aortic override. TOF/PA is an *extremely* heterogeneous lesion, not because of the intracardiac anatomy, but because of the variability of the pulmonary artery architecture. Simplistically, patients with TOF/PA fall into three subgroups: (*a*) confluent "true" (i.e., mediastinal) pulmonary arteries, normal to slightly small in caliber, supplied by the ductus arteriosus (see Fig. 17.1.4), (*b*) absent (or extremely diminutive; less than 2 mm) "true" pulmonary arteries with multiple aortopulmonary collateral arteries (MAPCAs), and (*c*) small mediastinal pulmonary arteries and MAPCAs with multiple segments of lung receiving "dual supply."

The first subgroup—those with normal or nearly normal central pulmonary arteries—may be managed in a fashion similar to TOF. The approach in the newborn period is to maintain patency of the ductus arteriosus with prostaglandin E_1, until either a palliative shunt is performed or, alternatively, complete correction can be performed in the newborn period (9). Left pulmonary artery stenosis at the ductal insertion site is common in this type of TOF/PA. If a shunt is performed, close monitoring of the left lung perfusion (by echocardiography and/or lung perfusion scan) is important in the 1 to 4 months after surgery. We prefer complete correction in the newborn period whenever possible. At the time of complete correction, some have suggested using pedicled pericardium and a flap of the left atrial appendage to establish continuity between the right ventricle and the distal pulmonary arteries (10); however, a right ventricular-pulmonary artery conduit is typically necessary (11, 12). If complete neonatal repair is undertaken, the distal end of the conduit can be incorpo-

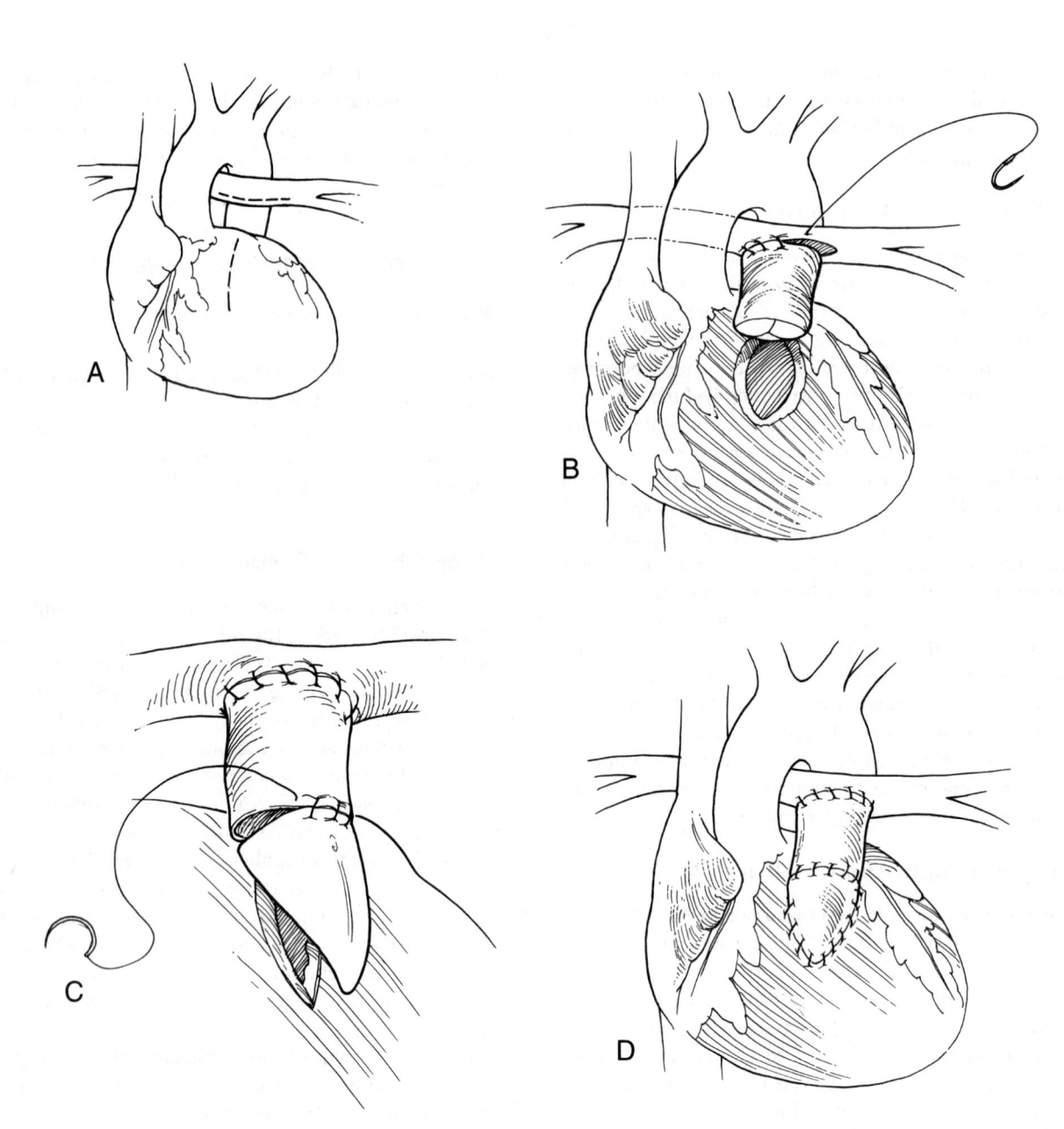

Figure 17.1.4. Repair of tetralogy of Fallot with pulmonary atresia. Pulmonary valve atresia can take one of two forms: either short segment pulmonary atresia in which the pulmonary artery is in physical continuity with the infundibulum, or long segment pulmonary atresia in which the pulmonary artery is discontinuous with the heart as is shown in **A**. Note the incisions in the central main pulmonary artery and in the blind-ended right ventricular infundibulum. In **B** a homograft valved conduit is anastomosed to the central pulmonary arteries. An appropriate sized infundibulotomy is performed by incising and resecting muscle in the free wall of the infundibulum and the homograft is then anastomosed to the infundibulotomy using a proximal hood to augment the anastomosis and prevent distortion of the valve itself, as shown in **C**. The completed reconstruction of the right ventricular outflow tract is shown in **D**. Tetralogy of Fallot with pulmonary atresia can also be repaired without a valved homograft by using either direct anastomosis of the pulmonary artery to the infundibulum with patch augmentation or a nonvalved conduit. Free pulmonary insufficiency should be expected when a valved conduit is not used. The variability in pulmonary artery architecture is not shown in this figure (11–13).

rated is such a way to "plasty" the left pulmonary artery origin. The VSD can be closed through the ventriculotomy that is used to attach the proximal end of the conduit.

The approach to the second and third subgroups is much more individualized, depending on the particular anatomy of the pulmonary arterial tree. It generally involves establishing forward flow into the "true" pulmonary arteries in the mediastinum, followed by angiography to determine the segments of lung that are supplied by (a) the "true" pulmonary arteries, (b), MAPCAs alone, or (c) both. Segments supplied by MAPCAs may need to be "unifocalized" into the "true" pulmonary artery confluence (13), whereas segments that have proximal stenoses but are supplied by the "true" pulmonary arteries may require balloon angioplasty. The initial surgical procedure that establishes flow into the "true" pulmonary arteries may be a shunt, a direct connection of the back of the aorta to the tiny central pulmonary arteries, or a right ventricle to pulmonary artery conduit.

Once the total cross-sectional area of the pulmonary vasculature is adequate to accept a full cardiac output (i.e., enough segments of lung supplied from the right ventricle via the "true" pulmonary arteries without pulmonary hypertension), then the VSD can be closed with acceptable right ventricle pressure (14). It is beyond the scope of this chapter to review the details of these new, complex approaches; the reader is referred to some of the recent references on the topic (11, 12, 15) (see also Chapter 29, *Cardiac Catheterization in the Critically Ill Cardiac Patient*).

Tetralogy of Fallot with Absent Pulmonary Valve

Tetralogy of Fallot with absent pulmonary valve (TOF/APV) includes dysgenesis of the pulmonary valve, annular stenosis, and pulmonary insufficiency. This constellation of anatomic findings is occasionally confused with tetralogy of Fallot with pulmonary atresia because of similarities in terminology (*pulmonary atresia* versus *absent pulmonary valve*). However, the pulmonary artery architecture and pathophysiology are vastly different. Perhaps better terminology would be to consider these patients as having "absent pulmonary valve syndrome"; nearly 100% also have the intracardiac features of TOF, although rare cases of absent pulmonary valve syndrome with an intact ventricular septum have been reported. Massive enlargement of the main and branch pulmonary arteries is common to all forms of the syndrome, as in utero pulmonary regurgitation results in pulsatile and increased pulmonary blood flow (Fig. 17.1.5). In addition to the mediastinal abnormalities of the pulmonary arteries with bizarre branching patterns at the hilum, the intraparenchymal pulmonary vessels are abnormal as well, with abnormal segmental arteries and elastic laminae (16). Finally, the airway itself is typically abnormal, with areas of tracheobronchial malacia in the mediastinum, and occasionally reduced numbers of bronchial generations (16).

Patients can be divided into two groups depending on age and severity of symptoms. The first group is comprised of neonates with severe cardiorespiratory distress, whereas the second group includes older patients who survive the immediate neonatal period (and are much more similar physiologically to TOF). The neonatal group presents typically within hours of birth with marked respiratory distress, cyanosis, and air trapping due to tracheobronchial compression. The hypoxemia is usually caused by a combination of right-to-left shunting at the VSD as well as pulmonary venous desaturation from ventilation-perfusion mismatch. Tracheal intubation and mechanical ventilation may not improve gas exchange, but high positive end-expiratory pressure (PEEP) may help to stent open "floppy" airways. Prone positioning is occasionally helpful in relieving some of the tracheal compression (17). Early repair of this subgroup is necessary, with anterior and posterior plication of the pulmonary arteries, closure of the VSD, and transannular patching of the right ventricular outflow tract (18–21) (Fig. 17.1.6). Many surgeons currently place a homograft valve or monocusp to minimize the pulmonary regurgitation and continued pulmonary artery pulsatile flow in the immediate postoperative period. Despite a technically adequate repair, many of these symptomatic neonates have continued pulmonary difficulties, nearly all have some degree of bronchospasm into infancy and childhood, and some require tracheostomy, long-term ventilation, and PEEP.

Tetralogy of Fallot with Complete Atrioventricular Canal

Although the repair of isolated TOF or complete atrioventricular canal (CAVC) can be accomplished with acceptable mortality risks, the combination of the two lesions

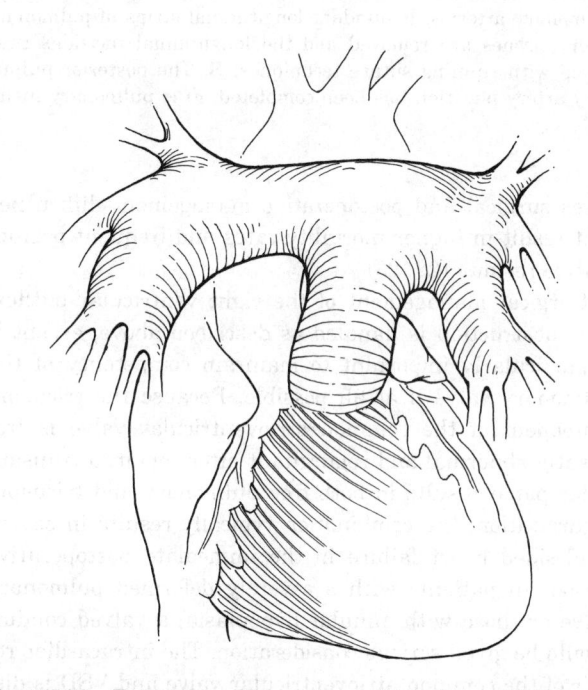

Figure 17.1.5. External cardiac anatomy of tetralogy of Fallot with absent pulmonary valve. Note the mildly hypoplastic pulmonary valve annulus with vestigial nonfunctioning valve tissue only, and the massively dilated main and central, right and left pulmonary arteries. The aneurysmal changes in the pulmonary arteries may extend into the secondary pulmonary artery branches or even into the distal bed. Tracheobronchial obstruction secondary to the massive pulmonary arteries commonly accompanies this lesion. The intracardiac anatomy is similar to that of simple tetralogy of Fallot.

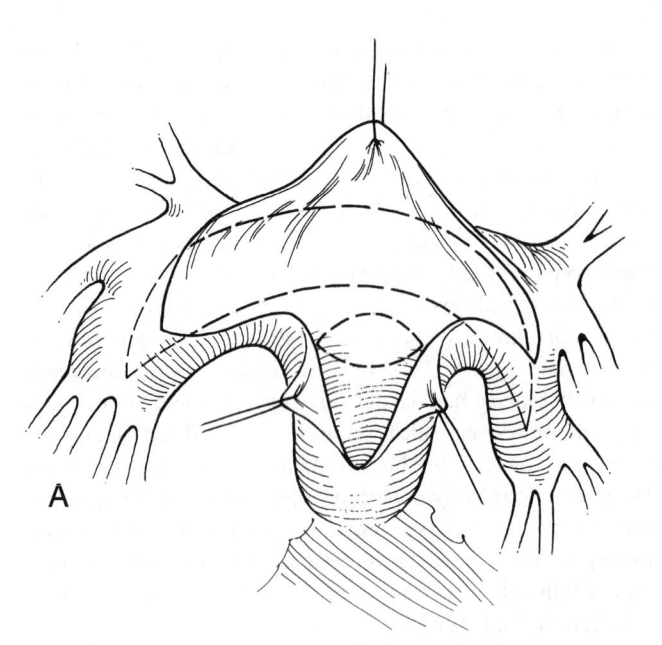

Figure 17.1.6. Repair of tetralogy of Fallot with absent pulmonary valve. **A.** An important component of the repair is plication of the aneurysmal pulmonary arteries. This proceeds by longitudinal anterior incisions in the aneurysmal segments extending commonly onto the secondary pulmonary artery branches. Once this has been done, an incision can be made in the posterior wall of the pulmonary arteries. Redundant longitudinal strips of pulmonary artery tissues are removed and the longitudinal incisions then closed with running suture techniques. **B.** The posterior pulmonary artery plication has been completed. Free pulmonary insufficiency will result if the absent pulmonary valve itself is not addressed. In older infants and children with this syndrome who are stable and asymptomatic at the time of repair, pulmonary insufficiency may be reasonably well tolerated. However, in young infants who are unstable with both cardiac and pulmonary involvement, the best results have been achieved by using a monocusp or by placing a valved homograft in the pulmonary position. In all cases, the repair is completed by closing the typical malalignment ventricular septal defect.

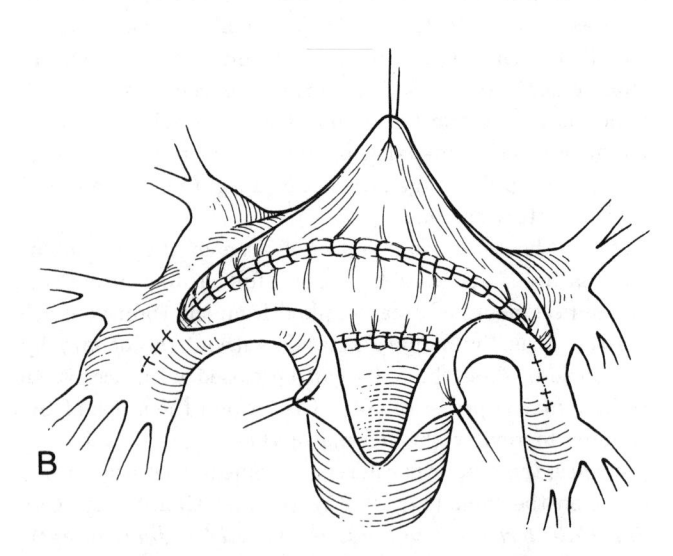

poses surgical and postoperative management difficulties that result in higher mortality rates and frequent postoperative residua (22, 23).

Surgical management of the right ventricular outflow tract obstruction is handled as described above, except it is particularly important to maintain competency of the pulmonary valve if at all possible. Because the tricuspid component of the common atrioventricular valve is frequently abnormal and regurgitant after repair, a transannular patch results in both free pulmonary and tricuspid regurgitation; the combination typically results in severe right-sided heart failure in the immediate postoperative period. In patients with a severely deformed pulmonary valve or those with annular hypoplasia, a valved conduit should be given serious consideration. The intracardiac repair of the common atrioventricular valve and VSD is discussed in Chapter 15.5, *Common Atrioventricular Canal.*

As in both isolated CAVC and TOF, postoperative residual defects must be sought, including residual VSD, right ventricular outflow tract obstruction, atrioventricular valve regurgitation, and conduction disturbances. Right-sided heart dysfunction is extremely common, given the abnormalities of the right-sided atrioventricular valve, infundibular incision, and pulmonary regurgitation (if present). As discussed for isolated TOF, leaving a patent foramen ovale is particularly helpful in these children with borderline right ventricle function.

REFERENCES

1. Miura T, Nakano S, Shimazaki Y, et al. Evaluation of right ventricular function by regional wall motion analysis in patients after correction of tetralogy of Fallot. J Thorac Cardiovasc Surg 1992;104:917–923.
2. Cullen S, Shore D, Redington A. Characterization of right ventricular diastolic performance after complete repair of tetralogy of Fallot: restrictive physiology predicts slow postoperative recovery. Circulation 1995;91:1782–1789.
3. Elzenga NJ, von Suylen RJ, Frohn-Mulder I, et al. Juxtaductal pulmonary artery coarctation: an underestimated cause of branch pulmonary artery stenosis in patients with pulmonary atresia or stenosis and a ventricular septal defect. J Thorac Cardiovasc Surg 1990;100:416–424.
4. Pass RH, Mayer JE Jr, Jonas RA, et al. Course in the intensive care unit after right ventriculotomy and neonatal repair of congenital heart disease [Abstract]. J Am Coll Cardiol 1997;29:107A.
5. Uva MS, Lacour-Gayet F, Komiya T, et al. Surgery for tetralogy of Fallot at less than six months of age. J Thorac Cardiovasc Surg 1994;107:1291–1300.
6. Gustafson RA, Murray GF, Warden HE, et al. Early primary

repair of tetralogy of Fallot. Ann Thorac Surg 1988;45: 235–241.
7. Groh MA, Meliones JN, Bove EL, et al. Repair of tetralogy of Fallot in infancy. Circulation 1991;84 (Supp III):III-206–III-212.
8. Lang P, Chipman CW, Siden H, et al. Early assessment of hemodynamic status after repair of tetralogy of Fallot: a comparison of 24 hour (ICU) and 1 year postoperative data in 98 patients. Am J Cardiol 1982;50:795–799.
9. Hennein H, Mosca R, Urcelay G, et al. Intermediate results after complete repair of tetralogy of Fallot in neonates. J Thorac Cardiovasc Surg 1995;109:332–344.
10. Kitagawa T, Katoh, I, Chikugo F, et al. Technique for constructing the pulmonary trunk for tetralogy of Fallot with pulmonary atresia. Ann Thorac Surg 1995;59:1245–1248.
11. Rome JJ, Mayer JE, Castañeda AR, Lock JE: Tetralogy of Fallot with pulmonary atresia. Rehabilitation of diminutive pulmonary arteries. Circulation 1993;88[Part 1]:1691–1698.
12. Reddy VM, Liddicoat JR, Hanley FL. Midline one-stage complete unifocalization and repair of pulmonary atresia with ventricular septal defect and major aortopulmonary collaterals. J Thorac Cardiovasc Surg 1995;109:832–845.
13. Puga FJ, Leoni FE, Julsrud PR, et al. Complete repair of pulmonary atresia, ventricular septal defect, and severe peripheral arborization abnormalities of the central pulmonary arteries. J Thorac Cardiovasc Surg 1989;98:1018–1029.
14. Shimazaki Y, Lio M, Nakano S, et al. Pulmonary artery morphology and hemodynamics in pulmonic valve atresia with ventricular septal defect before and after repair. Am J Cardiol 1991;67:744–748.
15. Pagani F, Cheatham J, Beekman R, et al. The management of tetralogy of Fallot with pulmonary atresia and diminutive pulmonary arteries. J Thorac Cardiovasc Surg 1995;110: 1521–1533.
16. Rabinovitch M, Grady S, David I, et al. Compression of intrapulmonary bronchi by abnormally branching pulmonary arteries associated with absent pulmonary valves. Am J Cardiol 1982;50:804–813.
17. Heinemann MK, Hanley FL. Preoperative management of neonatal tetralogy of Fallot with absent pulmonary valve syndrome. Ann Thorac Surg 1993;55:172–174.
18. Ilbawi M, Fedorchik J, Muster A, et al. Surgical approach to severely symptomatic newborn infants with tetralogy of Fallot and absent pulmonary valve. J Thorac Cardiovasc Surg 1986;91:584–589.
19. Snir E, deLeval M, Elliott M, et al. Current surgical technique to repair Fallot's tetralogy with absent pulmonary valve syndrome. Ann Thorac Surg 1991;51:979–982.
20. Watterson K, Malm T, Karl T, Mee R. Absent pulmonary valve syndrome: operation in infants with airway obstruction. Ann Thorac Surg 1992;54:1116–1119.
21. Kron IL, Johnson AM, Carpenter MA, et al. Treatment of absent pulmonary valve syndrome with homograft. Ann Thorac Surg 1988;46:579–581.
22. Ilbawi M, Cua C, DeLeon S, et al. Repair of complete atrioventricular septal defect with tetralogy of Fallot. Ann Thorac Surg 1990;50:407–412.
23. Vargas FJ, Coto EO, Mayer JE, et al. Complete atrioventricular canal and tetralogy of Fallot: surgical considerations. Ann Thorac Surg 1986;42:258–263.

17.2 Pulmonary Atresia with Intact Ventricular Septum Pulmonary Stenosis

Gil Wernovsky, MD, and Frank L. Hanley, MD

ANATOMY

In pulmonary atresia with intact ventricular septum (PA/IVS), complete obstruction of right ventricular outflow is found due to atresia of the pulmonary valve (platelike or membranous obstruction). Associated with this finding is an intact ventricular septum and variable hypoplasia of the right ventricle and tricuspid valve (sometimes referred to as "hypoplastic right heart syndrome" [Fig. 17.2.1]). The main pulmonary artery is present, usually somewhat smaller than normal, and pulmonary blood flow is supplied by a patent ductus arteriosus (PDA). The tricuspid valve is proportionately small, and it may be deformed. The tricuspid valve is frequently stenotic and/or regurgitant and sometimes grossly incompetent. A high association of coronary artery sinusoids and fistulae is seen in patients with a particularly small right ventricle and tricuspid valve annulus (1); these may represent the predominant source of blood flow to the coronary arteries, and greatly determine surgical management strategies (2–5).

Because PA/IVS is an extremely heterogeneous and rare lesion, our ability is limited in drawing conclusions regarding outcome from most published series with small numbers of patients with variable anatomy. However, it seems clear that patients with small right ventricles tend to have small tricuspid valves, an absent infundibulum, and coronary artery abnormalities, which places them at high risk for long-term survival. On the other hand, patients with nearly normal sized right ventricles typically do not have coronary anomalies. These patients have a well-developed infundibulum and a favorable prognosis.

PATHOPHYSIOLOGY

Preoperative physiology is similar to other forms of functional single ventricle with duct-dependent pulmonary blood flow (see Chapter 18, *Single Ventricle Lesions*). Complete mixing of the systemic and pulmonary venous return is seen, and the arterial oxygen saturation serves as a good estimate of the pulmonary to systemic flow ratio. The additional possible egress of blood from the right ventricle is

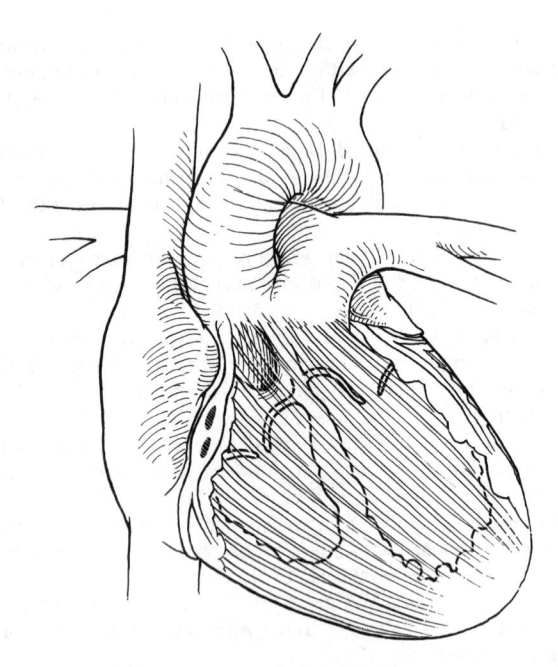

Figure 17.2.1. Anatomy of pulmonary atresia with intact ventricular septum. Typical morphologic features include a markedly hypertrophied and hypoplastic right ventricle, an atretic pulmonary valve with a well-developed main pulmonary artery, and normally developed branch pulmonary arteries. The right atrium is enlarged and hypertrophied and an atrial septal defect is present. The tricuspid valve is also invariably dysplastic and Ebstein's anomaly may occasionally exist. Coronary artery anomalies are common and include stenoses and fistula formation between the coronary arteries and the right ventricular cavity. The severity of the right ventricular hypoplasia varies widely, ranging from essentially normal right ventricular size to almost complete absence of the right ventricle. It is thought that pulmonary atresia is an acquired lesion in utero, and the degree of right ventricular hypoplasia is more severe with early intrauterine valve closure. The coronary artery fistulae can be minor or extensive, and the existence and degree of fistula formation varies directly with the degree of right ventricular hypoplasia. In its most severe form the entire myocardial circulation is derived from the right ventricle via fistulae with no connection of the coronary arteries to the aorta.

(a) to the aorta via sinusoids in the coronary circulation and (b) to the right atrium via a regurgitant tricuspid valve. Depending on the available egress, the right ventricle may develop high pressures during systole, up to 150 mm Hg or greater.

PREOPERATIVE EVALUATION

Electrocardiogram/Chest Radiograph

As opposed to many newborns with complex congenital heart disease, who typically have a normal electrocardiogram (ECG) despite significant intracardiac pathology, patients with PA/IVS have characteristic ECG findings. The QRS axis in the frontal plane may be a little more leftward than usual (0 to 90 degrees), but the pathognomonic features on the surface ECG are diminished right ventricular forces and left ventricular hypertrophy. The chest radiograph typically reveals a normal heart size, unless significant tricuspid regurgitation is present, which results in right atrial enlargement. The intensity of the pulmonary vascular markings is dependent on the size of the ductus arteriosus and the pulmonary vascular resistance.

Echocardiography/Catheterization

Echocardiography is sufficient to establish the basic diagnosis. Ductal patency can be confirmed and the degree of right ventricular hypertension estimated by a Doppler gradient across the regurgitant tricuspid valve. Abnormal color Doppler flow patterns into the right ventricle may be suggestive of coronary artery fistulae or sinusoids. The tricuspid annulus and degree of stenosis or regurgitation can be measured. Finally, the presence and size of the infundibulum, inflow, and body of the right ventricle can be determined.

Cardiac catheterization is almost always indicated in the newborn evaluation of PA/IVS. In addition to a complete hemodynamic assessment with measurement of right ventricular pressure, coronary artery angiography is crucial in the initial management of this disease. The combination of aortic root aortography (typically antegrade with balloon occlusion) and right ventricular angiography are typically sufficient to define the coronary artery branching pattern and distribution. Right ventricular dependent coronary circulation (RVDCC) exists when sufficiently large areas of myocardium are perfused only from the high pressure right ventricle (2). Typically multiple connections exist between the coronary arteries and the right ventricle, although the coronaries from the sinuses of Valsalva in the aortic root may also supply a large portion of myocardium. Despite the presence of sinusoids and/or fistulae, if the distribution of the coronary arteries from the aortic sinuses of Valsalva is adequate (without multiple stenoses or areas of myocardium solely perfused from the right ventricle) (2), a staged approach toward a "two-ventricle" repair is typically undertaken, especially with a nearly normal-sized right ventricle, tricuspid valve, and infundibulum. In cases of RVDCC, decompression of the right ventricle via a valvotomy or transannular patch would result in lowering the right ventricular pressure and hypoperfusion to large areas of myocardium, resulting in infarction and ventricular dysfunction.

SURGERY

Timing

Once the initial anatomic diagnoses are made, surgery takes place in the newborn period. For patients with RVDCC, a palliative Blalock-Taussig shunt, usually with concomitant duct ligation, is performed. The patient is managed similarly to other forms of single ventricle disorders and has further procedures (bidirectional Glenn, Fontan) at later dates (see Chapter 18, *Single Ventricle Lesions*) with acceptable results (6, 7). Patients with severe RVDCC and evidence of left ventricular dysfunction, ischemia, or arrhythmia may need to be considered for cardiac transplantation (2, 4, 5). However, if RVDCC is not present, a first stage procedure is performed with relief of the right ventricular outflow tract obstruction, usually coupled with a systemic-pulmonary artery shunt. The remainder of this discussion will focus on the management of patients following this approach.

Technique

The initial principle of this technique is to provide unobstructed pulmonary blood flow from the right ventricle (Fig. 17.2.2). In patients with a hypoplastic infundibulum, this typically requires a transannular patch rather than an isolated valvotomy. It is crucial that all obstruction is relieved to allow for regression of the significant hypertrophy present in the ventricle. Despite adequate relief of the right ventricular outflow tract obstruction, a persistent right-to-left shunt at the atrial level will persist in most patients. This is due to the combined effects of tricuspid stenosis, annular hypoplasia, and a diminutive and noncompliant right ventricle. In most cases, not enough blood flows antegrade through the right ventricle to provide adequate pulmonary blood flow and oxygen delivery; additional maneuvers to secure pulmonary blood flow include a small Blalock-Taussig shunt or prostaglandin to maintain patency of the ductus arteriosus (8).

If the right ventricular outflow tract obstruction is adequately relieved and the tricuspid valve and right ventricle are of "adequate" size, within 2 to 3 months hypertrophy regresses, compliance improves, and the right ventricle can increase its contribution to pulmonary blood flow. The shunt can then be surgically taken down or coil embolized in the catheterization laboratory. The final stage in management involves closure of the atrial communication. Some patients continue to have moderate hypoplasia of the right ventricular cavity, despite adequate relief of the outflow tract obstruction (9, 10). In addition, tricuspid valve size may eventually limit the amount of the systemic venous return that can pass through the right ventricle. In these patients, a "one-and-a-half" ventricle repair can be performed, with atrial septal defect closure combined with a superior vena caval to right pulmonary artery shunt (bidirectional Glenn). In this approach, the right ventricle only needs to eject the systemic venous return from the inferior vena cava (11).

Mortality

Surgical mortality risk is highly dependent on the heterogeneous anatomy. Although mortality for shunt proce-

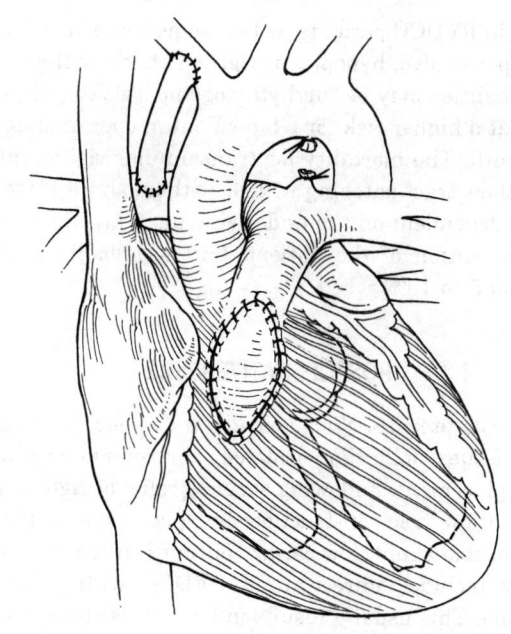

Figure 17.2.2 Typical surgical **palliation** in the neonatal period for pulmonary atresia with intact ventricular septum. Because of the variable morphology associated with pulmonary atresia with intact ventricular septum no single surgical procedure done in the neonatal period is appropriate for all patients. The goal of neonatal palliation is to provide both adequate oxygenation with a balanced pulmonary and systemic circulation and forward flow across the right ventricular outflow tract to encourage right ventricular development, with the ultimate goal of achieving a two-ventricle repair with completely separated systemic and pulmonary circulations. However, in cases with extremely small right ventricles or with major right ventricular to coronary artery fistulae, the right ventricle cannot be salvaged and the appropriate neonatal procedure is simply a modified Blalock-Taussig shunt. This situation may be present in 30 to 40% of patients with pulmonary atresia and intact ventricular septum. At the other end of the morphologic spectrum, some patients have a large compliant right ventricle, an adequate tricuspid valve, and no significant fistulae. These patients may achieve repair in the neonatal period with reconstruction of the right ventricular outflow tract only, with no need for an associated modified Blalock-Taussig shunt. It is likely that less than 10% of patients with pulmonary atresia and an intact ventricular septum will be candidates for an immediate reparative procedure.

As shown in this figure, the most common neonatal procedure involves creation of a modified Blalock-Taussig shunt to ensure appropriate and adequate pulmonary blood flow in association with right ventricular outflow tract reconstruction, most typically a right ventricular outflow tract patch extending from the infundibulum to the main pulmonary artery, to encourage forward flow across the right ventricular outflow tract, thereby promoting right ventricular development. This procedure is appropriate in patients with small noncompliant right ventricles that are not capable of providing adequate pulmonary blood flow in the neonatal period. In many cases, however, the patch provides decompression of the right ventricular hypertension, encouraging growth of the right ventricular chamber and involution of the severe right ventricular hypertrophy. In many cases, the right ventricle can be rehabilitated to the point where a two-ventricle repair ultimately can be achieved. A combination of the modified Blalock-Taussig shunt and right ventricular outflow tract patch reconstruction as shown may be appropriate in up to 50% of neonates with pulmonary atresia and intact ventricular septum.

dures (in RVDCC patients) is low, some concern exists that the hypertensive, hypoplastic right ventricle with coronary abnormalities may be "arrhythmogenic," making these patients at a higher risk for a later Fontan operation, or sudden death. The mortality for transannular right ventricular outflow tract patching with or without shunt placement is also dependent on the underlying anatomy and preoperative condition of the patient, but it probably is in the range of 5 to 10%.

POSTOPERATIVE ISSUES

See Chapter 18, *Single Ventricle Lesions,* for management issues following isolated aortopulmonary artery shunt placement. Following surgical relief of right ventricular outflow tract obstruction and placement of the Blalock-Taussig shunt, low cardiac output can occur. One possibility includes unrecognized RVDCC with myocardial ischemia. This usually results in low cardiac output immediately after surgery, ECG changes, ventricular arrhythmias, and segmental wall akineses or dyskineses on echocardiography. Large areas of myocardial ischemia following this procedure carry a grave prognosis.

A second form of low cardiac output can develop 1 to 3

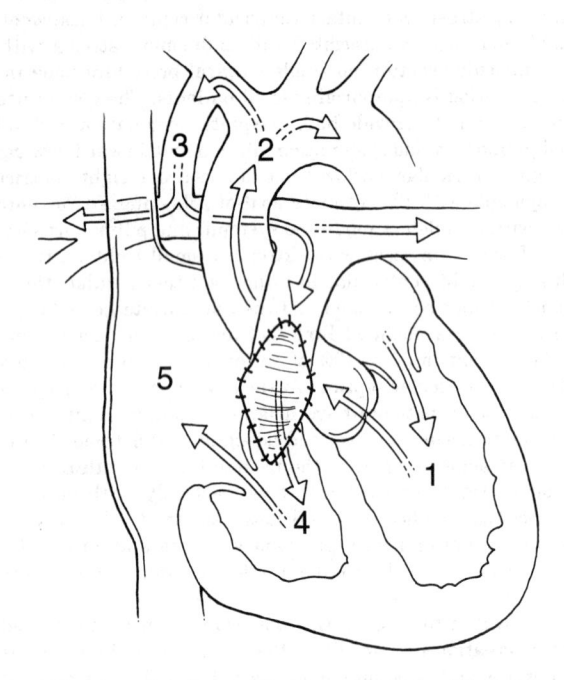

Figure 17.2.3. Circular shunt following neonatal palliation for pulmonary atresia with intact ventricular septum. When the repair involves placement of a systemic to pulmonary artery shunt and a transannular right ventricular outflow tract patch, an ineffective circular shunt becomes possible. The systemic to pulmonary artery connection in combination with the obligatory pulmonary insufficiency, associated tricuspid valve insufficiency, and atrial septal defect can result in flow patterns as shown (*arrows*) in this illustration. Blood from the left atrium enters the left ventricle (1), the aorta (2), then passes through the systemic to pulmonary artery shunt (3) into the pulmonary artery, then retrograde across the right ventricular outflow tract (4) and retrograde across the tricuspid valve into the right atrium (5), then across the right atrium back to the left atrium. See text for further description and physiologic implications.

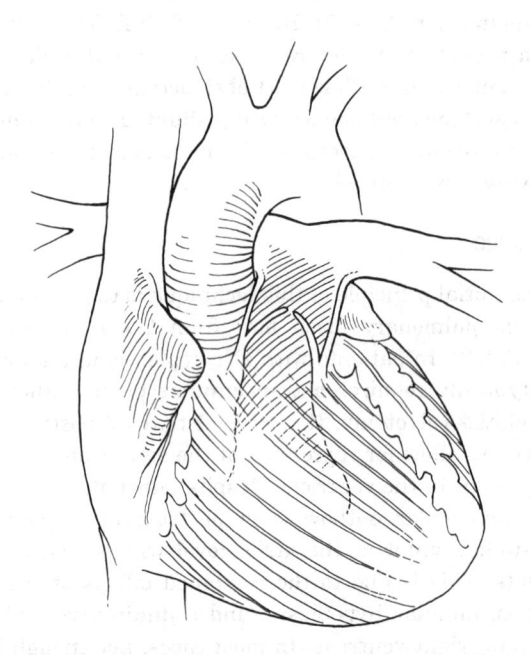

Figure 17.2.4. Anatomy of pulmonary valve stenosis. Typical features include a hypertrophied but well-developed right ventricle and infundibulum with a thickened doming pulmonary valve which may be tricuspid or bicuspid. The pulmonary artery system distal to the valve is usually normal.

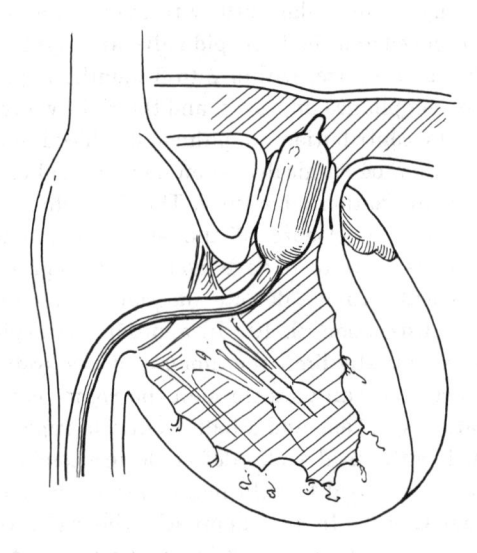

Figure 17.2.5. Balloon valvotomy is the treatment of choice for pulmonary valve stenosis. Results are excellent and dysmorphic changes in the pulmonary valve tissue may resolve with time following the procedure. The procedure is performed in the cardiac catheterization laboratory by the interventional cardiology team. Percutaneous access is typically gained through the femoral vein.

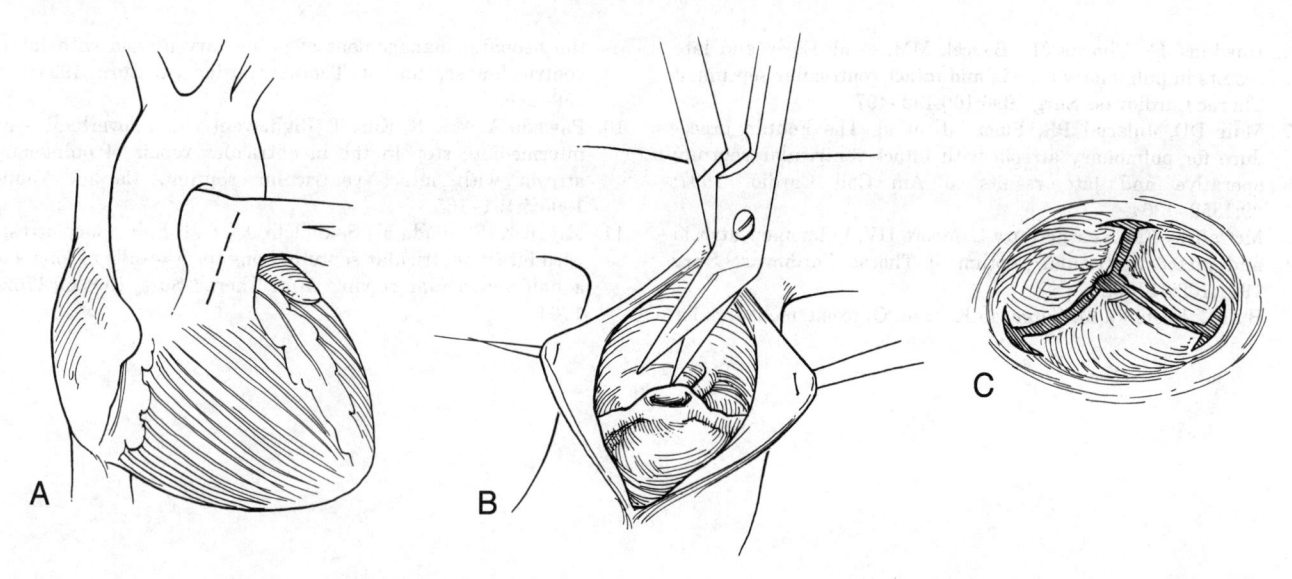

Figure 17.2.6. Surgical valvotomy for pulmonary stenosis. The procedure is performed on cardiopulmonary bypass with mild hypothermia and without the need for aortic cross-clamping. A longitudinal incision is made in the main pulmonary artery (**A**). After the pulmonary artery is opened, the fused commissures can often be identified within the doming and thickened pulmonary valve tissue (**B**). The fused commissures are opened using sharp dissection, and the leaflet edges may be mobilized when the tissue is particularly dysplastic (**C**). The pulmonary arteriotomy is then enclosed to complete the procedure.

days following surgery, resulting from a "circular shunt" (Fig. 17.2.3). By design, the transannular patch results in pulmonary regurgitation. Blood may flow from the Blalock-Taussig shunt retrograde through the right ventricular outflow tract into the right ventricle in diastole, and in patients with tricuspid regurgitation, retrograde into the right atrium in systole. This results in blood ejected from the left ventricle and aorta to return to the right atrium without adequate delivery of effective systemic blood flow. Patients with a large circular shunt can develop oliguria, metabolic acidemia, and systemic hypotension. Maneuvers to increase pulmonary vascular resistance and lower systemic vascular resistance may be helpful, but this physiology is particularly difficult to manage medically. Surgical maneuvers to narrow the shunt and/or minimize the tricuspid regurgitation may be necessary.

In patients with significant persistent hypoxemia, residual right ventricular outflow tract obstruction or severe tricuspid hypoplasia should be excluded.

POSTOPERATIVE CARE CHECKLIST

Postoperative care checklist includes:

- In shunt-dependent patients, balance the circulation (see Chapter 18, *Single Ventricle Lesions*).
- Monitoring for signs of ischemia with 12-lead ECG and/or echocardiography.
- Evaluate for signs of low cardiac output and "circular shunting."

PULMONARY VALVE STENOSIS

Isolated pulmonary valve stenosis (Fig. 17.2.4) typically coexists with a normal sized, hypertrophied right ventricle, a normal tricuspid valve, and normal distal pulmonary arteries. Balloon valvuloplasty has become the initial procedure of choice in most patients (Fig. 17.2.5) as described in Chapter 29, *Cardiac Catheterization in the Critically Ill Cardiac Patient*. In some patients with dysplastic pulmonary valves, surgical valvotomy may be necessary (Fig. 17.2.6). Following either procedure, a small right-to-left shunt may persist at the atrial level until right ventricular hypertrophy regresses and compliance improves.

REFERENCES

1. Hanley FL, Sade RM, Blackstone EH, et al. Outcomes in neonatal pulmonary atresia with intact ventricular septum—a multiinstitutional study. J Thorac Cardiovasc Surg 1993; 105:406–427.
2. Giglia TM, Mandell VS, Connor AR, et al. Diagnosis and management of right ventricle-dependent coronary circulation in pulmonary atresia with intact ventricular septum. Circulation 1992;86:1516–1628.
3. Gentles TL, Colan SD, Giglia TM, et al. Right ventricular decompression and left ventricular function in pulmonary atresia with intact ventricular septum: the influence of less extensive coronary anomalies. Circulation 1993;88(II):183–188.
4. Dyamenahalli U, Hanna BD, Sharratt GP. Pulmonary atresia with intact ventricular septum: management of the coronary arterial anomalies. Cardiology in the Young 1997;7:80–87.
5. Akiba T, Becker AE. Disease of the left ventricle in pulmonary atresia with intact ventricular septum. J Thorac Cardiovasc Surg 1994;108:1–8.

6. Hawkins JA, Thorne JK, Boucek MM, et al. Early and late results in pulmonary atresia and intact ventricular septum. J Thorac Cardiovasc Surg 1990;100:492–497.
7. Mair DD, Julsrud PR, Puga FJ, et al. The Fontan procedure for pulmonary atresia with intact ventricular septum: operative and late results. J Am Coll Cardiol 1997;29:1359–1364.
8. McCaffrey FM, Leatherbury L, Moore HV. Pulmonary atresia and intact ventricular septum. J Thorac Cardiovasc Surg 1991;102:617–623.
9. Bull C, Kostelka M, Sorenson K, et al. Outcome measures for the neonatal management of pulmonary atresia with intact ventricular septum. J Thorac Cardiovasc Surg 1994;107:359–366.
10. Pawade A, Mee R, Karl T. Right ventricular "overhaul"—an intermediate step in the biventricular repair of pulmonary atresia with intact ventricular septum. Cardiol Young 1995;5:161–165.
11. Miyaji K, Shimada M, Sekiguchi A, et al. Pulmonary atresia with intact ventricular septum: Long-term results of "one and a half ventricular repair." Ann Thorac Surg 1995;60:1762–1764.

Single Ventricle Lesions

Gil Wernovsky, MD, and Edward L. Bove, MD

GENERAL ANATOMY

A wide variety of anatomic lesions (Table 18.1), usually associated with atresia of an atrioventricular (AV) or semilunar valve, have the common physiology of complete mixing of the systemic and pulmonary venous return (see *Physiology*) (Figs. 18.1–18.3).

In addition, other patients are seen with borderline hypoplasia of an atrioventricular valve, outflow tract, and/or ventricular chamber in whom multiple surgical procedures can be considered to achieve a separated, "two-ventricle" circulation. An example of this type of lesion is Shone's syndrome, with multiple left-sided obstructive lesions including a supramitral ring, parachute mitral valve, subaortic stenosis, and coarctation of the aorta (1). Controversy exists whether patients with mild to moderate forms of Shone's syndrome or similar lesions (2) should be managed similar to patients with single ventricle, or alternatively, staged toward a separated, two-ventricular circulation (3, 4).

Finally, some patients have biventricular hearts with two ventricles of normal size, which cannot be repaired by means of conventional methods because of malattachments, overriding or straddling of an atrioventricular valve(s) over the ventricular septum, or a ventricular septal defect (VSD) that is remote from either great vessel. Although these patients may have ventricular chambers and atrioventricular valves suitable in size for "anatomic correction," the anatomy is such that a single ventricle management strategy must be undertaken. This includes, for example, patients with double outlet right ventricle with a "remote" VSD, patients with D-transposition of the great arteries with VSD and pulmonary stenosis, and tricuspid valve chordae that prohibit a Rastelli repair (see Chapter 19, *Other Conotruncal Lesions*), and so forth.

PHYSIOLOGY

In each of the anatomic lesions described above, there is complete mixing of the systemic and pulmonary venous return—typically at the atrial or ventricular level. The ventricular output is then divided between two parallel circuits. With complete mixing, pulmonary artery and aortic oxygen saturations are equal. The ventricular output is the *sum* of the pulmonary blood flow (Qp) and the systemic blood flow (Qs). The relative proportion of the ventricular output to either the pulmonary or systemic vascular bed is determined by the relative resistance to flow into the two circuits.

In nearly all hearts with single ventricle physiology, one of the two outflows is obstructed; it is extremely rare to have no obstruction to either pulmonary or systemic blood flow, or obstruction to both circuits. Patients can thus be thought of in two basic categories: those with obstruction to pulmonary blood flow (lesions with pulmonary atresia or stenosis, including tetralogy of Fallot (TOF) with pulmonary atresia or heterotaxy) and those with obstruction to systemic blood flow (hypoplastic left heart syndrome and various types of single left ventricle with transposition).

Resistance to pulmonary flow is determined by

1. Degree of subvalvar or valvar pulmonary obstruction
2. Pulmonary arteriolar resistance
3. Pulmonary venous and left atrial pressure

The left atrial pressure is in part determined by the volume of pulmonary blood flow entering the left atrium and the relative degree of restriction to outflow through the left atrioventricular valve and atrial septum.

Resistance to systemic flow is determined by

1. Presence of anatomic obstructive lesions (subaortic obstruction, aortic valve stenosis, arch hypoplasia, coarctation)
2. Systemic arteriolar resistance

BALANCING THE CIRCULATION

An acceptable balance between the pulmonary and systemic output provides enough pulmonary flow for adequate oxygen delivery to prevent acidosis without an excessive volume load to the single ventricle. Assuming a pulmonary venous saturation of 95 to 100% and a mixed venous oxygen saturation of 55 to 60%, **an arterial oxygen saturation of 75 to 80% represents a Qp/Qs ratio of approximately 1:0**. This typically results in mild ventricular volume overload (the Qp *plus* the Qs equals approximately two "cardiac outputs"), minimal AV valve regurgitation, and normal systemic blood flow.

Table 18.1. Anatomic Lesions Associated with Single Ventricle Lesions

Anatomy	Complete Intracardiac Mixing	
	Preoperative	Postoperative
Variations of Single Left Ventricle		
Tricuspid Valve Atresia		
Normally related great arteries (Fig. 18.1)	Yes	Yes
Transposed great arteries[a]	Yes	Yes
Double Inlet Left Ventricle	Yes	Yes
Normally related great arteries ("Holmes heart")	Yes	Yes
Transposed great arteries[a]	Yes[b]	Yes
Malaligned Complete Atrioventricular Canal with Hypoplastic Right Ventricle	Yes	Yes
Pulmonary Atresia with Intact Ventricular Septum (see Chapter 17.2)	Yes	Variable[b]
Variations of Single Right Ventricle		
Mitral Valve Atresia		
Hypoplastic left heart syndrome (Fig. 18.2)	Yes	Yes
Double outlet right ventricle	Yes	Yes
Aortic Valve Atresia		
Hypoplastic left heart syndrome	Yes	Yes
With large ventricular septal defect and normal left ventricle size	Yes	Variable[b]
Malaligned Complete Atrioventricular Canal with Hypoplastic Left Ventricle	Yes	Yes
Heterotaxy syndromes—typically with pulmonary stenosis or atresia—asplenia or polyspenia	Yes	Yes
Two-Ventricle Hearts with Potential Single Ventricle Physiology		
Tetralogy of Fallot with Pulmonary Atresia (see Chapter 17.1)	Yes	Variable[b]
Truncus Arteriosus (see Chapter 15.7)	Yes[c]	No
Total Anomalous Pulmonary Venous Return (see Chapter 15.6)	Yes[c]	No

[a] In tricuspid atresia or double inlet left ventricle with transposed great arteries ({S,D,D} or {S,L,L}), right ventricular hypoplasia, subaortic obstruction, arch hypoplasia, and coarctation frequently coexist.
[b] Single ventricle physiology pertains to postoperative patients with systemic to pulmonary artery shunts or following pulmonary artery banding, although two-ventricle repairs with normal series circulation or partial repairs with incomplete mixing are possible in certain anatomic subtypes.
[c] Streaming can result in incomplete mixing.

Transitional Circulation

After birth, there is a fall in pulmonary vascular resistance (PVR) and a subsequent increase in the pulmonary blood flow (PBF) from the combined ventricular output. As the PVR continues to fall with time, an increasing proportion of the combined ventricular output is committed to the lungs. The normal homeostatic mechanisms to improve systemic output result in increases in both stroke volume and heart rate. However, the normal fall in PVR over the first few hours to days of life, in the absence of a significant obstruction to pulmonary blood flow, gradually results in elevated pulmonary blood flow at the expense of systemic blood flow. As the Qp:Qs ratio approaches 2.0, the single ventricle becomes progressively volume overloaded, with mildly elevated end-diastolic and atrial pressures. The neonate may show signs of tachypnea or frank respiratory distress. The greater proportion of pulmonary venous return in the mixed ventricular blood results in an elevated systemic arterial oxygen saturation (approximately 85%), and visible cyanosis may be mild or absent.

Prior to surgical intervention (see below), a number of ventilatory and pharmacologic maneuvers can be used to "balance" the circulation (Qp:Qs ~ 1), resulting in adequate oxygen delivery and systemic blood flow. However, in many of these patients, ventilatory and pharmacologic management only temporizes the need for surgical intervention. See Chapter 12, *Preoperative Care*, for more details on diagnosis, stabilization, and management of the newborn with duct-dependent lesions.

Patients with "unbalanced" single ventricle physiology can be grouped into two physiologic extremes: hypoxemia and congestive heart failure.

Inadequate Pulmonary Blood Flow (Hypoxemia)

The newborn with single ventricle physiology and inadequate oxygen saturation may have limited pulmonary

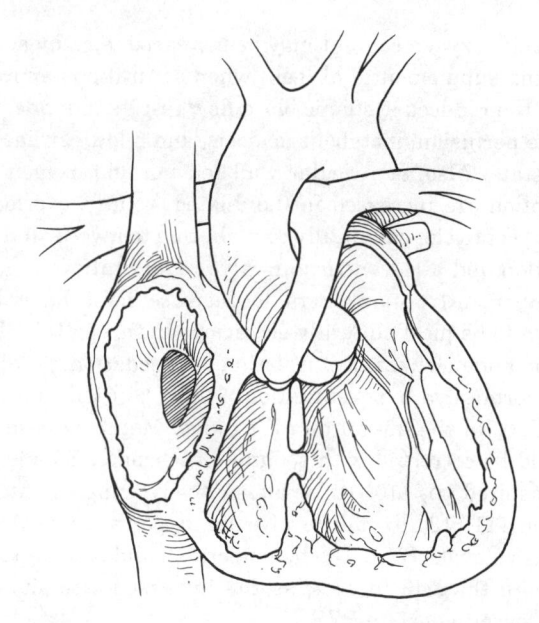

Figure 18.1. Anatomy of tricuspid atresia. The various forms of tricuspid atresia represent a common form of a single ventricle. This illustration shows type 1b tricuspid atresia. Note the normally related great vessels and the pulmonary hypoplasia with a restrictive communication between the normally developed left ventricle and the vestigial right ventricle. Complete absence of the tricuspid valve is seen, and a large atrial septal defect allows the only exit of blood from the right atrium. This particular form of tricuspid atresia represents a form of single ventricle that is generally not duct dependent.

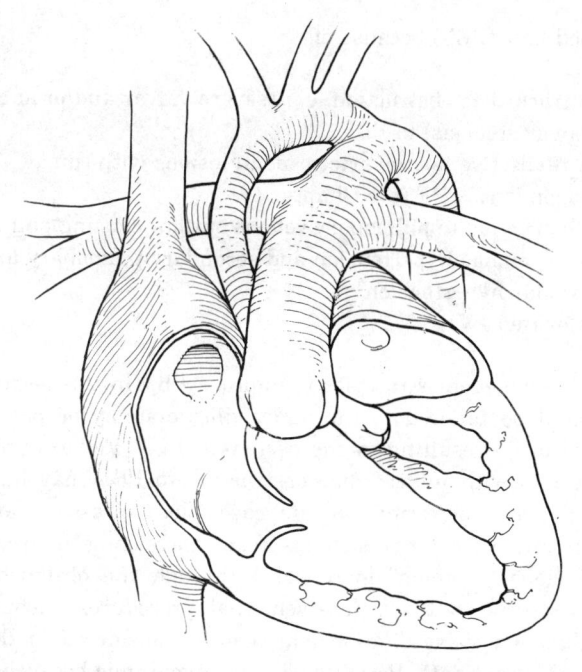

Figure 18.2. Anatomy of hypoplastic left heart syndrome. Hypoplastic left heart syndrome is one of the most common forms of single ventricle. Typical features include severe hypoplasia or atresia of the mitral and aortic valves and a severely underdeveloped left ventricle. The ascending aorta is markedly hypoplastic with a discrete coarctation in the periductal region. A large ductus arteriosus is present with an enlarged and dilated pulmonary valve and main pulmonary artery. The right ventricle is dilated and hypertrophied, and an atrial septal defect is present. This anatomy results in the typical single ventricle physiology of a mixed circulation with parallel systemic and pulmonary artery circuits. This lesion illustrates the concept of the ductus-dependent systemic circulation. The entire systemic output is dependent on flow through the ductus arteriosus.

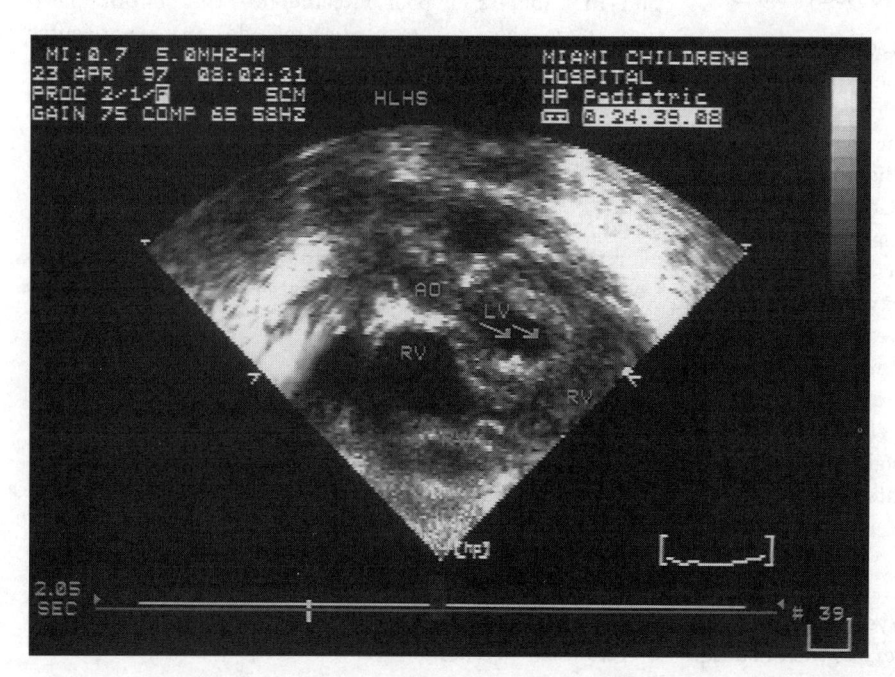

Figure 18.3. Subcostal view of a neonate with hypoplastic left heart syndrome. A small hypertrophied left ventricle (*LV*) is seen (*double arrows*), from which the aorta (*AO*) arises. RV, right ventricle.

blood flow (PBF) because of:

- Intracardiac obstruction (e.g., severe valvar and/or subvalvar stenosis) to PBF
- A restrictive ductus arteriosus in lesions with "duct-dependent" PBF (see Chapter 12)
- Obstruction to pulmonary venous outflow causing pulmonary venous hypertension and secondary pulmonary arteriolar hypertension
- Elevated PVR

Management strategies to improve PBF in this setting should be tailored to the underlying anatomy or pathophysiology resulting in the decreased PBF. For example, patients with intracardiac obstruction to PBF may have maneuvers performed to increase blood pressure and systemic vascular resistance (e.g., increasing inotropic infusions), "forcing" more blood through the obstructed intracardiac outflow. Interventional procedures such as pulmonary valve dilation may also be considered in this group of patients. Patients who are hypoxemic because of an obstructive left-sided atrioventricular valve and restrictive atrial septal defect (ASD) (5) may have transcatheter dilation of the atrial septum performed (6, 7). Patients thought to be hypoxemic because of elevated PVR should have ventilatory maneuvers performed to decrease PVR (increased F_{IO_2}, hyperventilation/alkalosis, nitric oxide, and so forth). Most intravenous pulmonary vasodilators are nonspecific; variable and sometimes labile responses of both the pulmonary and systemic vascular bed may occur, resulting in unpredictable results in this patient population.

Excessive Pulmonary Blood Flow (Congestive Heart Failure)

A more common scenario in nonoperated patients with single ventricle is a progressive increase in pulmonary blood flow with a concomitant reduction of systemic blood flow. When severe, this results in systemic hypoperfusion, metabolic acidosis, and shock. Once establishment of a patent ductus arteriosus is confirmed (see Chapter 12), maneuvers should be used to minimize systemic vascular resistance and maximize pulmonary vascular resistance. Patients with a relatively high arterial oxygen saturation (e.g., more than 90%) generally have a severe "steal" of the combined ventricular output into the pulmonary vascular circuit. In these "overcirculated" patients, excessive inotropic support (particular at alpha-doses) should be minimized (8) and afterload reduction (e.g., sodium nitroprusside) may be especially helpful in patients with elevated systemic vascular resistance and an adequate blood pressure.

It is important to emphasize that patients with single ventricle physiology and *high* arterial oxygen saturations actually may have *decreased* oxygen delivery to the tissues. Although oxygen content may be increased (e.g., by administering supplemental oxygen) when saturations approach 90%, the reduced systemic blood flow results in inadequate tissue perfusion, metabolic acidosis, and a low cardiac output state. Also, ventricular wall tension and oxygen consumption are increased in the dilated, volume overloaded single ventricle, potentially contributing to myocardial dysfunction and atrioventricular valve regurgitation.

Importantly, maneuvers to *increase* PVR have been shown to be most clinically efficacious in this setting. Intubation and mechanical ventilation with sedation, paralysis, and permissive hypoventilation (9) can be used to elevate the P_{CO_2} to the 40–50 mm Hg range. Metabolic acidemia should be corrected with sodium bicarbonate. Supplemental inspired CO_2 (10–12) or alternatively, supplemental nitrogen (11, 13) to induce alveolar hypoxia, may also be used to elevate PVR. The hematocrit should be maintained at more than 40 to 45%, as the increased viscosity may also serve to elevate PVR.

It is important to emphasize that preoperative patients with marked overcirculation and systemic hypoperfusion should not undergo lengthy periods of "medical management" of their unstable physiology. Patients with marked overcirculation and hypoperfusion should undergo relatively urgent surgical management to achieve a more favorable physiology.

PRINCIPLES OF NEWBORN SURGICAL MANAGEMENT

Patients with functional single ventricle, in most cases, will ultimately undergo various modifications of the Fontan operation (see below) as their ultimate surgical palliation. Risk factors for poor outcome after the Fontan operation have been shown to include (a) ventricular hypertrophy causig diastolic dysfunction (14), (b) elevated PVR or pulmonary artery pressure (15–18), (c) pulmonary artery distortion (18–20), (d) atrioventricular valve regurgitation (21, 22), and (e) ventricular systolic dysfunction (23). Surgical and medical management of newborns with single ventricle must minimize these potential risk factors over the long term. Thus, all surgical procedures for patients with single ventricle are geared toward the following general goals:

1. Unobstructed systemic blood flow (to minimize ventricular hypertrophy)
2. Limited PBF (to minimize ventricular volume load and the risk of pulmonary artery hypertension)
3. Unobstructed pulmonary venous return (to minimize left atrial and secondary pulmonary artery hypertension)
4. Minimize likelihood of pulmonary artery distortion
5. Avoid dysrhythmias

Single Ventricle Lesions 275

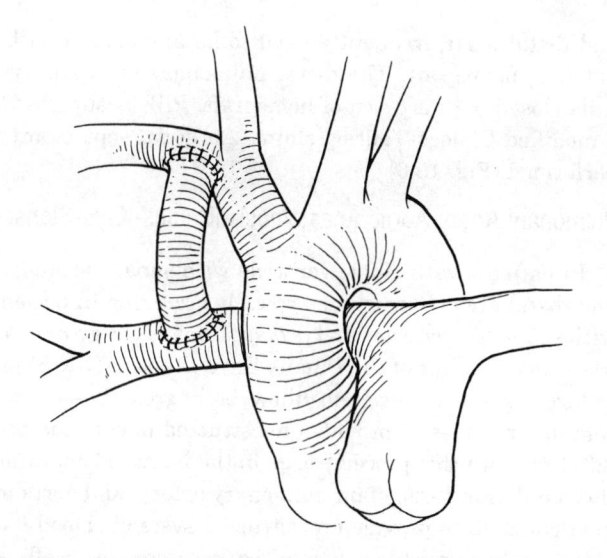

Figure 18.4. Surgical palliation for neonates with forms of single ventricle that have duct dependent or markedly reduced antegrade pulmonary blood flow. The modified Blalock-Taussig shunt is shown. Cardiopulmonary bypass is typically not necessary when this procedure is performed. The surgeon's preference determines whether a median sternotomy or right thoracotomy incision is used. The procedure consists of a Goretex® tube graft placed between the right subclavian artery and the right pulmonary artery. Tube graft size is chosen to create an appropriate resistance such that the systemic and pulmonary blood flows will be balanced following the procedure. This procedure can be performed in isolation or as part of a more complex reconstruction. Blood flow through the graft into the pulmonary circuit can be regulated in a number of ways, including the choice of the graft diameter itself and also by the proximal anastomosis position. If the proximal anastomosis is placed more centrally (e.g., on the ascending aorta), increased pulmonary blood flow will be achieved. Placing the systemic anastomosis on the innominate artery or on the subclavian artery will reduce the amount of blood flow into the pulmonary circuit. Such maneuvers are utilized to achieve the necessary delicate balance of systemic and pulmonary blood flow in newborn infants with single ventricle physiology.

Systemic-Pulmonary Artery Shunt

Historically, a number of connections between the systemic and pulmonary circulation have been used in single ventricle lesions with restricted PBF. Currently, a modified Blalock-Taussig shunt is the most common procedure used to secure PBF in this group of lesions (Fig. 18.4). Depending on the size of the patient and pre-existing pulmonary arteriolar resistance, a 3.0–4.0 mm Goretex® tube is placed from the brachiocephalic vessels (usually the proximal subclavian artery) to the pulmonary artery. In some groups, a "central" shunt from the ascending aorta is preferred. Other types of systemic-pulmonary shunts such as the Waterston and Potts shunt are associated with a higher risk of pulmonary artery hypertension and pulmonary artery distortion, and they are generally discouraged.

Pulmonary Artery Banding

In patients with no restriction to systemic blood flow and little to no restriction to PBF, a pulmonary artery band can be placed (without cardiopulmonary bypass) to limit PBF and pressure (Fig. 18.5). Care must be taken not to distort the branch pulmonary arteries and/or the pulmonary valve. Importantly, by decreasing the pulmonary blood flow, the acute reduction in the volume load on the ventricle results in immediate geometric changes of the ventricle, including an increase in wall thickness and decrease in cavity dimension (24). These changes may result in the acute development of subaortic stenosis if systemic outflow is dependent on a relatively small ventricular septal defect. Long-standing pulmonary artery banding has been associated with progressive subaortic stenosis (25),

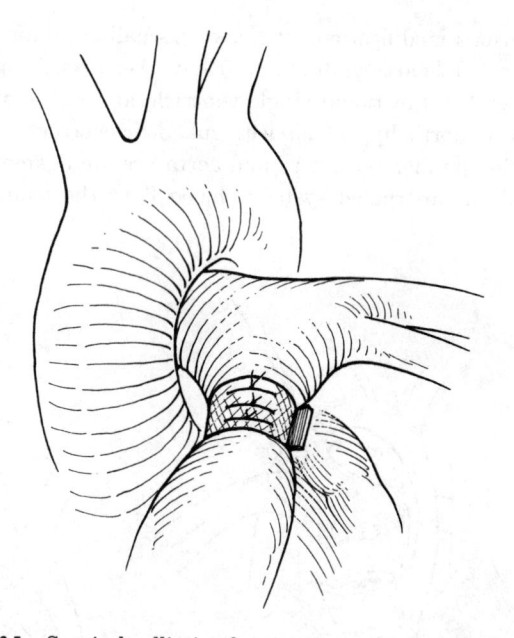

Figure 18.5. Surgical palliation for neonates and infants with single ventricle physiology and increased pulmonary blood flow and no obstruction to systemic blood flow. A pulmonary artery band is shown. Cardiopulmonary bypass is usually not necessary. This procedure is performed through a median sternotomy or lateral thoracotomy, depending on the surgeon's preference. Material used for the pulmonary artery band is critical because abrasive materials can erode into the pulmonary artery. The band is placed around the main pulmonary artery, taking care to avoid impinging on the branch pulmonary arteries and on the pulmonary valve itself. The band is gradually tightened until an oxygen saturation of between 75 and 85% in the systemic circulation is achieved. If lung disease or other factors exist, which suggest that the oxygen saturation is not a reliable indicator of the tightness of the band, then pressures proximal and distal to the band itself can be determined intraoperatively. A typical band gradient in a newborn infant would range between 40 and 60 mm Hg under conditions of general anesthesia. It is critical that the band itself be sutured to the adventitia of the main pulmonary artery to prevent distal migration of the band causing obstruction of the branch pulmonary arteries.

potential deformity and regurgitation of the pulmonary valve (26), and an increased risk for an eventual Fontan operation (27, 28).

In addition, precise adjustment of the diameter of the band may be difficult, particularly in small neonates. A band that is too loose may not alleviate symptoms or adequately protect the pulmonary vasculature; a band that is too tight may result in unacceptable hypoxemia, especially during the rapid growth phase of the neonate or young infant. For these reasons, some centers have elected to create pulmonary atresia by dividing the main pulmonary artery, oversewing the proximal pulmonary at the valve level, closing the distal pulmonary artery with a patch, and placing a systemic to pulmonary shunt to secure reliable pulmonary blood flow.

Stage I Norwood

Various modifications of Norwood's palliation for hypoplastic left heart syndrome (35) have been used for children with a functional single ventricle and aortic atresia or severe aortic hypoplasia with subaortic obstruction (36–38). The pulmonary artery and aorta are amalgamated to provide unobstructed systemic blood flow; the transverse and distal aorta frequently need to be augmented with a patch of homograft. The distal pulmonary artery is typically closed with a patch of homograft. PBF is supplied by a modified Blalock-Taussig shunt. An atrial septectomy is performed (Fig. 18.6).

Pulmonary Artery-Aortic Anastomosis (Damus-Kaye-Stansel)

In patients with single ventricle with subaortic stenosis and distal arch obstruction–typically occurring in patients with *single left ventricle* and *transposition of the great arteries*—modifications of the Damus-Kaye-Stansel (D-K-S) procedure have been used to allow both great vessels and semilunar valves to provide unobstructed flow to the body (29–33). With this procedure, as in the Norwood operation, the semilunar roots, main pulmonary artery, and aorta are amalgamated to provide unobstructed systemic blood flow; distal arch augmentation may be necessary as well. An atrial septectomy is performed if restriction of the left atrioventricular valve is found, and a modified Blalock-Taussig shunt is placed to provide adequate PBF. The neoaortic (native pulmonary) valve frequently has trivial to mild insufficiency following this procedure, but hemodynamically significant insufficiency is uncommon (26, 34).

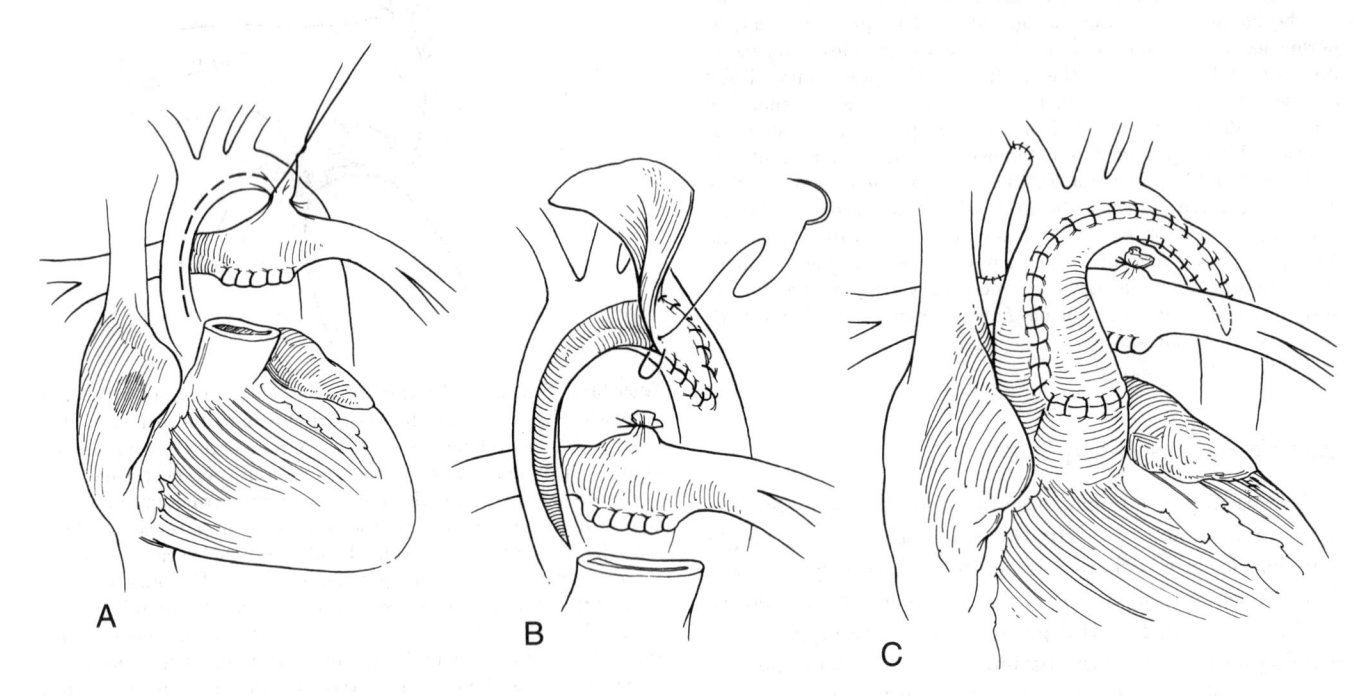

Figure 18.6. Stage I reconstruction for hypoplastic left heart syndrome. The purpose of the stage I reconstruction for hypoplastic left heart syndrome is to establish reliable, unobstructed outflow to the systemic circulation and to balance the systemic and pulmonary circulations. This is achieved by ligating and dividing the ductus arteriosus and detaching the central and branch pulmonary arteries from the main pulmonary artery as shown in **A**. The hypoplastic aorta is then opened from the descending aorta retrograde to the level of the aortic valve and augmented with a patch of homograft arterial wall. The augmented aorta is then connected to the cardiac end of the main pulmonary artery stump as shown in **B** and **C**. This achieves unobstructed outflow from the single right ventricle through the pulmonary valve to the aorta and systemic vascular bed. In addition, an atrial septectomy is performed to ensure unobstructed pulmonary venous outflow, and the pulmonary circulation is supplied through the use of a right-sided modified Blalock-Taussig shunt.

Immediate Postoperative Management

Immediate postoperative management following stage I palliation, pulmonary artery banding, or systemic to pulmonary artery shunt (single ventricle physiology) is similar to the physiology of the parallel circulation discussed above. Although postoperative management is similar, perioperative strategies must also take into account the effects on myocardial function and the pulmonary vascular resistance from the procedure itself (see Chapter 14, *Cardiopulmonary Bypass*). Following the D-K-S and Norwood procedures, pulmonary vascular resistance is typically transiently elevated and can be labile. In addition, the effects of myocardial ischemia from aortic cross clamping can lead to globally depressed cardiac output in the first 12 to 24 hours after surgery (39).

Postoperative evaluation should assess all aspects of the specific procedure used; evaluation after a Norwood palliation for hypoplastic left heart syndrome must be much more extensive than following a shunt for single ventricle with pulmonary atresia. The patient with either *low systemic cardiac output*, excessive *cyanosis* (oxygen saturation less than 75%), or relatively *high (more than 85 to 88%) oxygen saturations* must have the repair and postoperative physiology carefully evaluated.

Low Cardiac Output

A low cardiac output syndrome can occur in the first 24 to 48 hours after Norwood or D-K-S surgery, with typical findings of tachycardia, hypotension, oliguria, and metabolic acidosis. In addition to standard monitoring (see Chapter 11, *Invasive and Noninvasive Monitoring*), many centers have recently advocated intermittent measurement of mixed venous oxygen saturation following stage I surgery, typically in the superior vena cava. The arterial-venous oxygen saturation difference (A-V DO_2) is a sensitive predictor of low systemic blood flow and inadequate oxygen delivery (13, 40, 41); an A-V DO_2 more than 40 to 50% suggests advanced low cardiac output and inadequate tissue delivery of oxygen.

The patient with evidence of low systemic blood flow requires immediate attention and evaluation of the potential cause(s). Low systemic cardiac output may be caused by (a) globally decreased ventricular output (poor pump performance), (b) elevated Qp:Qs (adequate pump performance with maldistribution of flow), and (c) atrioventricular valve regurgitation (adequate pump performance with large regurgitant fraction with or without maldistribution of flow).

The combination of echocardiography to evaluate ventricular and atrioventricular valve function and measurement of the A-V DO_2 to evaluate the Qp:Qs is important in establishing the cause of the low cardiac output and rationally directing therapy. The patient with globally depressed function may best benefit from increasing inotropic support, whereas the patient with adequate pump function but a high Qp:Qs best benefits from maneuvers to increase the PVR and/or lower systemic vascular resistance.

Cyanosis

The differential diagnosis of excessive cyanosis includes:

1. Pulmonary venous desaturation (pneumothorax, pleural effusion, pulmonary edema, pneumonia, infection)
2. Systemic venous desaturation (anemia, high oxygen consumption states, low systemic cardiac output)
3. Decreased pulmonary blood flow (elevated PVR, pulmonary venous hypertension, restrictive atrial septal defect, pulmonary artery distortion, a physically "small" [or restrictive] systemic-to-pulmonary artery shunt)

Pulmonary venous desaturation is typically evaluated by chest radiograph and auscultation. As discussed, intermittent measurement of the mixed venous oxygen saturation is helpful in the differential diagnosis of low cardiac output; a low mixed venous oxygen saturation in the face of clinical evidence of adequate cardiac output is typically due to anemia or increased oxygen extraction. Once excessive pulmonary or systemic venous desaturation has been ruled out as a cause of unexplained cyanosis, echocardiography or cardiac catheterization may be necessary to identify the anatomic (shunt-related) or physiologic (PUR-related) causes of a decreased Qp:Qs ratio.

Elevated Oxygen Saturations

The patient who is "too pink" with a parallel circulation (oxygen saturation ~90%) typically has low PVR and pulmonary blood flow far in excess of systemic blood flow. This can result in inadequate systemic perfusion, renal dysfunction, and an inability to wean the patient from mechanical ventilation. In children palliated with left-sided obstructive lesions (e.g., Norwood procedure), *arch obstruction* must be ruled out, as distal obstruction will force more blood through the shunt and increase Qp at the expense of Qs.

SEPARATING THE CIRCULATION

Cavopulmonary connections (bidirectional Glenn, hemi-Fontan), and the modified Fontan operation will be discussed below.

General Principles

The eventual goal of surgical palliation for single ventricle lesions is to separate the systemic and pulmonary circuits, resulting in a normal (or near-normal) oxygen saturation. Cavopulmonary or atriopulmonary connections are used to divert systemic venous return directly into the pulmonary vascular bed—providing more "effective" pulmonary blood flow and reducing the volume load on the single ventricle. Following these procedures, the single ventricle only ejects blood to the systemic circuit with pulmonary blood flow derived by "passive flow" into the pulmonary vascular bed (at the expense of higher central venous pressure).

Bidirectional Glenn/Hemi-Fontan

Interim palliation with a bidirectional Glenn shunt has been increasingly used in the past decade, typically in infants (4 to 9 months of age) (42–48). Usually using cardiopulmonary bypass, the superior vena cava is divided with the cardiac end oversewn (Fig. 18.7). The cephalic end is anastomosed end to side to the ipsilateral pulmonary artery, with pulmonary artery augmentation as indicated.

Alternatively, the potential or eventual pathway for inferior vena cava blood to enter the pulmonary arteries may be constructed with a temporary "dam" separating the orifice of the superior vena cava (SVC) from the right atrium. This procedure is known as the "hemi-Fontan" (44).

Physiology and Indications for Surgery

Following the bidirectional Glenn procedure, the pulmonary blood flow is *obligate*, and it represents the brachiocephalic arterial outflow from the heart; all SVC return must pass through the lungs to reach the heart (in the absence of decompressing venous collaterals, see below). The *principle physiologic advantage of conversion to a bidirectional Glenn shunt* (drainage of the superior vena cava to the pulmonary artery and the inferior vena cava to the systemic ventricle) at an early age *is the reduction of the volume work of the single ventricle and a predictable Qp:Qs of approximately 0.6–0.7*. This ratio may be higher in young infants because of the relative size of the head and the upper extremities as opposed to size in older children (49), but in general, the aortic oxygen saturation is typically in the 75 to 85% range (42, 43, 46, 48). Contrary to the complete Fontan operation, ventricular filling is not absolutely dependent on pulmonary venous return, because inferior vena caval flow is still diverted directly to the single ventricle, which maintains preload.

Immediate reduction in the volume load of the single ventricle by removing the aortopulmonary shunt decreases the work of the single ventricle, and it may have positive long-term effects on atrioventricular valve and myocardial function. Beneficial effects in myocardial perfusion may also be found as diastolic pressure and coronary pressure increase when the systemic to pulmonary shunt is removed. The effects, however, of acute volume unloading on VSD size in patients who have a bulboventricular foramen and are dependent on an unrestricted VSD for systemic ventricular outflow remain unclear. As mentioned above (see *Pulmonary Artery Banding*), unloading of the systemic ventricle (24) can result in restrictive VSD physiology (50, 51), and therefore careful assessment should be performed of the subaortic area in patients with these anatomic subtypes (typically single left ventricle with transposition of the great arteries).

Arterial oxygen saturations following construction of a bidirectional Glenn shunt tend to be lower in very young (less than 3 months) patients. Although some patients as young as 4 weeks of age have had satisfactory bidirectional Glenn shunt creation (44, 47), in general, patients under 3 months of age have a higher incidence of early cyanosis, pulmonary artery thrombosis, and vascular congestion (44, 47); therefore, a delay of the procedure until the infant is older than 3 months of age is generally recommended. By 6 months of age the mortality risk approaches 0% in many centers (42, 43, 46, 52, 75).

An additional advantage of the early construction of a bidirectional Glenn shunt is the opportunity to address distortion of the pulmonary arteries from previous bands or shunts, to allow more satisfactory distribution of pulmonary artery blood flow and growth of the pulmonary vascular bed. Also, an intermediate bidirectional Glenn shunt or hemi-Fontan procedure allows for relative ease of completion of the Fontan operation (52, 53) and a perceived lower incidence of effusions and morbidity. Whether these salient benefits should be applied to all patients with single ven-

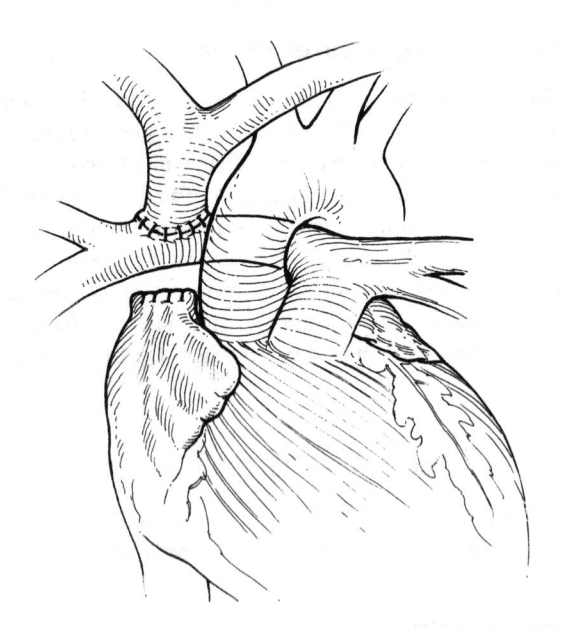

Figure 18.7.1. Bidirectional superior cavopulmonary anastomosis (Bidirectional Glenn). The superior vena cava is transected at the level of the right pulmonary artery, the cardiac end is oversewn, and the cephalad portion of the superior vena cava is anastomosed end-to-side into the proximal right pulmonary artery.

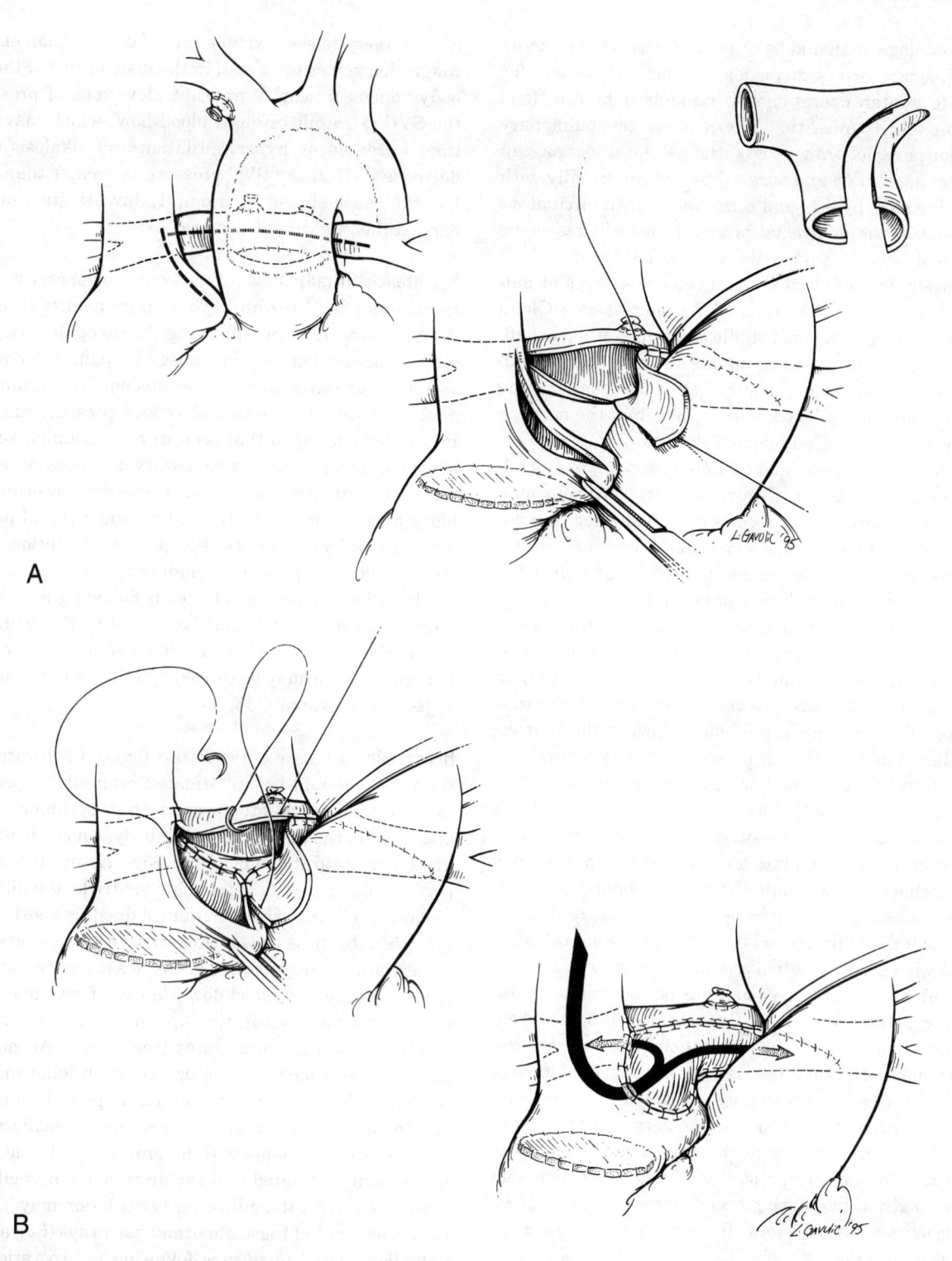

Figure 18.7.2. The technique of the hemiFontan procedure. The central pulmonary arteries are opened widely and an incision is made in the base of the right atrial appendage **(A)**. Although not shown in this illustration, the atrial incision does not cross the cavoatrial junction to avoid injuring the artery to the SA node. A patch of pulmonary allograft material is used to augment the pulmonary arteries (center). The atrial and pulmonary artery incisions are joined **(B)**. The final appearance of the hemiFontan connection are shown on the right. The patch used to separate the superior vena cava to pulmonary artery connection from the heart is shown within the right atrium. At the time of the Fontan procedure, the atrial patch is removed from within the right atrium leaving a wide connection for the inferior vena cava into the pulmonary arteries. (Adapted with permission from Bove EL, Mosca RS. Surgical repair of the hypoplastic left heart syndrome. Prog Pediatr Cardiol 1996;5:23–35.)

tricle physiology or should be reserved for selected patients with pulmonary artery distortion or other risk factors for a compete Fontan operation (54) remains unknown. It is important to recognize that intermediate cavopulmonary connections are not without risk; the patient undergoes an additional anesthetic and surgical procedure, usually with cardiopulmonary bypass and occasionally with circulatory arrest, and in the additional procedure may increase the incidence of late sinus node dysfunction (55, 56).

The usefulness of eliminating accessory sources of pulmonary blood flow at the time of the bidirectional Glenn remains controversial, with studies showing either beneficial, detrimental, or no effects on late outcome and morbidity (57–63). There have been suggestions that maintaining additional pulmonary blood flow—either from the aorta or ventricle—to increase pulmonary blood flow may improve development of the pulmonary vascular bed in young children or minimize the risk of pulmonary arteriovenous malformations; however, other reports have suggested that additional sources of pulmonary blood flow can cause increased pleural effusions and congestive heart failure following creation of the bidirectional Glenn.

While the azygous vein is usually ligated at the time of the bidirectional Glenn to decrease a source of decompression of the upper systemic veins, we have noted that in situations where the azygous vein is not ligated, the oxygen saturations remain acceptable following the bidirectional Glenn, and significant hypoxemia rarely occurs.

An intermediate cavopulmonary connection appears to be the ideal interim palliation, as it minimizes the volume overload and facilitates the subsequent Fontan operation. In addition, any other procedures necessary to minimize later morbidity (e.g., pulmonary arterioplasty, valvuloplasty, and so forth) may be performed concurrently.

Although the bidirectional Glenn (or hemiFontan) is associated with good palliation and midterm growth and development are satisfactory, the late development of progressive cyanosis is common. Cyanosis can progress from pulmonary arteriovenous malformations (64) or from collateral venous drainage (see below). However, older age alone can be associated with progressive cyanosis as a relatively lower proportion of the cardiac output is directed to the head and the upper extremities in older patients (49). In addition, the greater proportion of venous return from the lower extremities during exercise may result in unacceptable oxygen saturations as these patients become more active at school age.

Postoperative Issues

Elevated SVC Pressure Patients with clinical signs of significantly *elevated SVC pressure* (upper extremity plethora and edema) may have obstruction at the anastomosis, distal pulmonary artery distortion, or marked elevations in PVR. In these patients, it is not uncommon immediately after surgery to see a visible line of demarcation of venous congestion across the chest, in the distribution of the upper body venous return. Significant elevations of pressure in the SVC can limit cerebral blood flow, which may be further decreased by hyperventilation and alkalosis used to decrease PVR. If the SVC pressure is greater than 18 mm Hg, the cause should be promptly investigated, including early catheterization if necessary.

Hypertension/Bradycardia Transient postoperative *hypertension and bradycardia* have been frequently observed in the first 24 to 72 hours following the cavopulmonary shunt (43). Hypertension may be caused by pain, catecholamine secretion, or intracranial hypertension. We speculate that acute elevation of the central venous pressure may result in a reflex similar to that seen in head trauma, such that systemic hypertension is necessary to preserve adequate cerebral perfusion. Therefore, aggressive lowering of the blood pressure may adversely affect the cerebral perfusion pressure and vasodilators should be used cautiously especially when SVC pressure is markedly elevated. Transient bradycardia is also typically seen following a cavopulmonary connection, and it may be caused by the acute reduction of the volume load of the single ventricle, intercranial hypertension, or may be caused by injury to the sinus node or its arterial supply (55, 56).

Hypoxemia Excessive *hypoxemia* (oxygen saturations less than 75%) should be investigated promptly, especially in infants, where a greater proportion of systemic output is dedicated to the upper half of the body, which should result in oxygen saturations closer to 85%. As in all procedures performed in patients with single ventricle, the differential diagnosis of excessive or unexplained cyanosis can be grouped into three broad categories: (*a*) pulmonary venous desaturation, (*b*) systemic venous desaturation, and (*c*) decreased pulmonary blood flow. Causes of systemic and pulmonary venous desaturation are similar to those following newborn palliative procedures (see above). An additional cause of pulmonary venous desaturation following a bidirectional Glenn shunt or hemi-Fontan procedure is the development of pulmonary arteriovenous malformations, particularly in patients with heterotaxy syndrome (64–67). It has been postulated that the diversion of normal hepatic venous flow from the pulmonary circulation may be related to development of these abnormal pathways (64), and some have been noted to regress following incorporation of hepatic venous flow into the lungs (67). These pulmonary arteriovenous malformations typically cause gradual hypoxemia *months to years* following the surgical procedure, rather than in the immediate postoperative period.

Finally, decreased pulmonary blood flow may be caused by decompressing venous collaterals, an undiagnosed contralateral (usually left) SVC, or a baffle leak (if the intracardiac orifice of the SVC has been patch closed during the hemi-Fontan procedure) (52). Factors related to the development of decompressing venous collaterals include bilateral superior vena cava (68), a higher early postoperative transpulmonary gradient, and elevated superior vena caval pressure (68, 69). Successful transcatheter coil embolization of these vessels can be accomplished with good results.

Fontan Operation

The multiple technical modifications of the Fontan operation (70) in the past two decades (including conduits, atriopulmonary connections, intermediate cavopulmonary connections, extra cardiac conduits [71, 72], and the recent use of adjustable atrial defects (73) or fixed fenestrations in the intra-atrial baffle [74]), combined with improved patient selection and postoperative management, have reduced the operative mortality to less than 10% in many centers, with acceptable perioperative and midterm morbidity (17, 18, 53, 75–83). The long-term outcomes, however, continue to be in question (84). Because of the significant improvement in early mortality, attention has now been directed to decreasing the morbidity of the Fontan operation and improving the potential for long-term durability of the Fontan circulation.

Multiple modifications of the Fontan operation have recently been devised in hopes of improving late outcomes (72, 85–89). The intra-atrial lateral tunnel (Fig. 18.8) has supplanted the direct atrial-pulmonary anastomosis because of the salient hydrodynamics of blood flow (87, 90, 91) in more constricted atrial pathways, which do not allow for stasis and hydraulic energy loss as blood flows passively into the pulmonary vascular bed. Also, the lateral tunnel may result in a decreased incidence of late tachyarrhythmias (92, 93). Pulmonary blood flow (94) after most modifications of the Fontan operation may preferentially be distributed to the right lung possibly because the heart sits in the left chest and partially compresses the left lower lobe. Because gravity provides blood flow primarily to the lower lobes after the Fontan operation, preferential distribution to the right side may be a natural consequence of this anatomic feature (95, 96).

An additional recent modification of the Fontan operation is the use of an extra cardiac conduit (Fig. 18.9) from

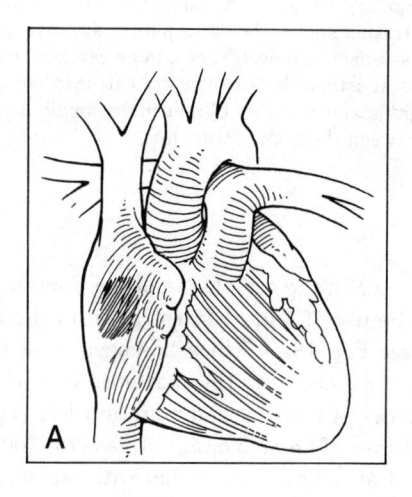

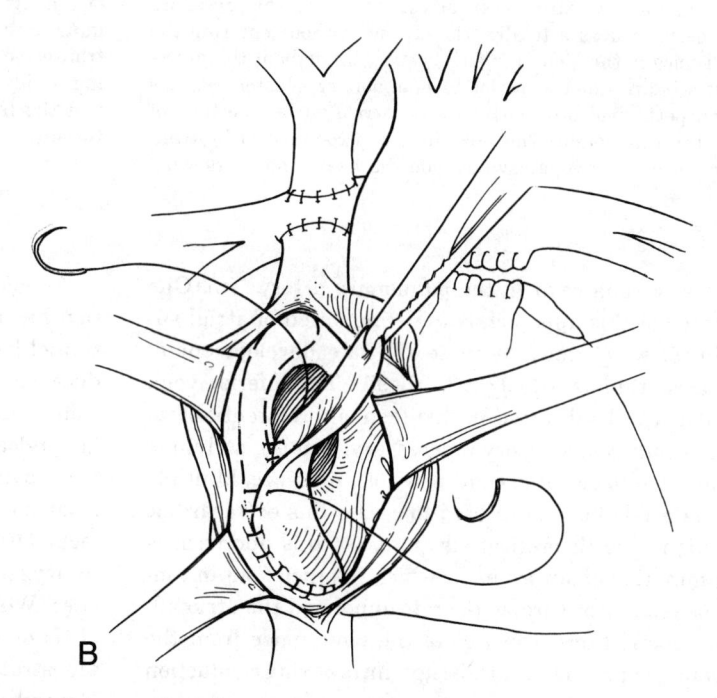

Figure 18.8. Fontan procedure. The lateral tunnel cavopulmonary modification of the Fontan procedure is shown. This currently represents one of the most popular forms of achieving the Fontan circulation. In many cases a superior cavopulmonary shunt has already been performed. If this is not the case it is performed simultaneously with the remainder of the lateral tunnel connection. **A**, Preoperative single ventricle with parallel circulation. **B**, The lateral tunnel proceeds with the performance of a right atriotomy using cardiopulmonary bypass and cardioplegic arrest with moderate hypothermia. A Goretex® patch is sewn around the orifice of the inferior vena cava and then along the lateral wall of the right atrium proceeding toward the superior vena cava. The patch is completed by sewing the upper end around the orifice of the superior vena cava, which has been connected to the right pulmonary artery, thereby creating an intra-atrial tunnel between the inferior vena cava and the pulmonary artery system. As shown in **B**, a fenestration can be placed in the Goretex® patch to allow right-to-left shunting (see text).

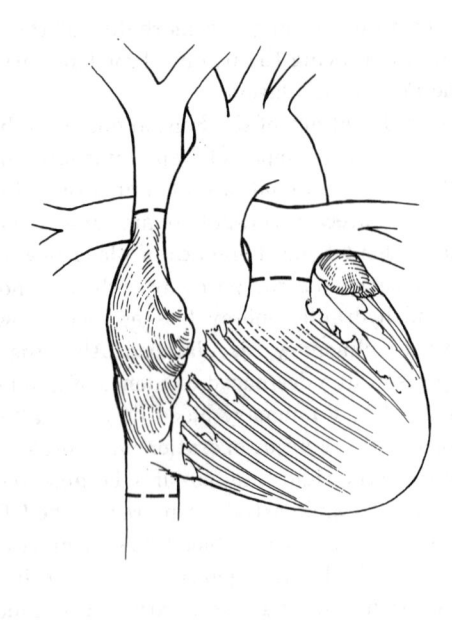

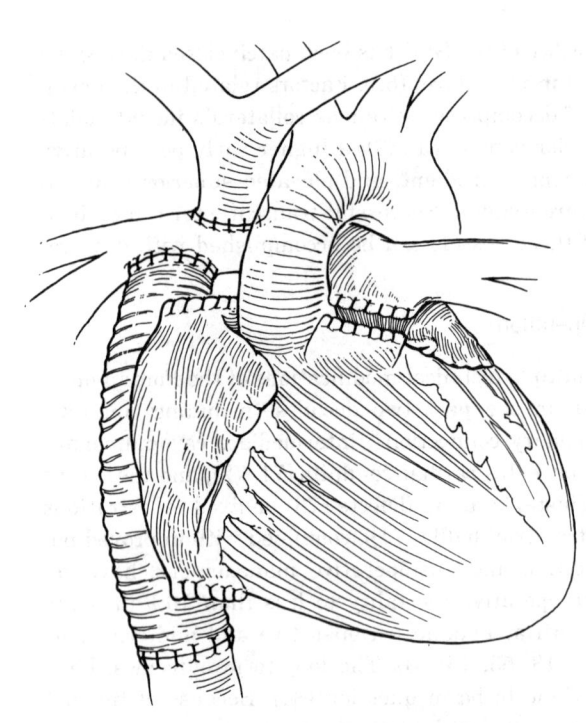

Figure 18.9. Fontan procedure. Another modification of the Fontan operation is the use of an extracardiac conduit Fontan. In this procedure cardiopulmonary bypass is required; however, only mild hypothermia and no cardioplegic arrest is needed. The procedure can be performed as a totally "closed" one without entering the heart. Typically the heart remains beating throughout the procedure. If a bidirectional superior cavopulmonary anastomosis has not been performed previously this is carried out at the time of the Fontan completion. The procedure is accomplished by transecting the inferior vena cava outside the heart and oversewing the cardiac end. An appropriately sized Goretex® conduit is then anastomosed end-to-end to the inferior vena cava. The conduit is then tailored appropriately and anastomosed to the undersurface of the right pulmonary artery as a completely extracardiac conduit. In the illustration shown the main pulmonary artery is also transected and oversewn. A fenestration can be achieved by creating a side-to-side anastomosis between the extracardiac conduit and the free right atrial wall, or by placing a small restrictive Goretex® tube between these two structures.

the inferior vena cava to the pulmonary artery (72). One advantage of this approach is the elimination of atrial suture lines, which may decrease the late development of atrial arrhythmias (81, 92, 93, 97–99). The inferior vena caval flow can be directed in this fashion preferentially to the right pulmonary artery if necessary, and the atrium is not subjected to elevated central venous pressure. Multiple graft materials have been used to create this extracardiac connection. The theoretical advantage of this approach is the elimination of suture lines, which in other Fontan connections (e.g., intracardiac lateral tunnel and the atriopulmonary connections) can isolate the sinus node from the atrioventricular node and disrupt intra-atrial conduction in addition to contributing to sinus node dysfunction. These suture lines have been shown to participate in reentrant circuits and atrial flutter and fibrillation late following the Fontan operation (81, 98). Whether extracardiac conduits will completely eliminate the predisposition for arrhythmia over the long term is still uncertain. In addition, the impact of longitudinal growth on the fixed-length extracardiac conduit as well as the potential for thrombus formation is still unknown.

A major advance in the completion of the Fontan operation has been the use of a fixed fenestration in the lateral tunnel baffle (see Fig. 18.7), which has been shown to reduce mortality (18), decrease the incidence of early effusions following the procedure, and maintain left ventricular preload in times of hemodynamic stress (74, 100, 101). Hemodynamic studies have shown that with temporary occlusion of such fenestrations (or adjustable atrial septal defects) (100–106), the cardiac output falls, although the rise in oxygen saturation maintains oxygen delivery to the tissues. Whether these fenestrations will spontaneously close (107) or whether benefit is found in maintaining an open fenestration permanently remains a controversial point. Nevertheless, isolated reports indicate that treatment of prolonged effusions and protein losing enteropathy by *creating* a fenestration in some patients with a previously intact atrial baffle (108), suggest a positive feature is found in maintaining left ventricular preload and/or minimizing central venous pressure in these patients.

Perfusion management techniques may also decrease early morbidity following the Fontan operation. Modified ultrafiltration, which eliminates extra tissue water following bypass, has resulted in a significant decrease in blood utilization and development of postoperative effusions following both hemi-Fontan and Fontan operations (75).

Although the long-term durability of the Fontan operation (84) and the late development of protein losing enteropathy remains a concern (80), most patients have been shown to have good or excellent functional results (76, 77).

Postoperative Issues

Postoperative management must be specifically tailored to the preoperative anatomy and physiology, as well as the specific type of surgical procedure performed, but in general it is directed toward *optimizing cardiac output at the lowest central venous pressure possible.*

Mechanical Ventilation Mechanical *positive pressure ventilation* with increased mean airway pressures may adversely affect PVR and ventricular filling; early institution of spontaneous ventilation may improve hemodynamics in the awake patient (109). During mechanical ventilation "physiologic" (3–5 cm H_2O) positive end-expiratory pressure (PEEP) is generally well tolerated, does not significantly affect PVR or cardiac output, and may improve oxygenation by reducing areas of microatelectasis, re-establishing functional residual capacity, and improving ventilation/perfusion matching.

Although attempts should be made to establish spontaneous ventilation and extubation as soon as possible after surgery, patients who require prolonged mechanical ventilation may benefit from nontraditional ventilation strategies such as pressure-support, negative pressure ventilation (109b), or high-frequency jet ventilation (109a).

Low Cardiac Output *Low cardiac output* (Table 18.2) after surgery should prompt immediate investigation of the repair and physiology. In addition to postoperative echocardiography (see Chapter 28, *Principles of Echocardiography*) "physiologic" right atrial (RA) and left atrial (LA) catheters are invaluable in the diagnosis and management of these patients (see Chapter 11, *Invasive and Noninvasive Monitoring*). Low cardiac output may be caused by:

1. Inadequate preload; typically due to hypovolemia (low RA and LA pressures)
2. Elevated PVR (low LA and high RA pressures)
3. Anatomic obstruction in the systemic venous pathway (low LA and high RA pressures)
4. Pump failure (high LA and high RA pressures)

Low cardiac output in the face of **high** *LA pressure is an ominous sign*; it may be caused by tamponade, ventricular dysfunction, loss of atrioventricular synchrony, atrioventricular valve regurgitation, or ventricular outflow obstruction (e.g., subaortic stenosis). Prompt investigation of the surgical repair, including catheterization and angiography,

Table 18.2. Differential Diagnosis of Low Cardiac Output after Fontan

RA_p	LA_p	Cause(s)
Low	Low	Hypovolemia
High	Low	↑ Pulmonary vascular resistance, baffle obstruction, pulmonary artery hypoplasia, or branch stenoses
High	High	Ventricular dysfunction, atrioventricular valve stenosis or regurgitation, arrhythmia, outflow obstruction, tamponade

is indicated in the patient with advanced low cardiac output, if the combination of electrocardiographic monitoring, echocardiography (110), and intracardiac pressure monitoring do not readily identify the cause.

Arrhythmias Significant *arrhythmias*, especially those with *loss of atrioventricular synchrony* (e.g., junctional ectopic tachycardia), are particularly poorly tolerated in this patient population. With progressive tachycardia continued hemodynamic deterioration usually occurs; frequently, it is difficult to determine if the arrhythmia is a *result* of poor hemodynamics or its *cause*. Given the high incidence of perioperative sinus node dysfunction (55, 56), atrial pacing may be necessary in the immediate postoperative period. Transthoracic atrial and ventricular pacing wires are therefore placed in all patients undergoing a Fontan operation. See Chapter 30, *Diagnosis and Management of Cardiac Arrhythmias,* for details on perioperative arrhythmia management. Common late arrhythmias include atrial flutter and sinus node dysfunction (55, 56, 93, 97, 111–113).

Cyanosis Evaluation of excessive *cyanosis* following the Fontan procedure is similar to that outlined above for the patient following neonatal palliation or the bidirectional Glenn shunt: evaluation of systemic venous desaturation, pulmonary venous desaturation, or decreased pulmonary blood flow. *Systemic venous desaturation* may be caused by low systemic cardiac output, anemia, or increased oxygen consumption states. In patients with fenestrated baffles, low cardiac output or anemia causing an extremely low mixed venous saturation will result in excessive peripheral desaturation, as the blood crossing the fenestration is lower in oxygen content than usual. Causes of *pulmonary venous desaturation* following the Fontan procedure include pneumothorax, pleural effusions, pneumonia, atelectasis, and, importantly, pre-existing pulmonary arteriovenous malformations, such as those that can occur following a Kawashima procedure or following a long-standing cavopulmonary shunt. In addition to an intentional fenestration or adjustable atrial septal defect, *decreased pulmonary blood flow* may also be caused by high PVR (in patients with the potential for right-to-left shunting), additional baffle leaks, a "too large" atrial septal defect or fenestration, or decompressing venous collaterals to the pulmonary venous atrium.

Effusions Duration and frequency of *pleural and pericardial effusions*, typically the most frequent postoperative problem requiring prolonged hospitalization, have been recently reduced with the use of baffle fenestrations (100), adjustable atrial septal defect, and modified ultrafiltration (75). Drainage catheters, with appropriate replacement of intravascular volume, electrolytes, protein, and immunoglobulins are necessary in cases of prolonged drainage. Patients with prolonged drainage (e.g., more than 2 to 3 weeks) should undergo cardiac catheterization to rule-out potentially correctable causes, such as baffle obstruction, innominate vein thrombosis, pulmonary artery distortion, and so forth.

Thrombosis Finally, following the Fontan operation, patients (especially those with low cardiac output) can be at increased risk for venous thrombosis (114–116) and central nervous system complications. Anticoagulation with heparin or warfarin, or antiplatelet medications may be useful in this subgroup of patients. Coagulation abnormalities (80, 117) and acute liver dysfunction (118) have been described in patients following the Fontan operation. The reported incidence of adverse neurologic sequelae after the Fontan operation is approximately 2 to 3% (77, 119–121).

REFERENCES

1. Shone JD, Sellers RD, Anderson RC, et al. The developmental complex of "parachute mitral valve," supravalvular ring of left atrium, subaortic stenosis, and coarctation of the aorta. Am J Cardiol 1963;11:714–725.
2. Cohen MS, Jacobs ML, Weinberg PM, et al. Morphometric analysis of unbalanced common atrioventricular canal using two-dimensional echocardiography. J Am Coll Cardiol 1996; 28:1017–1023.
3. Bolling SF, Iannettoni MD, Dick, II, et al. Shone's anomaly: operative results and late outcome. Ann Thorac Surg 1990; 49:887–893.
4. Delius R, Rademecker M, deLeval M, et al. Is a high-risk biventricular repair always preferable to conversion to a single ventricle repair? J Thorac Cardiovasc Surg 1996;112: 1561–1569.
5. Canter CE, Moorhead S, Huddleston CB, et al. Restrictive atrial septal communication as a determinant of outcome of cardiac transplantation for hypoplastic left heart syndrome. Circulation 1993;88(II):456–460.
6. Grady RM, Canter CE, Bridges ND. Transcatheter ASD creation in infants with left heart obstruction [Abstract]. J Am Coll Cardiol 1994;484A.
7. Perry SB, Lang P, Keane JF, et al. Creation and maintenance of adequate interatrial communication in left atrioventricular valve atresia or stenosis. Am J Cardiol 1986;58: 622–626.
8. Riordan CJ, Randsbaek F, Storey JH, et al. Inotropes in the hypoplastic left heart syndrome: effects in an animal model. Ann Thorac Surg 1996;62:83–90.
9. Chang AC, Zucker HA, Hickey PR, et al. Pulmonary vascular resistance in infants after cardiac surgery: role of carbon dioxide and hydrogen ion. Crit Care Med 1995;23:568–574.
10. Jobes DR, Nicolson SC, Steven JM, et al. Carbon dioxide prevents pulmonary overcirculation in hypoplastic heart syndrome. Ann Thorac Surg 1992;54:150–151.
11. Reddy VM, Liddicoat JR, Fineman JR, et al. Fetal model of single ventricle physiology: hemodynamic effects of oxygen, nitric oxide, carbon dioxide, and hypoxia in the early postnatal period. J Thorac Cardiovasc Surg 1996;112:437–449.
12. Mora GA, Pizarro C, Jacobs ML, et al. Experimental model of single ventricle: influence of carbon dioxide on pulmonary vascular dynamics. Circulation 1194;90:II-43–II-46.
13. Riordan CJ, Randsbaek F, Storey JH, et al. Effects of oxygen, positive end-expiratory pressure, and carbon dioxide on oxygen delivery in an animal model of the univentricular heart. J Thorac Cardiovasc Surg 1996;112:644–654.
14. Cohen AJ, Cleveland DC, Dyck J, et al. Results of the Fontan procedure for patients with univentricular heart. Ann Thorac Surg 1991;52:1266–1271.
15. Kaulitz R, Ziemer G, Luhmer I, et al. Modified Fontan operation in functionally univentricular hearts: preoperative risk factors and intermediate results. J Thorac Cardiovasc Surg 1996;112:658–664.
16. Mair DD, Hagler DJ, Julsrud PR, et al. Early and late results of the modified Fontan procedure for double-inlet left ventricle: the Mayo Clinic experience. J Am Coll Cardiol 1991;18:1727–1732.
17. Knott-Craig C, Danielson G, Schaff H, et al. The modified Fontan operation: an analysis of risk factors for early postoperative death or takedown in 702 consecutive patients from one institution. J Thorac Cardiovasc Surg 1995;109:1237–1243.
18. Gentles TL, Mayer JE Jr, Gauvreau K, et al. Fontan operation in 500 consecutive patients: factors influencing early and late outcome. J Thorac Cardiovasc Surg 1997;114: 376–391.
19. Mayer JE Jr, Bridges ND, Lock JE, et al. Factors associated with marked reduction in mortality for Fontan operations in patients with single ventricle. J Thorac Cardiovasc Surg 1992;103:444–452.
20. Senzaki H, Isoda T, Ishizawa A, et al. Reconsideration of criteria for the Fontan operation. Influence of pulmonary artery size on postoperative hemodynamics of the Fontan operation. Circulation 1994;89:1196–1202.
21. Bartmus DA, Driscoll DJ, Offord KP, et al. The modified Fontan operation for children less than 4 years old. J Am Coll Cardiol 1990;15:429–435.
22. Imai Y, Takanashi Y, Hoshino S, et al. Modified Fontan procedure in ninety-nine cases of atrioventricular valve regurgitation. J Thorac Cardiovasc Surg 1997;113:262–269.
23. Mayer JE Jr. Risk factors for modified Fontan operations. In: Jacobs ML, Norwood WI, eds. Pediatric cardiac surgery. Boston: Butterworth-Heinemann, 1992;70–82.
24. Rychik J, Jacobs ML, Norwood WI. Acute changes in left ventricular geometry after volume reduction operation. Ann Thorac Surg 1995;60:1267–1274.
25. Serraf A, Conte S, Lacour-Gayet F, et al. Systemic obstruction in univentricular hearts: surgical options for neonates. Ann Thorac Surg 1995;60:970–977.
26. Jenkins KJ, Hanley FL, Colan SD, et al. Function of the anatomic pulmonary valve in the systemic circulation. Circulation 1991;84(Suppl III):173–179.
27. Franklin RCG, Spiegelhalter DJ, Filho RIR, et al. Double-inlet ventricle presenting in infancy. III. Outcome and poten-

tial for definitive repair. J Thorac Cardiovasc Surg 1991; 101:924–934.
28. Malcic I, Sauer U, Stern H, et al. The influence of pulmonary artery banding on outcome after the Fontan operation. J Thorac Cardiovasc Surg 1992;104:743–747.
29. Lui RC, Williams WG, Trusler GA, et al. Experience with the Damus-Kaye-Stansel procedure for children with Taussig-Bing hearts or univentricular hearts with subaortic stenosis. Circulation 1993;88(II):170–176.
30. Karl TR, Watterson KG, Sano S, et al. Operations for subaortic stenosis in univentricular hearts. Ann Thorac Surg 1991;52:420–428.
31. Rychik J, Murdison KA, Chin AJ, et al. Surgical management of severe aortic outflow obstruction in lesions other than the hypoplastic left heart syndrome: use of a pulmonary artery to aorta anastomosis. J Am Coll Cardiol 1991;18:809–816.
32. Gates R, Laks H, Elami A, et al. Damus-Stansel-Kaye procedure: current indications and results. Ann Thorac Surg 1993;56:111–119.
33. van Son JAM, Reddy VM, Haas GS, et al. Modified surgical techniques for relief of aortic obstruction in {S,L,L} hearts with rudimentary right ventricle and restrictive bulboventricular foramen. J Thorac Cardiovasc Surg 1995;110:909–915.
34. Chin AJ, Barber G, Helton JG, et al. Fate of the pulmonic valve after proximal pulmonary artery-to-ascending aorta anastomosis for aortic outflow obstruction. Am J Cardiol 1988;62:435–438.
35. Norwood WI, Lang P, Castañeda AR, et al. Experience with operations for hypoplastic left heart syndrome. J Thorac Cardiovasc Surg 1981;82:511–519.
36. Jacobs M, Rychik J, Murphy J, et al. Results of Norwood's operation for lesions other than hypoplastic left heart syndrome. J Thorac Cardiovasc Surg 1995;110:1555–1562.
37. Forbess J, Cook N, Roth S, et al. Ten-year institutional experience with palliative surgery for hypoplastic left heart syndrome: risk factors related to stage I mortality. Circulation 1995;92:II-262–II-266.
38. Bove E, Lloyd T. Staged reconstruction for hypoplastic left heart syndrome: contemporary results. Ann Surg 1996;224:387–395.
39. Wernovsky G, Wypij D, Jonas RA, et al. Postoperative course and hemodynamic profile after the arterial switch operation in neonates and infants: a comparison of low-flow cardiopulmonary bypass and circulatory arrest. Circulation 1995;92:2226–2235.
40. Riordan CJ, Randsbaek F, Storey JH, et al. Balancing pulmonary and systemic arterial flows in parallel circulations: the value of monitoring system venous oxygen saturations. Cardiology in the Young 1997;7:74–79.
41. Rossi AF, Sommer RJ, Lotvin A, et al. Usefulness of intermittent monitoring of mixed venus oxygen saturation after stage I palliation for hypoplastic left heart syndrome. Am J Cardiol 1994;73:1118–1123.
42. Priidijan AK, Mendelsohn AM, Lupinetti FM, et al. Usefulness of the bidirectional Glenn procedure as staged reconstruction for the functional single ventricle. Am J Cardiol 1993;71:959–962.
43. Chang AC, Hanley FL, Wernovsky G, et al. Early bidirectional cavopulmonary shunt in young infants: postoperative course and early results. Circulation 1993;88:149–158.
44. Bradley SM, Mosca RS, Hennein HA, et al. Bidirectional superior cavopulmonary connection in young infants. Circulation 1996;94:II-5–II-11.
45. McElhinney DB, Reddy VM, Moore P, et al. Bidirectional cavopulmonary shunt in patients with anomalies of systemic and pulmonary venous drainage. Ann Thorac Surg 1997;63:1676–1684.
46. Hawkins JA, Shaddy RE, Day RW, et al. Mid-term results after bidirectional cavopulmonary shunts. Ann Thorac Surg 1993;56:833–837.
47. Reddy VM, Liddicoat J, Hanley F. Primary bidirectional superior cavopulmonary shunt in infants between 1 and 4 months of age. Ann Thorac Surg 1995;59:1120–1126.
48. Albanese SB, Carotti A, Di Donato RM, et al. Bidirectional cavopulmonary anastomosis in patients under two years of age. J Thorac Cardiovasc Surg 1992;104:904–909.
49. Gross GJ, Jonas RA, Castaneda AR, et al. Maturational and hemodynamic factors predictive of increased cyanosis after bidirectional cavopulmonary anastomosis. Am J Cardiol 1994;74:705–709.
50. Matitiau A, Geva T, Colan SD, et al. Bulboventricular foramen size in infants with double-inlet left ventricle or tricuspid atresia with transposed great arteries: influence on initial palliative operation and rate of growth. J Am Coll Cardiol 1992;19:142–148.
51. Donofrio MT, Jacobs ML, Norwood WI, et al. Early changes in ventricular septal defect size and ventricular geometry in the single left ventricle after volume-unloading surgery. J Am Coll Cardiol 1995;26:1008–1015.
52. Jacobs ML, Rychik J, Rome JJ, et al. Early reduction of the volume work of the single ventricle: the hemi-Fontan approach. Ann Thorac Surg 1996;62:456–461.
53. Jacobs ML, Norwood WI. Fontan operation: influence of modifications on morbidity and mortality. Ann Thorac Surg 1994;58:945–952.
54. Lambert JJ, Spicer RL, Waldman JD, et al. The bidirectional cavopulmonary shunt. J Thorac Cardiovasc Surg 1990;100:22–30.
55. Manning P, Mayer J, Wernovsky G, et al. Staged operation to Fontan increases the incidence of sinoatrial node dysfunction. J Thorac Cardiovasc Surg 1996;111:833–840.
56. Cohen MI, Wernovsky G, Jacobs ML, et al. Early and late sinus node dysfunction, a frequent sequelae after a staged Fontan [Abstract]. Circulation 1997;(Suppl I) 96:I-301.
57. Kobayashi J, Matsuda H, Nakano S, et al. Hemodynamic effects of bidirectional cavopulmonary shunt with pulsatile pulmonary blood flow. Circulation 1991;84 (Suppl III):III-219–III-225.
58. Day RW, Baker CM, Caton JR, et al. Bidirectional cavopulmonary shunt with an additional source of pulmonary flow: an interim or final stage of palliation. Cardiol Young 1997;7:63–70.
59. Mainwaring RD, Lamberti JJ, Uzark K, et al. Bidirectional Glenn: is accessory pulmonary blood flow good or bad? Circulation 1995;92:II-294–II-297.
60. Mainwaring RD, Lamberti JJ, Moore JW. The bidirectional Glenn and Fontan procedures—integrated management of the patient with a functionally single ventricle. Cardiol Young 1996;6:198–207.
61. Webber SA, Horvath P, LeBlanc JG, et al. Influence of competitive pulmonary blood flow on the bidirectional superior cavopulmonary shunt: a multi-institutional study. Circulation 1995;92:II-279–II-286.
62. Frommelt MA, Frommelt PC, Berger S, et al. Does an additional source of pulmonary blood flow alter outcome after a bidirectional cavopulmonary shunt? Circulation 1995;92:II-240–II-244.
63. Uemura H, Yagihara T, Kawashima Y, et al. Use of the bidirectional Glenn procedure in the presence of forward flow from the ventricles to the pulmonary arteries. Circulation 1995;92:II-228–II-232.

64. Srivastava D, Preminger T, Lock J, et al. Hepatic venous blood and the development of pulmonary arteriovenous malformations in congenital heart disease. Circulation 1995; 92:1217–1222.
65. Bernstein HS, Brook MM, Silverman NH, et al. Development of pulmonary arteriovenous fistulae in children after cavopulmonary shunt. Circulation 1995;92:II-309–II-314.
66. Amodeo A, Di Donato R, Carotti A, et al. Pulmonary arteriovenous fistulas and polysplenia syndrome. J Thorac Cardiovasc Surg 1994;107:1378–1379.
67. Shah MJ, Rychik J, Fogel MA, et al. Pulmonary AV malformations after superior cavopulmonary connection: resolution after inclusion of hepatic veins in the pulmonary circulation. Ann Thorac Surg 1997;63:960–963.
68. Magee AG, McCrindle BW, Benson LN, et al. Systemic venous collaterals after the bidirectional cavopulmonary anastomosis prevalence and risk factors. Cardiol Young 1996;6:S11.
69. McElhinney DB, Reddy VM, Hanley FL, et al. Systemic venous collateral channels causing desaturation after bidirectional cavopulmonary anastomosis: evaluation and management. J Am Coll Cardiol 1997;30:817–824.
70. Fontan F, Baudet E. Surgical repair of tricuspid atresia. Thorax 1971;26:240–248.
71. Laschinger JC, Redmond JM, Cameron DE, et al. Intermediate results of the extracardiac Fontan procedure. Ann Thorac Surg 1996;62:1261–1267.
72. Marcelletti C, Corno A, Giannico S, et al. Inferior vena cava–pulmonary artery extracardiac conduit: a new form of right heart bypass. J Thorac Cardiovasc Surg 1990;100:228–232.
73. Laks H, Ardehali A, Grant PW, et al. Modifications of the Fontan procedure: superior vena cava to left pulmonary artery connection and inferior vena cava to right pulmonary artery connection with adjustable atrial septal defect. Circulation 1995;91:2943–2947.
74. Bridges ND, Lock JE, Castañeda AR. Baffle fenestration with subsequent transcatheter closure: modification of the Fontan operation for patients at increased risk. Circulation 1990;82:1681–1689.
75. Koutlas TC, Gaynor JW, Nicolson SC, et al. Modified ultrafiltration reduces postoperative morbidity after cavopulmonary connection. Ann Thorac Surg 1997;64:37–43.
76. Gentles TL, Gauvreau K, Mayer JE Jr, et al. Functional outcome after the Fontan operation: factors influencing late morbidity. J Thorac Cardiovasc Surg 1997;114:392–403.
77. Wernovsky G, Stiles KM, Gauvreau K, et al. Cognitive development following the Fontan operation [Abstract]. Circulation 1995;(Suppl I):I-121.
78. Cetta F, Feldt R, O'Leary P, et al. Improved early morbidity and mortality after Fontan operation: the Mayo Clinic experience, 1987 to 1992. J Am Coll Cardiol 1996;28:480–486.
79. Uemura H, Yagihara T, Kawashima Y, et al. Surgery for congenital heart disease: what factors affect ventricular performance after a Fontan-type operation? J Thorac Cardiovasc Surg 1995;110:405–415.
80. Cromme-Dijkhuis AH, Hess J, Hahlen K, et al. Specific sequelae after Fontan operation at mid- and long-term followup. J Thorac Cardiovasc Surg 1993;106:1126–1132.
81. Gandhi S, Bromberg B, Rodefeld M, et al. Lateral tunnel suture line variation reduces atrial flutter after the modified Fontan operation. Ann Thorac Surg 1996;61:1299–1309.
82. Nir A, Driscoll DJ, Mottram CD, et al. Cardiorespiratory response to exercise after the Fontan operation: a serial study. J Am Coll Cardiol 1993;22:216–220.
83. Farrell PE, Chang AC, Murdison KA, et al. Outcome and assessment after the modified Fontan procedure for hypoplastic left heart syndrome. Circulation 1992;85:116–122.
84. Fontan F, Kirklin JW, Fernandez G, et al. Outcome after a "perfect" Fontan operation. Circulation 1990;81:1520–1536.
85. Van de Wal H, Tanke R, Roef M. The modified Senning operation for cavopulmonary connection with autologous tissue. J Thorac Surg 1994;108:377–380.
86. Carotti A, Iorio FS, Amodeo A, et al. Total cavopulmonary direct anastomosis: a logical approach in selected patients. Ann Thorac Surg 1993;56:963–964.
87. De Leval M, Dubini G, Migliavacca F, et al. Use of computational fluid dynamics in the design of surgical procedures: application to the study of competitive flows in cavopulmonary connections. J Thorac Cardiovasc Surg 1996;111: 502–513.
88. De Leval MR, Kilner P, Gewillig M, et al. Total cavopulmonary connection: a logical alternative to atriopulmonary connection for complex Fontan operations. J Thorac Cardiovasc Surg 1988;96:682–695.
89. Julsrud PR, Danielson GK. A modification of the Fontan procedure incorporating anomalies of systemic and pulmonary venous return. J Thorac Cardiovasc Surg 1990;100:233–239.
90. Sharma S, Goudy S, Walker P, et al. In vitro flow experiments for determination of optimal geometry of total cavopulmonary connection for surgical repair of children with functional single ventricle. J Am Coll Cardiol 1996;27:1264–1269.
91. Van Haesdonch J, Mertens L, Sizaire R, et al. Comparison by computerized numeric modeling of energy losses in different Fontan connections. Circulation 1995;92:II-322–II-326.
92. Fishberger SB, Wernovsky G, Gentles TL, et al. Factors influencing the development of atrial flutter following the Fontan operation. J Thorac Cardiovasc Surg 1997;113:80–86.
93. Gelatt M, Hamilton RM, McCrindle BW, et al. Risk factors for atrial tachyarrhythmias after the Fontan operation. J Am Coll Cardiol 1994;24:1735–1741.
94. Del Torso S, Milanesi O, Bui F, et al. Radionuclide evaluation of lung perfusion after the Fontan procedure. Int J Cardiol 1988;20:107–116.
95. Rebergen SA, Ottenkamp, Doornbos J, et al. Postoperative pulmonary flow dynamics after Fontan surgery: assessment with nuclear magnetic resonance velocity mapping. J Am Coll Cardiol 1993;21:123–131.
96. Fogel MA, Weinberg PM, Rychik J, et al. Caval contribution to flow in the branch pulmonary arteries of Fontan patients using a novel application of magnetic resonance presaturation pulse [Abstract]. Circulation 1996;94(Suppl I):I-181.
97. Kurer CC, Tanner CS, Vetter VL. Electrophysiologic findings after Fontan repair of functional single ventricle. J Am Coll Cardiol 1991;17:174–181.
98. Rodefeld M, Bromberg B, Schuessler R, et al. Atrial flutter after lateral tunnel construction in the modified Fontan operation: a canine model. J Thorac Cardiovasc Surg 1996;111: 514–526.
99. Balaji S, Gewillig M, Bull C, et al. Arrhythmias after the Fontan procedure. Circulation 1991;84(Supp III):III-162–III-167.
100. Bridges ND, Mayer JE Jr, Lock JE, et al. Effect of baffle fenestration on outcome of the modified Fontan operation. Circulation 1992;86:1762–1769.
101. Kopf GS, Kleinman CS, Hijazi ZM, et al. Fenestrated Fontan operation with delayed transcatheter closure of atrial septal defect. J Thorac Cardiovasc Surg 1992;103:1039–1048.
102. Bridges ND, Lock JE, Mayer JE, et al. Cardiac catheterization and test occlusion of the interatrial communication after

102. [reference continues] the fenestrated Fontan operation. J Am Coll Cardiol 1995;25:1712–1717.
103. Kuhn MA, Jarmakani JM, Laks H, et al. Effect of late postoperative atrial septal defect closure on hemodynamic function in patients with a lateral tunnel Fontan procedure. J Am Coll Cardiol 1995;26:259–265.
104. Laks H, Pearl JM, Haas GS, et al. Partial Fontan: advantages of an adjustable interatrial communication. Ann Thorac Surg 1991;52:1084–1095.
105. Kuhn MA, Permut LC, Laks H, et al. Hemodynamic effects of adjustable ASD closure in Fontan patients [Abstract]. J Am Coll Cardiol 1994;February:105A.
106. Harake I, Kuhn MA, Jarmakani JM, et al. Acute hemodynamic effects of adjustable atrial septal defect closure in the lateral tunnel Fontan procedure. J Am Coll Cardiol 1994; 23:1671–1676.
107. Pearl JM, Laks H, Barthell S, et al. Spontaneous closure of fenestrations in an interarterial gore-tex patch: application to the Fontan procedure. Ann Thorac Surg 1994;57:611–614.
108. Rychik J, Rome JJ, Jacobs ML. Late surgical fenestration for complications after the Fontan operation. Circulation 1997;96:33–36.
109. Penny DJ, Redington AN. Doppler echocardiographic evaluation of pulmonary blood flow after the Fontan operation: the role of the lungs. Br Heart J 1991;66:372–374.
109a. Meliones JN, Bove EL, Dekeon MK, et al. High-frequency jet ventilation improves cardiac function after the Fontan operation. Circulation 1991;84(Suppl III):364–368.
109b. Shekerdemian LS, Shore DF, Lincoln C, et al. Negative-pressure ventilation improves cardiac output after right heart surgery. Circulation 1996;(Suppl II):49–55.
110. Stumper O, Sutherland GR, Geuskens R, et al. Transesophageal echocardiography in evaluation and management after a Fontan operation. J Am Coll Cardiol 1991;17:1152–1160.
111. Gardiner HM, Dhillon R, Bull C, et al. Prospective study of the incidence and determinants of arrhythmia after total cavopulmonary connection. Circulation 1996;94:II-17–II-21.
112. Fishberger SB, Wernovsky G, Gentles TL, et al. Factors that influence the development of atrial flutter after the Fontan operation. J Thorac Cardiovasc Surg 1997;113:80–86.
113. Kavey RW, Gaum WE, Byrum CJ, et al. Loss of sinus rhythm after total cavopulmonary connection. Circulation 1995;92:II-304–II-308.
114. Kaulitz R, Ziemer G, Bergmann F, et al. Artial thrombus after the Fontan-operation: predisposing factors, treatment and prophylaxis. Cardiol Young 1997;7:37–43.
115. Fyfe DA, Kline CH, Sade RM, et al. Transesophageal echocardiography detects thrombus formation not identified by transthoracic echocardiography after the Fontan operation. J Am Coll Cardiol 1991;18:1733–1737.
116. Rosenthal DN, Friedman AH, Kleinman CS, et al. Thromboembolic complications after Fontan operations. Circulation 1995;92:II-287–II-293.
117. Jahangiri M, Shore D, Kakkar V, et al. Coagulation factor abnormalities after the Fontan procedure and its modifications. J Thorac Cardiovasc Surg 1997;113:989–993.
118. Matsuda H, Covino E, Hirose H, et al. Acute liver dysfunction after modified Fontan operation for complex cardiac lesions. J Thorac Cardiovasc Surg 1988;96:219–226.
119. Mathews K, Bale JF, Clark EB, et al. Cerebral infarction complicating Fontan surgery for cyanotic congenital heart disease. Pediatr Cardiol 1986;7:161–166.
120. Miller G, Eggli K, Contant C, et al. Postoperative neurologic complications after open heart surgery on young infants. Arch Pediatr Adolesc Med 1995;149:764–768.
121. Miller G, Mamourian A, Tesman J, et al. Long-term MRI changes in brain after pediatric open heart surgery. J Child Neurol 1994;9:390–397.

Other Conotruncal Lesions

19.1 Transposition of the Great Arteries

Gil Wernovsky, MD, and Richard A. Jonas, MD

D-TRANSPOSITION OF THE GREAT ARTERIES

Transposition of the great arteries (TGA) is a lethal and relatively frequent malformation accounting for 5 to 7% of all congenital cardiac malformations (1). Without treatment about 30% of these infants die in the first week of life, 50% within the first month, 70% within 6 months, and 90% within the first year (2). Today, aggressive medical and surgical interventions in the neonate can provide 90% or better early and midterm survival, and for many, the prospect of a vigorous adolescent and adult life. The incidence is reported to vary from 20.1 to 30.5 per 100,000 live births with a strong (60 to 70%) male preponderance (1–3). Although earlier epidemiologic and genetic surveys suggested some other associations, for example, increased prevalence in infants with diabetic mothers or prenatal exposure to sex hormone therapy, such has not been confirmed (4).

Anatomy

Transposition of the great arteries is defined as the aorta arising from the anatomic right ventricle (RV) and the pulmonary artery (PA) arising from the anatomic left ventricle (LV) (Fig. 19.1.1). The most common form of transposition occurs when the ventricles are normally positioned and the aorta is malposed **anteriorly and rightward** above the right ventricle, aligned with the RV via the infundibulum (D-transposition, D-TGA).

Associated anomalies include:

- Ventricular septal defect (VSD, approximately 40%)
- Coarctation or interrupted aortic arch (10%)
- Left ventricular outflow tract obstruction (LVOTO, 5 to 10%)
- Coronary branching abnormalities (33%)

Ventricular septal defect is the most frequent coexisting anomaly. It can be small, large, or (rarely) multiple, and it can be located anywhere in the septum. The distribution of anatomic subtypes (5) includes membranous (33%); atrioventricular canal (5%); muscular (27%); outlet septum, malalignment type (30%); and outlet septum, conus deficiency type (5%). The typical membranous defect lies adjacent to the membranous septum and tricuspid annulus at the anteroseptal tricuspid valve commissure, and it is situated between the conal (outlet) septum above and the muscular ventricular septum below. Defects in this location may spontaneously close or become smaller with time. Most muscular defects are in the midseptum, others occur in the posterior inflow, apical, or high anterior septum; muscular defects, rarely, are multiple. Spontaneous decrease in size with eventual closure has been documented frequently, particularly with an initially small, slit-shaped muscular inlet or trabecular defect. Atrioventricular canal (inlet septum) types of VSDs may be associated with coexisting atrioventricular valve or conduction tissue anomalies (6–8). This type of defect provides the potential for the tricuspid valve or orifice to straddle the ventricular septum, and it is sometimes associated with a hypoplastic right ventricle.

Of particular surgical importance are the malalignment (outlet) septal defects. Anterior (rightward) malalignment defects are associated with varying degrees of overriding of the pulmonary annulus onto the right ventricle. With increasing degrees of overriding, a series of anomalies are encountered that culminate, effectively, in double-outlet right ventricle with subpulmonary defect (see Chapter 19.2, *Double Outlet Right Ventricle*). Lev et al. (9) suggested that these represent a morphologic spectrum of hearts (Taussig-Bing anomaly). The VSD is an anterior defect, often with a muscular posterior rim, but it sometimes extends posteriorly to the tricuspid annulus (perimembranous extension). The subaortic stenosis caused by the anterior malalignment of the infundibular septum is frequently associated with **aortic arch hypoplasia, coarctation**, or **complete interruption of the aortic arch** (10, 11). Posterior (leftward) malalignment is associated with varying degrees of subpulmonary stenosis, annular hypoplasia, or pulmonary valvar atresia (12).

Obstruction to pulmonary blood flow is possible at multiple levels in patients with TGA; it is present in about 25% of all patients; 20% of the patients with TGA/intact ventricular septum (IVS) (but only 5% have important hemodynamic obstructions) and in 30% of patients with TGA/VSD. Gradients measured preoperatively across the left ventricular outflow tract by Doppler echocardiography or during cardiac catheterization can overestimate the degree of anatomic obstruction because of the greatly increased pulmonary blood flow in children with transposition of the great arteries, especially with an associated VSD (13).

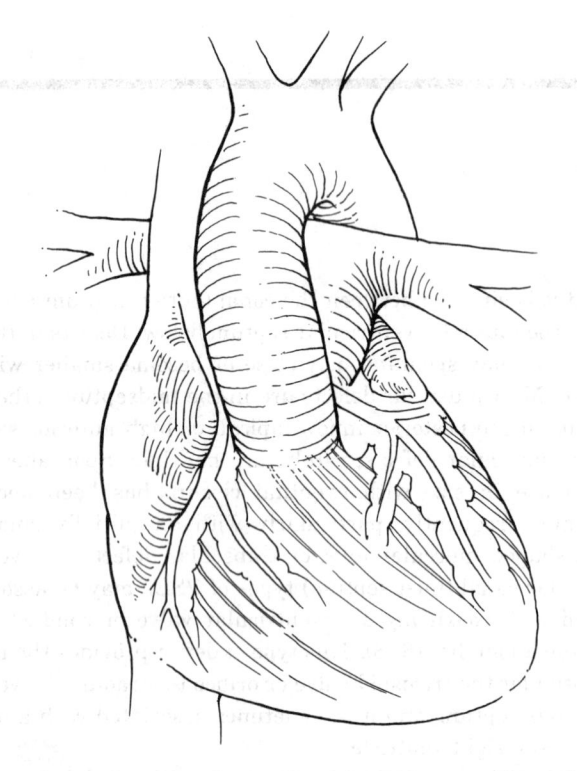

Figure 19.1.1. The external anatomy of simple d-transposition of the great arteries (TGA) is shown. The aorta and main pulmonary arteries are of approximately equal size. The aorta is anterior and slightly to the right side, arising from the infundibulum of the right ventricle. The main pulmonary artery arises from the left ventricle, and continuity of mitral valve to pulmonary valve fibrous is seen. Various coronary artery patterns may be present. A foramen ovale or ostium secundum atrial septal defect, and patent ductus arteriosus are typically present in the newborn infant.

In TGA/IVS, a dynamic type of obstruction is common (14), usually mild and not readily apparent on an autopsy specimen without careful analysis (15). Angiography and echocardiography clearly demonstrate a dynamic leftward bulging of the basal muscular ventricular septum toward the lower pressure left ventricle, which narrows the left ventricular outflow tract during systole, but opens widely during diastole. This systolic septal bulge reflects the reversal of the normal transseptal ventricular systolic pressure relationships seen in TGA. Dynamic obstruction is rarely noted in the neonate with elevated pulmonary artery resistance and left ventricular pressure, because the left ventricle assumes systemic systolic pressure and geometry (16). Following atrial level repair (Senning or Mustard), cardiac catheterization or Doppler echocardiography frequently reveals mild to moderate (10 to 40 mm Hg) systolic pressure differences across the subpulmonary outflow tract.

Fixed obstruction develops in some infants; it initially appears as a patch of endocardial thickening on the septal bulge but later can evolve into a sharp fibrous ridge or a discrete membrane, analogous to membranous subaortic stenosis, along the line of systolic mitral valve contact. Less commonly, fixed subpulmonary obstruction is caused by a tunnel-like subpulmonary fibromuscular ridge that extends across the outflow tract and onto the base of the anterior mitral leaflet (13, 17). Pulmonary valve stenosis and annular hypoplasia are rare in patients with TGA/IVS (18); when present it is almost always associated with combined subvalvar obstructive lesions.

Other uncommon forms of subpulmonary stenosis result from (*a*) malattachment of the anterior mitral valve to the muscular outlet septum by anomalous fibrous or chordal tissue (which can be associated with varying degrees of left ventricular hypoplasia); (*b*) redundant tricuspid valve tissue ("pouch") protruding through the VSD; (*c*) subpulmonic membrane; (*d*) aneurysm of the membranous septum; and (*e*) hypertrophy of the muscle of Moulaert.

Until recently, the extensive anatomic variability of the **coronary arteries** in hearts with TGA was only of academic interest. Shaher and Puddu described the multiple variations in the origin and epicardial course of the coronary arteries as early as 1966 (19). This marked diversity has been confirmed in other pathologic and surgical series. In normally related great arteries, the fixed interrelationship between the aorta and pulmonary trunk likely minimizes the abnormalities of the origin and distribution of the coronary arteries. However, the variable interrelationship of the aorta and pulmonary trunk in TGA, as well as the variability in the size and orientation of the conal septum, probably accounts for the greater variation in the origin and distribution of the epicardial coronary arteries in TGA. The coronary arteries appear to take the "shortest route" to a sinus in the aortic root. For example, when the aorta is more posterior (as in side-by-side great arteries), the circumflex coronary artery or even the entire left coronary artery system may arise from the posterior facing sinus, whereas the right coronary artery arises from the aorta anteriorly—a distribution similar to normally related great arteries.

The two aortic sinuses of Valsalva adjacent to the aorticopulmonary septum which "face" the pulmonary artery contain the ostia of the coronary arteries in more than 99% of cases (20, 21); these are termed the "septal or facing sinuses." When the great arteries are directly anterior-posterior, the facing sinuses are directed **leftward** and **rightward**. When the great arteries are directly side-by-side, the facing sinuses are directed **anteriorly** and **posteriorly**. When the aorta is anterior to and rightward of the pulmonary artery (the typical interrelationship), the facing sinuses are **leftward-anterior** and **rightward-posterior** (Fig. 19.1.2).

As in hearts with normally related great arteries, the three major coronary arteries are (*a*) the **right coronary artery**—defined as the coronary artery that passes in the

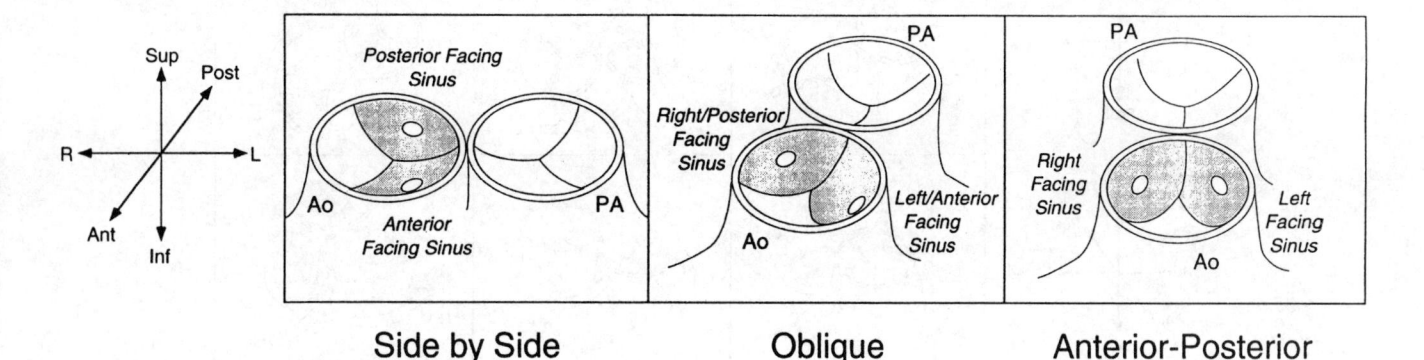

Figure 19.1.2. Nomenclature of the aortic sinuses that contain the coronary ostia, based on the interrelationship of the great arteries. *Ant*, anterior; *Ao*, aorta; *Inf*, inferior; *L*, left; *PA*, pulmonary artery; *Post*, posterior; *R*, right; *Sup*, superior. (Modified from Wernovsky G, Sanders SP. Coronary artery anatomy and transposition of the great arteries. Coron Artery Dis 1993;4:148–157. Reproduced with permission from *Coronary Artery Disease*, Philadelphia: Current Science Publishing.)

right atrioventricular groove, (*b*) the **circumflex coronary artery**—defined as the coronary artery that passes in the left atrioventricular groove, and (*c*) the **anterior descending artery**—the coronary artery that parallels the interventricular septum on the anterior surface of the heart. In addition to the variability in distal distribution, the proximal portion of each of the three major branches may pursue an intramural course, usually between the two great vessels. In these cases, the media of the aortic and coronary walls are attached without interposed adventitia (Fig. 19.1.3).

Pathophysiology and Initial Management

The dominant physiologic abnormalities in the newborn with TGA are a deficiency of oxygen supply to the tissues and an excessive right and left ventricular workload. The systemic and pulmonary circulations function in parallel rather than in series; hence, the greatest portion of the output of each ventricle is recirculated to that ventricle (Fig. 19.1.4). Particularly in TGA/IVS, only a relatively small proportion of blood is exchanged by intercirculatory shunts between the two circulations to eventually reach the appropriate vascular bed. The systemic and pulmonary arterial oxygen saturations are thus dependent on one or more of the following anatomic paths for this exchange: intracardiac (patent foramen ovale, atrial septal defect [ASD], VSD) and extracardiac (patent ductus arteriosus [PDA], bronchopulmonary collateral circulation).

Intercirculatory Mixing

The net volume of blood passing from the pulmonary circulation (left atrium, left ventricle, pulmonary arteries) to the systemic circulation (right atrium, right ventricle, aorta) represents the anatomic left-to-right shunt and is, in fact, the effective systemic blood flow (i.e., oxygenated pulmonary venous return perfusing the systemic capillary bed) (Fig. 19.1.4). Conversely, the net volume of blood passing from the systemic circulation to the pulmonary circulation represents the anatomic right-to-left shunt and is, in fact, the effective pulmonary blood flow (systemic venous return perfusing the pulmonary capillary bed). The effective pulmonary blood flow, effective systemic blood flow, and net anatomic right-to-left and net anatomic left-to-right shunts are each equal to each other, and this volume is the **intercirculatory mixing: the flow in TGA on which survival depends**. The net volume exchanged between systemic and pulmonary circulations must be equal over a given short interval of time, because any major differences will result in a depletion of the blood volume of one circulation at the expense of overloading the other.

The volumes of anatomic right-to-left and left-to-right shunted blood (i.e., "effective blood flows") that participate in functional gas exchange at the pulmonary and systemic capillary levels are relatively small in comparison with the large volumes of blood circulating (total systemic and pulmonary blood flow) or recirculating (physiologic left-to-right and right-to-left shunt flows) within each circulation. The physiologic left-to-right shunt represents the volume of the pulmonary venous blood recirculating through the lungs without having passed through the body, and the physiologic right-to-left shunt is the volume of systemic venous blood re-entering the systemic circulation without having passed through the lungs.

The extent of intercirculatory mixing in TGA depends on the number, size, and position of the anatomic communications, and on the total blood flow through the pulmonary circuit. In the neonate with an intact ventricular septum and a closed or closing ductus arteriosus, severe hypoxemia secondary to inadequate mixing at the foramen ovale level is usually present. When the interatrial or interventricular shunting sites are of adequate size, the level

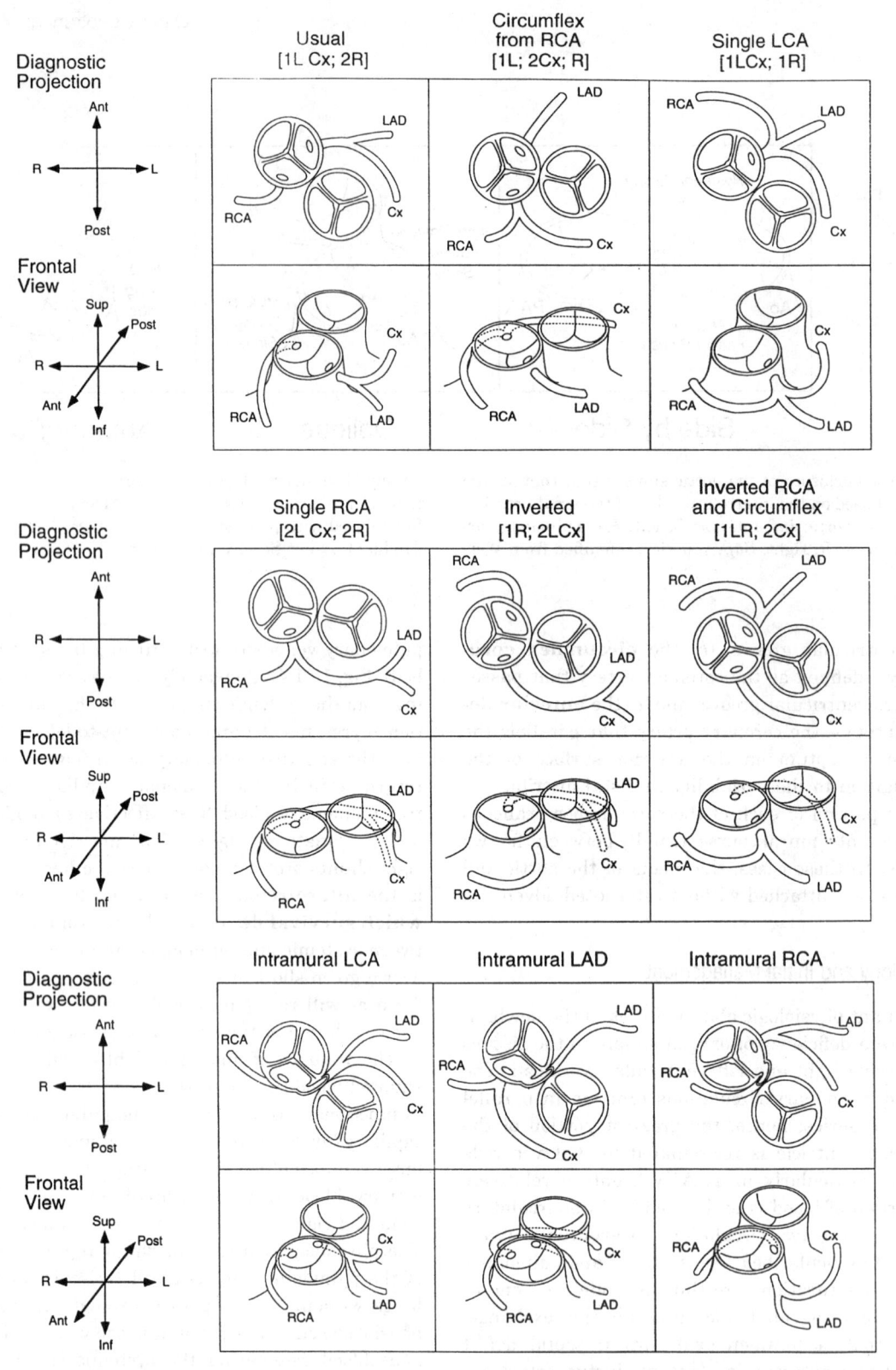

Figure 19.1.3. Coronary artery distribution in transposition of the great arteries (TGA). *Upper panels* (diagnostic projection) is a diagram of the origin and proximal course as visualized by two-dimensional echocardiography and caudally angulated aortography. The *lower panels* show the same coronary artery distribution as viewed anteriorly ("surgeon's view"–frontal projection). Note that the circumflex coronary artery, or even the entire left coronary artery system, is more likely to pursue a "retropulmonary" course (*dashed lines*) when the great arteries are in a side-by-side relationship (shown). An intramural course (*shaded*) of the proximal coronary artery exists in less than 3% of cases, but it has been associated with higher risk for transfer during an arterial switch operation. Alternative terminology in brackets is shown as popularized by Quagebeur and Kirklin et al (5). *Ant*, anterior; *Cx*, circumflex coronary artery; *Inf*, inferior; *L*, left; *LAD*, left anterior descending coronary artery; *Post*, posterior; *R*, right; *RCA*, right coronary artery; *Sup*, superior. (Modified from Wernovsky G, Sanders SP. Coronary artery anatomy and transposition of the great arteries. Coron Artery Dis 1993;4:148–157. Reproduced with permission from Coronary Artery Disease, Philadelphia: Current Science Publishing.)

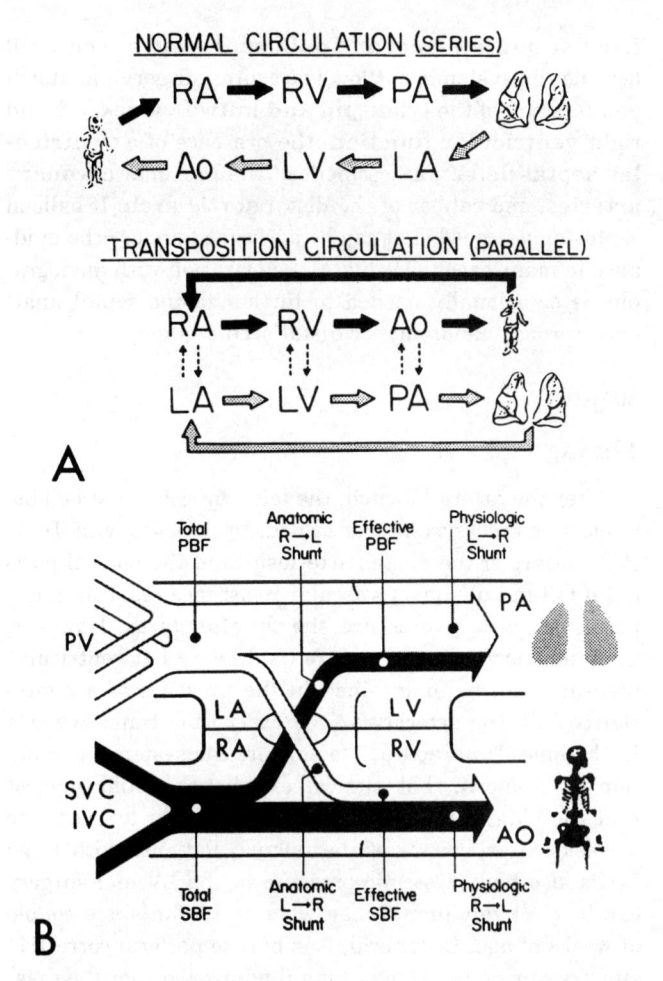

Figure 19.1.4. Circulation in transposition of the great arteries (TGA). **A.** Systemic and pulmonary circulation pathways: in series, with normally related great arteries; in parallel, with TGA. *Solid arrows*, relatively unoxygenated blood; *stippled arrows*, oxygenated blood; *dashed arrows*, intercirculatory shunts. **B.** Circulation schema demonstrating flows and shunts in infants with TGA/IVS. Note that the anatomic left-to-right shunt constitutes the effective SBF, and the anatomic right-to-left shunt constitutes the effective PBF (see text). *AO*, aorta; *IVC*, inferior vena cava; *LA*, left atrium; *LV*, left ventricle; *L → R*, left-to-right; *RA*, right atrium; *RV*, right ventricle; *R → L*, right-to-left; *PA*, pulmonary artery; *PBF*, pulmonary blood flow; *PV*, pulmonary veins; *SBF*, systemic blood flow; *SVC*, superior vena cava. (Adapted with permission from Paul MH, Wernovsky G. Transposition of the great arteries. In: Emmanouilides GC, Riemenschneider TA, Allen HD, et al (eds). Moss and Adams' heart disease in infants, children, and adolescents, including the fetus and young adult. Baltimore: Williams & Wilkins, 1995;1154–1225.)

of arterial oxygen saturation is influenced primarily by the pulmonary:systemic blood flow ratio, with a high pulmonary blood flow resulting in relatively high arterial oxygen saturation, as long as the ventricles can adequately maintain the high output state. If the pulmonary blood flow is decreased by subpulmonary or pulmonary stenosis or elevated pulmonary vascular resistance, the arterial oxygen saturation will be lowered in spite of adequately sized anatomic shunting sites (14, 22–25).

The physiologic mechanisms that precisely control the equalization of interchange between the two circulations remain speculative. The shunting patterns appear to be determined by local pressure gradients, which in turn are influenced by respiratory cycle phase, compliance of the cardiac chambers, heart rate, and the volume of blood flow and the vascular resistance in each of the circulations. With TGA/IVS, the interatrial shunt is from right atrium to left atrium during ventricular diastole, because left ventricular resistance to filling is less than right ventricular. The shunt is from left atrium to right atrium in ventricular systole, because the left atrium is less distensible than the right, and the net pressure in the left atrium is higher during ventricular systole. The pattern is affected by spontaneous respiration with the interatrial right-to-left (systemic-to-pulmonary) shunt increasing during inspiration when the systemic venous return increases and pulmonary venous return decreases. The effects on intercirculatory mixing from positive pressure mechanical ventilation have not been fully studied.

Management of Profound Hypoxemia

In neonates with TGA/IVS, the combination of a low arterial Po_2 (e.g., less than 20 mm Hg), an elevated Pco_2 (despite adequate chest motion and ventilation), and metabolic acidosis (with or without pulmonary edema on the chest radiograph) is a marker for **severely decreased effective pulmonary and systemic flows** ("poor mixing") and requires urgent attention. The initial management of the severely hypoxemic patient with TGA includes (*a*) ensuring adequate mixing between the two parallel circuits and (*b*) maximizing the mixed venous oxygen saturation.

Once the diagnosis of TGA is made, maintaining patency of the ductus arteriosus with prostaglandin E_1 (PGE_1) will increase pulmonary blood flow and intercirculatory mixing—if pulmonary vascular resistance is lower than systemic vascular resistance and there is an atrial communication. **In patients who do not respond to opening the ductus arteriosus with PGE_1 with an increased arterial oxygen saturation, the foramen ovale should be emergently enlarged by balloon atrial septostomy, and ventilatory maneuvers should be employed to decrease pulmonary vascular resistance and increase pulmonary blood flow.** (Balloon atrial septostomy remains an elective procedure in patients with adequate oxygen delivery. Many find it helpful to perform a balloon atrial septostomy—even in the stable patient on prostaglandin—so that PGE_1 can be discontinued and surgery can take place on a more elective basis.)

Despite the above maneuvers, some patients remain hypoxemic even with an open ductus arteriosus, an adequate sized atrial communication, and hyperventilation. In these patients, it is important to emphasize that **most systemic blood flow is the re-circulated systemic venous return**. In the presence of poor mixing, significant improvements in oxygen delivery can be made by **increasing the mixed venous oxygen saturation**, which is the major determinant of systemic arterial oxygen saturation. Maneuvers include **decreasing** oxygen consumption (muscle relaxants, sedation, mechanical ventilation) **and improving oxygen delivery** (increasing cardiac output with inotropic agents or increasing oxygen carrying capacity by treating anemia). Coexisting causes of pulmonary venous desaturation (e.g., pneumothorax) should be sought and treated. Increasing the fraction of inspired oxygen to 100% will have little effect on the arterial P_{O_2}, unless this serves to lower pulmonary vascular resistance and increase total pulmonary blood flow.

Preoperative Evaluation

As the arterial switch operation has gained widespread acceptance as the surgical procedure of choice for TGA (with or without a VSD), this discussion will focus on initial management and postoperative care following anatomic repair. For complete discussion of other surgical procedures, such as atrial redirection procedures (Senning and Mustard), the reader is referred to other texts on the subject (26).

Echocardiography/Catheterization

Echocardiography alone is sufficient to establish the diagnosis and plan surgery for most patients (Fig. 19.1.5). The examination should focus on adequacy of **the left ventricular outflow tract and pulmonary valve** (which will become the systemic outflow tract after surgery), anatomy and function of the **tricuspid and mitral valves**, left and right **ventricular function**, the presence of a **ventricular septal defect**, assessment of the proximal **coronary arteries**, and caliber of the distal **aortic arch**. If balloon septostomy is needed, it can be performed under echo guidance in many cases. Cardiac catheterization with angiography is occasionally needed to further define septal anatomy, coronary anatomy, or distal arch anatomy.

Surgery

Timing

After the arterial switch, the left ventricle must be able to eject against systemic afterload. In patients with TGA/IVS, closure of the ductus arteriosus and the normal postnatal fall in pulmonary vascular resistance result in a low pulmonary artery pressure shortly after birth. However, the pulmonary artery pressure (and hence left ventricular pressure) can be maintained in the presence of a nonrestrictive ductus arteriosus. The exact time frame when a LV becomes "unprepared" to support the systemic circulation is unknown, but clinical experience would suggest that the LV remains adequately prepared for at least 2 to 4 weeks after closure of the ductus. Patients with large VSDs also have systemic pressure in the LV and surgery can be electively undertaken when the infants is a couple of weeks of age. In general, it is best to perform corrective surgery during the same hospital admission that the diagnosis is made (26, 27).

Technique

A median sternotomy is performed and an external inspection of the heart is done to confirm coronary artery anatomy (Fig. 19.1.6). The patient is placed on cardiopulmonary bypass; the operation is typically done using predominantly low-flow hypothermic cardiopulmonary bypass with a limited period of deep hypothermic circulatory arrest if necessary. The great vessels are transected and the internal orifices of the coronary arteries are inspected. The coronary arteries are translocated posteriorly to the neoaorta. The originally posterior branch pulmonary arteries are brought anterior to the aorta (Lecompte maneuver) and the aortic reconstruction is completed with a circumferential suture line above the new coronary anastomoses. At this point, the right atrium is typically opened and the atrial septal defect and/or ventricular septal defect(s) are repaired. The pulmonary artery reconstruction is then performed. The coronary donor sites are typically "filled in" with a patch of autologous pericardium. Finally, continuity between the right ventricle and pulmonary arteries is established with a circumferential suture line.

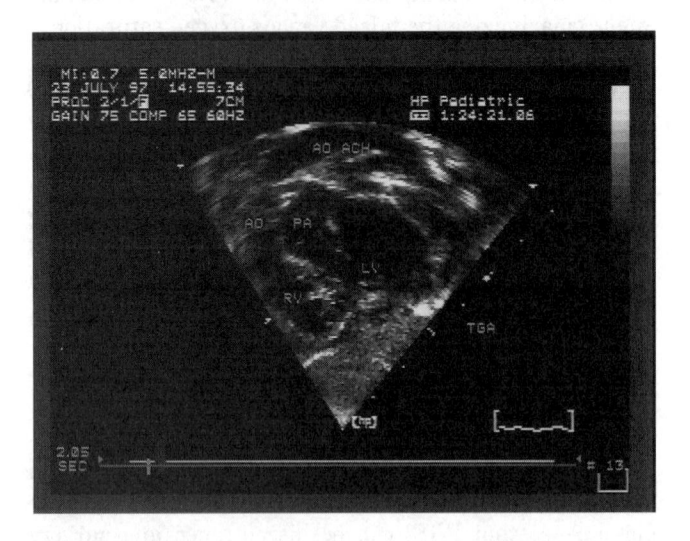

Figure 19.1.5. Subcostal view from a neonate with d-transposition of the great arteries (TGA). The aorta (*AO*) is seen to arise from the right ventricle (*RV*) and the pulmonary artery (*PA*), which is to the left of the aorta, to arise from the left ventricle (*LV*). This view also illustrates the aortic arch (*AO ACH*).

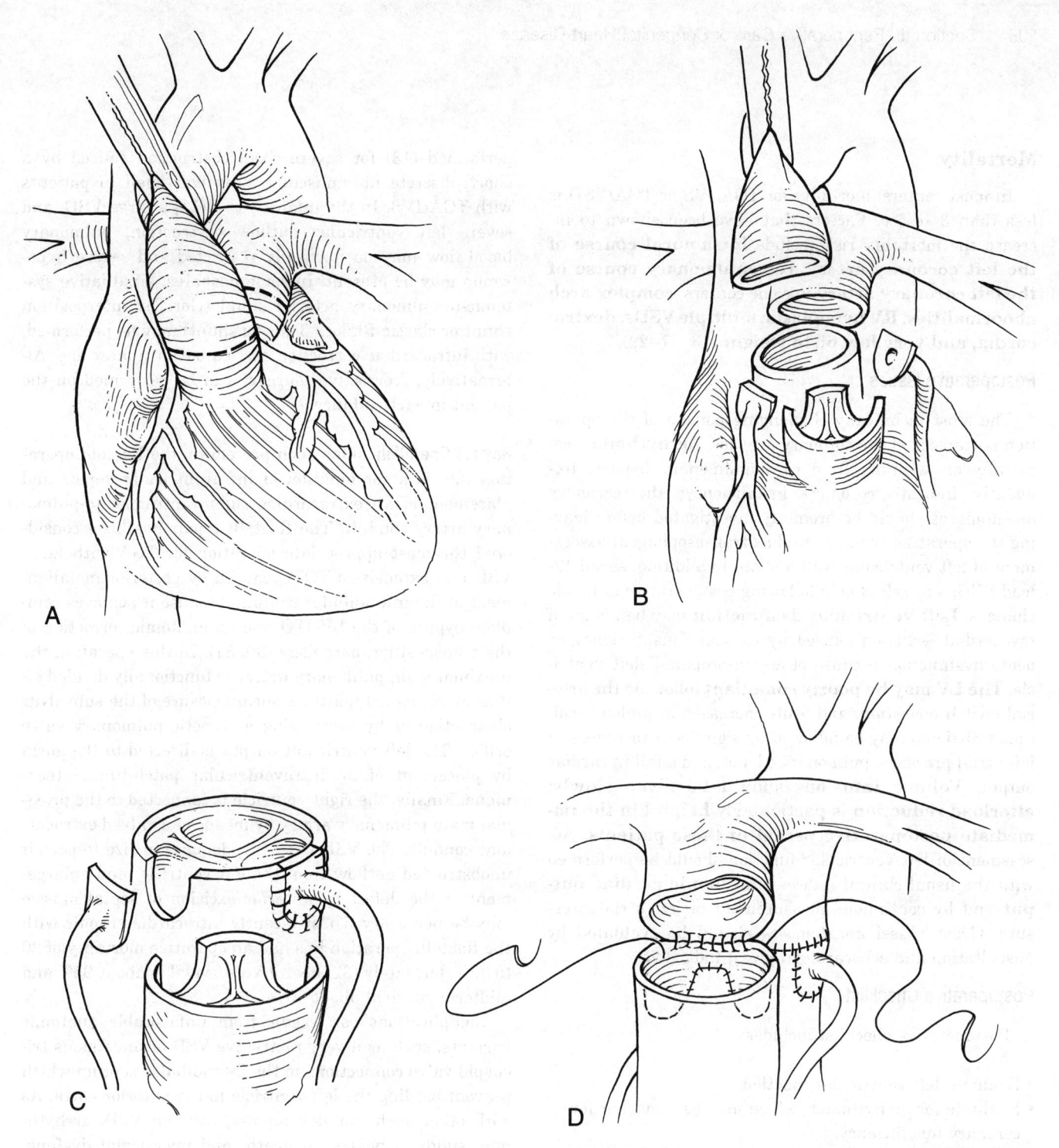

Figure 19.1.6. Arterial switch operation for d-transposition of the great arteries (TGA). **A.** The external anatomy is shown. The procedure is performed using cardiopulmonary bypass and either moderate or deep hypothermia with or without circulatory arrest. The *broken lines* show the sites of transection for the two great vessels. **B.** The aorta and main pulmonary arteries have been surgically transected and the coronary ostia have been removed from the native aortic root. **C.** The coronary buttons are in the process of being transferred to the neoaortic root. **D.** The coronary transfer has been completed and the neoarotic root has been anastomosed to the ascending aorta. The coronary explantation sites on the neopulmonary root have been repaired with a patch and the neopulmonary artery is in the process of antomosis to the distal main pulmonary artery. Note, the distal pulmonary artery has been moved anterior to the ascending aorta as described by Lecompte. In this illustration, the most typical coronary artery pattern is shown with the left/anterior facing sinus of Valsalva giving rise to the left main coronary artery, which branches into the anterior descending and the circumflex arteries. The right/posterior facing sinus gives rise to the right coronary artery. The procedure also involves closing the atrial septal defect and dividing the patent ductus arteriosus. The most critical part of the arterial switch operation is the transfer of the coronary arteries from their original position on the transposed aorta to their new position on the neoaortic root (the native pulmonary artery).

Mortality

In most centers, mortality for TGA/IVS or TGA/VSD is less than 3 to 5%. Factors that have been shown to increase the mortality risk include **intramural course of the left coronary artery, retropulmonary course of the left coronary artery** in some centers, **complex arch abnormalities, RV hypoplasia, multiple VSDs, dextrocardia, and very low birth weight** (13, 27–29).

Postoperative Issues

The most technically challenging portion of the operation is transfer of the coronary arteries. **Arrhythmias**, especially on weaning from cardiopulmonary bypass, frequently indicate coronary insufficiency; the coronary anastomoses should be promptly investigated before leaving the operating room, as well as transesophageal assessment of left ventricular wall motion. In addition, serial 12-lead ECGs are valuable in following postoperative ischemic changes. **Left ventricular dysfunction** may be a sign of myocardial ischemia caused by coronary insufficiency or acute dysfunction because of an "unprepared" left ventricle. **The LV may be poorly compliant** following the arterial switch operation, and acute increases in preload (volume infusions) may be followed by significant increases in left atrial pressure, pulmonary edema, and a fall in cardiac output. **Volume infusions should be given slowly; afterload reduction is particularly helpful in the immediate postoperative period in these patients.** Assessment of left ventricular function should be performed with the usual clinical indices of **systemic cardiac output** and by continuous measurement of left atrial pressure. Great vessel anastomoses should be evaluated by auscultation and echocardiography if indicated.

Postoperative Checklist

Postoperative checklist includes:

- Evaluate left ventricular function.
- Evaluate for arrhythmias, which may be a marker for coronary insufficiency.
- Evaluate for supravalvular aortic and pulmonary stenosis by echocardiography.
- Rule out residual ASD or VSD, if initially present.

Surgery for d-TGA/VSD/LVOTO—the Rastelli and "REV" Operations

Anatomic Considerations

Direct surgical relief of severe left ventricular outlet tract obstruction can be difficult, and it depends primarily on the anatomic type and severity of obstruction, which usually is directly related to the state of the interventricular septum and its alignment with the infundibular septum. Transpulmonary or transmitral resection has been performed (13) for severe fixed obstruction caused by a short, discrete fibromuscular subvalvar shelf in patients with TGA/IVS. In the infant with TGA, a large VSD, and severe left ventricular outflow obstruction, pulmonary blood flow may be markedly restricted and severe hypoxemia may be present. In some neonates, a palliative systemic-to-pulmonary arterial shunt (Gor-Tex interposition shunt or classic Blalock-Taussig shunt) may be performed, with intracardiac correction carried out at a later age. Alternatively, "corrective" surgery can be performed on the patient in early infancy.

Rastelli Operation One such procedure, the Rastelli operation (30) is a combination of intraventricular repair and placement of an extracardiac right ventricular-to-pulmonary artery conduit. The Rastelli repair has been considered the most appropriate operation for TGA with large VSD and extensive LVOTO caused by posterior malalignment of the infundibular septum, because it achieves complete bypass of the LVOTO and an anatomic correction of the transposition pathology (30, 31). In this operation the proximal main pulmonary artery is functionally divided either by pledgeted mattress suture closure of the subvalvar obstruction or by oversewing a stenotic pulmonary valve orifice. The left ventricular output is directed to the aorta by placement of an intraventricular patch-tunnel technique. Finally, the right ventricle is connected to the proximal main pulmonary artery by means of a valved extracardiac conduit. The VSD must be adequate in size to permit unobstructed outflow from the left ventricle, and enlargement of the defect by anterior excision of septal muscle may be necessary. Until recently intracardiac repair with the Rastelli operation has had an operative mortality of 20 to 30%, but lately (32) operative survival is about 95% and midterm survival about 90%.

Complications can result from unfavorable anatomic variants, such as a very restrictive VSD or anomalous tricuspid valve connections to the infundibular septum which prevent baffling the left ventricle to the anterior aorta. As with other such complex repairs, residual VSD, arrhythmia, sudden unexpected death, and myocardial dysfunction may complicate the postoperative course. As with all extracardiac conduiting operative techniques, there is concern about the functional longevity of the valved conduit. Improved results have been achieved with fresh or cryopreserved homograft valved conduits compared with the previously used Dacron conduits containing heterograft valves.

"REV" An interesting alternative "corrective" technique, termed "REV" (Reparation l'Etage Venticularie) by Lecompte (33–35), has been used recently for patients with TGA and LVOTO. The REV procedure appears to have some advantages over the Rastelli operation (i.e., application in younger patients and avoidance of a prosthetic extracardiac conduit; and avoidance of intracardiac tunnel obstruction). This operation requires a high, anterior right ventricular incision and a radical excision of the outlet septum to create an unobstructed anterior right ventricular cavity; establishing a short and direct intraventricular tunnel from the LV to the aorta; closure of the pulmonary artery orifice; and reimplantation of the transected (and usually anteriorly translocated) pulmonary artery directly onto the right ventricular outflow cavity without a prosthetic conduit. Recent operative survival in one series has been reported at 90%, without observation of progressive subaortic obstruction during follow-up (36). A comparative study of the "traditional" Rastelli operation with the newer REV approach in one series suggested that the REV allows complete repair earlier in infancy, is feasible in patients with anatomic contraindications to the Rastelli operation, and it may reduce both the need for reoperation and the prevalence of residual pulmonary outflow tract obstruction (32). However, the lifelong implications of pulmonary regurgitation following this newer operative approach require continued investigation. Furthermore, tension on the pulmonary artery reconstruction can lead to early right ventricular outflow tract obstruction.

Postoperative Checklist

Postoperative checklist includes:

- Evaluate left ventricular function.
- Rule out conduit obstruction or branch pulmonary artery distortion.
- Monitor for arrhythmias, particularly complete heart block or junctional ectopic tachycardia.
- Evaluate for subaortic stenosis (restrictive VSD) by echocardiography.
- Rule out residual VSD or ASD.

L-Transposition of the Great Arteries

Anatomy

L-Transposition of the great arteries (L-TGA) includes (a) ventricular inversion or "L-looped" ventricles (anatomic right ventricle on the left and anatomic left ventricle on the right), and (b) the great vessels are transposed (aorta arising from anatomic left-sided right ventricle and pulmonary artery arising from anatomic right-sided left ventricle) (Fig. 19.1.7). In L-TGA **("corrected TGA")**, about half of the patients have functionally one single pumping chamber and this condition is discussed elsewhere (see Chapter 18, *Single Ventricle Lesions*). **In the other half, this combination of ventricular inversion (atrioventricular discordance) and transposition of the great arteries (ventriculoarterial discordance) without associated cardiac anomalies results in normal arterial oxygen content, hence the term "corrected."** The "correction" of the circulation results because systemic venous blood passes from the right atrium through the mitral valve into the left ventricle and then to the main pulmonary artery; pulmonary venous blood passes from the left atrium through the tricuspid valve to the right ventricle and then to the aorta. Unfortunately, the "corrected" condition

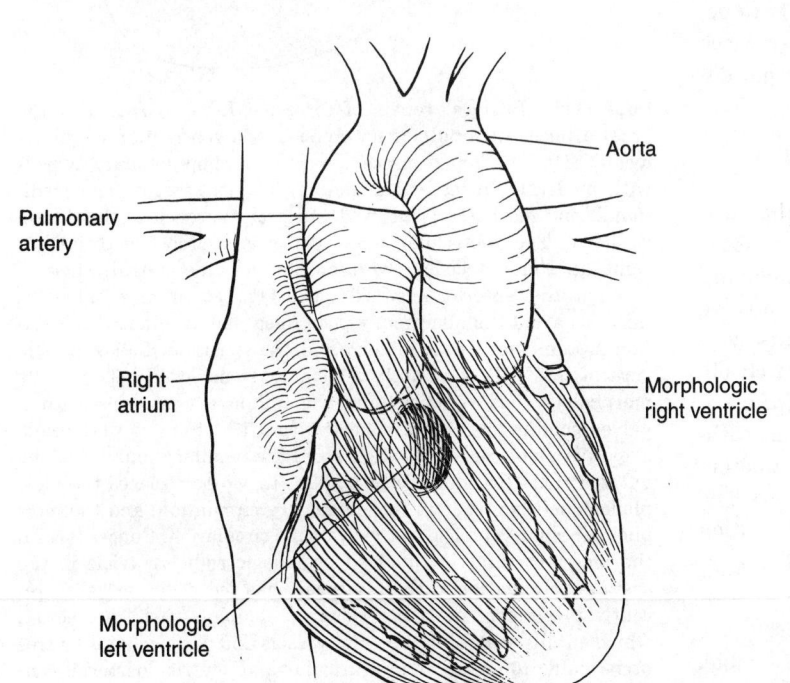

Figure 19.1.7. External anatomy of "corrected" L-transposition of the great arteries. In this lesion is seen atrioventricular discordance and ventriculoarterial discordance. The lesion is caused by embryologic L-looping of the ventricles. As a result, the morphologic left ventricular chamber is connected to the right atrium and pulmonary artery, positioned posteriorly and to the right. The morphologic right ventricle is connected to the left atrium and aorta, positioned anteriorly and to the left. Corrected transposition is rarely an isolated lesion. Commonly associated defects include ventricular septal defect and valvar or subvalvar pulmonary stenosis, either in isolation or together. The atrioventricular discordance results in abnormalities of the conduction system, and a high incidence of heart block.

rarely exists in isolation, and the overwhelming majority of hearts have associated structural and functional abnormalities. The four most commonly seen anomalies are:

- Ventricular septal defect (~80%)
- Subpulmonary and valvar pulmonary stenosis or atresia (~80%)
- Anatomic abnormalities of the systemic tricuspid valve (frequently "Ebsteinoid")
- Abnormal course of the conduction system, with a high incidence of spontaneous (1 to 2% per patient per year) or surgically induced (up to 50%) complete heart block

Pathophysiology

The specific preoperative physiology is determined by the associated anatomic abnormalities. The most frequent association, ventricular septal defect and pulmonary stenosis (due to a posteriorly malaligned infundibular septum) is physiologically similar to **tetralogy of Fallot**. The VSD is typically large and thus, the **degree of pulmonary obstruction determines whether the patient will have signs of congestive heart failure (minimal PS), cyanosis (significant PS), or be asymptomatic and "balanced."** In addition, congestive heart failure may be caused by regurgitation of the systemic atrioventricular valve, complete heart block, or any combination of the above.

Preoperative Evaluation

Electrocardiography (ECG)

Prior to medical, catheter, or surgical intervention, all patients should undergo a 12-lead ECG, specifically to determine the PR interval. Spontaneous complete heart block can occur, with a frequency of about 1 to 2% per patient per year (37).

Echocardiography/Catheterization

Echocardiography will definitively define the discordance between the atria, ventricles, and great vessels. The location, number, and size of the VSD(s), pulmonary stenosis, and anatomic abnormalities of the tricuspid valve can easily be visualized. It is unusual for patients with L-TGA and two normal-sized ventricles to have arch obstruction, unless there is significant deformity of the tricuspid (systemic atrioventricular) valve (38). Cardiac catheterization may be important for physiologic parameters (e.g., shunt size, pulmonary hypertension, and so on). The risk of inducing heart block during cardiac catheterization (transient or permanent) is in the range of 5 to 10%.

Surgery

Surgical management of L-TGA is extremely variable, and it depends on the type, number, and severity of associated lesions. Traditional classic "repair" typically consisted of VSD closure and relief of pulmonary outflow obstruction; important long-term sequelae have included complete heart block, progressive tricuspid (systemic atrioventricular valve) regurgitation, and right (systemic) ventricular dysfunction (39–43). These findings have prompted some centers to manage many of these patients in a similar fashion to those with a single ventricle, with an ultimate Fontan operation (see Chapter 18, *Single Ventricle Lesions*). Recently, numerous surgical series have reported favorable early results with anatomic correction—the "double

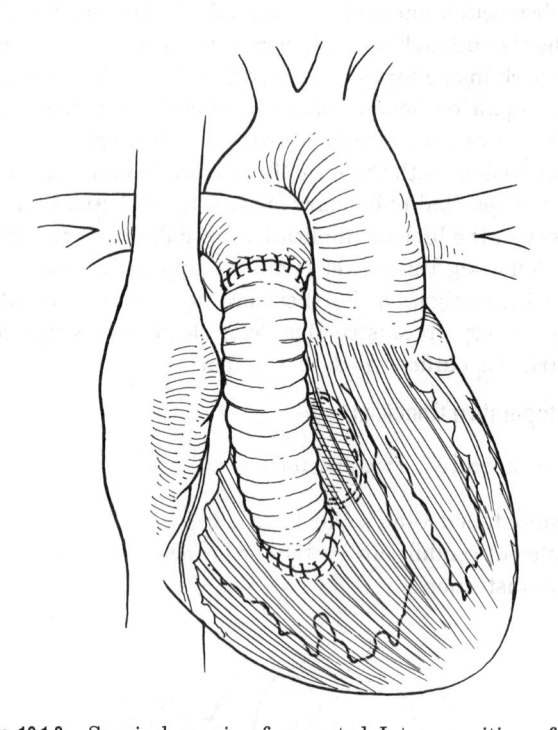

Figure 19.1.8. Surgical repair of corrected L-transposition of the great arteries with pulmonary stenosis and ventricular septal defect (VSD). The repair procedure uses cardiopulmonary bypass with moderate hypothermia and cardioplegic arrest. The traditional, and most widely utilized, surgical approach to this lesion is shown. The ventricular septal defect is approached through a right atriotomy incision, working through the mitral valve or through the anterior/leftward aorta. Particular care must be taken to avoid the abnormally positioned and attenuated conduction system that exists in corrected transposition. Following closure of the VSD, continuity is commonly achieved between the morphologic left ventricle and the pulmonary arteries with a valved conduit, as shown. The left ventriculotomy is performed, avoiding major coronary arteries and the papillary muscles of the left ventricle. It should be noted that this repair places the morphologic left ventricle in the pulmonary circulation, and the morphologic right ventricle in the systemic circulation. Concerns with the long-term function of the morphologic right ventricle in the systemic circulation with this repair has led some surgeons recently to perform the more complex "double switch" procedure, which entails switching the great vessels and performing an intraatrial baffle to create atrioventricular and ventriculoarterial concordance.

switch" operation or a combination of the Rastelli and Senning operations (44–48).

Technique—"Classic" Repair

The technique for VSD closure must be modified to reduce the risk of complete heart block (Fig. 19.1.8). If the defect is approached through the right atrium and mitral valve, sutures must be placed on the left side (morphologic right ventricular side) of the defect to reduce the risk of complete heart block. Because this is technically difficult, it is often useful to approach the VSD through the anterior and leftward aortic valve, so that the patch naturally comes to lie on the left side of the ventricular septum. Relief of subpulmonary stenosis and left atrioventricular (AV) valve abnormalities must be customized to the individual patient, but left ventricular-pulmonary artery conduits are frequently necessary. **All patients should have temporary pacing wires placed on the atrium and ventricle at the time of surgery.** Permanent wires should be placed if there is any sign of preoperative or intraoperative second or third degree block.

Technique—"Anatomic" Repair

In patients without significant obstruction to pulmonary blood flow, an atrial redirection operation (Senning or Mustard) is performed to baffle systemic venous return to the tricuspid valve and pulmonary venous return to the mitral valve. The VSD is closed, directing left ventricular outflow to the pulmonary valve, and an arterial switch operation is performed. In patients with significant valvar or subpulmonary obstruction, the VSD is closed directing LV outflow to the anterior and rightward aorta, and a right ventricle-pulmonary artery conduit is placed (Figs. 19.1.9, 19.1.10).

Timing

In asymptomatic patients, even those with significant structural abnormalities, operation is often delayed because of the risk of inducing complete heart block, the need for conduit placement in many circumstances, and the need for surgical plasty or replacement of the tricuspid valve in some patients. Decisions about the timing of surgery are further influenced by the lack of progression of associated defects (such as pulmonary stenosis) in most of these patients (49). In the "classic" repair, severe pulmonary stenosis is typically not amenable to direct surgical relief, and it often requires an LV-pulmonary artery conduit. Thus, surgery may be

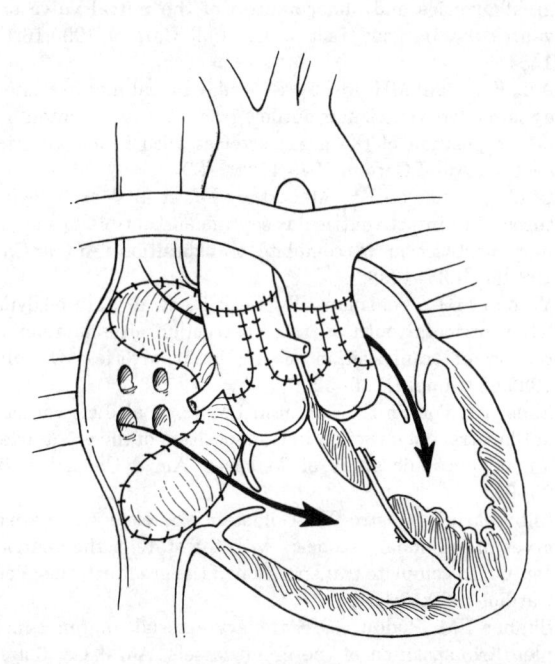

Figure 19.1.9. The "double switch" operation. For patients with congenitally corrected transposition of the great vessels without left ventricular outflow tract obstruction, the arterial switch can be combined with the Senning procedure to achieve atrioventricular and ventricular arterial concordance. The advantage of this repair is that the left ventricle is placed in the systemic circulation. Note that a patch closure of a large ventricular septal defect has also been performed.

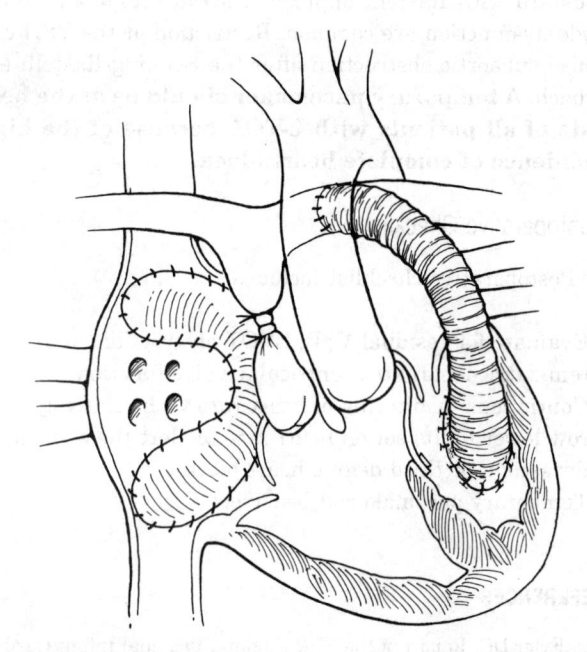

Figure 19.1.10. The combined Rastelli and Senning procedure. This procedure is performed for patients with congenitally corrected transposition of the great vessels in association with a ventricular septal defect (VSD) and left ventricular outflow tract obstruction, the most common form of congenitally corrected L-transposition of the great vessels. Note the atrial level baffle that creates atrioventricular concordance and the patch closure of the VSD, which allows the left ventricle to eject through the VSD to the aorta. The pulmonary artery has been ligated and a conduit has been placed from the right ventricle to the pulmonary artery.

furthered delayed to allow the largest possible conduit to be placed. Also, left-sided tricuspid valve incompetence requires replacement in as many as 15 to 20% of patients; surgery may be delayed so that a "big enough" prosthesis be placed.

Mortality

As L-TGA is a relatively rare form of congenital heart disease, large series of patients with analysis of risk factors for mortality are not available.

Postoperative Issues

Postoperative care in L-TGA is specifically geared toward the type of operation that was applied to "correct" the circulation. In patients who have a ventricular septal defect closed, the usual assessment for residual VSD should be undertaken. Also, as most patients also have some degree of left (pulmonary) ventricular outflow tract obstruction, assessment should be made to assure adequate relief of the obstruction. If the systemic tricuspid valve was surgically repaired or replaced, assessment of valve function via a left atrial line is crucial. Patients who undergo an "anatomic" repair (double switch or Senning/Mustard with Rastelli approach), atrial ectopy and sinus node dysfunction are common. Restriction at the VSD can cause subaortic obstruction after the Senning/Rastelli approach. **A temporary pacemaker should be at the bedside of all patients with L-TGA because of the high incidence of complete heart block.**

Postoperative Checklist

Postoperative checklist includes:

- Evaluate for residual VSD, LVOT obstruction, and systemic (tricuspid) atrioventricular valve function.
- Continuous monitoring of heart rate with relatively narrow lower limits set on heart rate to alert the clinician for second or third degree heart block.
- Temporary pacemaker at bedside.

REFERENCES

1. Fyler DC. Report of the New England Regional Infant Cardiac Program. Pediatrics 1980;65(Suppl):377.
2. Liebman J, Cullum L, Belloc NB. Natural history of transposition of the great arteries—anatomy and birth and death characteristics. Circulation 1969;40:237–262.
3. Pexeider T, Rousseil MP, Prados-Frutos JC. Prenatal pathogenesis of the transposition of the great arteries. In: Vogel M, Buhlmeyer K (eds). Transposition of the great arteries 25 years after Rashkind balloon septostomy. New York: Springer-Verlag, 1992;11–27.
4. Fuhrmann W. A family study in transposition of the great vessels and in tricuspid atresia. Humangenetiuk 1968; 6:148–157.
5. Kirklin JW, Barratt-Boyes BG. Complete transposition of the great arteries. In: Kirklin JW, Barratt-Boyes BG (eds). Cardiac surgery. New York:Churchill Livingstone, 1993;1383–1467.
6. Milanesi O, Ho SY, Thiene G, et al. The ventricular septal defect in complete transposition of the great arteries: pathologic anatomy in 57 cases with emphasis on subaortic, subpulmonary, and aortic arch obstruction. Hum Pathol 1987; 18:392–396.
7. Moene RJ, Oppenheimer-Dekker A, Bartelings MM, et al. Ventricular septal defect with normally connected and with transposed great arteries. Am J Cardiol 1986;58:627–632.
8. Moene RJ, Oppenheimer-Dekker A. Congenital mitral valve anomalies in the transposition of the great arteries. Am J Cardiol 1982;49:1972–1978.
9. Lev M, Bharati S, Meng L, et al. A concept of double-outlet right ventricle. Thorac Cardiovasc Surg 1972;64:271–281.
10. Moene RJ, Oppenheimer-Dekker A, Bartelings MM. Anatomic obstruction of the right ventricular outflow tract in transposition of the great arteries. Am J Cardiol 1983;51:1701–1704.
11. Moene RJ, Ottenkamp J, Oppenheimer-Dekker A, et al. Transposition of the great arteries and narrowing of the aortic arch. Br Heart J 1985;53:58–63.
12. Kurosawa H, Van Mierop LHS. Surgical anatomy of the infundibular septum in transposition of the great arteries with ventricular septal defect. J Thorac Cardiovasc Surg 1986;91: 123–132.
13. Wernovsky G, Jonas RA, Colan SD, et al. Results of the arterial switch operation in patients with transposition of the great arteries and abnormalities of the mitral valve or left ventricular outflow tract. J Am Coll Cardiol 1990;16:1446–1454.
14. Aziz KU, Paul MH, Idriss FS, et al. Clinical manifestations of dynamic left ventricular outflow tract stenosis in infants with d-transposition of the great arteries with intact ventricular septum. Am J Cardiol 1979;44:290–297.
15. Chui I, Anderson RH, Macartney FJ, et al. Morphologic features of an intact ventricular septum susceptible to subpulmonary obstruction in complete transposition. Am J Cardiol 1984;53:1633–1638.
16. Yacoub MH, Arensman FW, Keck E, et al. Fate of dynamic left ventricular outflow tract obstruction after anatomic correction of transposition of the great arteries. Circulation 1983;68 (Suppl II):56–62.
17. Sansa M, Tonkin IL, Bargeron LM Jr, et al. Left ventricular outflow tract obstruction in transposition of the great arteries: an angiographic study of 74 cases. Am J Cardiol 1979;44: 88–95.
18. Silberbach M, Castro WL, Goldstein MA, et al. Comparison of types of pulmonary stenosis with the state of the ventricular septum in complete transposition of the great arteries. Pediatr Cardiol 1989;10:11–15.
19. Shaher RM, Puddu GC. Coronary arterial anatomy in complete transposition of the great vessels. Am J Cardiol 1966; 17:355–361.
20. Gittenberger-de Groot AC, Sauer U, Oppenheimer-Dekker A, et al. Coronary arterial anatomy in transposition of the great arteries: a morphologic study. Pediatr Cardiol 1983;4(Suppl I): 15–24.
21. Smith A, Arnold R, Wilkinson JL, et al. An anatomical study of the patterns of the coronary arteries and sinus nodal artery in complete transposition. Int J Cardiol 1986;12:295–304.

22. Mair DD, Ritter DG, Ongley PA, et al. Hemodynamics and evaluation for surgery of patients with complete transposition of the great arteries and ventricular septal defect. Am J Cardiol 1971;28:632–640.
23. Mair DD, Ritter DG. Factors influencing intercirculatory mixing in patients with complete transposition of the great arteries. Am J Cardiol 1972;30:653–658.
24. Mair DD, Ritter DG. Factors influencing systemic arterial oxygen saturation in complete transposition of the great arteries. Am J Cardiol 1973;31:742–748.
25. Rudolph AM. Congenital diseases of the heart. Chicago: Year Book, 1974.
26. Paul MH, Wernovsky G. Transposition of the great arteries. In: Emmanouilides GC, Riemenschneider TA, Allen HD, et al. (eds). Moss and Adams' heart disease in infants, children, and adolescents, including the fetus and young adult. Baltimore: Williams & Wilkins, 1995;1154–1225.
27. Wernovsky G, Mayer JE Jr, Jonas RA, et al. Factors influencing early and late outcome of the arterial switch operation for transposition of the great arteries. J Thorac Cardiovasc Surg 1995;109:289–302.
28. Wernovsky G, Freed MD. Transposition of the great arteries: the arterial switch operation-results and outcome. In: Freedom RA (ed). Congenital heart disease. Philadelphia: Current Science, 1997.
29. Mayer JE Jr, Sanders SP, Jonas RA, et al. Coronary artery pattern and outcome of arterial switch operation for transposition of the great arteries. Circulation 1990;82 (Suppl IV):139–145.
30. Rastelli GC, McGoon DC, Wallace RB. Anatomic correction of transposition of the great arteries with ventricular septal defect and subpulmonary stenosis. J Thorac Cardiovasc Surg 1969;58:545–552.
31. Moulton AL, DeLeval MR, Macartney FJ, et al. Rastelli procedure for transposition of the great arteries, ventricular septal defect, and left ventricular outflow tract obstruction. Br Heart J 1981;45:20–28.
32. Vouhe PR, Tamisier D, Leca F, et al. Transposition of the great arteries, ventricular septal defect, and pulmonary outflow tract obstruction. J Thorac Cardiovasc Surg 1992;103:428–436.
33. Borromee L, Lecompte Y, Batisse A, et al. Anatomic repair of anomalies of ventriculoarterial connection associated with ventricular septal defect. II. Clinical results in 50 patients with pulmonary outflow tract obstruction. J Thorac Cardiovasc Surg 1988;95:96–102.
34. Lecompte Y, Neveux JY, Leca F, et al. Reconstruction of the pulmonary outflow tract without prosthetic conduit. J Thorac Cardiovasc Surg 1982;84:727–733.
35. Lecompte Y. The REV (réparation á l'etage ventriculaire) procedure: technique and clinical results. Cardiology in the Young 1991;1:63–70.
36. Lecompte Y, Bourlon K, Hisatomi K, et al. Anatomic repair for complex transposition. In: Vogel M, Buhlmeyer K (eds). Transposition of the great arteries: 25 years of Rashkind balloon atrial septostomy. New York: Springer-Verlag, 1992; 129–135.
37. Huhta JC, Maloney JD, Ritter DG, et al. Complete atrioventricular block in patients with atrioventricular discordance. Circulation 1983;67:1374–1377.
38. Celermajer DS, Cullen S, Deanfield JE, et al. Congenitally corrected transposition and Ebstein's anomaly of the systemic atrioventricular valve: association with aortic arch obstruction. J Am Coll Cardiol 1991;18:1056–1058.
39. Dimas AP, Moodie DS, Sterba R, et al. Long-term function of the morphologic right ventricle in adult patients with corrected transposition of the great arteries. Am Heart J 1989;118:526–530.
40. Connelly M, Liu P, Williams W, et al. Congenitally corrected transposition of the great arteries in the adult: functional status and complications. J Am Coll Cardiol 1996;27:1238–1243.
41. Termignon J, Leca F, Vouhe P, et al. "Classic" repair of congenitally corrected transposition and ventricular septal defect. Ann Thorac Surg 1996;62:199–206.
42. van Son J, Danielson G, Huhta J, et al. Late results of systemic atrioventricular valve replacement in corrected transposition. J Thorac Cardiovasc Surg 1995;109:642–653.
43. McGrath LB, Kirklin JW, Blackstone EH, et al. Death and other events after cardiac repair in discordant atrioventricular connection. J Thorac Cardiovasc Surg 1985;90:711–728.
44. Ilbawi MN, DeLeon SY, Backer CL, et al. An alternative approach to the surgical management of physiologically corrected transposition with ventricular septal defect and pulmonary stenosis or atresia. J Thorac Cardiovasc Surg 1990; 100:410–415.
45. Yamagishi M, Imai Y, Hoshino S, et al. Anatomic correction of atrioventricular discordance. J Thorac Cardiovasc Surg 1934;105:1067–1076.
46. Di Donato RM, Troconis CJ, Marino B, et al. Combined Mustard and Rastelli operations. J Thorac Cardiovasc Surg 1992;104:1246–1248.
47. Imai Y, Sawatari K, Hoshino S, et al. Ventricular function after anatomic repair in patients with atrioventricular discordance. J Thorac Cardiovasc Surg 1994;107:1272–1283.
48. Karl TR, Weintraub RG, Brizard CP, et al. Senning plus arterial switch operation for discordant (congenitally corrected) transposition. Ann Thorac Surg 1997;64:495–502.
49. Lundstrom U, Bull C, Wyse R, et al. The natural and "unnatural" history of congenitally corrected transposition. Am J Cardiol 1990;65:1222–1229.

19.2 Double Outlet Right Ventricle

Gil Wernovsky, MD, and Frank L. Hanley, MD

ANATOMY

"Double outlet right ventricle" (DORV) describes a ventricular-arterial alignment rather than a specific type of congenital heart disease (Fig. 19.2.1) (1, 2). DORV is thus a heterogeneous group of lesions with variable physiology and surgical options. The great vessels each are supported by an infundibulum (conus), and failure of the proper alignment of the conotruncus with the ventricular septum results in a spectrum anatomic subtypes.

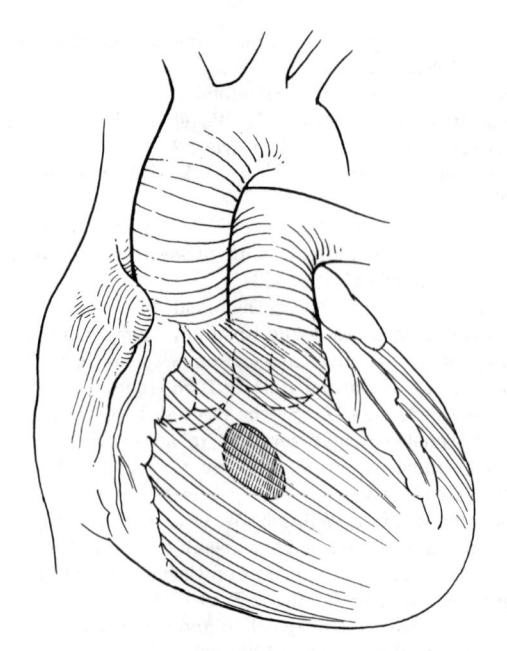

Figure 19.2.1. Anatomy of double outlet right ventricle. The external cardiac anatomy of the double outlet right ventricle with subaortic ventricular septal defect (VSD) is shown. Note that both great vessels arise from the right ventricular cavity. The great vessels are side-by-side and parallel. This is a result of the presence of subaortic conus, which causes the aorta to lie more anterior and to be aligned with the right ventricle. As a result, the two valves are at the same level and there is aortic valve/mitral valve discontinuity. Double outlet right ventricle is always associated with a VSD. It should be emphasized that double outlet right ventricle encompasses a wide morphologic spectrum. At one end of the spectrum, the double outlet right ventricle with subaortic VSD shares many features in common with tetralogy of Fallot. At the other end of the spectrum, double outlet right ventricle with subpulmonary VSD shares many features in common with transposition of the great vessels. Although the categorization of types of double outlet right ventricle is based on the relationship of the VSD to the two semilunar valves, it is important to recognize that the most important morphologic factor that determines the different types of double outlet right ventricle is not variation in the position of the VSD itself, but rather the varying orientation of the great vessels based on the degree of rotation of the conontruncus.

Four basic DORV types exist, which are based on the relationship of the conotruncal ventricular septal defect (VSD) with the great vessels:

1. Subaortic VSD (Fig. 19.2.1), with or without pulmonary stenosis
2. Subpulmonary VSD, with or without subaortic stenosis and/or arch obstruction
3. "Doubly committed" VSD
4. Remote VSD

Additional anomalies occur frequently, including right or left ventricular hypoplasia, straddling atrioventricular valves, mitral stenosis or atresia, multiple VSDs, and heterotaxy.

PHYSIOLOGY AND SURGICAL OPTIONS

The subaortic VSD type of DORV is physiologically similar to tetralogy of Fallot (Figs. 19.2.1 and 19.2.2). The VSD directs left ventricular outflow to the aorta; the degree of subpulmonary stenosis (sub-PS) determines whether the patient has symptoms of congestive heart failure (little to no sub-PS), cyanosis (moderate to severe sub-PS), or is "balanced" (see also Chapter 17.1, *Tetralogy of Fallot*). Surgical repair involves closure of the VSD to "baffle" the left ventricular outflow to the aorta, with relief of the pulmonary outflow tract obstruction as determined by the anatomy (Fig. 19.2.2).

In addition to the postoperative sequelae of tetralogy repair (see Chapter 17.1), the postoperative evaluation must exclude subaortic obstruction caused by a physically small VSD or the VSD baffle itself (3). The surgical mortality risk for this repair is similar to that of tetralogy of Fallot (4, 5).

The subpulmonary VSD type of DORV (sometimes referred to as "Taussig-Bing anomaly") (6) is physiologically similar to D-transposition of the great arteries. The VSD directs left ventricular outflow back to the pulmonary artery, whereas the systemic venous return recirculates to the aorta. Because of the large VSD and abundant intercirculatory mixing (see Chapter 19.1, *Transposition of the Great Arteries*), cyanosis may be absent and symptoms of congestive heart failure predominate. Subaortic stenosis and arch obstruction typically complicate this anatomic subtype (7). Surgical repair involves closure of the VSD to baffle the left ventricular outflow to the pulmonary root, with an arterial switch operation with or without arch augmentation (8). The posterior translocation of the native aorta to the neopulmonary root can cause proximal arch obstruction as well (9). In addition to the postoperative sequelae of the arterial switch operation with VSD closure (see Chapter 19.1), subaortic obstruction, subpulmonic obstruction, and arch obstruction must be ruled out. The surgical mortality risk for this lesion approaches 10% (5, 10).

For both the doubly committed VSD and remote VSD types of DORV, complex repairs must be considered. It is frequently impossible to baffle the left ventricular outflow to either great vessel without significant intracardiac obstruction; in these patients staged management to an eventual Fontan operation should be considered (4).

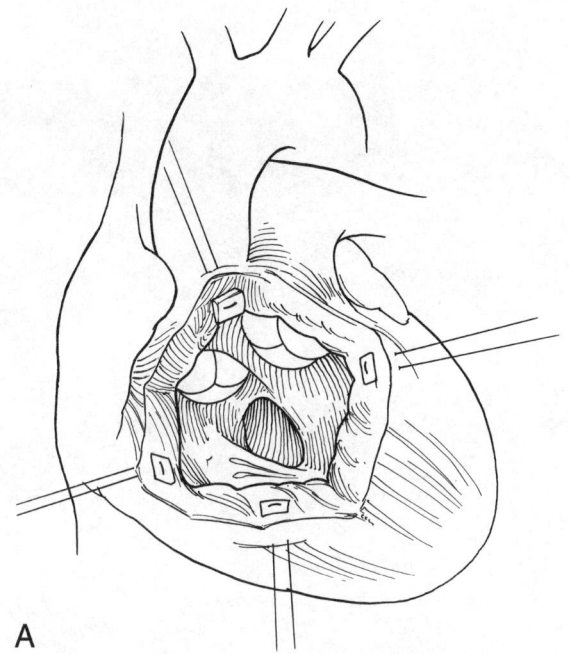

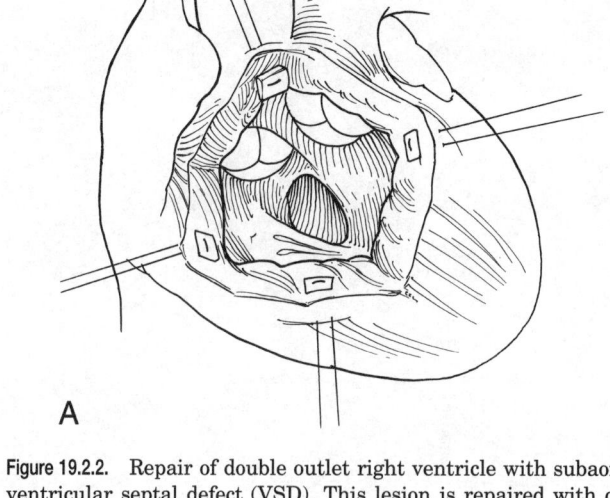

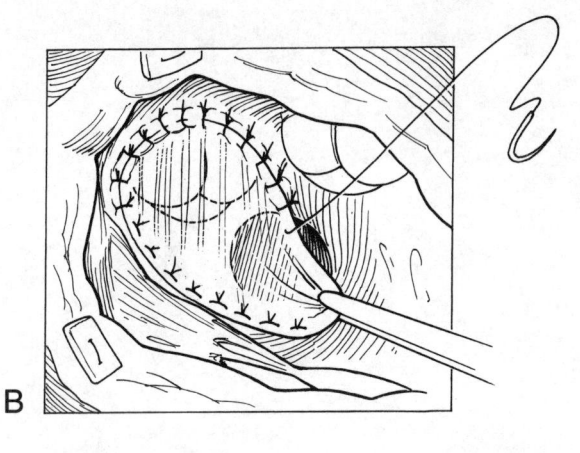

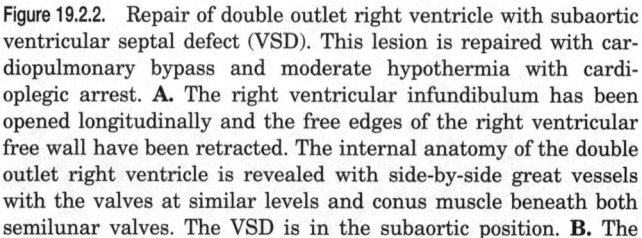

Figure 19.2.2. Repair of double outlet right ventricle with subaortic ventricular septal defect (VSD). This lesion is repaired with cardiopulmonary bypass and moderate hypothermia with cardioplegic arrest. **A.** The right ventricular infundibulum has been opened longitudinally and the free edges of the right ventricular free wall have been retracted. The internal anatomy of the double outlet right ventricle is revealed with side-by-side great vessels with the valves at similar levels and conus muscle beneath both semilunar valves. The VSD is in the subaortic position. **B.** The repair proceeds by placing a baffle around the anterolateral and inferior rims of the ventricular septal defect thereby closing the VSD and creating left ventricular-to-aortic continuity. Depending on the status of the development of the subpulmonary conus, the infundibular incision can be patched or closed primarily. It should be emphasized that other forms of double outlet right ventricle are repaired with a completely different operation; for example, double outlet right ventricle with subpulmonic VSD is typically repaired with an arterial switch procedures and VSD closure.

REFERENCES

1. Bostrom MPG, Hutchins GM. Arrested rotation of the outflow tract may explain double-outlet right ventricle. Circulation 1988;77:1258–1265.
2. Van Praagh R, Layton WM, Van Praagh S. The morphogenesis of normal and abnormal relationships between the great arteries and the ventricles: pathologic and experimental data. In: Van Praagh R, Takao A (eds). Etiology and morphogenesis of congenital heart disease. Mount Kisco: Futura, 1980; 271–316.
3. Serraf A, Lacour-Gayet F, Houyel L, et al. Subaortic obstruction in double outlet right ventricles: surgical considerations for anatomic repair. Circulation 1993;88(II):177–182.
4. Kleinert S, Sano T, Weintraub RG, et al. Anatomic features and surgical strategies in double-outlet right ventricle. Circulation 1997;96:1233–1239.
5. Aoki M, Forbess JM, Jonas RA, et al. Result of biventricular repair for double-outlet right ventricle. J Thorac Cardiovasc Surg 1994;107:338–350.
6. Van Praagh R. What is the Taussig-Bing malformation? Circulation 1968;37:445–449.
7. Parr GVS, Waldhausen JA, Bharati S, et al. Coarctation in Taussing-Bing malformation of the heart. J Thorac Cardiovasc Surg 1983;86:280–287.
8. Mavroudis C, Backer C, Muster A, et al. Taussig-bing anomaly: arterial switch versus Kawashima intraventricular repair. Ann Thorac Surg 1996;61:1330–1338.
9. Muster AJ, Berry TE, Ilbawi MN, et al. Development of neocoarctation in patients with transposed great arteries and hypoplastic aortic arch after Lecompte modification of anatomical correction. J Thorac Cardiovasc Surg 1987;93:276–280.
10. Serraf A, Lacour-Gayet F, Bruniaux J, et al. Anatomic repair of Taussig-Bing hearts. Circulation 1991;84(Suppl III):200–205.

Miscellaneous Lesions

20.1 Mitral Valve Disease

Anthony C. Chang, MD, and Jeffrey Jacobs, MD

Although isolated mitral valve stenosis or mitral valve insufficiency is relatively uncommon, its treatment remains challenging (1, 2). Most congenital abnormalities of the mitral valve apparatus are associated with other congenital cardiac lesions, but mitral valve disease in children can also be secondary to an inflammatory state (e.g., rheumatic heart disease or infectious endocarditis) or associated with syndromes (e.g., Marfan) and collagen vascular disease.

ANATOMY

The normal mitral valve apparatus (3) is composed of five parts (Fig. 20.1.1; see color plate 20.1.1B): (*a*) valvular leaflets, (*b*) annulus, (*c*) chordae tendinae, (*d*) papillary muscles, and (*e*) the left ventricular wall.

The mitral valve has two leaflets: an anterior or aortic leaflet that makes up one third of the circumference of the mitral valve orifice and a posterior or mural leaflet that makes up the other two thirds. The leaflets are separated by two commissurae: anterolateral and posteromedial commissurae. The mitral annulus is a D-shaped structure that comprises part of the fibrous skeleton of the heart. The leaflet tissue is attached to the papillary muscles by thin chordae tendinae. Chordae from both papillary muscles attach to both leaflets. Two papillary muscles exist in the normal heart: the anterolateral and the posteromedial papillary muscles. The papillary and chordal anchoring of the ventricular wall and annulus is thought to contribute to left ventricular systolic functions; therefore, surgeons usually attempt to preserve this subvalvular apparatus during mitral valve replacement.

Types of Mitral Valve Stenosis

Mitral stenosis can be caused by pathology in the supravalvar, valvar, or subvalvar regions of the mitral valve apparatus. A combination of stenotic lesions at two or all three of these levels can be present (4, 5).

Supravalvar Mitral Stenosis

In **cor triatriatum**, which is a lesion resulting from failure of the common pulmonary vein to be incorporated into the left atrium, a membrane with a small opening divides the left atrium into two: one with the left atrial appendage and the foramen ovale below the membrane and the other which receives the pulmonary veins (6). The pulmonary venous chamber may then communicate with the right atrium through a patent foramen ovale. This lesion is also associated with anomalous pulmonary venous drainage.

In **supravalvar mitral ring**, a ring of fibrous connective tissue above the mitral valve can also cause left atrial outlet obstruction. It is associated with **Shone complex**, which is an anatomic constellation with parachute mitral valve, subaortic stenosis, aortic stenosis, and coarctation of the aorta (7).

In both cor triatriatum and supravalvar mitral ring, the left atrium is divided into two compartments. In cor triatriatum, the posterior compartment contains the pulmonary veins whereas the anterior compartment contains the left atrial appendage and the mitral valve orifice. In supravalvar mitral membrane, however, the posterior compartment contains the pulmonary veins and the left atrial appendage whereas the anterior compartment contains only the mitral valve orifice.

Valvar Mitral Stenosis

Valvar mitral stenosis can involve the leaflets, the annulus, or both.

In commissural fusion, the mobility of the mitral valve leaflets can be severely limited by fusion of the commissurae. This problem is often associated with subvalvar pathology. Excessive dysplastic tissue, including mitral valve leaflet and chordal tissue, can obliterate the interchordal spaces. In mitral valve annular hypoplasia, the mitral valve annulus is small, and this can be associated with other hypoplastic left-sided structures. In double orifice mitral valve, an occasionally excessive leaflet tissue may bridge the mitral orifice joining the anterior and posterior leaflets, thus creating an accessory mitral orifice (8, 9). This accessory orifice can be associated with stenosis or insufficiency, but it also can be an incidental echocardiographic finding.

Subvalvar Mitral Valve Stenosis

Three forms of subvalvar mitral valve stenosis have been described: (*a*) parachute mitral valve (single papillary muscle), (*b*) hammock mitral valve (multiple papillary muscles), and (c) absence of one or both papillary muscles. Any of these lesions may be associated with stenosis at the valvar or supravalvar level.

In parachute mitral valve, all chordae of the mitral valve insert into one papillary muscle (10). This one papillary muscle exists because of either the fusion of the two papillary muscles or the failure of one of the papillary muscles to form. The interchordal spaces are obliterated by excess valvar and subvalvar tissue. The mitral orifice in hammock mitral valve is obstructed by intermixed chordae and multiple abnormal papillary muscles, which are implanted just below the mural mitral valve leaflet (11). The anterior leaflet is attached to chordae tendinae that cross the mitral orifice to reach the posterior papillary muscle apparatus, producing the hammock appearance. Other names for the hammock mitral valve include hypertrophied papillary muscles, obstructive papillary muscles, and mitral arcade (12, 13). With absence of papillary muscles, multiple chordae are attached to the ventricular wall. These chordae can cause mitral stenosis by obliterating the mitral valve orifice with imperforate interchordal spaces.

Types of Mitral Valve Regurgitation

Carpentier et al. (14, 15) have classified the anatomic lesions of mitral valve regurgitation into three groups according to the motion of the leaflets (normal, prolapsed, or restricted). Among causative reasons for mitral valve regurgitation occurrence include annular dilation and deformation, cleft malformation, isolated leaflet defect, and prolapsed mitral leaflet with absence of chordae tendinae or elongation of chordae tendinae or papillary muscles, or abnormal papillary muscles.

Associated Lesions

Mitral valve disease is associated with subaortic and aortic stenosis, coarctation of the aorta, and ventricular septal defect (VSD).

PATHOPHYSIOLOGY

Mitral Stenosis In mitral valve stenosis, progressive elevation in left atrial pressure leads to pulmonary venous hypertension and reflex pulmonary arteriolar vasoconstriction. In addition, outlet obstruction from the left atrium leads to reduced cardiac output but usually with preservation of left ventricular function.

For any given area of mitral valve in mitral stenosis, the pressure gradient is determined by cardiac output and heart rate. Thus, tachycardia shortens diastolic filling time, which can further compromise filling to the left ventricle. In addition, any pressure gradient between the left atrium and left ventricle may be less (for the degree of stenosis) if the left ventricular end-diastolic pressure is elevated.

The pulmonary hypertension observed with mitral valve stenosis appears to be more readily reversible compared with that seen with chronic left-to-right shunts (16). The cause is backward transmission of the elevated left atrial pressure and reflex pulmonary arteriolar vasoconstriction. In patients with mitral valve stenosis, an associated left-to-right shunt (e.g., VSD), however, can accelerate the progression of pulmonary vascular disease.

Mitral Regurgitation In mitral valve regurgitation, progressive dilation of the left atrium is seen at low pressure, but eventual elevation in left atrial pressure leads to pulmonary venous hypertension and pulmonary arteriolar vasoconstriction. In addition, the regurgitant volume creates a volume overload on the left ventricle that can lead to progressive left ventricular dysfunction.

Eccentric hypertrophy of the left ventricle is seen as well as annular dilation as a sequelae of the chronic volume overload. The pathophysiologic states of chronic mitral valve regurgitation progress from an initial compensated state to a later decompensated state, which is characterized by (a) increasing end-systolic and end-diastolic left ventricular volumes, (b) increasing left atrial pressure, and (c) reduced forward stroke volume. Because emptying of the left ventricle in mitral valve regurgitation includes a regurgitant volume that is decompressed into the left atrium, the ejection fraction should be supernormal if the left ventricular performance is intact. A normal ejection fraction can be an ominous sign that heralds left ventricular dysfunction. The resultant deterioration of left ventricular function with chronic mitral valve regurgitation may not be reversible even with mitral valve surgery (17).

Clinical Course

The clinical presentation of mitral valve stenosis and regurgitation depends on the severity of the lesion (degree of obstruction, regurgitation, or both) and presence of any associated lesions.

In mitral valve stenosis, the presentation of severe mitral valve stenosis and hypoplastic left heart variants is discussed elsewhere in this text. Those infants with less severe mitral valve stenosis will present beyond the neonatal period with failure to thrive, recurrent pneumonias, tachypnea, chronic cough, and wheezing. Atrial dysrhythmias can also occur (18, 19). Older children and young adults can present with exercise intolerance, dyspnea or orthopnea, pulmonary edema, hemoptysis, and atrial fibrillation.

Infants and young children with severe mitral valve regurgitation can also present with manifestations of low cardiac output and congestive heart failure including failure to thrive, tachypnea, pneumonias, wheezing, and feeding intolerance. In older children, the presentation depends on the acuteness of onset. Acute mitral valve regurgitation will present with pulmonary edema and heart failure, whereas chronic mitral valve regurgitation may remain asymptomatic for a prolonged period until ventricular failure appears with associated dyspnea, weakness, and chronic fatigue.

Medical management of children with congenital anomalies of the mitral valve is essentially the conventional treatment of heart failure. Components of this treatment include diuretics such as furosemide and digoxin. In addition, any atrial dysrhythmias should be aggressively treated. Anticoagulation therapy may be necessary in patients with chronic atrial fibrillation. Afterload reducing agents (such as intravenous phosphodiesterase inhibitors) and inotropic agents are efficacious in children with mitral valve regurgitation, but they are not recommended in children with isolated mitral valve stenosis as these agents can induce tachycardia and thus reduce left ventricular filling.

SURGERY

Preoperative Evaluation

Physical Examination

In patients with mitral valve stenosis, physical examination will reveal a mid-diastolic rumbling murmur heard best at the apex. The opening snap often associated with acquired rheumatic mitral stenosis is usually absent in cases of congenital mitral valve stenosis because the valve leaflets are relatively immobile. A loud pulmonary component of the second heart sound (P_2) and right ventricular heave will be present in patients with pulmonary hypertension. Severe mitral valve stenosis can be associated with decreased peripheral pulses.

In mitral valve regurgitation, physical examination will reveal a pansystolic murmur loudest at the apex and radiating toward the left axilla and back. Increased pericardial activity and a diffuse apical impulse may be palpated. The first heart sound is diminished. As with mitral valve stenosis patients, the pulmonary component of the second heart sound (P_2) will be increased in patients with pulmonary hypertension.

Chest Roentgenogram

In mitral valve stenosis, the chest radiograph can show evidence of left atrial enlargement including elevation of the left main stem bronchus on the anteroposterior projection. Pulmonary venous congestion and right ventricle enlargement may also be present.

In mitral valve regurgitation, the chest radiograph reveals both left atrial and left ventricular enlargement. Pulmonary vascular markings are increased. Right ventricular enlargement may also be present in cases of pulmonary hypertension.

Electrocardiography

With mitral valve stenosis, the electrocardiography (ECG) can show left atrial enlargement with wide notched P waves in lead II and a posteriorly directed P wave in the anterior precordial leads. Atrial tacchydysrhythmias may be present. Right ventricular hypertrophy is consistent with associated pulmonary hypertension.

Mitral valve regurgitation can manifest both left atrial and left ventricular enlargement. Right ventricular hypertrophy is consistent with associated pulmonary hypertension.

Echocardiography

Two-dimensional echocardiography with color flow Doppler interrogation is the modality of choice to evaluate mitral valve pathology. Detailed information can be obtained about all components of the mitral valve apparatus. Leaflet morphology and mobility can be assessed, annulus size can be measured, and chordae tendinae and papillary muscles can be examined in detail.

The level and anatomic substrate of mitral stenosis can be defined by echocardiography. Transvalvar gradient of mitral valve stenosis can be calculated except in cases of an interatrial communication, because this communication allows decompression of the left atrium and thus the gradient will be underestimated. Pulmonary artery pressure can also be estimated using a tricuspid regurgitation jet and the Bernoulli equation (see Chapter 28, *Principles of Echocardiography*). There can be left-to-right bowing of the interatrial septum due to elevated left atrial pressure. Similarly, the anatomic substrate of mitral valve regurgitation can be assessed while quantifying the degree of regurgitation (Fig. 20.1.2; see color plate 20.1.2.) (20).

Preoperative transesophageal echocardiography often permits an even more detailed assessment of mitral valve pathology than transthoracic echocardiography, especially in older patients with suboptimal transthoracic windows. In addition, three-dimensional echocardiography has been demonstrated to be useful in delineating the mitral valve apparatus.

Cardiac Catheterization

For patients with mitral valve stenosis, cardiac catheterization is indicated when the diagnosis is unclear after echocardiography as well as in patients with multiple associated anomalies or pulmonary hypertension. If performed, findings would include a pressure gradient between the a wave pressure of the left atrium and the end-diastolic pressure of the left ventricle as well as elevated left atrial and pulmonary artery pressures. Cardiac catheterization also may play a therapeutic role with balloon valvuloplasty of mitral stenosis (see below).

Magnetic resonance imaging (MRI) can visualize congenital anomalies of the left atrium and mitral valve including cor triatriatum and supravalvar mitral ring.

Balloon Angioplasty For patients with mitral valve stenosis, this interventional procedure was first reported to be successful in patients with rheumatic mitral stenosis (21) and then in children with congenital mitral valve stenosis with varying rates of success (22). This procedure involves a trans-septal technique (with catheter placed into the left atrium and left ventricle from a right atrial approach). The drop in pulmonary vascular resistance after this procedure can be immediate (23). Evaluation of this technique for congenital mitral valve stenosis has been limited. In cases of congenital mitral valve stenosis, the highest likelihood of success with balloon angioplasty is with stenosis confined to the valve leaflets and the poorest results have been with patients who have stenosis involving the subvalvar mitral apparatus. Complications include mitral valve regurgitation, injury to the mitral valve, and thromboembolic events.

Surgical Procedure

Timing

Timing of surgery for mitral valve stenosis should be determined not solely by severity of heart failure but also by degree of pulmonary artery hypertension (24). For mitral valve regurgitation, timing of surgery may be more difficult to determine because progression of left ventricular failure can be subtle.

Technique

The heart can be exposed for mitral valve surgery through a median sternotomy, right thoracotomy, or left thoracotomy. Several cardiac incisions can be used to expose the mitral valve. The standard approach is with an incision into the lateral left atrium posterior to the interatrial groove. This incision is carried posterior to the superior and inferior vena cavae. Dissection of the interatrial groove will improve exposure. A second approach is the superior approach through the dome of the left atrium between the aorta and superior vena cavae. A third approach is the trans-septal approach through the right atrium and atrial septum.

Mitral Valve Repair A detailed discussion of all of the valve repair techniques available is beyond the scope of this text (see Figs. 20.1.3 and 20.1.4; see color plates 20.1.3 and 20.1.4). Carpentier and others have described numerous valvuloplasty techniques for stenotic and/or regurgitant valves. The choice of technique depends on the anatomic substrate of the lesion. Valvuloplasty techniques are available to repair all major components of the mitral valve apparatus: (a) leaflet resection and repair; (b) annulus remodeling (Fig. 20.1.5); (c) choral shortening, transfer, fenestration, and replacement; and (d) papillary muscle elongation, shortening, and splitting. Other techniques for mitral valve stenosis include excision of mitral valve excresences, splitting of the solitary papillary muscle unit, and fenestrating the interchordal spaces (25). Satisfactory repair can now be performed in almost 80% of cases of mitral valve regurgitation, but the results of repair for stenotic and mixed lesions are less favorable (26, 27).

Mitral Valve Replacement A variety of mechanical prosthetic valves are now available with three basic designs being most common: (a) the caged-ball valve (Fig. 20.1.6), (b) the tilting disc valve (Fig. 20.1.7), and (c) the bileaflet valve (Fig. 20.1.8).

The most commonly used design in the United States is the bileaflet valve. In older children with an annulus size of 20 mm or greater, the technique of mitral valve replacement is identical to that of adults. St. Jude Medical manufactures its standard bileaflet valve in odd numbered annular sizes 19 to 33 mm. The most appropriate prosthetic valve for the smaller child is the low-profile bileaflet valve. This valve can be sutured in the supra-annular position in smaller children. St Jude produces the St. Jude HP (hemodynamics plus) valve in sizes 17 to 25 mm for these patients (Fig. 20.1.8). This valve design places the sewing cuff somewhat supra-annular so that the effective orifice area at the annular level is larger. Thus, a size 17 mm HP valve allows for an orifice at the annulus equivalent to a standard 19 mm St. Jude valve.

Heterograft valves have two distinct disadvantages in smaller children: these calcify and degenerate at an accelerated rate and their transvalvar gradients are excessive in the smaller sizes. Bioprosthetic valves in the mitral valve position require long-term anticoagulation.

Warfarin is used to maintain prothrombin time international normalized ratios (INR) between 2.5 and 3.5. Thromboembolic and hemorrhagic complications occur at the rate of approximately 0.3 to 4 events per patient year with mechanical valves in the mitral valve position (28).

Other Surgical Procedures

Minimally Invasive Surgery Several minimally invasive approaches have recently been described for mitral valve surgery. Cosgrove (29) has described a small parasternal incision from the inferior border of the right second costal cartilage to the superior edge of the right fifth costal carti-

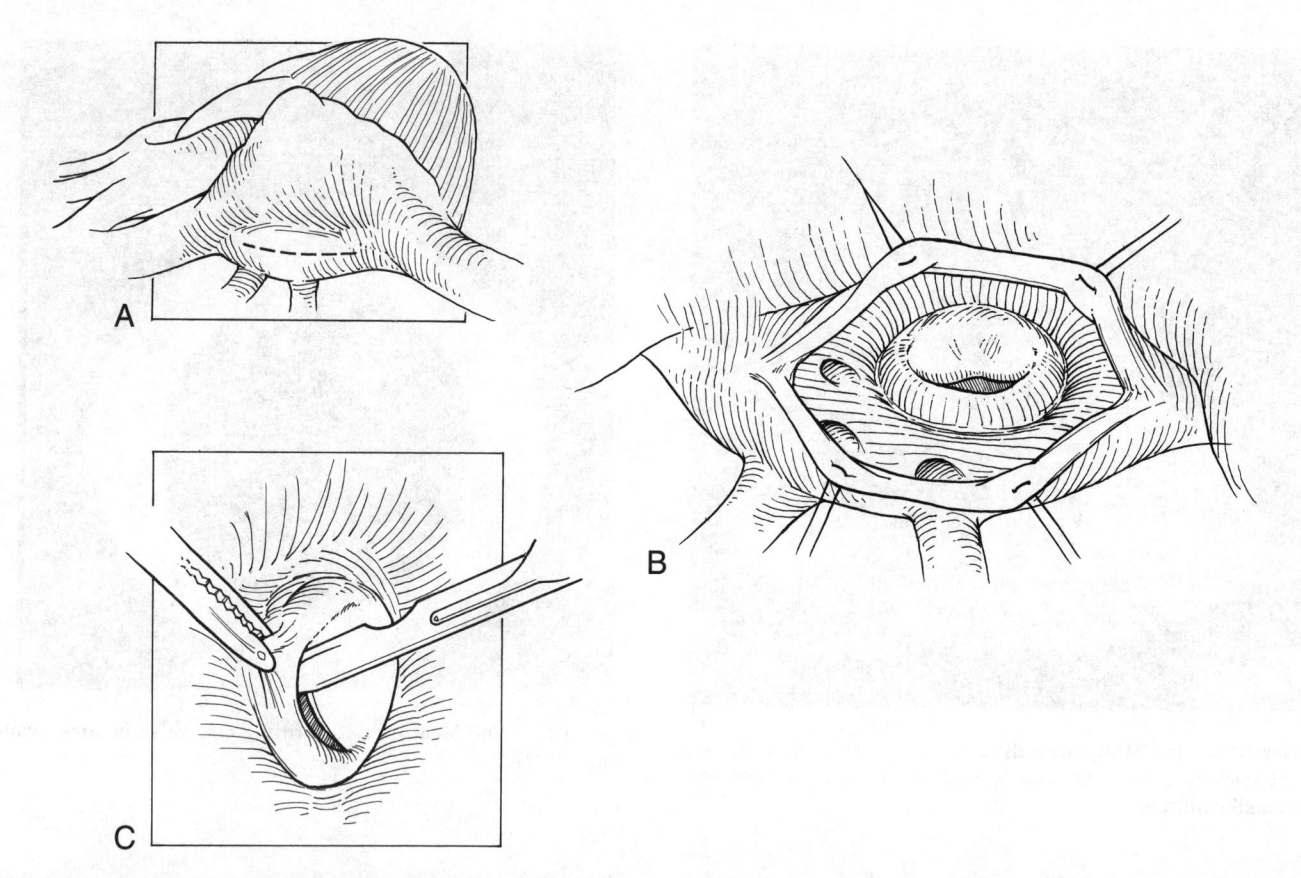

Figure 20.1.5. Repair of congenital mitral valve stenosis. Regardless of the specific valve pathology, the surgical approach to the mitral valve is typically through an incision in the interatrial groove just anterior to the right pulmonary veins. The procedure is performed using cardiopulmonary bypass and moderate hypothermia. Cardioplegic arrest of the heart is usually indicated. The typical incision is shown in **A**. Retraction of the incised atrial wall reveals the left atrial chamber and mitral valve as shown in **B**. In this case, dysplastic changes of the leaflet tissue are seen with underdevelopment of the commissurae. Commissurotomies are performed conservatively using sharp dissection. The maneuver both enlarges the valve orifice and increases the mobility of the valve leaflets. Once this is performed, the subvalvar mechanism of the mitral valve apparatus can be inspected. Over-aggressive commissurotomies should be judiciously avoided because significant mitral regurgitation can occur.

lage. Colvin (30) has described a mini-thoracotomy approach with cardiopulmonary bypass via the femoral vessels and with the aorta cross clamped internally with a patented balloon occlusion cannula. Potential advantages of minimally invasive approaches to cardiac surgery include less incisional pain and discomfort, reduced length of stay because of reduced surgical trauma, increased patient mobility, and decreased reliance on post discharge rehabilitation services (31). These approaches can achieve the often conflicting goals of reducing operative trauma while improving access to remote intracardiac structures such as the mitral valve (32).

Mortality

For mitral valvuloplasty, the mortality rate is reported to be less than 5% in more recent series (33, 34). For mitral valve replacement, the mortality rate is higher, especially when replacement is performed in the infants at the supraannular position (35).

Postoperative Management

Postoperative care of patients after mitral valve surgery should emphasize understanding of the left atrial and left ventricular compliance changes before and after intervention with a vigilance for pulmonary hypertension.

Ideal monitoring consists of arterial, central venous pressure, and pulmonary artery and left atrial pressure lines. In addition, atrial and ventricular temporary pacing wires are sometimes placed.

Specific Postoperative Problems

Low Cardiac Output

In mitral valve stenosis patients after surgery, the compliance of the left ventricle may remain suboptimal and thus cardiac output can be decreased in the initial postoperative period. In mitral valve regurgitation, adaptation of the ventricular volume overload can also lead to low cardiac output after surgery because the potential for blood to

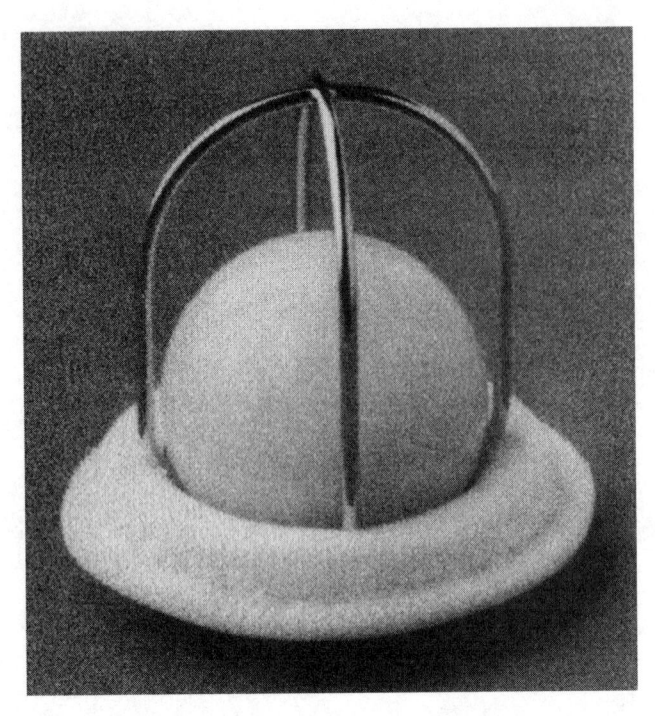

310 Section III. Perioperative Care of Congenital Heart Disease

Figure 20.1.6. The Starr-Edwards caged-ball valve is one of the earliest mechanical valve designs. Its high profile makes it less useful in small children.

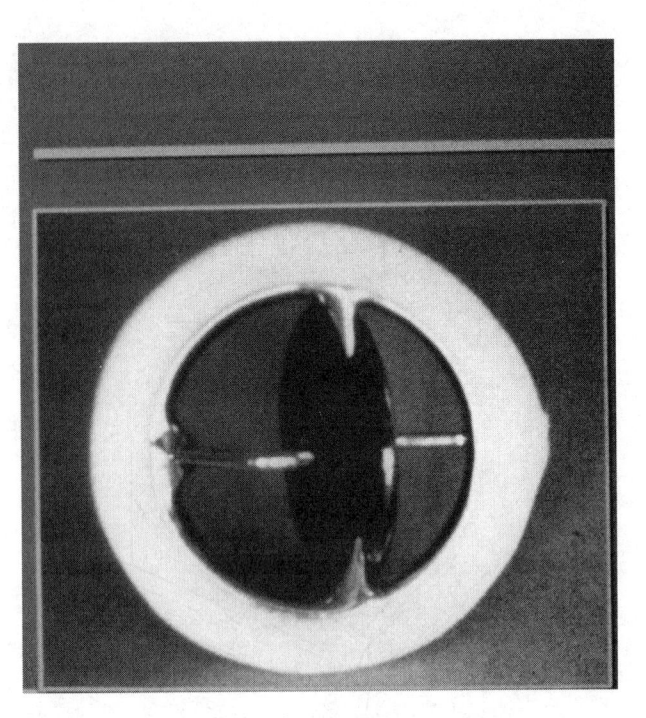

Figure 20.1.7. The Medtronic Hall tilting disc valve became available in 1977.

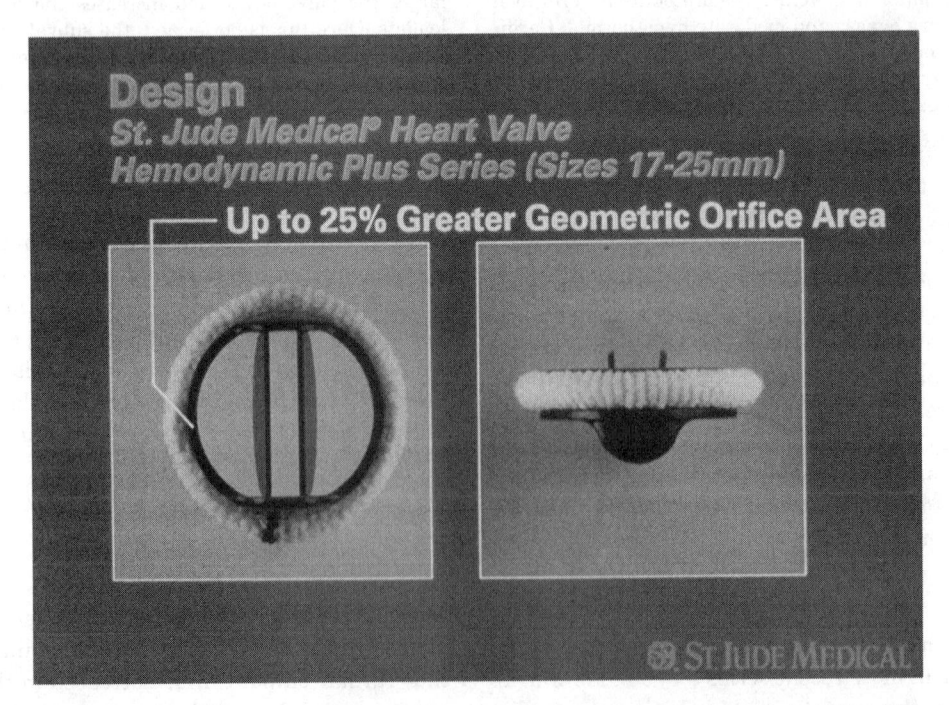

Figure 20.1.8. The most appropriate prosthetic valve for the smaller child is the low-profile bileaflet valve. This valve, which is manufactured by St. Jude Medical, can be sutured in the supra-annular position in smaller children.

decompress into a low pressure chamber (when the valve was regurgitant) is lost when the valve is repaired or replaced.

Postoperative therapy consists of maintenance of optimal heart rate with either sequential pacing or with isoproterenol because cardiac output in this lesion can be more heart rate dependent compared with others. Filling pressure to the left ventricle should be maintained at 15 mm Hg or greater to accommodate for the poorly compliant left ventricle. This underfilling of the left ventricle can be further exacerbated in the presence of pulmonary hypertension and right heart dilation. Overaggressive volume replacement should be avoided for both mitral valve stenosis and regurgitation patients; in the former, rapid volume administration can lead to excessive and rapid left atrial pressure elevation, which can then precipitate a pulmonary hypertensive crisis and in the latter, excessive volume can increase the degree of any residual regurgitation caused by annular dilation.

Appropriate afterload reduction can improve cardiac output in patients with poor left ventricular function after mitral valve repair or replacement for mitral valve regurgitation. If cardiac output is severely depressed, mechanical assist may be necessary.

Elevated Left Atrial Pressure

Intraoperative transesophageal echocardiography after separation from cardiopulmonary bypass allows rapid assessment of the surgical result and identification of poor surgical results prior to leaving the operating room. Causative factors for elevated left atrial pressure after mitral valve repair can include (a) residual left atrioventricular valve regurgitation, (b) residual left atrioventricular valve stenosis, (c) pulmonary hypertension (leading to dilation of the right ventricle and flattening of the left ventricle), and (d) left ventricular dysfunction. Common problems such as pericardial effusion (leading to tamponade) as well as atrioventricular dyssynchrony should always be ruled out.

Timely diagnosis of the cause for the left atrial pressure elevation will dictate therapy. Reoperation may be necessary in selected cases.

Pulmonary Hypertension

Pulmonary hypertensive crises are not uncommon after mitral valve surgery, especially in patients with long-standing mitral valve stenosis. In infants who have had a valve replacement in the supra-annular position, the relatively large valve prosthesis may impede flow to the ventricle and create a hypertensive left atrial chamber and further promote pulmonary hypertensive crises. (See Chapter 32, *Pulmonary Hypertension*, for additional information.)

Prosthetic Valve Problems

Issues regarding proper function of the mechanical valve should be attended to vigorously. Anticoagulation with intravenous heparin may be initiated during the postoperative period when bleeding has ceased. Chronic therapy usually includes warfarin, but aspirin and Persantine may be considered as an alternative therapy after the first few months. Treatment for thrombosis of the prosthetic valve is dependent on duration of time after surgery; it can include streptokinase or even tissue plasminogen activator (36).

Other than thrombosis, problems with the prosthetic valve can also arise secondary to tissue entrapment within the valve leaflets. This unusual complication can present by intermittent left atrial pressure elevation and absence of prosthetic valve click. Prompt transthoracic and even transesophageal echocardiographic examination of the valve should be performed whenever valve malfunction is suspected.

POSTOPERATIVE CARE CHECKLIST

Postoperative care checklist includes:

- Attention to prosthetic valve issues such as anticoagulation and potential malfunction.
- Avoid aggressive volume resuscitation and maintain an appreciation for left atrial and ventricular compliance changes before and after surgery.
- Vigilance for pulmonary hypertension.

REFERENCES

1. Davachi F, Moller JH, Edwards JE. Diseases of the mitral valve in infancy. Circulation 1971;43:565–572.
2. Lewis DA, Tweddell JS. Valve repair and replacement in children. Curr Opin Cardiol 1997;12:63–69.
3. Perloff JK, Roberts WC. The mitral apparatus. Circulation 1972;46:227–237.
4. Ruckman RN, Van Praagh R. Anatomic types of congenital mitral stenosis: report of 49 autopsy cases with consideration of diagnosis and surgical implications. Am J Cardiol 1978; 42:592–601.
5. Carpentier A, Branchini B, Cour JE et al. Congenital malformations of the mitral velve in children. J Thorac Cardiovasc Surg 1976;72:854–866.
6. Oglietti J, Cooley DA, Izquierdo JP, et al. Cor triatriatum: operative results in 25 patients. Ann Thorac Surg 1983;35: 415–420.
7. Shone JD, Sellers RD, Anderson RC, et al. The developmental complex of parachute mitral valve, supravalvar ring of the left atrium, subaortic stenosis, and coarctation of the aorta. Am J Cardiol 1963;11:714–725.
8. Bano-Rodrigo A, Van Praagh S, Trowitzsch E, et al. Double orifice mitral valve: a study of 27 postmortem cases with developmental, diagnostic and surgical considerations. Am J Cardiol 1988;61:152–160.

9. Bano-Rodrigo A, Van Praagh S, Trowitzsch E, et al. Double orifice mitral valve: a study of 27 postmortem cases with developmental, diagnostic, and surgical considerations. Am J Cardiol 1988;61:152–160.
10. Glancy DL, Chang MY, Dorney ER, et al. Parachute mitral valve: further observations and associated lesions. Am J Cardiol 1971;27:309–317.
11. Davachi R, Moller JH, Edwards JE. Diseases of the mitral valve in infancy: anatomic analysis of 55 cases. Circulation 1971;43:565–579.
12. Matsushima A, Park J, Szule M, et al. Anomalous atrioventricular valve arcade. Am Heart J 1991;121:1824–1826.
13. Layman T, Edwards J. Anomalous mitral arcade. Circulation 1967;35:389–395.
14. Carpentier A. Mitral valve reconstructive surgery. In: Jamieson SW, Shumway NE, eds. Operative Surgery, 4th ed. London: Butterworths, 1986;404–416.
15. Carpentier A, Branchini B, Cour JC, et al. Congenital malformations of the mitral valve in children. J Thorac Cardiovasc Surg 1976;72:854–863.
16. Dev V, Shrivastava S. Time course of changes in pulmonary vascular resistance and the mechanism of regression of pulmonary arterial hypertension after balloon mitral valvuloplasty. Am J Cardiol 1991;67:439–442.
17. Benmimoun EG, Friedli B, Rutishauser W, et al. Mitral valve replacement in children. Comparative study of pre and postoperative hemodynamics and left ventricular function. Br Heart J 1982;48:117–124.
18. Daoud G, Kaplan S, Perrin EV, et al. Congenital mitral stenosis. Circulation 1963;27:185–196.
19. Collins-Nakai RL, Rosenthal A, Castaneda AR, et al. Congenital mitral stenosis: a review of twenty years experience. Circulation 1977;56:1039–1047.
20. Wu YT, Chang AC, and Chin AJ. Semiquantitative assessment of mitral regurgitation by Doppler color flow imaging in patients aged <20 years. Am J Cardiol 1993;71(8):727–732.
21. Kveselis DA, Rochini AP, Beekman RB, et al. Balloon angioplasty for congenital and rheumatic mitral stenosis. Am J Cardiol 1986;57:348–350.
22. Spevak PJ, Bass JL, Ben-Shachar G, et al. Balloon angioplasty for congenital mitral stenosis. Am J Cardiol 1990;66:472–476.
23. Levine MJ, Weinstein JS, Diver DJ, et al. Progressive improvement in pulmonary vascular resistance after percutaneous mitral valvuloplasty. Circulation 1989;79:1061–1067.
24. Carabello BA, Crawford FA. Medical progress: valvular heart disease. N Engl J Med 1997;337:32–39.
25. Bolling S, Iannettoni M, Dick M, et al. Shone's anomaly: operative results and late outcome. Ann Thorac Surg 1990;49:887–893.
26. Carpentier A, Branchini B, Cour C, et al. Congenital malformations of the mitral valve. Pathology and surgical treatment. J Thorac Cardiovasc Surg 1976;72:854–862.
27. Stellin G, Bortolotti U, Mazzucco A, et al. Repair of congenitally malformed mitral valve in children. J Thorac Cardiovasc Surg 1988;95:480–487.
28. Cohn LH, Lipson W. Selection and complications of cardiac valvular prostheses. In: Bave AE, Geha AS, Hammond GL, et al, eds. Glenn's thoracic and cardiovascular surgery, 6th ed. Stamford, CT: Appleton and Lange, 1996;2046.
29. Cosgrove DM. Cleveland Clinic Foundation, Cleveland, Ohio. Minimally invasive mitral valve procedure: minithoracotomy. Adult Cardiac Surgery Symposium. 77th Annual AATS meeting, Washington, DC: May 4, 1997.
30. Colvin SB. New York University Medical Center, New York, NY. Minimally invasive mitral valve procedure: minithoracotomy with Port-Access. Adult Cardiac Surgery Symposium. 77th Annual AATS meeting, Washington, DC: May 4, 1997.
31. Cohn LH. Brigham and Women's Hospital, Boston, Massachusetts. Minimally invasive aortic valve procedure: Right paramedian approach. Adult Cardiac Surgery Symposium. 77th Annual AATS meeting, Washington, DC: May 4, 1997.
32. Burke RP, Michielon G, Wernovsky G. Video-assisted cardioscopy in congenital heart operations. Ann Thorac Surg 1994;58:864–868.
33. Barbero-Marcial M, Riso A, DeAlbuquerque AT, et al. Left ventricular apical approach for the surgical treatment of congenital mitral stenosis. J Thorac Cardiovasc Surg 1993;106:105–110.
34. Coles J, Williams W, Watanabe T, et al. Surgical experience with reparative techniques in patients with congenital mitral valvular anomalies. Circulation 1987;76(Suppl III):III-117–III-122.
35. Adatia I, Moore P, Jonas RA, et al. Clinical course and hemodynamic observations after aupraannular mitral valve replacement in infants and children. J Am Coll Cardiol 1997;29:1089–1094.
36. Renzulli A, Vitale N, Caruso A, et al. Thrombolysis for prosthetic vale thrombosis: indications and results. J Heart Valve Dis 1997;6:212–218.

20.2 Anomalous Origin of the Left Coronary Artery from the Pulmonary Artery (ALCAPA)

Anthony C. Chang, MD, and Frank L. Hanley, MD

A rare lesion, is one in which the left coronary artery originates from the pulmonary artery also known by the eponym Bland-White-Garland syndrome (1). Its presentation can be from cardiogenic shock in the infant to cardiomyopathy in the adult (2).

ANATOMY

As a result of the primordial maldevelopment so that the left coronary system becomes attached to the pulmonary artery bud, the left coronary artery originates from near the main pulmonary artery (Fig. 20.2.1). Cases in which the right coronary artery or both coronary arteries

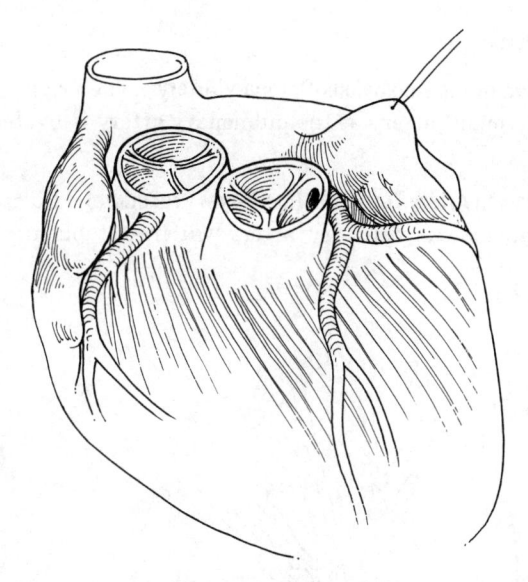

Figure 20.2.1. Anatomy of anomalous origin of the left coronary artery from the pulmonary artery. The origin of the left coronary artery from the pulmonary artery can vary in its position. In this illustration the coronary ostium is in the left lateral position, remote from the aortic root. The variation in origin of the coronary from the pulmonary artery has implications with regard to the most appropriate type of surgical repair. The right coronary artery is typically larger than normal in this lesion because it provides varying degrees of collateral flow to the left ventricular coronary circulation. The left ventricle typically suffers from ischemic injury, with a dilated poorly functioning chamber and varying degrees of infarction. Ischemic mitral valve dysfunction with insufficiency is common.

arise anomalously from the pulmonary artery have also been described (3). This is usually an isolated lesion.

PATHOPHYSIOLOGY

As pulmonary vascular resistance and pulmonary artery falls in the first few weeks of life, the left coronary artery fills with desaturated blood under less pressure, which leads to progressive myocardial ischemia and ventricular dilation. The right coronary artery, originating from the aorta, becomes the main source of coronary supply.

Via collaterals, blood flows from the right coronary artery to the left coronary artery, and it can even flow retrograde into the pulmonary arteries. Although the degree of left-to-right shunt is relatively small, the areas of the myocardium normally supplied by the left coronary artery are underperfused by this "steal" phenomenon and become ischemic. With time, the left-sided chambers become progressively dilated. In addition, ischemia to the papillary muscle can lead to mitral regurgitation.

Clinical Course

Neonates and infants often present with congestive heart failure and/or difficulty feeding (colicky pains secondary to myocardial ischemia), although a few patients can present as asymptomatic adults (4). Sudden death and angina can occur older children. Pulmonary hypertension can be found in the occasional adult patient who presents late with this defect (5).

SURGERY

Preoperative Evaluation

Physical Evaluation

Infants may have signs of low cardiac output and congestive heart failure, such as pallor, tachycardia, and respiratory distress. Cardiac auscultation may reveal gallop. A systolic murmur of mitral regurgitation may be present near the apex.

Chest Roentgenogram

Cardiomegaly with interstitial edema is usually present.

Electrocardiography

Classic findings include deep and wide Q waves in leads I, avL, and V_{4-6} consistent with anterolateral infarction (6).

Echocardiography

With color Doppler echocardiography used by an experienced practitioner, the lesion can be readily identified (7). The right coronary artery is dilated and the left coronary artery is seen deriving from the pulmonary artery. The echocardiogram shows typically dilated chambers similar to dilated cardiomyopathy and sometimes mitral regurgitation as well. Echogenicity may be seen from papillary muscles and endocardial surface from ischemia and fibrosis.

Cardiac Catheterization

Cardiac catheterization may be indicated if diagnosis is uncertain. Hemodynamic data usually show the elevated left ventricular end-diastolic pressure and left atrial pressure. It should be noted that the risk of cardiac catheterization may be significant given the left ventricular dysfunction.

Surgical Procedure

Timing

Surgery should be performed at the time of diagnosis because medical treatment is futile with a mortality rate of almost 90% (8). In most patients moderate to severe depression is found in left ventricular function, thus necessitating preoperative inotropic support. In addition, mechanical ventilation may need to be instituted, although special attention should be directed to the risk of anesthesia and intubation in the presence of severe myocardial dysfunction and low cardiac output.

Technique

Ligation of the Anomalous Coronary Artery The origin of the left coronary artery at the pulmonary artery is ligated (9).

Subclavian Artery Turndown (the Meyer Procedure) Ligation of the anomalous coronary artery with reestablishment of

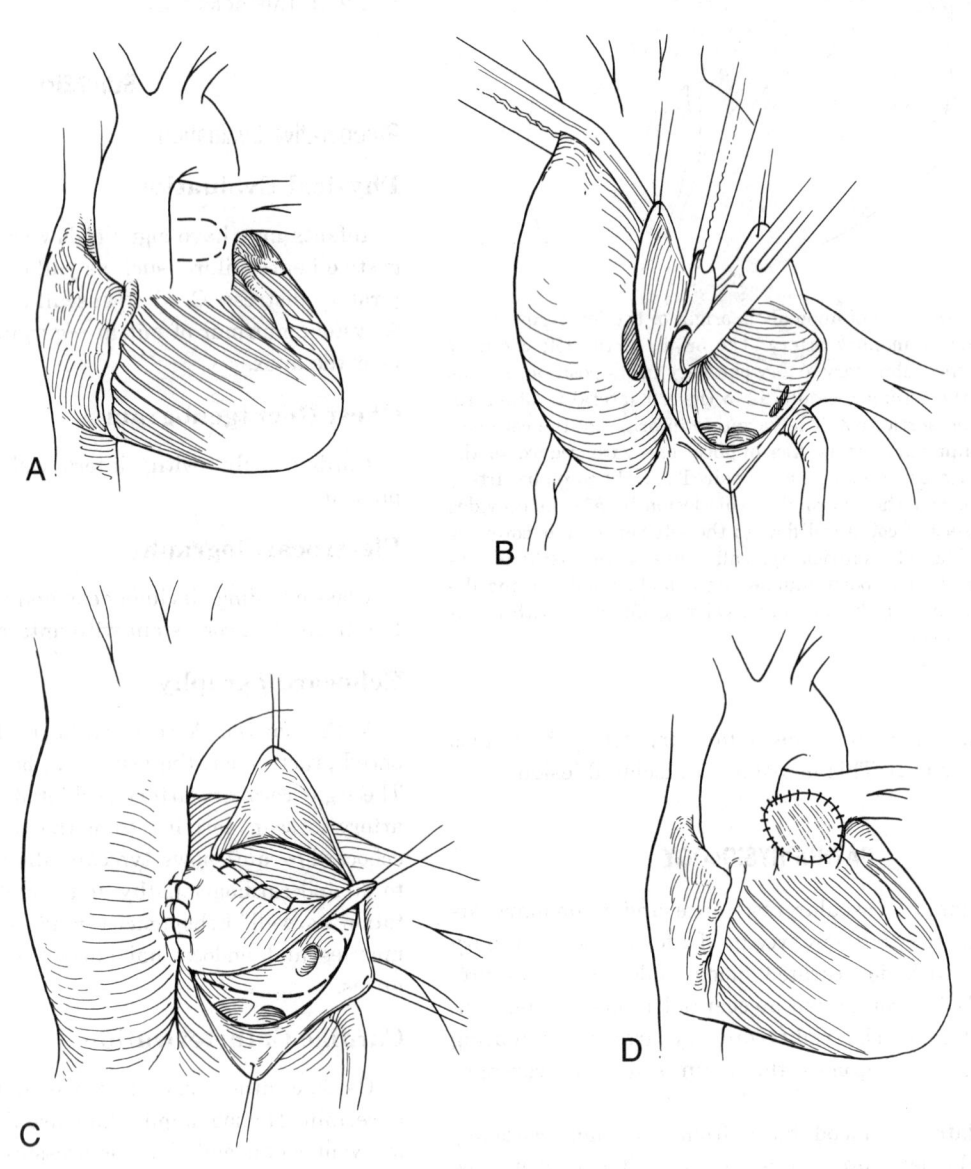

Figure 20.2.2. Repair of anomalous origin of left coronary artery from pulmonary artery using the Takeuchi procedure. Regardless of the repair technique, exquisite detail to left ventricular myocardial protection is critical to successful repair. Cardiopulmonary bypass with moderate hypothermia is used. Cardioplegia solution is delivered into both the aortic root and the pulmonary artery root. Other special maneuvers are also carried out during cardiopulmonary bypass. In cases with the left coronary artery arising in a position remote from the aortic root, the procedure of choice, direct coronary reimplantation into the aortic root, may not be feasible. In such cases, the Takeuchi procedure is a commonly performed reconstructive technique. **A.** This complex procedure involves creating an anterior flap in the free wall of the main pulmonary artery. **B.** An aortopulmonary window is then created between the adjacent sides of the aorta and pulmonary artery. **C.** The flap of anterior pulmonary artery wall is then sewn around the coronary ostium in the pulmonary artery sinus, thereby creating a tunnel between the aorta and the abnormal coronary ostium. **D.** A pericardial patch is used to reconstruct the defect in the anterior wall of the pulmonary artery, where the flap originated.

flow is done via a subclavian artery graft in an end-to-end or end-to-side fashion (10).

The Takeuchi Operation Via a surgically created aortopulmonary window, a tunnel is fashioned between the aorta and the coronary ostium of the anomalous left coronary artery within the pulmonary artery (Fig. 20.2.2). This surgery results in the aorta supplying blood to the left coronary artery (11).

Direct Reimplantation of the Left Coronary Artery In a technique resembling the coronary artery translocation for the arterial switch operation (12), the pulmonary artery is transected above the valve and the coronary button is fashioned and directly reimplanted to the aorta.

Mortality

The mortality rate of the ligation with or without graft techniques was considerably higher than with the Takeuchi operation (27 to 33% versus 0% early mortality) (13–15). In addition, long-term patency of early anastomotic technique is about 50% (16). The Takeuchi operation can lead to supravalvar pulmonary stenosis. Results of the coronary reimplantation technique has a mortality rate of 0% (17).

Postoperative Management

Postoperative care of patients after surgery for this defect involves surveillance for low cardiac output, which can worsen after the first few hours. Overly aggressive fluid resuscitation and catecholamine use should be avoided. Mechanical support should be readily available if the clinical status dictates its use.

Ideal monitoring consists of arterial, central venous pressure, left atrial pressure, and pulmonary artery lines (for thermodilution cardiac output if indicated). In addition, atrial and ventricular temporary pacing wires are placed.

Specific Postoperative Problems

Low Cardiac Output

When intraoperative ischemia secondary to cardiopulmonary bypass is added to preoperative ventricular dysfunction, poor cardiac output secondary to poor ventricular function as well as moderate to severe left atrioventricular valve regurgitation is expected. Even with surgery resulting in oxygenated blood supplying the myocardium, residual left ventricular dysfunction and increased left ventricular end-diastolic volume persist for months after surgery (18). Given this premise, however, it is still of paramount importance to obtain an electrocardiogram to rule out persistent myocardial ischemia, although its interpretation may be difficult.

Therapy includes aggressive afterload reduction (with phosphodiesterase inhibitors) to decrease wall stress of the left ventricle as well as the severity of mitral regurgitation. Metabolic derangements such as hypokalemia, hypocalcemia, and acidosis should be avoided to minimize ventricular ectopy. Anticoagulation therapy after surgical bleeding ceases may be indicated if left ventricular dysfunction is severe. In selected patients, mechanical support with left ventricular assist device (19) or extracorporeal membrane oxygenation may be needed to support the circulation. Mitral valve replacement has been reported as therapy for persistent mitral valve insufficiency even after reimplantation of the anomalous coronary artery (20).

Ventricular Dysrhythmias

(See Chapter 30, *Diagnosis and Management of Arrhythmias*.)

POSTOPERATIVE CARE CHECKLIST

Postoperative care checklist includes:

- Avoid aggressive volume resuscitation or excessive catecholamines.
- Institute early afterload reduction with attention to blood pressure.
- Monitor metabolic parameters closely to avoid likelihood of ventricular arrhythmias.
- Mechanical support team should be alerted.

REFERENCES

1. Bland EF, White PD, Garland J. Congenital anomalies of the coronary arteries: report of an unusual case associated with cardiac hypertrophy. Am Heart J 1933;8:787–790.
2. Daniels C, Bacon J, Fontana ME, et al. Anomalous origin of the left main coronary artery from the pulmonary trunk masquerading as peripartum cardiomyopathy. Am J Cardiol 1997;79:1307–1308.
3. Heifetz SA, Robinowitz M, Mueller KH, et al. Total anomalous origin of the coronary arteries from the pulmonary artery. Pediatr Cardiol 1986;7:11–18.
4. Purut CM, Sabiston DC. Origin of the left coronary artery from the pulmonary artery in the older adult. J Thorac Cardiovasc Surg 1991;102:566–570.
5. Christensen ED, Johansen JB, Thayssen P, et al. Treatment of anomalous origin of the left coronary artery from the pulmonary artery in adulthood. Cardiology 1996;87:260–262.
6. Johnsrude CL, Perry JC, Cecchin F, et al. Differentiating anomalous left main coronary artery originating from the pulmonary artery in infants from myocarditis and dilated cardiomyopathy by electrocardiogram. Am J Cardiol 1995;75:71–74.
7. Karr SS, Parness IA, Spevak PJ, et al. Diagnosis of anomalous left coronary artery by Doppler color flow mapping: distinction

from other causes of dilated cardiomyopathy. J Am Coll Cardiol 1992;19:1271–1275.
8. Vouhe PR, Baillot-Vernant F, Trinquet F, et al. Anomalous left coronary artery from the pulmonary artery in infants. J Thorac Cardiovasc Surg 1987;94:192–199.
9. Shrivastava S, Castaneda AR, Moller JH. Anomalous left coronary artery from pulmonary trunk: long-term follow-up after ligation. J Thorac Cardiovasc Surg 1978;76:130–134.
10. Stephenson LW, Edmunds LH, Friedman S, et al. Subclavian-left coronary artery anastomosis (Meyer operation) for anomalous origin of the left coronary artery from the pulmonary artery. Circulation 1981;64(Suppl II):130–133.
11. Takeuchi S, Imamura H, Katsumoto K, et al. New surgical method for repair of anomalous left coronary artery from pulmonary artery. J Thorac Cardiovasc Surg 1979;78:1–11.
12. Laborde F, Marchand M, Leca F, et al. Surgical treatment of anomalous origin of the left coronary artery in infancy and childhood: early and late results in 20 consecutive cases. J Thorac Cardiovasc Surg 1981;82:423–428.
13. Bunton R, Jonas RA, Lang P, et al. Anomalous origin of left coronary artery from pulmonary artery: ligation vs establishment of a two coronary artery system. J Thorac Cardiovasc Surg 1987;93:103–108.
14. Kesler KA, Pennington DG, Nouri S, et al. Left subclavian-left coronary artery anastomosis for anomalous origin of the left coronary artery. J Thorac Cardiovasc Surg 1989;98:25–29.
15. Backer CL, Stout MJ, Zales VR, et al. Anomalous origin of the left coronary artery: a twenty year review of surgical management. J Thorac Cardiovasc Surg 1992;103:1049–1058.
16. Berdjis F, Takahashi M, Wells WJ, et al. Anomalous left coronary artery from the pulmonary artery. J Thorac Cardiovasc Surg 1994;108:17–20.
17. Alexi-Meskishvili V, Hetzer R, Weng Y, et al. Anomalous origin of the left coronary artery from the pulmonary artery: early results with direct aortic reimplantation. J Thorac Cardiovasc Surg 1994;108:354–362.
18. Rein AJJT, Colan SD, Parness IA, et al. Regional and global left ventricular function in infants with anomalous origin of the left coronary artery from the pulmonary trunk: preoperative and postoperative assessment. Circulation 1987;75:115–123.
19. Chang AC, Hanley FL, Weindling S, et al. Left heart support with a ventricular assist device in an infant with acute myocarditis. Crit Care Med 1992;20:712–715.
20. Yam MC, Menahem S. Mitral valve replacement for severe mitral regurgitation in infants with anomalous left coronary artery from the pulmonary artery. Pediatr Cardiol 1996;17:271–274.

20.3 Ebstein's Anomaly of the Tricuspid Valve

Anthony C. Chang, MD, and Frank L. Hanley, MD

First described by Dr. Wilhelm Ebstein in 1866, Ebstein's anomaly is a rare congenital heart defect in which the tricuspid valve attachments are abnormally displaced downward toward the right ventricular apex. Ebstein's anomaly has a wide clinical spectrum, and it can manifest clinically in many ways, including the fetus with hydrops in utero, the neonate with severe cyanosis and circulatory collapse, the child with mild cyanosis, and the adult with minimal or no symptoms (1, 2). Ebstein's anomaly is associated with maternal lithium use (3).

ANATOMY

Ebstein's anomaly occurs as a result of a maldevelopment of the tricuspid valve, a structure that normally forms as a result of a "delamination" process of the inner layer of right ventricular myocardium (4) (Fig. 20.3.1). The septal and posterior leaflets are displaced downward whereas the anterior leaflet is not displaced but is redundant (or "sail-like"). Lastly, the chordae tendinae and the papillary muscles of the tricuspid valve can also be abnormal.

The so-called "atrialized" right ventricle describes the proximal inlet portion of the right ventricle that is above the displaced tricuspid valve. The "functional" right ventricle is the remaining part of the right ventricle that lies below the displaced tricuspid valve. In addition to the usual regurgitation, the abnormal tricuspid valve can also be stenotic or even imperforate.

Associated Lesions

Ebstein's anomaly is associated with atrial septal defect, pulmonary atresia or stenosis, patent ductus arteriosus, and corrected transposition of the great arteries. In addition, an increased incidence is seen of pre-excitation syndrome.

PATHOPHYSIOLOGY

The severe tricuspid regurgitation leads to (a) a dilated right atrium with right-to-left shunting at the atrial level and decreased pulmonary blood flow, and (b) compromised left ventricular filling from encroachment by the dilated right ventricle. In some patients, tricuspid regurgitation leads to mild to moderate cyanosis and minimal volume overload to the right ventricle.

Usually an interatrial communication (patent foramen ovale or atrial septal defect) is seen that creates right-to-left shunting at the atrial level and results in cyanosis. In addition, several mechanisms can lead to decreased or absent antegrade flow to the pulmonary arteries in the neonate with Ebstein's anomaly: (a) anatomic pulmonary stenosis or atresia, (b) subpulmonary obstruction due to the abnormal tricuspid valve tissue, (c) elevated pulmonary vascular resistance during the newborn period, and (d) tricuspid regurgitation so severe that the ability of the right

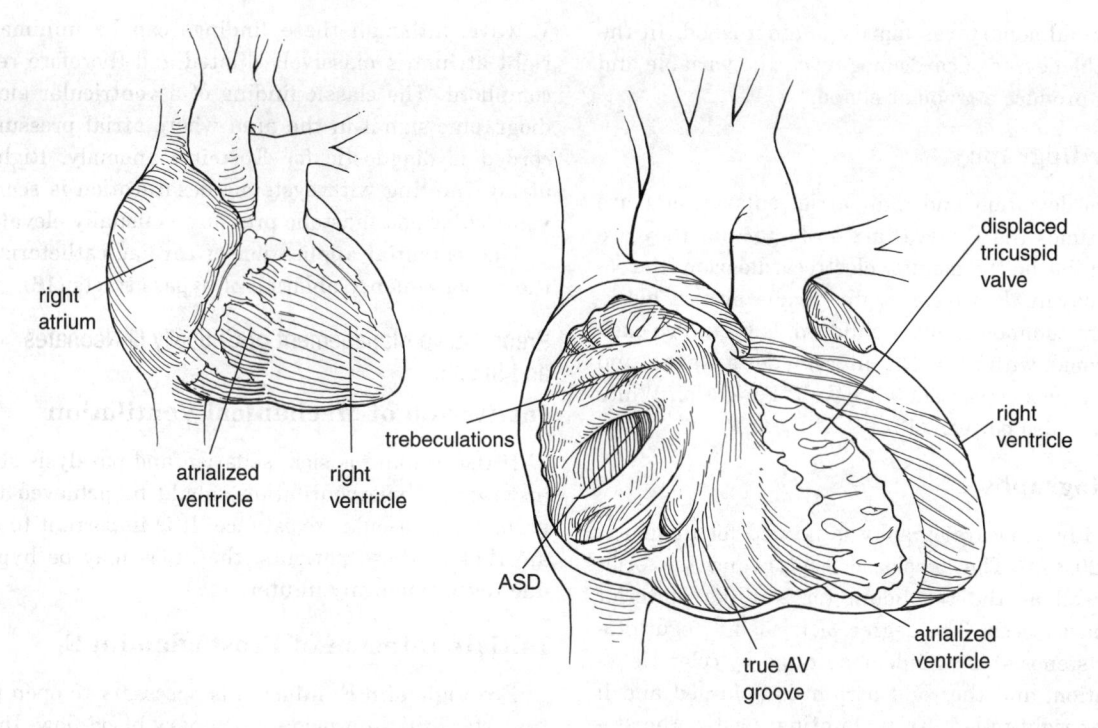

Figure 20.3.1. External cardiac and internal cardiac anatomy of Ebstein's anomaly. **A.** The enlarged right atrium, the atrialized portion of the right ventricle, which is typically thin walled and dilated, and the small right ventricular chamber. **B.** A cross section through the right atrium and right ventricle. Note the hypertrophied trebeculations in the right atrial chamber, the presence of an atrial septal defect (ASD), the absence of the tricuspid valve in the true atrioventricular groove, the thin portion of atrialized right ventricle, the displaced abnormal tricuspid valve within the right ventricular cavity, and the small right ventricular chamber.

ventricle to eject blood to the pulmonary circulation is impaired (the so-called "functional" or "pseudo" pulmonary atresia) (5). The tricuspid regurgitant volume leads to a severely dilated right ventricle and this in turn compromises filling and function of the left ventricle, which may have pathologic fibrosis (6).

Clinical Course

Cyanosis is the most common presentation in infancy (7). Cyanosis in the absence of other symptoms can be managed conservatively because hypoxemia may improve once pulmonary vascular resistance falls (see above). Neonates with severe tricuspid regurgitation, however, can present within a few hours of life with both cyanosis and congestive heart failure with circulatory collapse and metabolic acidosis. As a result of sustained atrial enlargement and/or coexisting conduction bypass tracts, supraventricular tachydysrhythmias can also be a presenting problem. The mortality rate is high (almost 20%) when patients present as neonates (8).

If the patient survives beyond the neonatal period, it appears that median age of survival is about 13 years (9). The older child can exhibit dyspnea on exertion and fatigability consistent with congestive heart failure. In addition, supraventricular tachydysrhythmias (10) can be a significant cause for death in older patients. Neurologic complications, such as cerebrovascular accidents and brain abscesses as well as infective endocarditis can also occur. Lastly, left ventricular dysfunction occurs due to the dilated right ventricle and resultant right-to-left bowing of the interventricular septum (11, 12).

SURGERY

Preoperative Evaluation

Physical Examination

In neonates and older infants, cyanosis is usually present. Regurgitant systolic murmur, caused by tricuspid regurgitation and located to the left of the sternum, can also be heard. Right ventricular delayed emptying can lead to a widely split S_2 as well as a gallop rhythm.

In older patients, cyanosis is also present in varying degrees. As in neonates, a holosystolic systolic murmur along the left sternal border as well as a gallop rhythm can be auscultated.

Chest Roentgenogram

In the neonate, cardiomegaly can be extreme; it is principally due to the massively enlarged right atrium. In addition, usually pulmonary vascularity is diminished. In the older child, the degree of cardiomegaly can be variable and at times can produce a globular shape.

Electrocardiography

Right axis deviation and right atrial enlargement are present. At times the P waves are so large that they are easily discernible on the monitor electrocardiogram (the so-called "himalayan" P waves). Right bundle branch block, which is more common in older children, is seen. Pre-excitation syndrome, with short PR interval, delta waves, and wide QRS complex consistent with Wolff-Parkinson-White syndrome, can also be seen (13).

Echocardiography

Usually only echocardiography is needed for diagnosis (14) (Fig. 20.3.2). The displaced septal and posterior leaflets as well as the redundant (or sail-like) anterior leaflet are easily seen. The degree of tricuspid regurgitation (and/or stenosis) is well demonstrated by color Doppler examination, and the right atrium is enlarged and it demonstrates right-to-left atrial shunting. Lastly, the status of pulmonary blood flow needs to be established.

Cardiac Catheterization

Previously considered a higher risk, cardiac catheterization is usually not indicated, but it may be performed to assess patency of the pulmonary valve (15). Characteristic findings include elevated right atrial pressure with a tall V wave, although these findings can be minimal if the right atrium is massively dilated and therefore relatively compliant. The classic finding of a ventricular electrocardiographic signal in the area where atrial pressure is recorded is diagnostic for Ebstein's anomaly. Right-to-left atrial shunting with systemic desaturation is seen. Right ventricular end-diastolic pressure is usually elevated.

One potential application of cardiac catheterization is the radiofrequency ablation of bypass tracts (16).

Preoperative Management of Critically Ill Neonates and Infants

Institution of Mechanical Ventilation

If the neonate is sick, sedation and paralysis should be instituted. Hyperventilation should be achieved to lower pulmonary vascular resistance. It is important to appreciate that in these patients, the lungs may be hypoplastic due to cardiomegaly in utero (17).

Initiate Infusion of Prostaglandin E_1

Prostaglandin E_1 infusion is necessary to open the ductus arteriosus to provide pulmonary blood flow. In certain neonates, weaning off prostaglandin E_1 is tolerated once pulmonary vascular resistance falls.

Measures to Lower Pulmonary Vascular Resistance

See Chapter 32, *Pulmonary Hypertension*, for additional information.

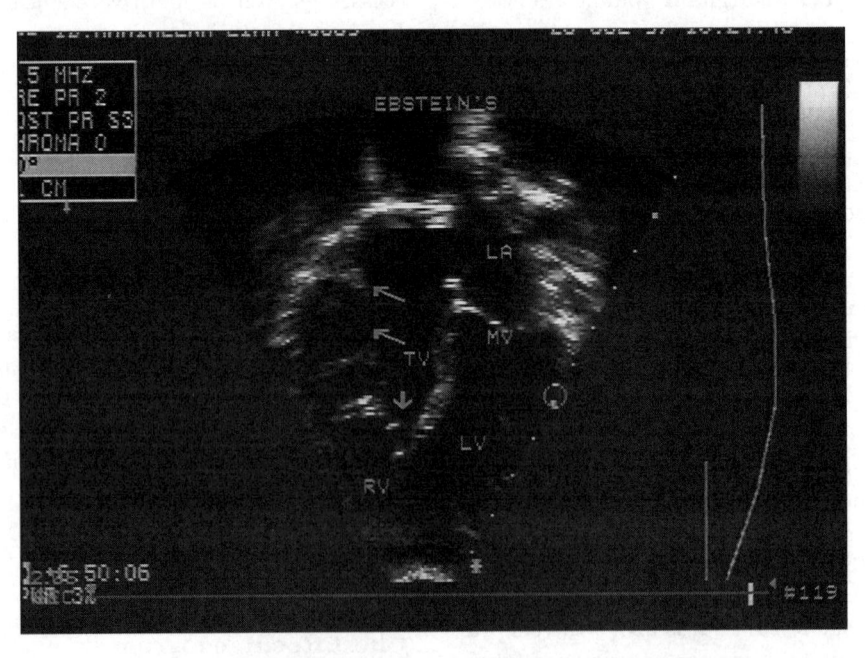

Figure 20.3.2. Apical four-chamber view in a child with Ebstein's anomaly. The septal leaflet of the triscupid valve is displaced downward toward the apex of the right ventricle (RV) (*arrow*). LA, left atrium; LV, left ventricle; MV, mitral valve; TV, tricuspid valve.

Correction of Metabolic Acidosis

Poor cardiac output can lead to metabolic acidosis; relief of acidosis will improve myocardial dysfunction. In addition, metabolic acidosis is also a stimulus for an undesired increase in pulmonary vascular resistance.

Appropriate Use of Inotropic Agents

Low cardiac output in this defect is caused both by decreased pulmonary blood flow and by decreased compliance of the left ventricle, which is encroached on by the dilated right ventricle. Avoid use of epinephrine if possible because it can further increase pulmonary vascular resistance.

Avoid Excessive Volume Infusions

Overzealous fluid administration can lead to further annular dilation and aggravate the tricuspid regurgitation. Despite the tricuspid regurgitation, the central venous pressure can be low (less than 10 mm Hg) because the right atrium is compliant.

Note. Central venous lines should be inserted with particular caution because the patient may be at higher risk due to tachyarrhythmias and a thin-walled, dilated right atrium that may perforate.

Surgical Procedures

Timing

Neonates who present critically ill have a very poor prognosis, with mortality up to 75% (18). When renal, neurologic, and pulmonary status are stable, surgery should be performed without further delay. Surgery is indicated in the symptomatic older child with congestive heart failure or severe cyanosis (oxygen saturation less than 80%), and it may be indicated in the child with cardiomegaly, paradoxical embolism, or intractable dysrhythmias.

Techniques

The results of surgical intervention in the neonate with Ebstein's anomaly has been poor.

Systemic-Pulmonary Shunt A systemic-to-pulmonary shunt to provide a source of pulmonary blood flow carries a high mortality (19).

Palliative Surgery One promising palliative surgery consists of plication of right atrial tissue, atrial septectomy, insertion of an aortopulmonary shunt, and patch closure of the tricuspid valve annulus (thus surgically creating tricuspid atresia) with the coronary sinus below the patch (20). This surgical strategy commits the neonate to future single ventricle palliations that include either a bidirectional cavopulmonary anastomosis (21) or a Fontan operation.

Orthotopic Cardiac Transplantation An alternative approach is orthotopic cardiac transplantation (22). See Chapter 21, *Pediatric Heart and Lung Transplantation*.

In children with noncritical Ebstein's anomaly, several other surgical options exist.

Tricuspid Valvuloplasty or Replacement Through a median sternotomy and under cardiopulmonary bypass, the atrial septal defect is closed. A decision is made intraoperatively regarding the necessity of tricuspid valve replacement (Fig. 20.3.3). Plication of excessive right atrial tissue may be undertaken. Tricuspid valve valvuloplasty consists of plastic reconstruction of both the valve and the right ventricle (23) or a variation that consists of plication of the atrialized right ventricle, posterior tricuspid annuloplasty, and right atrial reduction (24). Tricuspid valve replacement consists of initial excision of the tricuspid valve tissue, followed by securing the prosthetic valve to the atrioventricular ring with placement of the prosthetic valve above the coronary sinus to decrease the likelihood of heart block (25).

Recently, a new technical modification by Carpentier et al. with vertical plication of the right ventricle and reimplantation of the tricuspid valve leaflets has been successful (26). In some patients, interruption of coexisting accessory bypass tracts is performed. Significant improvement in exercise tolerance has been reported after tricuspid valve surgery (27).

Fontan Operation The Fontan operation is reserved for older children in whom the right ventricle cannot be salvaged as a functional ventricle (28). See Chapter 18, *Single Ventricle Lesions*, for additional information.

Mortality

In most centers, mortality for palliative surgery for Ebstein's anomaly is high, although Starnes (20) reported no deaths in five neonates in his series. In older children, surgery for the tricuspid valve ranges from 0 to 25% in this patient population with the mortality rate for replacement usually higher than that for annuloplasty (29–31).

Postoperative Management

The neonates with Ebstein's anomaly who underwent the palliative surgery described above can be among the most critically ill neonates in the cardiac intensive care setting. In other children, postoperative care is individualized to the type of surgery. Ideal monitoring consists of arterial and central venous pressure lines. In addition, atrial and ventricular temporary pacing wires are particularly useful in patients with this lesion.

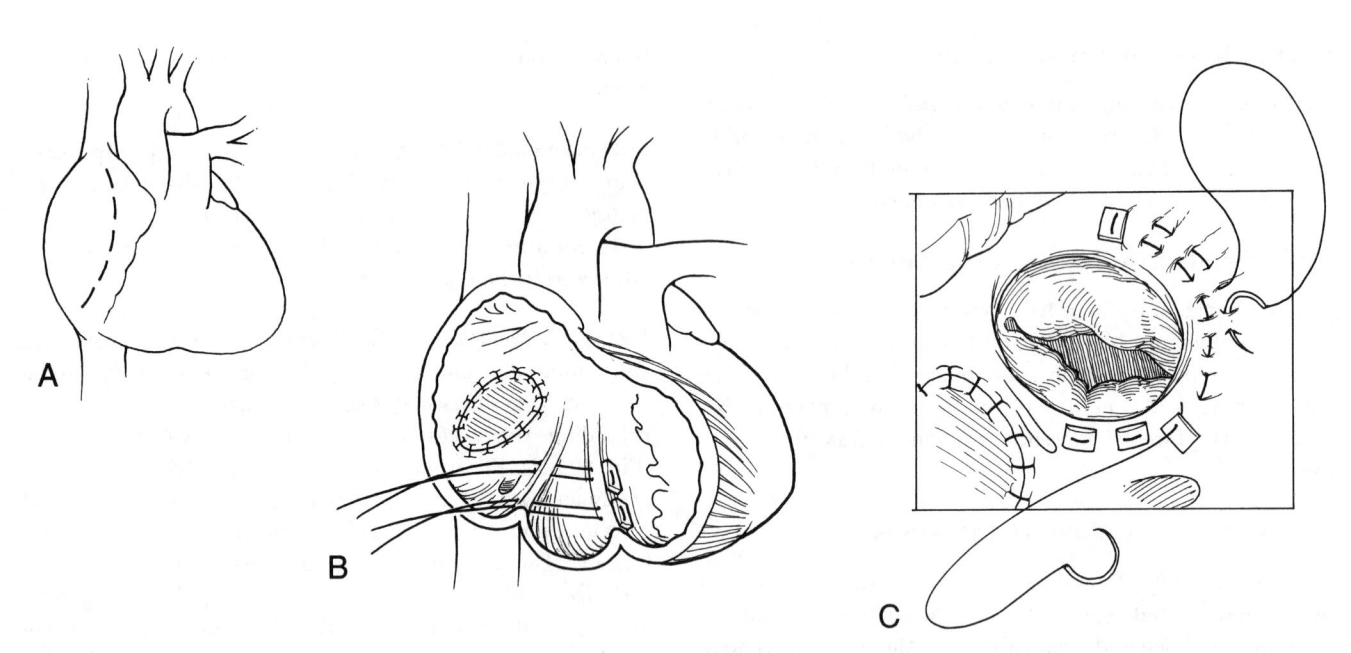

Figure 20.3.3. Repair of Ebstein's anomaly. Cardiopulmonary bypass with moderate hypothermia and cardioplegic is used. **A.** The external anatomy and site of the right atrial incision are shown. **B.** The atrial septal defect has been repaired with a patch and the atrialized portion of the right ventricle is plicated with pledgetted sutures. This reduces the volume of the dilated atrialized ventricle and creates a ridge of tissue against which the large sail-like anterior tricuspid valve leaflet can abut to improve competence of the abnormal tricuspid valve. **C.** An annuloplasty at the level of the valve annulus is performed to further improve competency of the abnormal valve by reducing the valve orifice.

Specific Postoperative Problems

Low Cardiac Output

In critically ill neonates after the palliative surgery, tricuspid valve regurgitation leads to right ventricular dilation and the left ventricle may not be able to adequately fill and provide sufficient cardiac output. In addition, as a result of the palliative operation, a potential "circular" shunt can occur: blood can traverse from the aortopulmonary shunt downward through the pulmonary valve, back into the right atrium from tricuspid regurgitation, to the left atrium via an interatrial communication, and out the left ventricle and aorta. This ineffective circulation can lead to metabolic acidosis. Inotropic support with judicious use of volume is the mainstay of therapy.

Pulmonary Insufficiency

In the neonate with severe Ebstein's anomaly, lung hypoplasis can complicate this disease; and it is underappreciated (32). Attention needs to be directed to maintaining ventilation at functional residual capacity and avoiding unnecessary overdistension and hyperinflation.

Residual Tricuspid Regurgitation

In both the neonate and child with residual tricuspid regurgitation, inotropic support with afterload reduction and judicious volume support can ameliorate the tricuspid regurgitation.

Postoperative Dysrhythmias

Postoperative dysrhythmias can occur with any of the above surgeries because of the intrinsic abnormalities of the conduction system in this defect. Supraventricular tachycardia is not uncommon. Ventricular tachycardia and fibrillation have led to mortality in postoperative patients (33). In addition, the incidence of heart block appears to be higher with tricuspid valve replacement (versus annuloplasty), and it has been reported to be as high as 20% after tricuspid valve replacement (34). See Chapter 30, *Diagnosis and Management of Cardiac Arrhythmias*, for additional information.

POSTOPERATIVE CARE CHECKLIST

Postoperative care checklist includes:

- Appreciation for right ventricular volume overload and failure with left ventricular compliance compromise.
- Institute measures to reduce pulmonary vascular resistance.
- Attention to supraventricular and ventricular arrhythmias.

- If mechanical valve is placed, anticoagulation needs to be initiated.

REFERENCES

1. Hornberger LK, Sahn DJ, Kleinman CS, et al. Tricuspid valve disease with significant tricuspid insufficiency in the fetus: diagnosis and outcome. J Am Coll Cardiol 1991;17:167–173.
2. Celermajer DS, Bull C, Till JA, et al. Ebstein's anomaly: presentation and outcome form fetus to adult. J Am Coll Cardiol 1994;23:170–176.
3. Nora JJ, Nora AH, Toews WH. Lithium, Ebstein's anomaly, and other congenital heart defects. Lancet 1974;2:594.
4. Van Mierop LHS, Gessner IH. Pathogenic mechanisms in congenital cardiovascular malformations. Prog Cardiovasc Dis 1972;15:67–75.
5. Smallhorn JF, Iukawa T, Benson L, et al. Noninvasive recognition of functional pulmonary atresia by echocardiography. Am J Cardiol 1984;54:925–926.
6. Celermajer DS, Dodd SM, Greenwald SE, et al. Morbid anatomy in neonates with Ebstein's anomaly of the tricuspid valve: pathophysiologic and clinical implications. J Am Coll Cardiol 1992;19:1049–1053.
7. Mayer FE, Nadas AS, Ongley PA. Ebstein's anomaly: presentation of 10 cases. Circulation 1957;16:1057–1069.
8. Celermajer DS, Cullen S, Sullivan ID, et al. Outcome in neonates with Ebstein's anomaly. J Am Coll Cardiol 1992;19:1041–1046.
9. Kumar AJ, Fyler DC, Mettinen OS, et al. Ebstein's anomaly: clinical profile and natural history. Am J Cardiol 1971;28:84–95.
10. Kumar AE, Fyler DC, Miettinen OS, et al. Ebstein's anomaly: clinical profile and natural history. Am J Cardiol 1971;28:84–95.
11. Benson LN, Child JS, Schwaiger M, et al. Left ventricular geometry and function in adults with Ebsteins anomaly of the tricuspid valve. Circulation 1987;75:353–359.
12. Saxena A, Fong LV, Tristam M, et al. Left ventricular function in patients >20 years of age with Ebstein's anomaly of the tricuspid valve. Am J Cardiol 1991;67(2):217–219.
13. Smith WM, Gallagher JJ, Kerr CR, et al. The electrophysiologic basis and management of symptomatic recurrent tachycardia in patients with Ebstein's anomaly of the tricuspid valve. Am J Cardiol 1982;49:1223–1234.
14. Shiina A, Sewawrd JB, Edwards WD, et al. Two-dimensional echocardiographic spectrum of Ebstein's anomaly: detailed anatomic assessment. J Am Coll Cardiol 1984;3:356–370.
15. Freedom RM, Culham G, Moes F, et al. Differentiation of functional and structural pulmonary atresia: role of aortography. Am J Cardiol 1978;41:914–920.
16. Cappato R, Hebe J, Weib C, et al. Radiofrequency current ablation of accessory pathways in Ebstein's anomaly. J Am Coll Cardiol 1993;21(SupplA):172A.
17. Lang D, Obenhoffer R, Cook A, et al. Pathologic spectrum of malformations of the tricuspid valve in prenatal and neonatal life. J Am Coll Cardiol 1991;17:1161–1167.
18. Watson H. Natural history of Ebstein's anomaly of tricuspid valve in childhood and adolescence: an international cooperative study of 505 cases. Br Heart J 1974;36:417–427.
19. Roberson DA, Silverman NH. Ebstein's anomaly: echocardiographic and clinical features in the fetus and neonate. J Am Coll Cardiol 1989;14:1300–1307.
20. Starnes VA, Pitlick PT, Berstein D, et al. Ebstein's anomaly appearing in the neonate. J Thorac Cardiovasc Surg 1991;101:1082–1087.
21. McCredie RM, Oakley C, Mahoney EB, et al. Ebstein's disease: diagnosis by electrode catheter and treatment by partial bypass of the right side of the heart. N Engl J Med 1962;267:174–179.
22. Cabanero J, de Buruaga JS, Gomez JA, et al. Heart transplant in Ebstein's anomaly with endocardial fibroelastosis. Am Heart J 1992;124:532–534.
23. Carpentier A, Chauvaud S, Mace L. A new reconstructive operation for Ebstein's anomaly of the tricuspid valve. J Thorac Cardiovasc Surg 1988;96:92–101.
24. Danielson GK, Maloney JD, Devloo RAE. Surgical repair of Ebstein's anomaly. Mayo Clin Proc 1979;54:185–192.
25. Westaby S, Karp RB, Kirklin JW. Surgical treatment in Ebstein's malformation. Ann Thorac Surg 1982;34:388–395.
26. Carpentier A, Chauvaud S, Mace L, et al. A new reconstructive operation for Ebstein's anomaly of the tricuspid valve. J Thorac Cardiovasc Surg 1988;96:92–101.
27. Maclellan-Torbert SG, Driscoll DJ, Mottram CD, et al. Exercise tolerance in patients with Ebstein's anomaly. J Am Coll Cardiol 1997;29:1615–1622.
28. Marcelletti C, Duren DR, Schuilenburg RM, et al. Fontan's operation for Ebstein's anomaly. J Thorac Cardiovasc Surg 1980;79:63–70.
29. Mair DD, Seward JB, Driscoll DJ, et al. Surgical repair of Ebstein's anomaly: selection of patients and early and late operative results. Circulation 1985;72(Suppl II)II-70–II-76.
30. Quaegebeur JM, Sreeram N, Fraser AG, et al. Surgery for Ebstein's anomaly: the clinical and echocardiographic evaluation of a new technique. J Am Coll Cardiol 1991;17:722–728.
31. Danielson GK, Driscoll DJ, Mair DD, et al. Operative treatment of Ebstein's anomaly. J Thorac Cardiovasc Surg 1992;104:1195–1202.
32. Satomi G, Momoi N, Kikuchi N, et al. Prenatal diagnosis and outcome of Ebstein's anomaly and tricuspid valve dysplasia in relation to lung hypoplasia. Echocardiography 1994;11:215–219.
33. Danielson GK, Furster V. Surgical repair of Ebstein's anomaly. Ann Surg 1982;196:499–506.
34. Peterffy A, Bjork VO. Surgical treatment of Ebstein's anomaly: early and late results in seven consecutive cases. Scand J Thorac Cardiovasc Surg 1979;13:1–7.

20.4 Rings and Slings

Anthony C. Chang, MD, and Frank L. Hanley, MD

Rings and slings are usually isolated lesions that involve vascular structures, causing encirclement or encroachment on the esophagus and/or trachea to cause symptoms.

ANATOMY

Rings and slings are lesions that form as a result of abnormal development of the embryonic double arch, and they are best described by the Edwards double arch model (1).

Types of Vascular Rings

Double Aortic Arch

The double aortic arch is formed as a result of failure of either the right or the left arch to regress (Fig. 20.4.1). Usually, the right arch is the larger of the two and the left arch is the smaller. The left arch can even be atretic. A carotid and subclavian artery originates from both arches.

Right Aortic Arch with Aberrant Left Subclavian Artery

A right aortic arch with aberrant left subclavian artery results from persistence of the right fourth aortic arch. The ring is formed when the left subclavian artery courses behind the esophagus.

Pulmonary Artery Sling

With a pulmonary artery sling the left pulmonary artery has its origin from the proximal right pulmonary artery; during its leftward course to the left lung, it courses posteriorly to the trachea (2). The ligamentum arteriosum completes the vascular ring around the trachea (Fig. 20.4.2). The left pulmonary artery can be hypoplastic. A high incidence is found of complete tracheal rings, which are usually associated with decreased airway diameter and can be isolated or be a long segment (3).

Associated Lesions

Rings and slings can be associated with bronchial or tracheal stenosis or hypoplasia, right aortic arch, tetralogy of Fallot, and atrioventricular canal.

PATHOPHYSIOLOGY

The trachea and the esophagus are encircled by the vascular structures and respiratory and feeding difficulties arise.

In vascular rings, because both the esophagus and the trachea are encircled by the vascular structures, the infant

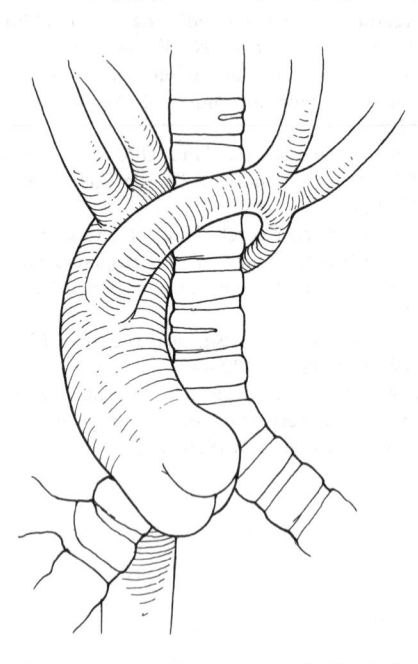

Figure 20.4.1. Anatomy of double aorta arch. Typically, right arch is larger than the left arch. The trachea and esophagus are encircled by the ring formed by the two arches.

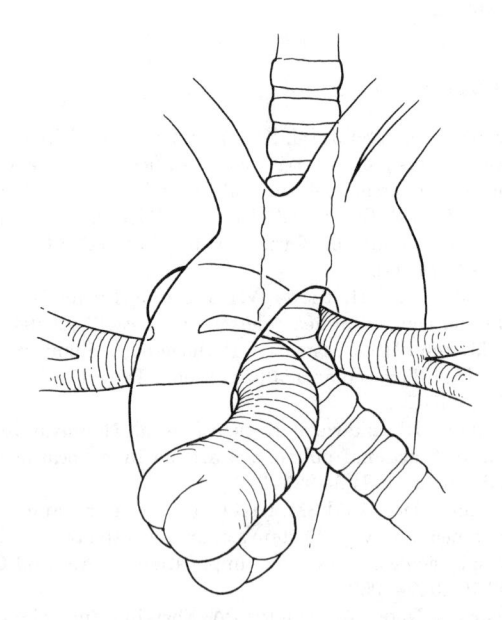

Figure 20.4.2. The anatomy of pulmonary artery sling is shown. The left pulmonary artery arises from the origin of the right pulmonary artery. The artery then passes between the trachea and esophagus. The left pulmonary artery may be moderately hypoplastic.

may have both feeding and respiratory difficulties. Pulmonary artery sling, on the other hand, presents with only respiratory problems.

Clinical Course

The infants present with tracheal compressions symptoms such as stridor, apnea, reactive airway disease, recurrent infections, noisy breathing, or persistent cough. Symptoms referable to esophageal compression are less common, but they include choking with feeding, emesis, and dysphagia.

SURGERY

Preoperative Evaluation

Physical Examination

Usually few physical findings are present. With compromise to the trachea, scattered wheezing may be present. In addition, respiratory distress can occur with neck hyperextension.

Chest Roentgenogram

Tracheal deviation suggesting a right aortic arch is seen. Tracheal narrowing or bowing and abnormal aeration of the lung parenchyma (4) may be seen as well. Hyperinflation of the right lung may be observed in infants with pulmonary artery slings.

Barium esophagram, which can be virtually diagnostic, may show characteristic patterns of indentations (right, left, and posterior for vascular rings and anterior for pulmonary artery sling).

Electrocardiography

Electrocardiograms are usually normal.

Echocardiography

Echocardiography imaging is useful to delineate the vascular ring anatomy (5, 6). Magnetic resonance imaging (MRI), especially with three-dimensional reconstruction, is superior to ultrasound in delineating vascular ring anatomy with fibrotic cords or interruption of structures. The tracheal anatomy should be carefully assessed with computerized tomography or MRI prior to surgery, especially for pulmonary artery sling. A bronchoscopy can also be indicated (7).

Cardiac Catheterization

An aortogram is rarely indicated.

Surgical Procedure

Timing

Surgery is indicated with presence of symptoms.

Technique

Vascular Rings Via a left posterolateral thoracotomy, either the smaller left arch (in double aortic arch) or the liga-

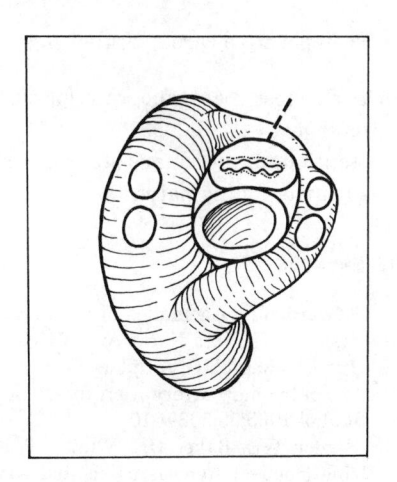

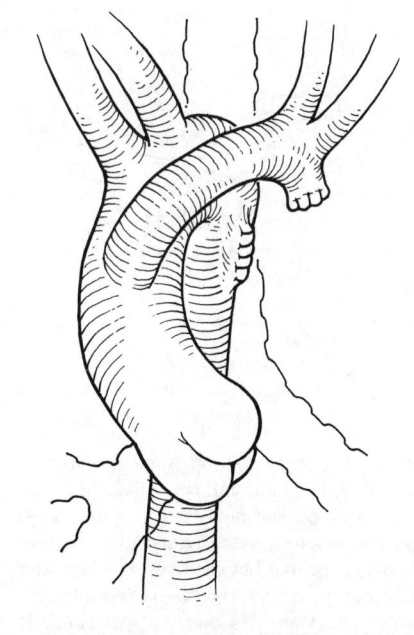

Figure 20.4.3. Repair of double aortic arch. Exposure is through a left thoracotomy in the typical case with hypoplastic left arch. The left arch is identified and divided at the segment connecting the left subclavian artery to the descending aorta. The ligament artenosum is also divided and adhesions, which may contribute to compression of the trachea and esophagus, are also released.

mentum (in right aortic arch with aberrant left subclavian artery) is divided to disrupt the continuity of the vascular ring (Fig. 20.4.3). The smaller left arch is divided between the left subclavian artery and the junction of the left arch with the descending thoracic aorta. In patients with a dominant left arch, a right thoracotomy needs to be performed (8).

Pulmonary Artery Sling In pulmonary artery sling, the left pulmonary artery is detached from its origin and reanastomosed to the main pulmonary artery via a median sternotomy and under cardiopulmonary bypass (although it can also be performed via a left thoracotomy) (Fig. 20.4.4). This reimplantation technique has been complicated by left pulmonary artery stenosis on follow-up (9). Jonas et al. have described a technique involving tracheal transection and mobilizing the left pulmonary artery forward, thus obviating the need for vascular anastomosis (10). The presence and extent of tracheal narrowing dictates the surgery required for the trachea, from no resection to tracheoplasty with autologous pericardium (11). Vascular rings have been divided using video-assisted thorascopic techniques (12).

Mortality

Operative mortality for all vascular rings has been reported to be less than 5% (13) and currently approaches 0% (14). Residual pulmonary dysfunction is not uncommon (15). For pulmonary artery slings, previous reports noted a high mortality rate (50%) with high incidence of residual tracheal or bronchial narrowing and left pulmonary artery stenosis (16), but recent reports indicating no mortality are more favorable.

Postoperative Management

Postoperative care of patients after these operative procedures is usually uneventful. Early extubation is usually done in the operating room.

Specific Postoperative Problems

Residual Lung Disease

Tracheomalacia can coexist with vascular rings, and it may partially explain residual respiratory symptoms even months after surgical division. Residual tracheal or bronchial narrowing is common after repair for pulmonary artery slings as well. In addition, a recurrent left laryngeal nerve can be injured. Attention to respiratory status as well as humidity, chest physiotherapy, and suctioning should aid in recovery. Prolonged intubation and mechanical ventilation can be a postoperative issue in the presence of tracheomalacia.

Mediastinal Complications

See Chapter 23, *Pulmonary Issues*, for additional information.

POSTOPERATIVE CARE CHECKLIST

Postoperative care checklist includes:

- Check chest roentgenogram for common intrathoracic problems.
- Attention to pulmonary status, particularly with pulmonary artery sling patients.

REFERENCES

1. Edwards JE. Anomalies of the derivatives of the aortic arch system. Med Clin North Am 1948;52:925–949.
2. Jue KL, Raghib G, Amplatz K, et al. Anomalous origin of the left pulmonary artery from the right pulmonary artery. Am J Radiol 1965;95:598–610.
3. Berdon WE, Baker DH, Wung JT, et al. Complete cartilage ring tracheal stenosis associated with anomalies left pulmonary artery: the ring-sling complex. Radiology 1984;152:47.
4. Pickhardt PJ, Siegel MJ, Gutierrez FR. Vascular rings in symptomatic children: frequency of chest radiographic findings. Radiology 1997;203:423–442.
5. Bissett GS, Strife JL, Kirks DR, et al. Vascular rings; MR imaging. AJR 1987;149:251–256.
6. Yeager SB, Chin AJ, Sanders SP. Two-dimensional echocardiographic diagnosis of pulmonary artery sling in infancy. J Am Coll Cardiol 1986;7:625–629.

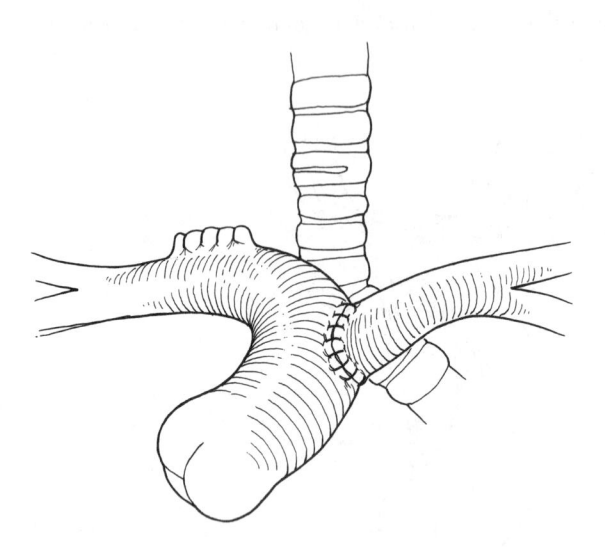

Figure 20.4.4. Repair of pulmonary artery sling. A mediansternotomy approach is advocated. Cardiopulmonary bypass may or may not be necessary depending on the details of the anatomy. In either case, the left pulmonary artery is divided at its origin and removed from its abnormal course between the trachea and esophagus. The left pulmonary artery is then reimplanted into the main pulmonary artery in its normal position. It should be noted that intrinsic tracheal abnormalities are common in this lesion. Tracheal resection and reanamosis may be indicated.

7. Hinton AE, O'Connell JM, van Besouw JP, et al. Neonatal and pediatric fiberoptic laryngocopy and bronchoscopy using the laryngeal mask airway. J Laryngol Otol 1997;111:349–353.
8. McFaul R, Millard P, Nowicki E. Vascular rings necessitating right thoracotomy. J Thorac Cardiovasc Surg 1981;82: 306–312.
9. Sade RM, Rosenthal AM, Fellows K, et al. Pulmonary artery sling. J Thorac Cardiovasc Surg 1975;69:333.
10. Jonas RA, Spevak PJ, McGill T, et al. Pulmonary artery sling: primary repair by tracheal resection in infancy. J Thorac Cardiovasc Surg 1989;97:548–550.
11. Backer CL, Idriss FS, Holinger LD, et al. Pulmonary artery sling: results of surgical repair in infancy. J Thorac Cardiovasc Surg 1992;103:683.
12. Burke RP, Chang AC. Video assisted-thorascopic division of a vascular ring in an infant: a new operative technique. J Cardiol Surg 1994;9:132–133.
13. Wychulis AR, Kincaid OW, Weidman WH, et al. Congenital vascular rings: surgical considerations and results of operation. Mayo Clin Proc 1971;46:182–188.
14. Backer CL, Ilbawi MN, Idriss FS, et al. Vascular anomalies causing tracheoesophageal compression. J Thorac Cardiovasc Surg 1989;97:725–731.
15. Marmon LM, Bye MR, Haas JM, et al. Vascular rings and slings: long-term follow-up of pulmonary function. J Ped Surg 1984;19:683–690.
16. Sade RM, Rosenthal A, Fellows K, et al. Pulmonary artery sling. J Thorac Cardiovasc Surg 1975;69:333–346.

Part C: Other Topics Relating to Cardiac Surgery
Pediatric Heart and Lung Transplantation 21

Pierre C. Wong, MD, and Vaughn A. Starnes, MD

Pediatric heart transplantation is now performed throughout the world in neonates, infants, and children for both severe congenital heart disease and cardiomyopathy. Current 30-day perioperative mortality for all children is approximately 15 to 20% (1) and the 1- and 5-year actuarial survival is 75 to 80% and 60 to 75%, respectively, with institutional variation (1–6). Experience with pediatric heart-lung and lung transplantation has also grown substantially in recent years. The 1- and 5-year survival rates for heart-lung transplant recipients are approximately 60 and 40% in children; the 24-month survival for double lung transplant recipients is about 60% (1, 7). The leading cause of early death in these patients is infection whereas obliterative bronchiolitis (chronic rejection) accounts for many late deaths following transplant. Satisfactory results for heart-lung and lung transplantation have also been obtained in infants (8). This chapter provides an introduction to pediatric heart and lung transplantation, with an emphasis on perioperative management.

PATIENT SELECTION FOR TRANSPLANTATION
General Considerations

The challenge of organ transplantation is to maximize survival and improve quality of life. Transplantation is not a cure; it carries known attrition rates because of acute and chronic rejection, infection, and other complications. It would not be prudent to prematurely transplant organs in patients who still had potentially years of good quality life with their failing organs. It would also be suboptimal, however, to wait too long to list a patient for transplantation—poor pretransplant clinical status significantly increases the likelihood of an adverse postoperative outcome and may even preclude transplantation (1, 9, 10). Timely intervention is even more important currently because the increasing shortage of donor organs almost guarantees a longer waiting period, sometimes in excess of 1 year. As a general rule, potential candidates should have decreased quality of life and limited potential for long-term survival, with an estimated remaining life span of no more than 1 to 2 years. Unfortunately, this determination is not always easy. When in doubt, a suggested policy has been to list a patient for transplantation too early rather than too late.

Once referred for transplantation, patients undergo a comprehensive evaluation involving relevant medical subspecialists and extensive laboratory testing (Table 21.1). Not all patients referred for transplantation will be accepted because several contraindications do exist (11); over the years, however, these contraindications have become more relative than absolute (Table 21.2).

Patients listed for heart transplantation are designated either status I or status II, with status I patients taking precedence whenever a donor becomes available. To qualify as status I, patients must be hospitalized in the intensive care unit and be receiving mechanical support or intravenous inotropic therapy. Infants less than 6 months of age are the exception—they are automatically designated status I regardless of their medical condition. Status II is composed of all other heart transplant candidates not fulfilling the criteria for status I. These patients are generally less critically ill than status I patients, and presumably the need for transplantation is not as urgent. For lung and heart-lung transplant candidates, only status II exists. Consequently, the waiting time for these organs tends to be longer than that for a heart alone, and potential recipients should be evaluated and listed earlier.

Indications for Heart Transplantation

Pediatric heart transplant candidates fall into two general categories: (*a*) patients with cardiomyopathy (primary and secondary) and (*b*) patients with congenital heart disease (CHD). In the early days of pediatric heart transplantation, most patients received a transplant for cardiomyopathy and most of these patients were school-age or older. This trend has changed considerably in the 1990s, with an ever-increasing number of heart transplants being performed in younger patients, and in a greater proportion in children with CHD (12).

In addition to the general contraindications listed in Table 21.2, another risk factor specific for heart transplantation is elevated pulmonary vascular resistance (PVR) (13). This condition can cause the unprepared donor right ventricle to fail—leading to a low output state and increased risk of postoperative morbidity and mortality (14). Several studies have clearly demonstrated a significantly increased risk of mortality when PVR exceeds 2.5 Wood units or when indexed PVR exceeds 6 WU·m^2 (15, 16). It appears that pulmonary vasoreactivity, however, rather than a single PVR measured at baseline, is more important in determining suitability for transplantation (12, 17–19). Some

Table 21.1. Pretransplant Testing

Primary Medical and Psychosocial Evaluations
  Surgeon
  Cardiologist
  Pulmonologist
  Transplant Coordinator
  Social Worker
Ancillary Medical Evaluations (if necessary)
  Infectious diseases
  Psychiatry
  Nephrology
  Neurology
  Gastroenterology
Blood Tests
  ABO type
  Electrolytes, blood chemistries (including liver/renal function tests)
  Complete blood count/differential
  Viral serologies (HIV; CMV; EBV; hepatitis A, B, C; herpes simplex, etc.)
  HLA typing
  Panel reactive antibody (PRA)
Other testing (as indicated)
  Chest roentgenogram
  Cardiac catheterization
  Echocardiogram
  Electrocardiogram
  Pulmonary function testing (PFT)
  Chest CT scan
  Head CT scan

CT, computed tomography; CMV, cytomegalovirus; EBV, Epstein-Barr virus; HIV, human immunodeficiency virus.

Table 21.2. Contraindications to Transplantation

Recent or recurrent malignancy
Serious active or recurrent infection (e.g., human immunodeficiency virus, hepatitis B)
Significant systemic disease (e.g., diabetes, systemic lupus erythematosus)
Chromosomal, metabolic, or genetic abnormality with poor long-term prognosis
Other organ system disease (hepatic, renal, neurologic)
Psychosocial instability

patients with an indexed PVR greater than 6 WU · m² will demonstrate a marked reduction in pulmonary resistance when treated with pulmonary vasodilators such as nitric oxide, nitroprusside, or prostaglandin E_1 (PGE_1) (12, 20–24); this reduced PVR accurately predicts the resultant PVR after transplantation (14, 25). Other patients will not initially respond to vasodilator challenge in the catheterization laboratory, but they subsequently exhibit dramatic reduction in PVR following 3 to 7 days of intravenous (IV) therapy with inotropes (dobutamine, dopamine) and vasodilators (nitroprusside, amrinone) (26). When a high, fixed PVR (more than 6–8 WU · m²) is present that is nearly or completely unresponsive to vasodilators, many centers will not consider the patient a suitable candidate for heart transplantation. Heart-lung transplantation (or rarely, heterotopic transplantation) becomes the only alternative.

Cardiomyopathy

The term "cardiomyopathy" refers to a disease process afflicting cardiac muscle and interfering with normal myocardial function. It results from many causes, some representing primary myocardial disease (congenital or acquired), whereas others are manifestations of more global, systemic disease with secondary myocardial involvement (see Chapter 31, *The Failing Myocardium*).

Because of the unpredictable natural history observed in children with dilated cardiomyopathy, presently no widely accepted clinical or laboratory criteria exist that could help distinguish children who should be listed for transplantation. Ultimately the decision for transplantation in the pediatric patient has remained an individualized process, with multiple factors—including weight gain, quality of life, number of hospitalizations and medications, and clinical course—involved in the decision-making process. One important risk factor, elevated pulmonary vascular resistance, which signifies a more advanced stage of disease, is associated with a higher risk of mortality following transplantation for cardiomyopathy (3). Prolonged increase in pulmonary artery pressures may eventually result in a fixed, elevated PVR. Early and significant elevation is also seen in the setting of restrictive cardiomyopathy (15). Therefore, pulmonary hypertension in the setting of cardiomyopathy necessitates aggressive medical management, and perhaps early referral for transplantation.

Congenital Heart Disease

Patients with CHD considered for transplantation can be divided into two subgroups. The first subgroup is composed of patients with complex CHD for which no good anatomic surgical repair exists. It has been estimated that perhaps 10% of all patients born with CHD in the United States fit this description (27).

Transplantation has already been performed as therapy for many types of complex CHD (28, 29). In some, it serves as the sole, definitive operation. In others, palliative surgery is first performed to stabilize the patient and therefore serve as a "bridge" to subsequent cardiac transplantation (30, 31). A list of anatomic lesions that can be considered for cardiac transplantation is provided in Table

Table 21.3. Potentially Transplantable Congenital Heart Lesions

Hypoplastic left ventricle syndrome and variants
Severe Shone's syndrome
Severe Ebstein's anomaly of tricuspid valve
Atrioventricular septal defects with unbalanced ventricles
Complex d-transposition with intervening atrioventricular valve tissue
Pulmonary atresia/intact ventricular septum, sinusoids, myocardial dysfunction
Anomalous left coronary artery with irreversible myocardial dysfunction
Multiple cardiac tumors with concomitant myocardial dysfunction

21.3. For these defects, considerable debate exists about the medical and surgical management; every institution has its own management philosophy and definition of operability (20, 32). Substantial anatomic variability seen in many of the lesions further complicates the decision.

The prototype lesion in this group—and the one for which transplantation is most compelling—is hypoplastic left heart syndrome (HLHS). In such patients, enthusiasm for the reconstructive surgical alternative, the Norwood procedure, is mixed. This repair is currently offered in only a few large centers, with a wide variation in reported results (27, 33, 34). At best, collective short and long-term experience with the Norwood repair has been marginal, and therefore transplantation has become a realistic alternative. Results of transplantation for HLHS have been good (27, 35); because of lack of donor availability, however, a significant proportion (up to 40%) either die before transplantation or become too sick to undergo transplantation.

Even less experience is currently available with transplantation for other forms of complex CHD, such as vere Ebstein's anomaly. As more data accumulate, it seems likely that transplantation will become an increasingly accepted alternative for those complex CHD lesions with generally unfavorable short to long-term surgical outcomes. Even patients with visceral heterotaxy (asplenia) and complex CHD can receive a transplant with acceptable results; contrary to expectations, they have neither an increased propensity for infection nor a decreased risk of rejection (36).

The second subgroup of CHD patients considered for transplantation consists of those who have previously undergone surgical repair, but subsequently have developed an irreversible and uncorrectable abnormality of anatomy, physiology, or myocardial function. Examples in this group include patients with a failed Fontan operation (4), complex CHD with severe atrioventricular (AV) valve regurgitation, and right ventricle (RV) dysfunction following Norwood procedure for HLHS or after atrial switch procedure (Mustard or Senning). In these clinical situations, the challenge is to determine the optimal time for transplantation. Even less information is available about myocardial dysfunction in this setting; unlike dilated cardiomyopathy, however, these patients are even less likely to have reversible myocardial dysfunction. It is unclear whether these patients are at higher risk because of the history of previous cardiac surgery and exposure to blood products (which can lead to formation of anti-HLA antibodies). One report documented significantly poorer survival following cardiac transplantation for this group of patients as compared with children with dilated cardiomyopathy; most deaths were caused by intractable rejection (37). Other centers, however, have reported no difference in long-term post-transplant survival between patients with dilated cardiomyopathy and those with CHD (38, 39).

Indications for Lung and Heart-Lung Transplantation

Cumulative experience with pediatric lung transplantation has grown dramatically in the past few years (1). Potential candidates for lung transplantation include those patients with untreatable pulmonary vascular or parenchymal pathology (40–42); indications for pediatric lung transplantation are given in Table 21.4. Lung transplantation can also be performed in conjunction with cardiac re-

Table 21.4. Indications for Lung and Heart-Lung Transplantation

Indications for Lung Transplantation
  Diseases of pulmonary parenchyma
    Cystic fibrosis
    Severe bronchopulmonary dysplasia
    Idiopathic pulmonary fibrosis
    Rheumatoid lung
    Desquamative interstitial pneumonitis
    Congenital diaphragmatic hernia
    Obliterative bronchiolitis (idiopathic, post-transplant)
    Surfactant B deficiency
    Emphysema
  Diseases of pulmonary vasculature
    Severe primary pulmonary hypertension
    Diffuse branch pulmonary artery stenosis or hypoplasia
    Congenital pulmonary vein stenosis
    Diffuse pulmonary arteriovenous fistulae causing severe cyanosis
    Eisenmenger's with repairable congenital heart disease
Indications for Heart-Lung Transplantation
  Cardiomyopathy with long-standing, irreversible pulmonary hypertension
  Severe, unrepairable congenital heart disease with significant pulmonary abnormalities
    Irreversible pulmonary vascular disease (Eisenmenger's)
    Abnormally small or absent central pulmonary arteries (e.g., tetralogy of Fallot)
    Associated pulmonary vein stenosis
  Severe pulmonary vascular/parenchymal disease and coexisting myocardial dysfunction

pair (e.g., in patients with Eisenmenger's syndrome due to a reparable form of CHD). This technique has been performed successfully for simple cardiac lesions using both single and double lung transplantation (43, 44). Preliminary results with lung transplantation and cardiac repair in more complex forms of CHD (e.g., tetralogy of Fallot with pulmonary atresia) have been marginal (40, 45).

Newer techniques have been developed to further address the donor organ shortage seen in pediatric patients. Specifically these techniques include single lung and lobar (including living donor-related lobar) transplantation. Single lung transplantation has been proposed as an alternative to conventional double lung transplantation for conditions such as primary pulmonary hypertension, pulmonary fibrosis, and emphysema (40, 46, 47). No consensus of opinion exists, but given the progressive, bilateral nature of most pediatric pulmonary diseases, and the potential requirements for growth in the pediatric patient, double lung transplantation appears to be the preferred option (39). Lobar transplantation (both cadaveric and living-related) represents a new and intriguing option for pediatric patients (48, 49). Cadaveric lobar transplants have been successfully performed in patients with Eisenmenger's syndrome, primary pulmonary hypertension, and congenital diaphragmatic hernia. Living-related lobar transplantation has been used primarily in patients with cystic fibrosis. In this procedure, a lower lobe is harvested from each of two living-related donors; both lobes are sequentially transplanted into the recipient. This form of transplantation carries the advantage of obviating a long waiting time because of donor shortages; intermediate-term results have been encouraging (50, 51).

Candidates for heart-lung transplantation can be divided into three separate groups (see Table 21.4). In general, these patients have severe pulmonary parenchymal or vascular disease accompanied by uncorrectable myocardial anatomic or functional abnormalities. When deciding between lung versus heart-lung transplantation in patients with pulmonary disease, the critical issue is usually the status of left ventricular function. Decreased right ventricular function in these patients, especially in the setting of pulmonary hypertension, is not a contraindication; studies have shown excellent potential for long-term RV function recovery after lung transplantation alone (52, 53).

PREOPERATIVE CARE FOR PATIENTS UNDERGOING TRANSPLANTATION

Although most patients are well enough to await transplantation as an outpatient, a subset—the status I heart transplant candidates—require intensive care prior to transplantation. Because this group of patients is at significantly higher risk for post-transplant morbidity and mortality (2), good pretransplant management is vital to achieve a greater likelihood of a successful outcome. This strategy includes maintaining stable hemodynamic and ventilatory status, maximizing nutritional support (either by enteral supplements or total parenteral nutrition), and preventing iatrogenic complications and nosocomial infections. Some patients will have strict fluid restrictions, but even with these exigencies it is vital to provide as much caloric support as possible. Routine but meticulous surveillance of all organ systems is needed, particularly the renal and hepatic systems.

If significant myocardial dysfunction is present, anticoagulation (with heparin or warfarin) may be required to prevent formation of intracardiac thrombi. When myocardial dysfunction is severe, however, mechanical circulatory support may be necessary as a bridge to transplantation. A variety of mechanical devices have been developed and successfully used for adult patients, including intra-aortic balloon pump, univentricular and biventricular assist devices, and the total artificial heart (54–58). Options for mechanical assist in pediatric patients, however, are more limited (see Chapter 22, *Mechanical Support of the Myocardium*).

Patients with HLHS pose particular challenges prior to transplantation. Among the pretransplant management goals in these patients is appropriate balance of the pulmonary:systemic flow ratio, using measures designed to increase pulmonary vascular resistance (see Chapter 18, *Single Ventricle Lesions*). Because PGE_1 is also a potent pulmonary vasodilator, several groups have reported the alternative of stenting of the ductus arteriosus in the cardiac catheterization laboratory (59, 60). In addition, banding of the pulmonary artery has also been suggested as a means of controlling pulmonary blood flow (61). Although successful transplantation after 5 months has been reported for HLHS (60), significant deterioration usually begins after 2 to 3 weeks or even sooner. Patients with HLHS and restrictive atrial septum represent an even higher risk subset for transplantation (60, 62).

SURGICAL ASPECTS OF TRANSPLANTATION

Donor and Recipient Considerations

Heart transplant candidates are listed by blood type and desired donor weight range. For infant heart transplants, donors weighing up to 300% more than the recipient can be successfully used (24); for older recipients, however, body weight of the donor should be 50 to 100%. A large donor-to-recipient size mismatch appears to be well-tolerated (63), but a donor weighing less than 25% of the recipient should not be used (24). Recent studies have shown that the transplanted heart grows proportionately with the body, and output is sufficient to sustain normal organ growth (64). It is preferable to use an oversized donor heart in recipients with pre-existing elevated PVR. Lung and heart-lung recipients are listed by blood type and desired height. Donor and recipient lungs must be closely matched to avoid significant under or oversizing of the lungs.

Maximal acceptable ischemic time varies with institution, but it is usually 6 to 8 hours for a heart transplant (up to 10 hours in some institutions) and 6 hours for a lung or heart-lung transplant. Cardiopulmonary bypass is used in virtually all cases of pediatric thoracic transplantation.

Technique of Heart Transplantation

Orthotopic heart transplantation technique is shown in Figure 21.1. Transesophageal echocardiography is used to assess atrial and arterial anastomoses as well as ventricular function (65). A variation of the technique is bicaval superior vena cava and inferior vena cava (SVC/IVC) anastomosis, which leaves intact the donor right atrium, thereby improving cardiovascular dynamics, minimizing possible injury to the sinus node, and reducing the risk of atrial arrhythmias (66–68).

In patients with CHD, abnormalities of systemic and pulmonary venous return, as well as malposition of the great arteries, can pose challenges in the implantation of an anatomically normal donor heart. However, virtually all anatomic problems can be solved using creative surgical techniques, which include rerouting of venous and arterial pathways and augmentation of arterial stenoses (69–72). During organ harvesting, it is helpful to include as much of both donor vena cavae (including innominate vein) and great arteries as possible (73).

Technique of Lung and Heart-Lung Transplantation

Single lung transplantation is performed via thoracotomy, and it can be done without cardiopulmonary bypass. In double lung transplantation, exposure is provided by a median sternotomy or a transverse submammary "clamshell" incision (the latter is often used to maximize operative exposure, especially with areas of the thorax that are difficult to reach). Recipient lung main stem bronchus, pulmonary artery, and pulmonary vein are clamped and transected distally. Donor graft is inspected for size matching with the recipient, and if too large, the donor lung is trimmed. Pulmonary vein is first anastomosed, then the bronchus, and finally artery. To correct for size discrepancies in the artery and vein, the larger vessel can be tapered to size. If a size discrepancy exists between donor and re-

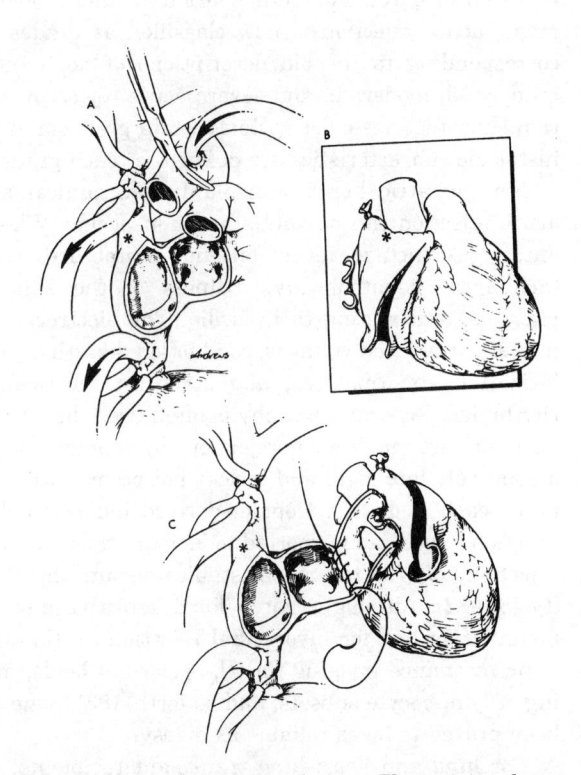

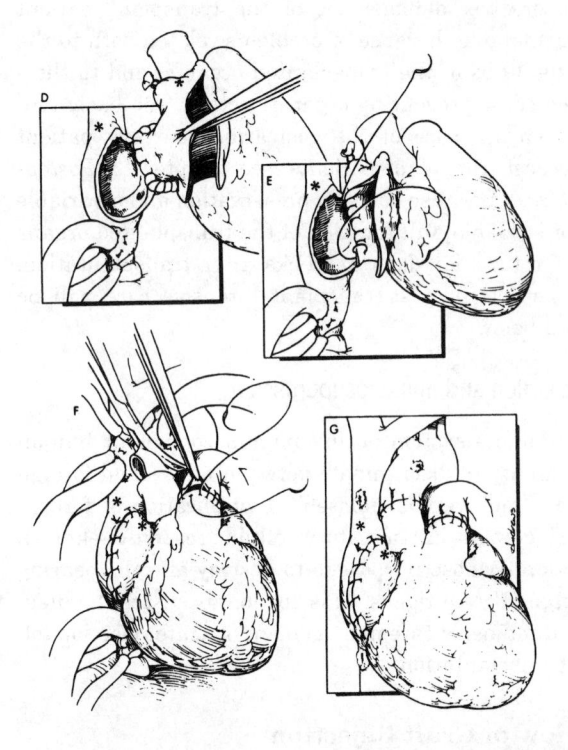

Figure 21.1. Cardiac transplantation technique. The recipient heart is excised leaving a remaining atrial cuff just anterior to the superior and inferior vena cavae and pulmonary veins, and a small posterior rim of residual atrial septum. The pulmonary artery and aorta are transected well above the sinuses of Valsalva. The donor atria and great arteries are trimmed and anastomosed to the appropriate connections. *Asterisks* denote the location of the sinoatrial nodes in the donor heart and recipient tissue. (Reprinted with permission from Cooley DA. Techniques in cardiac surgery, 2nd ed. Philadelphia: WB Saunders, 1984:372.)

cipient bronchi, the smaller bronchus is "telescoped" into the larger bronchus. Omental wraps are not generally used, although a pericardial or pericardial fat pedicle can be used (74). In a double lung transplant, the two sides are anastomosed in sequence. On completion of the anastomoses, the lungs are ventilated, the heart vented, and rewarming begun. Bronchoscopy can also be performed to examine the bronchial anastomoses.

Heart-lung transplantation technique is relatively straightforward. Either a midline sternotomy or clamshell incision can be used, depending on the patient's cardiopulmonary anatomy and history of previous thoracic surgery. Careful dissection is performed to isolate and protect pedicles of pericardium containing the phrenic nerves. The trachea is clamped just above the carina, and transected distally. The entire heart and lungs are removed en bloc, leaving only a right atrial cuff. Donor heart and lungs are inspected for size and, if necessary, the lungs are trimmed for fit. The graft is placed in the thoracic cavity, with the donor lungs inserted below the pericardial pedicles. The trachea is anastomosed, followed by the right atrial and aortic anastomoses.

POSTOPERATIVE CARE IN TRANSPLANTATION

Postoperative management of the transplant patient can be demanding because of problems related both to the unique qualities of the transplanted organ(s) and to therapy directed at preventing organ rejection. The basic tenets that govern care of the postcardiac surgery patient apply to post-transplant patients (see Chapter 13, *Postoperative Care*). Because of organ preservation and a variable period of ischemia, full function of the transplanted organs may not return for days to weeks after transplantation. Special aspects of post-transplant intensive care will be discussed below.

Graft Rejection and Immunosuppression

The immune system of any immunocompetent human has the ability to discriminate between native and foreign tissue, or "self" versus "nonself." Identification of foreign tissue triggers an inflammatory cellular response—known as rejection—whose purpose is to destroy all cells bearing the foreign HLA antigens. This section discusses the diagnosis and intensive care management of acute rejection following transplantation.

Overview of Graft Rejection

Rejection is classified as hyperacute, acute, and chronic. *Hyperacute rejection* occurs within minutes to hours after transplantation; it results from preformed donor-specific antibodies (e.g., HLA class I or blood groups ABO antibodies) that fix complement. This process rapidly destroys the graft. Hyperacute rejection is uncommon because recipients are now carefully screened before surgery for the presence of preformed antibodies. *Acute rejection* usually occurs within days to months following transplant; afterward the risk diminishes significantly, although it never completely disappears. This form of rejection involves cell-mediated immunity; inflammatory cell infiltration of the graft (lymphocytes, macrophages, and so forth) produces progressive organ dysfunction and necrosis. It is the rejection process most commonly seen in the post-transplant intensive care setting, and it will be discussed in this section. *Chronic rejection* is generally a slower, more protracted process involving smooth muscle obliteration of coronary arteries (in transplanted hearts) or bronchioles (in transplanted lungs); typically this process occurs over months to years.

Although clinical suspicion of acute rejection can be present, definitive diagnosis rests on obtaining histologic evidence of cellular infiltration in the graft. Tissue samples must be obtained by the appropriate technique: either myocardial, transbronchial, or open lung biopsy. To facilitate diagnosis uniformity, the International Society of Heart and Lung Transplantation has developed precise, widely accepted histologic classification schemata of acute rejection (75, 76). For both heart and lung biopsy specimens, acute rejection is now classified as grades 0 to 4, corresponding to the old descriptions of no, minimal to mild, mild, moderate, and severe acute rejection. In addition subcategories exist within certain grades and specific histologic characteristics are defined for each grade.

For pediatric heart transplantation, clinical signs of acute rejection can be subtle and nonspecific. When present, signs include fever, fatigue, irritability, vomiting, tachypnea, hepatomegaly, coolness of the skin or diphoresis, and resting tachycardia. The electrocardiogram may show reduced voltages, conduction disturbances, repolarization abnormalities, and atrial or ventricular dysrhythmias. Echocardiography is often used, but it remains an imperfect monitor for rejection. Systolic dysfunction is a relatively late sign, and it does not occur until rejection is at least moderate. Doppler-derived indices of diastolic function have been purported to be more sensitive for early rejection (77–79), but recent studies dispute their reliability (80–82). Although search for a sensitive and specific noninvasive test for myocardial rejection continues (magnetic resonance imaging [MRI], epicardial leads, monitoring of lymphocyte subsets, and so forth) (83), none has yet been proved to be as reliable as biopsy.

For lung and heart-lung transplant recipients, clinical signs for rejection can also be subtle: fever, decreased activity, tachypnea, arterial desaturation, wheezing, fine crackles, and resting tachycardia. Chest roentgenogram may show a hazy interstitial pattern, which may be focal but is usually diffuse. Pleural effusions can also be present. The difficulty lies in the nonspecific nature of pulmonary infiltrates, which could also represent rejection, infection, atelectasis, or pulmonary edema. Transbronchial biopsy is usually necessary to obtain further information (84). Pulmonary function testing is the most sensitive noninvasive method of rejection surveillance. Detecting pulmonary rejection in the young infant, however, relies heavily on clinical data. If the diagnosis is unclear, a trial dose of IV steroids is sometimes given. If the patient improves and the pulmonary infiltrates resolve, retrospective diagnosis of rejection can be made. In heart-lung transplant patients, myocardial biopsy is not a good method of surveillance because asynchronous pulmonary and cardiac rejection can be seen (85), with myocardial rejection occurring far less frequently than pulmonary rejection. Rejection surveillance in heart-lung patients, therefore, parallels that of lung transplant patients.

Intensive Care Management of Graft Rejection

Most heart and lung transplant patients with mild to moderate rejection will be clinically stable, and not in need of ICU management. Immunosuppressive therapy should begin immediately when the diagnosis of rejection is made. Pulse steroid therapy using IV methylprednisolone (15 mg/kg/d) is given for 3 days for mild to moderate rejection with only mild organ dysfunction. If the rejection episode is recurrent (i.e., refractory), or if organ dysfunction is more pronounced, antilymphocyte antibody therapy is begun (Table 21.5). The murine monoclonal antibody to CD3 receptors, OKT3, has been shown to reverse significant episodes of resistant rejection in up to 90% of patients with cardiac rejection. Methotrexate therapy has been used successfully in children and adults for acute refractory rejection (86, 87). Nonpharmacologic therapies used with some success in organ transplantation include total lymphoid irradiation (88, 89) and photopheresis (90–92), although minimal experience exists with the latter therapy in pediatric patients.

Intensive care for such patients also includes vigorous nutritional, ventilatory, and hemodynamic support until rejection is successfully reversed and graft function returns. In heart transplant patients this includes standard therapy for the failing heart: mechanical ventilation, inotropic support, afterload reduction, and judicious use of diuretics for pulmonary edema. If cardiac function is severely compromised, temporary mechanical circulatory support may be necessary. For transplanted lungs, severe rejection may require mechanical ventilation to maintain normal oxygenation and gas exchange; in extreme cases, even high frequency jet ventilation or extracorporeal membrane oxygenation (ECMO) may be necessary. As part of therapy, patients will become profoundly immunosuppressed, and painstaking precautions must be taken to prevent nosocomial infections. This includes reverse isolation, routine surveillance cultures, and appropriate antibiotic therapy. Adequate nutritional support is critical. As the rejection process resolves, graft function should return and intensive support can be weaned. In some cases of severe rejection, however, graft damage is so extensive and permanent that effective function is no longer possible—retransplantation is the only option.

Immunosuppressive Therapy

Immunosuppression is the cornerstone of post-transplant management. The goal is to achieve a level of immunosuppression sufficient to prevent organ rejection while not subjecting recipients to substantial risk for overwhelming infection. Treatment begins on the day of transplantation prior to the operation. Following transplantation, intensive immunotherapy is continued and adjusted daily. It is important to become familiar with the pharmacologic properties and potential toxicities of these agents.

An overview of the common immunosuppressive agents used in pediatric transplantation is given in Table 21.5. Several of the newer drugs, such as mycophenolate mofetil and rapamycin, have not been included because of lack of pediatric experience. Most centers employ a triple drug combination of corticosteroids, cyclosporine, and azathioprine in patients older than 1 year, but about half of the centers use only the latter two drugs for infants (93). Some centers prefer to use antilymphocyte antibodies such as OKT3 or antithrombocyte globulin (ATG) as initial therapy (also known as induction therapy). These agents rapidly induce a state of profound immunosuppression, which permits slower or delayed initiation of nephrotoxic immunosuppressive agents. The value of induction therapy is uncertain because some studies have demonstrated no significantly increased freedom from rejection (94). Moreover, some suggest that this therapy strategy may predispose patients to increased infection, humoral rejection (an uncommon form of acute rejection), and post-transplant lymphoproliferative disease (95).

Cardiovascular Management

Post-transplant patients usually return from the operating room with monitoring lines in place; these lines generally include a central line, an arterial line, and a pulmonary artery catheter for measurement of cardiac output and pulmonary artery pressures. Chest and mediastinal tubes are present. In the case of a heart and heart-lung transplant, external atrial and ventricular pacing wires are also usually placed.

Inotropic agents (e.g., dobutamine, dopamine, milrinone) are usually necessary in the immediate postoperative period. The transplanted heart has depleted myocar-

Table 21.5. Immunosuppressive Agents

Drug	Dosage	Action	Monitoring	Side Effects	Comments
Cyclosporine A	IV: 3–5 mg/kg/d divided q 12 h PO: Initial dose 3x IV dose divided q 8–12 h	Inhibits interleukin-2 synthesis	RIA/HPLC (whole blood trough) 350–600 RIA 150–400 HPLC	Nephrotoxicity (elevated blood urea nitrogen/creatinine), hypertension, neurotoxicity (tremors, seizures), hirsutism, gingival hyperplasia, hepatotoxicity, malignancy	Mainstay of immunosuppression in many programs Erythromycin, diltiazem, fluconazole increase levels Phenobarbital, phenytoin, metaclopramide decrease levels
Corticosteroids (Methylprenisolone, Prednisone)	IV: (Methylprenisolone): 5 mg/kg q 8 h (1st day), followed by 0.5 mg/kg IV q 12 h PO: (Prednisone): 0.1–0.5 mg/kg bid	Generalized immunosuppression; impaired production of interleukin 1 and 2	Serum glucose, cholesterol	Hypertension, hyperglycemia, cushingoid appearance, impaired tissue healing, hypercatabolism	Some centers discontinue steroid therapy after 6 mo–1 y post-transplant.
Azathioprine	IV/PO: 1–3 mg/kg/d (qhs)	Forms defective cell proteins; blocks T-cell functions; depresses white cell count/function	Hold if white blood cells < 4000 or ANC < 1500	Myelosuppression, hepatotoxicity, pancreatitis, aphthous stomatitis	Long-term use associated with increased risk of malignancy
Tacrolimus (FK-506)	IV: 0.01–0.05 mg/kg/d PO: 0.1–0.4 mg/kg/d divided q 12 h	Similar to cyclosporine	Whole blood (trough): 10–20 ng/mL	Nephrotoxicity, neurotoxicity, glucose intolerance, hypertension, gastrointestinal upset, anemia	Approximately 100 times more powerful than cyclosporine Effective "rescue" therapy in cyclosporine-resistant cases of rejection Pediatric experience limited, but encouraging
OKT3	IV: 0.1–0.2 mg/kg/d for 10–14 d (max daily dose 10 mg/d)	Monoclonal antibody against lymphocyte CD3 receptor Eliminates lymphocytes from body	T-lymphocyte subsets CBC, CXR	Anaphylaxis, pulmonary edema, fever, tachycardia, chills, headache Predisposition to infection, possibly to humoral rejection and malignancy	Pretreat with corticosteroids and antihistamines Induces state of profound immunosuppression Can be used as induction therapy, also as treatment of severe, life-threatening rejection
Antithymocyte globulin (ATG)	IV: 15 mg/kg/d for 7–10 d	Nonspecific, heterologous antilymphocyte antibodies Eliminates lymphocytes from body	T-lymphocyte subsets	Serum sickness reactions (fever, urticaria, hypotension), glomerulonephritis	Same as OKT3

ANC, absolute neutrophil count; CBC, complete blood count; CXR, chest X-ray; HPLC, high pressure liquid chromatography; RIA radioimmunoassay.

dial catecholamine stores (96–98), leading to an even greater dependence on inotropic agents. With time, inotropic agents can be weaned, although heart and heart-lung patients are sometimes slow to recover normal cardiac function and may require a prolonged period of inotropic support. When severe myocardial dysfunction is present, external mechanical cardiac support (assist device, balloon counterpulsation, or ECMO) may be necessary.

Systemic Hypertension

Systemic hypertension can be seen as a side effect of cyclosporine and tacrolimus, and it is also felt to be secondary to renal artery vasoconstriction and impaired fluid homeostasis (99–101).

Nifedipine, a calcium channel antagonist, effectively treats this type of hypertension, and it does not significantly alter cyclosporine levels. It can be administered orally or sublingually (the latter has a more rapid onset of action). Alternatively, angiotensin-converting enzyme inhibitors (ACE), such as captopril and enalapril (which has an intravenous preparation) can be used. Although intravenous hydralazine, nitroprusside, and the phosphodiesterase inhibitors (e.g., amrinone and milrinone) can be used for short-term treatment of acute systemic hypertension, long-term antihypertensive therapy usually requires a calcium channel antagonist or ACE inhibitor.

Pulmonary Hypertension

Pulmonary hypertension can be a significant postoperative problem complicating heart, heart-lung, and lung transplantation. This condition can result from pre-existing pulmonary vascular disease caused by long-standing CHD or cardiomyopathy, or from transient postoperative pulmonary vasoconstriction due to sequelae from cardiopulmonary bypass such as atelectasis, endothelial dysfunction, and so forth (102). When severe, pulmonary hypertensive crises can be life-threatening. Treatment includes the usual ventilatory maneuvers to lower pulmonary vascular resistance—hyperventilation, hyperoxygenation, sedation—and administration of vasodilators such as PGE_1 (103), prostacyclin, nitroprusside, and inhaled nitric oxide (104) (see Chapter 32, *Pulmonary Hypertension*). In the setting of pulmonary hypertension, the unprepared right ventricle may require inotropic support until PVR decreases or the donor right ventricle adapts to accommodate the elevated afterload.

Dysrhythmias

In postoperative heart and heart-lung transplant patients, cardiac diastolic function and passive filling are usually impaired (105, 106), and therefore cardiac output is even more dependent on adequate heart rate with atrioventricular synchrony. In heart transplant recipients with residual donor right atrial tissue (standard atrial anastomosis), the electrocardiogram will normally show two P waves, corresponding to recipient and donor sinus nodes; this can be easily mistaken for atrial tachydysrhythmias.

Because sinus node dysfunction of the implanted heart can be present, intravenous isoproterenol or external atrial pacing is often necessary to maintain an adequate heart rate. Return of sinus node function can require several days to weeks. Occasionally normal sinus node function does not return and a permanent atrial or ventricular pacemaker would need to be implanted (7). Without vagotonic influence, baseline heart rate is at times increased and significantly less beat-to-beat variability is seen. Cardiac denervation, however, also renders anticholinergic agents, such as atropine sulfate, ineffective.

Both supraventricular and ventricular dysrhythmias can be seen following heart transplantation (95, 107, 108). Standard antidysrhythmia management applies to these situations (see Chapter 30, *Diagnosis and Management of Cardiac Arrhythmias*), but the actions of antidysrhythmic drugs can be altered in the denervated heart. For example, digoxin will have no AV nodal effect, and adenosine should be used at a low dose because the denervated heart is particularly sensitive to this agent (109). Monitoring for potential drug interactions—especially with cyclosporine—is necessary. Lastly, arrhythmias can be a sign of acute cardiac rejection or coronary disease (110).

Other Considerations

Pericardial effusion presence does not signal rejection, but sometimes the effusion becomes large enough to produce hemodynamic compromise and pericardiocentesis becomes necessary (21, 111). Heart-lung transplantation patients usually do not develop pericardial effusions because the entire donor pericardium is removed during harvesting.

Pulmonary and Ventilatory Management

Post-transplant patients return to the ICU intubated and mechanically ventilated. In heart-lung and lung transplant patients, the transplanted lungs may not initially exhibit normal gas exchange because of ventilation or perfusion abnormalities caused by lung injury from the previous period of ischemia, or from pulmonary contusions or atelectasis following surgical manipulation. Eventually these abnormalities resolve and pulmonary function should return to normal.

Mechanical Ventilation of the Transplanted Patient

Oxygenation and ventilation normalization is the overriding goal in patients after transplantation so that ventilator support can be discontinued as soon as possible. Although this is a generally accepted postoperative principle, it takes on an even greater significance in post-transplant patients because endotracheal intubation and mechanical ventilation can impair the normal mechanisms of pulmonary clearance and, therefore, increase the risk of infection in an immunocompromised patient (112). It is also important to remember that some transplant patients will have become accustomed to a relatively higher preoperative arterial CO_2 concentration (e.g., cystic fibrosis patients) or may have lost their hypoxic respiratory drive stimulus because of chronic hypoxemia (e.g., cyanotic congenital heart disease). These patients will require a higher arterial P_{CO_2} to maintain an effective respiratory drive, and a higher P_{CO_2} should be accepted when weaning them to extubation. It is not uncommon to see such a patient breathing comfortably after extubation with a P_{CO_2} of 50–60 torr.

Some lung transplant patients who were already malnourished prior to transplantation have difficulty weaning to extubation. This is secondary to poor ventilatory muscle strength, incisional pain (especially following a clamshell incision), and to altered lung inflation mechanics following denervation (e.g., ablation of the Hering-Breuer reflex). Such patients may require respiratory muscle training by means of ventilator "sprinting," which is composed of short periods during which there is minimal ventilator support and the patient generates most of the respiratory effort, alternating with longer periods when ventilatory support is increased and the patient rested. To evaluate progress, serial measurements of negative inspiratory force or maximal inspiratory pressure are useful. Occasionally, diaphragmatic paresis or even paralysis requires diaphragmatic plication. When patients require mechanical ventilation for long periods of time, a tracheostomy can also be considered. This procedure protects the subglottic area and assists in the weaning from mechanical ventilation; however, the risk of pulmonary infection can increase.

In patients with transplanted lungs, issues of pulmonary management tend to dominate postoperative care. Several factors contribute to the complexity of management: (*a*) transplanted lungs are even more susceptible to infection because of previous surgical manipulation, impaired mucociliary clearance (6), and lung denervation, which has eliminated the cough reflex; (*b*) transplanted lungs are vulnerable to acute rejection; and (*c*) transplanted lungs no longer have normal lymphatic drainage, when combined with ischemic damage, results in a tendency to retain fluid (113, 114).

Vigorous pulmonary toilet is required to mobilize and remove secretions. Regular tracheal cultures should be obtained for infection surveillance. Bronchoscopy and bronchoalveolar lavage (BAL) are sometimes necessary to clean out the airways, especially with a narrowed bronchial anastomosis. If suspicion of rejection or infection exists, transbronchial biopsies and cultures should be obtained during bronchoscopy.

Management of the transplanted lung is also made more difficult by a myriad of potential pathologic processes. When a pulmonary opacification is seen on chest x-ray, the differential diagnosis includes reperfusion injury, pulmonary contusion, acute rejection, infection, atelectasis, pulmonary edema, pleural effusion, and pulmonary vein obstruction (115). Clinical data often suggest one possibility over the others, but any uncertainty requires an aggressive approach to diagnosis. This includes bronchoscopy, BAL, and transbronchial biopsy (116, 117), computed tomography scan to evaluate for pleural effusion and parenchymal disease, and transesophageal echocardiography (TEE) to examine the pulmonary veins.

Several other factors are to be considered in the pulmonary management of lung transplant recipients. Following implantation of transplanted lungs, persistent pleural effusions or air leaks may require chest tubes for several weeks. Pleural effusions occur because of a donor–recipient mismatch in the size of the lungs; when the donor lungs do not completely fill the pleural cavity of the recipient, transudative fluid seeps in to fill the space. Other patients may have persistent air leaks lasting 1 or more weeks. Eventually these leaks should seal and the tubes can be removed. Finally, some lung transplant recipients can develop stenosis at the site of a bronchial anastomosis; when severe, these stenoses can compromise gas exchange. To open these areas, some centers have successfully placed balloon-expandable stents using a combination of bronchoscopy and fluoroscopy (118–120).

Infectious Disease Management

Because of immunosuppression, marginal nutritional status, and surgical breaching of the normal protective barriers, transplant patients are especially vulnerable to infections (both nosocomial and opportunistic) in the immediate postoperative period. Infection remains one of the most common causes of postoperative mortality following transplant (121, 122). The strategy against infection includes routine surveillance cultures from all potential sites of infection, regular replacement of indwelling catheters, and strict isolation. Most serious infections occur within the first 3 to 6 months following transplant, when immunosuppression is at its peak.

Immunocompromised patients are susceptible to all forms of infections—bacterial, viral, fungal, and parasitic (Table 21.6). In the setting of immunosuppression, any temperature elevation potentially indicates an active infection. If an infection is suspected, an aggressive investigation should be instituted. When patients are clinically ill, broad-spectrum anti-infective therapy can be initiated be-

Table 21.6. Infectious Pathogens Causing Disease in Transplant Patients

Bacterial
  Gram positive
    Staphylococcus (aureus, epidermidis)
    Streptococcus
  Gram negative
    Enterobacter
    Escherichia coli
    Klebsiella
    Hemophilus
  Other
    Mycobacterium spp
    Mycoplasma
    Legionella
    Nocardia
Viral
  Cytomegalovirus (CMV)
  Herpesvirus (herpes simplex, varicella-zoster)
  Respiratory syncytial virus (RSV)
  Influenza
  Parainfluenza
  Adenovirus
  Epstein-Barr virus (EBV)
Fungal
  Candida
  Aspergillus
  Cryptococcus
  Coccidioides
  Mucor
Parasitic
  Pneumocystis carinii
  Toxoplasma gondii

fore culture results are available. Coverage should be narrowed as soon as possible because of potential medication toxicity (e.g., renal damage from amphotericin) and the risk of superinfection.

Cytomegalovirus (CMV) is one of the most frequent and important post-transplant infections. It is also known as the "40-day fever" because infection tends to occur between 1 to 3 months after transplant. It occurs both as a primary infection—newly acquired from blood product transfusion or a CMV-positive donor—or as reactivation of a previous infection. Risk of CMV disease is highest in CMV-negative recipients who receive an organ from a CMV-positive donor; however, reactivation can also occur in the CMV-positive recipient.

A variety of invasive diseases are produced, involving lung, liver, gastrointestinal, hematologic, neurologic, and ocular systems. Patients can often have fever, rash, and hematologic abnormalities (leukopenia, thrombocytopenia, atypical lymphocytosis). Primary infections tend to be the worst (123), although severe reactivation disease has also been reported (124). Diagnosis can be made by CMV inclusion bodies retrieved from suspected sites; positive CMV culture results; or positive CMV IgM serology (125). For treatment of invasive CMV, IV ganciclovir has been used successfully (126). A dose of 10 mg/kg/d in two divided doses is given for clinical CMV infection. CMV prophylaxis (ganciclovir 5 mg/kg/d given once per day) and IV gamma globulin (127) for those patients at risk for development of primary or reactivation disease can also be used.

Fluid and Renal Management

All transplant patients who have been on cardiopulmonary bypass will have some degree of capillary leak. This is especially true in the transplanted lung, which suffers from a variable period of ischemia and impaired lymphatic drainage. It is therefore important to avoid fluid overload. After returning from the operating room, patients should be kept on two-thirds to three-fourths maintenance fluids for the first few days. Fluids can be liberalized cautiously later, especially if the patient is extubated and ready to take oral feedings. Diuretics can be used to optimize fluid balance. In malnourished patients, serum albumin can be low and IV albumin infusions can be given to increase oncotic pressure; this may also increase the effectiveness of diuretic therapy.

Numerous factors can compromise renal function. Both low cardiac output and cyclosporine induce prerenal arteriolar vasoconstriction that can decrease urine output and cause prerenal azotemia (characteristically with cyclosporine a high blood urea nitrogen [BUN]:creatinine ratio is seen). Other medications, e.g., aminoglycosides and amphotericin B, can act alone or in concert with cyclosporine to decrease renal function. Even excessive use of some of the loop diuretics (furosemide, ethacrynic acid) could cause nephrotoxicity. Because of its importance, renal function must be monitored closely before and after transplantation. Any indication of renal compromise may necessitate temporary reduction (or even discontinuation) of potentially nephrotoxic drugs. In the case of severe oliguria or anuria, peritoneal or hemodialysis may be required (128, 129).

Nutritional and Gastrointestinal Management

Postoperative nutrition must be maximized in the transplant patient, for the following reasons: (*a*) thoracic surgical patients have tremendous caloric needs, which are augmented by the often-malnourished preoperative state (130); (*b*) high-dose corticosteroids aggravate the catabolic state, impairing wound healing; and (*c*) poor nutrition further increases the high risk of infection. Whatever the circumstances, some type of nutritional support should be initiated as soon as possible. Nutrition can be provided by either the enteral or parenteral route, although enteral feedings are preferable. A variety of high calorie liquid preparations are available to accommodate any number of dietary exigencies (e.g., low protein, low sodium, high fat, elemental formula, and so forth). If the enteral route is not available, total parenteral nutrition can be used for nutritional support. A high dextrose concentration in the hyperalimentation fluid, when administered in conjuction with IV intralipids, generally provides sufficient calories with an acceptable amount of fluid intake. Because patients are being treated with IV corticosteroids, some can develop significant hyperglycemia and glycosuria with either enteral or parenteral nutrition, and insulin therapy is sometimes required for control.

Normal gastric and intestinal motility are necessary for proper enteral nutrition. Immediately following surgery, motility can be diminished but it generally resumes within several days. Because some transplant patients— especially those with heart-lung and lung transplants— have had their vagal gastric innervation interrupted during the operation, these patients have impaired gastric motility and may require a motility agent (e.g., metoclopramide or cisapride). Some patients develop gastroesophageal reflux (which is potentially hazardous for transplanted lungs), and these patients require gastrostomy with or without fundoplication. Occasionally gastric motility will be so impaired that jejunal feedings are required, either through nasogastric tube or gastrostomy.

Hepatic function should be monitored routinely following transplant. The liver usually sustains few adverse effects from the operation but one or several of the many drugs administered to the patient (alone or in combination) can be hepatotoxic. Elevated liver transaminases can be one of the first signs of CMV hepatitis. An elevated bilirubin may indicate biliary obstruction, possibly from cholelithiasis (131). Pancreatitis can occur following steroid, azathioprine, or cyclosporine therapy (132); however, elevations of serum amylase and lipase are occasionally seen in the absence of clinical pancreatitis.

Neurologic Management

Seizures can occur after transplantation (133–135), and they can be secondary to high cyclosporine levels, but they can occur even when levels are normal. The cause for seizures is often unclear but presumably because of a lowered seizure threshold (from cyclosporine) in combination with the epileptogenic effects of other medications. Hypomagnesemia has also been implicated. Workup for seizures includes computed tomography scan or magnetic resonance imaging, EEG, and lumbar puncture to evaluate for infection.

When no clear cause for seizures is found, treatment should be given if they are recurrent. Phenobarbital, phenytoin, and carbamazepine are effective anticonvulsants, although they can alter cyclosporine levels. Benzodiazepines (especially lorazepam) induce immediate relief of seizures, but they also produce sedation and respiratory depression. Valproic acid has no significant effect on cyclosporine levels, and in general it has excellent anticonvulsant activity; because of potential liver toxicity, however, liver function tests must be followed closely. Stroke and hypoxic-ischemic encephalopathy, presumably related to hypoperfusion or embolic events during surgery, are also known to occur (136).

Pain management is a concern with post-transplant patients, especially those who have undergone the clamshell incision. Intrathecal morphine can be useful for local analgesia in the immediate postoperative period. Pain control with morphine or another narcotic (e.g., oxycodone, meperidine) is sometimes necessary.

Adjustment disorders and even depression can be seen in some patients who have a prolonged ICU stay (137). These disorders can usually be treated with psychiatric therapy and mild anxiolytics (e.g., benzodiazepines). Occasionally more potent antidepressant medications are necessary (e.g., haloperidol). These should be administered with the guidance of a psychiatrist.

LONG-TERM FOLLOW-UP OF TRANSPLANTATION

In patients after heart transplantation, the leading causes of death are graft failure, acute rejection, infection, and graft coronary artery disease. Most pediatric heart transplant patients enjoy excellent quality of life following transplantation, although decreased growth has been an issue in patients on long-term steroid therapy (138–141). After 1 to 2 years post-transplant, corticosteroids are tapered to minimal doses (or even discontinued), reducing their adverse effects on body growth. As the period from transplantation lengthens, risks of infection and acute rejection decrease, but a risk of rejection remains in some long-term survivors (142).

Graft coronary artery disease (GCAD) is the manifestation of chronic rejection in the transplanted heart, and it can be difficult to diagnose. Pathologically diffuse intimal thickening is present with eventual luminal obliteration. The cause of GCAD is unknown, but an association appears to be present with an increased frequency of acute cellular rejection; hyperlipidemia and postoperative CMV have also been implicated (143). The incidence in pediatric patients is probably between 7 and 15% (144, 145). Because of denervation, the patient will not have typical anginal symptoms. Noninvasive methods of diagnosis, including exercise testing, thallium scintigraphy, and positron emission tomography (PET scanning) have been used with marginal success.

Coronary angiography has been considered the gold standard but given the diffuse nature of the disease, even this modality tends to underestimate its severity. No effective therapy currently exists for GCAD; the disease is generally too diffuse for coronary angioplasty or bypass surgery. Retransplantation is the only treatment.

In pediatric heart-lung and lung recipients, pulmonary function tests are initially decreased but they improve steadily over the initial 6 months following transplant. A mild restrictive pattern is seen, which improves over time (31, 146). Gas exchange is usually normal. The adult experience has shown normal right-sided hemodynamics, normal function, and good exercise tolerance in uncomplicated postlung transplant patients (45, 141). Similar long-term data regarding pulmonary function and quality of life in pediatric patients are still forthcoming. Some question remains whether transplanted lung tissue will grow in young children, or whether the lung just becomes more emphysematous to accommodate increasing chest size. Preliminary data suggest that lung growth does indeed occur after transplantation (144).

Obliterative bronchiolitis (OB) is the manifestation of chronic rejection in the transplanted lung. The incidence in adults surviving more than 6 months is approximately 35 to 40% (43, 147), whereas in the pediatric population the reported prevalence ranges between 20 and 40% (40, 106, 148). Fibrotic narrowing and eventually complete obliteration of the bronchioles can occur. Dyspnea and cough are the first clinical signs. The cause of OB is presumably immunologically mediated—similar to GCAD—with repeated acute rejection and possibly CMV also implicated (149). In addition, local infection by other organisms may participate in its genesis. The earliest laboratory sign of OB is small airways obstruction, as demonstrated by pulmonary function testing. The chest x-ray can be surprisingly normal, but high resolution computed tomography scan can show small areas of consolidation or bronchiectasis (150, 151). Transbronchial biopsy, when positive, confirms the diagnosis but the yield is low, even with multiple specimens (152). Open lung biopsy remains the definitive test but this procedure carries many risks. Management is difficult; augmented immunosuppression and total lymphoid irradiation have been reported to arrest the progression of OB in some patients (153, 154); in some patients, however, retransplantation is the only option. Results of retransplantation have not been encouraging, with a 2-year survival of only about 30 to 50% (1, 155).

In all post-transplant patients, post-transplant lymphoproliferative disease (PTLD), a form of lymphoma, is a common malignancy occurring in approximately 10% of pediatric transplant recipients. It is associated with Epstein-Barr virus, probably from reactivation of a latent infection (156). It presents with fever, lymphadenopathy, malaise, anemia, and gastroenteritis (157, 158). When suspected, the diagnosis should be pursued with imaging techniques (computed tomography scan, magnetic resonance imaging) and lymph node biopsy, if feasible. Immediate reduction in immunosuppression and IV acyclovir therapy are generally effective, but some patients will require additional chemotherapy and radiation therapy.

REFERENCES

1. Rouge RC, Naftel DC, Costanzo-Nordin MR, et al. Pretransplantation risk factors for death after heart transplantation: a multiinstitutional study. J Heart Lung Transplant 1993; 12:549–562.
2. Bailey LL, Gundry SR, Razzouk AJ, et al. Bless the babies: one hundred fifteen late survivors of heart transplantation during the first year of life. J Thorac Cardiovasc Surg 1993;105:805–815.
3. Sarris GE, Smith JA, Bernstein D, et al. Pediatric cardiac transplantation: the Stanford experience. Circulation 1994;90(Part 2):II-51–II-55.
4. Addonizio LJ, Hsu DT, Douglas JF, et al. Cardiac transplantation in children after "failed" Fontan operations [Abstract]. J Heart Lung Transplant 1992;12:s93.
5. Slaughter MS, Braunlin E, Bolman RM III, et al. Pediatric heart transplantation: results of 2- and 5-year follow-up. J Heart Lung Transplant 1994;13:624–630.
6. Herve P, Silbert D, Cerrina J, et al. Paris-Sud Lung Transplant Group. Impairment of bronchial mucociliary clearance in long-term survivors of heart/lung and double lung transplantation. Chest 1993;103:59–63.
7. Chinnock RE, Torres VI, Jutzy RV, et al. Cardiac pacemakers in pediatric heart transplant recipients: incidence, indications, and associated factors. Pacing Clin Electrophysiol 1996;19:26–30.
8. Starnes VA, Oyer PE, Bernstein D, et al. Heart, heart-lung and lung transplantation in the first year of life. Ann Thorac Surg 1992;53:306–310.
9. Costard-Jäckle A, Hill I, Schroeder JS, et al. The influence of preoperative patient characteristics on early and late survival following cardiac transplantation. Circulation 1991; 84(Suppl III):III-329–III-337.
10. Addonizio LJ, Hsu DT, Fuzesi L, et al. Optimal timing of pediatric heart transplantation. Circulation 1989;80(Suppl III):III-84–III-89.
11. Evans RW, Maier AM. Outcome of patients referred for cardiac transplantation. J Am Coll Cardiol 1986;8:1312–1317.
12. Hosenpud JD, Novick RJ, Breen TJ, et al. The registry of the International Society for Heart and Lung Transplantation: twelfth official report—1995. J Heart Lung Transplant 1995;14:805–815.
13. Erickson KW, Costanzo-Nordin MR, O'Sullivan J, et al. Influence of preoperative transpulmonary gradient on late mortality after orthotopic heart transplantation. J Heart Transplant 1990;9:526–537.
14. Griepp RB, Stinson EB, Dong E Jr, et al. Determinants of operative risk in human heart transplantation. Am J Surg 1971;122:192–197.
15. Addonizio LJ, Gersony WM, Robbins RC, et al. Elevated pulmonary vascular resistance and cardiac transplantation. Circulation 1987;76:V52–V55.
16. Costard-Jäckle A, Fowler MB. Influence of preoperative pulmonary artery pressure on mortality after heart transplantation: testing of potential reversibility of pulmonary hypertension with nitroprusside is useful in defining a high risk group. J Am Coll Cardiol 1992;19:48–54.
17. Zales VR, Pahl E, Backer C, et al. Pharmacologic reduction

of pulmonary vascular resistance pretransplant predicts outcome following pediatric cardiac transplantation. [Abstract]. J Heart Lung Transplant 1993;12:s-93.
18. Gajarski RJ, Towbin JA, Bricker T, et al. Intermediate follow-up of pediatric heart transplant recipients with elevated pulmonary vascular resistance index. J Am Coll Cardiol 1994;23:1682–1687.
19. Kleinert S, Weintraub RG, Wilkinson JL, et al. Pulmonary vascular resistance in children with end-stage cardiomyopathy [Abstract]. J Heart Lung Transplant 1996;15:s70.
20. Deeb GM, Bolling SF, Buynn TP, et al. Amrinone versus conventional therapy in pulmonary hypertensive patients awaiting cardiac transplantation. Ann Thorac Surg 1989;48: 665–669.
21. Hauptman PJ, Couper GS, Aranki SF, et al. Pericardial effusions after cardiac transplantation. J Am Coll Cardiol 1994;23:1625–1629.
22. Murali S, Uretsky BF, Reddy S, et al. Reversibility of pulmonary hypertension in congestive heart failure patients evaluated for cardiac transplantation: comparative effects of various pharmacologic agents. Am Heart J 1991;122:1375–1381.
23. Kieler-Jensen N, Ricksten SE, Stenqvist O, et al. Inhaled nitric oxide in the evaluation of heart transplant candidates with elevated pulmonary vascular resistance. J Heart Lung Transplant 1994;13(3):366–375.
24. Semigran MJ, Cockrill BA, Kacmarek R, et al. Nitric oxide is an effective pulmonary vasodilator in cardiac transplant candidates with pulmonary hypertension [Abstract]. J Heart Lung Transplant 1992;12:s67.
25. Bourge RC, Kirklin JK, Naftel DC, et al. Analysis and predictors of pulmonary vascular resistance after cardiac transplantation. J Thorac Cardiovasc Surg 1991;101:432–445.
26. O'Connell JB, Bourge RC, Costanzo-Nordin MR, et al. Cardiac transplantation: recipient selection, donor procurement, and medical follow-up. Circulation 1992;86:1061–1079.
27. Penkoske PA, Rowe RD, Freedom RM, et al. The future of heart and heart-lung transplantation in children. J Heart Transplant 1984;3:233–238.
28. Macoviak JA, Baldwin JC, Ginsburg R, et al. Orthotopic cardiac transplantation for univentricular heart. Ann Thorac Surg 1988;45:85–86.
29. Hehrlein FW, Netz H, Moosdorf R, et al. Pediatric heart transplantation for congenital heart disease and cardiomyopathy. Ann Thorac Surg 1991;52:112–117.
30. Bove EL. Transplantation after first-stage reconstruction for hypoplastic left heart syndrome. Ann Thorac Surg 1991; 52:701–707.
31. Starnes VA, Griffin ML, Pitlick PT, et al. Current approach to hypoplastic left heart syndrome: palliation, transplantation, or both? J Thorac Cardiovasc Surg 1992;104:189–195.
32. Chiavarelli M, Bailey LL. Neonatal heart transplantation: indications and results. In: Kaye MP, O'Connell JB. Heart and lung transplantation 2000. Austin: RG Landes Company, 1993.
33. Jonas RA. Intermediate procedures after first-stage Norwood operation facilitate subsequent repair. Ann Thorac Surg 1991;52:696–700.
34. Norwood WI Jr. Hypoplastic left heart syndrome. Ann Thorac Surg 1991;52:688–695.
35. Chiavarelli M, Gundry SR, Razzouk AJ, et al. Cardiac transplantation for infants with hypoplastic left-heart syndrome. JAMA 1993;270:2944–2947.
36. Boucek MM, Mathis CM, Lebeck L, et al. Cardiac transplantation in infants and children with anatomic and functional absence of the spleen (asplenia) [Abstract]. J Heart Lung Transplant 1993;12:s92.
37. Ardehali A, Laks H, Drinkwater D, et al. Heart transplantation for congenital heart diseases [Abstract]. J Am Coll Cardiol 1994;24:8A.
38. Webber SA, Fricker FJ, Michaels M. Orthotopic heart transplantation in children with congenital heart disease. Ann Thorac Surg 1994;58:1664–1669.
39. Hsu DT, Quaegebeur JM, Michler RE, et al. Heart transplantation in children with congenital heart disease. J Am Coll Cardiol 1995;26:743–749.
40. Marshall SE, Kramer M, Lewiston NJ, et al. Selection and evaluation of recipients for heart-lung and lung transplantation. Chest 1990;98:1488–1494.
41. Pasque MK, Cooper JD, Kaiser LR, et al. Improved techniques for bilateral lung transplantation: rationale and initial clinical experience. Ann Thorac Surg 1990;49:785–791.
42. Spray TL. Projections for pediatric heart-lung and lung transplantation. J Heart Lung Transplant 1993;12:s337–S343.
43. Spray TL, Mallory GB, Canter CB, et al. Pediatric lung transplantation: indications, techniques, and early results. J Thorac Cardiovasc Surg 1994;107:990–1000.
44. Fremes SE, Patterson MD, Williams WG, et al. Single lung transplantation and closure of patent ductus arteriosus for Eisenmenger's syndrome. J Thorac Cardiovasc Surg 1990; 100:1–5.
45. Bridges ND, Mallory GB Jr, Huddleston CB, et al. Lung transplantation in children and young adults with cardiovascular disease. Ann Thorac Surg 1995;59:813–821.
46. Cooper JD, Patterson GA, Trulock EP, et al. Results of single and bilateral lung transplantation in 131 consecutive recipients. J Thorac Cardiovasc Surg 1994;107:460–471.
47. Pasque MK, Kaiser LR, Dresler CM, et al. Single lung transplantation for pulmonary hypertension: technical aspects and immediate hemodynamic results. J Thorac Cardiovasc Surg 1992;103:475–482.
48. Starnes VA, Barr ML, Cohen RG. Lobar transplantation: indications, technique, and outcome. J Thorac Cardiovasc Surg 1994;108:403–411.
49. Theodore PR, Starnes VA. Reduced-size lung transplantation: clinical experience. In: Kern JA, Kron IL, eds. Reduced-size lung transplantation. Austin: RG Landes 1993:76–87.
50. Cohen RG, Barr ML, Schenkel FA, et al. Living-related donor lobectomy for bilateral lobar transplantation in patients with cystic fibrosis. Ann Thorac Surg 1994;57:1423–1428.
51. Starnes VA, Barr ML, Schenkel FA, et al. Cardiopulmonary physiology in adult and pediatric bilateral lobar transplantation recipients: one year follow-up [Abstract]. J Heart Lung Transplant 1996;15:39A.
52. Ritchie M, Waggoner AD, Dávila-Román VG, et al. Echocardiographic characterization of the improvement in right ventricular function in patients with severe pulmonary hypertension after single-lung transplantation. J Am Coll Cardiol 1993;22:1170–1174.
53. Scuderi LJ, Bailey SR, Calhoon JH, et al. Echocardiographic assessment of right and left ventricular function after single-lung transplantation. Am Heart J 1994;127:636–642.
54. Farrar DJ, Hill JD, Gray LA Jr, et al. Heterotopic prosthetic ventricles as a bridge to cardiac transplantation. N Engl J Med 1988;318:333–340.
55. Pennington DG, McBridge LR, Knater KR, et al. Bridging

to heart transplantation with circulatory support devices. J Heart Transplant 1989;8:116–123.
56. Farrar DJ, Hill JD, and Thoratec Ventricular Assist Device Principal Investigators. Recovery of major organ function in patients awaiting heart transplantation with Thoratec ventricular assist devices. J Heart Lung Transplant 1994;1125–1132.
57. Joyce LD, Emery RW, Eales F, et al. Mechanical circulatory support as a bridge to transplantation. J Thorac Cardiovasc Surg 1989;98:935–941.
58. Copeland JG, Pavie A, Duveau D, et al. Bridge to transplantation with the CardioWest total artificial heart: the international experience 1993 to 1995. J Heart Lung Transplant 1996;15:95–99.
59. Ruiz CE, Gamra H, Zhang HP, et al. Brief report: stenting of the ductus arteriosus as a bridge to cardiac transplantation in infants with the hypoplastic left-heart syndrome. N Engl J Med 1993;328:1605–1608.
60. Slack MC, Kirby WC, Towbin JA, et al. Stenting of the ductus arteriosus in hypoplastic left heart syndrome as an ambulatory bridge to cardiac transplantation. Am J Cardiol 1994;74:636–637.
61. Razzouk AJ, Bailey LL. Infant heart transplantation. In: Emmanouilides GC, Riemenschneider TA, Allen HD, et al., eds. Moss and Adams Heart disease in infants, children, and adolescents including the fetus and young adult. Baltimore: Williams & Wilkins 1995:510–516.
62. Canter CE, Huddleston CB, Spray TL. Restrictive atrial communication limits applicability of cardiac transplantation for hypoplastic left heart syndrome [Abstract]. Circulation 1992;86:i–237.
63. Fullerton DA, Gundry SR, Alonso de Begona J, et al. The effects of donor-recipient size disparity in infant and pediatric heart transplantation. J Thorac Cardiovasc Surg 1992;104:1314–1319.
64. Zales VR, Wright KL, Muster AJ, et al. Ventricular volume growth after cardiac transplantation in infants and children. Circulation 1992;86(Suppl II):II-272–II-275.
65. Kaye DM, Bergin P, Buckland M, et al. Value of postoperative assessment of cardiac allograft function by transesophageal echocardiography. J Heart Lung Transplant 1994;13:165–172.
66. Dreyfus G, Jebara V, Mihaileanu S, et al. Total orthotopic heart transplantation: an alternative to the standard technique. Ann Thorac Surg 1991;52:1181–1184.
67. Leyh RG, Jahnke AW, Kraatz E, et al. Cardiovascular dynamics and dimensions after bicaval and standard cardiac transplantation. Ann Thorac Surg 1995;59:1495–1500.
68. Brandt M, Harringer W, Hirt SW, et al. Bicaval vs right atrial anastomosis in heart transplantation: influence on late occurrence of atrial arrhythmia [Abstract]. J Heart Lung Transplant 1996;15:s51.
69. Menkis AH, McKenzie FN, Novick RJ, et al. Special considerations for congenital heart diseases. J Heart Lung Transplant 1990;9:608–617.
70. Doty DB, Renlund DG, Caputo GR, et al. Cardiac transplantation in situs inversus. J Thorac Cardiovasc Surg 1990;99:493–499.
71. Chartrand C, Guerin R, Kangah M, et al. Pediatric heart transplantation: surgical considerations for congenital heart diseases. J Heart Transplant 1990;9:608–617.
72. Mayer JE, Perry S, O'Brien P, et al. Orthotopic heart transplantation for complex congenital heart disease. J Thorac Cardiovasc Surg 1990;99:484–492.
73. Cooper MM, Fuzesi L, Addonizio LJ, et al. Pediatric heart transplantation after operations involving the pulmonary arteries. J Thorac Cardiovasc Surg 1991;102:386–395.
74. Spray TL, Huddleston CB. Pediatric lung transplantation. Chest Surg Clin North Am 1993;3:123–143.
75. Billingham ME, Cary NRB, Hammond ME, et al. A working formulation for the standardization of nomenclature in the diagnosis of heart and lung rejection: heart rejection study group. J Heart Transplant 1990;6:587–593.
76. Yousem SA, Berry GJ, Cagle PT, et al. Revision of the 1990 working formulation for the classification of pulmonary allograft rejection: lung rejection study group. J Heart Lung Transplant 1996;15:1–15.
77. Valantine HA, Fowler MB, Hunt SA, et al. Changes in Doppler echocardiographic indexes of left ventricular function as potential markers of acute cardiac rejection. Circulation 1987;76:V-86–V-92.
78. Desreunnes M, Corcos T, Cabrol A, et al. Doppler echocardiography for the diagnosis of acute cardiac allograft rejection. J Am Coll Cardiol 1988;12:63–70.
79. Valantine HA, Yeoh TK, Gibbons R, et al. Sensitivity and specificity of diastolic indexes for rejection surveillance: temporal correlation with endomyocardial biopsy. J Heart Lung Transplant 1991;10:757–765.
80. Ayres NA, Pignatelli R, Towbin J, et al. Relationship of echo with biopsy following cardiac transplantation in pediatric patients [Abstract]. J Am Coll Cardiol 1993;21:36A.
81. Ciliberto GR, Mascarello M, Gronda E, et al. Acute rejection after heart transplantation: noninvasive echocardiographic evaluation. J Am Coll Cardiol 1994;23:1156–1161.
82. Ruiz CE, Zhang HP, Larsen RL, et al. Poor determination of rejection by echocardiography after paediatric heart transplantation: a comparative study with endomyocardial biopsy [Abstract]. Eur Heart J 1994;16(Suppl):463.
83. Valantine HA, Hunt SA. Clinical and non-invasive methods of diagnosing rejection after heart transplantation. In: Rose ML, Yacoub MH, eds. Immunology of heart and lung transplantation. London: Edward Arnold, 1995:219–231.
84. Starnes VA, Theodore J, Oyer PE, et al. Pulmonary infiltrates after heart-lung transplantation: evaluation by serial transbronchial biopsies. J Thorac Cardiovasc Surg 1989;98:945–950.
85. Griffith BP, Hardesty RL, Trento A, et al. Asynchronous rejection of the heart and lungs following cardiopulmonary transplantation. Ann Thorac Surg 1985;40:488–493.
86. Costanzo-Nordin M, Grusk B, Siver M, et al. Reversal of recalcitrant cardiac allograft rejection with methotrexate. Circulation 1988;78:III47–57.
87. Chinnock R, Emery J, Larsen R, et al. Methotrexate therapy for complex graft rejection in pediatric heart transplant recipients. J Heart Lung Transplant 1995;14:726–733.
88. Salter MM, Kirklin JK, Bourge RC, et al. Total lymphoid irradiation in the treatment of early or recurrent heart rejection. J Heart Lung Transplant 1992;11:902–912.
89. Kirklin JK, George JF, McGiffin DC, et al. Total lymphoid irradiation: is there a role in pediatric heart transplantation? J Heart Lung Transplant 1993;12:S293–S300.
90. Costanzo-Nordin MR, Hubbell EA, O'Sullivan EJ, et al. Phopheresis versus corticosteroids in the therapy of heart transplant rejection. Preliminary clinical report. Circulation 1992;86:II242–II250.
91. Barr ML, Berger CL, Wiedermann JG, et al. Photochemotherapy for the prevention of graft atherosclerosis in cardiac

transplantation [Abstract]. J Heart Lung Transplant 1993;12:s85.
92. Dall'Amico R, Livi U, Montini G, et al. Photopheresis as adjuvant treatment of heart transplant (Htx) patients with multiple rejections [Abstract]. J Heart Lung Transplant 1996;13:s81.
93. Kaye MP. Pediatric thoracic transplantation: the world experience. J Heart Lung Transplant 1993;12:S344–S350.
94. Johnson MR, Mullen M, O'Sullivan J, et al. Risk/benefit ratio of perioperative OKT3 in cardiac transplantation. Am J Cardiol 1994;74:261–266.
95. Little RE, Kay GN, Epstein AE, et al. Arrhythmias after orthotopic cardiac transplantation: prevalence and determinants during initial hospitalization and late follow-up. Circulation 1989;80:III-140–III-146.
96. Mohanty PK, Sowers JR, Thames MD, et al. Myocardial norepinephrine, epinephrine and dopamine concentrations after cardiac autotransplantation in dogs. J Am Coll Cardiol 1986;7:419–424.
97. Drake AJ, Stanford C. Effect of cardiac denervation on catecholamine levels in dog heart. J Physiol (Lond) 1982; 324:14P.
98. Yusuf S, Theodoropoulos S, Mathias CJ, et al. Increased sensitivity of the denervated transplanted human heart to isoprenaline both before and after beta adrenergic blockade. Circulation 1987;75:696–704.
99. Kaye D, Thompson J, Jennings G, et al. Cyclosporin therapy after cardiac transplantation causes hypertension and renal vasoconstriction without sympathetic activation. Circulation 1993;88:1101–1109.
100. Textor SC, Canzanello VJ, Taler SJ, et al Cyclosporin-induced hypertension after transplantation. Mayo Clin Proc 1994;69:1182–1193.
101. Braith RW, Mills RM Jr, Wilcox CS, et al. Breakdown of blood pressure and body fluid homeostasis in heart transplant recipients. J Am Coll Cardiol 1996;27:375–383.
102. Kimblad PO, Sjöberg T, Steen S. Pulmonary vascular resistance related to endothelial function after lung transplantation. Ann Thorac Surg 1994;58:416–420.
103. Aoe M, Trachiotis GD, Okabayashi K, et al. Administration of prostaglandin E1 after lung transplantation improves early graft function. Ann Thorac Surg 1994;58:655–661.
104. Adatia I, Lillehei C, Arnold JH, et al. Inhaled nitric oxide in the treatment of postoperative graft dysfunction after lung transplantation. Ann Thorac Surg 1994;57:1311–1318.
105. Young JB, Leon CA, Short HD, et al. Evolution of hemodynamics after orthotopic heart and heart-lung transplantation: early restrictive patterns persisting in occult fashion. J Heart Transplant 1987;6:34–43.
106. Young JB, Winters WL, Bourge R, et al. Task force 4: function of the heart transplant recipient. J Am Coll Cardiol 1993;22:31–41.
107. Jacquet L, Ziady G, Stein K, et al. Cardiac rhythm disturbances early after orthotopic heart transplantation: prevalence and clinical importance of the observed abnormalities. J Am Coll Cardiol 1990;16:832–837.
108. Scott CD, Dark JH, McComb JM. Arrhythmias after cardiac transplantation. Am J Cardiol 1992;70:1061–1063.
109. Ellenbogen KA, Thames MD, DiMarco JP, et al. Electrophysiological effects of adenosine in the transplanted human heart. Evidence of supersensitivity. Circulation 1990;81: 821–828.
110. Park JK, Hsu DT, Hordof AJ, et al. Arrhythmias in pediatric heart transplant recipients: prevalence and association with death, coronary artery disease, and rejection. J Heart Lung Transplant 1993;12:956–964.
111. Vandenberg BF, Mohanty PK, Craddock KJ, et al. Clinical significance of pericardial effusion after heart transplantation. J Heart Transplant 1988;7:128–134.
112. Schowengerdt K, Naftel D, Selb P, et al. Infection after pediatric heart transplantation: a multi-institutional, multivariable analysis [Abstract]. J Heart Lung Transplant 1996; 15:s71.
113. Siegelman SS, Sinha SBP, Veith FJ. Pulmonary reimplantation response. Ann Surg 1973;177:30–36.
114. Prop JM, Ehrie MG, Crapo JD, et al. Reimplantation response in isografted rat lungs. J Thorac Cardiovasc Surg 1984;87:702.
115. Paradis, IL, Duncan SR, Dauber JH, et al. Distinguishing between infection, rejection and the adult respiratory distress syndrome after human lung transplantation. J Heart Lung Transplant 1992;11:S232–S236.
116. Starnes VA, Theodore J, Oyer PE, et al. Pulmonary infiltrates after heart-lung transplantation: evaluation by serial transbronchial biopsies. J Thorac Cardiovasc Surg 1989; 98:945–950.
117. Sibley RK, Berry GJ, Tazelaar HD, et al. The role of transbronchial biopsies in the management of lung transplant recipients. J Heart Lung Transplant 1993;12:308–324.
118. Spatenka J, Khagani A, Irviong JD, et al. Gianturco self-expanding metallic stents in treatment of tracheobronchial stenosis after single lung and heart-lung transplantation. Eur J Cardiothorac Surg 1991;5:648–652.
119. Shennib H, Massard G. Airway complications in lung transplantation. Ann Thorac Surg 1994;57:506–511.
120. Armitage JM, Kurland G, Michaels M, et al. Critical issues in pediatric lung transplantation. J Thorac Cardiovasc Surg 1995;109:60–65.
121. Grossi P, De Maria R, Caroli A, et al. Infections in heart transplant recipients: the experience of the Italian heart transplantation program. J Heart Lung Transplant 1992; 11:847–866.
122. Miller LW, Schlant RC, Kobashigawa J, et al. Task force 5: complications. J Am Coll Cardiol 1993;22:41–54.
123. Miller LW, Naftel DC, Bourge RC, et al. Infection following cardiac transplantation: a multi-institutional analysis [Abstract]. J Heart Lung Transplant 1992;11:192.
124. Dummer JS, White LT, Ho M, et al. Morbidity of cytomegalovirus infection in recipients of heart or heart-lung transplants who received cyclosporine. J Infect Dis 1985;152: 1182–1191.
125. Drew WL. Diagnosis of cytomegalovirus infection. Rev Infect Dis 1988;10(Suppl 3):468–476.
126. Keay S, Petersen E, Icenogle T, et al. Ganciclovir treatment of serious cytomegalovirus infection in heart and heart-lung transplant recipients. Rev Infect Dis 1988;10:563–572.
127. Jonsyn G, Radovancevic B, Abou-Awdi NL, et al. Immunoglobulin plays a major role in antiviral prophylaxis in CMV mismatched cardiac transplant recipients [Abstract]. J Heart Lung Transplant 1995;14:s64.
128. Armitage JM, Fricker FJ, del Nido P, et al. A decade (1982 to 1992) of pediatric cardiac transplantation and the impact of FK 506 immunosuppression. J Thorac Cardiovasc Surg 1993;105:464–473.
129. Vricella LA, Alonso de Begona J, Gundry SR, et al. Aggressive peritoneal dialysis for treatment of acute kidney failure after neonatal heart transplantation. J Heart Lung Transplant 1992;11:320–329.
130. Frazier OH, Van Buren CT, Poindexter SM, et al. Nutri-

130. tional management of the heart transplant recipient. J Heart Transplant 1985;4:450–452.
131. Peterseim DS, Pappas TN, Meyers CH, et al. Management of biliary complications after heart transplantation. J Heart Lung Transplant 1995;14:623–631.
132. Aziz S, Bergdahl L, Baldwin L. Pancreatitis after cardiac and cardiopulmonary transplantation. Surgery 1985;97:653–660.
133. Grigg MM, Costanzo-Nordin MR, Celesia GG, et al. The etiology of seizures after cardiac transplantation. Transplant Proc 1988;20(Suppl 3):937–944.
134. Atkinson K, Biggs J, Darveniza P, et al. Cyclosporine-associated central-nervous system toxicity after allogenic bone marrow transplantation. N Engl J Med 1984;310:527.
135. Beamn M, Parvin S, Veitch PS, Walls J. Convulsions associated with cyclosporine A renal transplant recipients. Br Med J 1985;290:139–140.
136. Kichuk MR, Cargan AL, Hsu DT, et al. Neurologic events in pediatric heart transplant recipients [Abstract]. J Heart Lung Transplant 1996;15:s71.
137. Craven J. Toronto Lung Transplant Group Psychiatric aspects of lung transplant. Can J Psychiatry 35:759–764.
138. Baum D, Bernstein D, Starnes VA, et al. Pediatric heart transplantation at Stanford: results of a 15-year experience. Pediatrics 1991;88:203–214.
139. Backer CL, Zales VR, Harrison HL, et al. Intermediate term results of infant orthotopic cardiac transplantation from two centers. J Thorac Cardiovasc Surg 1991;101:826–832.
140. Pennington DG, Noedel N, McBride LR, et al. Heart transplantation in children: an international survey. Ann Thorac Surg 1991;52:710–715.
141. Chapelier A, Vouhé P, Macchiarini P, et al. Comparative outcome of heart-lung and lung transplantation for pulmonary hypertension. J Thorac Cardiovasc Surg 1993;106:299–307.
142. Winters GL, Costanzo-Nordin MR, O'Sullivan EJ, et al. Predictors of late acute orthotopic heart transplant rejection. Circulation 1989;80:III-106–III-110.
143. Yacoub M, Rose M. Accelerated coronary sclerosis. In: Rose ML, Yacoub MH, eds. Immunology of heart and lung transplantation. London: Edward Arnold, 1993:289–299.
144. Haverich A, Dammenhayn L, Demertzis L, et al. Lung growth after experimental pulmonary transplantation. J Heart Lung Transplant 1991;16:288–295.
145. Pahl E, Zales VR, Fricker FJ, et al. Posttransplant coronary artery disease in children: a multicenter national survey. Circulation 1994;90(Part 2):II-56–II-60.
146. Noyes BE, Kurland G, Orenstein DM, et al. Experience with pediatric lung transplantation. J Pediatr 1994;124:261–268.
147. Tamm M, Sharples L, Dennis C, et al. Obliterative bronchiolitis in 120 consecutive heart-lung transplants [Abstract]. Am Rev Respir Dis 1993;147:a197.
148. Whitehead B, Rees P, Sorensen K, et al. Incidence of obliterative bronchiolitis after heart-lung transplantation in children. J Heart Lung Transplant 1994;13:903–908.
149. Dark JH. Clinical diagnosis of rejection and the development of obliterative bronchiolitis after lung transplantation. In: Rose ML, Yacoub MH. Immunology of heart and lung transplantation. London: Edward Arnold, 1993:276–288.
150. Halvorsen RA, DuCret RP, Kuni CC, et al. Obliterative bronchiolitis after lung transplantation. Diagnostic utility of aerosol ventilation lung scanning and high resolution CT. Clin Nucl Med 1991;16:256–258.
151. Lentz D, Bergin CJ, Berry GJ, et al. Diagnosis of bronchiolitis obliterans in heart-lung transplantation patients: importance of bronchial dilatation on CT. Am J Roentgenol 1992;159:463–467.
152. Kramer MR, Stoehr C, Whang JL, et al. The diagnosis of obliterative bronchiolitis after heart-lung and lung transplantation: low yield of transbronchial biopsy. J Heart Lung Transplant 1993;12:675–681.
153. Corris PA, Fishwick D, Parry G, et al. The role of total lymphoid irradiation (TLI) in the treatment of obliterative bronchiolitis (OB) [Abstract]. J Heart Lung Transplant 1994;13:s54.
154. Dusmet M, Maurer J, Winton T, et al. Methotrexate in the treatment of bronchiolitis obliterans syndrome [Abstract]. J Heart Lung Transplant 1996;15:s102.
155. Adams DH, Cochrane AD, Khaghani A, et al. Retransplantation in heart-lung recipients with obliterative bronchiolitis. J Thorac Cardiovasc Surg 1994;107:450–459.
156. Ho M, Jaffe R, Miller G, et al. The frequency of Epstein-Barr virus infection and associated lymphoproliferative syndrome after transplantation and its manifestations in children. Transplantation 1988;45:719–727.
157. Armitage JM, Kormos RL, Stuart RS, et al. Posttransplant lymphoproliferative disease in thoracic organ transplant patients: ten years of cyclosporine-based immunosuppression. J Heart Lung Transplant 1991;10:877–887.
158. Chen JM, Barr ML, Chadburn A, et al. Management of lymphoproliferative disorders after cardiac transplantation. Ann Thorac Surg 1993;56:527–538.

Mechanical Support of the Myocardium

Mohan Reddy, MD, and Frank L. Hanley, MD

In children with reversible cardiac or pulmonary dysfunction, prolonged extracorporeal support is now a well-established modality with significant improvement in survival of otherwise unsalvageable cases. Since the technology of extracorporeal membrane oxygenation (ECMO) has been in use for neonatal pulmonary dysfunction, it has become the initial support method of choice for extracorporeal support. However, with the introduction of pediatric centrifugal pumps (Bio-Medicus, Minneapolis, MN), their use as ventricular assist devices (VADs) soon followed. The choice between ECMO and a VAD is often institution and surgeon dependent. However, with experience, it is now possible to define certain guidelines for the choice of mechanical support.

MECHANICAL SUPPORT METHODS

At present four methods of mechanical support of the failing heart exist. The feasibility and success of these methods is considerably different in pediatric patients than for adult patients; therefore, the preferred method of mechanical assistance is different in these patient groups (see Table 22.1).

Although the intra-aortic balloon pump (IABP) is the most extensively used mechanical assistance, its application has been limited in pediatric patients. The IABP uses the principle of counterpulsation. The balloon is positioned in the upper thoracic aorta. It deflates at the beginning of systole, thereby decreasing the afterload, and inflates at the beginning of diastole, thereby increasing the diastolic perfusion. The augmentation of cardiac output by this technique is limited to only 15 to 20%. This technique, almost invariably used in conjunction with inotropic support, is extensively used in adults with a high success rate. The size of the balloon has precluded the use of this device in children. With the use of smaller balloons in children aged more than 5 years the limited success achieved with this device was outweighed by the morbidity of femoral artery complications associated with balloon size and difficulty with insertion. In addition the higher heart rates in children pose difficulty with synchronization and notably the IABP does not provide right-side heart support. However, this device may still have some role in older children with less severe reversible myocardial dysfunction.

Currently, ECMO and VADs have become the mainstay of mechanical support and on occasion are used as a bridge to transplant in the pediatric population. The rest of this chapter focuses on these two modalities of mechanical cardiac and cardiopulmonary support. The total artificial heart as it exists today has not been used in children.

INDICATIONS FOR MECHANICAL SUPPORT

In general, cardiac and pulmonary dysfunction should be deemed reversible within reason before patients are placed on mechanical support. In patients who cannot be weaned from bypass and in patients with postoperative low cardiac output, residual structural lesions should be ruled out, using pressure and oximetry data from indwelling intracardiac catheters, and transesopheal echocardiography and/or surface echocardiography. Cardiac catheterization is indicated in some patients postoperatively for decision making. After ruling out any residual structural lesions medical management is maximized. If cardiac output is not adequate despite the use of multiple inotropic agents or if the dose of epinephrine exceeds 0.3 μg/kg/min in conjunction with other agents then mechanical support should be seriously considered. It should be emphasized that the adequacy of medical support must be individualized. Sometimes temporary improvement or ability to wean from bypass with medical management may soon be followed by continuing deterioration. In such circumstances early initiation of mechanical support is warranted rather than continued persistence with medical therapy. In patients with coexistent post-bypass pulmonary dysfunction, lung injury, or pulmonary hemorrhage the threshold should be low for early initiation of mechanical support. In addition, in patients with single ventricle physiology (Norwood or Damus procedures with systemic to pulmonary shunt), early and aggressive initiation of mechanical support is warranted. Our own personal bias in patients with stage I single ventricle repairs is to initiate mechanical support if inotropic support exceeds a combination of dopamine at 10 μg/kg/min and epinephrine at 0.2 μg/kg/min. In addition, when indicated, other appropriate pharmacotherapy consisting of afterload reduction and bicarbonate and calcium supplementation should be initiated and other metabolic parameters should be optimized before deciding to initiate mechanical assistance. It is important to realize the benefit of early initiation of mechanical assistance. Therefore, an aggressive early management and continuous assessment of the patient's status will avoid delays

Table 22.1. Methods of Mechanical Assistance

Children	Adults
ECMO	IABP
VAD	VAD
IABP	TAH
TAH	ECMO

ECMO, extracorporeal membrane oxygenation; IABP, intra-aortic balloon pump; TAH, total artificial heart; VAD, ventricular assist device.

and improve outcomes of mechanical assistance. Instead of viewing mechanical assistance as a salvage, it may be a better approach to pre-empt the deterioration of the hemodynamic situation by early initiation of mechanical assistance.

The following are common indications for prolonged extracorporeal support in patients with congenital heart disease:

Inability to wean from cardiopulmonary bypass
Postoperative
   Low cardiac output
   Cardiac arrest
   Intractable dysrhythmias: intractable ventricular tachycardia (VT) or junctional ectopic tachycardia with hemodynamic compromise
   Pulmonary hypertension not responsive to medical therapy and nitric oxide
Nonsurgical reversible myocardial injury
   Acute myocarditis or cardiomyopathy
Bridge to transplantation
Pre or postoperative pulmonary dysfunction
   Persistent pulmonary hypertension in neonates
   Pulmonary hemorrhage
   Post-bypass pulmonary dysfunction
   Neonatal respiratory distress or meconium aspiration in a child with congenital heart disease.

ECMO VERSUS VAD

In the past ECMO was the method most commonly employed for prolonged extracorporeal support largely because the technology existed and was already in use by the neonatologists to treat patients with isolated pulmonary problems. In addition the support methods in use for adult cardiac population, namely the IABP, existing ventricular assist devices, and the total artificial heart (TAH) were unsuitable for pediatric patients because of size constraints. The introduction of centrifugal and pneumatic pumps has eliminated this constraint. After isolated reports of these pumps used as VADs, many institutions now have reasonable experience with both ECMO and VADs. Experience from our and other institutions permits us to draw some general guidelines in choosing the type of mechanical assistance that most specifically addresses the physiologic deficiency. Figure 22.1 illustrates these guidelines.

The guidelines given above are general and based on experience and literature review. A VAD can be used even in patients weighing less than 5 kg. However, the choice of the device must be individualized to a given situation. Although the patient's size and the indication for use are important in the selection of the device, equally important is the presence of intracardiac communication (patent foramen ovale or atrial septal defect) and single ventricle physiology. In addition, sometimes when a VAD is used to support a ventricle, the dysfunction of the other ventricle may be unmasked. In such situations, a bi-VAD (two VADs, one for the right ventricle and one for the left ventricle, used in series) is indicated or the support method may have to be changed to ECMO.

A comparison of ECMO and VADs is given in Table 22.2. Although both modalities are effective, because of their simplicity and the need for less aggressive anticoagulation VADs are being increasingly used even in children weighing less than 5 kg.

DEVICE APPLICATION

As emphasized earlier, prior to application of mechanical support it is mandatory that any residual correctable lesions be ruled out and medical therapy be optimized. In addition every effort should be made to assess the patient's neurologic status prior to initiation of mechanical support. A thorough clinical examination and head ultrasound (in neonates and infants) to rule out intracranial bleeding and evidence of cerebral damage is essential. However, this

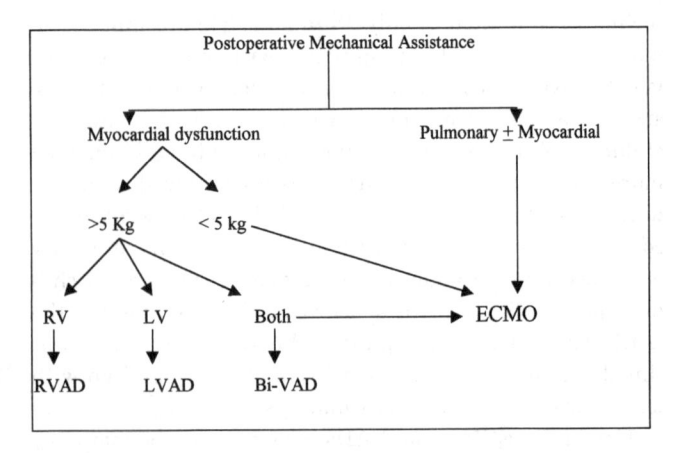

Figure 22.1. Postoperative mechanical assistance guidelines.

Table 22.2. Comparison of ECMO and VAD

	ECMO	VAD
Type of pump	Roller	Centrifugal or pneumatic
Oxygenator	Yes	No
Circuit	Complex, priming volume higher	Simple, priming volume small
Air embolism risk	Small	Higher
Anticoagulation	ACT about 180–200	ACT about 140–160
Cannulation	Neck/direct cardiac if chest open	Always direct, sternum left open
Patent foramen ovale	Little effect	Potential for desaturation

ACT, active clotting factor; ECMO, extracorporeal membrane oxygenation; VAD, ventricular assist device.

may not be possible in the operating room and in such a situation the decision should be based on the patient's preoperative status and intraoperative course.

In the operating room when a decision is made to place the patient on mechanical support, cannulae used for standard cardiopulmonary bypass are utilized. Every effort is made to control all surgical bleeding. If the patient can be weaned from bypass for a short period of time, heparin is reversed and clotting factors are administered to correct coagulation abnormalities. Then the patient is placed on mechanical support with limited anticoagulation using heparin.

When a decision is made in the postoperative period to provide mechanical assistance, then the cannulation is generally performed in the neck for ECMO and in the mediastinum for VADs. Whenever mediastinal cannulation is performed the chest is left open. Occasionally in older children the sternum is left open but the skin is closed.

MANAGEMENT OF PATIENTS ON MECHANICAL SUPPORT

In most centers patients on ECMO are managed by the neonatology-pediatric services and the patients on VADs are managed by the cardiac surgery-cardiology team, although multidisciplinary involvement is essential to success in all cases. Patients on ECMO are generally minimally ventilated as opposed to patients on VADs whose ventilation should be optimized. Patients in both groups are on minimal inotropic support, and are completely sedated and paralyzed until they are about to be weaned from mechanical support.

The mechanics of ECMO are similar to cardiopulmonary bypass. An obligatory volume displacement roller pump is usually used. The venous drainage is gravity dependent, and a small venous reservoir (bladder) and an oxygenator are present in the circuit. The commonly used VAD in pediatric patients is a centrifugal pump (Biomedicus), which pumps blood by imparting kinetic energy to the blood by rotating it at high speed in the pump head. There is no obligatory volume displacement by the pump. Therefore, it is both preload and afterload sensitive. Venous return to the pump is active and not dependent on gravity. These differences in device function make a considerable impact on the postoperative management.

Monitoring

Postoperative monitoring includes:

- ECG
- Core temperature
- Left atrial catheter for monitoring pressure
- Right atrial catheter(s) for monitoring pressure and infusing inotropes and other drugs
- Pulmonary artery catheter/thermistor/oximetry to measure pressure, cardiac output, or mixed venous oxygen saturation
- Systemic arterial catheter to measure pressure and blood gases
- Pulse oximeter
- Urinary catheter

Management

The percentage of total cardiac output provided by the mechanical support depends on the degree of myocardial dysfunction. Mean systemic arterial pressure should be maintained at 40 mm Hg or greater in neonates and young infants and about 60 mm Hg in older children. In patients on a VAD the atrial pressures are always maintained over 5 mm Hg to prevent any air from being sucked into the circuit. This is especially critical in patients on left ventricular assist because of the fatal consequences of coronary and systemic arterial embolism. Right atrial pressure, which is generally used to monitor the volume status, is maintained between 5 and 10 mm Hg. In patients placed on a left VAD whose right atrial pressure is inappropriately high, right ventricular dysfunction should be suspected.

In patients with single ventricle physiology with shunt

dependency, the shunt may be temporarily occluded during the period of ECMO to prevent pulmonary overcirculation, left heart distension, and pulmonary edema.

The usual clinical indicators of good cardiac output should be monitored. Blood gases, urine output, and mixed venous oxygen saturation are measured periodically. Cardiac output can be monitored with a pulmonary artery thermistor.

Systemic anticoagulation is achieved with heparin and the activated clotting time (ACT) is kept in the range of 140 to 160 seconds. The ACT is checked every 30 minutes initially and every 3 hours thereafter. Patients are also monitored for disseminated intravascular coagulopathy and hemolysis. Hematocrit is maintained at about 30%. Core temperature is maintained between 35°C and 37°C.

Daily clinical neurologic evaluation should be performed and periodically head ultrasound is repeated in neonates and infants. If necessary a head computerized tomographic scan is performed. A significant change in neurologic status may some times mandate discontinuation of mechanical support.

See Table 22.3 for guidelines on troubleshooting for patients on VAD. These guidelines are specific for a patient on a left ventricular assist device. Guidelines for patients on right ventricular assist devices or biventricular devices would vary slightly although following the same principles.

Weaning

A decision to wean from mechanical support is made after assessing the cardiac function by hemodynamic parameters and echocardiographic evaluation by transesophageal echocardiography. Inotropic support is optimized and the amount of mechanical support is gradually decreased by decreasing the device flow. After observing the hemodynamics at "idle" flow and assessing the ventricular function the mechanical support is completely withdrawn. Following this the patient should be closely monitored for signs of low cardiac output. Often the chest is left open for a day or more after weaning from the mechanical support.

Complications

The most common complications are bleeding and embolism. Mild to moderate mediastinal bleeding, which is common, is often caused by anticoagulation or coagulopathy. Surgical bleeding should always be aggressively addressed. Occasionally bleeding directly or indirectly is fatal. Excessive bleeding necessitating massive transfusions often results in pulmonary and multiorgan dysfunction.

Neurologic events such as intracranial hemorrhage or cerebral embolism are not uncommon, and they are one of the major indications for withdrawal of support. In addition, these events can result in significant long-term neurologic residual deficit. Other complications include renal failure, multisystem organ dysfunction, infections, and mechanical circuit complications.

OUTCOME

Cumulative data from the Extracorporal Life Support Organization (ELSO) registry indicates that the overall survival rate of ECMO in postcardiotomy patients is about 46%. Most of these patients are free of any long-term sequelae. Our experience and that of others is similar. Our data indicate that survival is significantly better (68%) when ECMO is initiated either in the operating room or within 12 hours of surgery, which underscores the need for early and aggressive initiation of mechanical support.

The survival and complications with VADs are similar in various institutional experiences. The risk of bleeding appears to be less and the potential for air embolism is greater.

Table 22.3. Trouble Shooting Patients on Left Ventricular Assist Device

Low LA pressure: hypovolemia, RV failure, excessive mechanical support
High LA pressure: inadequate pump support, volume overload, obstruction to cannula
Low RA pressure: hypovolemia, patent foramen ovale/atrial septal defect
High RA pressure: volume overload, RV dysfunction
Inability to maintain adequate pump flow: hypovolemia, malpositioned cannulae, thrombosis of cannulae or pump, kinking of cannulae or tubing
Metabolic acidosis: inadequate support, hypovolemia, organ damage (liver, bowel)
Hypoxia: pulmonary problem, patent foramen ovale/atrial septal defect
Excessive bleeding: Heparin overdose, DIC, dislodgment of cannulae, surgical suture line bleeding.

LA, left atrial; RA, right atrial; RV, right ventricle.

SUGGESTED READINGS

1. Anderson HL, Attori RJ, Custer JR, et al. Extracorporeal membrane oxygenation for pediatric cardiopulmonary failure. J Thorac Cardiovasc Surg 1990;99:1011–1019.
2. Golding LR, Jacobs G, Groves LK, et al. Clinical results of mechanical support of the failing heart. J Thorac Cardiovasc Surg 1982;83:597–601.
3. Kanter KR, Pennington G, Weber TR, et al. Extracorporeal membrane oxygenation for postoperative cardiac support in children. J Thorac Cardiovasc Surg 1987;93:27–35.
4. Kart TR, Sano S, Horton S, et al. Centrifugal pump left heart assist in pediatric cardiac operations. Indications, techniques, and results. J Thorac Cardiovasc Surg 1991;102:624–630.
5. Klein MD, Shaheen KW, Whittlesey GC, et al. Extracorporeal membrane oxygenation for circulatory support of children

after repair of congenital heart defects. J Thorac Cardiovasc Surg 1990;100:498–505.
6. Meliones JN, Custer JR, Shedecor S, et al. Extracorporeal life support for cardiac assist in pediatric patients. Reviews of ELSO registry data. Circulation 1991;84:III168–III172.
7. Pennington DG, Merjavy JP, Swartz MT, et al. Clinical experience with a centrifugal pump ventricular assist device. Trans Am Soc Artif Intern Organs 1992;29:93–99.
8. Pollock JC, Charlton MC, Williams WG, et al. Intraaortic balloon pumping in children. Ann Thorac Surg 1980;29:522–528.
9. Veasy LG, Blalock RC, Orth JL, et al. Intraaortic balloon pumping in infants and children. Circulation 1983;68:1095–1100.
10. Rogers AJ, Trento A, Siewers RD, et al. Extracorporeal membrane oxygenation for postcardiotomy cardiogenic shock in children. Ann Thorac Surg 1989;47:903–906.
11. Weinhaus L, Canter C, Noetzel M, et al. Extracorporeal membrane oxygenation for circulatory support after repair of congenital heart defects. Ann Thorac Surg 1989;48:206–212.
12. Costa RJ, Chard RB, Nunn GR, et al. Ventricular assist devices in pediatric cardiac surgery. Ann Thorac Surg 1995;60:S536–S538.
13. del Nido PJ, Armitage JM, Fricker FJ, et al. Extracorporeal membrane oxygenation as a bridge to pediatric heart transplantation. Circulation 1994;90:II66–II69.
14. Warnecke H, Berdjis F, Henning E, et al. Mechanical left ventricular support as a bridge to cardiac transplantation in children. Eur J Cardiothorac Surg 1991;S:330–333.
15. Black MD, Coles JG, Williams WG, et al. Determinants of success in pediatric cardiac patients undergoing extracorporeal membrane oxygenation. Ann Thorac Surg 1995;60:133–138.
16. Walters HL, Hakimi M, Rice MD, et al. Pediatric cardiac surgical ECMO: multivariate analysis of risk factors for hospital death. Ann Thorac Surg 1995;60:329–336.
17. Kulik TJ, Moler FW, Palnisano JM, et al. Outcome associated factors in pediatric patients treated with extracorporeal membrane oxygenator after cardiac surgery. Circulation 1996;94:II63–II68.
18. Joyce LD, Kiser JC, Eales F, et al. Experience with generally accepted centrifugal pumps: personal and collective experience. Ann Thorac Surg 1996;61:287–290.
19. Noon GP, Ball JW Jr, Short HD. Bio-Medicus centrifugal pump ventricular support for postcardiotomy cardiac failure: a review of 129 cases. Ann Thorac Surg 1996;61:291–295.
20. Argenziano M, Rose EA. The continuing evolution of mechanical ventricular assistance. Curr Probl Sur 1997;34:317–386.

Part D: Issues in Other Systems
Pulmonary Issues

23

Christopher JL Newth, MB, ChB, and Jurg Hammer, MD

PULMONARY PHYSIOLOGY OF THE PEDIATRIC PATIENT

The cardiovascular and respiratory systems are closely integrated in mammals for respiratory gas transport to and from tissues to keep pace with metabolic demands. This intimate association implies that the performance level of one system directly affects the demands of the other. Cardiovascular disease can often lead to respiratory failure because of the profound effect the cardiovascular function has on gas exchange, solute and water movement, and pulmonary mechanics. Conversely, respiratory failure can lead to cardiac failure, and it may be difficult to discern which is the primary problem.

Anatomically, the lungs begin as an outpouching of the primitive gut during the fourth week of gestation. At about this time cardiac formation begins. By the process of successive budding of the original diverticulum, all the airways an individual will ever have are laid down by 4 months of gestation. In contrast, alveolar budding begins at about the fifth month of gestation. At birth, the alveoli are still relatively primitive, but obviously they can sustain ventilation. Alveoli multiply rapidly, both before and after birth, and the process is probably completed between 5 to 7 years of age.

Although the adult pattern of blood supply to the lungs is achieved before the end of the second gestational month, structural and morphometric studies have shown that the intra-acinar arteries do not develop until shortly after birth. Thereafter, these vessels multiply rapidly, complementing the growth of alveoli in the postnatal period (1). The relative immaturity of the pulmonary microcirculation underlies significant differences in the physiology of the endothelium of the newborn and adult lungs, including functions related to water and solute exchange and handling of vasoactive hormones.

In many ways, the infant and young child are similar to the exercising adult. The adult has a large capacity for exercise, demonstrating that the respiratory and cardiovascular systems have considerable reserve for increasing the uptake and transport of respiratory gas to and from the tissues. Nevertheless, these limits may be reached quickly when more than one stress is imposed on a system. This is particularly true in the infant, whose normal resting state is already one of high respiratory and cardiovascular activity, compared with that of the resting adult (2). Oxygen consumption normalized to body surface area or weight is considerably higher in the infant than in the adult because of the larger surface area-to-body weight ratio and higher energy requirements for growth (3). Cardiac output related to weight or surface area in the infant is also high compared with that of the adult (4), and experimental evidence suggests that the reserve for further increasing cardiac output is limited (5).

As might be anticipated with a high metabolic rate, alveolar ventilation per unit of lung volume in the infant is high when compared with that of the adult (2). The sternum is soft and affords an unstable base for the highly compliant ribs. In addition, the ribs are horizontally placed and the intercostal muscles poorly developed, so that bucket-handle motion on which thoracic respiration depends is largely eliminated. Under these circumstances, diaphragmatic ventilation becomes extremely important. Any disease or physiologic function that impairs diaphragmatic function (such as postoperative phrenic nerve paralysis) predisposes the infant to respiratory failure. Stress will more quickly exhaust the energy-producing enzymes of the relatively few type I muscle fibers, and rapid eye movement (REM) sleep (the predominant sleep state of the young infant) decreases reserve because the proportion of ventilation performed by the diaphragm increases dramatically in this sleep state (6). In addition, conductance in both peripheral and central airways (7) is low, as is lung compliance. Both of these factors are related to a degree to the smaller numbers of alveolar septae (and thus, lower elastic recoil) in the infant lung (8). Consequently, infants have little tolerance for compromise of their lung mechanics (9). Gas exchange studies have shown that the infant has a large alveolar-arterial oxygen difference. This has been attributed to ventilation-perfusion inequality by some and a shunt by others (10). Functional residual capacity is probably less than closing volume (8) until the child reaches 3 to 4 years of age. At this age, the intra-alveolar pores of Kohn and the bronchoalveolar canals of Lambert develop (11), and for the first time, gas exchange beyond obstructed airways can be maintained by collateral ventilation. These phenomena may contribute to the (normal) lower arterial oxygen tension in the young child (12) compared with the adult.

Assessment of Pulmonary Function

The perioperative course of the cardiothoracic patient is frequently complicated by respiratory compromise from various reasons (Table 23.1). Precise assessment of ventilatory adequacy must be based on serial clinical examinations and laboratory studies, and much emphasis has to be placed on arterial blood gases (or their indirect measurement). In addition, with recent technologic developments it is now possible to perform bedside pulmonary function measurements in even the sickest of infants. Although it is generally true that pulmonary function testing does not establish a diagnosis, it reveals patterns of abnormality that are highly characteristic of certain diseases. In the perioperative care of cardiac patients, the major goals of pulmonary function testing are to:

1. Understand the underlying pulmonary pathophysiology
2. Aid with the diagnosis
3. Assess therapeutic responses
4. Provide a guide to changes in a patient's condition, which allow timely intervention

Infant lung function testing generally requires the use of sedation, and neuromuscular blockade when patients are on mechanically assisted ventilation. The latter situation also requires that no leak occur around the endotracheal tube in order to obtain good quality studies. This can be achieved in most cases with either a cuffed endotracheal tube (ETT) or with uncuffed tubes with pharyngeal packing (13). The basic concepts of infant pulmonary function testing will be introduced, but for more detailed information the reader is referred to original papers and reviews (14–17).

Thoracoabdominal Asynchrony

Thoracoabdominal asynchrony and paradoxic breathing, often referred to as "chest wall retractions," are characteristic signs of respiratory distress and respiratory muscle dysfunction in infants and young children. This phenomenon can be easily detected, quantified, and monitored by esophageal pressure monitoring or less invasively by phase angle analysis of the Lissajous figure (18) using uncalibrated respiratory inductance plethysmography. Such electromechanical measurements provide objective means to follow changes in the severity of upper and lower airway obstruction and the response to therapy reliably and with less inconvenience to the patient than clinical, radiologic, or arterial blood gas monitoring (19–21). Diaphragmatic paralysis can be easily detected at the bedside by the generation of characteristic loop patterns (22). Nevertheless, these methods require further critical evaluation to clarify their predictive and diagnostic value (e.g., during weaning from mechanical ventilation).

Respiratory Mechanics

Measurement of respiratory mechanics is essentially an analysis of the static forces that are responsible for lungs and chest wall stability and of the dynamic forces that result in movement of gases. Compliance is a measure of the distensibility or elasticity of the respiratory system, and it is defined as the change in lung volume per unit change in pleural pressure. Resistance is measured by relating gas flow to the corresponding driving pressure, and it represents the resistive properties of the airways, lung tissue, and chest wall. Total respiratory system compliance can be subdivided into lung and chest wall components. It must be emphasized that compliance is a function not only of the elastic properties of the respiratory system, but also of its volume. In other words, the value obtained is different at various lung volumes, dependent on the shape of the pressure-volume curve. Sudden changes in compliance often reflect the opening and closing of individual lung units rather than changes in lung tissue and surface tension characteristics (23).

A number of innovative approaches have been designed to assess compliance and resistance directly in ventilated infants (17, 24–26). Calculation of lung compliance in-

Table 23.1. Causes of Respiratory Compromise in the Cardiac Patient

Central	Compromise from anesthesia of sedation
	Hypoxic encephalopathy
	Apnea of prematurity
Upper Airway	Vocal cord paralysis
	Postextubation subglottic edema
	Vascular compression
	Laryngotracheobronchomalacia
	Blocked endotracheal or tracheostomy tubes
Lung	Infection
	Pulmonary edema
	Atelectasis
	Pneumothorax of pleural effusion
	Acute respiratory distress syndrome or sepsis
	Bronchopulmonary dysplasia
	Secondary surfactant deficiency (cardiopulmonary bypass)
	Reperfusion injury
	Transplant rejection
Cardiovascular	Congestive heart failure
	Cyanotic lesions
	Anemia
Neuromuscular	Diaphragmatic paralysis
	Respiratory muscle weakness (malnutrition)
	Malnutrition
	Neuromuscular blockade (incomplete reversal postoperative)
Chest Wall	Flail chest
	Kyphoscoliosis
	Clam shell chest incision

volves measurement of esophageal pressure as a quantification of pleural pressure (27). This technique is minimally invasive by virtue of the need for an esophageal catheter and the accuracy of such measurements in intubated infants and children is open to debate (28, 29). Total respiratory system compliance is determined by measuring airway pressure during a brief airway occlusion at end-inspiration (during which time, mouth pressure and alveolar pressure are the same) and fitting a straight line to the flow-volume curve obtained during the subsequent passive exhalation (30, 31). A passive exhalation is achieved either by invoking the Hering-Breuer inflation reflex or by use of neuromuscular blockade. Dynamic compliance could be simply calculated from ventilator settings by dividing tidal volume by the total change in pressure necessary to deliver that volume. However, dynamic compliance changes with alteration of mechanical ventilation settings including respiratory frequency, and inspiratory and end-expiratory pressures.

Increased pulmonary blood flow and pulmonary edema are possible mechanisms for pulmonary dysfunction after cardiac surgery. Respiratory failure is common after neonatal cardiac surgery requiring prolonged ventilatory support (32). Pulmonary vascular congestion (including lymphatic congestion) or interstitial edema causes a decrease in lung compliance. At greater degrees of vascular engorgement or when interstitial edema progresses to alveolar edema, pulmonary resistance increases. Although many infants have abnormal lung compliance in the postoperative period, those infants with respiratory failure also have greatly increased resistance. Lung function measurements can be helpful in the management of ventilatory support and timing of its withdrawal (33). In infants with underlying pulmonary disease such measurements can quantitate the extent of a restrictive or obstructive alteration in lung mechanics and assess the benefit of therapeutic interventions. It is important to note that in the case of intubated patients, such measurements include the physical properties of the endotracheal tube. Normal data for intubated infants lie in the range of 0.8–1.2 mL.cm H_2O^{-1}.kg^{-1} for total respiratory system compliance and 0.04–0.08 cm H_2O mL^{-1}.sec^{-1} (up to 0.1 cm H_2O/mL/sec with ETT less than 3.5 mm internal diameter [ID]) for resistance (34).

Maximal Expiratory Flow-Volume Curves

Measurement of maximal expiratory flow-volume (MEFV) relationships is a sensitive test to assess abnormalities in the tracheobronchial tree, and it contributes greatly to the diagnosis and treatment of lung disease. The forced deflation technique is regarded as the "gold standard" to generate MEFV curves in intubated infants and small children who are unable to perform a voluntary forced exhalation (35, 36). In this technique, the lungs are inflated to total lung capacity (defined as +40 cm H_2O inspiratory pressure) at which point the intubated airway is suddenly exposed to negative pressure (usually −40 cm H_2O), resulting in rapid lung deflation to residual volume. Forced vital capacity (FVC) and expiratory flows at various subdivisions are measured by an interposed pneumotachograph. This procedure is usually performed with 100% oxygen and with the individual under neuromuscular blockade or heavy sedation.

Forced expiratory maneuvers are critically dependent on their ability to produce flow limitation conditions in the airways. Only if it is certain that flow is effort independent (i.e., an increase in effort does not cause additional increase in flow) at a particular lung volume, can change in flow rates after a therapeutic maneuver (e.g., bronchodilator) be attributed to differences in airway conductance rather than effort. Effort independence has been shown to occur in intubated animals and infants with normal airways using negative airway opening pressures of −40 cm H_2O during the forced deflation maneuver (36–38).

Normal values for FVC lie in the range of 55–70 mL.kg^{-1} and for maximal expiratory flow at 25% FVC around 24–38 mL.kg^{-1}.sec^{-1}. Because it has become standard of care to use inhaled bronchodilators for a variety of diseases in intubated and ventilated patients, their effectiveness can now easily be documented (39). Pattern recognition of the characteristic flow-volume curves of obstructive versus restrictive pulmonary diseases can be helpful in identifying the underlying pathophysiology (14, 40).

Functional Residual Capacity

Technical difficulties involved in lung volume measurements have limited such measurements to research institutions. Nevertheless, determination of lung volumes is an important part of infant pulmonary function testing, and it helps in assessment of respiratory disorders and in evaluating responses to therapy. Knowledge of functional residual capacity (FRC) is essential if mechanical ventilation is to be rationally applied (41–43). Lung volume is also an important variable when lung mechanics are measured (44) because *specific compliance* and *specific resistance* are normalized by lung volume (i.e., FRC).

Several techniques can be used to measure FRC, of which helium (He) dilution (a closed-circuit method) (45), nitrogen (N_2) washout (in its modern form, an open-circuit method) (46), and sulphahexafluoride (SF6) washin-washout (47, 48) are the most widely used in intubated infants.

Pulmonary Diffusing Capacity and Pulmonary Blood Flow

Pulmonary diffusing capacity and pulmonary blood flow tests can be used to determine noninvasively the capillary blood volume of the lungs (from the diffusing capacity, D_Lco) and the blood flow in the lung capillaries, which passes alveoli and can therefore participate effectively in gas exchange ($Q_P$eff). These tests can be performed either as single-breath or rebreathe techniques in the intensive care unit (ICU), and FRC or other lung volumes can be obtained at the same time. Carbon monoxide, which binds tightly to hemoglobin, is commonly used for diffusing capacity measurements, and a soluble gas such as acetylene or Freon 22 for effective pulmonary blood flow. These tests have been applied to infants in the ICU (49–51) as research tools, and they have provided some valuable physiologic information but their roles in routine clinical measurements are not yet defined.

BRONCHOSCOPY

Traditionally, bronchoscopy in pediatric patients has been undertaken with rigid instruments that allowed excellent optics but limited access to the lower airways. The introduction of ultrathin flexible bronchoscopes allows visualization of more distal generations of airways even in premature neonates. However, the small size of pediatric airways still presents some limitations to bronchoscopists. For example, the ultrathin (less than 3 mm diameter) flexible (and directable) bronchoscopes used in infants may not have an operating channel to allow suction, and the smallest bronchoscope to allow a transbronchial biopsy is currently a 3.4 mm diameter bronchoscope that is equipped with a 1–2 mm operating channel (52). In these situations, the rigid bronchoscope still plays a vital role (Fig. 23.1).

Rigid bronchoscopy is usually performed in the operating room, and it has the advantage of providing better quality optics, together with the ability to ventilate the patients, suction, biopsy, and apply laser therapy at any time. However, rigid bronchoscopes lack the directional control of flexible instruments, and they cannot be passed through an endotracheal tube, which limits their use in critically ill patients. In the ICU, flexible bronchoscopy can be easily and safely performed at the bedside through an ETT if necessary (with relatively little interference to mechanical ventilation if a Bodai connector is used). In this situation, the bronchoscope can be used to provide information on function, anatomy, and infection of the airways (Table 23.2). In nonintubated patients the procedure is usually well tolerated with light sedation (e.g., midazolam, propofol, ketamine) and topical anesthesia (lidocaine 1%) to the oropharynx, vocal cords, and carina to attenuate cough and gag reflexes. Video recording of the procedure is beneficial for documentation, review, and teaching purposes.

Bronchoscopic procedures are superseding open lung biopsy as the investigation of choice for diagnosing lung pathology in transplant recipients and other immunocompromised patients. Transbronchial biopsy is well established in lung transplant recipients for detecting rejection (53). In immunocompromised patients, bronchoalveolar lavage (BAL) is almost as sensitive as open lung biopsy in detecting opportunistic infections (54–56) with a low incidence of false-positive results. Various authors

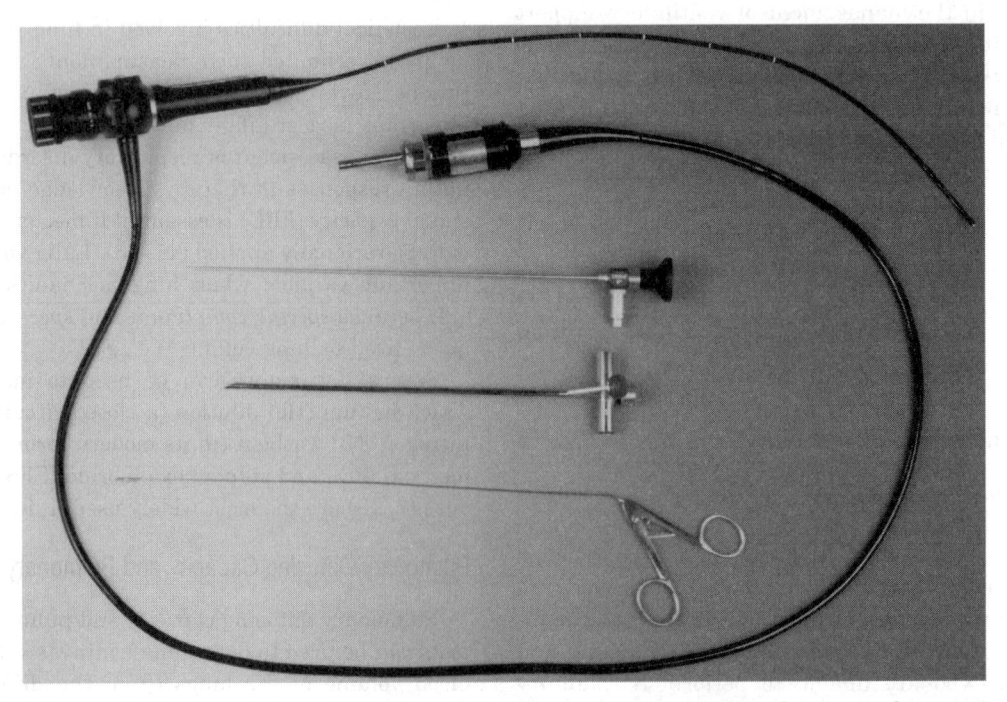

Figure 23.1. Photograph showing a 3.5 mm flexible bronchoscope and a 3.5 mm rigid bronchoscope with extraction forceps.

Table 23.2. Indications for Bronchoscopy in the Cardiac Patient

Diagnostic
  Unexplained upper airway obstruction (stridor)
  Hoarseness or weak cry
  Evaluation of airway trauma (prolonged intubation)
  Suspected vocal cord paralysis
  Persistent atelectasis
  Pneumonia or infiltrates in compromised host
  Recurrent or persistent pneumonia
  Chronic cough
  Persistent wheezing
  Congenital anomalies (e.g., vascular ring, tracheoesophageal fistula)
  Assessment of extrinsic airway compression
  Inspection of bronchial suture lines in heart-lung transplant
Therapeutic
  Difficult endotracheal intubation
  Acute lobar atelectasis
  Guide to surgical interventions

have reported identification of specific infectious agents in 40 to 71% of cases (57–59). BAL is well tolerated, and it is not associated with the high incidence of pneumothorax and prolonged mechanical ventilation seen following open lung biopsy (60, 61). Lung biopsy (either open or transbronchial) should now be regarded as a second line investigation for those patients in whom BAL does not reveal a specific pathogen.

Bronchoscopy has also been extended to the neonatal age group, where it is of value in the diagnosis of various congenital malformations, as well as acquired airway disorders (62). Ultrathin bronchoscopes (down to 1.8 mm external diameter) allow bronchoscopy to be performed in neonates as small as 700 g (63, 64), although the small size of these bronchoscopes causes some limitation of image quality, and the lack of guidewires in the smallest bronchoscopes allows only limited directional control. Bronchoscopic techniques have been used to manage airway obstruction caused by tracheal granulations and strictures, and to treat lobar atelectasis. Availability of small diameter bronchoscopes also allows for endoscopic intubation with endotracheal tubes as small as 2.5 mm ID in infants with dysmorphic airways. Availability of laryngeal mask airways or specially designed face masks (64a), coupled with flexible fiberoptic bronchoscopy, means that control of all but the most difficult airways is readily assured.

Bronchoscopy also provides access via the operating channel for lasers, allowing treatment of a wide variety of airway diseases, including granulomata, cystic lesions, and even tracheoesophageal fistulae (65, 66). Modern laser light sources can be projected along a 400–600 μm quartz fiber that can be passed through any bronchoscope with a suction port. Foreign bodies cannot be removed safely with flexible fiberoptic bronchoscopes, but the flexible instrument can be used at the bedside quickly to exclude the presence of a foreign body, thus avoiding transport of a potentially unstable patient to the operating room.

Complications of bronchoscopy include transient desaturation and hypoventilation, pyrexia, pneumothorax, pulmonary artery perforation, and laryngeal perforation, but in general the technique causes far less morbidity and mortality than open lung biopsy (67, 68)—often the only other available diagnostic tool for many disorders.

SPECIFIC PROBLEMS IN CHILDREN WITH CONGENITAL HEART DISEASE

Infants with congenital cardiac anomalies often manifest with respiratory symptoms secondary to cardiac dysfunction increasing the work of breathing and impairing gas exchange. The oxygen cost of breathing can become extraordinary and cause respiratory fatigue and failure, especially when oxygen requirements are already elevated as during fever, agitation, or by metabolism stimulating intravenous catecholamines. Mechanical ventilation may be required to unload the failing heart from the increased work of breathing.

The mechanism responsible for pulmonary compromise depends on the specific pathophysiologic alteration produced by each anomaly (Fig. 23.2). Lesions associated with increased pulmonary blood flow or pulmonary artery pressure (e.g., ventricular septal defect [VSD], complete [AV]-canal, patent ductus arteriosus [PDA], atrial septal defect [ASD]) have raised vascular pressures within the lung causing fluid to accumulate in the interstitium and alveoli. Respiratory compliance is decreased as a result of the peribronchial lymphatic and interstitial engorgement and ultimately pulmonary edema, which renders the lungs stiff. Airway resistance is increased by compression of bronchial airways by peribronchial edema or engorged vessels (69–71). Bronchial compression by enlarged pulmonary arteries can cause lobar atelectasis, which further increases ventilation-perfusion mismatch. Respiratory problems from lesions obstructing the inflow or outflow of the systemic ventricle are caused by pulmonary venous and lymphatic congestion leading to pulmonary edema. Respiratory symptoms are usually more severe than those of shunt lesions. This is especially true for children with obstructed pulmonary venous return, severe coarctation, or aortic stenosis. Increased pulmonary venous return may lead to left ventricular volume overload, increased left atrial pressure, and pulmonary congestion and edema, resulting in similar alterations of respiratory mechanics. In pulmonary edema, positive pressure ventilation alone, along with subsequent expansion of collapsed lung units, will reduce intrapulmonary shunting and decrease pulmonary vascular resistance.

Alteration of Respiratory Mechanics by Cardiac Anomalies

Large L--> R Shunt
- ASD
- VSD
- PDA
- Single ventricle
- Aortopulmonary window
- Truncus arteriosus

Inflow or Outflow Obstruction of the Systemic Ventricle
- Coarctation
- Aortic stenosis/atresia
- Mitral stenosis/atresia
- Obstruction to pulmonary venous return

Vascular airway compression
- Vascular ring
- Pulmonary artery sling
- Anomalous origin of the innominate artery
- Absent pulmonary valves

↓ Increased pulmonary blood flow → Pulmonary venous congestion

↓ Extrinsic airway compression

→ Interstitial and/or alveolar edema → **Respiratory compliance reduced**

→ Enlarged pulmonary arteries / Engorged peribronchial vessels / Peribronchial edema → **Respiratory resistance increased**

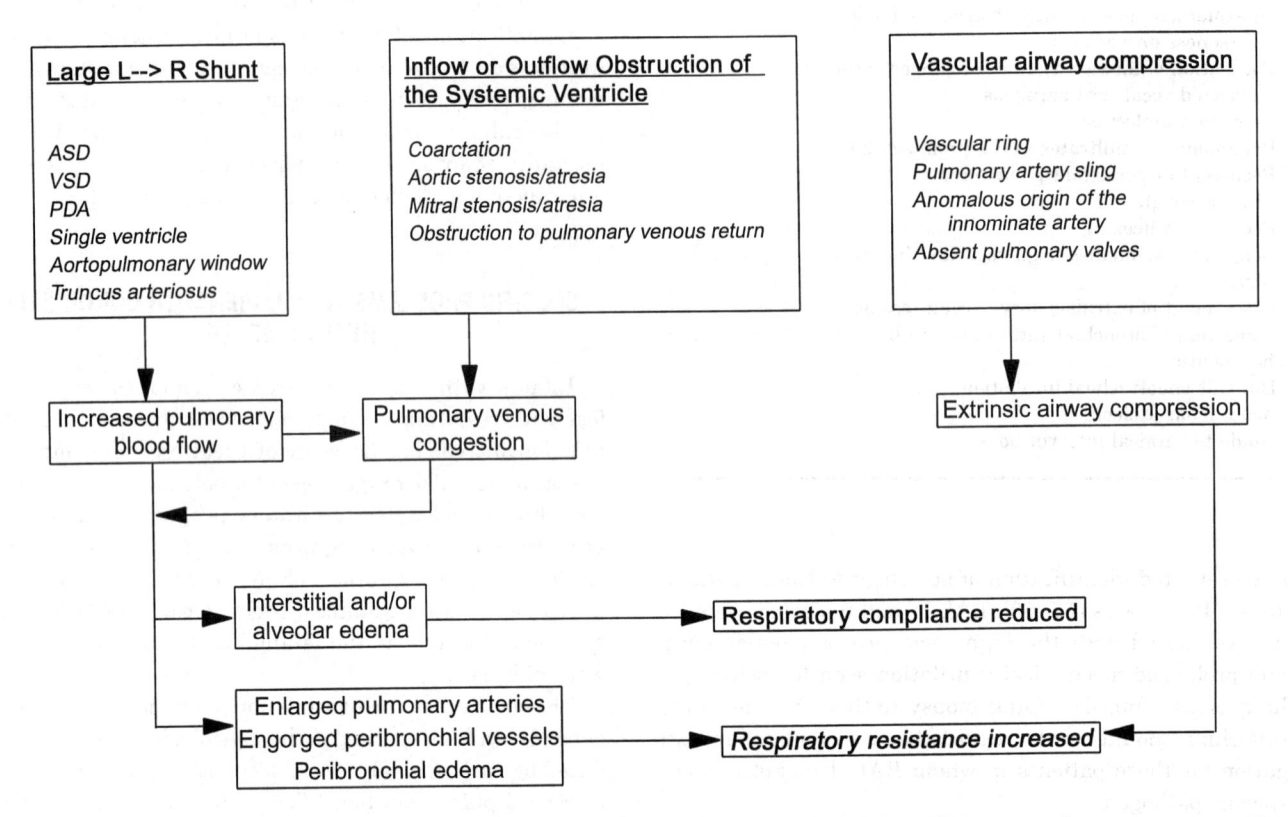

Figure 23.2. Alteration of respiratory mechanics by cardiac anomalies. *ASD*, atrial septal defect; *PDA*, patent ductus arteriosus; *VSD*, ventricular septal defect.

Malformations associated with decreased pulmonary blood flow (e.g., pulmonary atresia, tetralogy of Fallot [TOF]) can have increased lung compliance and abnormal ventilation-perfusion relationships because of reduced hydrostatic pressure (72). In such lesions, positive pressure ventilation can further reduce pulmonary blood flow by increasing pulmonary vascular resistance. Low cardiac output to the point of myocardial failure is another reason for respiratory compromise and its effects on lung function are similar to that of increased pulmonary blood flow.

During cardiopulmonary bypass, the lungs may be partially or completely atelectatic for lengthy periods, compromising lung mechanics for a variable time after resuming ventilation. Hence, cardiopulmonary bypass increases lung stiffness in children with decreased or normal pulmonary blood flow. Needless to say, the beneficial effects of corrective surgery in infants with increased pulmonary blood flow outweigh any transient detrimental effects of cardiopulmonary bypass (73).

Postoperatively, respiratory disadvantages and prolonged mechanical ventilation are related to the duration of cardiopulmonary bypass and intraoperative cardiac ischemia, the age of the patient, and presence of preoperative pulmonary compromise (74). Other factors involved in postoperative respiratory compromise include inspissated secretions, bronchospasm, mucosal edema, or interstitial bulk impeding gas flow. Increased pulmonary blood volume and pulmonary edema can cause pulmonary dysfunction after cardiac surgery. Pulmonary vascular congestion and interstitial edema decrease lung compliance. Greater degrees of alveolar edema or vascular engorgement result in compression of small airways, which increases pulmonary resistance. Fluid imbalance and secondary surfactant deficiency after cardiopulmonary bypass additionally impair pulmonary function. As a result, the increased work of breathing or the ventilation-perfusion mismatching can prolong the requirement for mechanical ventilatory support. Premature extubation with subsequent respiratory decompensation is expected to prolong ventilator dependence (75). It may be difficult at times to determine the relative contribution of cardiac and pulmonary systems to postoperative respiratory compromise.

SPECIFIC LESIONS

Absent Pulmonary Valve

Aneurysmal dilation of the main pulmonary arteries in infants with absent pulmonary valve causes compression of the lower trachea and the main stem bronchi. In its most severe form, vascular compression occurs also distally in intrapulmonary bronchi as a result of abnormal pulmonary artery branching determined during fetal life. Instead of single segmental arteries, tufts of pulmonary arteries encircle and compress the intrapulmonary bronchi (76, 77). Infants with the severe form of the absent pulmonary valve syndrome present in the newborn period with respiratory distress and signs typically associated with obstructive lung disease such as wheezing and air trapping (78). The severity of the intrapulmonary bronchial compression precludes a successful outcome from surgical and medical therapy and these patients frequently die in the newborn period (79). Pulmonary function testing may be helpful in determining the presence of central and peripheral airway obstruction pre- and postoperatively (Fig. 23.3; see color plate 23.3). Those children presenting outside the newborn period can often be successfully managed medically and surgically (80).

In the respiratory management of these children it is essential to maintain normal or increased systemic arterial oxygen tension and normal or low carbon dioxide tension. This prevents pulmonary artery constriction. Because of the anatomic cause of obstructive small airway disease, bronchodilator therapy is unlikely to be effective, and it should be guided by the results of pulmonary function tests. Elevated positive end-expiratory pressures or prone ventilation may help keep obstructed airways patent during ventilatory support or nasopharyngeal mask continuous positive airway pressure (CPAP), but this obviously cannot be a long-term solution.

Vascular Rings

Stridor appearing at birth is the major respiratory symptom in infants with vascular rings. Stridor is usually present in both inspiration and expiration, and it increases with effort and during feedings. Other less common symptoms include cough, recurrent bronchopulmonary infections, life-threatening reflex apneas, and dysphagia.

Endotracheal intubation is rarely necessary in the preoperative phase and surgical correction usually results in immediate improvement of the respiratory symptoms. Long-term follow-up studies of patients after surgical repair have shown residual lung function abnormalities in more than 50% of cases, even in those with complete resolution of symptoms (81, 82). Respiratory flow-volume loops demonstrate a distinctive plateau as a result of inspiratory and expiratory flow reduction. Long-term function abnormalities have been attributed to either residual tracheomalacia, local tracheostenosis, or an increased incidence of reactive airways disease. Severe tracheomalacia is a challenging problem.

Upper Airway Obstruction

Upper airway obstruction is defined as an obstruction occurring between the nares and the carina. Such obstructive lesions are usually characterized by difficulty in inhaling air, resulting in inspiratory stridor. Many causes are seen of upper airway obstruction in infants, whereas only a few are observed in the perioperative care of cardiac patients (Table 23.3).

Airways of infants and young children are large relative to those of an adult. However, the absolute diameter is small so that narrowing (secondary to inflammation and edema or congenital narrowing) of any part, and in particular the subglottic region, causes a much greater reduction in the cross-sectional area in the neonate than in an adult. Because an inverse fourth-power relationship of the airway radius to resistance exists, such a decrease in cross-sectional area in the young child, as in the neonate, results in relatively large increases in airway resistance to breathing, and thus, respiratory work.

During inspiration against a fixed obstruction in the extrathoracic trachea, large negative intrapleural pressures (relative to the atmospheric pressure around the neck) can be generated immediately below the obstruction by even small infants. The subsequent dynamic narrowing of the extrathoracic trachea, the cartilage of which is relatively soft in infants, leads to inspiratory stridor. As a result of the increased negative pleural pressure, the sternum and

Table 23.3. Stridor in the Perioperative Cardiac Infant

Common
  Postextubation subglottic edema
  Subglottic stenosis—acquired or congenital
  Vocal cord dysfunction
  Laryngomalacia (infantile larynx)
  Tracheomalacia
Rare
  Congenital upper airway anomalies (choanal atresia, tracheal stenosis)
  Micrognathia, large tongue
  Adenoidal and tonsillar hypertrophy
  Laryngeal cysts, webs, hemangiomas
  Laryngotracheobronchitis—viral croup
  Spasmodic croup
  Epiglottis
  Foreign body aspiration
  Allergic reactions
  Psychogenic

rib cage, which are compliant in young children, can be deformed. This is responsible for the classic signs of retraction of suprasternal tissues, sternum, and costal cartilages. This may be pronounced in cardiac patients because of higher chest wall compliance following sternotomies. Increased lung water resulting in increased lung stiffness can add further load on the respiratory muscles. During exhalation, the opposite occurs with the extrathoracic trachea tending to "balloon." Thus, the obstruction to airflow is greater during inhalation than during exhalation. Exaggerated respiratory efforts are associated with pulsus paradoxus.

In acute upper airway obstruction, hypoxemia from $\dot{V}/\dot{Q}$ mismatch is the earliest important arterial blood gas abnormality, and it occurs out of proportion to carbon dioxide retention from alveolar hypoventilation (83, 84). Several mechanisms may contribute to $\dot{V}/\dot{Q}$ mismatch, either singly or in combination. If a lesion is associated with a disease in which widespread tracheal or laryngeal inflammation are seen (e.g., laryngotracheitis or croup), there may be copious secretions. If ability to produce an effective cough to clear the airways is impaired, retention of these secretions can lead to subclinical plugging of bronchioles and small bronchi, and thus $\dot{V}/\dot{Q}$ mismatch. Occasionally, these secretions can block a larger bronchus and cause overt atelectasis, often of the right upper lobe, or if the heart is enlarged, the left lower lobe because of some compression of the left main stem bronchus. Laryngeal and tracheal irritation in an inflammatory process can cause reflex bronchoconstriction in more distal airways. This will lead to ventilation maldistribution. Patients with acute upper airway obstruction sometimes present with frank pulmonary edema (85). In less severe cases of upper airway obstruction, subclinical increases in lung water could cause flooding of some alveoli and, thus, hypoxemia secondary to $\dot{V}/\dot{Q}$ mismatch.

Any infant presenting with a congenital heart lesion who has evidence of upper airway obstruction should be carefully evaluated for congenital malformations of the upper airway, including choanal stenosis or atresia, bilateral vocal cord paralysis, laryngeal cysts, and congenital complete tracheal rings (associated with vascular ring). Assuming that no preoperative lesion is present, the appearance of upper airway obstruction in the postoperative phase is usually associated either with complications of the endotracheal tube or as a lesion acquired from the surgical procedure. The latter usually relates to damage to the left recurrent laryngeal nerve during the course of surgery for relief of coarctation of the aorta or patent ductus arteriosus. This will cause either a transient or permanent left vocal cord paralysis. On inspiration, the flaccid left vocal cord will become adducted across the midline toward the abducted right vocal cord. The net effect is inspiratory airflow obstruction, which commonly requires intubation for relief in an infant. If the nerve damage is permanent, over time such a vocal cord becomes "frozen" in its resting position, and it will cease to adduct with subsequent less airflow obstruction. Alternatively, if the damage to the left recurrent laryngeal nerve is transient, the situation will correct itself with time.

Endotracheal tube complications usually arise from incorrect choice of its size for perioperative management, or inadequate analgesia and sedation during the postoperative weaning process, whereby the infant struggles while intubated, causing subglottic trauma from the ETT with subsequent edema. Some infants are particularly difficult to sedate (e.g., infants with Down's syndrome) and require either heavier sedation or more analgesia. It is sometimes not recognized that certain infants (e.g., Down's syndrome, achondroplasia, Ellis van Creveld) have narrow subglottic regions requiring a smaller endotracheal tube for their size (86, 87). The experienced physician should recognize the absence of a leak prior to surgery, and change the endotracheal tube down to a more appropriate size. Presence of a leak prior to going on bypass is sufficient to assume that despite the lack of a leak after bypass because of accumulation of extravascular fluid, the subglottic edema will regress with the rest of the body tissue edema and the patient will not suffer any complications in the subglottic area. However, the development of postextubation stridor is unpredictable, and no reliable predictor of swelling before extubation exists (88). Risk factors associated with the development of postextubation stridor are patient age, traumatic intubation, duration of intubation, Down's syndrome, and absence of a leak prior to extubation (85, 89, 90).

Management of upper airway obstruction depends to a large extent on the underlying cause (Fig. 23.4). If the patient is globally fluid overloaded, continued judicious use of diuretics is appropriate. Racemic epinephrine (RE) use will be successful only in cases involving subglottic edema. Its use is based on the topical vasoconstrictor (α-adrenoceptor) effect when applied to the inflamed, edematous mucosa of the subglottic region. RE is composed of equal parts of the D- and L-isomers of epinephrine. The L-isomer is about 15 to 20 times more potent than the D form, and theoretically, a 2.25% solution of RE is equipotent with the 1.0% L-epinephrine that could be used instead. Nebulized phenylephrine solution (0.25%) has similar activity (91). RE delivered by intermittent positive pressure breathing (IPPB) has been associated with a decreased intubation rate (92). It has also been demonstrated that delivery of RE by IPPB is no more effective than that delivered by a powered nebulizer and face mask to a spontaneously breathing child (93). RE appears safe when given as a 0.5 mL of 2.25% solution in 3.5 mL water (1:8 dilution) to infants and up to 2.0 mL of 2.5% solution in 2 mL water (1:1 dilution) in children. The dose can be repeated hourly, but

Management of postextubation stridor

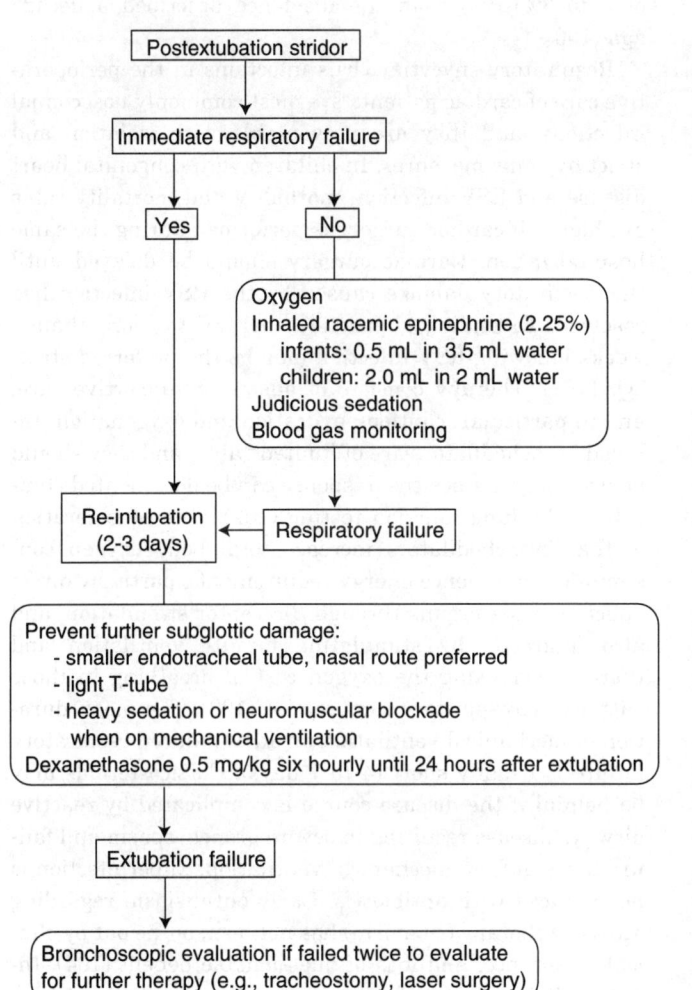

```
Postextubation stridor
         ↓
Immediate respiratory failure
    ↓           ↓
   Yes          No
    ↓           ↓
              Oxygen
              Inhaled racemic epinephrine (2.25%)
                 infants: 0.5 mL in 3.5 mL water
                 children: 2.0 mL in 2 mL water
              Judicious sedation
              Blood gas monitoring
    ↓           ↓
    ←──── Respiratory failure
Re-intubation
(2-3 days)
    ↓
Prevent further subglottic damage:
  - smaller endotracheal tube, nasal route preferred
  - light T-tube
  - heavy sedation or neuromuscular blockade
     when on mechanical ventilation
Dexamethasone 0.5 mg/kg six hourly until 24 hours after extubation
    ↓
Extubation failure
    ↓
Bronchoscopic evaluation if failed twice to evaluate
for further therapy (e.g., tracheostomy, laser surgery)
```

Figure 23.4. Management of postextubation stridor.

Table 23.4. Uncuffed Endotracheal Tube Size for Upper Airway Obstruction

Age	Size (ID)
< 6 months	3.0 mm
> 6 months–2 years	3.5 mm
> 2–5 years	4.0 mm
> 5 years	4.5 mm

ID, internal diameter.

if recurrent doses are needed, or carbon dioxide retention ensues, the patient should be reintubated with a smaller endotracheal tube (Table 23.4).

The clinical importance of acute upper airway obstruction derives from the fact that some cases can progress rapidly and if not treated appropriately and quickly may further progress to cause severe hypoxia and even cardiorespiratory arrest. If a child with subglottic edema needs to be reintubated, a smaller endotracheal tube has to be used to prevent additional trauma. The nasal route is preferred to optimize securement and tube stabilization. The child should be weaned from the ventilator and kept in a head box or with a light T-tube delivering humidified oxygen at the appropriate concentration. This prevents the infant from "tonguing" the tube and minimizes shifting of the ETT with head movements, thus decreasing the risk of trauma and further subglottic edema. Alternatively, the child can be heavily sedated or placed under neuromuscular blockade and receive mechanical ventilatory assistance. In most cases of simple subglottic edema, extubation can be successfully undertaken after a resting period of 72 hours. It is not necessary to await the reappearance of a leak around the endotracheal tube. The benefit of corticosteroids in this situation is debatable. Tibballs et al. (94) have shown steroids to be beneficial in shortening the time of intubation in infants and children intubated for subglottic edema (croup). Alternatively, Tellez et al. (88) have shown prophylactic steroids to be of no benefit in preventing subglottic edema following extubation. Pending the appearance of an appropriately controlled trial, we recommend that dexamethasone 0.5 mg/kg be given 6 hourly intravenously to such patients for 24 hours prior and continued for 24 hours following extubation.

Bronchopulmonary Dysplasia

For the purpose of this discussion, we defined bronchopulmonary dysplasia (BPD) as chronic obstructive lung disease of infancy characterized clinically by persistent respiratory distress and usually oxygen dependency after supplemental oxygen and ventilator management in the newborn period. The disease is characterized pathologically by:

1. Interstitial fibrosis and a decreased number of alveolar units
2. Increased lung water due to abnormal permeability of the alveolar-capillary membrane
3. Small airway constriction and overdistension, related to chronic inflammation, airway edema, and airway collapsibility
4. Elevated pulmonary vascular resistance due to structural fibrotic changes

Right-to-left shunting may occur through the foramen ovale and patent ductus arteriosus. Pulmonary vascular reactivity is increased because of excessive muscularization of the pulmonary arterioles. Both tracheomalacia and bronchomalacia occur in the older BPD infant, and they are responsible for acute cyanotic spells.

Cardiac abnormalities can be difficult to recognize clinically in the infant with BPD because they produce symptoms similar to the underlying disease. Furthermore, such lesions contribute to the pathophysiology of BPD by worsening hypoxemia or increasing pulmonary blood flow (95). Major problems encountered in the perioperative management of cardiac patients with BPD are growth failure, recurrent superinfections, and bronchial hyperreactivity, necessitating high caloric nutrition, appropriate antibiotic treatment, inhaled bronchodilators, and corticosteroids, respectively. Systemic corticosteroid use should be limited to episodes of acute exacerbations with bronchospasm because of their potential for severe side effects. Conversely, infants with severe disease may be steroid dependent. Diuretics are commonly used to combat chronically increased lung water, which contributes to the alteration of respiratory mechanics and the impairment of gas exchange. Other problems are pulmonary hypertension and cor pulmonale. The mainstay of therapy is the treatment of hypoxia to promote growth and control pulmonary hypertension. Weaning of mechanical ventilation is a tedious process and the commonly used methods are (a) slow weaning of synchronized intermittent mandatory ventilation (SIMV), (b) sprinting, or (c) pressure support ventilation.

Tracheostomy can reduce the work of breathing, and it allows long-term ventilation of infants with severe BPD. Gastroesophageal reflux is a common problem, and it may require gastrostomy tube placement together with a Nissen fundoplication to prevent further lung damage from chronic aspiration.

RESPIRATORY SYNCYTIAL VIRUS INFECTION

Respiratory syncytial virus (RSV) is the most serious pathogen for respiratory disease in infants and young children. Clinical manifestations range from mild upper respiratory tract infections to severe lower respiratory disorders such as bronchiolitis and pneumonia. Apnea is a common presentation of the newborn or premature infant. Infants with underlying congenital heart disease (in particular, cardiac patients with pulmonary hypertension), bronchopulmonary dysplasia, immunodeficiency, or prematurity are at higher risk for severe and prolonged disease. A number of infants are so severely affected that they develop respiratory failure requiring intubation and assisted ventilation. Development of acute respiratory distress syndrome can complicate and prolong the disease course (96). However, disease mortality rate is usually low with complete recovery (97, 98) even in children with pulmonary hypertension. Present RSV mortality rates in pediatric patients with congenital heart disease are much less (on the order of 3 to 8%) (99) than the incidence described a decade ago (100).

Respiratory snycytial virus infections in the perioperative care of cardiac patients are most commonly nosocomial infections, and they are preventable with isolation and strict hygienic measures. In children with congenital heart disease and RSV infection, morbidity and mortality rates are higher if cardiac surgery is performed during the same hospitalization. Cardiac surgery should be delayed until the respiratory damage caused by the RSV infection has resolved. Extending supportive therapy to more than 5 weeks following RSV infection may be the preferred strategy (101). Therapy consists of adequate supportive care, and in particular, cautious hydration and oxygenation. Inhaled bronchodilators are of limited value, and they should be used only if a positive response can be documented clinically or by lung function testing (102). One consideration is that bronchodilators increase total body oxygen consumption (and hence energy requirement), partly by direct effect on other organs through β-receptor stimulation, and also indirectly by stimulating minute ventilation and thereby increasing the oxygen cost of breathing in those with cardiorespiratory compromise (103). The mean duration of mechanical ventilation for RSV-induced respiratory failure is usually short (4 to 7 days). Corticosteroids may be helpful if the disease course is complicated by reactive airways disease resulting in severe bronchospasm and failure to wean from mechanical ventilation. Superinfection is not reduced with antibiotics. Early enthusiasm regarding antiviral therapy (ribavirin) has not been borne out by clinical experience, and it is of questionable benefit (104). Inhaled nitric oxide is of questionable therapeutic benefit in infants with RSV infection, but its role needs to be further elucidated. In a study of 12 infants, we found statistically significant bronchodilation in only four infants using doses of nitric oxide up to 60 parts per million. The clinical significance of these data are unclear (Patel N, Hammer J, Newth CJL; personal observations). The rare patient who fails conventional ventilation secondary to severe RSV infection can be successfully managed with extracorporeal membrane oxygenation (ECMO) (105).

NONCARDIOGENIC PULMONARY EDEMA

Acute respiratory distress syndrome (ARDS) is a syndrome of acute hypoxemic respiratory failure following a variety of insults that may or may not have directly injured the lungs. It is defined clinically by (106) (a) acute disease onset, (b) Pao_2/Fio_2 ratio 200 mm Hg or less, (c) bilateral infiltrates on chest radiograph, and (d) absence of clinical evidence of left atrial hypertension (i.e., noncardiogenic pulmonary edema).

Typically, patients with heart disease are excluded from studies of ARDS because elevated pulmonary venous pressure and vascular resistance may contribute to pulmonary edema. Its occurrence in children is 8 to 10 cases per 1000 pediatric ICU admissions with a mortality rate of about 40 to 60% (107, 108).

The clinical course of ARDS can be divided into four stages:

1. Acute injury
2. Latent period 6 to 72 hours following the initial insult
3. Acute respiratory failure
4. Chronic physiologic abnormalities

In the acute phase, interstitial and intra-alveolar edema can be seen as hazy bilateral infiltrates on chest radiographs. Intrapulmonary shunting with hypoxemia and a decrease in compliance are the principal alterations in gas exchange and pulmonary mechanics, respectively. Transition to the chronic phase is smooth and characterized by the development of fibrotic lung disease and obstructive airway disease. Patients can progress to intractable respiratory failure or recover after long-term ventilation.

Therapy consists of supportive care. Cardiovascular support may be required in the form of inotropes and afterload reducing agents. The overall goal of fluid therapy in the initial phase is to maintain adequate oxygen delivery with the lowest effective intravascular volume, which is usually achieved by administrating 70% of maintenance fluid, with additional volume for cardiac or nutritional support. Guidance of inotropic support and fluid management can be facilitated by pulmonary artery catheters used to assess cardiac output and pulmonary capillary wedge pressure. Nevertheless, such invasive monitoring in small infants and children is potentially more hazardous than in adults and central venous pressure and invasive arterial blood pressure monitoring is often sufficient to assess overall cardiac function. Secondary infection, especially gram-negative bacterial pneumonia and sepsis, is a major cause of mortality and requires appropriate antibiotic treatment.

Conventional mechanical ventilation is commonly applied in pressure control mode using a decelerating gas flow pattern and an increased inspiratory:to expiratory (I:E) ratio up to 1:1 to improve oxygenation and ventilation (109). Little experience has been acquired with inverse I:E ratio ventilation in infants. Positive end-expiratory pressure (PEEP) improves oxygenation by recruitment of collapsed or poorly ventilated alveolar units (110). Adverse effects are barotrauma, air leak, and decreased cardiac output. Prone nursing improves oxygenation and oxygen delivery in some infants with ARDS (111, 111a). Modern ventilator strategies involve the use of permissive hypercapnia, which is based on the recognition that compensated hypercapnia has few serious adverse effects and may reduce ventilator-induced injury (112, 113). Theoretic benefits of newer ventilatory strategies such as high-frequency ventilation, ECMO, or partial liquid ventilation also include the reduction of secondary injury to the lung. High-frequency ventilation has been demonstrated to be effective in the treatment of ARDS (114), whereas the role of ECMO needs to be defined. In a recent study, the survival rate for children with ARDS treated with ECMO was 41% (115). Virtually no information is found on survival rate for cardiac patients going on ECMO support for pulmonary parenchymal disease. The diagnostic requirement for noncardiogenic edema usually excludes cardiac patients from a diagnosis of ARDS. The National Institutes of Health fast entry criteria for ECMO support are: PaO_2 less than 40 mm Hg for more than 2 hours, with FIO_2 1.0; slow entry criteria are: PaO_2 less than 50 mm Hg, with FIO_2 0.6 or more, PEEP 5 cm H_2O or greater, and pulmonary shunt more than 30%; but different ECMO entry criteria have been used in other studies. Perfluorocarbon-associated gas exchange (partial liquid ventilation) is currently under clinical investigation in infants with ARDS after animal models have shown striking responses to this treatment (116, 116a). A variety of specific therapies have been proposed including surfactant replacement (117, 118) and inhaled nitric oxide (119–122). Preliminary results suggest that either may be a useful adjuvant therapy, but it remains unclear whether they can reduce morbidity and mortality.

PHRENIC NERVE LESIONS

Phrenic nerve injury is a recognized complication of cardiothoracic surgery for lesions requiring dissection in close proximity to the nerve, and it results in diaphragmatic paresis or paralysis. It is attributed to insults such as nerve transection, nerve stretch, electrocautery trauma, or cold injury from topical cardiac hypothermia. Postoperative prevalence has been estimated to be between 0.5 to 2.2%; however, an incidence of up to 10% has been described in children under 2 years of age (123, 124). Phrenic nerve injury is most commonly observed after Blalock-Taussig shunt construction, atrial septectomy, pulmonary artery banding, PDA ligation, and coarctation repair. Diaphragmatic paralysis can also occur congenitally as a result of diaphragmatic malformation (eventration, muscle fiber aplasia), or it can be acquired by birth trauma.

Infants and young children are especially susceptible to respiratory compromise from diaphragmatic paralysis because of greater reliance on the diaphragm for ventilation, high chest wall compliance (125), weak intercostal musculature, and small bronchi, which are easily obstructed by retained secretions. These changes are particularly marked in the supine position. Thoracoabdominal asynchrony wastes energy distorting the rib cage rather than inspiring air, reduces ventilatory efficiency, and predisposes to the development of respiratory fatigue. Diagnosis of phrenic nerve injury should be considered whenever there is unexplained persistent atelectasis, paradoxic breathing, or inability to wean from ventilatory support in the early postoperative period. Clinical signs of diaphragmatic dysfunction can be difficult to diagnose (particularly when unilateral and in infants) because of the presence of chest tubes and assisted ventilation. Much can be learned from simple inspection. Optical markers placed on the chest wall amplify the visual perception of asynchronous or paradoxic breathing. Inspiratory indrawing of the lateral chest is known as Hoover's sign (126), and it is typically observed in infants with diaphragmatic paralysis. Diaphragmatic paralysis should be suspected with progressive elevation of a hemidiaphragm on serial chest radiographs, but this sign can be inconsistent on mechanical ventilation. Diagnosis is usually confirmed by fluoroscopy or ultrasonography while the infant is breathing spontaneously (i.e., on CPAP) by demonstrating immobility or paradox motion of the affected hemidiaphragm. Obstructing the infant's airway during a couple of inspiratory efforts facilitates the detection of an upward (paradoxic) moving hemidiaphragm. Direct percutaneous phrenic nerve stimulation can be used at the bedside; it allows early diagnosis because it does not require a spontaneously breathing patient (121). In our opinion, the simplest and least invasive technique, which allows little room for interpretive errors in this setting, is the generation of characteristic figure-of-8 loop patterns on respiratory inductive plethysmography (22).

Most injuries gradually resolve spontaneously over time and permanent sequelae from persistent paralysis or long-term intubation are rare (127). Phrenic nerve injuries in children aged older than 1 year can usually be managed conservatively. Controversy remains concerning the appropriate timing of surgical plication in infants and young children. Surgical plication has been demonstrated to reduce the number of days on mechanical ventilation, with extubation possible within 2 to 6 days of plication (128–130). Hence, early plication has been advocated as soon as the diagnosis of phrenic nerve injury is made. However, others have shown that spontaneous recovery is common within the first 2 to 3 weeks, and they advocate plication only if the patient is unable to wean for a determined amount of time (e.g., 2 to 6 weeks) (131–134). Intraoperative recognition of severe or irreversible damage to the phrenic nerve in a neonate should probably mandate immediate plication. Bilateral plication for bilateral diaphragmatic paralysis cannot be recommended from the current experience (135).

Problems Related to the Pleural Space

Disorders of the pleura constitute an important cause of morbidity during the perioperative care of infants with cardiac disease. Their prompt recognition and appropriate management can prevent cardiorespiratory compromise.

Pneumothorax

Intrapleural accumulation of air results whenever the pleural space develops a communication with the atmosphere, either from a chest wall defect or from alveolar rupture (i.e., cardiopulmonary resuscitation, mechanical ventilation, and so forth). Air can also escape into the perivascular space and dissect centrifugally along the perivascular plane rupturing into the mediastinum with subsequent rupture into the pleural space.

Irrespective of the underlying cause, massive or continuous air leak is more likely to occur on positive pressure ventilation (c.f., negative pressure, spontaneous ventilation), and it can elevate the intrapleural pressure above the atmospheric level causing a tension pneumothorax. This results in a mediastinal shift to the contralateral side impeding venous return, cardiac output, and ventilation. Hypoxemia, hypercapnia, tachycardia, hypotension, and narrowing of pulse pressure occur and immediate intervention is required to prevent a cardiac arrest from tamponade. In small infants, auscultation can be unreliable because breath sounds from the remaining expansible lung areas are easily transmitted across the small newborn chest on mechanical ventilation. Serial chest x-rays are essential during the mechanical assistance of ventilation of newborn and older infants, particularly if interstitial emphysema, pneumomediastinum, or hyperlucency of any lung zone exist. Periodic physical examinations and accurate interpretation of cardiorespiratory monitoring systems together with arterial blood gas analysis are important for early clinical recognition.

Chest tubes for pneumothoraces are usually left in place for approximately 3 days. Treatment of a persistent (more than 2 to 3 weeks) bronchopleural fistula requires pleurodesis with a sclerosing agent or pleurectomy. Absorption of a loculated pneumothorax is theoretically facilitated by oxygen breathing, which increases the pressure gradient of nitrogen between pleura and venous blood. In clinical practice, breathing 100% oxygen may not be appropriate, and resolution of a pneumothorax by this technique can still be inordinately slow.

Pleural Effusions (Transudate, Exudate)

Pleural membranes are permeable to liquid and a small amount of liquid is normally present within the pleural space. The majority of liquid (about 90%), which is filtered out of the arterial capillaries, is reabsorbed at the venous end. The rest is returned via the lymphatics. An increase in capillary hydrostatic pressure as seen in congestive heart failure, or an increase in right-sided cardiac pressure, venous hypertension, SVC obstruction, and overhydration can result in transudates with the appearance radiologically of pleural effusions. Exudates are commonly caused by increased capillary permeability, and they originate from nonspecific inflammation (e.g., ARDS following shock or reperfusion injury), infections, toxins, and pulmonary infarction. Blood vessel rupture in the lungs or the thoracic cage is responsible for blood in the pleural space.

Physical and chemical characteristics of pleural liquid differentiate transudate (protein less than 3 g/100 mL, low-density liprotein (LDH) less than 200 IU) from exudate (protein more than 3 g/100 mL, LDH more than 200 IU), which is important to diagnose the cause accurately and plan for therapy. Depending on the ability of the thorax to reabsorb fluid, a pleural effusion can be asymptomatic for days or weeks if pleural fluid accumulates slowly. At some point, sufficient fluid gathers to cause cardiorespiratory compromise requiring chest tube placement for drainage.

Chylothorax

Traumatic disruption of the thoracic duct and lymphatics results in the accumulation of chyle. Postoperative chylothorax occurs in approximately 1 of every 200 patients who undergo pediatric cardiothoracic procedures (136, 137). Variations in lymphatic pathways and the presence of accessory lymphatic channels account for chylous effusions resulting from operative approaches that do not even expose the main thoracic duct (138, 139). Chyle is usually sterile, contains predominantly lymphocytes, has a protein content between half and the same as plasma, and a fat content exceeding that of plasma. The characteristic milky appearance of chyle can be observed without feedings. Conversely, chyle can appear clear if the infant has not been fed in many days.

The mainstay of initial therapy for chylothoraces is pleural space evacuation and diet modification using either total parenteral nutrition (enteric rest) or enteral low-fat, solid food or enteral elemental diet supplemented with intravenous lipid emulsion. Medium-chain triglyceride formulae (e.g., Portagen, Pregestimil, Mead Johnson Nutritionals, Evansville, IN) can be used for oral feedings as they pass directly into the portal system (140). Nonoperative therapy, which is successful in most patients, occurs after 7 to 30 days of total gut rest (141). Systemic venous hypertension or increased right-sided cardiac pressure hindering spontaneous closure of the traumatized lymphatic vessels is associated with the failure of conservative therapy (142). Operative intervention such as the placement of a pleuroperitoneal shunt, thoracic duct ligation, or pleurodesis should be considered after 4 to 6 weeks of unsuccessful conservative therapy because continuous loss of chyle results in lymphocyte depletion and susceptibility to opportunistic infections (143).

REFERENCES

1. Rabinovitch M, Reid LM. Quantitative structural analysis of the pulmonary vascular bed in congenital heart defects. In: Pediatric cardiovascular disease. Philadelphia: FA Davis, 1981.
2. Cook CD, Herry RB, O'Brian D, et al. Studies of respiratory physiology in the newborn infant. I. Observations on normal premature and fullterm infants. J Clin Invest 1955;34: 975–982.
3. Kennaird DL. Oxygen consumption and evaporative water loss in infants with congenital heart disease. Arch Dis Child 1976;51:34–41.
4. Rudolph AM. Congenital diseases of the heart. Chicago: Year Book Medical Publishers, 1974.
5. Romero TE, Friedman WF. Limited left ventricular response to volume overload in the neonatal period: a comparative study with the adult. Pediatr Res 1979;13:910–915.
6. Keens TG, Bryan AC, Levison H, et al. Development of fatigue-resistant muscle fibers in the human diaphragm and intercostal muscles. Physiologist 1977;20:50.
7. Hogg JC, Williams J, Richardson JB, et al. Age as a factor in the distribution of lower airway conductance and in the pathologic anatomy of obstructive lung disease. N Engl J Med 1970;282:1283–1287.
8. Mansell A, Bryan AC, Levison H. Airway closure in children. J Appl Physiol 1972;33:711–714.
9. Roussos C, Macklem PT. The respiratory muscles. N Engl J Med 1982;307:786–797.
10. Nelson NM, Prod'hom LS, Cherry RB, et al. Pulmonary function in the newborn infant: the alveolar-arterial oxygen gradient. J Appl Physiol 1963;18:534–538.
11. Boyden EA. Notes on the development of the lung in infancy and early childhood. Am J Anat 1967;121:749–762.
12. Bryan AC, Mansell AL, Levison H. Development of the mechanical properties of the respiratory system. In: Hodson WA. Development of the lung. New York: Marcel Dekker, 1977;445–468.
13. Deakers TW, Reynolds G, Stretton M, et al. Cuffed endotracheal tubes in pediatric intensive care. J Pediatr 1994; 125:57–62.
14. Hammer J, Newth CJL. Infant lung function testing in the intensive care unit. Intensive Care Med 1995,21:744–752.
15. England SJ. Current techniques for assessing pulmonary function on the newborn and infant: advantages and limitations. Pediatr Pulmonol 1988;4:48–53.
16. Sly PD, Brown KA, Bates JHT, et al. Noninvasive determination of respiratory mechanics during mechanical ventilation of neonates: a review of current and future techniques. Pediatr Pulmonol 1988;4:39–47.
17. American Thoracic Society/European Respiratory Society. Respiratory mechanics in infants: physiologic evaluation in health and disease. Am Rev Respir Dis 1993;147:474–496.
18. Sivan Y, Deakers TW, Newth CJL. Thoracoabdominal asynchrony in acute upper airway obstruction in small children. Am Rev Respir Dis 1990;142:540–544.

19. Hammer J, Newth CJL, Deakers TW. Validation of the phase angle technique as an objective measure of upper airway obstruction. Pediatr Pulmonol 1995;19:167–173.
20. Sivan Y, Deakers TW, Newth CJL. Thoracoabdominal asynchrony in acute upper airway obstruction in small children. Am Rev Respir Dis 1990;142:540–544.
21. Allen JL, Wolfson MR, McDowell K, et al. Thoracoabdominal asynchrony in infants with airflow obstruction. Am Rev Respir Dis 1990;141:337–342.
22. Hammer J, Deakers TW, Newth CJL. Lissajous figure analysis in infants with thoracoabdominal asynchrony due to neuromuscular disease [Abstract]. Am J Respir Crit Care Med 1994;149:A36.
23. Ratjen F, Zinman R, Stark S, et al. Effect of changes in lung volume on respiratory system compliance in newborn infants. J Appl Physiol 1989;67:1192–1197.
24. Zin WA, Pengelly LD, Milic-Emili J. Single-breath method for measurement of respiratory mechanics in anesthetized animals. J Appl Physiol 1982;52:1266–1271.
25. Olinsky A, Bryan MH, Bryan AC. A simple method of measuring total respiratory system compliance in newborn infants. S Afr Med J 1976;50:128–130.
26. Guslits BG, Wilkie RA, England SJ, et al. Comparison of methods of measurement of compliance of the respiratory system in children. Am Rev Respir Dis 1987;136:727–729.
27. Mead J, Whittenberger JL. Physical properties of human lungs measured during spontaneous respiration. J Appl Physiol 1952;5:779–796.
28. LeSouëf PN, Lopes JM, England SJ, et al. Influence of chest wall distortion on esophageal pressure. J Appl Physiol 1983;55:353–358.
29. Heaf DP, Turner H, Stocks J, et al. The accuracy of esophageal pressure measurements in convalescent and sick intubated infants. Pediatr Pulmonol 1986;2:5–8.
30. Mortola JP, Fisher JT, Smith B, et al. Dynamics of breathing in infants. J Appl Physiol 1982;52:1209–1215.
31. LeSouëf PN, England SJ, Bryan AC. Passive respiratory mechanics in newborns and children. Am Rev Respir Dis 1984;129:727–729.
32. Downes JJ, Nicodemus HF, Pierce WS, et al. Acute respiratory failure in infants following cardiovascular surgery. J Thorac Cardiovasc Surg 1970;59:21–37.
33. DiCarlo JV, Raphaely RC, Steven JM, et al. Pulmonary mechanics in infants after cardiac surgery. Crit Care Med 1992;20:22–27.
34. Hammer J, Numa A, Patel N, et al. Normal values for pulmonary function in intubated infants [Abstract]. Am J Respir Crit Care Med 1995;151:A439.
35. Motoyama EK. Pulmonary mechanics during early postnatal years. Pediatr Res 1977;11:220–223.
36. Hammer J, Newth CJL. Effort and volume dependence of forced-deflation flow-volume relationships in intubated infants. J Appl Physiol 1996;80:345–350.
37. Newth CJL, Amsler B, Anderson GP, et al. The effects of varying inflation and deflation pressures on the maximal expiratory deflation flow-volume relationship in anesthetized rhesus monkeys. Am Rev Respir Dis 1992;144:807–813.
38. Hammer J, Sivan Y, Deakers TW, et al. Flow limitation in anesthetized rhesus monkeys: a comparison of rapid thoracoabdominal compression and forced deflation techniques. Pediatr Res 1996;39:539–546.
39. Mallory GB, Motoyama AK, Koumbourlis AC, et al. Bronchial reactivity in infants in acute respiratory failure with viral bronchiolitis. Pediatr Pulmonol 1989;6:253–259.
40. Motoyama EK, Fort MD, Klesh KW, et al. Early onset of airway reactivity in premature infants with bronchopulmonary dysplasia. Am Rev Respir Dis 1987;136:50–57.
41. Shannon DC. Rational monitoring of respiratory function during mechanical ventilation of infants and children. Intensive Care Med 1989;15:13–16.
42. Richardson CP, Jung AL. Effects of continuous positive airway pressure on pulmonary function and blood gases of infants with respiratory distress syndrome. Pediatr Res 1978;12:771–774.
43. East TD, In't Veen JC, Pace NL, et al. Functional residual capacity as a noninvasive indicator of optimal positive end-expiratory pressure. J Clin Monit 1988;4:91–98.
44. Sivan Y, Deakers TW, Newth CJ. Effect of positive end-expiratory pressure on respiratory compliance in children with acute respiratory failure. Pediatr Pulmonol 1991;11:103–107.
45. Heldt GP, Peters RM. A simplified method to determine functional residual capacity during mechanical ventilation. Chest 1978;74:492–496.
46. Sivan Y, Deakers TW, Newth CJ. An automated bedside method for measuring functional residual capacity by N_2 washout in mechanically ventilated children. Pediatr Res 1990;28:446–450.
47. Vilstrup CT, Bjorklund LJ, Larsson A, et al. Functional residual capacity and ventilation homogeneity in mechanically ventilated small neonates. J Appl Physiol 1992;73:276–283.
48. Schulze A, Schaller P, Töpfer A, et al. Measurement of functional residual capacity by sulfur hexafluoride in small-volume lungs during spontaneous breathing and mechanical ventilation. Pediatr Res 1994;35:494–499.
49. Koch G. Alveolar ventilation, diffusing capacity and the A-a PO_2 difference in the newborn infant. Respir Physiol 1968;4:168–192.
50. Bose CL, Lawson EE, Greene A, et al. Measurement of cardiopulmonary function in ventilated neonates with respiratory distress syndrome using rebreathing methodology. Pediatr Res 1986;20:316–320.
51. Cotton EK, Cogswell JJ, Cropp GJ. Measurements of effective pulmonary blood flow in the normal newborn human infant. Pediatrics 1971;47:520–528.
52. Stokes DC. Is there room for another pediatric bronchoscope? Pediatr Pulmonol 1992;12:201–202.
53. Higenbottam T, Stewart S, Penketh A, et al. Transbronchial lung biopsy for the diagnosis of rejection in heart-lung transplant patients. Transplantation 1988;46:532–539.
54. McCubbin MM, Trigg ME, Hendricker CM, et al. Bronchoscopy with bronchoalveolar lavage in the evaluation of pulmonary complications of bone marrow transplantation in children. Pediatr Pulmonol 1992;12:43–47.
55. Abadco DL, Amaro-Galvez R, Rao M, et al. Experience with flexible fiberoptic bronchoscopy with bronchoalveolar lavage as a diagnostic tool in children with AIDS. Am J Dis Child 1992;146:1056–1059.
56. Winthrop AL, Waddell T, Superina RA. The diagnosis of pneumonia in the immunocompromised child: use of bronchoalveolar lavage. J Pediatr Surg 1990;25:878–880.
57. Stover DE, White DA, Romano PA, et al. Diagnosis of pulmonary disease in acquired immunodeficiency syndrome (AIDS). Am Rev Respir Dis 1984;130:659–662.
58. Pattishall EN, Noyes BE, Orenstein DM. Use of bronchoalveolar lavage in immunocompromised children with pneumonia. Pediatr Pulmonol 1988;5:1–5.
59. Bye MR, Bernstein L, Shah K, et al. Diagnostic bronchoal-

veolar lavage in children with AIDS. Pediatr Pulmonol 1987;3:425–428.
60. Early GL, Williams TE, Kilman JW. Open lung biopsy: its effect on therapy in the pediatric patient. Chest 1985;87:467–469.
61. Doolin EJ, Luck SR, Sherman JO, et al. Emergency lung biopsy: friend or foe of the immunocompromised child? J Pediatr Surg 1986;21:485–487.
62. Lindahl H, Rintala R, Malinen L, et al. Bronchoscopy during the first month of life. J Pediatr Surg 1992;27:548–550.
63. Finer NN, Muzyka D. Flexible endoscopic intubation for the neonate. Pediatr Pulmonol 1992;12:48–51.
64. Schinwell ES. Ultrathin fiberoptic bronchoscopy of airway toilet in neonatal pulmonary atelectasis. Pediatr Pulmonol 1992;13:48–49.
64a. Frei FJ, aWengen DF, Reitishauser M, et al. The airway endoscopy mask: useful device for fiberoptic evaluation and intubation of the paediatric airway. Paediatr Anaesth 1995;5:319–324.
65. Ward RF. Treatment of tracheal and endobronchial lesions with the potassium titanyl phosphate laser. Ann Otol Rhinol Laryngol 1992;101:205–208.
66. Schittenbecher PP, Mantel K, Hofmann U, et al. Treatment of congenital tracheoesophageal fistula by endoscopic laser coagulation: preliminary report of three cases. J Pediatr Surg 1992;27:26–28.
67. Foglia RP, Shilyansky J, Fonkalsrud EW. Emergency lung biopsy in immunocompromised pediatric patients. Ann Surg 1989;210:90–92.
68. Snyder CL, Ramsay NK, McGlave PB, et al. Diagnostic open-lung biopsy after bone marrow transplantation. J Pediatr Surg 1990;25:871–877.
69. Davies CJ, Cooper SG, Fletcher ME, et al. Total respiratory compliance in infants and young children with congenital heart disease. Pediatr Pulmonol 1990;8:155–161.
70. Ishii M, Matsumoto N, Fuyuki T, et al. Effects of hemodynamic edema formation on peripheral versus central airway mechanics. J Appl Physiol 1985;59:1578–1584.
71. Hordof AJ, Mellins RB, Gersony WM, et al. Reversibility of chronic obstructive airways disease in infants following repair of ventricular septal defect. J Pediatr 1977;90:187–191.
72. Lister G, Talner NS. Management of respiratory failure of cardiac origin. In: Gregory GA, ed. Clinics in critical care medicine: respiratory failure in the child. New York: Churchill Livingstone, 1981.
73. Lanteri CJ, Kano S, Duncan AW, et al. Changes in respiratory mechanics in children undergoing cardiopulmonary bypass. Am J Respir Crit Care Med 1995;152:1893–1900.
74. Kanter RK, Bove LE, Tobin JR, et al. Prolonged mechanical ventilation of infants after open heart surgery. Crit Care Med 1986;14:211–214.
75. Macklem PT. Perspective: the respiratory muscles. Chest 1984;85:60S.
76. Rabinovitch M, Grady S, David I, et al. Compression of intrapulmonary bronchi by abnormally branching pulmonary arteries associated with absent pulmonary valves. Am J Cardiol 1982;50:804–813.
77. Momma K, Ando M, Takao A. Fetal cardiac morphology of tetralogy of Fallot with absent pulmonary valve in the rat. Circulation 1990;82:1343–1351.
78. Bove EL, Shaher RM, Alley R, et al. Tetralogy of Fallot with absent pulmonary valve and aneurysm of the pulmonary artery: report of two cases presenting as obstructive lung disease. J Pediatr 1972;81:339–343.
79. Fischer DR, Neches WH, Beerman LB, et al. Tetralogy of Fallot with absent pulmonic valve: analysis of 17 patients. Am J Cardiol 1984;53:1433–1437.
80. Dunnigan A, Oldham HN, Benson DW. Absent pulmonary valve syndrome in infancy. Surgery reconsidered. Am J Cardiol 1981;48:117–122.
81. Marmon LM, Bye MR, Haas JM, et al. Vascular rings and slings: long-term follow-up of pulmonary function. J Pediatr Surg 1984;19:683–690.
82. Anand R, Dooley KJ, Williams WH, et al. Follow-up of surgical correction of vascular anomalies causing tracheobronchial compression. Pediatr Cardiol 1994;15:58–61.
83. Costigan DC, Newth CJL. Respiratory status of children with epiglottitis with and without an artificial airway. Am J Dis Child 1983;137:139–141.
84. Newth CJL, Levison H, Bryan AC. The respiratory status of children with croup. J Pediatr 1972;81:1068–1073.
85. Travis KW, Todres DI, Shannon DC. Pulmonary edema associated with croup and epiglottitis. Pediatrics 1977;59:695–698.
86. Sherry KM. Post-extubation stridor in Down's syndrome. Br J Anaesth 1983;55:53–54.
87. Aboussouan LS, O'Donovan PB, Moodie DS, et al. Hypoplastic trachea in Down's syndrome. Am Rev Respir Dis 1993;147:72–75.
88. Tellez DW, Galvis AG, Storgion SA, et al. Dexamethasone in the prevention of postextubation stridor in children. J Pediatr 1991;118:289–294.
89. Koka BV, Jeon ID, Andre JM, et al. Postintubation croup in children. Anesth Analg 1977;56:501–505.
90. Kemper KJ, Benson MS, Bishop MJ. Predictors of postextubation stridor in pediatric trauma patients. Crit Care Med 1991;19:352–355.
91. Lenney W, Milner AD. Treatment of acute viral croup. Arch Dis Child 1978;53:704.
92. Adair JC, Ring WH, Jordan WS, et al. Ten-year experience with IPPB in the treatment of acute laryngotracheobronchitis. Anesth Analg 1971;50:649.
93. Oh TH, Downes JJ. Comparison of intermittent positive pressure breathing (IPPB) and powered nebulizer to administer racemic epinephrine in croup. In: Abstract of Scientific Meetings. New Orleans: American Society of Anesthesiologists, 1977:149–150.
94. Tibbals J, Shann FA, Landau LI. Placebo-controlled trial of prednisolone in children intubated for croup. Lancet 1992;340:745–748.
95. Abman SH, Accurso FJ, Bowman CM. Unsuspected cardiopulmonary abnormalities complicating bronchopulmonary dysplasia. Arch Dis Child 1984;59:966–970.
96. Hammer J, Numa A, Neuth CJL. Acute respiratory distress syndrome caused by respiratory syncytial virus. Pediatr Pulmonol 1997;23:176–183.
97. Stretton M, Ajizian SJ, Mitchell I, et al. Intensive care course and outcome of patients with respiratory syncytial virus. Pediatr Pulmonol 1992;13:143–150.
98. Moler FW, Khan AS, Meliones JN, et al. Respiratory syncytial virus morbidity and mortality estimates in congenital heart disease patients: a recent experience. Crit Care Med 1992;20:1406–1413.
99. Moler FW, Khan AS, Meliones JN, et al. Respiratory syncytial virus morbidity and mortality estimates in congenital heart disease patients: a recent experience. Crit Care Med 1992;20:1406–1413.
100. MacDonald NE, Hall CB, Suffin SC, et al. Respiratory syncy-

tial viral infection in infants with congenital heart disease. N Engl J Med 1982;307:397–400.
101. Khong A, Wong PC, Samara Y, et al. Impact of respiratory syncytial virus on cardiac surgery for congenital heart disease: postoperative course and outcome. Pediatr Cardiol 1995;16:256.
102. Hammer J, Numa A, Newth CJL. Albuterol responsiveness in infants with respiratory failure due to respiratory syncytial virus infection. J Pediatr 1995;127:485–490.
103. Newth CJL, Amsler B, Richardson BP, et al. The effects of bronchodilators on spontaneous ventilation and oxygen consumption in rhesus monkeys. Pediatr Res 1997;42:157–162.
104. Meert KL, Sarnaik AP, Gelmini MJ, et al. Aerosolized ribavirin in mechanically ventilated children with respiratory syncytial virus lower respiratory tract disease: a prospective, double-blind, randomized trial. Crit Care Med 1994;22:566–572.
105. Khan JY, Kerr SJ, Tometzki A, et al. Role of ECMO in the treatment of respiratory syncytial virus bronchiolitis: collaborative report. Arch Dis Child Fetal Neonatal Ed 1995;73:91–94.
106. Bernard GR, Artigas A, Brigham KL, et al; and the Consensus Committee. The American-European Consensus Conference on ARDS. Definition, mechanisms, relevant outcomes, and clinical trial coordination. Am J Respir Crit Care Med 1994;149:818–824.
107. Timmons OD, Havnes PL, Fackler JC. Predicting death in pediatric patients with acute respiratory failure. Pediatric Critical Care Study Group. Extracorporeal Life Support Organization. Chest 1995;108:789–797.
108. Davis SL, Fuhrman DP, Costarino AT. Adult respiratory distress syndrome in children: associated disease, clinical course, and predictors of death. J Pediatr 1993;123:35–45.
109. Boros SJ, Matalon SV, Ewald R. The effect of independent variations in I:E ratio and end-expiratory pressure during mechanical ventilation of hyaline membrane disease: the significance of mean airway pressure. J Pediatr 1977;91:794–798.
110. Gattinoni L, Pelosi P, Crotti S, et al. Effects of positive end-expiratory pressure on regional distribution of tidal volume and recruitment in adult respiratory distress syndrome. Am J Respir Crit Care Med 1995;151:1807–1814.
111. Murdoch IA, Storman MO. Improved arterial oxygenation in children with the adult respiratory distress syndrome: the prone position. Acta Pediatr 1994;83:1043–1046.
111a. Numa AH, Hammer J, Newth CJL. Effect of prone and supine positions on functional residual capacity, oxygenation and respiratory mechanics in ventilated infants and children. Am J Respir Crit Care Med 1997;156:1185–1189.
112. Hickling KG, Walsh J, Henderson S, et al. Low mortality rate in adult respiratory distress syndrome using low-volume, pressure-limited ventilation with permissive hypercapnia: a prospective study. Crit Care Med 1994;22:1568–1578.
113. Feihl F, Perret C. Permissive hypercapnia. How permissive should we be? Am J Respir Crit Care Med 1994;150:1722–1737.
114. Arnold JH, Truog RD, Thompson JE, et al. High-frequency oscillatory ventilation in pediatric respiratory failure. Crit Care Med 1993;21:272–278.
115. Pearson GA, Grant J, Field D, et al. Extracorporeal life support in pediatrics. Arch Dis Child 1993;68:94–96.
116. Leach CL, Fuhrman BP, Morin FC, et al. Perfluorocarbon-associated gas exchange (partial liquid ventilation) in respiratory distress syndrome: a prospective, randomized, controlled study. Crit Care Med 1993;21:1270–1278.
116a. Leach CL, Greenspan JS, Rubenstein SD, et al. Partial liquid ventilation with perflubron in premature infants with severe respiratory distress syndrom. N Engl J Med 1996;335:761–767.
117. Lewis JF, Jobe AH. Surfactant and the adult respiratory distress syndrome. Am Rev Respir Dis 1993;147:218–233.
118. Perez-Benavides F, Riff E, Franks C. Adult respiratory distress syndrome and artificial surfactant replacement in the pediatric patient. Pediatr Emerg Care 1995;11:153–155.
119. Finer NN, Etches PC, Kamstra B, et al. Inhaled nitric oxide in infants referred for extracorporeal membrane oxygenation: dose response. J Pediatr 1994;124:302–308.
120. Rossaint R, Falke KJ, Lopez F, et al. Inhaled nitric oxide for the adult respiratory distress syndrome. N Engl J Med 1993;328:399–405.
121. Rossaint R, Gerlach H, Schmidt-Ruhnke H, et al. Efficacy of inhaled nitric oxide in patients with severe ARDS. Chest 1995;107:1107–1115.
122. Germain JF, Mercier JC, Casadevall I, et al. Is there a role for inhaled nitric oxide in pediatric ARDS? Pediatr Pulmonol Suppl 1995;1:110–112.
123. Molk Q, Ross-Russell R, Mulvey D, et al. Phrenic nerve injury in infants and children undergoing cardiac surgery. Br Heart J 1991;65:287–292.
124. Kunovsky P, Gibson GA, Pollock JC, et al. Management of postoperative paralysis of diaphragm in infants and children. Eur J Cardiothorac Surg 1993;7:342–346.
125. Papastamelos C, Panitch HB, England SE, et al. Developmental changes in chest wall compliance in infancy and early childhood. J Appl Physiol 1995;78:179–184.
126. Hoover CF. The functions of the intercostal muscles. JAMA 1919;73:17–20.
127. Hong-Xu Z, D'Agostino RS, Pitlick PT, et al. Phrenic nerve injury complicating closed cardiovascular surgical procedures for congenital heart disease. Ann Thorac Surg 1985;39:445–449.
128. Mearns AJ. Iatrogenic injury to the phrenic nerve in infants and young children. Br J Surg 1977;64:558–560.
129. Shoemaker R, Palmer G, Brown JW, et al. Aggressive treatment of acquired phrenic paralysis in infants and small children. Ann Thorac Surg 1981;32:251–259.
130. Hamilton JR, Tocewicz K, Elliott MJ, et al. Paralysed diaphragm after cardiac surgery in children: value of plication. Eur J Cardiothorac Surg 1990;4:487–490.
131. Smith CD, Sade RM, Crawford FA, et al. Diaphragmatic paralysis and eventration in infants. J Thorac Cardiovasc Surg 1986;91:490–497.
132. Lynn AM, Jenkins JG, Edmonds JF, et al. Diaphragmatic paralysis after pediatric cardiac surgery: a retrospective analysis of 34 cases. Crit Care Med 1983;11:280–282.
133. Langer JC, Filler RM, Coles J, et al. Plication of the diaphragm for infants and young children with phrenic nerve palsy. J Ped Surg 1988;23:749–751.
134. Kunovsky P, Gibson GA, Pollock JC, et al. Management of postoperative paralysis of diaphragm in infants and children. Eur J Cardiothorac Surg 1993;7:342–346.
135. Stewart S, Alexson C, Manning J. Bilateral phrenic nerve paralysis after the Mustard procedure. J Thorac Cardiovasc Surg 1986;92:138–141.
136. Cenese PG, Vecchini R, D'Anico DF, et al. Postoperative chylothorax: six cases in 2,500 operations with a survey of the world literature. J Thorac Cardiovasc Surg 1975;69:966–971.

137. Higgins CB, Mulder DG. Chylothorax after surgery for congenital heart disease. J Thorac Cardiovasc Surg 1971;61: 411–418.
138. Joyce LD, Lindsay WG, Nicoloff DM. Chylothorax after median sternotomy for intrapericardial cardiac surgery. J Thorac Cardiovas Surg 1976;71:476–480.
139. Pollard WM, Schuchmann GF, Bowen TE. Isolated chylopericardium after cardiac operations. J Thorac Cardiovasc Surg 1981;81:943–946.
140. Frazer AC. Differentiation in the absorption of olive oil and oleic acid in the rat. J Physiol (Lond) 1943;102:306–312.
141. Nguyen DM, Shum-Tim D, Dobell AR, et al. The management of chylothorax/chylopericardium following pediatric cardiac surgery: a 10-year experience. J Cardiol Surg 1995; 10:302–308.
142. Bond SJ, Guzetta PC, Snyder ML, et al. Management of pediatric postoperative chylothorax. Ann Thorac Surg 1993; 56:469–473.
143. Murphy MC, Newman BM, Rodgers BM. Pleuroperitoneal shunts in the management of persistent chylothorax. Ann Thorac Surg 1989;48:195–200.

Neurologic Disorders

Adre J. du Plessis, MBChB, MPH

Children with heart disease are susceptible to neurologic impairment from a wide spectrum of causes. Primarily, however, this predisposition relates to the risk for disturbances in cerebral oxygen supply and demand. The population of children requiring cardiac intensive care (i.e., children with acute cardiac decompensation or needing postoperative critical care) may be at particular risk for neurologic injury.

Earlier reports (1–4) of the neurologic complications of congenital heart disease (CHD) emphasized the role of sustained and cumulative exposure to pathophysiologic factors such as chronic cyanosis, polycythemia, and right-to-left shunts arising from the often prolonged period of uncorrected cardiac anatomy. Infants with cyanotic CHD and chronic hypoxia were found to have a progressive impairment in cognitive performance that correlated with increasing age at repair of the cardiac defect (5). Previous surgical constraints in the young infant necessitated repeated palliative procedures prior to final repair, often extending exposure to the injurious effects of chronic cyanosis and polycythemia. Advances in surgical technique and intraoperative support strategies have had a significant impact on the risks for neurologic injury in this population. First, these advances have allowed corrective heart surgery in increasingly younger infants (6, 7), thereby reducing exposure to risk factors described (see above). However, the very techniques that have facilitated such early cardiac repair in infants may themselves be associated with neurologic risk, and recent focus has been on identifying mechanisms of neurologic injury in the intraoperative and early postoperative periods. Another important impact of these surgical advances has been a dramatic reduction in the mortality rate of CHD. As a consequence, the quality of functional, and particularly neurologic, outcome has become an important "next frontier" in the management of many congenital heart conditions.

PREOPERATIVE NEUROLOGIC DYSFUNCTION

Despite the earlier surgical repair of many congenital heart defects, certain mechanisms, both congenital and acquired, continue to impair neurologic function in the preoperative period. Developmental cardiac anomalies are associated with an increased prevalence of *brain dysgenesis*, ranging from 10 to 29% (8–10). Such disturbances in brain development may present with acute neonatal problems (e.g., seizures) or with long-term sequelae (e.g., mental retardation and epilepsy). In addition, infants with CHD are at increased risk for acquired antenatal and perinatal brain injury (both hemorrhagic and ischemic), as demonstrated by a recent brain ultrasound study (see below) (11).

NEONATAL INTRACRANIAL HEMORRHAGE

Intracranial, particularly intra-periventricular, hemorrhage (IVH-PVH) is one of the most common neurologic complications in the newborn (12). Several risk factors for IVH-PVH have been identified. Prematurity predisposes to IVH-PVH because of the structural and physiologic vulnerability of the immature periventricular germinal matrix. In a recent study (13), the incidence of IVH-PVH was found to be 20% in infants younger than 34 weeks gestation and decreased to 3.5% at term (13). Risk of IVH-PVH increases when hemodynamic instability is superimposed on the delicate microvascular substrate of the immature brain. Therefore, conditions such as perinatal asphyxia, postnatal hypoxia, or fluctuations in blood pressure, as may occur in the infant with hemodynamically unstable CHD, increase the risk of IVH-PVH (12). In term infants with CHD, up to 24% may develop IVH-PVH in the newborn period (11). Coagulation disturbances are another important antecedent to IVH-PVH (12). Fibrinolytic activity is normally increased in the immature germinal matrix (14). During CPB, systemic fibrinolytic activity may be enhanced (15), and, together with anticoagulation use, might inhibit the ability to prevent or contain IVH-PVH.

The trend toward performing cardiac surgery in ever younger and less mature infants, together with the widespread use of bedside cranial ultrasound (CUS) in the newborn, has raised difficult management issues. However, no clearly established management strategies currently exist for the newborn with intracranial hemorrhage requiring cardiac surgery. We use the guidelines discussed below in our cardiac intensive care unit to (*a*) determine the need for preoperative CUS, and (*b*) plan the timing of cardiac surgery in infants with intracranial hemorrhage documented by CUS.

Indications for Preoperative Cranial Ultrasound (CUS)

We exclude IVH-PVH by CUS in all premature infants with a birth weight less than 1500 g and newborn infants with preoperative neurologic dysfunction, coagulation disturbances, or hemodynamic instability causing significant metabolic acidosis. Infants with certain cardiac diagnoses may be at particular risk, such as those with hypoplastic left syndrome (HLHS) in whom up to 25% have intracranial hemorrhage at autopsy (16). Coarctation of the aorta, with its associated intracranial vascular malformations and hypertension, constitutes another high-risk group (12, 17). Although the risk period for the development of IVH-PVH in infants with CHD has not been delineated, 90% of IVH-PVH in the newborn population overall occurs within the first 3 days of life (12).

Timing and Management of Cardiac Surgery in Infants with Intracranial Hemorrhage

Despite the apparent risks for extending IVH-PVH during cardiopulmonary bypass (CPB) and infant cardiac surgery (i.e., marked cerebral perfusion changes and anticoagulation), prospective data do not exist to address the question of optimal timing of surgery. Infants undergoing extracorporeal membrane oxygenation (ECMO) provide the closest precedent. Minor subependymal hemorrhage carries low risk of extension during ECMO (18, 19). However, most centers would consider intraventricular (particularly with ventricular dilation) or intraparenchymal hemorrhage as contraindications to ECMO. Despite the similarities between CPB and ECMO, several important differences are evident, such as the fluctuations in temperature and perfusion pressure (even circulatory arrest), degree of anticoagulation, cannulation site, and duration of exposure to bypass circuits. Such differences prevent direct application of the ECMO experience to the infant with IVH-PVH destined for cardiac surgery. We base decisions for the optimal timing of CPB in infants with IVH-PVH on (a) severity of the cardiac illness (which may directly affect the risk for hemorrhage extension), (b) likely complexity of surgery, and (c) severity of preoperative IVH-PVH. Hemorrhage confined to the subependymal region should not delay any type of surgery. In infants with intraventricular or intraparenchymal hemorrhage, we attempt to delay CPB for at least 7 days, if the cardiac condition permits. One potential future option for infants with more extensive IVH-PVH in urgent need of surgery is the use of antifibrinolytic agents (20) and proteinase-inhibitors (21). This approach has been described in patients undergoing ECMO (20, 21), but it has not been evaluated in infants with intracranial hemorrhage undergoing CPB. Finally, in infants with extensive IVH-PVH in urgent need of intervention, procedures that may be suboptimal but do not require cardiopulmonary bypass (e.g., balloon angioplasty of coarctation, pulmonary artery banding) should be considered.

INTRAOPERATIVE NEUROLOGIC INJURY

Neurologic complications presenting in the early postoperative period are likely in large part caused by processes triggered during the intraoperative period.

Etiology-Mechanisms

The etiology of brain injury occurring with cardiac surgery may be multifactorial; however, the topography of the neuropathology (4, 8, 16, 22) (i.e., laminar cortical necrosis, and periventricular white matter injury) (23), points to hypoxia-ischemia/reperfusion (HI/R) injury as the primary pathogenetic mechanism. The exact timing of such intraoperative brain injury remains uncertain. However, the support techniques used to facilitate intracardiac repair (i.e., periods of arrested or attenuated bypass perfusion) likely constitute high risk periods for cerebral HI/R injury.

Current Neuroprotective Strategies

To reduce this risk for HI/R injury, cerebral protection techniques have aimed at pre-emptive suppression of cerebral metabolism by means of hypothermia and drugs (e.g., barbiturates) in anticipation of impaired intraoperative cerebral oxygen supply (24). In addition to cerebral metabolic suppression, hypothermia may have important neuroprotective effects on neurotransmitter systems implicated in excitotoxic neuronal damage (25–30). Despite current neuroprotective strategies, substantial neurologic morbidity persists in the early postoperative period (see below) (31, 32).

Optimal support strategy during the intracardiac periods of surgery (i.e., continuous low flow CPB [LF-CPB] versus deep hypothermic circulatory arrest [DHCA]) remains controversial (33–36). This question was the focus of a recent randomized clinical trial (Boston Circulatory Arrest Study) (37) that compared the incidence of neurologic complications following the two strategies (i.e., predominant LF-CPB versus predominant DHCA) in a population of infants undergoing the arterial switch operation for transposition of the great arteries. Assignment to and duration of DHCA were associated with a significantly greater incidence of perioperative neurologic dysfunction, specifically seizures (37), as well as worse psychomotor development at 1 year of age than infants assigned to continuous LF-CPB (38).

Intraoperative acid-base management follows one of two strategies (i.e., α-stat or pH-stat). The biochemical rationale underlying the two strategies is discussed in detail elsewhere (see Chapter 14, *Cardiopulmonary Bypass*). Although each strategy has theoretic benefits and limitations for cerebral protection (39, 40), the optimal strategy has not been determined prospectively in children. At a cerebrovascular level, the more hypercarbic pH-stat method causes vasodilation (41) and "luxury perfusion" (42) (i.e., cerebral blood flow in excess of cerebral oxygen demand). This enhanced cerebral perfusion theoretically promotes homogeneity of brain cooling; in addition, a more hypercarbic approach may decrease cerebral "steal" through systemic-pulmonary collaterals from the head and neck vessels (43). However, cerebral hypercarbic vasodilation can potentially increase the cerebral microvascular exposure to microembolic phenomena in the CPB perfusate. In addition, the pH-stat method can impair autoregulation (42), increasing the risk of ischemia during periods of LF-CPB. During cooling, cerebral autoregulation is preserved at lower temperatures with α-stat versus pH-stat technique (44); ultimately, however, autoregulation fails at deep hypothermia with both techniques (45). Both hypothermia and hypocarbia can impair tissue oxygen delivery by increasing oxyhemoglobin affinity (46). The relative hypercarbia and enhanced CBF of the pH-stat method counteracts such mechanisms.

Studies in a piglet model have examined the cerebral effects of these acid-base strategies (47–49). Aoki et al. (47) demonstrated a more rapid recovery of cerebral high-energy phosphates and intracellular pH with the pH-stat versus α-stat technique used prior to DHCA. Hiramatsu et al. (48) suggested that the early recovery of cerebral high-energy phosphates might be improved using the pH-stat strategy during both pre-DHCA cooling and post-DHCA rewarming. Skaryak et al. (49) found that the use of pH-stat during cooling, followed by a brief period of α-stat prior to DHCA, improved cerebral metabolic recovery after DHCA.

Several prospective studies have examined the neurologic effects of acid-base strategy in adult cardiac surgery (50–52). Bashein et al. (50) found no significant neuropsychologic outcome differences between the two acid-base strategies. Two subsequent studies have demonstrated a worse neurologic and cognitive outcome after the pH-stat technique (51, 52). However, at the moderate levels of hypothermia used during cardiac surgery (i.e., minimal temperature of 28 to 30°C) the distinction between the two strategies may be minimal. No published prospective clinical data compare the two strategies in children, in whom deep hypothermia use will induce more widely divergent cellular and vascular cerebral effects. In a retrospective study of infants undergoing deep hypothermic circulatory arrest, the α-stat strategy appeared to be less neuroprotective (53). A randomized clinical trial is currently in progress at Boston Children's Hospital comparing the neurologic and developmental sequelae of these two strategies in infants.

Future Neuroprotective Strategies

Recent studies aimed at both cerebral vascular as well as cerebral cellular mechanisms have potential importance for the development of future neuroprotective strategies. Perfusion (continuous or intermittent) with asanguinous oxygenated crystalloid ("cerebroplegia") (54–57) solution may allow more profound ("ultraprofound") (55) hypothermia while obviating the rheologic and reperfusion complications of cold whole blood. This technique has demonstrated improved preservation of cerebral high-energy phosphates and cerebral function recovery following DHCA (54). Selective cerebral perfusion techniques aim to maintain continuous perfusion to the brain during periods of circulatory arrest to the rest of the body. These approaches have been described in both animal and adult human studies and may be either antegrade (through the carotid system) (58, 59) or retrograde (through the central veins) (60–62). Utility and safety of these selective cerebral perfusion techniques have not been evaluated in children.

At a parenchymal cellular level, a number of neuroprotective agents directed against the injurious cascades triggered by hypoxia-ischemia have recently been developed, and they are currently under investigation (63–65). These include excitotoxin antagonists (66–68), free radical inhibitors and scavengers (69, 70), antileukocyte adhesion molecules (71, 72), and calcium channel blockers (73, 74), among others.

POSTOPERATIVE NEUROLOGIC COMPLICATIONS

Overview

From a neurologic perspective, the early postoperative period is important for a variety of reasons. A recent multicenter survey found that up to 20% of children undergoing cardiac surgery will present with neurologic dysfunction during this early period following surgery (31, 32). Such dysfunction is likely caused, in large part, by injury triggered by intraoperative events. In addition, however, the increased risk of cardiorespiratory instability and potential impairment of cerebrovascular autoregulation during this period may predispose to further neurologic injury. As our ability to identify infants at risk for such intra- and postoperative injury increases this will become an important period for the initiation of future neuroprotective therapies.

Neurologic dysfunction in the postoperative period can emanate from injury at any level of the neuroaxis (Fig. 24.1). For example, an apparent delayed postoperative recovery of consciousness with persistent ventilator dependence from suspected cerebral dysfunction (75) might be closely mimicked by dysfunction at the lower end of the neuroaxis (i.e., the neuromuscular junction) from prolonged use of neuromuscular blocking agents (76–82). In such a case, distinction between these two levels requires careful neurologic examination augmented by neurophysi-

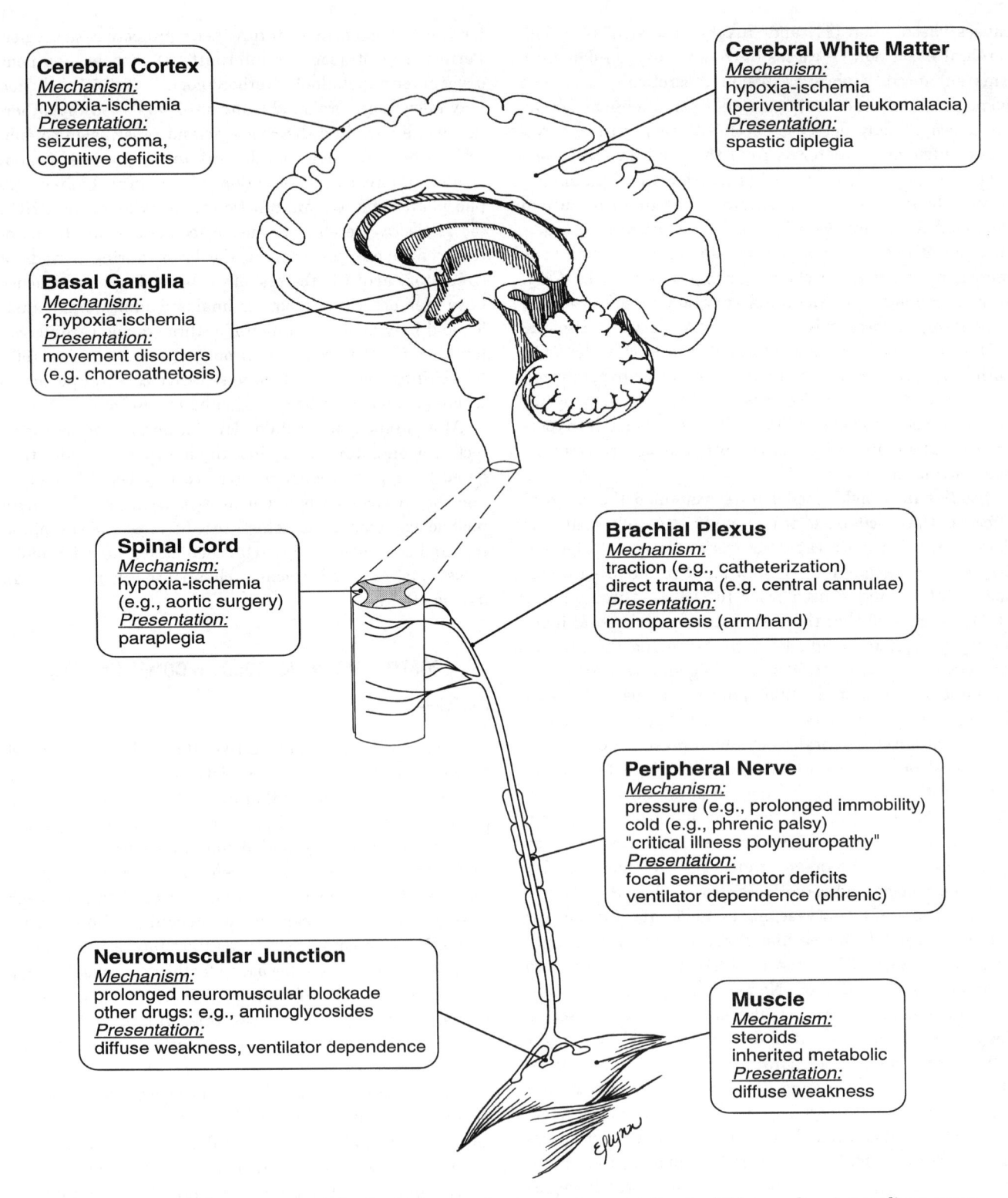

Cerebral Cortex
Mechanism:
hypoxia-ischemia
Presentation:
seizures, coma, cognitive deficits

Cerebral White Matter
Mechanism:
hypoxia-ischemia (periventricular leukomalacia)
Presentation:
spastic diplegia

Basal Ganglia
Mechanism:
?hypoxia-ischemia
Presentation:
movement disorders (e.g. choreoathetosis)

Spinal Cord
Mechanism:
hypoxia-ischemia (e.g., aortic surgery)
Presentation:
paraplegia

Brachial Plexus
Mechanism:
traction (e.g., catheterization)
direct trauma (e.g. central cannulae)
Presentation:
monoparesis (arm/hand)

Peripheral Nerve
Mechanism:
pressure (e.g., prolonged immobility)
cold (e.g., phrenic palsy)
"critical illness polyneuropathy"
Presentation:
focal sensori-motor deficits
ventilator dependence (phrenic)

Neuromuscular Junction
Mechanism:
prolonged neuromuscular blockade
other drugs: e.g., aminoglycosides
Presentation:
diffuse weakness, ventilator dependence

Muscle
Mechanism:
steroids
inherited metabolic
Presentation:
diffuse weakness

Figure 24.1. Diagram showing neuroaxis levels of injury, mechanisms and presentation in children undergoing cardiac surgery.

ologic testing with a peripheral nerve stimulator. Widespread use of paralyzing and sedating medications in the postoperative patient limit the bedside neurologic examination. However, a growing number of adjunctive diagnostic techniques now allow interrogation of neurologic function (Table 24.1), structure (Table 24.2), and perfusion (Table 24.3) in these patients.

Neurologic syndromes presenting in the early postoperative period are often transient in their acute expression. However, long-term outcome of such apparently reversible dysfunction has seldom been studied systematically. In one recent prospective study (38), transient early postoperative seizures were predictive of a worse later developmental outcome.

POSTOPERATIVE SEIZURES

Incidence

Seizures are among the most common manifestations of neurologic dysfunction in the early period following cardiac surgery. Reported frequency of clinical seizures following CPB ranges from 4 to 15% (37, 83–86). Because the behavioral expression of seizures in the young infant can be subtle (see below) and escape bedside detection, this incidence range is likely an underestimate. Using continuous video-electroencephalography recording, Newburger et al. (37) detected electrographic seizure activity in 26% of infants following DHCA, whereas clinically evident seizures were observed in only 11%.

Mechanisms

Although numerous causes may underlie seizure activity in the child with CHD, those originating from hypoxic-ischemic injury, either focal (i.e., cerebrovascular accident) (87–90) or generalized (following diffuse cerebral hypoperfusion) are of particular concern. In addition to seizures of known cause, a substantial number of postoperative seizures remain idiopathic and are commonly referred to as "postpump seizures."

Presentation

Bedside diagnosis of seizures in the young infant can be challenging, because clinical signs are often subtle or even occult (91–93). This is particularly likely in the encephalopathic or sedated patient and, of course, in infants receiving neuromuscular blocking agents. In these infants striking electrographic seizure activity can occur without obvious behavioral accompaniment (92, 94, 95); often the only clinical manifestations are paroxysmal autonomic changes (tachycardia, hypertension, pupillary dilation) (91).

Table 24.1. Functional Neurodiagnostic Studies Relevant to Cardiac Intensive Care

Diagnostic Techniques	Indications	Limitations
Cerebral Cortex Electroencephalogram (EEG)	Diagnosis of seizures (esp. if sedated, paralyzed) Evaluation/prognostication in stupor-coma Evaluation for brain death	Does not exclude inferomedial seizure focus Sensitive to drugs and artifact in ICU
Visual Pathways Visual evoked potentials (VEP)	Evaluation of visual pathways and occipital cortex Prognostication in hypoxic-ischemic encephalopathy	Limited normative data for newborn or young infant Sensitive to artifact in ICU
Brainstem Auditory evoked potentials (BAEP)	Evaluation of auditory neural pathways Evaluation (indirect) of brainstem above upper medulla	Does not exclude lower medullary lesion Sensitive to artifact in ICU
Spinal Cord Somatosensory evoked potentials (SSEP)	Evaluation of spinal cord (posterior columns), brainstem, and somatosensory cortex	Does not exclude anterior spinal injury Sensitive to artifact in ICU
Peripheral Nerve and Muscle Electromyography and nerve conduction (EMG/NCV)	Evaluation of lower motor unit Anterior horn cells (e.g., anterior spinal cord ischemia) Peripheral nerve (e.g., phrenic, brachial plexus palsy) Neuromuscular junction (e.g., residual paralysant drug effect) Muscle (e.g., myopathies)	Sensitive to artifact in ICU

ICU, Intensive care unit.

Table 24.2. Structural Neurodiagnostic Studies Relevant to Cardiac Intensive Care

Diagnostic Technique		Characteristics/Limitations
Brain Ultrasound (US)	Technique	Portable, repeated studies in unstable infant
	Limitation	Requires open fontanelle
	Anatomy	Basal ganglia, thalamus, periventricular white matter, ventricles
	Limitation	Poor imaging of peripheral parenchyma (esp. cortex), subarachnoid and subdural spaces, posterior fossa
	Pathology	Intra/periventricular hemorrhage, ischemia, hydrocephalus Focal and multifocal injury
	Limitation	Small white matter lesions (< 1.0 cm) may be missed
Computerized Tomography (CT)	Technique	Higher spatial resolution than US
	Limitations	Not portable, ionizing, expensive
	Anatomy	Entire brain parenchyma and cerebrospinal fluid spaces
	Limitation	Lower tissue definition than MRI
	Pathology	Hemorrhage, ischemia, major dysgenesis
	Limitation	Less sensitive to acute periventricular leukomalacia than US (more sensitive to late periventricular leukomalacia than US)
Magnetic Resonance Imaging (MRI)	Technique	Best available tissue definition, nonionizing
	Limitations	Not portable, expensive, ferromagnetic constraints (e.g., pacemakers, valves, ventilators)
	Anatomy	Entire brain parenchyma, cerebrospinal fluid spaces and spinal cord Best technique for posterior fossa

	Pathology	Dysgenesis (small and large); myelination maturation
		Ischemia: Focal, global, or "watershed"
		  Early, acute detection (esp. diffusion-weighted MRI)
		Hemorrhage: Best technique for dating hemorrhage
		  Distinguishes hemorrhagic infarct from primary hemorrhage

Postpump seizures are a unique clinical entity, and they constitute the most common seizure type in the early post-bypass period. The commonly held tenet that these seizures reflect intraoperative HI/R injury is by no means established. In fact, these seizures differ in several ways from other forms of hypoxic-ischemic seizures. First, their onset (i.e., 24 to 48 hours post-bypass) is later than that of seizures occurring, for example, after birth asphyxia (96, 97). In addition, although only 50% of infants with postasphyxial seizures have a normal outcome (96, 98, 99), postpump seizures were generally considered benign, transient events with little prognostic significance for future neurologic outcome. This latter notion has been challenged recently (see below) (37).

These postpump seizures occur during an apparent period of susceptibility and follow a typical clinical course. Their onset is usually in the second 24 postoperative hours, although some occur earlier. They often occur serially for hours to several days, and progression to status epilepticus is not uncommon. Motor manifestations (when evident) are usually focal (86) or multifocal.

Bedside electroencephalography (EEG) can be a valuable diagnostic technique and help to direct management. First, EEG will detect cerebral ictal discharges and thus distinguish true seizures from infant behavior patterns that closely mimic seizures. Second, a highly focal EEG abnormality should raise the question of a focal structural lesion, such as an infarct (89, 90), in which case brain imaging may be indicated. Finally, anticonvulsants and other central nervous system depressant drugs may control only the clinical manifestations of seizure activity; the otherwise undetected persistence of electrographic seizures will be evident on EEG.

Management

The therapeutic approach to postpump seizures is best dictated by their typical clinical course. A tendency toward repeated seizures and the risk of status epilepticus require that rapid therapeutic blood levels be pursued with adequate doses of intravenous anticonvulsant drugs (ACD). Reversible disturbances in blood glucose,

Table 24.3. Brain Perfusion Studies Relevant to Cardiac Intensive Care

Diagnostic Technique	Indications/Limitations
Doppler Ultrasound	
Transcranial Doppler (TCD)	Portable, noninvasive
	Measures cerebral blood flow velocity and resistive index
	Limitations: No anatomic data
	Measures velocity not volumetric flow
Duplex Doppler	Selected region-of-interest flow in large arteries and veins
Power Doppler	Regional flow, including small (0.5–1.0 mm) neonatal vessels
Magnetic Resonance Angiography (MRA)	Evaluation of vascular anatomy
	Limitations: Not portable; ferromagnetic constraints (see Table 2)
	Limited anatomic resolution
Contrast Angiography	Most detailed evaluation of vascular anatomy and patency
	Limitations: Not portable, ionizing radiation
	Invasive, contrast injection
Radioisotope Scans	Global and regional (limited) cerebral perfusion
	Brain death evaluation
	Limitations: Limited portability; ionizing radiation (minor)
Single Photon Emission Computed Tomography (SPECT)	Regional cerebral perfusion and function
	More sensitive to postacute ischemic lesions than computed tomography or magnetic resonance imaging (Fig. 24.4)
	Limitations: Flow-function uncoupled during acute ischemia
	Ionizing radiation (minor)
Near Infrared Spectroscopy (NIRS)	Portable, continuous, real-time, noninvasive
	Evaluation of cerebral hemodynamics and oxygenation
	Limitations: Limited clinical experience and validation

magnesium (100), and calcium (101) should be corrected while ACD therapy is commencing. Guidelines for selection and dosing of ACD, as outlined in Table 24.4, will establish seizure control in virtually all cases (96).

Major parenteral anticonvulsants (Table 24.4) all have potential cardiac and respiratory depressant effects if used incorrectly. During infusion of these agents, careful cardiorespiratory monitoring is thus mandatory, particularly in the postoperative patient. Excessively rapid or large doses of phenobarbital (PB) can have direct myocardial depressant effects. Data are lacking for safe blood levels in infants with early postoperative seizures and with recent myocardial exposure to surgery, hypothermia, CPB, and DHCA. Almost 80% of neonatal seizures will be controlled with PB monotherapy according to the guidelines in Table 24.4 (102, 103). Only once a PB level of 40 µg/mL has been achieved should phenytoin (DPH) be added to the regimen. Cardiotoxic effects of DPH (i.e., bradyarrhythmias and myocardial depression) (104) are caused by the diluent propylene glycol, and they are related primarily to the rate of infusion (Table 24.4).

Phenytoin should be avoided in patients with conduction defects and bradyarrhythmias (105).

Within several seizure-free days, the ACD regimen can be reduced to a single maintenance agent, usually PB. In view of the apparent circumscribed period of vulnerability to "postpump" seizures, early withdrawal of ACD may be considered (Table 24.4).

The role of persistent electrographic seizures in causing or extending brain injury remains controversial (106). Their potential for causing disturbances in systemic (107) and cerebral hemodynamics (108) and metabolism (109), including the release of neurotoxic excitatory amino acids (110) supports the use of anticonvulsants for these electrographic seizures. However, such clinically silent EEG seizures can remain refractory to standard ACD approaches; the high doses often required to suppress such EEG seizures can expose the infant to hemodynamic side effects.

Seizures associated with stroke differ from postpump seizures in their clinical presentation and outcome. Specifically, their tendency toward subsequent epilepsy (88) (see below) necessitates consideration of longer term ACD therapy.

Table 24.4. Management of Postoperative Seizures

Measure blood glucose, electrolytes, calcium, and magnesium
If clinical seizure manifestations are:
  Unequivocal: commence anticonvulsant drug (ACD) therapy and record electroencephalogram (EEG)
  Equivocal: confirm by EEG; then commence ACD
Anticonvulsant Drug (ACD) Therapy
  Acute ACD Management
    Incremental steps for seizure activity that persists
      Lorazepam 0.05–0.1 mg/kg infusion over 2–5 min; repeat twice if seizures persist
      Phenobarbital (PB) 20 mg/kg loading dose over 10–15 min
        If seizures persist, repeat 5 mg/kg infusions at 10-min intervals to a maximal 40 mg/kg total dose
        In infants, 1 mg/kg dose will increase blood level approximately 1 µg/mL
        Aim: seizure control or blood level of 40 µg/mL
        Caution: myocardial depression with hypotension after large, rapid infusions
      Phenytoin (DPH) 20 mg/kg IV loading dose not exceeding 1 mg/kg/min
        Aim: seizure control or blood level of 20 µg/mL
        Caution: cardiac arrhythmias with rapid infusions nonlinear kinetics at higher total doses
  Maintenance ACD Management
    Phenobarbital 3–4 mg/kg/d (po or IV) divided bid
    Phenytoin 4–5 mg/kg/d (po or IV) divided bid
  ACD Discontinuation
    If seizure-free for 48 h, discontinue DPH and maintain PB monotherapy
    If seizure-free at hospital discharge and neurologic exam appropriate, wean PB.
    If seizures or other neurologic concerns persist, maintain PB at 3–4 mg/kg and re-evaluate with 6 weekly examinations +/− EEG

Outcome

Newburger et al. (37) followed a cohort of infants with EEG-documented postoperative seizures; by age 1 year none of these infants had developed epilepsy and none were receiving ACD (personal communication, JW Newburger, MD). However, infants with perioperative seizures were found to have a significantly worse neurodevelopmental outcome at age 1 year (37). Rarely, more serious neurologic syndromes, such as West syndrome (111), can develop in infants with apparent idiopathic postpump seizures. Risk for subsequent epilepsy among children with stroke as the cause for their seizures ranges from 19 to 28% (87, 88). This risk appears to increase with the age at stroke beyond the newborn period (when the risk appears low) (90) as well as the time to first seizure following stroke (88).

CEREBROVASCULAR ACCIDENTS (STROKE)

Incidence

Cerebrovascular accidents (strokes) occur in 2.5 per 100,000 children each year (112). Congenital heart disease, which is the leading known association of childhood stroke, is present in 25 to 30% of cases (87, 112, 113). In earlier autopsy studies, almost 20% of children with CHD demonstrated features of cerebrovascular injury (1, 4).

Mechanisms

Cardiogenic stroke (i.e., stroke associated with heart disease) can be classified on the basis of the likely thrombotic or embolic source, as (a) cardioembolic (i.e., probable intracardiac embolic source); (b) paradoxic (i.e., probable venous embolic source with a cardiac anatomy that permits embolus passage into the cerebral circulation); or (c) venous (i.e., cerebral vein thrombosis caused by central venous hypertension and venous stasis). A cardioembolic source can be difficult to document, because an intracardiac thrombus may not or no longer be detected by echocardiography (ECHO).

Risk factors for cardiogenic stroke can be conceptualized by considering Virchows triad (i.e., altered vascular surface, stasis, and hypercoagulability) and the risk of "paradoxic" embolization. These risk factors have changed over the past two decades. In earlier studies (1–4) the risk for stroke was related to the effects of long-standing heart defects, such as chronic hypoxia and polycythemia (1, 114–116), and uncorrected paradoxic pathways (e.g., right-to-left shunts). The shift toward earlier corrective surgery over the past two decades (see above) (7) has reduced the duration of exposure to such stroke risk factors. Consequently, recent focus has been on intra- and postoperative mechanisms of stroke.

A number of intraoperative mechanisms related to CPB can predispose to cerebral vaso-occlusion. Embolic phenomena (particulate or gaseous) (117, 118) may be generated during CPB and will bypass filtration by the pulmonary bed, entering the systemic arterial circulation directly. An earlier autopsy study (8) found a four to fivefold increase in cerebral embolic infarction following surgery for CHD. Since that report, advances in CPB apparatus and technique, including refinements in membrane oxygenators, in-line arterial filters, and anticoagulation, have reduced the incidence of macroembolization and large vessel occlusion (119). The impact of these advances on the incidence of microembolization and small-vessel disease is difficult to evaluate.

Because of the extensive interface between bypass blood and artificial surfaces, CPB may trigger an often marked inflammatory response. Complex physiologic cascades activated in the process (120, 121), including endothelial-leukocyte interactions (121–125), can further enhance the risk of ischemic injury. On withdrawal of CPB and resumption of the cardiac-driven circulation, emboli (particularly air emboli) may enter the arterial circulation from the surgical field.

In the postoperative period factors predisposing to stroke include stasis (intra- and extracardiac), altered vascular surfaces (native or prosthetic) and, in some situations, a potential procoagulant shift in the humoral clotting systems (126). Intracardiac stasis can result from localized areas of low flow (e.g., proximal segment of a ligated main pulmonary artery; see Fig. 24.2) (127, 128) or global ventricular dysfunction. Transient or sustained elevations of right heart and, hence, central venous pressure in the early postoperative period, will predispose to thrombosis locally in the right atrium and central veins (129–133). Prosthetic material in such areas of disturbed flow will increase the likelihood of thrombus formation, and the presence of a right-to-left shunt (native or iatrogenic) will compound the risk of paradoxic embolization (Fig. 24.3). Elevated right atrial pressure transmitted to the cerebral venous circulation will predispose to venous thrombosis, particularly in the dural venous sinuses (115). Elevated systemic venous pressure may contribute to protein-losing enteropathy (134), liver impairment (135), and pleural effusions, factors that can disturb the humoral coagulant systems (126). A number of the stroke risk factors mentioned can be present after the Fontan operation as highlighted in several recent reports (127, 136). We found a 2.6% incidence of stroke in a retrospective review of 645 patients following the Fontan operation; the risk extended over 3 years following the procedure (127). Rosenthal et al. (136) found a 20% incidence of thromboembolic complications overall among 71 patients following the Fontan procedure, the risk for which extended over 15 years; 3 of these patients (4%) developed strokes.

Presentation

Strokes originating during or immediately after cardiac surgery may escape clinical recognition for several days because of the effects of postoperative sedating and paralyzing agents. In the young infant, stroke often presents with focal seizures (87, 89, 90) or changes in mental status; focal motor deficits can be subtle (87). In older infancy and childhood stroke usually presents with acute focal motor deficits, and language or visual dysfunction.

Management

The therapeutic approach to stroke in the child with heart disease includes (*a*) preventive and (*b*) "rescue" strategies. Experience with rescue therapies remains confined to adult and experimental stroke; these rescue therapies are aimed at the salvage of potentially viable brain through techniques that aim to revascularize ischemic regions (thrombolytic therapy) (137, 138) or to curtail biochemical cascades triggered during HI/R (65). The current discussion will focus on the principles of stroke prophylaxis with antithrombotic agents. For a more detailed discussion of antithrombotic therapy see Chapter 5, *Cardiovascular Pharmacology*.

Preventive stroke therapy can be viewed as primary or secondary (139). Primary stroke prevention aims to identify and treat high-risk patients prior to a stroke, whereas secondary prevention aims at minimizing the risk of stroke

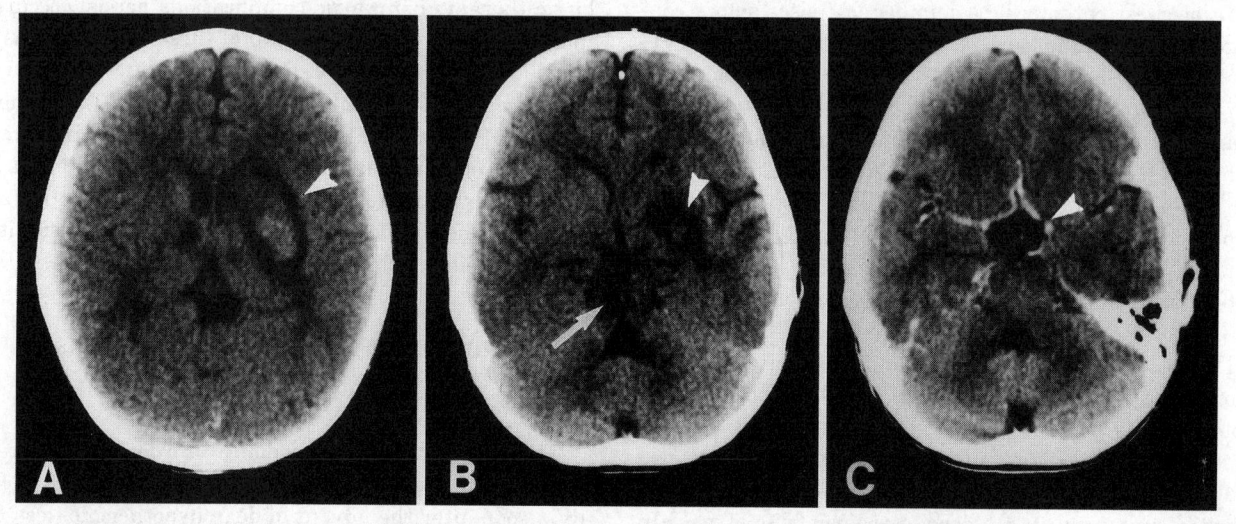

Figure 24.2. Cranial computed tomography (*CT*) in a 3-year-old boy with sudden onset right hemiparesis following a Fontan operation with a fenestrated cavocaval tunnel (**A, B**). Infarcts in the distribution of the left middle cerebral artery (*arrowhead*) and right midbrain (*arrow*). **C**. Contrast-enhanced CT shows occlusion of the left middle cerebral artery (*arrowhead*). du Plessis A, Chang A, Wessel D, et al. Cerebrovascular accidents following the Fontan procedure. Pediatr Neurol 1995;12(3):230–236.

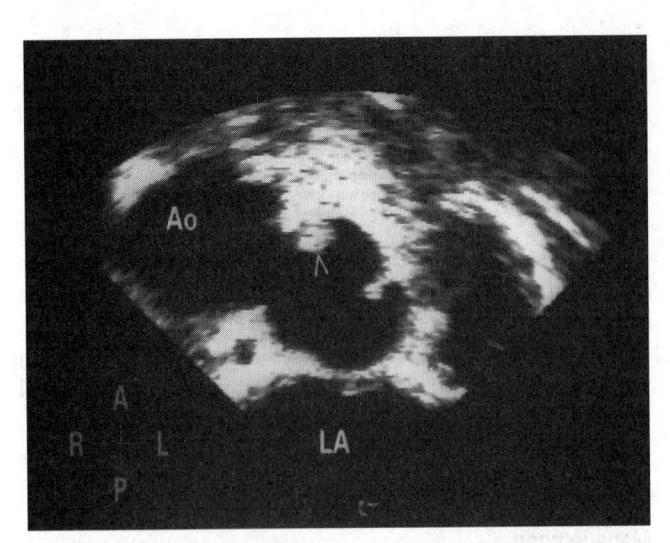

Figure 24.3. Transesophageal echocardiogram showing thrombus formation (*arrow*) in the proximal main pulmonary artery stump that had been ligated and oversewn at the Fontan operation. Ao, aorta; LA, left atrium. (Reprinted with permission from du Plessis A, Chang A, Wessel D, et al. Cerebrovascular accidents following the Fontan procedure. Pediatr Neurol 1995;12(3):230–236.)

recurrence. Consistent and universally accepted guidelines for both primary and secondary stroke prophylaxis in children are lacking, in large part because of poor definition of risk factors and lack of prospective studies. Consequently, current guidelines are largely empiric and anecdotal. Established indications for *primary stroke prophylaxis* in children include prosthetic heart valves, dilated cardiomyopathy, or intracardiac thrombus on echocardiogram. Certain combinations of factors can increase the risk for stroke, such as a right-to-left shunt and high right atrial pressure (130, 131) in patients requiring prolonged bedrest (e.g., because of chest catheters). A number of these factors converge in post-Fontan patients, particularly those with residual right-to-left shunts (fenestrated or adjustable ASD) (127). Clearly a need exists to delineate the role of antitrombotic treatment and its duration in the management of the post-Fontan patient. In other situations of suspected but undefined stroke risk, close ECHO surveillance can help to identify intracardiac thrombus prior to embolization. In adults, newer techniques such as indium-111 platelet scans have improved the prediction of embolic risk (140, 141).

The decision regarding whether and when to initiate secondary stroke prophylaxis with antithrombotic agents should aim to balance the risk for (*a*) recurrent cerebral embolization, and (*b*) potentiating secondary hemorrhage into an area of cerebral infarction. Embolus recurrence risks are unknown in childhood cardioembolic stroke. In adults (following myocardial infarction) this risk is highest in the early poststroke period (i.e., about 1% per day) (10 to 20% over the first 2 weeks) (142–144). Cardioembolic strokes are particularly susceptible to hemorrhagic transformation (145) and this risk is again highest during the early poststroke period. Even without anticoagulant therapy, hemorrhagic transformation occurs (often silently) in 20 to 40% of adults with cardioembolic strokes (145–149). Risk of significant clinical deterioration following hemorrhagic transformation is greater in the anticoagulated patient (148, 149).

Although it is difficult to predict which infarcts will undergo hemorrhagic transformation, certain guidelines exist. Seventy-five percent of infarcts destined to undergo hemorrhagic transformation do so within 48 hours after stroke onset (149). Large infarcts, particularly those larger than 30%, or one lobe, of a cerebral hemisphere are at greater risk of hemorrhagic transformation (148–150). Uncontrolled systemic hypertension, stroke caused by septic emboli (see below), and cerebral venous thrombosis are additional risk factors for hemorrhagic infarction.

Seizures are a common complication of stroke (87, 89, 90), and they may require anticonvulsant therapy. Important potential drug interactions exist between coumadin and anticonvulsants; phenobarbital and carbamazepine can decrease the coumadin effect, whereas phenytoin can either decrease or increase this effect. Close monitoring of the international normalized ratio (INR) or prothrombin time is mandatory during and particularly on cessation of ACD therapy, because these drug interactions are unpredictable.

Cerebrovascular disease associated with infective endocarditis (IE) warrants brief mention. Neurologic manifestations of IE are protean (151), and they include meningitis, brain abscess, and seizures. However, cerebrovascular complications are the most common, specifically septic embolism and hemorrhage. Despite advances in modern antibiotic therapy, neurologic complications persist, occurring in 33% of children with IE; half of these complications are embolic in origin (152). Cerebrovascular complications carry the highest mortality rate (up to 80 to 90%) primarily because of intracranial hemorrhage (151). The risk for, and mortality of, cerebral hemorrhage in this population contraindicates anticoagulant therapy. Prior to initiating anticoagulant therapy for cardiogenic stroke, the possibility of septic embolism should be excluded.

POSTOPERATIVE MOVEMENT DISORDERS

Incidence

The first reports of movement disorders following cardiac surgery appeared more than three decades ago (153–155), soon after the advent of deep hypothermic (less than 20°C) CPB. Since that time, more than 90 cases have been reported, a figure that likely underestimates the true incidence, for several reasons. Milder, transient dyskinesias are commonly ascribed to postoperative agitation and discomfort, and they are obscured by the effects of sedative and analgesic medication. In addition, the low single-center incidence leads to under reporting. Reported incidence following cardiac surgery has ranged from 0.5% (156) to as high as 19% in an earlier study (157). Despite the relatively low incidence in most series, these disorders present complex management issues and may be extremely distressing to patients and their families. In addition, recovery is often prolonged and incomplete, whereas severe cases face a significant mortality risk.

Although choreoathetosis is the most common and dramatic of these disorders, a spectrum of dyskinesias has been seen in the early postoperative period (e.g., oculogyric crises, parkinsonism) (158, 159). An age-related vulnerability to the occurrence and severity of these syndromes is apparent. Postoperative choreoathetosis is not seen in adults and is rare in the first 3 months of life. The age of reported cases ranges from 1.7 months to 10 years (mean age 25 months). In infants younger than 10 months the condition usually involves the distal extremities; it is less severe and more likely to improve. In children older than 1 year of age the dyskinesias tend to be both proximal and distal, more severe, and the patient is less likely to recover fully.

These movement disorders should be distinguished from dyskinesias related to medications such as dopamine-antagonist antiemetics (e.g., metoclopramide), opiate withdrawal (e.g., fentanyl) (160), and the short-acting benzodiazepines (161, 162).

Clinical Course

Postoperatively, a typical latency is seen to the onset of involuntary movements. In some cases partial or even complete return to the preoperative neurologic state has been reported to occur prior to the onset of dyskinesia (154, 157, 163). Abnormal movements begin between 2 to 7 days postoperatively, and they are usually heralded by an acute delirium with irritability (often extreme), confusion, disorientation, and insomnia. Striking truncal and extremity hypotonia is a frequent early finding. Concurrently, an apparent apraxia of oromotor and oculomotor activity develops. Speech and feeding are usually impaired and the infant is at risk for aspiration. The child's apparent inability to look at or to "recognize" familiar faces often leads to concerns of "blindness." However, preservation of visual reflexes (i.e., the doll's eye reflex and oculokinetic nystagmus) indicates a form of supranuclear ophthalmoplegia.

Initially, involuntary movements involve the distal extremities, with writhing athetoid activity, and orolingual and facial musculature, with grimacing and tongue thrusting. Involuntary motor activity intensity increases with stress, excessive stimulation, and pain, whereas natural or sedated sleep diminishes or abolishes the movements. In the more severe cases a period of progression ensues with involvement of the more proximal musculature and trunk, becoming in some cases frankly ballismic (i.e., with wild flailing of the extremities). This period of deterioration can persist for a period of 1 to 2 weeks, and it is usually followed by a plateau phase lasting days to weeks. Hereafter, gradual improvement commences, which can persist for weeks to months, or even years. Wong et al. (43) described two levels of severity. A mild transient form remains confined to the distal extremities and orofacial muscles, and it resolves within 6 months. The severe (often ballismic) form progresses to involve the proximal limb muscles and trunk and persists longer than 6 months.

This syndrome is so characteristic that the diagnosis is usually evident on purely clinical grounds. Laboratory investigations are generally useful only in excluding other conditions. Cases studied with electroencephalography have usually demonstrated normal or diffusely "slow" background activity. Neuroimaging has been unhelpful and in only a small minority of cases have focal abnormalities been noted, the most common abnormality being nonspecific diffuse atrophy. Functional brain imaging with single photon emission computed tomography (SPECT) (158) revealed a high incidence of focal perfusion defects in both the cortical and subcortical regions, even in the absence of focal abnormalities on computed tomography (CT) and magnetic resonance imaging (MRI) scan (Fig. 24.4; see color plate 24.4).

Published neuropathology data for these movement disorders are limited. Findings have ranged from "normal" (164), to extensive loss of pallidal ganglion cells (154) and "hypoxic neuronal degeneration and capillary proliferation" in the basal ganglia (165). Kupsky et al. (166) described neuronal loss, nerve fiber degeneration, and reactive astrocytosis in the globus pallidus, particularly the lateral nucleus.

Mechanisms

Putative mechanisms that have been proposed to underlie these postoperative movement disorders, have focused mainly on hypoxia-ischemia as the mediating event. However, autopsy studies have failed to demonstrate the typical neuropathologic patterns of either focal "stroke" or global cerebral ischemia. Deep hypothermic circulatory arrest has preceded most but not all of these cases (167). Wong et al. (43) found that all 11 patients with severe, persistent choreoathetosis and all but 1 of the 8 patients with a milder transient form of the disorder underwent DHCA. In addition they found that all severe, persistent choreoathetosis cases had cyanotic CHD; 9 of 11 had some form of pulmonary stenosis of whom 5 of 6 had sufficient angiographic data to demonstrate systemic-to-pulmonary collaterals from the head and neck vessels. This latter finding suggested the potential for a "steal" mechanism from the cerebral to the pulmonary circulation during CPB. Other proposed mechanisms have included nonhomogeneous or excessively rapid brain cooling during bypass, reperfusion injury, and hyperglycemia with lactic acidosis. Some authors have implicated deep hypothermia as the primary injurious factor (153, 154, 167). DeLeon et al. (167) suggested that CPB temperatures 25°C or lower, higher CPB flow rates, and cooling times longer than 1 hour in duration predisposed to choreoathetosis. These findings were not supported by the largest study to date (43), which found shorter cooling times (i.e., time from onset of CPB cooling to onset of circulatory arrest) in patients with persistent forms of choreoathetosis than among controls. Data from an immature rodent model demonstrating a transient expression of glutamate receptors in the globus pallidus have suggested that the age-related vulnerability to movement disorders following cardiac surgery might be related to maturational excitotoxic factors (168). In summary, the apparent selective vulnerability of the complex basal ganglia neurochemical pathways to intraoperative injury in these children remains unclear.

Management

Therapeutic approaches to these postoperative dyskinesias include preventive, pharmacologic, and supportive measures (Table 24.5). Currently, the most crucial management issue (i.e., prevention) remains an elusive goal, largely because of the absence of a defined and preventable cause. Wong et al. (43) identified risk factors for severe choreoathetosis and proposed guidelines for prevention including early corrective surgery, careful management of systemic-to-pulmonary collateral vessels, and avoidance of excessively rapid cooling on bypass. At our institution changing strategies focused on the abovementioned risk factors, together with a decrease in the use of DHCA, have been associated with a marked reduction in the incidence of postoperative movement disorders over the past 5 years (156). The pursuit of pharmacologic therapies aimed at controlling the involuntary movements once they occur has been equally frustrating. Agents traditionally effective in the treatment of other hyperkinetic dyskinesias have, for the most part, been disappointing in control of postoperative choreoathetosis. Approaches have included agents directed at dopamine receptor blockade (phenothiazines, butyrophenones), dopamine depletion (reserpine, tetrabenazine), stimulation of gamma-aminobutyric acid (GABA) receptors (benzodiazepines, barbiturates, baclofen), as well as an assortment of other drugs, including L-dopa, valproic acid, carbamazepine, phenytoin, diphenhydramine, adrenocorticotrophic hormone (ACTH), and chloral hydrate. This wide range of therapies highlights our current ignorance regarding the neurochemical mechanisms involved in these postoperative movement disorders. In essence, no agent has demonstrated consistent ability to suppress selectively the dyskinesia while preserving consciousness. Usually, involuntary movements have abated only at doses sufficient to cause deep sedation.

In the acute phase of dyskinesia, the following approach is suggested. For mild dyskinesias, specific sedating agents such as benzodiazepines or chloral hydrate may be adequate. In more severe dyskinesias, a cautious trial of a specific neuroleptic agent such as haloperidol can be started at low doses and increased gradually, provided that myocardial function remains adequate. In the absence of a clear, early response at nonsedating doses, or in the event of other side effects, neuroleptic agents should be replaced by more specific sedating agents. Paradoxically, several of the sedative (e.g., midazolam) (161, 162) and neuroleptic agents (e.g., haloperidol) used to treat these movement disorders can themselves be associated with iatrogenic dyskinesias. Of the benzodiazepines, longer acting agents such as clonazepam may be preferable, but an increase in pulmonary secretions should be anticipated. Supportive measures include minimizing sensory stimulation, avoidance of abrasions and aspiration (e.g., nasogastric feedings), and anticipation of increased caloric needs. Parental support is an important aspect of management.

Outcome

Overall, these movement disorders tend to improve, albeit often incompletely. In mild cases resolution of the involuntary movements can be expected. More severe cases

Table 24.5. Therapeutic Approach to Postoperative Movement Disorders

Pharmacologic Management
Mild dyskinesia: mild, nonspecific sedative agents (e.g., chloral hydrate)
Severe dyskinesia: trial of specific antidyskinesia agents (e.g., dopamine-blocker [haloperidol] at low dose)
If movements improve with preservation of consciousness, continue drug
If movements fail to improve, sedation excessive, or other side effects, switch to more specific sedative agents

Supportive Management
Reduce sensory stimulation
  External: use quiet dark room
  Internal: adequate analgesia, prevent constipation and esophagitis
Monitor stress points for abrasions and infection
Avoid aspiration (e.g., with nasogastric feedings)
Anticipate increased caloric demands
Parental support

have an associated mortality rate of up to 40% and, in survivors, a high incidence of persistent neurodevelopmental deficit, with only 10% of survivors recovering a normal neurologic examination. Common long-term residua include hypotonia and developmental delay, especially in expressive language.

BRAIN DEATH

Hypoxic-ischemic encephalopathy and coma are uncommon catastrophes in cardiac intensive care, and in severe cases may evolve to brain death. Brain death is defined as the *"irreversible* cessation of *all cerebral and brainstem function."* Somatic death is the inevitable and imminent consequence of brain death. Determination of irreversibility requires that (*a*) the proximate cause of coma is known, is irreversible, and can account for the loss of all brain function; (*b*), all potential reversible factors (e.g., pharmacologic, metabolic toxins, hypothermia, hypotension) have been considered and excluded as significant contributors; and (*c*) an appropriate observation period has been allowed to establish irreversibility. Absence of all cerebral and brainstem function is established primarily by bedside neurologic examination. Many clinicians remain uncomfortable diagnosing brain death on clinical criteria alone and consequently a number of "confirmatory" neurodiagnostic tests have been described, including EEG, radioisotope scans, and angiography. However, such tests themselves have limitations of sensitivity and specificity, particularly in the newborn and young infant.

Initially, brain death criteria (169) failed to distinguish between adults and children. However, maturational differences in neurologic vulnerability and expression of brain injury subsequently established the need for age-specific brain death criteria, and a multidisciplinary Task Force (170) developed the following guidelines for the diagnosis of brain death in children. Brain death should be diagnosed in *infants aged 7 days to 2 months* if, over an interval of at least 48 hours, two neurologic examinations are diagnostic and two EEGs are isoelectric; in *infants aged 2 months to 1 year*, if the same findings are separated by at least 24 hours, or if an initial diagnostic examination is accompanied by absent brain perfusion on cerebral angiography. *Children older than 1 year* are brain dead if two diagnostic neurologic examinations are separated by 12 hours; if hypoxia-ischemia is the cause, an observation period of 24 hours is recommended. In *children older than 1 year*, neurodiagnostic testing is not required if the cause of brain death is irreversible (e.g., prolonged cardiac arrest versus toxic or metabolic encephalopathy). However, such diagnostic testing can permit a decreased observation period if, for example, the EEG is isoelectric or angiography shows absent brain perfusion.

In the early newborn period, and particularly in the premature infant, the usual clinical, EEG, and circulatory criteria are potentially misleading (171, 172). These difficulties stem from the lack of experience in this age group (171), as well as the relatively low oxygen and cerebral blood flow requirements in the neonate, resulting in increased resilience to hypoxic-ischemic injury. These issues are particularly relevant to the cardiac intensive care unit, where ever-younger infants are increasingly represented and in whom hypoxia-ischemia is the predominant mechanism of brain death.

For the reasons mentioned the Task Force guidelines recommend delaying the diagnosis of brain death in preterm and young term newborns. A subsequent retrospective study (172) focusing on the difficulties of diagnosing brain death in the newborn concluded that term infants clinically brain dead for 2 days and preterm infants clinically brain dead for 3 days would not survive. In addition, it was suggested that the diagnosis could be established purely on clinical grounds and that the potential value of confirmatory neurodiagnostic studies was to decrease the period of observation.

Finally, although the complexity surrounding the diagnosis of brain death in children demands that stringent, objective criteria be met, in reality withdrawal of life support in the brain-injured comatose infant with heart disease is more often the result of decisions made by the family and caretakers that embrace the child's projected future quality of life.

CONCLUSION

Advances in the management of infants with CHD in recent decades have dramatically increased the survival of this population. However, the incidence of neurologic complications following cardiac surgery remains a concern. Detection, diagnosis, and management of neurologic dysfunction in the intensive care setting can be particularly challenging. Widespread use of sedating and paralyzing medications required for the optimal cardiorespiratory management of these patients depletes the diagnostic armamentarium of the clinician at the bedside. This diagnostic delay together with an incomplete understanding of the mechanisms of neurologic injury, restricts current therapy largely to the treatment of sequelae of neurologic injury. Future advances in cerebral diagnostic and monitoring techniques will enhance our understanding of the mechanisms and timing of neurologic injury, and facilitate more preventive interventions. Concurrently, novel neuroprotective agents are in development, aimed at limiting the extent of injury following a neurologic insult. These advances will allow the development of improved population-based preventive strategies, improved presymptomatic management of individual patients with identified risk, and more effective treatment of symptomatic neurologic injury.

REFERENCES

1. Berthrong M, Sabiston D. Cerebral lesions in congenital heart disease. Bulletin Johns Hopkins Hospital 1951;89:384.
2. Tyler R, Clark D. Cerebrovascular accidents in patients with congenital heart disease. Arch Neurol Psychiatry 1957;77:483–489.
3. Phornphutkul C, Rosenberg A, Nadas A, et al. Cerebrovascular accidents in infants and children with cyanotic congenital heart disease. Am J Cardiol 1973;32:329–334.
4. Terplan K. Brain changes in newborns, infants and children with congenital heart disease in association with cardiac surgery. Additional observations. J Neurosurg 1976;212:225.
5. Newburger J, Silbert A, Buckley L, et al. Cognitive function and age at repair of transposition of the great arteries in children. N Engl J Med 1984;310:1495–1499.
6. Castaneda A, Mayer J, Jonas R, et al. The neonate with critical congenital heart disease: repair—a surgical challenge. J Thorac Cardiovasc Surg 1989;98(5):869–875.
7. Benson D. Changing profile of congenital heart disease. Pediatrics 1989;83(5):790–791.
8. Terplan K. Patterns of brain damage in infants and children with congenital heart disease: association with catheterization and surgical procedures. Am J Dis Child 1973;125:175–185.
9. Jones M. Anomalies of the brain and congenital heart disease: a study of 52 necropsy cases. Pediatr Pathol Lab Med 1991;11:721–736.
10. Glauser T, Rorke L, Weinberg P, et al. Congenital brain anomalies associated with the hypoplastic left heart syndrome. Pediatrics 1990;85(6):984–990.
11. van Houten J, Rothman A, Bejar R. Echoencephalographic (ECHO) findings in infants with congenital heart disease (CHD). Pediatrics Res 1993;33(4):376A.
12. Volpe JJ. Intracranial hemorrhage. In: Volpe JJ, ed. Neurology of the Newborn. 3rd ed. Philadelphia: WB Saunders, 1994:373–463.
13. Heibel M, Heber R, Bechinger D, et al. Early diagnosis of perinatal cerebral lesions in apparently normal full-term newborns by ultrasound of the brain. Neuroradiology 1993;35:85–91.
14. Gilles F, Price R, Kevy S. Fibrinolytic activity in the ganglionic eminence of the premature brain. Biol Neonate 1971;18:426–432.
15. Giuliani R, Szwarcer E, Aquino E, et al Fibrin-dependent fibrinolytic activity during extracorporeal circulation. Thromb Res 1991;61:369–373.
16. Glauser T, Rorke L, Weinberg P, et al. Acquired neuropathologic lesions associated with the hypoplastic left heart syndrome. Pediatrics 1990;85(6):991–1000.
17. Young R, Liberthson R, Zalneraitis E. Cerebral hemorrhage in neonates with coarctation of the aorta. Stroke 1982;13(4):491–494.
18. Rudack D, Baumgart S, Gross G. Subependymal (grade 1) intracranial hemorrhage in neonates on extracorporeal membrane oxygenation. Clin Pediatr 1994;33(10):583–587.
19. von Allmen D, Babcock D, Matsumoto J, et al. The predictive value of head ultrasound in the ECMO candidate. J Pediatr Surg 1992;27(1):36–39.
20. Wilson J, Bower L, Fackler J, et al. Aminocaproic acid decreases the incidence of intracranial hemorrhage and other hemorrhagic complications of ECMO. J Pediatr Surg 1993;28(4):536–541.
21. Brunet F, Mira J, Belghith M, et al. Effects of aprotinin on hemorrhagic complications in ARDS patients during prolonged extracorporeal CO_2 removal. Int Care Med 1992;18:364–367.
22. Gilles F, Leviton A, Jammes B. Age-dependent changes in white matter in congenital heart disease [Abstract]. J Neuropathol Exp Neurol 1973;32:179.
23. Volpe JJ. Hypoxic-ischemic encephalopathy: neuropathology and pathogenesis. In: Volpe JJ, ed. Neurology of the newborn. 3rd ed. Philadelphia: WB Saunders, 1994:279–313.
24. Hickey P, Anderson N. Deep hypothermic circulatory arrest: a review of pathophysiology and clinical experience as a basis anesthetic management. J Cardiothorac Anesth 1987;1:137–155.
25. McDonald J, Chen C-K, Trescher W, et al. The severity of excitotoxic brain injury is dependent on brain temperature in immature rat. Neurosci Lett 1991;126:83–86.
26. Buchan A, Pulsinelli W. Hypothermia but not the N-methyl-D-aspartate antagonist, MK801, attenuates neuronal damage in gerbils subjected to transient global ischemia. J Neurosci 1990;10:311–316.
27. Busto R, Dietrich W, Globus M-T, et al. Small differences in intraischemic brain temperature critically determine the extent of ischemic neuronal injury. J Cereb Blood Flow Metab 1987;7:729–738.
28. Busto R, Globus M, Dietrich W, et al. Effect of mild hypothermia on ischemia-induced release of neurotransmitters and free fatty acids in rat brain. Stroke 1989;20:904–910.
29. Baker A, Zornow M, Grafe M, et al. Hypothermia prevents ischemia-induced increases in hippocampal glycine concentrations in rabbits. Stroke 1991;22:666–673.
30. Illievich U, Zornow M, Choi K, et al. Effects of hypothermia or anesthetics on hippocampal glutamate and glycine concentrations after repeated transient global cerebral ischemia. Anesthesiology 1994;80(1):177–186.
31. Ferry P. Neurologic sequelae of cardiac surgery in children. Am J Dis Child 1987;141:309–312.
32. Ferry P. Neurologic sequelae of open-heart surgery in children: an irritating question. American Journal of Diseases in Childhood 1990;144:369–373.
33. Rebeyka I, Coles J, Wilson G, et al. The effect of low-flow cardiopulmonary bypass on cerebral function: an experimental and clinical study. Ann Thorac Surg 1987;43:391–396.
34. Rossi R, van der Linden J, Ekroth R, et al. No flow or low flow? A study of the ischemic marker creatine kinase BB after deep hypothermia procedures. J Thorac Cardiovasc Surg 1989;98:193–199.
35. Swain J, McDonald T, Griffith P, et al. Low-flow hypothermic cardiopulmonary bypass protects the brain. J Throrac Cardiovasc Surg 1991;102:76–83.
36. Swain J, Anderson R, Siegman M. Low-flow cardiopulmonary bypass and cerebral protection: a summary of investigations. Ann Thorac Surg 1993;56(6):1490–1492.
37. Newburger J, Jonas R, Wernovsky G, et al. A comparison of the perioperative neurologic effects of hypothermic circulatory arrest versus low-flow cardiopulmonary bypass in infant heart surgery. N Engl J Med 1993;329:1057–1064.
38. Bellinger D, Jonas R, Rappaport L, et al. Developmental and neurologic status of children after heart surgery with hypo-

thermic circulatory arrest or low-flow cardiopulmonary bypass. N Engl J Med 1995;332:549–555.
39. Burrows F. Con: pH-stat management of blood gases is preferable to alpha-stat in patients undergoing brain cooling for cardiac surgery. J Cardiothorac Vasc Anesth 1995;9(2): 219–221.
40. Kern F, Greeley W. Pro: pH-stat management of blood gases is not preferable to alpha-stat in patients undergoing brain cooling for cardiac surgery. J Cardiothorac Vasc Anesth 1995;9(2):215–218.
41. Prough D, Stump D, Roy R, et al. Response of cerebral blood flow to changes in carbon dioxide tension during hypothermic cardiopulmonary bypass. Anesthesiology 1986;64:576–581.
42. Henriksen L. Brain luxury perfusion during cardiopulmonary bypass in humans. A study of the cerebral flow response to changes in CO_2, O_2, and blood pressure. Cereb Blood Flow Metab 1986;6:366–378.
43. Wong P, Barlow C, Hickey P, et al. Factors associated with choreoathetosis after cardiopulmonary bypass in children with congenital heart disease. Circulation 1992;86(Suppl II):II-118–II-126.
44. Murkin J, Farrar J, Tweed W, et al. Cerebral autoregulation and flow/metabolism coupling during cardiopulmonary bypass: the influence of $PaCO_2$. Anesth Analg 1987;66:825–832.
45. Greeley W, Ungerleider R, Smith L, et al. The effects of deep hypothermic cardiopulmonary bypass and total circulatory arrest on cerebral blood flow in infants and children. J Thorac Cardiovasc Surg 1989;97:737–745.
46. Dexter F, Hindman B. Theoretical analysis of cerebral venous blood hemoglobin oxygen saturation as an index of cerebral oxygenation during hypothermic cardiopulmonary bypass. Anesthesiology 1995;83:405–412.
47. Aoki M, Nomura F, Stromski M, et al. Effects of pH on brain energetics after hypothermic circulatory arrest. Ann Thorac Surg 1993;55:1093–1103.
48. Hiramatsu T, Miura T, Forbess J, et al. pH strategies and cerebral energetics before and after circulatory arrest. J Thorac Cardiovasc Surg 1995;109:948–958.
49. Skaryak L, Chai P, Kern F, et al. Blood gas management and degree of cooling: effects on cerebral metabolism before and after circulatory arrest. J Thorac Cardiovasc Surg 1995;110:1649–1657.
50. Bashein G, Townes B, Nessly M, et al. A randomized study of carbon dioxide management during hypothermic cardiopulmonary bypass. Anesthesiology 1990;72:3–6.
51. Stephan H, Weyland A, Kazmaier S, et al Acid-base management during hypothermic cardiopulmonary bypass does not affect cerebral metabolism but does affect blood flow and neurological outcome. Br J Anaesth 1992;69(1):51–57.
52. Murkin JM, Martzke JS, Buchan AM, et al. A randomized study of the influence of perfusion technique and pH management strategy in 316 patients undergoing coronary artery bypass surgery. II. Neurologic and cognitive outcomes. J Thorac Cardiovasc Surg 1995;110:349–362.
53. Jonas R, Bellinger D, Rappaport L, et al. Relation of pH strategy and developmental outcome after hypothermic circulatory arrest. J Thorac Cardiovasc Surg 1993;106:362–368.
54. Robbins R, Balaban R, Swain J. Intermittent hypothermic asanguinous cerebral perfusion (cerebroplegia) protects the brain during prolonged circulatory arrest. J Thorac Cardiovasc Surg 1990;99:878–884.
55. Bailes J, Leavitt M, Teeple E, et al. Ultraprofound hypothermia with complete blood substitution in a canine model. J Neurosurg 1991;74:781–788.
56. Steyn R, Jeffrey R. An adjunct to cerebral protection during circulatory arrest. Eur J Cardiovasc Surg 1993;7(8):443–444.
57. Crittenden M, Roberts C, Rosa L, et al. Brain protection during circulatory arrest. Ann Thorac Surg 1991;51(6):942–947.
58. Kazui T, Inoue N, Yamada O, et al. Selective cerebral perfusion during operation for aneurysms of the aortic arch. Ann Thorac Surg 1992;53:109–114.
59. Filgueiras C, Winsborrow B, Ye J, et al. A 31P-magnetic resonance study of antegrade and retrograde cerebral perfusion during aortic arch surgery in pigs. J Thorac Cardiovasc Surg 1995;110:55–62.
60. Usui A, Hotta T, Hiroura M, et al. Retrograde cerebral perfusion through a superior vena caval cannula protects the brain. Ann Thorac Surg 1992;53:47–53.
61. Safi H, Brien H, Winter J, et al. Brain protection via cerebral retrograde perfusion during aortic arch aneurysm repair. Ann Thorac Surg 1993;56:270–276.
62. Oohara K, Usui A, Murase M, et al. Regional cerebral tissue blood flow measured by the colored microsphere method during retrograde cerebral perfusion. J Thorac Cardiovasc Surg 1995;109:772–779.
63. Vannucci R. Current and potentially new management strategies for perinatal hypoxic-ischemic encephalopathy. Pediatrics 1990;85(6):961–968.
64. Palmer C, Vannucci R. Potential new therapies for perinatal cerebral hypoxia-ischemia. Clin Perinatol 1993;20(2): 411–432.
65. Ginsberg M. Emerging strategies for the treatment of ischemic brain injury. In: Waxman S, ed. Molecular and cellular approaches to the treatment of neurological disease. New York: Raven Press, 1993:207–237.
66. Albers G, Goldberg M, Choi D. N-methyl-D-aspartate antagonists ready for clinical trial in brain ischemia? Ann Neurol 1989;25:389–403.
67. Buchan A. Advances in cerebral ischemia: experimental approaches. Neurol Clin 1992;10(1):49–61.
68. Meldrum B. Protection against ischemic neuronal damage by drugs acting on excitatory neurotransmission. Cerebrovasc Brain Metab Rev 1990;2:27–57.
69. Hall E. The role of oxygen radicals in traumatic injury: clinical implications. J Emerg Med 1993;11(Suppl 1):31–36.
70. Soloniuk D, Perkins E, Wilson J. Use of allopurinol and deferoxamine in cellular protection during ischemia. Surg Neurol 1992;38(2):110–113.
71. Bowes M, Zivin J, Rothlein R. Monoclonal antibody to the ICAM-1 adhesion site reduces neurological damage in a rabbit cerebral embolism stroke model. Exp Neurol 1993; 119:215–219.
72. Clark W, Madden K, Rothlein R, et al. Reduction of central nervous system ischemic injury in rabbits using leukocyte adhesion antibody treatment. Stroke 1991;22:877–883.
73. Forsman M, Tubylewicz Olsnes B, Semb G, et al. Effects of nimodipine on cerebral blood flow and neuropsychological outcome after cardiac surgery. Br J Anaesth 1990;65: 514–520.
74. Valentino K, Newcomb R, Gadbois T, et al. A selective N-type calcium channel antagonist protects against neuronal cell loss after global cerebral ischemia. Proc Natl Acad Sci USA 1993;90:7894–7897.
75. Plum F, Posner J. Multifocal, diffuse, and metabolic brain diseases causing stupor or coma. In: Plum F, Posner J, eds. The diagnosis of stupor and coma. 3rd ed. Philadelphia: FA Davis, 1985:177–303.

76. Sheth R, Pryse-Phillips W, Riggs J, et al. Critical illness neuromuscular disease in children manifested as ventilatory dependence. J Pediatr 1995;126:259–261.
77. Gooch J, Suchyta M, Balbierz J, et al. Prolonged paralysis after treatment with neuromuscular junction blocking agents. Crit Care Med 1991;19(9):1125–1131.
78. Partridge B, Abrams J, Bazemore C, et al. Prolonged neuromuscular blockade after long-term infusion of vecuronium bromide in the intensive care unit. Crit Care Med 1990;18(10):1577–1582.
79. Rossiter A, Souney P, McGowan S, et al Pancuronium-induced prolonged neuromuscular blockade. Crit Care Med 1991;19(12):1583–1587.
80. Segredo V, Caldwell J, Matthay M, et al. Persistent paralysis in critically ill patients after long-term administration of vecuronium. N Engl J Med 1992;20:524–528.
81. Subramony S, Carpenter D, Seshadri R, et al. Myopathy and prolonged neuromuscular blockade after lung transplant. Crit Care Med 1991;19(12):1580–1582.
82. Danon M, Carpenter S. Myopathy with thick filament (myosin) loss following prolonged paralysis with vecuronium during steroid treatment. Muscle Nerve 1991;14:1131–1139.
83. Brunberg J, Reilly E, Doty D. Central nervous system consequences in infants of cardiac surgery using deep hypothermia and circulatory arrest. Circulation 1974;50(Suppl II):II-60–II-68.
84. Clarkson P, MacArthur B, Barrat-Boyes B, et al. Developmental progress after cardiac surgery in infancy using hypothermia and circulatory arrest. Circulation 1980;62:855–861.
85. Ehyai A, Fenichel G, Bender H. Incidence and prognosis of seizures in infants after cardiac surgery with profound hypothermia and circulatory arrest. JAMA 1984;252:3165–3167.
86. Miller G, Eggli K, Contant C, et al. Postoperative neurologic complications after open heart surgery on young infants. Arch Pediatr Adolesc Med 1995;149:764–768.
87. Lanska M, Lanska D, Horwitz S, et al. Presentation, clinical course and outcome of childhood stroke. Pediatr Neurol 1991;7:333–341.
88. Yang J, Park Y, Hartlage P. Seizures associated with stroke in childhood. Pediatr Neurol 1995;12:136–138.
89. Clancy R, Malin S, Laraque D, et al. Focal motor seizures heralding stroke in full-term infants. Am J Dis Child 1985;139:601–606.
90. Levy S, Abroms I, Marshall P, et al. Seizures and cerebral infarction in the full-term newborn. Ann Neurol 1985;17:366–370.
91. Mizrahi E. Neonatal seizures: problems in diagnosis and classification. Epilepsia 1987;28(Suppl 1):S46–S55.
92. Scher M, Painter M. Electroencephalographic diagnosis of neonatal seizures: issues of diagnostic accuracy, clinical correlation, and survival. In: Wasterlain C, Vert P, eds. Neonatal seizures. New York: Raven Press, 1990:15–25.
93. Shewmon D. What is a neonatal seizure? Problems in definition and quantification for investigative and clinical purposes. J Clin Neurophysiol 1990;7(3):315–368.
94. Clancy R, Legido A, Lewis D. Occult neonatal seizures. Epilepsia 1988;29(3):256–261.
95. Scher M, Painter M. Controversies concerning neonatal seizures. Pediatr Clin North Am 1989;36(2):281–310.
96. Volpe JJ. Neonatal seizures. In: Volpe JJ, ed. Neurology of the Newborn. 3rd ed. Philadelphia: WB Saunders, 1994:172–207.
97. Sarnat H, Sarnat M. Neonatal encephalopathy following fetal distress. Arch Neurol 1976;33:696–705.
98. Andre M, Matisse N, Vert P. Prognosis of neonatal seizures. In: Wasterlain C, Vert P, eds. Neonatal seizures. New York: Raven Press, 1990:61–67.
99. Bergman I, Painter M, Hirsch R, et al. Outcome in neonates with convulsions treated in an intensive care unit. Ann Neurol 1983;14:642–647.
100. Satur C, Jennings A, Walker D. Hypomagnesemia and fits complicating pediatric cardiac surgery. Ann Clin Biochem 1993;30:315–317.
101. Lynch B, Rust R. Natural history and outcome of neonatal hypocalcemic and hypomagnesemic seizures. Pediatr Neurol 1994;11:23–27.
102. Gal P, Toback J, Boer H, et al. Efficacy of phenobarbital monotherapy in treatment of neonatal seizures—relationship to blood levels. Neurology 1982;32:1401–1404.
103. Gilman J, Gal P, Duchowny M, et al. Rapid sequential phenobarbital treatment of neonatal seizures. Pediatrics 1989;83(5):674–678.
104. Earnest M, Marx J, Drury L. Complications of intravenous phenytoin for acute treatment of seizures. JAMA 1983;249:762–765.
105. Cranford R, Leppik I, Patrick B, et al. Intravenous phenytoin: clinical and pharmacological aspects. Neurology 1978;28:874–880.
106. Holmes G. Do seizures cause brain damage? Epilepsia 1991;32(Suppl 5):S14–S28.
107. Lou H, Friis-Hansen B. Arterial blood pressure elevations during motor activity and epileptic seizures in the newborn. Acta Pediatr Scand 1979;68:803.
108. Perlman J, Volpe J. Seizures in the preterm infant: effects on cerebral blood flow velocity, intracranial pressure, and arterial blood pressure. J Pediatr 1983;102:288.
109. Young R, Petroff O. Neonatal seizure: magnetic resonance spectroscopic findings. Semin Perinatol 1990;14(3):238–247.
110. Siesjo B, Wieloch T. Epileptic brain damage: pathophysiology and neurochemical pathology. In: Delgado-Escueta A, Ward A, Woodbury D, et al., eds. Adv Neurol 1986;44:813–847.
111. du Plessis A, Kramer U, Jonas R, et al. West syndrome following deep hypothermic cardiac surgery. Pediatr Neurol 1994;11(3):246–251.
112. Schoenberg B, Mellinger J, Schoenberg D. Cerebrovascular disease in infants and children: a study of incidence, clinical features, and survival. Neurology 1978;28:763–768.
113. Riela A, Roach E. Etiology of stroke in children. J Child Neurol 1993;8:201–220.
114. Komp D, Sparrow A. Polycythemia in cyanotic heart disease—a study of altered coagulation. J Pediatr 1970;76(2):231–236.
115. Cottrill C, Kaplan S. Cerebral vascular accidents in cyanotic congenital heart disease. Am J Dis Child 1973;125:484–487.
116. Martelle R, Linde L. Cerebrovascular accidents with the tetralogy of Fallot. Am J Dis Child 1961;101:206–209.
117. Caro J, Groome P, Flegel K. Atrial fibrillation and anticoagulation: from randomized trials to practice. Lancet 1993;341:1381–1384.
118. Moody D, Bell M, Challa V, et al. Brain microemboli during cardiac surgery or aortography. Ann Neurol 1990;28:477–486.
119. Nussmeier N, McDermott J. Macroembolization: prevention and outcome modification. In: Hilberman M, ed. Brain injury and protection during heart surgery. Boston: Martinus Nijhoff Publishing, 1988:85–108.
120. Lucchesi B. Complement activation, neutrophils, and oxygen

120. radicals in reperfusion injury. Stroke 1993;24(12)(Suppl 1):I41–I47.
121. Seghaye M, Duchateau J, Grabitz R, et al. Complement activation during cardiopulmonary bypass in infants and children. Relation to postoperative multiple system organ failure. J Thorac Cardiovasc Surg 1993;106(6):978–987.
122. Casey L. Role of cytokines in the pathogenesis of cardiopulmonary-induced multisystem organ failure. Ann Thorac Surg 1993;56(Suppl 5):S92–S96.
123. Elliott M, Finn A. Interaction between neutrophils and endothelium. Ann Thorac Surg 1993;56(6):1503–1508.
124. Jorens P, De Jongh R, De Backer W, et al. Interleukin-8 production in patients undergoing cardiopulmonary bypass. The influence of pretreatment with methylprednisolone. Am Rev Resp Dis 1993;148(4)(Pt 1):890–895.
125. Woods M, Greaves M, Smith G, et al. The fate of circulating megakaryocytes during cardiopulmonary bypass. J Thorac Cardiovasc Surg 1993;106(4):658–663.
126. Cromme-Dijkhuis A, Henkens C, Bijleveld C, et al. Coagulation factor abnormalities as possible thrombotic risk factors after Fontan operations. Lancet 1990;336:1087–1090.
127. du Plessis A, Chang A, Wessel D, et al. Cerebrovascular accidents following the Fontan procedure. Pediatr Neurol 1995;12(3):230–236.
128. Rosenthal D, Bulbul Z, Friedman A, et al. Thrombosis of the pulmonary artery stump after distal ligation. J Thorac Cardiovasc Surg 1995;110(5):1563–1565.
129. Nakazawa M, Nakanishi T, Okuda H, et al. Dynamics of right heart flow in patients after Fontan procedure. Circulation 1984;69(2):306–312.
130. Dobell A, Trusler G, Smallhorn J, et al. Atrial thrombi after the Fontan operation. Ann Thorac Surg 1986;42:664–667.
131. Putnam J, Lemmer J, Rocchini A, et al. Embolectomy for acute pulmonary artery occlusion following Fontan procedure. Ann Thorac Surg 1988;45:335–336.
132. Stumper O, Sutherland G, Geuskens R. Transesophageal echocardiography in evaluation and management after a Fontan procedure. J Am Coll Cardiol 1991;17(5):1152–1160.
133. Dajee H, Deutsch L, Benson L, et al. Thrombolytic therapy for superior vena caval thrombosis following superior vena cava-pulmonary anastamosis. Ann Thorac Surg 1984;38:637.
134. Hess J, Kruizinga A, Bijleveld C, et al. Protein-losing enteropathy after Fontan operation. J Thorac Cardiovasc Surg 1984;88:606–609.
135. Lemmer J, Coran A, Behrendt D, et al. Liver fibrosis (cardiac cirrhosis) five years after modified Fontan operation for tricuspid atresia. J Thorac Cardiovasc Surg 1983;86:757–760.
136. Rosenthal D, Friedman A, Kleinman C, et al. Thromboembolic complications after Fontan operations. Circulation 1995;92(Suppl II):287–293.
137. del Zoppo G, Ferbert A, Otis S, et al. Local intra-arterial fibrinolytic therapy in acute carotid territory stroke: a pilot study. Stroke 1988;19:307–313.
138. Mori E, Tabuchi M, Yoshida T, et al. Intracarotid urokinase with thromboembolic occlusion of the middle cerebral artery. Stroke 1988;19:802–812.
139. Anderson D. Cardioembolic stroke: primary and secondary prevention. Postgrad Med 1991;90(8):67–77.
140. Ezekowitz M, Burrow R, Heath P, et al. Diagnostic accuracy of indium-111 platelet scintigraphy in identifying left ventricular thrombi. Am J Cardiol 1983;51:1712–1716.
141. Stratton J, Richie J. Indium-111 platelet imaging of left ventricular thrombi. Predictive value for systemic emboli. Circulation 1990;81:1182–1189.
142. Group CES. Immediate anticoagulation of embolic stroke: brain hemorrhage and management options. Stroke 1984;15:779–789.
143. Group CES. Cardioembolic stroke, immediate anticoagulation, and brain hemorrhage. Arch Intern Med 1987;1987:636–640.
144. Force CET. Cardiogenic brain embolism. The second report of the Cerebral Embolism Task Force. Arch Neurol 1989;46:727–743.
145. Hart R, Easton J. Hemorrhagic infarcts. Stroke 1986;17:586–589.
146. Furlan A, Cavalier S, Hobbs R, et al. Hemorrhage and anticoagulation after nonseptic embolic brain infarction. Neurology 1982;32:280–282.
147. Horning C, Dorndorf W, Agnoli A. Hemorrhagic cerebral infarction—a prospective study. Stroke 1986;17:179–185.
148. Okada Y, Yamaguchi T, Minematsu K, et al. Hemorrhagic transformation in cerebral embolism. Stroke 1989;20:598–603.
149. Sherman D, Dyken M, Fisher M, et al. Antithrombotic therapy for cerebrovascular disorders. Chest 1992;102(4):529S–537S.
150. Yatsu F, Hart R, Mohr J, et al. Anticoagulation of embolic strokes of cardiac origin: an update. Neurology 1988;38:314–316.
151. Jones H, Sieker R. Neurologic manifestations of infective endocarditis. Brain 1989;122:1295–1315.
152. Saiman L, Prince A, Gersony W. Pediatric infective endocarditis in the modern era. J Pediatr 1993;122:847–853.
153. Bjork V, Hultquist G. Brain damage in children after deep hypothermia for open heart surgery. Thorax 1960;15:284–292.
154. Bjork V, Hultquist G. Contraindications to profound hypothermia in open-heart surgery. J Thorac Cardiovasc Surg 1962;44(1):1–13.
155. Bergouignan M, Fontan F, Trarieux M. Syndromes choreiformes de l'enfant au de'cours d'interventions cardio-chirurgicales sous hypothermic profounde. Rev Neurol 1961;105:48–59.
156. Wessel D, du Plessis A. Choreoathetosis. In: Jonas R, Newburger J, Volpe J, eds. Brain injury and pediatric cardiac surgery. Boston: Butterworth-Heineman, 1995:353–362.
157. Brunberg J, Doty D, Reilly E. Choreoathetosis in infants following cardiac surgery with deep hypothermia and circulatory arrest. J Pediatr 1974;84(2):232–235.
158. du Plessis A, du Plessis A, Chang A, Wessel D, et al. Cerebrovascular accidents following the Fontan procedure. Pediatr Neurol 1995;12(3):230–236.
159. Straussberg R, Shahar E, Gat R, et al. Delayed parkinsonism associated with hypotension in a child undergoing open-heart surgery. Devel Med Child Neurol 1993;35:1007–1014.
160. Lane J, Tennison M, Lawless S, et al. Movement disorder after withdrawal of fentanyl infusion. J Pediatr 1991;119:649–651.
161. Bergman I, Steeves M, Burckart G, et al. Reversible neurologic abnormalities associated with prolonged intravenous midazolam and fentanyl administration. J Pediatr 1991;119:644–649.
162. Sury M, Billingham I, Russell G, et al. Acute benzodiazepine withdrawal syndrome after midazolam infusions in children. Crit Care Med 1989;17:301–302.
163. Donaldson D, Fullerton D, Gollub R, et al. Choreoathetosis in children after cardiac surgery [Abstract]. Neurology 1990;40(Suppl 1):337.

164. Robinson R, Samuels M, Pohl K. Choreic syndrome after cardiac surgery. Arch Dis Child 1988;63:1466–1469.
165. Chaves E, Irene Scaltsas-Persson I. Severe choreoathetosis (CA) following congenital heart disease (CHD) surgery [Abstract]. Neurology 1988;38(Suppl):284.
166. Kupsky W, Drozd M, Barlow C. Selective injury of the globus pallidus in children with post-cardiac surgery choreic syndrome. Dev Med Child Neurol 1995;37:135–144.
167. DeLeon S, Ilbawi M, Arcilla R, et al. Choreoathetosis after deep hypothermia without circulatory arrest. Ann Thorac Surg 1990;50:714–719.
168. Greenamyre T, Penney J, Young A, et al. Evidence for transient perinatal glutamatergic innervation of globus pallidus. J Neurosci 1987;7:1022–1030.
169. Research. Guidelines for the determination of death. JAMA 1981;246:2184–2186.
170. Task Force for the Determination of Brain Death in Children. Guidelines for the determination of brain death in children. Ann Neurol 1987;22(1):616–617.
171. Volpe J. Brain death determination in the newborn. Pediatrics 1987;80:293–297.
172. Ashwal S, Schneider S. Brain death in the newborn. Pediatrics 1989;84(3):429–437.

Renal Issues

25

Martin J. Elliott, MD, and Ralph E. Delius, MD

Excessive fluid accumulation is one of the most clinically evident changes that occurs during cardiopulmonary bypass. The increase in body fluid is most marked in small babies of low weight or in patients undergoing long periods of bypass (1). This edema formation can lead to organ dysfunction, including impaired myocardial contractility and diminished pulmonary compliance. Judicious management of perioperative fluid status is important in minimizing the morbidity associated with cardiopulmonary bypass, particularly in the neonate. This issue becomes more complex and compelling in patients with postoperative renal insufficiency. This chapter focuses on the various strategies for treating renal failure and for minimizing extravascular fluid accumulation.

BASIC PRINCIPLES

Pathophysiology of Cardiopulmonary Bypass

Cardiopulmonary bypass has many effects on renal function and on hormones involved in fluid regulation and homeostasis.

Renal blood flow is diminished during nonpulsatile bypass, particularly to the renal cortex. Glomerular filtration rate (GFR) is also reduced during cardiopulmonary bypass. Antidiuretic hormone (ADH), or vasopressin, which is released by the posterior pituitary gland in response to hypovolemia or hypertonicity, is elevated in patients undergoing cardiopulmonary bypass (2). This elevation can persist for up to 48 hours into the postoperative period. Increased plasma renin activity and elevated aldosterone levels have also been documented following cardiopulmonary bypass (3). Atrial natriuertic factor (ANF), released by the heart in response to atrial distension, stimulates sodium and water excretion; it is decreased during cardiopulmonary bypass but increases after weaning from bypass support (3). However, the usual correlation between atrial pressures and ANF release is absent in the immediate postoperative period (4). In the immediate postoperative period these changes in ADH, aldosterone, and ANF result in a tendency for sodium and water retention.

Cardiopulmonary bypass also leads to a generalized inflammatory response. Exposure of blood to the nonendothelial surfaces of the bypass circuit appears to be the inciting element of the inflammatory response. This inflammatory response appears to be mediated in part by complement activation (5) and cytokine release (6). This in turn leads to activation of neutrophils, which adhere to the endothelium and release superoxides, lysozymes, and elastase (7). These factors can damage endothelial cells and lead to an increase in capillary permeability (8). In addition, studies suggest that immature animals may have inherently greater capillary permeability (9). Thus, the tendency for sodium and water retention in conjunction with an intense inflammatory response that results in increased capillary permeability leads to a strong predilection for fluid overload and edema.

Postoperative Fluid Management

Fluid administration during the first 24 hours after operation is primarily concerned with maintaining an optimal hemodynamic state. Normal parenteral fluid requirements in children are 100 mL/kg/d for the first 10 kg, 50 mL/kg/d for the next 10 kg, and 20 mL/kg/d for each kilogram above 20 kg.

On the first postoperative day with open heart surgery total fluid intake can be limited to 50% of the maintenance requirements because of hemodilution during cardiopulmonary bypass and the tendency to retain fluid and water postoperatively. Although a 10% dextrose solution is used for neonates, infants and children receive a 5% dextrose solution. Fluid intake on subsequent days is adjusted according to assessment of the patient's hydration status. Typically, patients are advanced to about 70% of maintenance requirements the second postoperative day and to 100% on the third day after surgery. Diuretics (usually furosemide in intermittent or continuous intravenous administration) are usually initiated the first postoperative morning to assist with fluid removal from the interstitial space and to counteract the sodium and fluid avid state of the postoperative patient.

Patients undergoing closed heart surgery have different fluid requirements because the pathophysiology of cardiopulmonary bypass is not superimposed on the postoperative state. Patients are usually given 75% of maintenance requirements on the first postoperative day, except in situations of preoperative heart failure or pulmonary edema, in which case fluid can be more restricted. For subsequent days the principles are similar to those used after open heart surgery. Most patients can be advanced to 100% of maintenance requirements on the second postoperative day. Diuretics are given based on clinical assessment of hydration status.

Expansion of the intravascular volume is often needed during the first 24 to 48 hours to maintain optimal preload. Typically colloid solutions (5–10 mL/kg) are used to minimize interstitial fluid overload. Packed red blood cells are ideal for intravascular volume expansion if the patient is anemic. Fresh frozen plasma can also be used, particularly in the bleeding patient. A 5% albumin solution can be used if the patient is not anemic or bleeding. Artificial colloid solutions (hetastarch, dextrans, gelatin derivatives) have been successfully used for volume expansion, but concerns about alterations in coagulation induced by these agents and their interference with cross matching have discouraged their use (10).

Postoperative Oliguria

A urine output of 0.5–1 mL/kg/hr usually reflects adequate renal perfusion and is an indirect measure of cardiac output and fluid status. Urine output that is less than this should be expeditiously addressed. First, technical factors such as a blocked urinary catheter should be excluded. Volume status of the patient should also be assessed by physical examination and evaluation of vital signs and filling pressures. A volume challenge with 10–20 mL/kg of colloid should be given if the patient is deemed to be hypovolemic. In addition, the diagnosis of postoperative residua or cardiac tamponade should be considered as this often leads to hemodynamic instability and oliguria. Cardiac function should also be optimized and appropriate inotropic agents or afterload reducing agents started if indicated. Dopamine (3–5 µg/kg/min) improves renal blood flow, and it may improve urine output (11). If oliguria persists after these steps a test dose of furosemide (1 mg/kg) can be given. In some children, ethacrynic acid (0.5–1.0 mg/kg) may be effective if furosemide fails. Failure to respond to these measures strongly suggests that renal failure has developed. Use of other diuretics is usually futile and merely serves to delay initiation of appropriate therapy.

ACUTE RENAL FAILURE

Diagnosis of acute renal failure is pragmatically defined as persistent oliguria despite adequate circulating volume, circulatory support, and aggressive diuretic therapy. Acute renal failure is said to occur in 4 to 8% of patients following open heart surgery for congenital heart defects (12, 13), although anecdotal data suggest that the incidence of acute renal failure is decreasing in most centers.

Younger children and patients who have had longer bypass times are particularly at risk (13). Children with cyanotic congenital heart disease or lesions that obstruct the left ventricular outflow tract also have a higher risk of postoperative renal failure (14). Multiple factors can contribute to renal failure, including hypoxia, acidosis, hypotension, nephrotoxic agents, and pre-existing renal anomalies. Hyperuricemia has also been implicated as a contributing factor to postoperative renal failure in congenital heart disease patients (15).

Determination of free water clearance (free H_2O clearance = urine output − [urine osmolality × urine output/plasma osmolarity]) and elevated urinary levels of β-2 macroglobulin, which have been touted as sensitive indicators of renal dysfunction in the postoperative patient, can occasionally be helpful (12, 16). Once renal failure has been identified then appropriate measures should be taken to manage the complications as related to the oliguric state.

Management of Acute Renal Failure

Supportive therapy is the first line for patients with postoperative renal failure, although some form of dialysis may be necessary in some cases (see below).

All drug dosages should be re-evaluated in light of diminished creatinine clearance. Metabolic acidosis should be treated with sodium bicarbonate. Tromethamine (THAM) can be substituted if the patient is hypernatremic. Fluids should be restricted (maintenance volume × 0.3 + urine output) until effective dialysis can be initiated. Adequate calories should be supplied once dialysis is established. Mortality rates appear to be improved in patients with acute renal failure receiving adequate calories compared with patients who are starved on the basis of the misguided notion that severe fluid and protein restriction may delay the need for dialysis (17, 18).

Potassium should be removed from all administered fluids and should not be given unless the serum levels are below 3.0 mmol/L. Hyperkalemia should be addressed promptly. Calcium antagonizes the myocardial effects of hyperkalemia by raising the threshold potential, which decreases the electrical irritability caused by elevated extracellular potassium levels. Strategies to promote transfer of potassium into the intracellular space such as giving sodium bicarbonate (1–2 mEq/kg) and glucose/insulin (0.5 g/kg glucose with 0.1 U/kg insulin) can also temporarily control hyperkalemia. Ion exchange resins effectively remove potassium from the patient until dialysis can be established, but they must be used cautiously as they can occasionally cause bowel obstruction or perforation in children. Magnesium-containing antacids should be discontinued. Formerly, aluminum-containing antacids were substituted for magnesium-containing antacids, which had the added benefit of decreasing intestinal absorption of phosphate. However, aluminum intoxication has been described in infants with renal failure (19).

DIALYSIS

Patients with oliguria and rising blood urea nitrogen (BUN) and creatinine as well as hyperkalemia, azotemia, acidosis, or excessive fluid overload will require dialysis. Many groups are aggressive about instituting dialysis, particularly in patients with diuretic-resistant volume overload (20, 21). Improvements in hemodynamic status as well as pulmonary function have been noted following initiation of peritoneal dialysis or continuous arteriovenous hemofiltration (20, 21). The available dialysis techniques include peritoneal dialysis, intermittent hemodialysis, or various forms of continuous hemofiltration or dialysis.

Peritoneal Dialysis

The peritoneum is the largest serous membrane in the body. Its membrane is semipermeable, and osmosis and diffusion across concentration gradients are the primary means by which solutes and fluid are exchanged across it. The surface area of the peritoneum is proportionally greater relative to total body mass in children compared with adults. Therefore, peritoneal dialysis is usually more efficient in neonates and infants than in larger children and adults. Hemodialysis may correct hyperkalemia or acidosis more rapidly in situations where these complications are immediately life threatening, although this benefit may be offset by the extra set-up time needed for hemodialysis.

Advantages of peritoneal dialysis compared with other forms of dialysis include (a) it is usually better tolerated hemodynamically; (b) easier to initiate; (c) does not require arterial or venous access; and (d) is more likely to be effective independent of the hemodynamic state. Disadvantages are related to septic and mechanical complications of the peritoneal dialysis catheter and that it may occasionally cause respiratory compromise.

Relative contraindications to peritoneal dialysis include recent abdominal surgery (less than 1 week); peritonitis from any cause, particularly necrotizing enterocolitis; uncorrected gastroschisis, omphalocele, or diaphragmatic hernia; or the presence of a ventriculoperitoneal shunt.

Technique

A peritoneal dialysis catheter can be placed at the time of the original operation or in the intensive care unit. Various types of catheters can be used. Some are intended solely for short-term use, whereas others with felt cuffs, such as the Tenkhoff catheter, can be used for short or long-term dialysis. The basic insertion technique is similar, with minor modifications, for all types of catheters (Table 25.1).

Commercial preparations of dialysate are usually used (Baxter Healthcare Corp., Deerfield, IL). Three concentra-

Table 25.1. Peritoneal Catheter Insertion

The following technique is used for insertion of an acute peritoneal dialysis catheter (Cook Inc., Bloomington, IN):
1. Ensure that the bladder is empty.
2. Provide adequate analgesia and sedation; 1% lidocaine can be used for local anesthesia.
3. Standard sterile technique is used. The physician placing the catheter and any assistants wear a cap, mask, gown, and gloves. Betadine and sterile drapes are used to prepare the abdomen.
4. Insertion site is chosen. In most cases the catheter will be placed midway between the umbilicus and the anterior superior iliac spine. If a surgical scar is present the catheter can be inserted in the midline 1 to 3 cm below the umbilicus.
5. Skin of the abdominal wall is elevated by an assistant. The physician then introduces an 16-gauge intravenous cannula into the peritoneal cavity. A "pop" is often perceived as the needle enters the peritoneal cavity. The needle is directed toward the pelvis, then withdrawn; peritoneal fluid often refluxes out the cannula. Warmed dialysate (20–30 mL/kg) is then placed in the peritoneal cavity through the cannula. This serves to distend the abdomen and allow easier placement of the dialysis catheter.
6. A guidewire is then introduced into the peritoneal cavity via the cannula. The cannula is then removed, leaving the guidewire in place. A stab incision using an 1 1 blade is made where the guidewire exits the skin.
7. Dilators, which are provided with the catheter insertion kit, are sequentially inserted over the guidewire. The catheter is then inserted and the guidewire removed. A purse string suture is placed around the catheter insertion site to minimize leaks and to secure the catheter.
8. A sterile dressing is then applied and an abdominal radiograph is obtained to confirm position.
9. Peritoneal catheters are treated with the utmost sterile technique at all times. The skin entry site should be examined for any signs of infection daily. An aliquot of the peritoneal dialysis effluent should be submitted for cell count and culture daily.

tions of dextrose are available: 1.5, 2.5, and 4.25 g/dL. Dextrose solution concentration is the primary determinant of the amount of ultrafiltration that occurs with each dialysis cycle. Dialysis is usually initiated with 1.5 g/dL solution and later changed if needed. All infused dialysate should be warmed prior to administration, and heparin (200 U/L) is usually added to the peritoneal dialysate. Other primary variables that can be adjusted are the volume of dialysate used per cycle (20–40 mL/kg) and the dwell time (length of time each cycle the fluid is allowed to remain in the peritoneal cavity). A typical starting regimen would be 20 mL/kg/cycle. Each cycle would last 1 hour, with 15 minutes for infusion, 30 minutes dwell time, and 15 minutes for drainage. These variables are adjusted if needed. If more rapid fluid removal is needed then a more concentrated solution or more rapid cycles may be needed. Another regimen that is gaining favor for neonates is the "rule of ten," 10 mL/kg/cycle, 10 minute infusion, 10 minute dwell, and 10 minute drain.

Additives to the dialysate can be adjusted as needed. Patients with severe metabolic acidosis may require bicarbonate be added to the dialysate. The development of hypokalemia is common, in which case potassium can be added to the dialysate. Hyperglycemia can be addressed by adding insulin to the dialysate. Frequent monitoring of fluid status and electrolytes is needed appropriately to adjust the dialysis regimen.

Complications

Peritonitis Peritonitis is one of the more frequent complications of peritoneal dialysis. The incidence of peritonitis is directly proportional to the time on dialysis. The most common causative organisms include *Staphylococcus aureus*, *S. epidermidis*, gram-negative organisms, or *Candida* species. Catheter-associated peritonitis should be suspected if the patient is febrile, peritoneal effluent becomes cloudy, the effluent has a white cell count greater than 100 neutrophils per milliliter, or the skin site is inflamed or exuding pus. If peritonitis is suspected an aliquot of effluent should be submitted for cell count with differential, Gram stain, and culture. Blood cultures can also be tested, but they are rarely positive.

Bacterial peritonitis can be treated either by removing the catheter and administering parenteral antibiotics or by leaving the catheter in place and adding antibiotics to the dialysate. A first generation cephalosporin in combination with an aminoglycoside should be initiated until culture results are available. A 7 to 10 day course of antibiotics is usually necessary. Fungal peritonitis invariably requires removal of the peritoneal catheter. Intravenous amphotericin B is required and hemodialysis or continuous arteriovenous hemofiltration will be necessary if dialysis is still needed.

Hyperglycemia The peritoneum of infants and young children allows more rapid absorption of the dextrose in the dialysate compared with older children or adults. Significant hyperglycemia can develop, especially in patients who are glucose intolerant because of stress or who are receiving parenteral hyperalimentation. Reducing the dextrose concentration or the number of cycles may be helpful, but this is often not feasible. Insulin (1 U regular/4 g dialysate dextrose) can be added to the dialysate. Careful monitoring of the blood glucose level is essential to prevent hypoglycemia.

Hypoproteinemia Protein, especially albumin, is lost into the dialysate more rapidly in pediatric patients. Nutritional support should address this loss of protein (0.3–0.5 g protein/kg/d). An albumin infusion is occasionally necessary.

Mechanical Catheter Problems Failure to adequately drain the effluent is the most common catheter problem. This can be caused by kinking, occlusion of the catheter by omentum, or by fibrin plugs. Kinking and occlusion by the omentum can sometimes be remedied by slightly repositioning or withdrawing of the catheter, although catheter replacement is often necessary. Fibrin plugs can sometimes be flushed with a heparin solution.

Leakage around the catheter is another fairly common mechanical complication, and it is a predisposing factor for peritonitis. Smaller dialysate volumes are occasionally helpful in reducing leakage. A purse string suture around the catheter site may also be helpful. If leakage persists, dialysis should be discontinued for 24 hours to allow tissues around the catheter to seal.

Intermittent Hemodialysis

Hemodialysis relies on the same principles as peritoneal dialysis, namely diffusion of solutes across a semipermeable membrane based on concentration gradients across the membrane. Hemodialysis usually entails blood flow through semipermeable hollow fibers that are bathed in dialysate that flows over the hollow fibers is in the direction opposite to that of the blood within the fibers. This effectively results in a countercurrent flow mechanism similar to that seen in the loop of Henle. Hemodialysis is an efficient means of solute or fluid removal and a 3 to 4 hour session every 2 to 3 days is often sufficient.

Hemodialysis has several disadvantages for the acutely ill congenital heart disease patient. Rapid fluid shifts and electrolyte changes can cause hemodynamic instability and cardiac arrhythmias. Two sites of vascular access are required in smaller patients, one for drainage and the other for reinfusion. Patients larger than 7–8 kg can often have a double lumen catheter placed in a central venous line. Hemodialysis also requires trained nurses and equipment that is specially adapted for the smaller patient. Hemodialysis is useful in those patients in whom renal function is slow to return and whose other organ system problems have resolved. It is also a reasonable option in patients who have a contraindication to peritoneal dialysis. Efficiency of hemodialysis can also be of benefit when fluid overload, hyperkalemia, or metabolic acidosis is acutely life threatening. Nevertheless, hemodialysis should be reserved for patients requiring long-term dialysis and for those patients with a contraindication to peritoneal dialysis or one of the forms of continuous hemofiltration.

Continuous Hemofiltration

Various forms of continuous hemofiltration or hemodialysis have been developed for critically ill patients with renal dysfunction or diuretic-resistant fluid overload. These continuous techniques have several advantages over peritoneal dialysis or intermittent hemodialysis in the critically ill patient. They are well tolerated hemodynamically, remove solutes efficiently, and offer considerable flexibility in fluid management. They can be used in neonates as small as 1 kg. Improvement in cardiac function and pulmonary gas exchange has been noted in postoperative pediatric heart patients following initiation of continuous hemofiltration (21). Although no absolute contraindications are found to continuous hemofiltration or hemodialysis, these techniques do require anticoagulation and vascular access with relatively large bore cannulas. Indications for these continuous techniques include acute renal failure, severe electrolyte or acid-base disturbance, or diuretic-resistant fluid overload regardless of renal function.

Principles

Ultrafiltration takes place when a hydrostatic pressure gradient is found across a semipermeable membrane. Solute transport across the membrane is convective; solutes, which are smaller than the size of pores in the membrane, are swept along as the solvent is forced across the membrane by the hydrostatic pressure gradient. Dialysis, in contrast, is independent of the hydrostatic pressure across the membrane. Dialysis requires a concentration gradient across a semipermeable membrane. The driving force for transfer of solutes across the membrane is diffusion down a concentration gradient. As discussed later, ultrafiltration and dialysis can be used in conjunction.

Techniques

Slow continuous ultrafiltration (SCUF) involves simple ultrafiltration. A SCUF circuit is seen in Figure 25.1A. Arteriovenous pressure gradient across the hemofilter is the sole force of filtration. This technique is useful for fluid removal only, as no attempt is made to alter or clear solutes.

Continuous arteriovenous hemofiltration with dialysis (CAVH-D) is similar to SCUF in that the arteriovenous pressure gradient across the hemofilter is the driving force for ultrafiltration. However, in CAVH the volume of ultrafiltrate is much greater and the ultrafiltrate is replaced with a premixed replacement fluid individually formulated for the patient (see Fig. 25.1B). Replacement fluid composition is similar to plasma. In this manner solutes are removed and fluid balance precisely controlled.

Continuous arteriovenous hemofiltration with dialysis (CAVH-D) incorporates the principles of ultrafiltration with dialysis. The circuit is similar to that used for CAVH (Fig. 25.1C). Dialysate is passed across the hemofilter in a direction opposite to the blood flow. Dialysate and ultrafiltrate are then collected together. This technique is efficient for solute removal, and it approaches that of intermittent hemodialysis. Replacement fluid may or may not be used with CAVH-D, depending on local preferences.

All three of these techniques have the disadvantage of requiring both arterial and venous access. To obviate the need for arterial access, a roller pump can be placed in the circuit to provide hydrostatic pressure. This modification is referred to as "continuous venovenous hemofiltration" (CVVH or CVVH-D). Vascular access is greatly simplified, particularly in larger patients in whom a double lumen cannula can be used for inflow and outflow. Use of a roller pump makes the process even more efficient, because the hydrostatic pressure is dependent only on the speed of the pump, and it can be manipulated independent of the arteriovenous gradient. However, the disadvantages of CVVH or CVVH-D are that the circuit is more complex, carries a risk of air embolus, and often requires an extra nurse to operate and monitor the roller pump. Use of CAVH or CVVH depends on the ability to gain adequate vascular access, arteriovenous pressure difference, and nursing staffing issues.

Use of any of these forms of continuous ultrafiltration with or without dialysis is fairly complex, and it should not be done "spur of the moment." Careful nursing training is necessary before CAVH or its variants can be implemented. However, practical manuals are available, and they are invaluable in setting up a program (22).

A generalized description of the techniques is given below:

1. Obtain arterial and venous access using the largest available cannulas. Inadequate arterial or venous access minimizes arteriovenous pressure difference and reduces ultrafiltration efficiency.
2. An appropriate hollow fiber filter should be chosen. Filters that are small and short are most efficient, and they have less tendency to clot. The filter should be rinsed with 2 L of heparinized saline before placing it in the circuit.
3. A heparin infusion is established and given in the arterial limb of the circuit. A typical starting dose is 5–7 U/kg/h. Heparin infusion rate is adjusted by checking activated clotting times (ACTs) from the venous limb of the circuit. No consensus exists on what constitutes adequate anticoagulation. Adequate anticoagulation of the circuit without significantly anticoagulating the patient is the goal. An ACT approximately 1.5 times base-

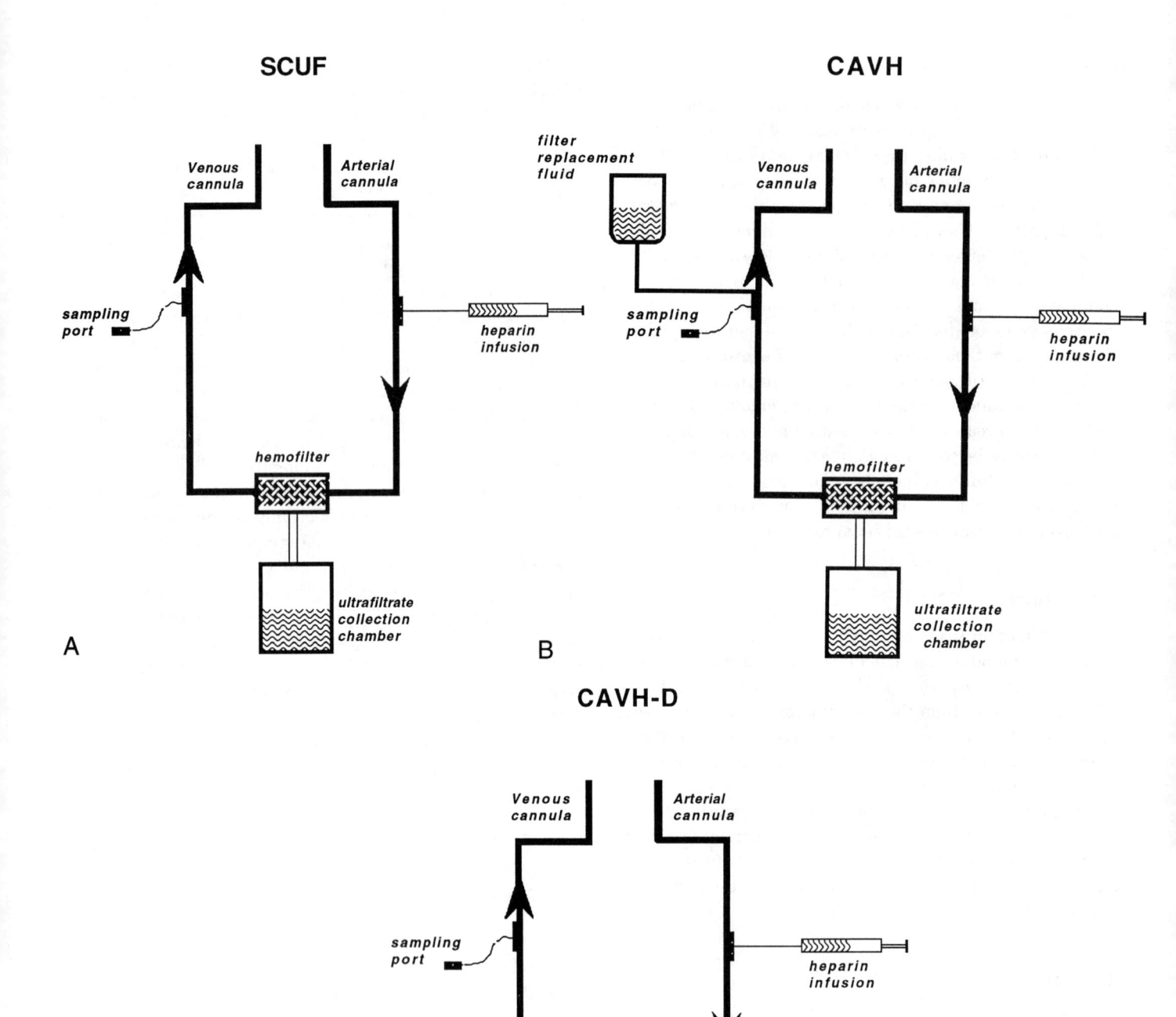

Figure 25.1. **A.** Schematic diagram of slow continuous ultrafiltration (*SCUF*). **B.** Schematic diagram of continuous arteriovenous hemofiltration (*CAVH*). Note that some groups prefer to infuse the filter replacement fluid on the arterial side of the circuit. **C.** Schematic diagram of continuous arteriovenous hemofiltration with dialysis (*CAVH-D*). Some groups also give filter replacement fluid when using dialysis. Note that the dialysate flows through the hemofilter opposite the direction of the blood flow.

line appears to be adequate. Patients with a baseline ACT greater than 200 seconds may not require heparin infusion.

4. Ultrafiltrate amount generated is dependent on several factors, including the hydraulic pressure of the blood flowing through the filter, negative hydrostatic pressure exerted by the ultrafiltrate column, and oncotic pressure, particularly as the blood reaches the outlet portion of the hemofilter. The ultrafiltrate column is often connected to a volume control pump, allowing exact control of the amount of ultrafiltrate generated. If dialysate is used the amount of fluid filtered is also dependent on the dextrose concentration of the dialysate. Dialysate is infused into ports in the hemofilter, with the dialysate flow direction opposite to that of blood flow.

5. Replacement fluid can be infused if CAVH or CVVH is performed. The composition of the replacement fluid is to some degree dependent on the needs of the patient. Various formulas have been used. Replacement fluid is usually reinfused into the venous limb of the circuit, but some groups have reported reinfusion on the arterial side, claiming to have less problems with filter clotting with this modification (22, 23).

Complications

Continuous hemofiltration techniques all share the disadvantages of requiring vascular access and anticoagulation. Filter clotting is common, and the filters typically require replacing every 12 to 48 hours. These techniques are powerful methods of fluid removal and dehydration can occur. Electrolyte abnormalities can also develop quickly, particularly with CAVH or CVVH because large volumes of replacement fluid are reinfused.

ULTRAFILTRATION

Cardiopulmonary bypass requires some degree of hypothermia in most applications, especially in pediatric cases in which warm heart preservation schemes are not feasible. Although hypothermia has the benefit of decreasing oxygen consumption, it can also lead to an increase in blood viscosity, vasoconstriction, and microvascular sludging. Hemodilution, which entails the use of a dilute blood or crystalloid prime in the cardiopulmonary bypass pump, is one strategy used to offset these effects of hypothermia. With hypothermia and reduced oxygen consumption, a low hematocrit is adequate to maintain oxygen delivery. With rewarming, however, oxygen consumption increases and a higher hematocrit is needed.

Ultrafiltration during cardiopulmonary bypass, which was first described by Romagnoli et al. in 1976 (24), can be used to remove excess fluid and raise the hematocrit during rewarming. Ultrafiltration during bypass was popularized in the mid-1980s by Magilligan and Oyama (25) and others, and it is now conventionally used for adult and pediatric patients. A modified form of perioperative ultrafiltration performed immediately after weaning has recently been developed that has several advantages over conventional ultrafiltration.

Conventional Ultrafiltration

With conventional ultrafiltration the hemofilter is incorporated into the bypass circuit. Typically the inlet is distal to the oxygenator and the outlet flows into the venous reservoir (Fig. 25.2). Ultrafiltration is performed during the rewarming period prior to weaning from cardiopulmonary bypass. This technique is effective in removing fluid from the bypass circuit, and it usually results in a rise in hematocrit. However, this technique is often inconsistent. Ultrafiltration often results in a fall in the venous reservoir level. One is then faced with terminating ultrafiltration be-

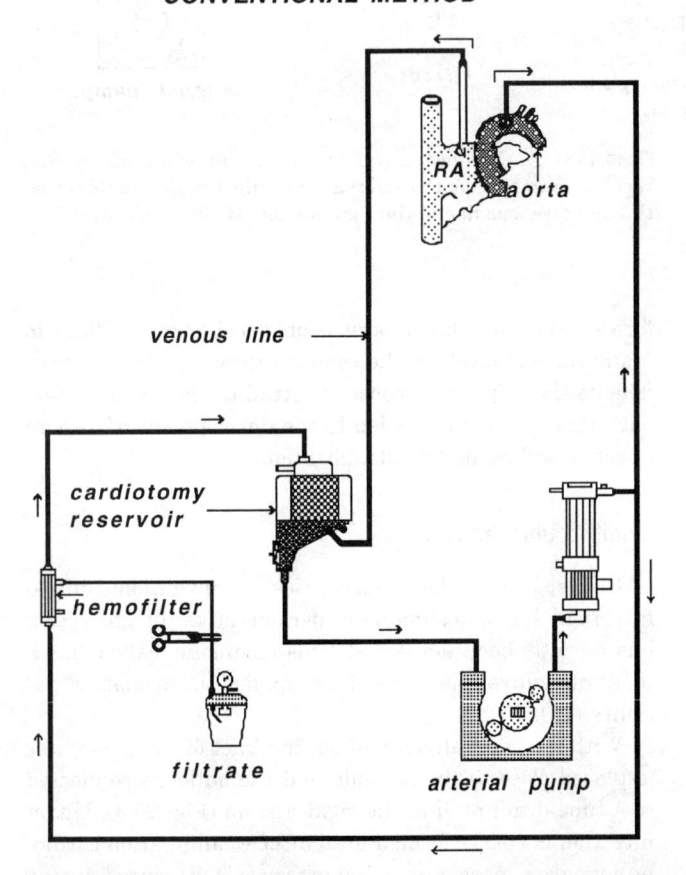

Figure 25.2. Standard ultrafiltration circuit while on bypass. No capability exists to filter while off bypass with this circuit. RA, right atrium.

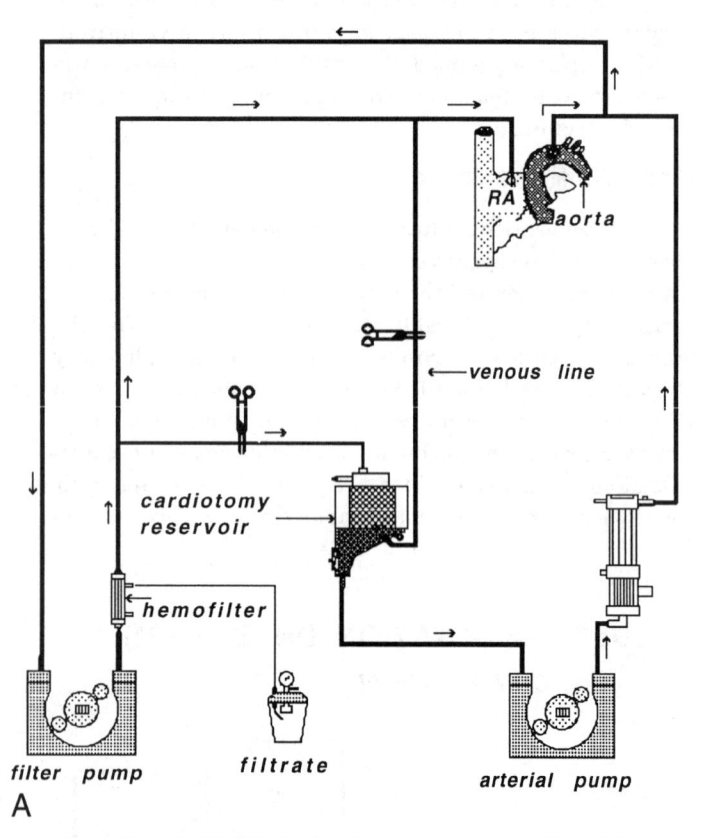

Figure 25.3. **A.** Modified ultrafiltration circuit while off bypass. Blood is drained from the arterial side of the circuit and reinfused through a venous line in the right atrium. **B.** Modified ultrafiltration circuit on bypass. Ultrafiltration can be performed while the patient is on bypass, just as is done with the conventional technique.

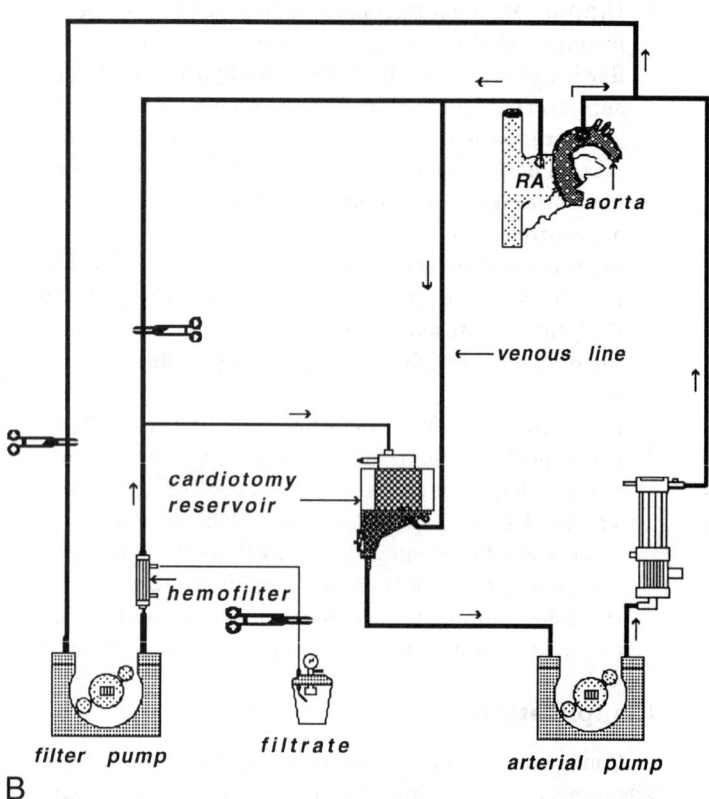

fore a reasonable hematocrit is obtained or giving fluid to maintain safe levels in the venous reservoir, which in turn defeats the original purpose of ultrafiltration. Frustration with this technique has led to the development of a more effective technique for ultrafiltration.

Modified Ultrafiltration

In response to the inadequacies of conventional ultrafiltration, a new technique of perioperative ultrafiltration has recently been developed. This technique, called "modified ultrafiltration," was first applied in pediatric patients (26).

With modified ultrafiltration, the inlet of the hemofilter is placed close to the cannula and the outlet is connected to a tube draining into the right atrium (Fig. 25.3). Ultrafiltration is not performed until after weaning from cardiopulmonary bypass. Left atrial pressure is measured during and after weaning from bypass. Optimum left atrial pressure is then determined and ultrafiltration initiated. Left atrial pressure is maintained at the desired level; if pressure falls, blood from the venous reservoir is pumped into the patient. This blood first goes through the ultrafilter before it is returned to the patient, removing excess water in the process. Ultrafiltration is continued until the desired hematocrit, usually 36 to 42%, is achieved.

Rarely does hemodynamic instability terminate ultrafiltration. In fact, the exact opposite usually happens—hemodynamics improve markedly during ultrafiltration. Prospective studies have demonstrated that during ultrafiltration blood pressure and cardiac index increase (Fig. 25.4), accompanied by a decrease in pulmonary vascular resistance. Systemic vascular resistance is unchanged (27). Another prospective study showed several other beneficial effects of modified ultrafiltration, including decreased total body water, decreased postoperative blood loss and requirements, and fewer days on the ventilator and in the intensive care unit (28). Some preliminary studies have even suggested that modified ultrafiltration may be neuroprotective by maintaining normal oxygen demand-

**Hemodynamic Consequences
of Modified Ultrafiltration**

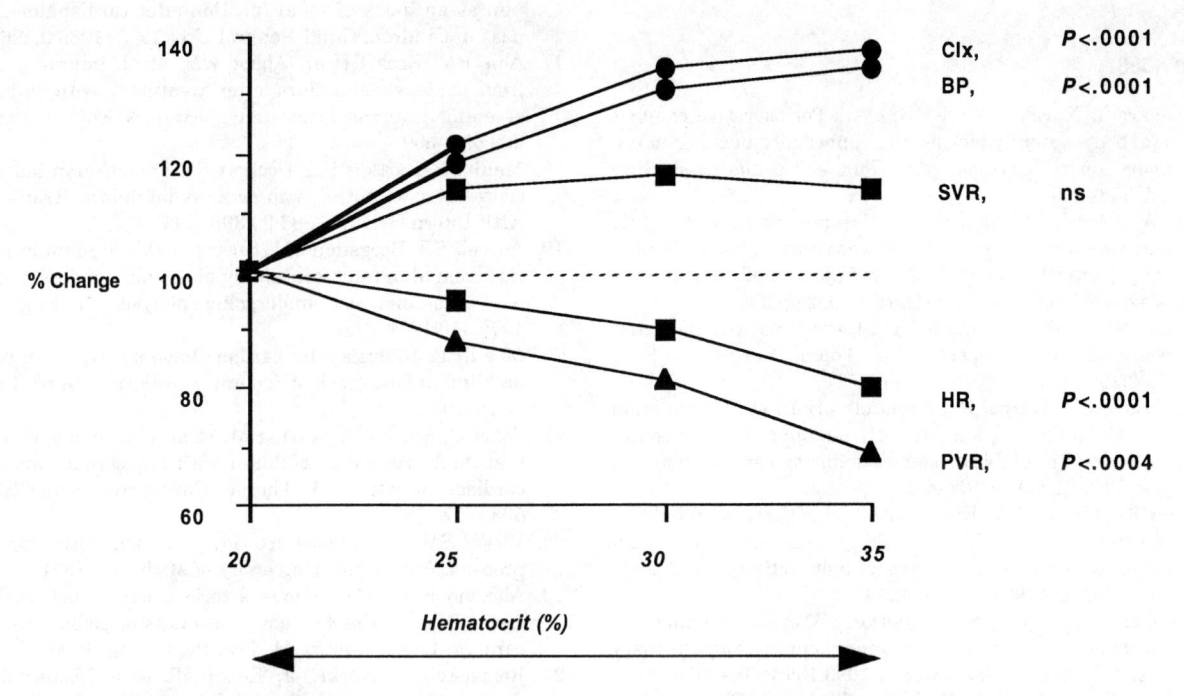

Figure 25.4. Hemodynamic changes during modified ultrafiltration after weaning from bypass. BP, blood pressure; CIx, cardiac index; HR, heat rate; PVR, pulmonary vascular resistance; SVR, systemic vascular resistance.

delivery relationships (29). Reasons for these salutary, and in some cases unexpected, effects are unclear, but several hypotheses have been offered, including decreased pulmonary and cardiac edema and perhaps most intriguingly, filtration of inflammatory mediators and other noxious substances (26).

HEMATURIA

Hemoglobinuria and hematuria are commonly seen after cardiopulmonary bypass. It is important to distinguish between hemoglobinuria and hematuria when evaluating a patient with pigmented urine after cardiopulmonary bypass.

Hemoglobinuria is caused by the hemolysis that often occurs during bypass support. Long bypass times, cardiotomy suction, and excessive occlusion of the roller pump can lead to hemolysis and elevated levels of free hemoglobin. Hemoglobinuria also often resolves within a few hours of cardiopulmonary bypass, but the implication of this finding is potentially significant. Hemoglobinuria could be the manifestation of a transfusion reaction. Direct and indirect Coombs' test should be obtained. Hemoglobin in the urine is potentially toxic to renal tubular function. Hemoglobin, which is a positively charged protein, can combine with negatively charged proteins (Temm-Harsfall proteins) in the renal tubules to form casts. Urine pH should be determined; if it is below 7 it should be alkalinized by giving intravenous bicarbonate (1–2 mEq/kg). Urine output should be brisk; mannitol (0.25–0.75 g/kg/dose) can be helpful in maintaining urine output and preventing occlusion of renal tubules by proteinaceous casts such as haptoglobin. When these hemoglobin binding proteins are saturated, free hemoglobin becomes present in the serum. Although some hemoglobin is cleared by the reticuloendothelial system, a large amount is filtered into the urine and excreted, leading to the characteristic red discoloration.

Urinalysis will reveal presence of red cells and confirm the diagnosis of the *hematuria*. Hematuria is usually self-limited and resolves within a few hours after bypass. However, hematuria could also be secondary to a thrombocytopenia or coagulopathy. Persistent hematuria should be evaluated by a renal ultrasound to rule out the possibility of an underlying tumor or congenital defect.

CONCLUSION

Several strategies have been developed to decrease the consequences of extracellular fluid accumulation. As the late 1990s approach, and worldwide mortality for congenital heart surgery approaches zero, physicians should be aware of these strategies and take efforts to minimize the morbidity associated with fluid overload.

REFERENCES

1. Maehara T, Novak I, Wyse RH, et al. Perioperative changes in total body water by bio-electrical impedance in children undergoing open heart surgery. Eur J Cardiothorac Surg 1992;5:258–265.
2. Wu W, Zbuzek VK, Bellevue C. Vasopressin release during cardiac operation. J Thorac Cardiovasc Surg 1980;79:83–90.
3. Burch M, Lum L, Elliott M, et al. Influence of cardiopulmonary bypass in children. Br Heart J 1992;68:309–312.
4. Dewar ML, Walsh G, Chiu RC, et al. Atrial natriuretic factor: response to cardiac operation. J Thorac Cardiovasc Surg 1988;96:266–270.
5. Wachtfogel YT, Harpel PC, Edmunds LH Jr, et al. Formation of C1s-C1-inhibitor, kallikrein-C1-inhibitor and plasmin-alpha 2-plasmin-inhibitor complexes during cardiopulmonary bypass. Blood 1989;73:468–471.
6. Stahl RF, Fisher CA, Kucich U, et al. Effects of simulated extracorporeal circulation on leukocyte elastase release, superoxide generation and procoagulant activity. J Thorac Cardiovasc Surg 1991;101:230–239.
7. Steinberg JB, Kapelanski DP, Olson JD, et al. Cytokine and complement levels in patients undergoing cardiopulmonary bypass. J Thorac Cardiovasc Surg 1993;105:1008–1016.
8. Smith EEJ, Naftel DC, Blackstone Eh, et al. Microvascular permeability after cardiopulmonary bypass. J Thorac Cardiovasc Surg 1987;94:225–233.
9. Mills AN, Haworth SG. Greater permeability of the neonatal lung. J Thorac Cardiovasc Surg 1991;101:909–916.
10. Huskisson I. Intravenous volume replacement: which fluid and why? Arch Dis Child 1992;67:649–653.
11. Hilberman M, Maseda J, Stinson EB, et al. The diuretic properties of dopamine in patients after open-heart operation. Anesthesiology 1984;61:489–494.
12. Kron IL, Joob AW, Van Meter C. Acute renal failure in the cardiovascular surgical patient. Ann Thorac Surg 1985;39:590–598.
13. Rigden SPA, Barratt TM, Dillon MJ, et al. Acute renal failure complicating cardiopulmonary bypass surgery. Arch Dis Child 1982;57:425–430.
14. Bourgeois BFD, Donath A, Paunier L, et al. Effect of cardiac surgery on renal function in children. J Thorac Cardiovasc Surg 1979;77:283–286.
15. Yip WCL, Tay JSH, Ho TF. Hyperuricemia as a cause of acute renal failure complicating cardiopulmonary bypass surgery [Letter]. Arch Dis Child 1983;58:159.
16. Fernandez F, de Miguel MD, Banio V, et al. Beta-2 microglobulin as an index of renal function after cardiopulmonary bypass in children. Child Nephrol Urol 1988–1989;9:326–330.
17. Able RM, Beck CH Jr, Abbot WM, et al. Improved survival from acute renal failure after treatment with intravenous essential L-amino acids and glucose. N Engl J Med 1973;288:695–699.
18. Mault JR, Bartlett RH, Dechert RE, et al. Starvation: a major contributor to mortality in acute renal failure. Trans Am Soc Artif Intern Organs 1983;29:390–395.
19. Adreoli SP, Bergstein JM, Sherrard DJ. Aluminum intoxication from aluminum-containing phosphate binders in children with azotemia not undergoing dialysis. N Engl J Med 1979;310:1079–1081.
20. Mee RBB. Dialysis after cardiopulmonary bypass in neonates and infants [Letter]. J Thorac Cardiovasc Surg 1992;103:1021–1022.
21. Zobel G, Stain JL, Kuttnig M, et al. Continuous extracorporeal fluid removal in children with low cardiac output after cardiac operation. J Thorac Cardiovasc Surg 1991;101:593–597.
22. Dirkes SM. Continuous arteriovenous hemofiltration: clinical protocol. Ann Arbor: University of Michigan, 1991.
23. Alexander SR. Continuous arteriovenous hemofiltration. In: Levin DL, Morriss FC, eds. Essentials of pediatric intensive care. St. Louis: Quality Medical Publishing, 1990.
24. Romagnoli A, Hacker J, Keats AS, et al. External hemoconcentration after deliberate hemodilution. In: Abstracts of scientific papers, p 269. Annual Meeting of the American Society of Anesthesiologists, San Francisco, October, 1976.
25. Magilligan DJ, Oyama C. Ultrafiltration during cardiopulmonary bypass: laboratory evaluation and initial clinical experience. Ann Thorac Surg 1984;37:183–189.
26. Elliott MJ. Ultrafiltration and modified ultrafiltration in pediatric open heart operations. Ann Thorac Surg 1993;56:1158–1522.
27. Naik SK, Balaji S, Elliott M. Modified ultrafiltration improves haemodynamics after cardiopulmonary bypass in children [Abstract]. J Amer Coll Cardiol 1993;19:37.
28. Niak SK, Knight A, Elliott MJ. A prospective randomized study of a modified technique of ultrafiltration during pediatric open heart surgery. Circulation 1991;84(Suppl III):422–431.
29. Skaryak LA, Kirshbom PM, DiBernardo, et al. Modified ultrafiltration improves cerebral metabolic recovery after circulatory arrest. J Thorac Cardiovasc Surg; 1995;109(4):744–752.

Perioperative Issues in Other Organ Systems 26

Eva Nozik Grayck, MD, Jon N. Meliones, MD, and Frank Kern, MD

HEMATOLOGIC ISSUES IN THE PERIOPERATIVE PERIOD

Normal mechanisms of clotting and thrombolysis will be briefly reviewed for the following discussions on postoperative bleeding after cardiopulmonary bypass (CPB) (1) and anticoagulation therapy.

Hemostasis requires both platelet adhesion and activation to form a platelet plug and coagulation cascade to form a stable fibrin clot. When the endothelium is injured Von Willebrand factor is exposed, which anchors the platelets to the vessel wall via the platelet receptor. Adhesion of platelets initiates platelet activation and subsequent degranulation, which releases products that increase platelet aggregation and activate the coagulation cascade. The coagulation cascade is composed of intrinsic, extrinsic, and common pathways that act synergistically to form a stable insoluble clot (see Fig. 26.1).

The coagulation cascade is balanced by the simultaneous activation of the fibrinolytic system. Several mediators, including kallikrein, convert plasminogen to plasmin. Plasmin is a proteolytic enzyme that dissolves fibrin, and it may also decrease platelet adhesion by reducing platelet receptors (1). The end result is clot dissolution.

Postoperative Bleeding

Effective hematologic management of the pediatric cardiac surgical patient requires an understanding of the normal mechanisms of clotting and thrombolysis described above as well as the post-bypass disturbances in hemostasis. In addition, neonates and infants have additional factors to consider when managing postoperative bleeding. With a thorough understanding of these principles, an appropriate strategy can be developed for the use of blood products in the perioperative period.

Risk Factors

Under normal conditions, the coagulation system and fibrinolysis are in balance to prevent the formation of blood clots. Exposure of blood to the nonendothelialized surface of the cardiopulmonary bypass circuit activates platelets and promotes clot formation. To prevent active coagulation during CPB patients must be anticoagulated with heparin.

Following CPB, numerous disturbances in hemostasis occur that can lead to excessive bleeding in the postoperative period (see Table 26.1). Alterations in hemostasis following bypass can also result from platelet abnormalities and complement activation. Fibrinolysis, manifest by elevated concentrations of fibrin degradation products and endogenous tissue plasminogen activator, produces further bleeding diathesis (2). Finally, underlying coagulation defects such as Von Willebrand's disease can predispose patients to excessive bleeding.

Cardiopulmonary bypass produces a greater risk of hemorrhage in neonates and infants because of extensive hemodilution, increased inflammatory response, and variable response to heparin. First, the disproportionate size of the circuit prime relative to blood volume in neonates and infants produces marked hemodilution (200 to 300% in neonates compared with 30% dilution in adults). This hemodilution effect results in a significant reduction in fibrinogen, clotting factors, and platelets, which increases the risk for bleeding. Second, post-CPB hemorrhage can be exaggerated in neonates and infants because CPB produces perhaps a more severe inflammatory response in these patients. In addition to exposure to the CPB circuit, deep hypothermic temperatures and circulatory arrest also produce an inflammatory response in neonates and infants (3). Inflammatory mediators increase the incidence of postoperative bleeding by altering vascular permeability, damaging capillaries, activating platelets, and inducing fibrinolysis. Finally, bleeding in neonates and infants is also complicated by age-dependent differences in heparin use required during bypass. Heparin requirements and effects during CPB are far less predictable in neonates compared with adult patients. Neonatal patients are susceptible to delayed clearance of heparin because of hepatic immaturity and direct effects of hypothermia on metabolism and excretion of heparin (3). On the other hand, higher doses of heparin may be necessary to compensate for the decreased activity associated with increased dilution of antithrombin III in a relatively larger pump prime.

In addition to factors related to CPB technology, neonates and infants are also at increased risk of bleeding because of issues related to their hepatic function and underlying heart disease. Neonates have immature synthetic function of the liver, which results in decreased levels of contact factors XII, XI, prekallikrein, and high molecular weight kininogen. This contributes to the prolonged activated partial thromboplastin time (APTT) observed during the first 6 months of life (4, 5). Hepatic dysfunction is also frequently present in pediatric cardiac patients as a consequence of low cardiac output, suboptimal hemodynamic profile after Fontan operation, or inferior vena caval ob-

Figure 26.1. Coagulation cascade. Ca, calcium; HMW, high molecular weight; PL, platelet.

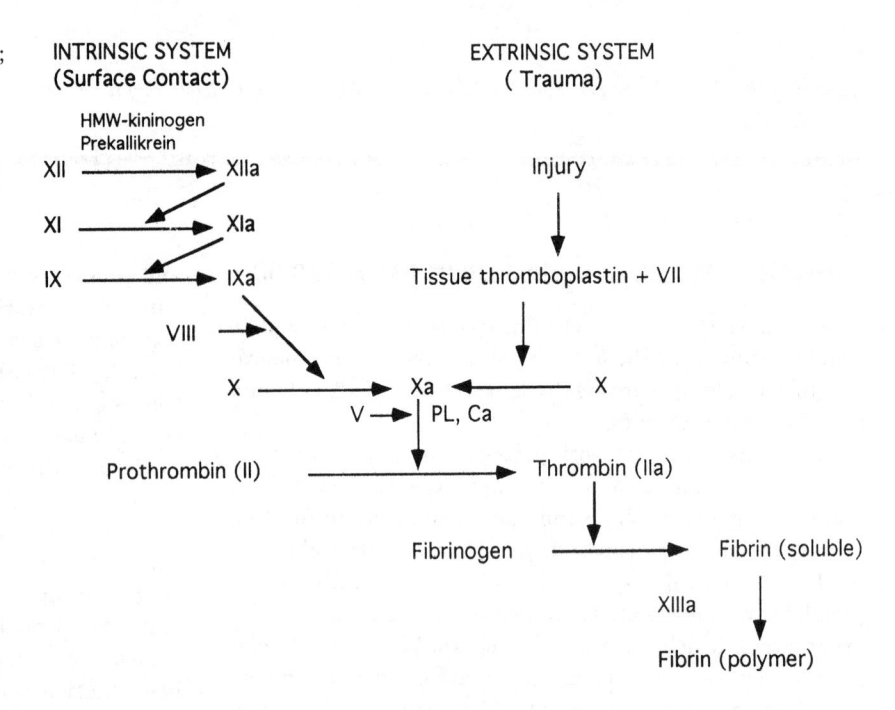

INTRINSIC SYSTEM (Surface Contact)

HMW-kininogen
Prekallikrein

XII → XIIa
XI → XIa
IX → IXa
VIII →
X → Xa ← X
V → PL, Ca
Prothrombin (II) → Thrombin (IIa)
Fibrinogen → Fibrin (soluble)
XIIIa ↓
Fibrin (polymer)

EXTRINSIC SYSTEM (Trauma)

Injury ↓
Tissue thromboplastin + VII

Table 26.1. Mean Coagulation Data for All Neonates

Assay[a]	PreCPB	1 min on CPB	Cold CPB	Warm CPB	Postprotamine	ICU
Fibrinogen	210 ± 52	91 ± 15[b]	92 ± 19[b]	105 ± 22[b]	159 ± 58[b]	183 ± 33
Factor 2	56 ± 14	28 ± 8[b]	29 ± 9[b]	32 ± 10[b]	56 ± 14	64 ± 13[e]
Factor 5	70 ± 21	0	0	0	40 ± 11[b]	48 ± 14[b]
Factor 7	55 ± 13	26 ± 6[b]	27 ± 7[b]	29 ± 8[b]	50 ± 14[c]	63 ± 24[e]
Factor 8	58 ± 26	0	0	0	36 ± 26[d]	73 ± 40[e]
Factor 9	39 ± 19	24 ± 10[d]	22 ± 7[d]	33 ± 13[e]	39 ± 23	61 ± 20[e]
Factor 10	53 ± 13	31 ± 9[b]	30 ± 8[b]	33 ± 10[b]	53 ± 16	55 ± 17
Platelets (k/mm³)	219 ± 57	64 ± 26[b]	65 ± 24[b]		93 ± 31[b]	161 ± 65[e]
Antithrombin 3	50 ± 17	29 ± 11[b]	28 ± 12[b]	31 ± 12[b]	51 ± 17	61 ± 21[e]
Heparin (units)	0.05 ± 0.09	0.37 ± 0.11[b]	0.39 ± 0.10[b]	0.39 ± 0.11[b]	0.08 ± 0.14	0.08 ± 0.09
ACT (seconds)	167 ± 20	> 700[b]	> 700[b]	> 700[b]	148 ± 22[e]	
PT (seconds)	13.4 ± 2.4	25.1 ± 3.1[b]	25.0 ± 7.1[b]	22.2 ± 5.3[b]	15.2 ± 1.6[e]	13.9 ± 1.7
PTT (seconds)	58.2 ± 16.7	> 90[b]	> 90[b]	> 90[b]	72 ± 18.8[d]	63.7 ± 14.1

[a] Fibrinogen, Factors 2, 5, 7, 8, 9, 10 and antithrombin 3 are in % activity.
[b] $P < 0.0001$, [c] $P < 0.01$, [d] $P < 0.002$, [e] $P < 0.05$
ACT, anticoagulation therapy; CPB, cardiopulmonary by pass; ICU, intensive care unit; PT, prothrombin time; PTT, partial thromboplastin time.

struction during cannulation. Second, cyanotic congenital heart disease can predispose patients to post-CPB bleeding. Platelet abnormalities are an important cause of postoperative bleeding in cyanotic patients because antecedent chronic hypoxia can lead to thrombocytopenia and platelet dysfunction (3). Abnormalities in platelet function are also associated with asplenia or polysplenia, which can occur with complex cyanotic heart disease. Prostaglandin E_1, often necessary in neonates with cyanotic heart disease, can interfere with platelet function, and it can contribute to bleeding. In addition to platelet dysfunction, cyanosis is also associated with decreased coagulation factor levels and disseminated intravascular coagulopathy, which can further contribute to the risk of hemorrhage after surgery.

Neonates and infants may have an increased incidence of postoperative bleeding secondary to the technical complexity of congenital heart surgical repair with its extensive reconstruction and numerous suture lines. In addition, reoperation, a relatively common occurrence in pediatric patients, requires resection through vascular scar tissue, which results in prolonged CPB and increased bleeding.

Treatment Strategy

Excessive bleeding can produce cardiovascular instability and impair oxygen delivery. In addition, multiple transfusions that are required to treat blood loss expose the patient to morbidity associated with hypocalcemia, blood-borne infections, and transfusion reactions. Laboratory tests in the management of postoperative bleeding can include hemoglobin and hematocrit, platelet count, prothrombin time, partial thromboplastin time, fibrinogen, and fibrin degradation products. Activated clotting time therapy should be obtained especially if "pump" blood was given back to the patient because this source of blood contains heparin. Optimal approach to postoperative bleeding is a systematic evaluation of the coagulation status with replacement therapy directed to the specific abnormalities detected.

Transfusion with packed red blood cells should be reserved for instances of low hematocrit or persistent bleeding, which produces a reduction in oxygen delivery. Selective therapy with platelets for thrombocytopenia or platelet dysfunction, cryoprecipitate for hypofibrinogenemia, or fresh frozen plasma (FFP) for factor deficiency should be considered. Platelet dysfunction is a common cause of bleeding following CPB, and administration of platelets should be considered if bleeding persists as a problem. Platelet and FFP transfusions should be done cautiously, however, because this therapy can dilute red blood cells and thereby inhibit clot formation (3). For neonates and infants, fresh whole blood has been recommended because it provides a balance of red blood cells, clotting factors, and platelets with minimal donor exposure (6). Effort to obtain fresh whole blood can be hindered by the standard protocols to test for blood-borne infections.

If bleeding continues despite the correction of the coagulopathy, a bleeding source that should be surgically treated must be considered. Whereas some patients with bleeding can be supported with blood products until hemostasis is achieved, patients with significant blood loss (more than 10 mL/kg/h) may necessitate an exploration in a timely fashion, either in the cardiac intensive care setting or in the operating room.

Various antifibrinolytic therapies have been evaluated to improve hemostasis following CPB. *Epsilon aminocaproic acid* (EACA) and *tranexamic acid* (TA) are two synthetic compounds that prevent breakdown of the fibrin clot by complexing with plasmin to prevent its fibrinolytic activity. EACA has been shown to produce a small but significant decrease in bleeding in adult patients and to decrease blood loss during bypass in children with congenital heart disease (1, 7, 8). Prophylactic use of TA also has been found to decrease bleeding with CPB (9). *Aprotinin* is a naturally occurring protease inhibitor that inhibits fibrinolysis by binding and inactivating plasmin and kallikrein; it also protects platelet function following CPB (10–13). Protective effects of aprotinin in adult cardiac surgery patients have been demonstrated by several investigators (14–17), and aprotinin has also been shown to be safe and efficacious in high risk patients undergoing reoperations or active infective endocarditis (18). In pediatric patients, however, aprotinin has not been shown to decrease bleeding as effectively as in adult patients; it also failed to improve platelet aggregation in 24 children placed on CPB (19). This study found no benefit in low or high dose aprotinin protocols (19). *Desmopressin*, also been in pediatric patients, has shown no beneficial effects on bleeding (20). Further investigations may elucidate the differences between adult and pediatric patients subjected to CPB and provide innovative therapies to minimize the requirements for blood product transfusions in the perioperative period.

Postoperative Anticoagulation

Some patients in the cardiac intensive care setting will be at increased risk of thrombosis and chronic anticoagulation may need to be initiated. These patients include those with prosthetic valves, aortopulmonary shunts, atrial fibrillation, systemic emboli, pulmonary hypertension, or cardiomyopathy. Patients who have undergone cavopulmonary anastomoses such as Fontan or bidirectional Glenn procedure are also at risk for thromboses; these patients also benefit from long-term anticoagulation (21).

Common long-term agents are warfarin, aspirin, and dipyridamole (see Chapter 5, *Cardiovascular Pharmacology*). Warfarin acts by interfering with vitamin K-dependent factors II, IV, IX, and X. When warfarin is begun, heparin may need to be continued until the vitamin K-dependent factors with long half-lives are inhibited. Aspirin is a cyclo-oxygenase inhibitor that decreases platelet aggregation. Dipyridamole is a phosphodiesterase inhibitor that increases cyclic adenosine monophosphate levels and also blocks platelet aggregation.

GASTROINTESTINAL ISSUES IN THE PERIOPERATIVE PERIOD

Perioperative Nutrition

Vigilance regarding nutrition for the pediatric cardiac patient in the intensive care setting is sometimes neglected but it is vitally important for adequate postoperative recovery, especially because some patients may have been malnourished secondary to their cardiac disease. Pediatric patients with congestive heart failure have been shown to have an increased oxygen consumption from 6.4 mL O2/kg/min to 9.4 mL O2/kg/min (22, 23).

In the cardiac intensive care setting, the goals of nutritional support are to minimize the catabolic effects that develop in response to the stress of surgery and to ensure a positive nitrogen balance for tissue repair. Basal metabolic rate is increased in critically ill infants and children compared with healthy children, and it is related to illness severity (24, 25). Substrate requirements also differ in critically ill patients, with 50% of oxygen consumption derived from utilization of fat. Providing 120–150 kcal/kg/d or higher may be necessary in the postoperative period to meet these nutritional requirements. Nutrition can be administered by the enteral or parenteral route.

Enteral Nutrition

The enteral route for nutrition is preferred because it can allow for complete nutritional support with minimal complications. Enteral feedings can be delivered orally or through tubes (via nasal or oral routes) to the stomach or duodenum.

Commonly used medications such as benzodiazepines or narcotics can cause decreased gastric emptying, and they may necessitate continuous transpyloric feeding with the addition of medications (such as metaclopramide or cisapride) to improve emptying (26). Although muscle relaxants do not affect the smooth muscle in the gastrointestinal tract, they are usually administered concurrently with benzodiazepines and narcotics, which can decrease gut motility. In addition, because patients requiring muscle relaxants are generally sicker and may have impaired gut perfusion, enteral feedings should therefore be instituted cautiously in these patients if parenteral nutrition is not used.

Absorption of carbohydrates, proteins, and fats can be impaired following cardiopulmonary bypass and surgery, thereby requiring adjustments in nutritional supplements. Loss of disaccharidase activity in brush border of intestinal mucosa impairs the ability to digest complex carbohydrates, whereas a high concentration of simple carbohydrates produces an osmotic load that can cause diarrhea (27). Diarrhea caused by an inability to absorb carbohydrates is easily detected by the presence of reducing substances in the stool. In addition, ischemic injury to the gut mucosa and its microvasculature following cardiopulmonary bypass can trigger an inflammatory response that alters permeability to proteins. Lastly, fat intolerance can occur in patients with disruption of the thoracic duct or high right atrial pressures. These patients will develop chylous effusions, which may clear when medium chain triglycerides are used as the primary source of fat. Medium chain triglycerides are absorbed by the gut and therefore do not require chylomicron formation and clearance by the thoracic duct for systemic absorption.

Certain cardiac operations are associated with specific gastrointestinal complications; examples are the Fontan procedure and protein-losing enteropathy, coarctation repair, and mesenteric arteritis; and Norwood procedure for hypoplastic left heart syndrome with reduced gut perfusion and resultant ischemia. These conditions all warrant a more judicious protocol for enteral feeding and use of more elemental formulas.

Parenteral Nutrition

Indications for total parenteral nutrition (TPN) use in postoperative cardiac patients include postoperative ileus, gut ischemia, malabsorption, or primary intestinal disorder. TPN is typically composed of amino acids, glucose, trace minerals and vitamins, and intralipids. Whereas TPN can be administered through a peripheral or central line, central access is required for glucose concentrations greater than 12.5%.

Use of TPN can be complicated by line infections, cholestasis, hypertriglyceridemia, and hepatic steatosis associated with excess glucose. Excess glucose administration can increase the respiratory quotient, which can play a small role in increasing ventilatory requirements. Intralipids are used in conjunction with TPN for additional calories in the form of fat. The earlier practice of intermittent bolus administration of 10% lipid emulsions was associated with pulmonary function impairment and pulmonary artery pressure increases; these undesired effects are particularly pertinent in the cardiac patient, but they were not seen with continuous infusions of 20% fat emulsions (28).

Gastrointestinal Ischemia

Gastrointestinal ischemia can develop in full-term neonates and infants with congenital heart disease. Clinical features include a tender distended abdomen, hypoactive bowel sounds, bloody stools, and malabsorption. Radiologic evaluation can show pneumatosis intestinalis, free air in the portal vein, or air or fluid levels in the bowel loops (29).

The pathogenesis of ischemic gut injury in cardiac patients is not completely understood. Significant differences are seen between mesenteric ischemia in full-term neonates with congenital heart disease and resultant systemic hypoperfusion and necrotizing enterocolitis in premature neonates (30). Studies attribute gut ischemia in cardiac patients to cold stress associated with hypothermic bypass, low cardiac output following left ventricular outflow tract obstruction, and decreased mesenteric blood flow as a consequence of diastolic steal with a large patent ductus arteriosus (31). An association is seen between gut ischemia and the presence of hypotension and apnea in patients on prostaglandin E for ductal-dependent lesions (32).

Gut ischemia has also been described after cardiac catheterization in neonates and infants with congenital heart disease, but a specific causal relationship with catheterization events or precatheterization condition was not defined (33, 34). Gastrointestinal rotavirus infection was reported in two patients who developed gut ischemia after catheterization; in these patients, it was likely that the diarrhea and dehydration following rotavirus infection decreased blood flow to the gut, impaired oxygen delivery, and increased the risk for developing enterocolitis (35).

One study reported an association between mesenteric ischemia and prostaglandins, umbilical artery catheter, acidosis, preoperative thrombocytopenia, young age, and hypoxemia but less evidence for association with sepsis, lower extremity hypotension, and renal or hepatic dysfunction (36). Rotavirus has also been isolated from postoperative patients with mesenteric ischemia, again implicating gastrointestinal viral infection in congenital cardiac patients with gut ischemia (37).

Medical management of gut ischemia is similar in cardiac patients and premature infants. The gastrointestinal tract is rested by discontinuing enteral feedings, applying nasogastric suction, and administering broad spectrum antibiotics. Surgical intervention is required for intestinal perforation or necrosis. Prognosis of cardiac patients with gastrointestinal ischemia is significantly worse than for premature neonates with necrotizing enterocolitis (30). High risk cardiac patients should therefore be observed carefully for signs and symptoms of gut ischemia and enteral feedings should not be initiated until hemodynamic stability has been achieved.

Gastrointestinal Bleeding

Gastrointestinal bleeding from stress ulcers can complicate the course of critically ill patients with congenital heart disease. Frequency of gastrointestinal hemorrhage in intensive care setting varies considerably, depending on the population and age of patients, prophylactic medications use, and extent of hemorrhage detected.

In a review of 698 patients in a pediatric intensive care unit, an upper gastrointestinal bleeding incidence of 6.4% was found, but with only 0.4% of this group being clinically significant (38). Another group reported a much higher incidence of 25% in a pediatric intensive care unit patient population and identified three risk factors: cardiovascular shock, surgery lasting longer than 3 hours, and severe trauma (39). Although many infants and children with complex cardiac lesions will have the first two risk factors, the incidence of upper gastrointestinal tract ulcer and bleeding is relatively uncommon in these patients. Multiorgan dysfunction including renal dysfunction, cardiac failure, hepatic dysfunction, and factors such as sepsis and steroid use can increase the risk of upper gastrointestinal tract bleeding in the congenital heart disease patient. Microscopic or occult blood in the gastrointestinal tract is common, and it does not necessarily predict the development of macroscopic bleeding (40).

Medical therapy for gastric ulcers and gastrointestinal hemorrhage includes antacids, H2 antagonists such as ranitidine, and sucralfate. Prophylaxis with three agents protects against hemorrhage with an overall rate of 5.7% significant gastrointestinal hemorrhage (versus 20% in untreated patients) (40). Antacids are inexpensive and effective, although their use can be complicated by diarrhea and electrolyte disturbances. Elevated gastric pH can increase the likelihood of bacterial colonization of the gastrointestinal tract and bacterial translocation resulting in blood-borne infections (40, 41). Enteral feedings also protect against gastrointestinal hemorrhage and bacterial translocation; this strategy provides additional incentive to advance from parenteral to enteral feedings whenever possible (38). Sucralfate is the drug of choice in hepatic and renal failure (42). Although endoscopy provides the definitive diagnosis for upper gastrointestinal tract bleeding, it is both invasive and expensive; the procedure should be reserved for selected patients in whom medical therapy has failed to control upper gastrointestinal tract bleeding. When major gastrointestinal hemorrhage occurs in patients with multisystem organ failure, the prognosis is usually poor.

INFECTIOUS ISSUES IN THE PERIOPERATIVE PERIOD

Among patients in the intensive care setting, infants and children have a higher incidence of nosocomial infections than adults (13.7 versus 4.8%) (43, 44). In pediatric patients, *Staphylococcus epidermitis*, *S. aureus*, enterococcus, and enteric gram-negative bacilli are important nosocomial pathogens in the perioperative period (45). Increased use of broad-spectrum antibiotics in these patients has also encouraged the development of multiple-resistant bacteria and fungi. Although the cause and type of infection varies, the development of nosocomial infections in the perioperative period can have devastating consequences. In this section we will describe the common infections that occur in perioperative cardiac patients.

Diagnosis of Postoperative Infections

Many infants and children will have episodes of fever in the perioperative period without evidence of infection. The clinical challenge is to determine which patients would be at high risk for infections and therefore be treated empirically. Patients who develop fever more than 48 hours after surgery and patients that develop high fevers (more than 39°C) should be considered at high risk. In addition, patients with hemodynamic instability (tachycardia, hypotension, decreased perfusion) or abnormal laboratory data such as elevated or depressed white blood cell count with a left shift or acidosis indicate a patient at high risk for a serious infection. The common site for infections include intravascular catheters, respiratory system, urinary tract, and mediastinum. Less common sites include endocarditis, sinuses, and central nervous system infections.

Initial evaluation in conditions suggestive of sepsis includes a thorough examination, laboratory assessment as described above, and cultures from a variety of sites (blood, tracheal, urinary, and wound). Empiric antibiotics may be indicated as described below.

Catheter Sepsis

Most patients receive prophylactic antibiotics prior to surgery and in the immediate perioperative period. When to terminate these antibiotics is dependent on the individual center, and it is often open to debate. In some institutions, antibiotic prophylaxis consists of a cephalosporin for 48 hours. Although some centers recommend antibiotic continuation as long as central catheters are in place, this approach can result in the selection of resistant organisms or fungal species. The primary method of reducing catheter-related sepsis is to decrease the duration of intravascular catheter (43, 45). A description of each catheter (site, duration, and culture data) should be routinely incorporated into each patient's assessment.

In adult intensive care patients, the incidence of catheter sepsis is low and ranges between 1 and 5% (44). The incidence of positive catheter tip cultures is higher in infants, approaching 16% (45). The reason for this increased incidence is not known, but the in situ time may be longer in neonates and children, which can be partially due to a general reluctance to routinely change catheters in pediatric patients. Risk factors for the development of positive catheter tip cultures include longer in situ time, younger age, and inotropic support (45). Although exchanging a catheter over a guidewire does not appear to reduce the risk for colonization, changing the catheter to a new site may decrease the incidence of infection (46).

Intravascular catheter location can vary in incidence of infection. Transthoracic catheters appear to have the lowest incidence of infections (0% in one series), whereas percutaneously placed pulmonary artery catheters have the highest incidence of infection (10.6%) (45). Peripheral, arterial, and central venous catheters were found to have 0.9, 3.9, and 5.9% positive tip cultures, respectively (45). Time limitation for the use of individual catheters differs depending on institutional preference. Some centers recommend changing intravascular catheters after 1 week of use. Parental nutrition use also increases the risk for catheter-related sepsis; one practice that may decrease the potential for infection may be to use a dedicated port for parental nutrition that is not routinely interrupted.

A staphylococcus species is the most frequent causative organism of catheter-related sepsis. When a catheter sepsis is suspected, blood cultures from both the catheter and the periphery should be obtained. The catheter should be removed if possible. Although catheter removal should be adequate treatment, clinical suspicion of endocarditis remains. In these cases, the initial antibiotic selection can be relatively broad if the source is not known.

In conditions where catheter cultures are positive, bacteria-specific therapy is initiated. If peripheral cultures are also positive, however, the question of endocarditis remains. Repeat peripheral cultures should be performed after initiation of therapy. If peripheral cultures remain positive for more than 48 hours after catheter removal and after initiation of appropriate antimicrobial therapy, the risk for endocarditis or infected thrombus is higher. These patients should undergo an echocardiogram and 4 to 6 weeks of antibiotic therapy should be strongly considered.

Pneumonitis

Development of pneumonitis is relatively uncommon in infants and children in the postoperative period. Patients at risk include those who have been intubated prior to the operation and those with a previous history of respiratory infections. Diagnosis of nosocomial pneumonia can be difficult, and it requires a constellation of symptoms and laboratory tests. Evidence for associated pneumonia after surgery includes the development of respiratory insufficiency or a requirement for increased respiratory support. Presence of localized infiltrate on chest roentgenogram is also strongly suggestive of pneumonitis. An endotracheal aspirate gram stain that has bacteria and many polymorphonuclear cells can be diagnostic of pneumonitis. A precedent pneumonia, viral or bacterial, can lead to a devastating acute respiratory distress syndrome after cardiopulmonary bypass.

Urinary Tract Infection

Urinary tract infection should be considered in any patient with a urinary catheter in place. An indwelling catheter with open drainage for more than 4 to 5 days results in a risk of infection close to 100%; use of a sterile and closed drainage system is strongly recommended to minimize the risk of bacteriuria. Diagnosis of a urinary tract infection requires a positive culture of a clean catheter urine specimen. Appropriate antibiotic therapy is directed at the offending organism.

Mediastinitis

Mediastinitis is a relatively uncommon (less than 1.0%) but devastating infection in infants and children after cardiac surgery (47, 48). The possibility of mediastinitis should always be considered in postoperative patients with unexplained fevers. Diagnosis can be difficult, and it requires a careful evaluation of the wound and sternum by experienced personnel. Occasionally, drainage occurs from the wound or instability of the sternum is seen. Fortunately, most of these wound infections are superficial and can be adequately treated with anti-staphylococcal antibiotics and with drainage and irrigation if necessary (48, 49). When the infection is more extensive, however, a more thorough debriding may be required. In these conditions, an early skin or muscle flap may be required to ensure healing (49).

REFERENCES

1. Hardy J-F, Desroches J. Natural and synthetic antifibrinolytics in cardiac surgery. Can J Anaesth 1992;39(4):353–365.
2. Slaughter T. The coagulation system and cardiac surgery. In: Estafanous FG, Barash PG, Reves JG, eds. Cardiac anesthesia: principles and clinical practice. Philadelphia: JB Lippincott, 1994:621–633.
3. Kern F, Gieser W, Farrell D. Extracorporeal circulation and circulatory assist devices in the pediatric patient. In Lake C, ed. Cardiac anesthesia. Philadelphia: WB Saunders, 1993: 151–179.
4. Andrew M, Paes B, Milner R, et al. Development of the human coagulation system in the full-term infant. Blood 1987; 70(1):165–172.
5. Kern F, Morana N, Sears J, et al. Coagulation defects in neonates during cardiopulmonary bypass. Ann Thorac Surg 1992;54:541–546.
6. Manno C, Hedberg K, Kim H, et al. Comparison of the hemostatic effects of fresh whole blood, stored whole blood, and components after open heart surgery in children. Blood 1991;77:930–936.
7. Vander Salm T, Ansell J, Okike O, et al. The role of epsilon-aminocaproic acid in reducing bleeding after cardiac operation: a double-blind randomized study. J Thorac Cardiovasc Surg 1988;95:538–540.
8. McClure P, Izsak J. The use of epsilon-aminocaproic acid to reduce bleeding during cardiac bypass in children with congenital heart disease. Anesthesiology 1974;40(6):604–608.
9. Horrow J, Hlavacek J, Strong M, et al. Prophylactic tranexamic acid decreases bleeding after cardiac operations. J Thorac Cardiovasc Surg 1990;99:70–74.
10. van Oeveren W, Jansen J, Bidstrup B, et al. Effects of aprotinin on hemostatic mechanisms during cardiopulmonary bypass. Ann Thorac Surg 1987;44:640–645.
11. van Oeveren W, Harder M, Roozendaal K, et al. Aprotinin protects platelets against the initial effect of cardiopulmonary bypass. J Thorac Cardiovasc Surg 1990;99:788–797.
12. Huang H, Ding W, Su Z, et al. Mechanism of the preserving effect of aprotinin on platelet function and its use in cardiac surgery. J Thorac Cardiovasc Surg 1993;106:11–18.
13. Wildevuur C, Eijsman L, Roozendaal K, et al. Platelet preservation during cardiopulmonary bypass with aprotinin. Eur J Cardiothorac Surg 1989;3:533–538.
14. Bidstrup B, Royston D, Sapsford R, et al. Reduction in blood loss and blood use after cardiopulmonary bypass with high dose aprotinin (trasylol). J Thorac Cardiovasc Surg 1989;97: 364–372.
15. Havel M, Teufelsbauer H, Knobl P. Effect of intraoperative aprotinin administration on postoperative bleeding in patients undergoing cardiopulmonary bypass operation. J Thorac Cardiovasc Surg 1991;101:968–972.
16. Royston D, Bidstrup B, Taylor K, et al. Effect of aprotinin on need for blood transfusion after repeat open-heart surgery. Lancet 1987;87(2):1289–1291.
17. Dietrich W, Spannagl M, Jochum M. Influence of high-dose aprotinin treatment on blood loss and coagulation patterns in patients undergoing myocardial revascularization. Anesthesiology 1990;73:1119–1126.
18. Bidstrup BP, Harrison J, Royston D, et al. Aprotinin therapy in cardiac operations: a report on use in 41 cardiac centers in the united kingdom. Ann Thorac Surg 1993;55:971–976.
19. Boldt J, Knothe C, Zickmann B, et al. Comparison of two aprotinin dosage regimens in pediatric patients having cardiac operations. J Thorac Cardiovasc Surg 1993;105:705–711.
20. Reynolds L, Nicolson S, Jobes DR, et al. Desmopressin does not decrease bleeding after cardiac operation in young children. J Thorac Cardiovasc Surg 1993;106:954–958.
21. Pridjian A, Mendelsohn A, Lupinetti F, et al. Usefulness of the bidirectional Glenn procedure as staged reconstruction for the functional single ventricle. Am J Cardiol 1993;71: 959–962.
22. Krauss A, Auld P. Metabolic rate of neonates with congenital heart disease. Arch Dis Child 1975;50:539.
23. Stocker F, Wilkoff W, Miettinen O, et al. Oxygen consumption in infants with heart disease. J Pediatr 1972;80:43–51.
24. Steinhorn D, Green T. Severity of illness correlates with alterations in energy metabolism in the pediatric intensive care unit. Crit Care Med 1991;19:1503–1509.
25. Tilden S, Watkins S, Tong T, et al. Measured energy expenditure in pediatric intensive care patients. American Journal of Diseases of Children 1989;143:490–492.
26. Smith-Wright D, Green T, Lock J, et al. Complications of vascular catheterization in critically ill children. Crit Care Med 1984;12(12):1015.
27. Lebenthal E, Lee P. Glucoamylase and disaccharidase activities in normal subjects and in patients with mucosal injury of the small intestine. J Pediatr 1980;97:389–393.
28. Gilbertson N, Kovar I, Cox D, et al. Introduction of intravenous lipid administration on the first day of life in the very low birth weight neonate. J Pediatr 1991;119:615–623.
29. Kliegman R, Fanaroff A. Necrotizing enterocolitis. N Engl J Med 1984;310:1093–1113.
30. Hebra A, Brown M, Hirschl R, et al. Mesenteric ischemia in hypoplastic left heart syndrome. J Pediatr Surg 1993; 28(4):606–611.
31. Allen H, Haney P. Left ventricular outflow obstruction and necrotizing enterocolitis. Radiology 1984;150:401–402.
32. Leung M, Chau K-T, Hui P-W, et al. Necrotizing enterocolitis in neonates with symptomatic congenital heart disease. J Pediatr 1988;113:1044–1046.
33. Cooke R, Meradji M, De Villeneuve V. Necrotizing enterocolitis after cardiac catheterization in infants. J Intervent Cardiol 1980;55:66–68.
34. Dickinson D, Galloway R, Wilkinson J, et al. Necrotizing enterocolitis after neonatal cardiac catheterization. Journal of Interventional Cardiology 1982;57:431–433.

35. Meliones J, Shope T, Rosenthal A, et al. Rotavirus-associated necrotizing enterocolitis after cardiac catheterization in infants. J Intervent Cardiol 1991;4(2):121.
36. Callow L, Meliones J, Deming M, et al. Necrotizing enterocolitis in neonates after surgery for left heart obstruction. Circulation 1990;82:III-417.
37. Meliones J, Shope T, Rosenthal A, et al. Rotavirus-associated necrotizing enterocolitis after cardiac catheterization in infants. J Intervent Cardiol 1991;4:121-124.
38. Lacroix J, Nadeau D, Laberge S, et al. Frequency of upper gastrointestinal bleeding in a pediatric intensive care unit. Crit Care Med 1992;1:35-45.
39. Cochran E, Phelps S, Tolley E, et al. Prevalence of, and risk factors for, upper gastrointestinal tract bleeding in critically ill pediatric patients. Crit Care Med 1992;20(11):1519-1523.
40. Lopez-Herce J, Dorao P, Elola P, et al. Frequency and prophylaxis of upper gastrointestinal hemorrhage in critically ill children: a prospective study comparing the efficacy of almagate, ranitidine, and sucralfate. Crit Care Med 1992;20(8):1082-1089.
41. Zobel G, Kuttnig M, Grubbauer H. Reduction of colonization and infection rate during pediatric intensive care by selective decontamination of the digestive tract. Crit Care Med 1991;19:1242-1246.
42. George DE, Glassman M. Peptic ulcer disease in children. Gastrointest Endosc Clin N Am 1994;4(1):23-35.
43. Donowitz L. High risk of nosocomial infection in the pediatric critical care patient. Crit Care Med 1986;14(1):26.
44. Collignon P, Soni N, Pearson I, et al. Sepsis associated with central vein catheters in critically ill patients. Intensive Care Med 1988;14:227-231.
45. Damen J, Van Der Tweel L. Positive tip cultures and related risk factors associated with intravascular catheterization in pediatric cardiac patients. Crit Care Med 1988;16:221.
46. Brun-Buisson C, Abrouk F, LeGrand P, et al. Diagnosis of central venous catheter-related sepsis. Catheters and Sepsis 1987;147:873.
47. Rutledge R, Applebaum R, Kim BJ. Mediastinal infection after open heart surgery. Surgery 1985;97:88-92.
48. Edwards M, Baker C. Median sternotomy wound infections in children. Pediatr Infect Dis J 1983;2:105-109.
49. Stiegel RM, Beasley M, Sink J, et al. Management of postoperative mediastinitis in infants and children by muscle flap rotation. Ann Thorac Surg 1988;46:45-46.

Section IV:

Special Cardiac Evaluation and Management in Cardiac Intensive Care

Perioperative Radiographic Studies

Richard I. Markowitz, MD, and Kenneth E. Fellows, MD

Portable plain films of the chest are indispensable to the perioperative management of congenital heart disease. Their routine use allows (a) documentation of the position of the numerous tubes and monitoring catheters used in cardiac patients, (b) monitoring of the vascular volume changes and other physiologic events that occur postoperatively, and (c) detection of complications (such as bleeding and pneumothorax) before they may be clinically manifest. Frequency of "routine" chest radiographs varies among institutions, and it depends on many factors, including complexity of heart disease and surgery, and the known or expected complications at the completion of the surgical repair.

Other imaging technology such as noncardiac ultrasound (US), computed tomography (CT), and magnetic resonance imaging (MRI) are less frequently needed in the perioperative period. Because it is a bedside technique, US can be helpful in marking pleural effusions before thoracentesis and in evaluating some abdominal complications (i.e., gastric outlet obstruction, abscess formation). CT and MRI may be helpful in documenting the extent of cerebral vascular accidents and other complications affecting the central nervous system (see Chapter 24, *Neurologic Disorders*) (1). MRI can also be useful in evaluating postoperative airway problems (2). Spiral CT is a new technique that allows rapid and precise two-dimensional or three-dimensional visualization of vessels following a peripheral injection of contrast material. This technique may become useful postoperatively for excluding anastomotic stenoses or leaks without the necessity for cardiac catheterization.

As the most frequently used radiographic study in the pediatric cardiac intensive care unit is the anterior-posterior (AP) chest radiograph, this chapter focuses on a systematic approach to interpretation of the preoperative and postoperative chest film, with emphasis on the radiographic diagnosis of complex congenital heart disease.

SYSTEMATIC APPROACH TO CHEST FILMS

It is necessary to approach chest radiographs systematically in an organized and thorough fashion so that clinically important information is not overlooked (3). Because it is human nature to focus on the most relevant areas first, usually the heart and lungs, this evaluation should be postponed until the bones, soft tissues, and abdominal organs have been studied. Only then should an organized review of the thoracic contents and invasive lines and tubes begin. A detailed check list is provided to encourage this systematic approach (Table 27.1).

As another rule of good practice, every evaluation must include comparison to preceding examinations because, in many instances, it is the change in size, position, or radiographic appearance that is most important for accurate diagnosis.

A substantial portion of the abdomen is often included on portable chest radiographs. Although not usually a primary focus of attention, important life-threatening complications, as well as important details, can be detected there. Position of the stomach as well as that of enteric drainage or feeding tubes should be noted. Liver and spleen sizes are difficult to accurately assess on plain films; however, gross enlargement or change in size can have clinical implication and therefore should be considered. Status of the bowel gas pattern is also important, and it is discussed in the section on necrotizing enterocolitis (NEC).

When surgery immediately follows cardioangiography, persistent excretion of contrast by the kidneys may be observed. A prolonged nephrogram effect, 12 to 24 hours after cardiac catheterization, indicated by a dense blush of the renal parenchyma, can be an indication of diminished renal perfusion. Although rare, true hydronephrosis can indicate an undetected renal or collecting system anomaly. Occasionally, opacification of the gallbladder can be detected several days after injection of radiopaque contrast material, particularly in infants with low cardiac output or decreased systemic perfusion who undergo high dose angiocardiography (4). This alternative hepatobiliary pathway of contrast excretion does not necessarily imply renal failure, but it can be a physiologic consequence of the patient's disease and age.

In the chest, heart, lung, mediastinum, bony thorax, and pleural spaces must all be evaluated (Table 27.1). One of the immediate postoperative concerns is to confirm that the various tubes and catheters placed intraoperatively have remained in position after the patient has been moved to the cardiac intensive care unit. Different institutions and individual surgeons have their favorite types and methods of device insertion. Therefore, one must learn where each kind of tube or monitoring lead is supposed to be according to the local practice. Figures 27.1 and 27.2 show examples of some of the tubes, catheters, and other

Table 27.1. Checklist for Radiographic Assessment

__ Situs	__ Pleural effusion	__ Spleen
__ Normal	__ Coils, stents	__ Stomach
__ Inverted	__ Mediastinum	__ Bowel
__ Ambiguous	__ Aortic arch	__ Kidneys
__ Heart	__ Thymus	__ Pneumoperitoneum
__ Size	__ Trachea/bronchi	__ Calcification
__ Shape	__ Calcification	__ Tubes and Lines
__ Position	__ Pneumomediastinum	__ Endotracheal tube
__ Prostheses (valves, stents)	__ Clips, coils, conduits	__ Nasogastric tube
__ Calcification	__ Thorax	__ Mediastinal tubes
__ Pneumopericardium	__ Ribs	__ Thoracotomy/pleural tubes
__ Lungs	__ Notching	__ Pericardial drain
__ Volume	__ Previous surgery	__ Intracardiac monitoring catheters
__ Atelectasis/consolidation	__ Spine	__ ECMO cannuale
__ Vascularity	__ Sternum	__ Cardiac pacer wires
__ Edema	__ Soft tissues	__ Other
__ Hemorrhage	__ Abdomen	__ Comparison to previous study
__ Pneumothorax	__ Liver	

ECMO, extracorporeal membrane oxygenation.

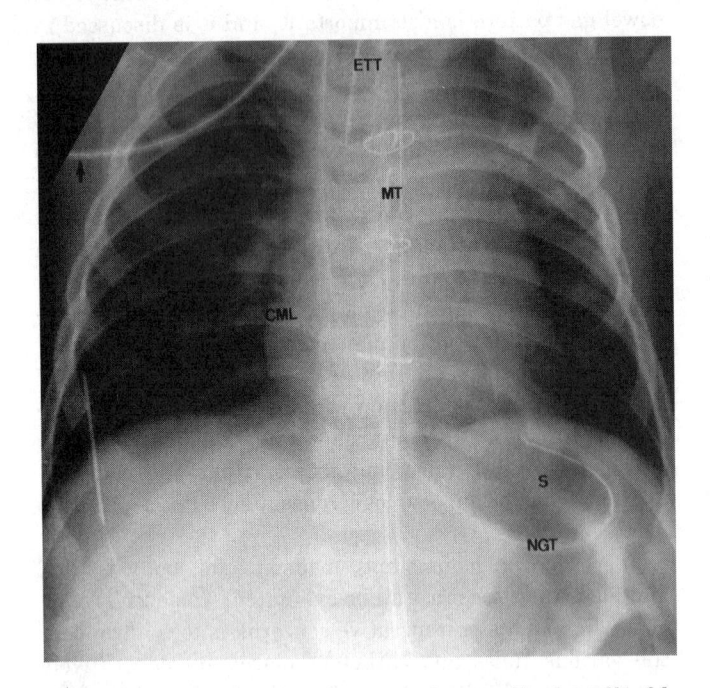

Figure 27.1. Postoperative arterior-posterior portable chest film following *VSD* repair. The midline wire sutures indicate a sternotomy incision has been used. Also seen is deformity of the left fourth and fifth ribs from a previous thoracotomy for coarctation repair. An extrathoracic wire (*arrow*) crosses the apex of the right lung. ETT, endotracheal tube; MT, mediastinal drainage tube; S, stomach; NGT, nasogastric tube; CML, cardiac monitoring line in the right atrium.

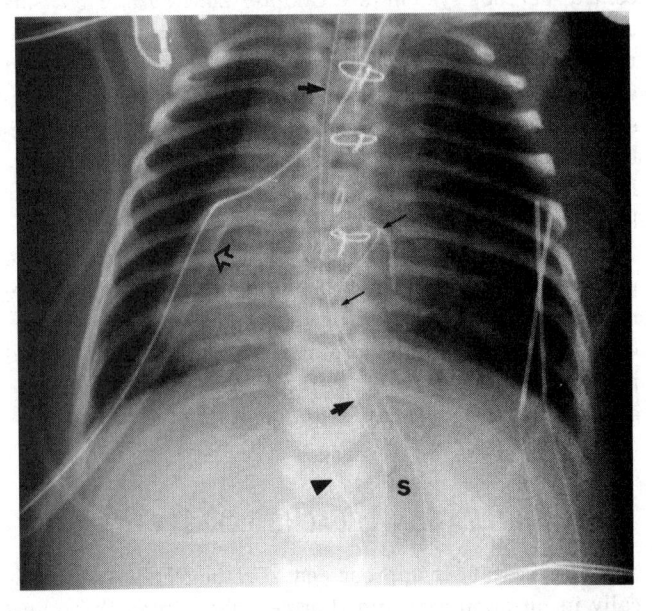

Figure 27.2. Postoperative arterior-posterior portable film in patient with polysplenia (situs ambiguous; note dextrocardia and stomach (*S*) in left upper quadrant). Large arrows, nasogastric tube; small arrows, intracardiac atrial monitoring lines; open arrow, mediastinal tube; arrow head, umbilical venous line.

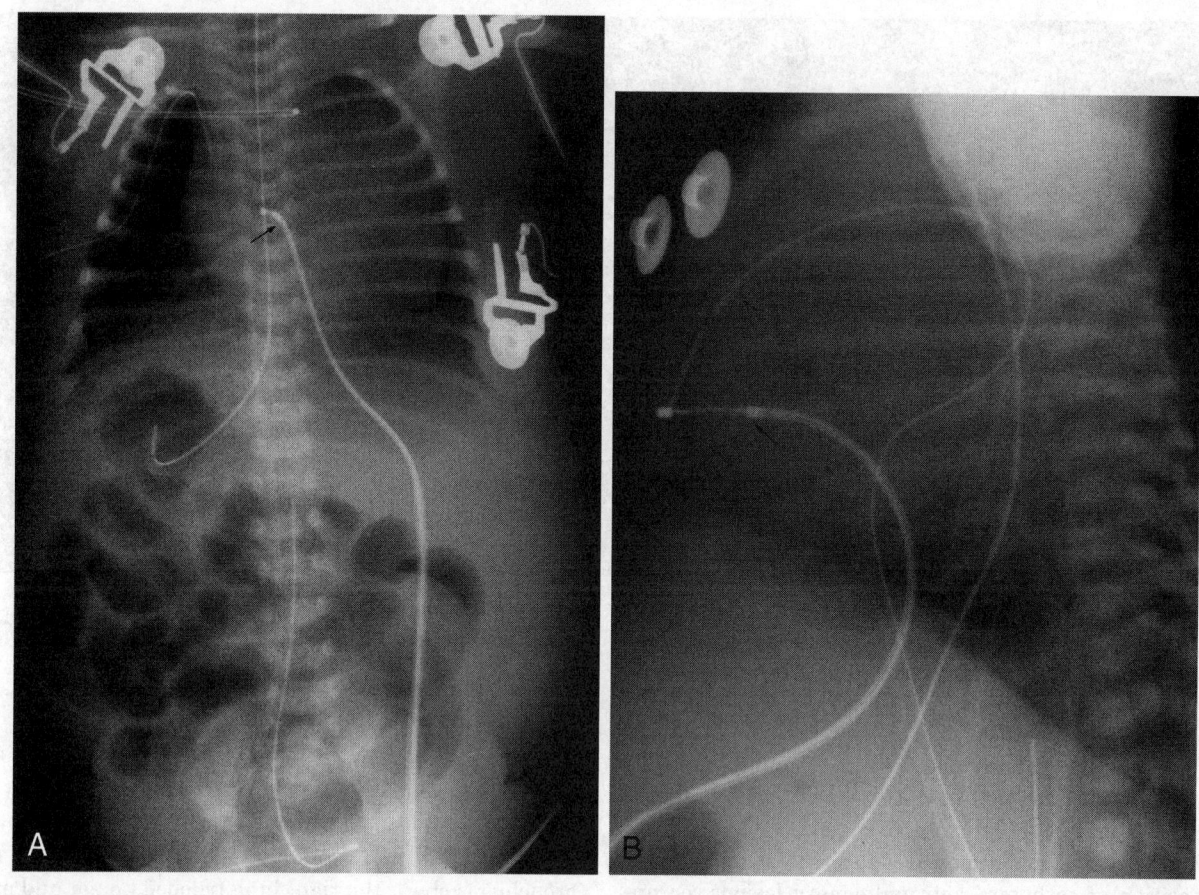

Figure 27.3. **A.** arterior-posterior portable chest in infant with asplenia (situs ambiguous; (**A** and **B**) note levocardia and stomach in right upper quadrant). A right chest tube (*small arrow*) was placed to evacuate a pneumothorax and a temporary cardiac pacing catheter was placed through the umbilicus (*large arrow*). **B.** Cross-table, portable lateral chest, same infant, shows the anterior location of the tips of both the chest tube (*small arrow*) and the pacing catheter (*large arrow*). Without the lateral film, the precise location of the pacing catheter would be difficult to identify with certainty. Also note the unusual catheter course through the umbilical vein; typical for patients with heterotaxy syndrome.

monitoring devices used. A single frontal projection *does not* disclose the anterior-posterior position of a tube. Thus, a cross-table lateral projection is necessary to tell if a given tube lies anteriorly or posteriorly (Fig. 27.3).

TECHNICAL CONSIDERATIONS

In contemporary intensive care units, portable chest films are made in one of two ways: (*a*) by conventional (analogue) techniques, or (*b*) by digital (computed radiographic) techniques (5). The former uses an x-ray beam acting on a film-screen combination in an x-ray cassette to create a direct or analogue image on the film. Computed radiography uses an x-ray beam to create a pattern on special electronic plates within a cassette; a pattern is then "read" by a computer, which, in turn, stores the digital image electronically as well as prints a digital recreation on film, simulating an ordinary (analogue) film (6). Although digital techniques slightly sacrifice detail or resolution, they have the advantage of virtually eliminating repeat x-ray exposures (for reasons of poor technical quality or film loss), and they facilitate the electronic transfer of the images to multiple sites (TV monitors or workstations) simultaneously at any time (5, 7). Potential advantages of digital radiography still to be realized are uniformly reduced x-ray doses and decreased expense (7). However, the trend is toward digital technology and most viewing of "portable films" in the future will be on multibank (TV monitor) workstations within the intensive care unit. These workstations will also be available in doctors' offices, on wards, and in conference rooms, so that the digital images can be reviewed anyplace and anytime. These "peripherally accessible communications systems" (PACS) are now well developed, and they only await price reductions and minor modifications to become commonly used throughout large medical centers and hospitals (7).

Whether analogue or digital, portable films on postoper-

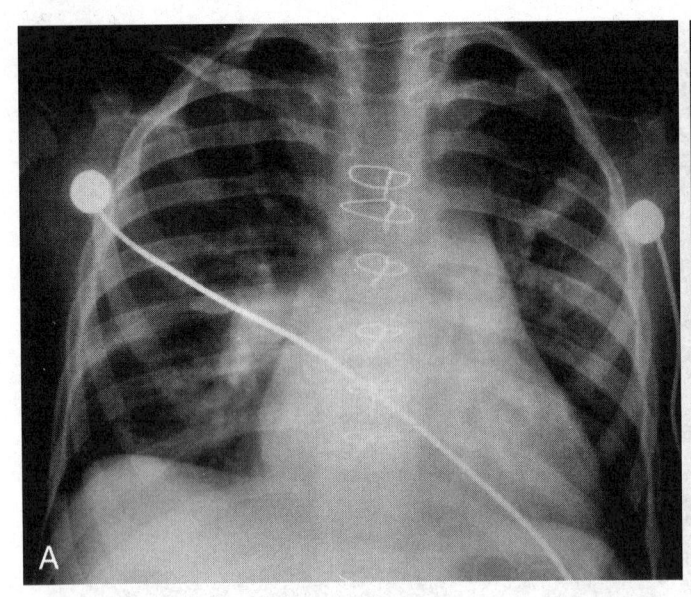

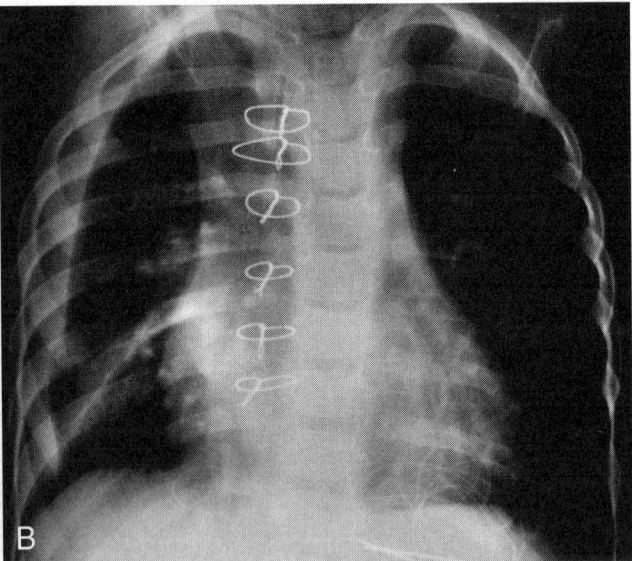

Figure 27.4. A. Frontal postoperative film shows cardiomegaly, patchy atelectasis (**A** and **B**), and is suggestive of right pleural fluid. **B.** Right lateral decubitus (*right side down*) view, same patient, confirms large pleural effusion layered between lung and chest wall.

ative patients are usually obtained in a supine, anterior-posterior (AP) projection. These AP views provide the most information and require minimal radiation exposure (8). Lateral views are sometimes needed for locating the precise position of catheters, intrapulmonary lesions, or unusual pleural fluid accumulations. Cross-table lateral views help define the presence or extent of air in the mediastinum and mediastinal air-fluid levels in suspected mediastinal abscesses. Similarly, lateral decubitus views are used to detect small pneumothoraces and to define the mobility of pleural fluid (Fig. 27.4). Often a tendency is seen to rely day after day on frontal (AP) films alone; when specific questions are not answered by the AP projections, or when the AP films are confusing in some aspect, and one or more lateral views should be obtained.

PREOPERATIVE FILMS AND ASSESSMENT

Preoperative frontal and lateral chest films are the necessary baseline studies for the accurate interpretation of all subsequent postoperative films. The most important aspects of preoperative films are the thoracoabdominal situs, size and shape of the heart, and status of the lungs and pulmonary vasculature (9). Notation of existing calcifications and bony abnormalities should also be made.

SITUS

Situs solitus is the normal or usual position of the thoracoabdominal organs. The bulk of the heart is in the left chest (levocardia), the stomach bubble (a marker of the splenic position) is in the left upper quadrant, and the liver with a large right lobe/small left lobe is in the right upper quadrant (Fig. 27.1). Additionally, the right main stem bronchus is short, the right lung trilobed (major and minor fissures); the left mainstream bronchus long, the left lung bilobed (no minor fissure). The mirror image or reverse of this is situs inversus (dextrocardia, stomach bubble and spleen in the right upper quadrant; left-sided liver having a large left lobe and small right lobe). Airways and lungs are also inverted, short main stem bronchus and minor fissure being left sided. Aortic arch can be right or left sided in both solitus or inversus states as it is not "situs" dependent.

A third possibility, situs ambiguous, exists in association with the heterotaxy syndromes asplenia and polysplenia (see Chapter 18, *Single Ventricle Lesions*). In situs ambiguous, the right and left-sided asymmetry of organogenesis is absent; as a result, the liver is more or less symmetrically lobulated and the spleen is either absent (asplenia) or reduced in volume to multiple small nodules (polysplenia). A stomach can be midline, right or left sided, and the heart position can be levocardia, dextrocardia, or centrally located (mesocardia). The lungs can be either both trilobed (in asplenia: bilateral minor fissures on plain films) or bilobed (Fig. 27.5), or mixed (as in normal). Total anomalous pulmonary venous drainage and univentricular hearts are also common in children who have visceral heterotaxy (10).

In addition to guarding against infectious complications from encapsulated organisms in patients with either as-

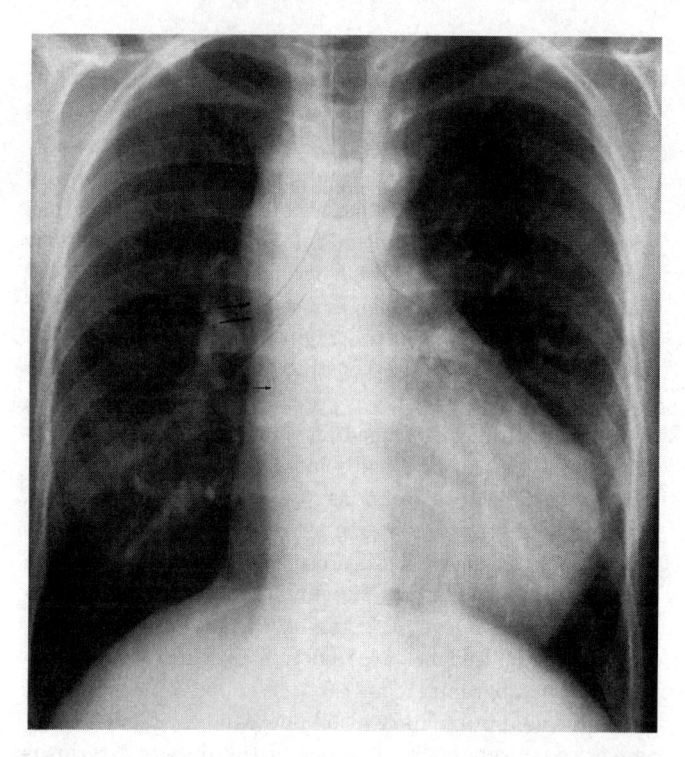

Figure 27.5. Frontal chest film in polysplenia. Enhanced tracheobronchial structures show symmetric (two left main stem) bronchi. Note also a prominent right aortic arch, and lateral to the right descending aorta (*arrow*), a parallel vertical density representing a dilated azygous vein (*double arrows*). Azygous continuation of an (interrupted) inferior vena cava is common in polysplenia.

plenia or polysplenia, intestinal complications such as small bowel obstruction and volvulus must be considered because all children with heterotaxy syndrome have some degree of intestinal malrotation.

CARDIAC SILHOUETTE

Cardiac size is an important piece of information that is most accurately and easily determined from chest films. A more precise estimation of heart size can be made from both frontal and lateral films, in which the inspiratory effort has been satisfactory (on the AP film, diaphragmatic apex at the level of the anterior fifth to sixth ribs, and the posterior ninth to tenth ribs) (11, 12). In newborns, a cardiothoracic ratio of 60% or less is normal; in infants and children, a cardiothoracic ratio of 45% or less. Heart size postoperatively may depend on its preoperative size, in addition to the surgery performed and multiple other postoperative factors. It is therefore necessary to accurately assess the "beginning" heart size. Preoperative shape of the cardiac silhouette is considerably less important than the size, and it will be frequently modified by subsequent surgery in many patients. For example, the thymus may be removed in neonates to aid surgical exposure.

Preoperative notation of the side of the aortic arch and, if right sided, exclusion of a vascular ring (either double aortic arch or right arch with aberrant left subclavian artery) are important (11). Vascular rings can be responsible for postoperative airway problems, particularly following extubation (9). Because of fluid or hematoma in the mediastinum after surgery, vascular rings can be obscured on postoperative films.

LUNGS

Because cardiovascular physiology is largely reflected by the pulmonary vasculature and because airway management is a large part of managing children following surgery for congenital heart disease, preoperative assessment of the pulmonary parenchyma is necessary to provide good postoperative care.

A number of pulmonary abnormalities may be present on preoperative films and cause confusion or additional problems following cardiac surgery. Asymmetry in lung size and perfusion should be noted. For instance, unilateral lung hypoplasia is characteristic of the scimitar syndrome, and it should not be confused with postoperative atelectasis. Similarly, postoperative unilateral pulmonary hypovascularity can be an indication of right or left branch pulmonary stenosis, which is either congenital (present on preoperative films) or iatrogenic (seen only on postoperative films). Most patients having large left-to-right shunts (Qp/Qs ratio greater than 2) frequently have hyperinflated lungs, as the distended pulmonary vessels compress small airways, causing air trapping (see Chapter 23, *Pulmonary Issues*) (13). This hyperinflation usually disappears immediately following surgical correction of the left-to-right shunt, and it should not be confused with postoperative hypoventilation.

Children with Qp/Qs ratios greater than 2 will have detectable vessels in the outer one third of the lungs (on frontal view), and dilation of vessels in the upper lobes so that equilibration is seen in size between upper and lower lobe vessels on films taken in the upright position (in normal patients, lower lobe vessels appear considerably larger on films because of the effect of gravity on pulmonary blood flow) (Fig. 27.6). This "equilibration" of flow is a radiographic sign of a large left-to-right shunt, and it should not be confused with the "redistribution" (constriction of lower lobe vessels and redirection of flow into dilated upper lobe vessels) of blood flow that occurs with pulmonary venous hypertension caused by myocardial dysfunction, mitral stenosis and/or regurgitation, obstructed pulmonary venous return, and other disease states (Fig. 27.7).

Other important factors need to be considered regarding the pulmonary vasculature (11). Enlarged vessels present preoperatively in children having large left-to-right shunts do not decrease or change dramatically in the early postoperative period; also, heart size often remains increased. It often takes many months for the pulmonary vessels and heart size to return to normal radiographically. Pulmonary interstitial edema, however, usually clears on films within the first 3 to 4 postoperative days after the obstruction has been relieved (as in obstructed total anomalous pulmonary venous return), or the volume overload has been corrected (following medical management or repair of a ventricular septal defect [VSD] or mitral regurgitation) (Fig. 27.8).

Unilateral prominence of the pulmonary vascularity may be the result of either a previous palliative procedure to augment pulmonary blood flow, or contralateral pulmonary arterial stenosis. Focally increased pulmonary vascularity can indicate a pulmonary arteriovenous fistula. In patients who have undergone a cavopulmonary shunt, especially the "classic" Glenn procedure, superior vena cava to right pulmonary artery anastomosis, multiple arteriovenous fistulae can develop in the basilar portion of the lung (usually right) and be large enough to cause changes on the chest radiograph (Fig. 27.9).

Diminished pulmonary blood flow can be difficult to recognize radiographically. Patency of the ductus arteriosus or other sources of collateral flow can compensate for severe pulmonary outflow obstruction, causing little alter-

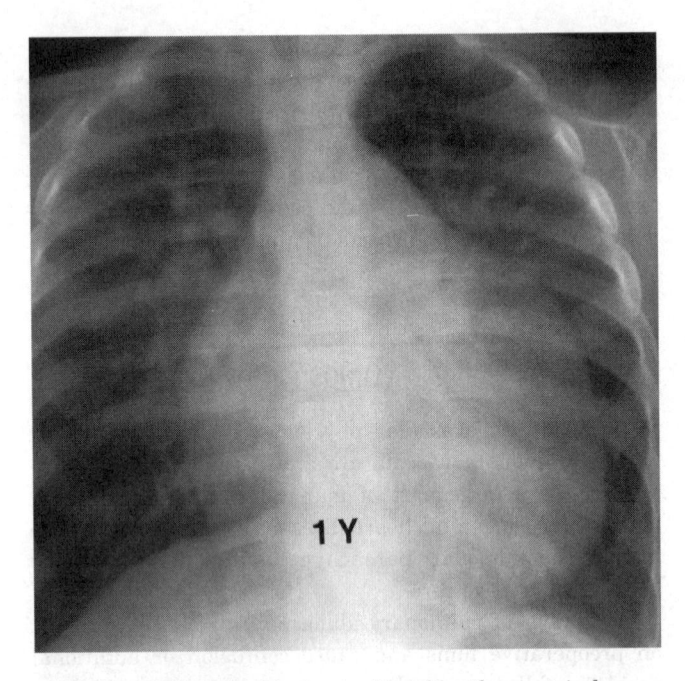

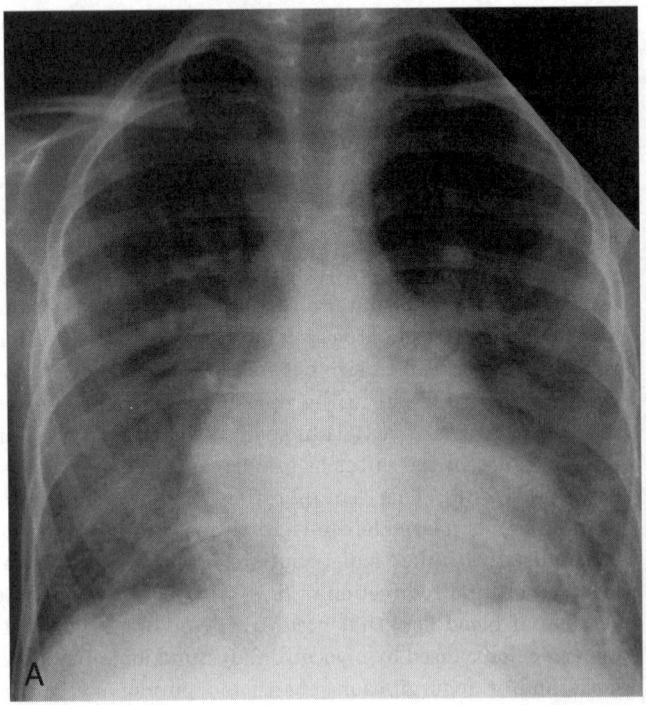

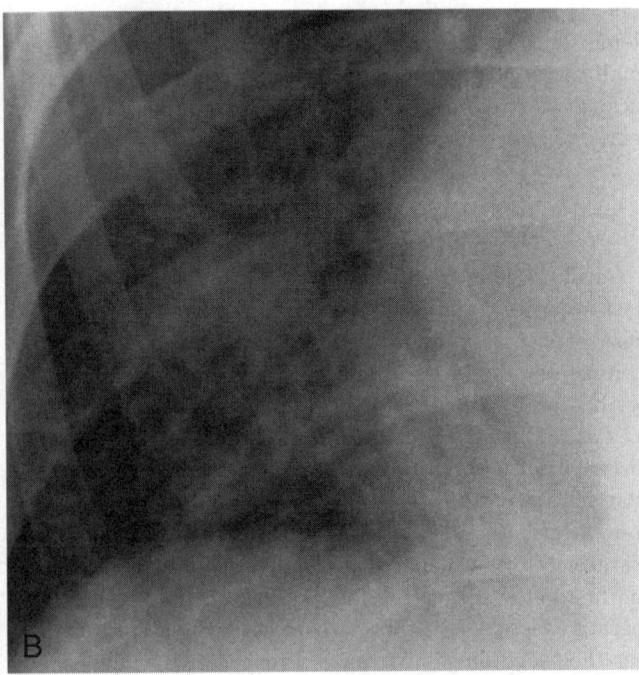

Figure 27.6. Frontal chest in 1-year-old child with a ventricular septal defect. Cardiomegaly is present and the pulmonary vessels are not only diffusely distended, but the upper lobe vessels are as large as the lower lobe vessels ("equilibration" of the shunt volume between the upper and lower lobes). These are signs of a large left-to-right shunt.

Figure 27.7. Frontal chest in 12-year-old with mitral stenosis and regurgitation. **A.** The heart (A and B) is enlarged and there is diffuse interstitial pulmonary edema [best seen as short, linear Kerley B lines in costophrenic sulci (magnified in **27.7B**)]. The upper lobe vessels are distended and the lower lobe vessels are inconspicuous (constricted); this is the pulmonary vascular "redistribution" seen in left atrial (or pulmonary venous) hypertension of any cause.

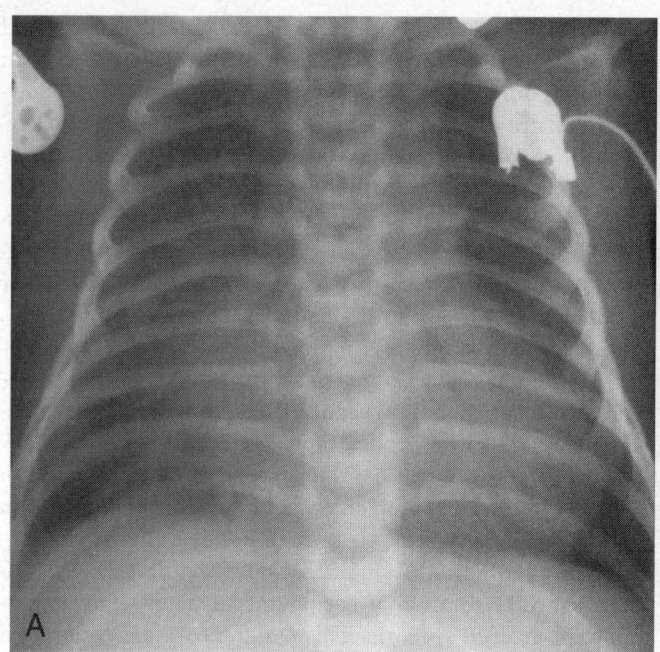

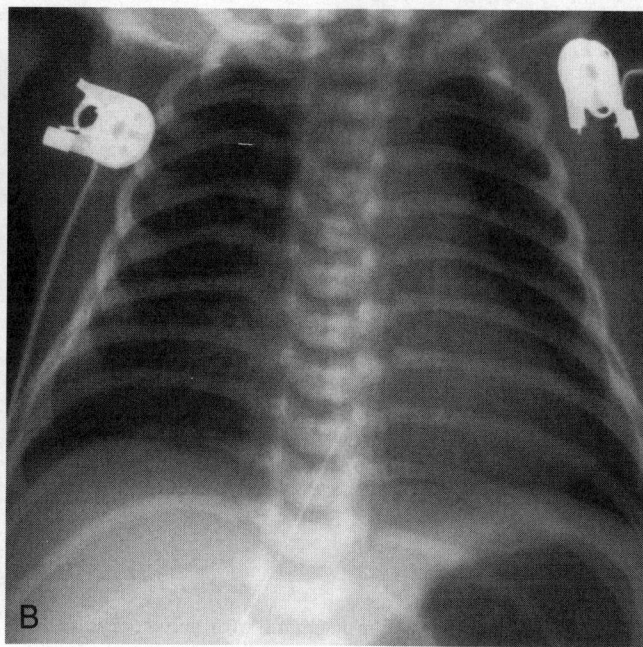

Figure 27.8. **A.** Preoperative frontal chest film in a neonate with symptomatic heart (**A** and **B**) failure because of a large shunt through a patent ductus arteriosus. Cardiomegaly and diffuse pulmonary edema are present. **B.** Postoperative chest film, 5 days after ligation of patent ductus arteriosus. Cardiomegaly has diminished and pulmonary edema has resolved.

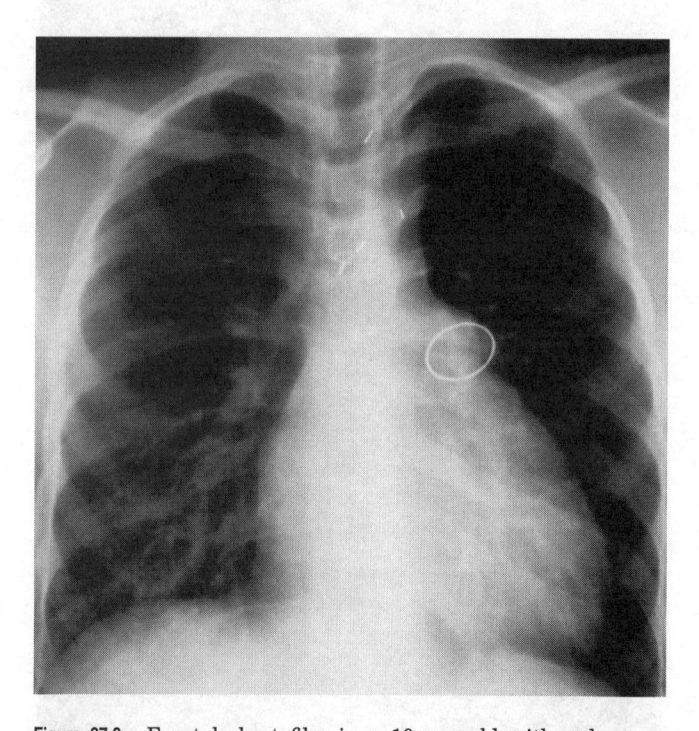

Figure 27.9. Frontal chest film in a 10-year-old with pulmonary atresia and ventricular septal defect. As a child, the patient had a Glenn (superior vena cava to right pulmonary artery) shunt, subsequently converted to a repair using a valved (metallic ring) right ventricular-pulmonary artery conduit. The nodular densities in the right lower lobe are characteristic of diffuse pulmonary arteriovenous fistulae seen in some patients following cavopulmonary anastomoses.

ation in the radiographic pattern of pulmonary vascularity. Lung hyperlucency without increased volume and thin vessels that fade away in the midlung zone can be indications of severely decreased pulmonary blood flow (Fig. 27.10).

CALCIFICATIONS

Sometimes in children between approximately 5 and 15 years old, a 1–2 mm calcification is seen over the proximal descending aorta on frontal chest films, indicating calcification of the ligamentum arteriosum; it excludes the presence of a patent ductus arteriosus. This solitary, pinpoint calcification is different from the multiple, curvilinear calcifications seen in the borders of hilar pulmonary arteries in older children who have longstanding pulmonary artery hypertension. Large plaques of cutaneous, pleural, or mediastinal calcification are usually iatrogenic and usually represent an extravasation of fluid containing high concentrations of calcium. In children having had previous right ventricular to pulmonary artery conduits, dense, irregular calcification of the conduit homograft may be seen in the retrosternal space (Fig. 27.11). Considerably less frequently, right ventricular outflow patches and even material used to close VSDs can calcify, typically without clinical significance.

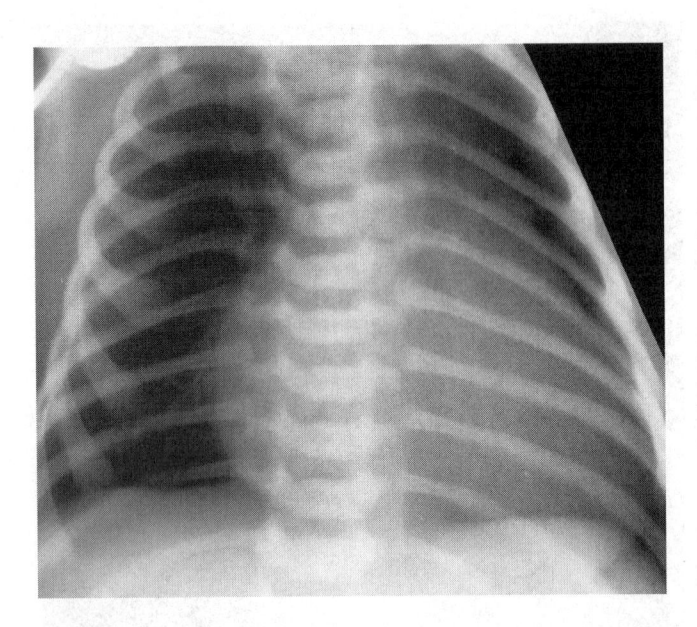

Figure 27.10. Frontal chest film in infant with pulmonary atresia and intact ventricular septum and a small patent ductus arteriosus. Severe cardiomegaly (from tricuspid regurgitation) is present and the lungs are oligemic (few vessels of decreased size).

BONY THORAX

Several thoracic osseous deformities are associated with congenital heart disease, such as the high incidence of scoliosis in cyanotic congenital heart disease and the rib notching that can accompany tetralogy of Fallot (collateral flow to oligemic lungs) or thoracic coarctation (collaterals to the descending aorta) (11). Butterfly vertebrae are associated with pulmonary stenosis in arteriohepatic dysplasia (Alagile's syndrome), and vertebral defects can seen in the VACTERL association (see Chapter 12, *Preoperative Care*). Iatrogenic abnormalities can result from previous thoracotomies (irregular cortical bone along rib margins), previous sternotomies (retrosternal soft tissue thickening, and wire sutures in the sternum itself), or long-term prostaglandin therapy, which causes generalized periosteal clavicle and rib thickening.

POSTCATHETERIZATION ASSESSMENT

Postcatheterization chest films are not routinely done in most institutions, although a rare exception may be in those patients in whom wedge pulmonary vein injections have been done to provide retrograde opacification of atretic pulmonary arteries. These wedge injections can leave segmental stains in the pulmonary parenchyma (Fig. 27.12), which signify interstitial extravasation of contrast material and represent an infarction of the involved lung parenchyma. Chest pain, pleural effusion, and mild hemoptysis can be a result of this complication.

Cardiac catheterizations, which include interventional procedures, are more likely to have sequelae visible on postprocedure chest films. For this reason, routine follow-up films are often obtained for several days following therapeutic catheter procedures (see Chapter 29, *Cardiac Catheterization in the Critically Ill Cardiac Patient*).

Coil embolization, most commonly used to occlude systemic-pulmonary artery collateral vessels and Blalock-Taussig shunts, is clearly visible on chest films. Number and location of these coils should be compared from film to film to ensure stable positioning.

Dilation of branch pulmonary arterial stenoses is a frequent interventional procedure that can have sequelae detectable on chest radiographs. Unilateral pulmonary edema lasting several hours or days can follow dilation of right or left branch pulmonary arteries. This overperfusion phenomenon is typically transient and usually without significant morbidity. A more serious finding is lobar infarction after dilation of peripheral lobar or segment pulmonary arterial stenosis. This can indicate dissection of a

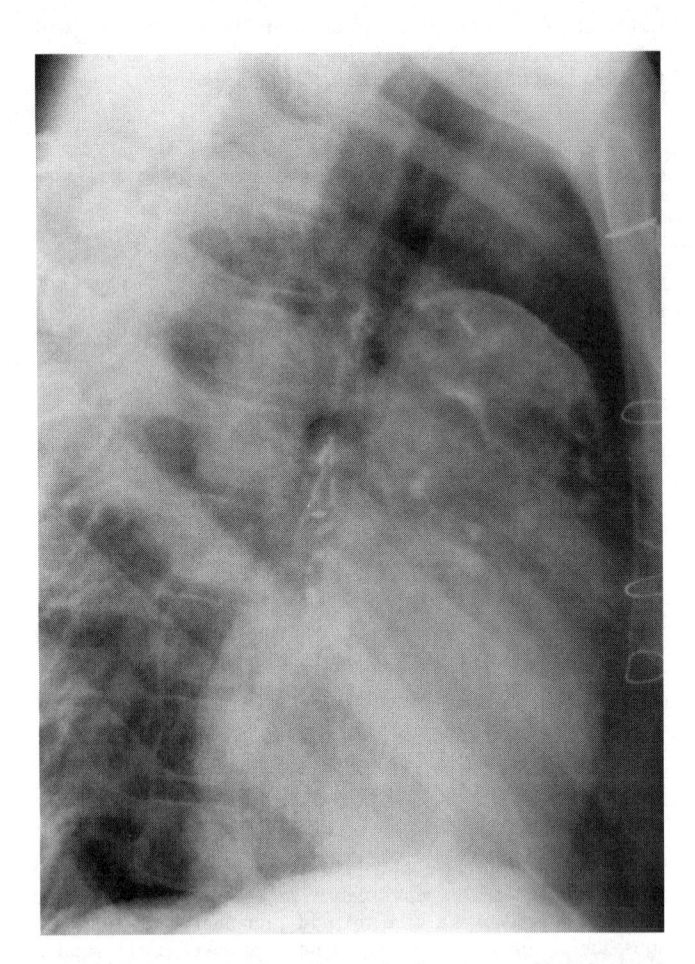

Figure 27.11. Lateral chest radiograph of a 14-year-old with tetralogy of Fallot who underwent repair utilizing a right ventricle to pulmonary artery homograft. Dense, retrosternal calcification is seen within the homograft.

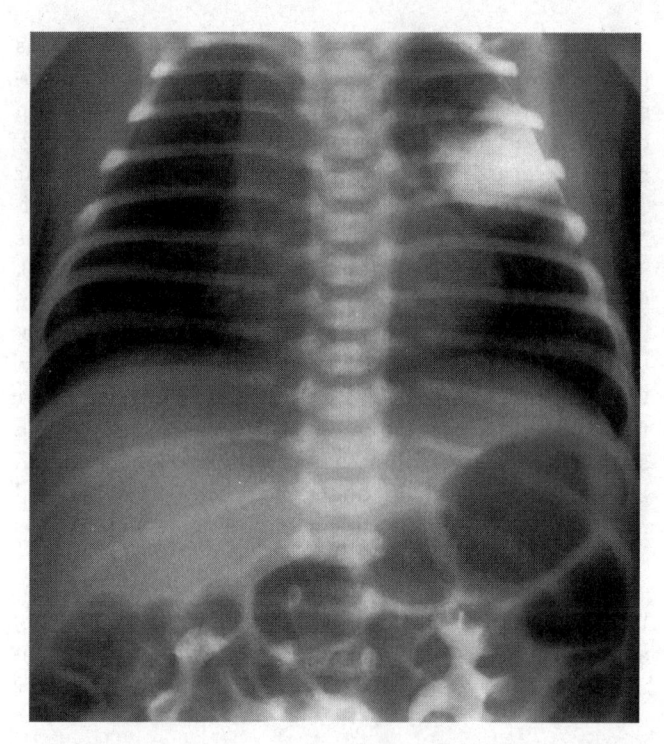

Figure 27.12. A 3-month-old infant with left pulmonary artery atresia. Postcatheterization chest film shows "stain" of contrast material in the parenchyma of the left upper lobe following a pulmonary venous wedge injection. This local extravasation of contrast media typically clears in 24 to 48 hours. A typical postcatheterization nephrogram can also be seen.

large pulmonary artery, which can hemorrhage, possibly fatally. Signs of pulmonary infarction and intraparenchymal bleeding on the chest radiographs include sudden opacification of a segment or lobe, sometimes associated with pleural fluid (transudate or blood), and often accompanied by chest pain and hemoptysis. Such findings may be indications for either urgent recatheterization or surgical pulmonary lobectomy.

Dilation of native or recurrent (postoperative) aortic coarctation can be complicated early by local hemorrhage and later by aneurysm formation. Signs for both will be a large left upper mediastinal mass on plain films; differentiation of hemorrhage from an aneurysm is possible when blood can be seen accumulating over the apex of the left lung, or when the mass increases rapidly in the first 24 to 28 hours after the procedure.

POSTOPERATIVE RADIOGRAPHIC ASSESSMENT

Radiographic evaluation of the chest plays an important role in clinical assessment and management in the immediate postoperative period, and it provides physiologic as well as anatomic information. Despite technical limitations imposed by the requirements of intensive care and the urgency of the situation, careful consideration is necessary to derive the most information.

CARDIAC SIZE AND BLOOD VOLUME

Although a radiograph is a display of the gross anatomy, physiologic implications exist to the size, shape, and position of the various organs. For example, a small heart size may imply diminished circulating blood volume, whereas an increasing heart size may correlate with intravascular fluid overload, pericardial effusion, valvular regurgitation, or impaired myocardial contractility. Before any conclusions about heart size can be drawn, the degree of pulmonary inflation, which greatly influences the transverse dimension of the cardiac shadow on the supine frontal projection, should be considered. Hyperinflation of the lungs diminishes heart size and underinflation (or an end-expiration film) accentuates it. Accurate comparison of one chest film to another requires that differences in lung inflation be carefully considered.

Heart and mediastinum positions are also affected by differences in the volumes of the right and left hemithoraces. For example, complete atelectasis of one lung or the surgical absence of a lung will cause the heart to shift toward that side. Similarly, lung opacification for any reason can obscure the cardiac margins to such an extent that an assessment of cardiac size cannot be determined. This is often the case in patients placed on extracorporeal membrane oxygenation (ECMO), wherein conventional ventilation of the lungs may be temporarily discontinued (see Chapter 22, *Mechanical Support of the Myocardium*).

Abdomen

Abdominal sequelae and complications of cardiothoracic surgery are unusual, but they include inadvertent insertion of drainage tubes or lines through the peritoneum, feeding tube malposition, ascites, and most seriously, necrotizing enterocolitis (NEC). Peritoneal insertion of drainage tubes can be manifest by the presence of a small pneumoperitoneum noted in the epigastric region on a supine radiograph. This is usually not a serious problem, and it most often resolves without treatment.

Radiopaque enteric tube position is easily determined radiographically. Failure to insert the tube fully into the stomach or tube buckling at the esophagogastric junction prevents adequate gastric drainage. Attempted feeding of large boluses through a tube that is not in the stomach can result in aspiration. On rare occasions, these tubes can be inserted into the trachea and parallel to the endotracheal tube.

Plain supine abdominal radiograph is insensitive in detecting small amounts of ascites, which are more easily detected by sonography performed at the bedside. Large amounts of intraperitoneal fluid will cause bulging of the flanks accompanied by centralization of gas within the floating bowel loops. Ascitic fluid composition is, of course, indeterminate radiographically.

One of the more frustrating clinical problems is NEC development. This complication typically occurs in neonates with unrecognized duct-dependent systemic blood flow in whom the ductus arteriosus begins to constrict, or neonates who have undergone extensive, complex reconstructive surgery, typically with the use of deep hypothermic circulatory arrest (14) (see Chapter 12, *Preoperative Care* and Chapter 18, *Single Ventricle Lesions*). This presumed ischemic insult to the bowel can be the result of a preceding or persistent low perfusion state (15). Often a "grace" period occurs during which the patient shows no sign or symptoms, only to present 48 to 72 hours later with distension, ileus, and gastrointestinal bleeding. In its worst form, this can progress to frank bowel necrosis, perforation, peritonitis, disseminated intravascular coagulopathy, sepsis, and death. Unfortunately, the earliest radiographic signs of generalized gaseous distension and slight separation of adjacent bowel loops can be nonspecific. Gas presence within the bowel wall, referred to as "pneumatosis intestinalis," is a more specific sign, but it is often transient and not a reliable indication of severity or prognosis. Because stool within the bowel lumen has a similar "bubbly" appearance, it can mimic pneumatosis intestinalis. Rings of gas surrounding a bowel loop or lines of gas parallel to a loop are better radiologic signs (Fig. 27.13). Overt free intraperitoneal air signifies bowel perforation, but decubitus views or a supine cross-table lateral projection may be necessary to detect small amounts of free air. One must be careful not to misinterpret dissection of air from a pneumomediastinum into the peritoneal cavity as a sign of NEC. Gas within the portal venous system (Fig. 27.13) is another helpful, but often transient, sign of bowel ischemia, which can be associated with a worse prognosis (16, 17).

Bowel obstruction secondary to other congenital anomalies is unusual in children with congenital heart disease, although, as a general rule, infants born with one congenital anomaly have a greater risk for having another. For

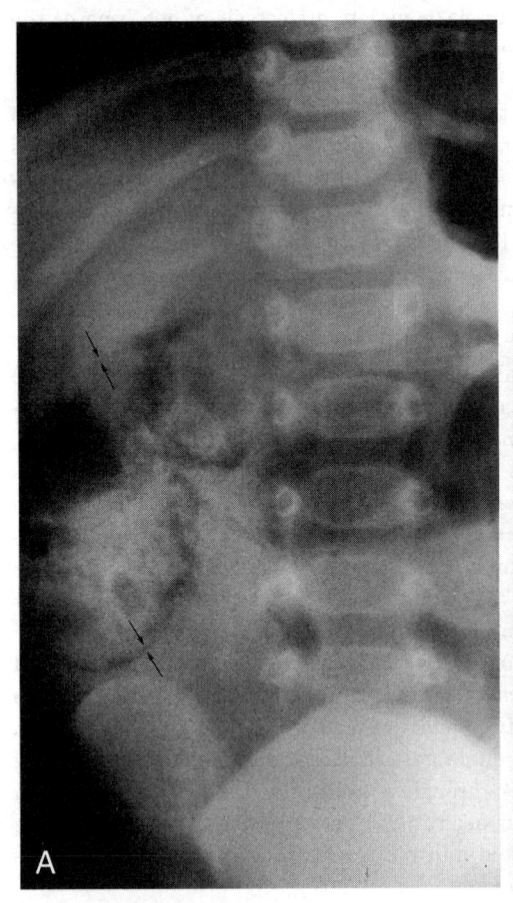

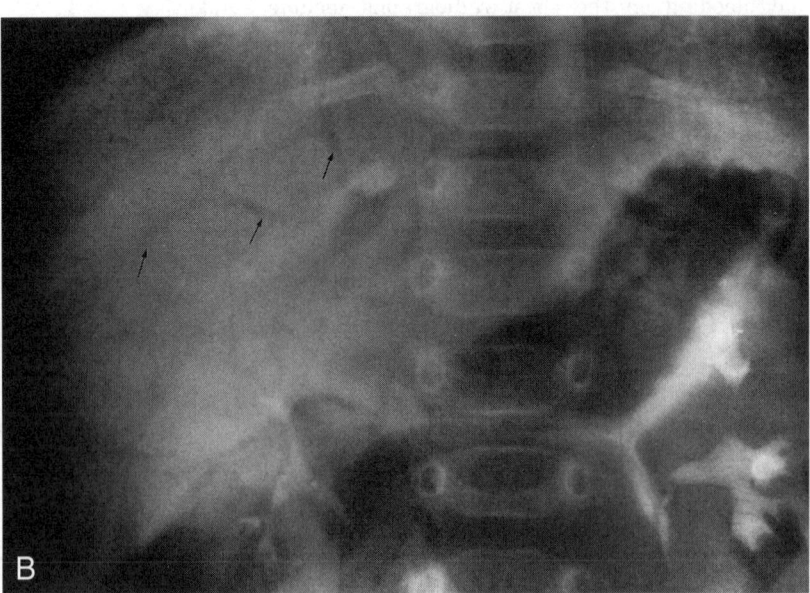

Figure 27.13. **A.** Supine abdominal film in an infant with hypoplastic left heart syndrome (**A** and **B**). Distinct intramural gas (pneumatosis intestinalis) (*arrows*) is seen in the ascending colon and hepatic flexure, which is indicative of necrotizing enterocolitis (*NEC*). **B.** Abdominal film 1 day later shows another manifestation of *NEC*, portal venous gas (*arrows*).

example, infants with trisomy 21 may have duodenal obstruction or colonic aganglionosis, in addition to congenital heart disease. Because repair of many cardiac defects is safely performed early in infancy, it is important that these newborns undergo a prompt and comprehensive assessment prior to operative repair to avoid unexpected postoperative complications. Patients with heterotaxy syndromes are also at risk for postoperative volvulus because of associated malattachment of the mesentery that accompanies asplenia and polysplenia (see above).

THORAX

The surgical incision itself can have radiographic manifestations that are of interest. Lateral thoracotomies always cause some detectable alteration in the relative position of the ribs as compared with the normal opposite side (Fig. 27.1). Old, healed thoracotomies can cause posterior fusion of the ribs. Unilateral rib notching can occur following thoracotomy in patients who have undergone palliative shunt procedures to enhance pulmonary blood flow. Whereas this was originally described as a consequence of the Blalock-Taussig procedure and attributed to collateral vessels supplying blood flow to the ipsilateral arm, it is now clear that this phenomenon represents an attempt to provide additional transpleural blood to the under-perfused lung via pleural adhesions created at the time of the original thoracotomy. This can be an important preoperative consideration when contemplating a second thoracotomy because of the greater risk of bleeding.

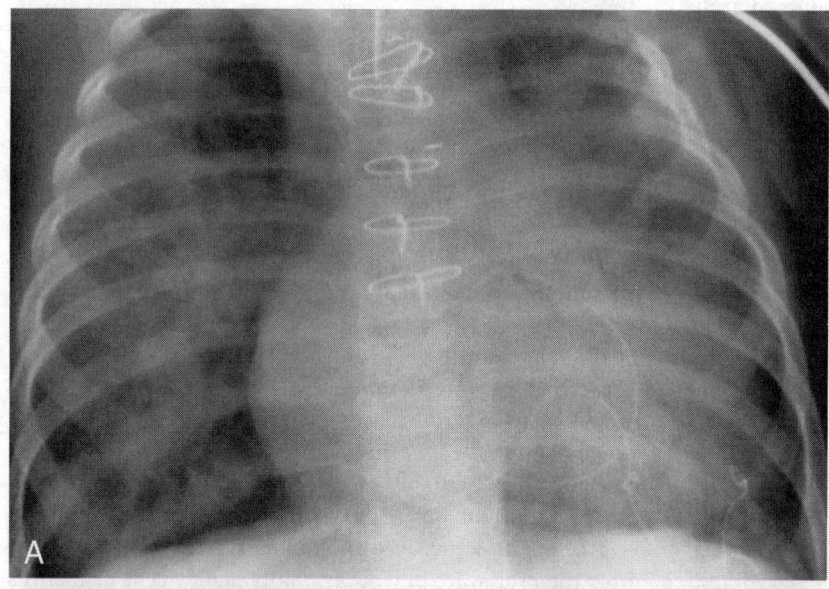

Figure 27.14. **A.** Postoperative supine chest film shows (**A** and **B**) air radiolucency sharply marginating the right mediastinal and cardiac borders, and extending over the hilum and medial aspect of the right lung, which is characteristic of a pneumothorax on supine films. **B.** Same patient following resolution of the pneumothorax.

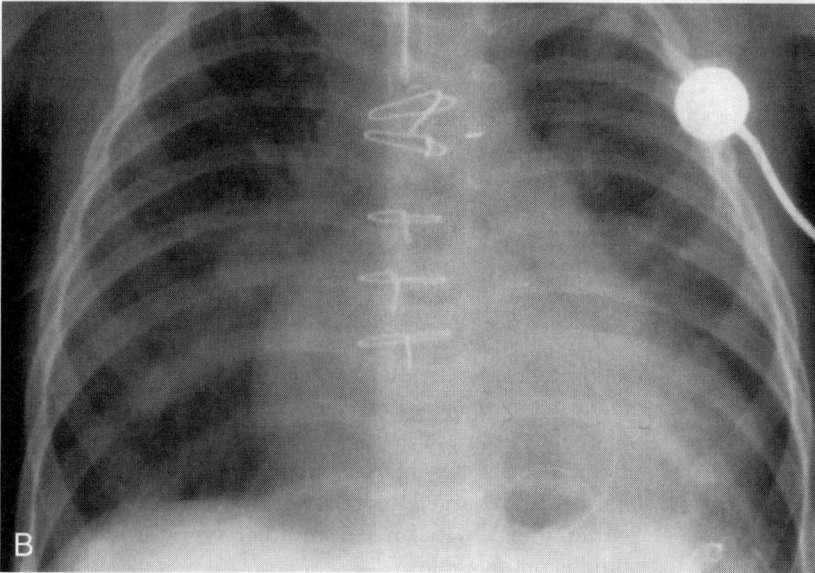

On occasion the surgeon may decide that primary closure of the median sternotomy is inadvisable and will close the incision with a sterile membrane. This is usually not apparent radiographically except for the recognition of mediastinal widening and subtle separation and lateral displacement of the medial ends of the clavicles. Likewise, a vertical band of lucency superimposed on the midchest can represent mild depression of the anterior chest wall at the incision site. Finally, presence of intracardiac catheters without sternal wires suggests recent surgery with delayed sternal closure.

Wound infection is usually impossible to detect on the frontal radiograph. Persistent soft tissue swelling and persistent gas behind the sternum on lateral radiographs are suspicious signs of wound infection (18). Contrast enhanced computed tomography is often helpful in defining a drainable fluid collection under these circumstances.

Pneumothorax is an infrequent occurrence immediately following median sternotomy, but it is more common after lateral thoracotomy. In the supine position small amounts of air will collect medially and inferiorly because these are the highest portions of the pleural space (Fig. 27.14). Extension of air laterally and inferiorly into a costophrenic sulcus has been termed the "deep sulcus" sign. Air surrounding the lung apex and extending inferiorly and laterally is usually noted when the patient is in the upright or semierect position. Diagnosis of tension pneumothorax should be suggested when a shift of the mediastinum toward the opposite side is seen, or when the ipsilateral hem-

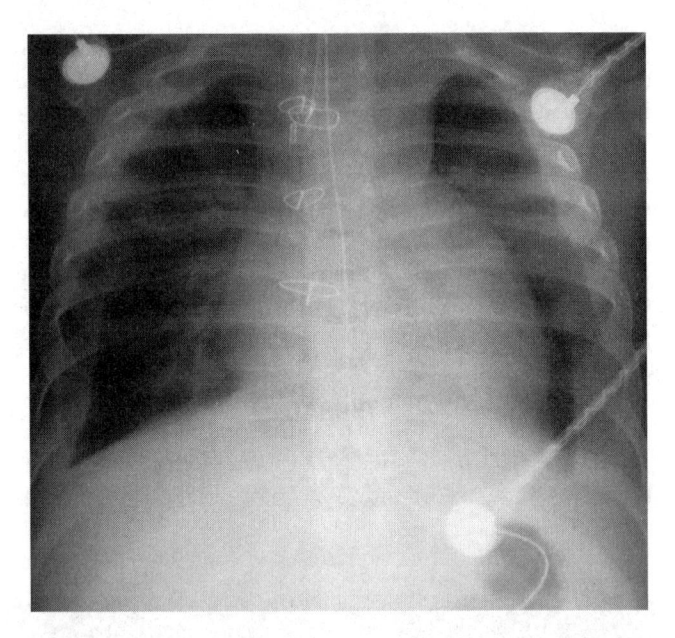

Figure 27.16. Frontal chest film 1 week after completion of Fontan operation. Large, bilateral pleural effusions are seen. Subsegmental atelectasis, probably compression from surrounding pleural fluid, is prominent in the right upper lobe and left lower lobe (behind the heart).

idiaphragm is markedly depressed and flattened (Fig. 27.15).

Fluid can develop within the pleural space for a variety of reasons. Elevated systemic venous pressure is likely to be associated with pleural effusions and, although a venous-lymphatic mechanism is postulated, the exact mechanism is probably more complex. Following the Fontan procedure or one of its modifications, pleural effusion is a common occurrence that usually starts several days after the procedure and occasionally lasts weeks or months (19) (Figs. 27.16, 27.17) (see Chapter 18, *Single Ventricle Lesions*). In young children, these effusions often collect in the subpulmonic position, although they are not "loculated" or restricted to that region. If allowed to go untreated, they can fill the entire pleural space. Recent work has suggested that performance of the procedure in two stages, partial exclusion of the hepatic venous drainage from the blood flow that goes directly to the lungs, or fenestration of the intra-atrial baffle are maneuvers that may lessen the severity and morbidity of the effusions (20).

Chylothorax is an infrequent complication in children following cardiovascular surgery, but it has been reported following various operations, typically surgery involving the aortic arch and following cavopulmonary connections. Delayed onset of symptoms can occur long after the patient has been discharged from the hospital. Radiographic differentiation of chylothorax from other types of intrapleural fluid is not possible.

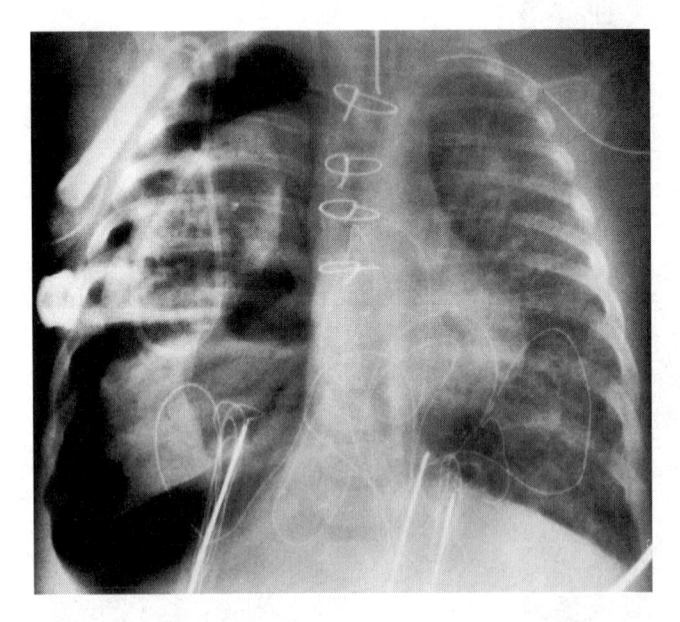

Figure 27.15. Postoperative right tension pneumothorax. The signs of elevated intrapleural pressure are collapse of the right lung, shift of the heart and mediastinum to the left, widened right intercostal spaces, and depression of the right hemidiaphragm.

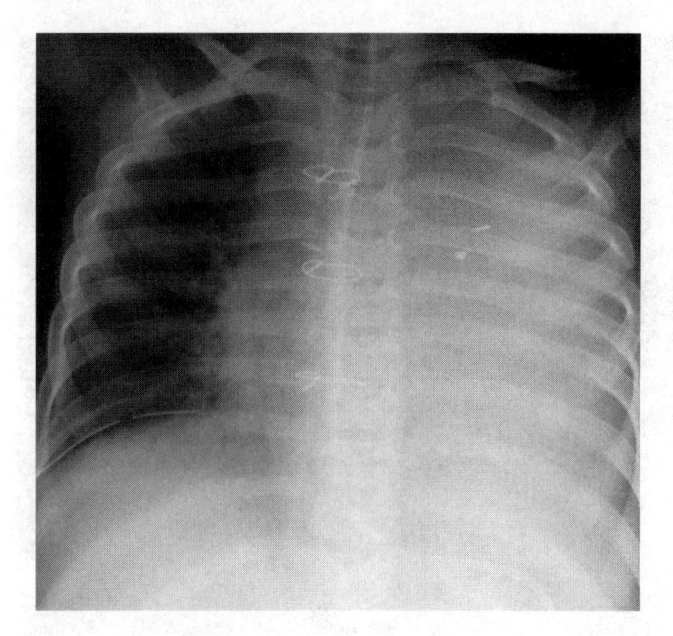

Figure 27.17. Frontal chest film 2 weeks after Fontan operation. The left chest is opacified by pleural fluid that has caused collapse of the left lung and shift of the heart and mediastinum to the right. A right chest tube is present at the right lung base.

AIRWAY AND LUNGS

Evaluation of the lungs includes consideration of the degree of general and regional pulmonary inflation. In the intubated patient, small lung volumes can be the result of insufficient mechanical ventilation instead of intrinsic lung disease. Similarly, hyperinflation can be iatrogenic rather than an indication of pathologic air trapping. Endotracheal tube position in mechanically ventilated patients is also critical: if the tube is placed too far into the tracheobronchial tree, one lung or lobe may not be adequately aerated; if the tube is situated too high it can become dislodged. It is also important to realize that with the tube affixed to the patient's face, as the neck is extended the tip of the endotracheal tube will rise superiorly, and conversely, as the patient's neck is flexed in the chin-to-chest position, the tip of the tube will move downward into the trachea or main bronchi (21).

Atelectasis caused by inspissation of mucus within a segmental bronchus is common. Collapse of one or more segments or lobes can also be the result of extrinsic compression by adjacent organs or fluid collections. Large pleural effusions typically cause this type of atelectasis (Fig. 27.17). The difference between "pneumonia" (i.e., infection) and atelectasis is not always evident based on a single radiograph. Change in radiography over time, as well as clinical parameters, strongly influences the diagnosis. Atelectasis can be diagnosed when clear volume loss is seen in a lobe or segment. As a group, patients with trisomy 21 with large left-to-right shunts have a higher frequency of both atelectasis and pneumonia. In these patients, the left lower and right middle lobes are most frequently affected. Aspiration, usually affecting the right upper and left lower lobes, can also be a cause of atelectasis or pneumonia in any patient.

Radiographic assessment of the lungs is not complete without consideration of "lung water content" or the presence or absence of pulmonary edema. Although many causes of pulmonary edema other than "congestive heart failure" exist, the net result of increased lung water has similar radiographic findings in most cases. Blurring of vessel margins within the lung and increased overall lung density, especially in the perihilar regions, are typical radiographic signs. Kerley B lines at the lung periphery indicate increased fluid within lymphatics of the subpleural interlobular septi (Fig. 27.7), but they are rarely seen in infants and children. Because the distribution of lung water is influenced by gravity, patient position determines where the edema is most severe. As demonstrated by CT, in the supine position, the lung bases (i.e., lower lobes) and dependent portions of the upper lobes will be most affected. Pulmonary hemorrhage can mimic edema or pneumonia, but its distribution tends to be less dependent on gravity.

Transient paralysis of diaphragmatic contraction has been reported in as many as 10% of patients who have had open heart surgery (22–25). While the patient remains on mechanical ventilation this dysfunction is usually not apparent, as minute ventilation is controlled and radiographs are taken during the inspiratory phase of the ventilator. However, the patient can have increased work of breathing once support is lowered or discontinued (see Chapter 23, *Pulmonary Issues*). Although under normal circumstances the hemidiaphragm on the side of the cardiac apex tends to be slightly lower than the opposite side, when this discrepancy is exaggerated or reversed, diaphragmatic dysfunction should be considered (Fig. 27.18). Such an appearance can also be caused by a unilateral subpulmonic effusion, or to unequal hemithoracic volumes in patients who have undergone previous lateral thoracotomies.

Progressive difficulty in ventilation because of decreased lung compliance in the absence of a cardiovascular factor may result from the so-called "acute respiratory distress syndrome" (ARDS). This acquired abnormality has been attributed to damage to the pneumocytes from a variety of causes including local hypoxia, infection, and other noxious agents that lead to depletion of surfactant and loss of lung compliance. Radiographic signs include progressive decrease in overall lung volume associated with a diffuse, homogeneous increase in lung density (often inappropriately described as "ground glass") and the presence of air bronchograms. Pleural effusions are not part of the radiographic pattern. Because of the difficulty in mechanical ventilation and ensuing hypoxemia and hypercarbia, increased pressures are often employed, which can lead to

Figure 27.18. Frontal chest film in an infant following repair of tetralogy of Fallot. An abnormality of right diaphragmatic function is suggested by elevation of the right hemidiaphragm and discoid atelectasis throughout the right lung, whereas the (functioning) left diaphragm is depressed and the left lung hyperinflated. Confirmation of unilateral diaphragmatic paresis (lack of motion) or paralysis (paradoxic motion) requires either fluoroscopic or ultrasonic demonstration.

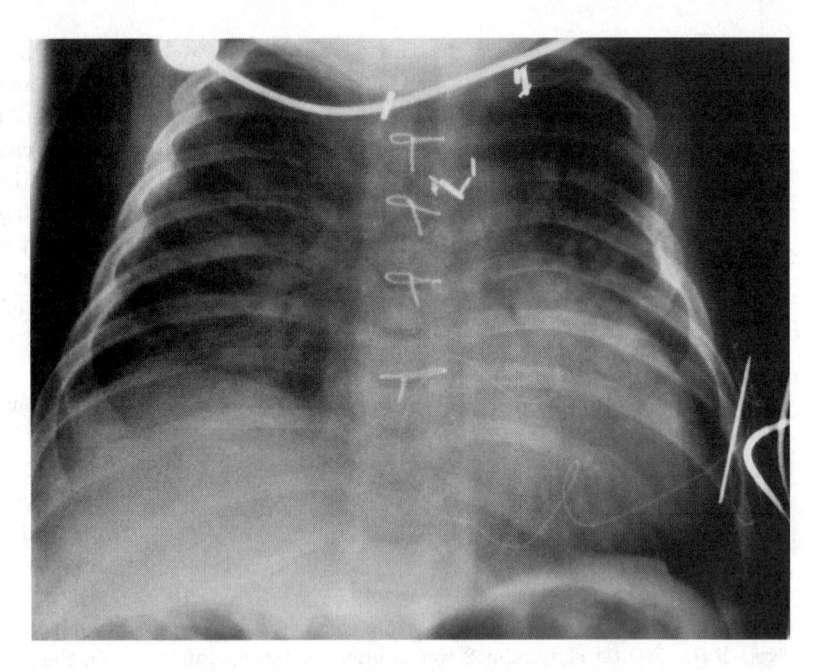

such "air-block" phenomena as pneumomediastinum, pneumothorax, pneumopericardium, pneumoperitoneum, and subcutaneous emphysema (discussed in a following section).

HEART AND GREAT VESSELS

Heart size on postoperative films depends on its preoperative size, intravascular blood volume following surgery, surgery performed and its effect on hemodynamics and myocardial function, and on bleeding or other fluid accumulations around the heart. In general, the first postoperative film taken within hours of surgery shows a heart smaller than preoperatively, typically because of hypovolemia, an acute reduction in the volume work of the heart (e.g., elimination of a large left-to-right shunt), and the effects of positive pressure ventilation. Characteristically, the heart is usually larger or "enlarged" on subsequent films after volume replacement and a reduction in mechanical ventilation. Creation of surgical systemic-to-pulmonary shunts invariably causes persistent cardiomegaly, whereas performance of cavopulmonary anastomosis (and its variations) typically is accompanied by little change or by an actual decrease in heart size on plain films (26). Persistent and severe postoperative cardiomegaly raises the possibility of several complications, most frequently overhydration or blood replacement, residual volume overload, pericardial effusion, valvular regurgitation, or myocardial dysfunction. Despite removal of the pericardium during most surgical procedures, hematomas can accumulate next to and around the heart, and they may simulate a hemopericardium. Mediastinal bleeding adjacent to the heart can occur when transthoracic intracardiac monitoring lines are removed. Pulmonary monitoring lines have a higher complication rate than atrial lines (27).

Pericardial effusions can simulate cardiac enlargement on plain films, but this complication typically occurs weeks to months postoperatively, not in the first few days. Postoperative pericardial effusion is rarely an isolated complication; it usually occurs along with pleural effusions following the Fontan procedure or in the postpericardiotomy syndrome. On single postoperative chest films, pericardial effusions, hemopericardium, and cardiomegaly appear similar; it is the rate of development that is differentiating. Hemopericardium usually develops in hours, pericardial effusion over days or weeks, and an enlarging heart caused by myocardial dysfunction over weeks to months.

Pneumopericardium (Fig. 27.19) is usually a transient phenomenon caused by air being trapped during the surgical procedure, and therefore it is seen in the first few postoperative days only. Persistence beyond 48 or 72 hours should signal a search for an air leak in the mediastinum.

Intravascular or intracardiac air is rarely detected on chest films, but it should always be looked for over the liver as a sign of necrotizing enterocolitis. Large bubbles of gas within the mediastinal great vessels or within cardiac chambers are invariably iatrogenic (associated with vigorous resuscitation), and they are usually a radiographic sign of impending death.

MEDIASTINUM

Pneumomediastinum is detectable as streaky, radiolucencies in the upper mediastinum that often extend into the soft tissues of the neck and upper thorax (subcutane-

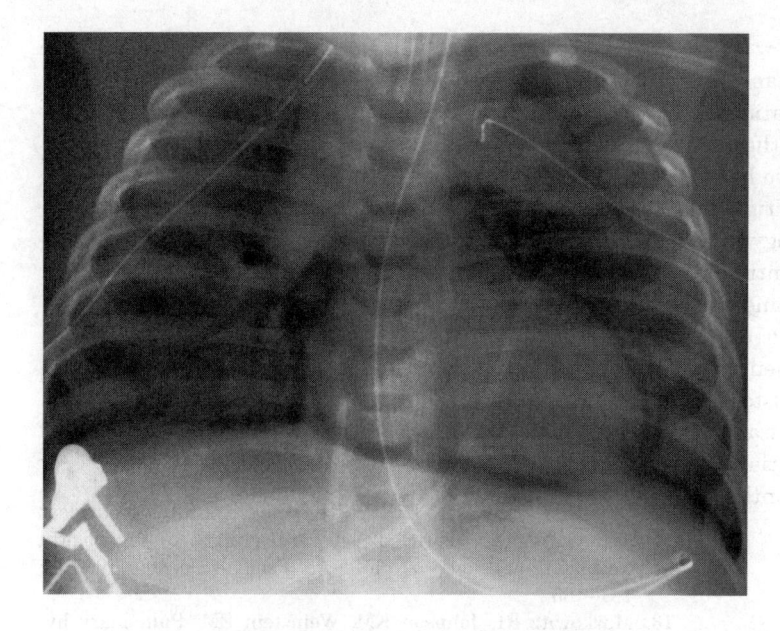

Figure 27.19. An infant with unoperated ventricular septal defect and congestive heart failure receiving preoperative mechanical ventilation. Bilateral chest tubes have been inserted for pneumothoraces (still present at lung apices). Additionally seen are pneumomediastinum (air outlines and elevates thymus, causing distinct, bilateral "sail signs") and a pneumopericardium (air silhouettes the heart and the thin left pericardium itself). A thin, small pericardial drainage tube is projected over the heart.

ous emphysema). It is usually caused by the retrograde dissection of air from overdistended or overventilated lungs along the pulmonary interstitium to the mediastinum, and (infrequently) along pulmonary vessels to the pericardium. Despite measures to alter ventilatory support at that point, air extension from the mediastinum into the abdomen (dissecting inferiorly from the mediastinum into the retroperitoneum) and from thoracic soft tissues into the abdominal wall are common. Such extension should not be mistaken for bowel rupture causing pneumoperitoneum.

Occasionally the mediastinum is narrower on postoperative films than it was preoperatively, usually because much of the thymus has been excised and the lungs are overinflated. Alternatively, the mediastinum can be widened postoperatively because the heart and great vessels have been altered, incised, patched, and otherwise changed, resulting in dilation, contour alteration, or blood and other fluid accumulation in their proximity. For instance, following Norwood palliation (26) in hearts having a single ventricle, the superior left mediastinum is often much more prominent because of the arch reconstruction and associated hematoma. Rapid (8 to 24 hours) and progressive mediastinal widening usually indicates ongoing postoperative bleeding, and it can be an indication for reoperation.

Aneurysms and pseudoaneurysms are additional causes of postoperative mediastinal and pericardiac masses. True

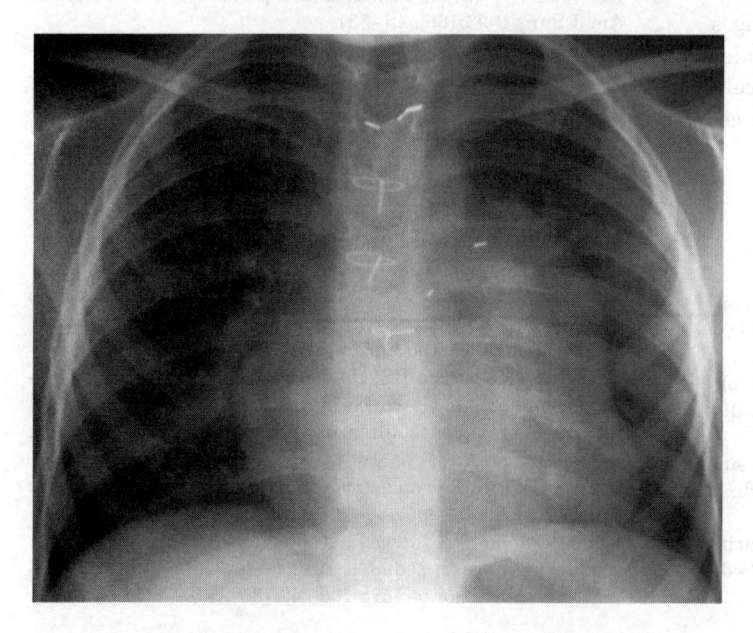

Figure 27.20. Frontal chest film 1 year after repair of tetralogy of Fallot in a 3-year-old. Generalized cardiomegaly and a prominent bulging of the right ventricular outflow tract patch are seen at the left upper cardiac border.

aneurysms (ballooning of the entire wall of an artery or cardiac chamber) are rare, but they can occur, for instance, in the left mediastinum after repair of aortic coarctation. Ultrasonography or other imaging is necessary in these cases to differentiate such a mass from a postoperative hematoma. Postoperative masses in the region of the right ventricular outflow tract following repair for tetralogy of Fallot can be caused by either dilation of the right ventricular patch material (Fig. 27.20) (28) or by a pseudoaneurysm of the patch (a leak at its margin causing an expanding hematoma) (29, 30). In our experience, pseudoaneurysms are easily visible in the first few postoperative days, and they enlarge over the ensuing days and weeks, whereas true patch aneurysms are small initially and enlarge slowly over the first few postoperative months, finally attaining a stable size at about 6 months.

CONCLUSION

Cardiac surgeons and pediatric cardiologists make many clinical decisions based on their bedside interpretation of films (31, 32). Involvement of a radiologist, in as timely a manner as possible, in the interpretation and decision process promotes improved care for patients. Although the clinician knows best the status and specific problems of any patient, and therefore searches out the most pertinent corresponding information on the films, this focus of attention can occasionally lead to tunnel vision. An experienced, but less biased interpreter of films, can detect impending complications and subtle abnormalities not initially evident to the clinical reviewers. It is helpful when clinicians involved in postoperative care and radiologists reviewing the radiographs on those patients have a close working relationship, so that information flows easily between them (3). This is best facilitated by having a film viewing device (film alternator or multibank video workstation) in the intensive care unit, where all recent images on each patient are aggregated, and where the clinicians and radiologists consult together.

REFERENCES

1. Ferry PC. Neurologic sequelae of open-heart surgery in children. An irritating question. Am J Dis Child 1990;144:369–373.
2. al-Ali F, Higgins CB, Gooding CA. MRI of tracheal and esophageal compression following surgery for congenital heart disease. J Comp Assist Tomogr 1994;18:39–42.
3. Henry DA, Jolles H, Berberich JJ, et al. The post-cardiac surgery chest radiograph: a clinically integrated approach. J Thorac Imaging 1989;4:20–41.
4. Markowitz RI, Malat J, Keller MS, et al. Gallbladder opacification in infants following high dose angiocardiography. Pediatr Radiol 1988;18:319–322.
5. Traver RD, Cohen M, Broderick NJ, Conces DJ Jr. Pediatric digital chest imaging. J Thorac Imaging 1990;5:31–35.
6. Glazer HS, Muka E, Sagel SS, et al. New techniques in chest radiography. Radiol Clin North Am 1994;32:711–727.
7. Witt RM, Cohen MD, Appledorn CR. Initial experience with a radiology imaging network to newborn and intensive care units. J Digit Imaging 1991;4:39–42.
8. Arroe M. The risk of x-ray examinations of the lungs in neonates. Acta Paediatr Scand 1991;80:489–493.
9. Crowley JJ, Oh KS, Newman B, et al. Telltale signs of congenital heart disease. Radiol Clin North Am 1993;31:573–582.
10. Heinemann MK, Hanley FL, Van Praagh S, et al. Total anomalous pulmonary venous drainage in newborns with visceral heterotaxy. Ann Thorac Surg 1994;57:88–97.
11. Amplatz K, Moller JH, Castaneda-Zuniga W. Radiology of congenital heart disease. New York: Thieme Medical Publishers, 1986:67–128.
12. Davidson A, Krull F, Kallfelz HC. Cardiomegaly—what does it mean? A comparison of echocardiographic to radiological cardiac dimensions in children. Pediatr Cardiol 1990;11:181–185.
13. Markowitz RI, Johnson KM, Weinstein EM. Pulmonary hyperinflation in infants with large left-to-right shunts. Invest Radiol 1988;23:354–358.
14. Leung MP, Chau KT, Hui PW, et al. Necrotizing enterocolitis in neonates with symptomatic congenital heart disease. J Pediatr 1988;113:1044–1046.
15. Allen HA, Haney PJ. Left ventricular outflow obstruction and necrotizing enterocolitis. Radiology 1984;150:401–402.
16. Kennedy J, Holt CL, Ricketts RR. The significance of portal vein gas in necrotizing enterocolitis. Am Surg 1987;53:231–234.
17. Kosloske AM, Musemeche CA, Ball WS Jr, et al. Necrotizing enterocolitis: value of radiographic findings to predict outcome. AJR 1988;151:771–774.
18. Carter AR, Sostman HD, Curtis AM, et al. Thoracic alterations after cardiac surgery. AJR 1983;140:475–481.
19. Norwood WI Jr, Jacobs ML, Murphy JD. Fontan procedure for hypoplastic left heart syndrome. Ann Thorac Surg 1992;54:1025–1029.
20. Norwood WI, Jacobs ML. Fontan's procedure in two stages. Am J Surg 1993;166:548–551.
21. Donn SM, Kuhns LR. Mechanism of endotracheal tube movement with change of head position in the neonate. Pediatr Radiol 1980;9:37–39.
22. Efthimiou J, Butler J, Woodham C, et al. Diaphragm paralysis following cardiac surgery: role of phrenic nerve cold injury. Ann Thorac Surg 1991;52:1005–1008.
23. Mok Q, Ross-Russel R, Mulvey D, et al. Phrenic nerve injury in infants and children undergoing cardiac surgery. Br Heart J 1991;65:287–292.
24. Watanabe T, Trusler GA, Williams WG, et al. Phrenic nerve paralysis after pediatric cardiac surgery. Retrospective study of 125 cases. J Thorac Cardiovasc Surg 1987;94:383–388.
25. Zhao HX, D'Agostino RS, Pitlick PT, et al. Phrenic nerve injury complicating closed cardiovascular surgical procedures for congenital heart disease. Ann Thorac Surg 1985;39:445–449.
26. Norwood WI Jr. Hypoplastic left heart syndrome. Ann Thorac Surg 1991;52:688–695.
27. Gold JP, Jonas RA, Lang P, et al. Transthoracic intracardiac monitoring lines in pediatric surgical patients: a ten-year experience. Ann Thorac Surg 1986;42:185–191.

28. Ascuitto RJ, Ross-Asciutto NT, Markowitz RI, et al. Aneurysms of the right ventricular outflow tract after repair of tetralogy of Fallot: role of radiology. Radiology 1988;167:115–119.
29. Castaneda AR. Classical repair of tetralogy of Fallot: timing, technique, and results. Semin Thorac Cardiovasc Surg 1990;2:70–75.
30. DiDonato RM, Jonas RA, Lang P, et al. Neonatal repair of tetralogy with and without pulmonary atresia. J Thorac Cardiovasc Surg 1991;101:126–137.
31. Hauser GJ, Pollack MM, Sivit CJ, et al. Routine chest radiographs in pediatric intensive care: a prospective study. Pediatrics 1989;83:465–470.
32. Sivit CJ, Taylor GA, Hauser GJ, et al. Efficacy of chest radiography in pediatric intensive care. AJR 1989;152:575–577.

Echocardiography

28.1 Principles of Echocardiography

Steven D. Colan, MD

BASICS OF ECHOCARDIOGRAPHY

Physics of Ultrasound and Instrumentation

An understanding of certain physical principles of ultrasound and ultrasound imaging can help the ultrasonographer obtain the best possible information from the echocardiographic exam. Ultrasound instrumentation relies on the piezoelectric properties of crystalline substances which are able to convert electrical energy to and from mechanical energy. The crystal functions as the transmitter, but the same crystal is also able to function as a receiver. It is important to recall that sound waves are actually physical compression waves, and as such can only be propagated within a medium, a property which distinguishes sound from electromagnetic waves. It is the interaction of the sound waves with the medium which permits ultrasound (at frequencies higher than 20,000 Hz) to be used for imaging and thermal purposes. The nature of this interaction also dictates the limits of ultrasound imaging.

Sound transmission depends on the physical properties, such as stiffness and density, of the medium in which it propagates; solids transmit sound more rapidly and with less energy loss than liquids or gases. When sound waves encounter an interface between substances with different mechanical properties, the change in transmission properties results in a variable transmission of the compression wave. The sound which is not conducted across the interface is reflected, with the amount of reflected energy being proportional to the difference in acoustic transmission properties between the two media. The acoustic interfaces between bone and tissue and those between gas and tissue, for example, are so extreme that virtually all sound is reflected. It is therefore not possible to image structures which lie beyond these interfaces. Consequently, ultrasound imaging can only be conducted through certain "windows," or portals, which avoid bone, lung, and bowel gas.

Imaging Modes: M-Mode and Sector Scan

Ultrasound imaging devices employ a pulse generator to send electrical pulses to the transducer, which responds by emitting a short burst of sound energy. The transducer then acts as a receiver, converting the reflected ultrasound energy into an electric signal which is transmitted to the image processor. This sequence, labeled a "pulse-echo cycle," is repeated at a high frequency, typically on the order of 1000 Hz (1000 cycles per second).

Since the duration of the incident signal is very brief (1 microsecond), most of the time is spent "listening" for the reflected signal. Each of these pulse-echo cycles is analyzed to determine the depth of reflecting interfaces. The instrument calculates the time required for the reflection to reach the transducer and based on the speed of sound in soft tissue (1530 m/sec), calculates the distance of the reflector from the transducer.

M-mode Echocardiography

M-mode is essentially one-dimensional imaging in which the position of the reflectors relative to the transducer are displayed as a function of time. Each pulse-echo sequence samples the reflecting structures along a single narrow beam (so-called "ice-pick" view of the heart). The extremely high sampling frequency (1000 Hz) permits excellent time resolution, which is particularly useful in event timing (such as accurate estimation of ejection time from the length of time during which the aortic valve is open). M-mode echocardiography, guided by the spatial information available from two-dimensional imaging, is now primarily used for evaluation of left ventricular size and function rather than for anatomic delineation.

Two-dimensional Echocardiography

Two-dimensional echocardiography and its images are constructed by rapidly sampling from multiple radial lines along an arc. This can be accomplished mechanically, by rotating the transducer head through an arc, but is now almost exclusively performed by using multiple active elements in a fixed head transducer. Each image, or frame, is displayed as a single image but in fact represents a composite of multiple uni-dimensional samples collected over time. The image display processor interpolates and smooths the image so that it appears uniform, but the manner in which the samples are obtained implies that the information density is far greater in the near field (where sample lines are closely spaced) than in the far field.

Multiple factors affect the information content of the two-dimensional images, including depth of **penetration, resolution,** and **interference.** Ultrasound beams are attenuated by tissue, and this attenuation ultimately defines the maximum usable depth of ultrasound in any given patient. Lower frequency ultrasound penetrates further than higher frequency ultrasound. Consequently, it is necessary to use 3.5 and 2.5 MHZ transducers in larger patients, whereas 7.5 and 5.0 MHZ transducers provide adequate penetration in small children. The magnitude of signal attenuation is dependent on the density of tissue and strength of reflectors, both of which are variable across the width of the image.

Resolution is usually evaluated as axial resolution, lateral resolution, and temporal resolution.

Axial resolution is the limit of the ability to discriminate between objects in the direction of the sound beam. The primary factor which determines axial resolution is pulse duration, that is, the length of the incident pulse of sound wave (with shorter pulses providing better axial resolution). Consequently, the best axial resolution is obtained from the higher frequency transducers.

Lateral resolution is the limit of the ability to discriminate objects oriented perpendicular to the sound beam and is determined primarily by the width of the sound beam and line density, both of which vary according to distance from the transducer. The number of elements in a transducer refers to the number of separately active piezoelectric crystals, and is usually between 48 and 128. Increasing the number of elements adds to the overall size of the transducer, to the expense of producing the transducer, and to the cost and complexity of the electronic configuration. The physical size of the transducer face (known as the transducer "footprint") is also an important determinant of lateral resolution since lateral resolution is proportional to the width of the acoustic aperture. Although larger transducers with a greater number of elements and channels provide improved lateral resolution, the physical access is usually limited by the size of the acoustic window or the size of the endocavitary instrument.

Temporal resolution refers to the ability to discriminate changing physiologic parameters in real time. It is determined primarily by sampling frequency. The M-mode sampling frequency of 1000 Hz is adequate to discriminate all time-variant functions of physiologic importance. Among the fastest moving cardiac structures are semilunar valves during opening and closure. In contrast, temporal resolution of two-dimensional imaging is far more limited. For example, a "sticking" prosthetic valve which has a step wise motion clearly visible on M-mode will appear closed and then open on sequential two-dimensional images.

The ultrasound operator is provided with enormous control over the imaging instrument. Some of the control features affect the image display but do not fundamentally alter the information content. For example, display brightness and contrast can compensate to a certain degree for the excessive ambient light sometimes encountered in the cardiac intensive care setting. In contrast, there are aspects of machine operation and image processing which do influence information content and to which the operator must be attentive. For example, the strength of the incident signal can be controlled directly; due to tissue attenuation, however, the strength of returning signals from the near field is greater than far field signals. The operator is therefore provided with adjustments called time-gain compensation (TGC), which allows the signal gain to be adjusted as a function of image depth. Diminishing the near field gain reduces the strength of the received signal, maintaining full utilization of the gray scale spectrum for improved contrast resolution and providing a more uniform image. Interference from very strong reflectors in the far field, such as the pleural interface, can be eliminated by reducing gain at the appropriate distance.

Limitations of Ultrasound

Inadequate acoustic access is the primary factor which limits diagnostic utility of echocardiography. Post-thoracotomy patients are particularly prone to have previously identified echocardiographic windows disappear. In a recent report, the frequency with which diagnostic errors can occur in the assessment of the aortic arch reconstruction in patients who undergo surgical palliation of hypoplastic left heart syndrome has been documented (1). This is one example of how the same examination techniques which were extremely reliable in the preoperative patient can become potentially misleading in the postoperative setting. Transesophageal imaging has therefore been useful in the cardiac intensive care unit, particularly since the availability of biplane probes which can be used in patients as small as 3 kg.

There are other sources of error which the echocardiographer must be aware to avoid artifacts and misrepresentation. For example, since structures oriented parallel to the direction of the insonating beam reflect ultrasound more poorly than structures perpendicular to the beam, a thin atrial septum may generate no reflection when imaged from the apex and thus create the false impression of an atrial septal defect. The examiner must rely on other additional imaging windows such as the subxiphoid view (from which a perpendicular imaging plane is possible). In addition, certain artifacts are common and can be recognized if the underlying physics are understood. As an example, images of the descending aorta often display what appears to be a second, identical structure immediately posterior to it. The source of this artifact is an intense secondary reflection by the anterior aortic wall of the echo returning from the posterior wall.

Furthermore, certain structures are acoustic sinks and disallow generation of image beyond them. Prosthetic valves, intravenous lines, and pacing leads are examples of common echo-dense structures that can block ultrasound. Lastly, the length of time required to generate each 2-dimensional image depends on the width and depth of the image and the use of color Doppler, which requires additional imaging time. Frame rates can easily drop below 10 frames per second for large images with full-frame color Doppler. Slow frame rates are a particular limitation in smaller patients due to more rapid heart rates. For infants with heart rates as high as 180 beats per minute or 3 beats per second, even a fairly high rate of 30 frames per second provides only 10 frames per beat with usually only 3 frames per systole, which is inadequate for accurate determination of function. Frame rate can be increased by reducing depth of image, narrowing the sweep angle, and restricting width of color imaging. The operator must pay attention to frame rate and heart rate to avoid inadequate sampling rate.

THE ECHOCARDIOGRAPHIC EXAMINATION

General Considerations

A sound understanding of cardiac anatomy and ultrasound imaging are prerequisites to an adequate echocardiographic examination. There are other factors which, if paid insufficient attention, can impede even the best cardiac ultrasonographer.

First, the hemodynamic and respiratory status of the patient should be carefully monitored at all times during the examination. It is not uncommon for all caretakers to be distracted by interesting or significant findings on the echocardiogram and fail to pay adequate attention to the overall status of the patient. Changes such as pressure on the thoracic cage or subxiphoid area secondary to the transducer, sedation, or position alterations can have impact on hemodynamic and/or ventilation status.

Second, all available clinical information about the patient should be reviewed and recorded in as much detail as possible. Many patients in the intensive care setting have central vascular or atrial monitoring lines in place, have had recent reparative cardiac or thoracic surgery, are receiving cardioactive medications, and/or have major disorders of fluid balance. The ultrasound findings cannot be correctly interpreted without this information.

Thirdly, only transducers appropriate for patient size must be employed. A common shortcoming in this regard is lack of availability of a 7.5-MHZ transducer for neonates.

Fourth, the physical ambience should be optimized towards a ideal echocardiographic examination. Ambient lighting in the intensive care unit should be reduced if at all possible. In addition, the patient position should be adjusted to reduce operator fatigue.

Fifth, a systematic and thorough anatomic approach should always be followed except in the case of a cardiorespiratory arrest which precludes a detailed examination. If the patient is stable, the crisis-oriented atmosphere of the intensive care unit all too often leads to a hurried examination in which anatomic features are examined in a sequence dictated by the questions originating from caretakers gathered around the bedspace. This scattered approach will frequently result in a failure to adequately image all cardiac structures.

Finally, the archival taped record of the examination must be recorded with attention to proper image display to permit unequivocal off-line interpretation. This is particularly important with respect to right-left orientation. The general rule which should be followed is to orient the transducer with respect to the long axis plane of the body, and to never right-left invert the image. The transducers always have an indicator marking the right side of the transducer. If this marker is always kept to the left side of the body, then right-left orientation can be unambiguously interpreted. The basic rules for the examination are:

1. Left-sided structures are displayed to the right of the screen
2. Superior structures are displayed toward the top of the screen
3. Anterior structures are displayed to the right and top of the screen

The Standard Views

The Subxiphoid View

Infants and young children nearly always have excellent acoustic access from the subxiphoid space. It is generally possible to simultaneously image the ventricles and proximal great vessels from this view, permitting their interrelationship to be defined, often better than from any other view.

Imaging is first performed with the transducer oriented right-left, sweeping from posterior to anterior structures. The initial image should include a cross-sectional abdominal view with identification of the relationship of the aorta, spine, inferior vena cava, and hemiazygous vein (Fig. 28.1.1) for determination of visceroatrial situs. The sequential images proceed anteriorly through the heart (Fig. 28.1.2) to the level of the coronal view of the right ventricular outflow tract and pulmonary valve (Fig. 28.1.3). Short axis (parasagittal) images are obtained by clockwise rotation of the transducer 90° (marker is directed posteriorly and inferiorly). The transducer is aligned with the inferior and superior vena cavae (Fig. 28.1.4) and the sweep is conducted from the extreme right, through the right ventricular outflow tract (Fig. 28.1.5), to the apex of the heart (Fig. 28.1.6). Inferior angulation permits confirmation of inferior vena cava continuity and patency (Fig. 28.1.7).

The Apical View

Apical images are far more limited in scope than either parasternal or subxiphoid images due to a more limited

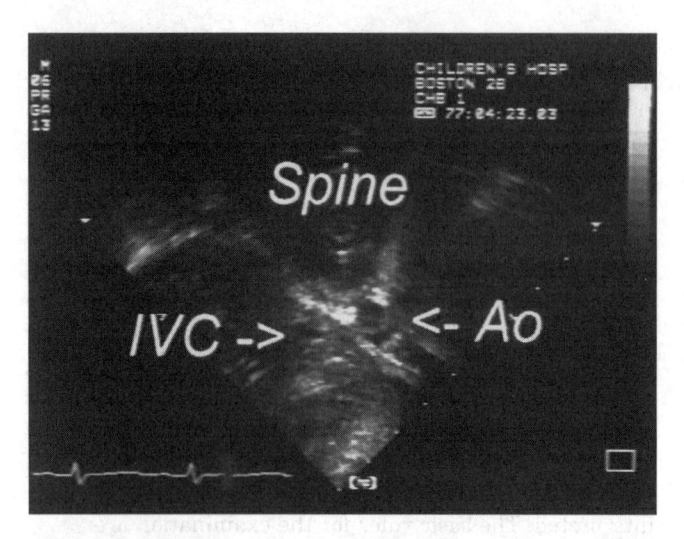

428　Section IV. Special Cardiac Evaluation and Management in Cardiac Intensive Care

Figure 28.1.1. Subcostal, transverse image, posterior and inferior. At this level the inferior vena cava (*IVC*), spine, and descending aorta (*Ao*) can be defined and their situs determined.

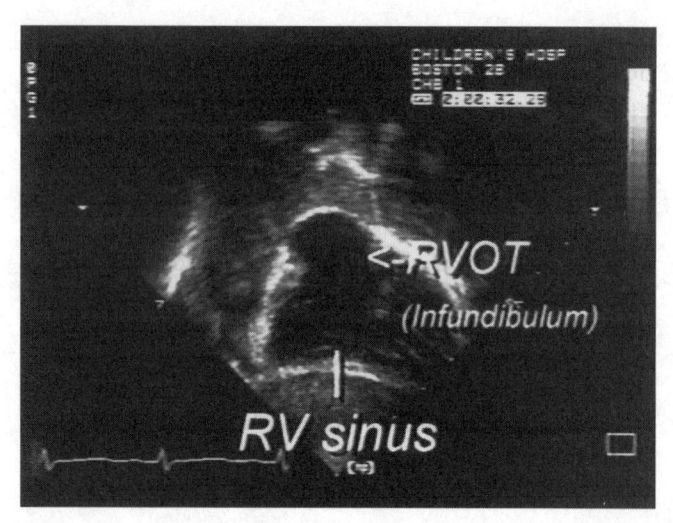

Figure 28.1.3. Subcostal, transverse image showing the anterior limit of sweep. A coronal image of the right ventricular (*RV*) sinus and outflow tract (*RVOT*) to the level of the pulmonary valve can usually be obtained.

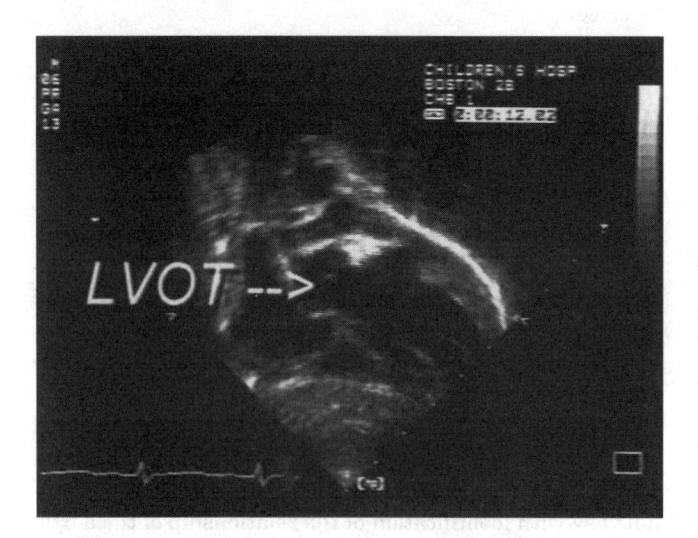

Figure 28.1.2. Subcostal, transverse image, midsweep. Imaging through the left ventricular outflow tract (*LVOT*) displays the interventricular septum in its midportion.

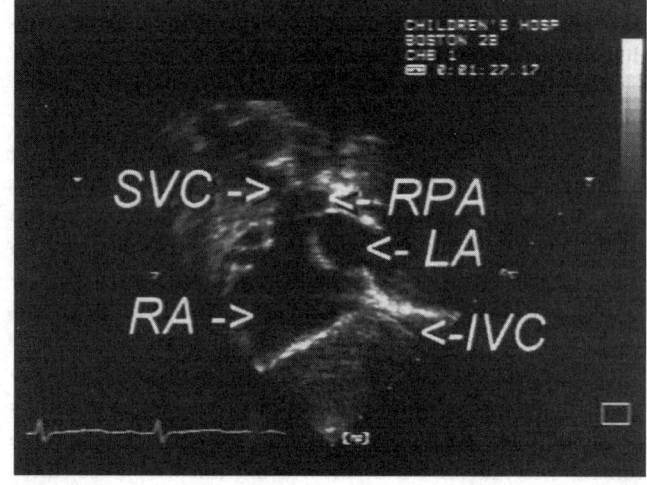

Figure 28.1.4. Subcostal, parasaggital image, rightward initial position. The inferior (*IVC*) and superior (*SVC*) vena cavae with the intervening sinus venous portion of the atrial septum between the right (*RA*) and left (*LA*) atria are usually best obtained from this view. The right pulmonary artery (*RPA*) can be seen as it passes posterior to the *SVC*.

window. In spite of the restricted ability to define anatomic relationships from this view, the best alignment with left ventricular inflow and outflow for Doppler assessment is usually obtained. Also, the apical ventricular septum is often best interrogated for ventricular septal defects and for apical thrombi.

The coronal image, sweeping from posterior to anterior, displays the four chambers of the heart simultaneously with the atrioventricular alignment (Fig. 28.1.8). Pulmonary venous inflow can be visualized and velocity samples obtained. Clockwise rotation of the transducer into a parasagital plane aligns the plane of insonation with the left ventricular outflow tract and proximal ascending aorta (Fig. 28.1.9).

The Parasternal View

Images obtained from the third or fourth intercostal space provide the most direct images of the ventricular outflow tracts, semilunar valves, and arterial roots.

The long axis view is obtained by aligning the transducer with the long axis plane of the ventricle (left hip to

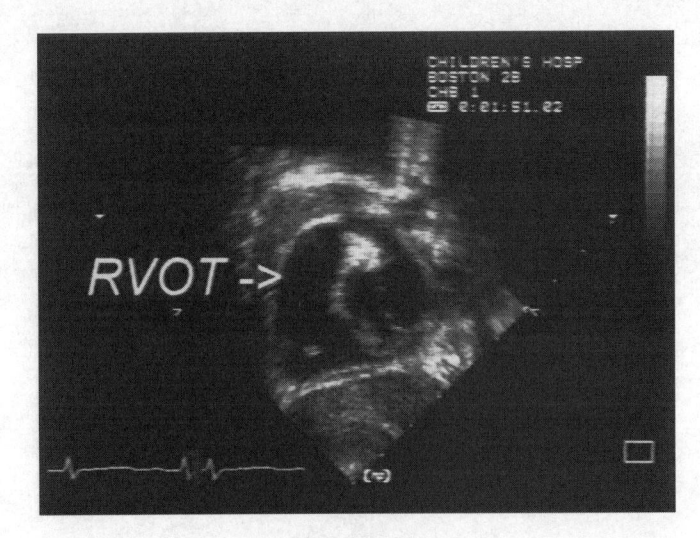

Figure 28.1.5. Subcostal, parasaggital image, midsweep. The right ventricular outflow tract (*RVOT*) and short axis image of the left ventricle are traversed at the midportion of this sweep.

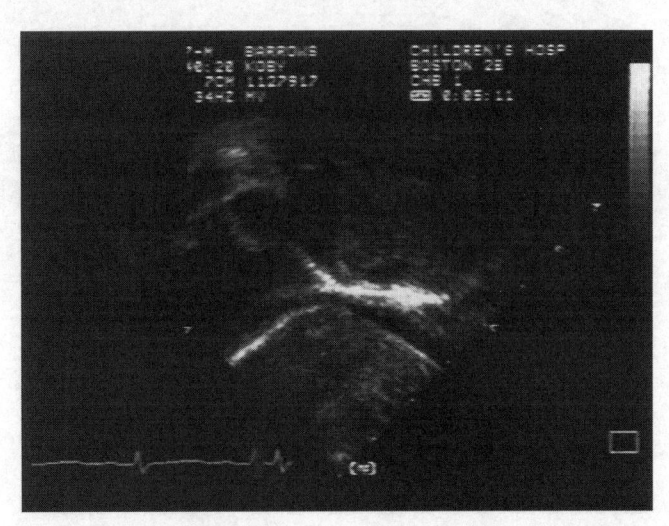

Figure 28.1.7. Subcostal, parasaggital image, downward angulation to visualize inferior vena caval continuity as it passes through the liver.

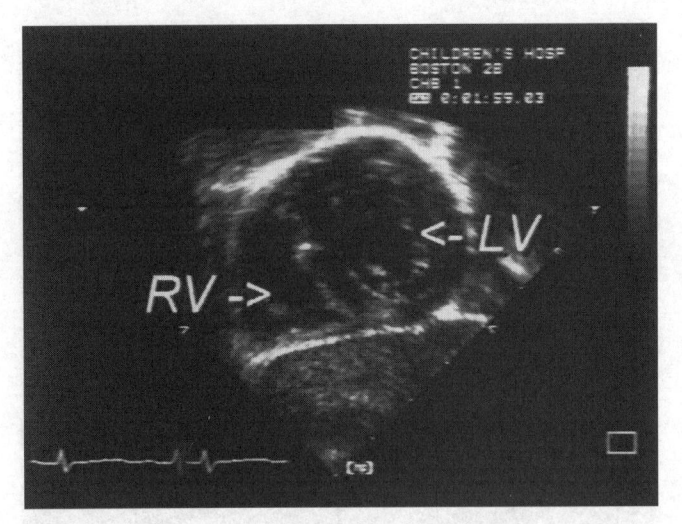

Figure 28.1.6. Subcostal, parasaggital image, leftward extent of sweep. The apical extent of the interventricular septum between the right (*RV*) and left (*LV*) ventricles should be interrogated for septal defects from this view.

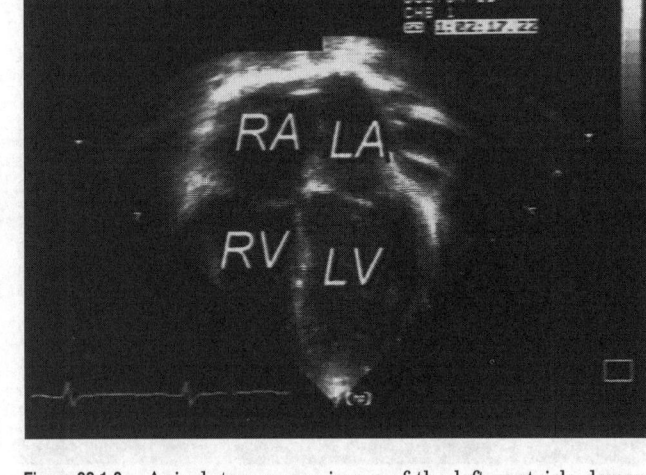

Figure 28.1.8. Apical, transverse image of the left ventricle demonstrating the mitral and tricuspid valves as well as the right (*RA*) and left atria (*LA*) and the right (*RV*) and left ventricles (*LV*).

right shoulder in levocardia). The rules outlined above indicate that the transducer marker should be positioned toward the left. This results in the apex displayed toward the left of the screen in levocardia (toward the right in dextrocardia), which is unfortunately the opposite of the practice in most laboratories. The aortic valve, mitral valve, and left ventricular outflow tract form the center position (Fig. 28.1.10). Imaging toward the right displays the tricuspid valve and right ventricular inflow (Fig. 28.1.11), and toward the left displays the pulmonary valve and main pulmonary artery (Fig. 28.1.12). Rotation into the orthogonal plane aligns the transducer with the short axis plane of the ventricle and the aortic valve in cross-section (Fig. 28.1.13). Apical angulation displays a series of short axis planes of the left ventricle and multiple levels of the ventricular septal (Fig. 28.1.14). Superior angulation, often with sliding the transducer up an interspace, brings the pulmonary bifurcation into view (Fig. 28.1.15).

The Suprasternal Notch and High Parasternal Views

These images are generally the least familiar to the non-echocardiographer and the most uncomfortable for the patient. Imaging is facilitated by placement of a pillow or rolled blanket under the shoulders with neck extension

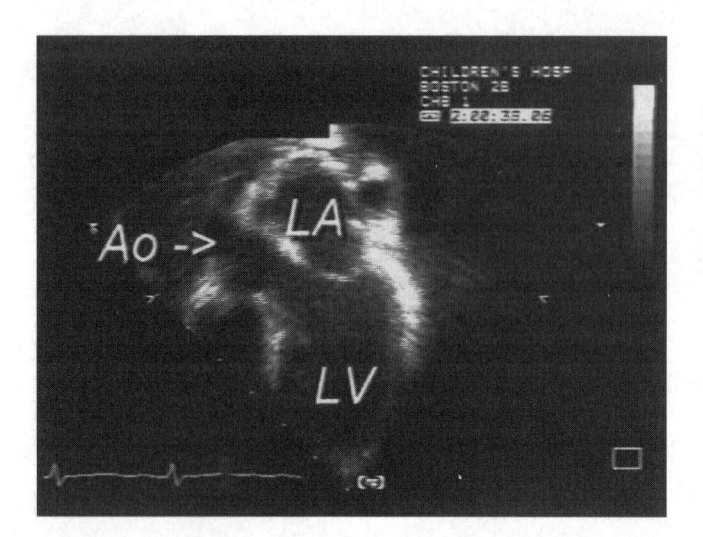

Figure 28.1.9. Apical, parasagital view of the left ventricular (*LV*) outflow tract, aortic valve, proximal ascending aorta (*Ao*), mitral inflow, and left atrium (*LA*). Note the descending aorta posterior to the *LA*.

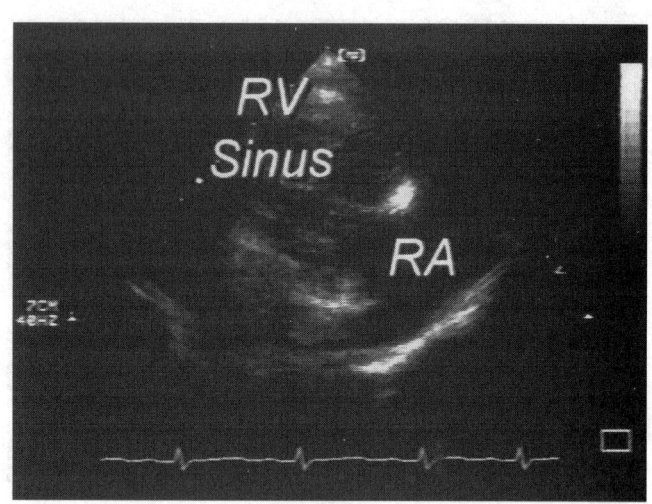

Figure 28.1.11. Parasternal image with the imaging plane aligned with the long axis of the heart. Rightward angulation provides images of the right atrium (*RA*), tricuspid valve, and right ventricular inflow (*RV Sinus*).

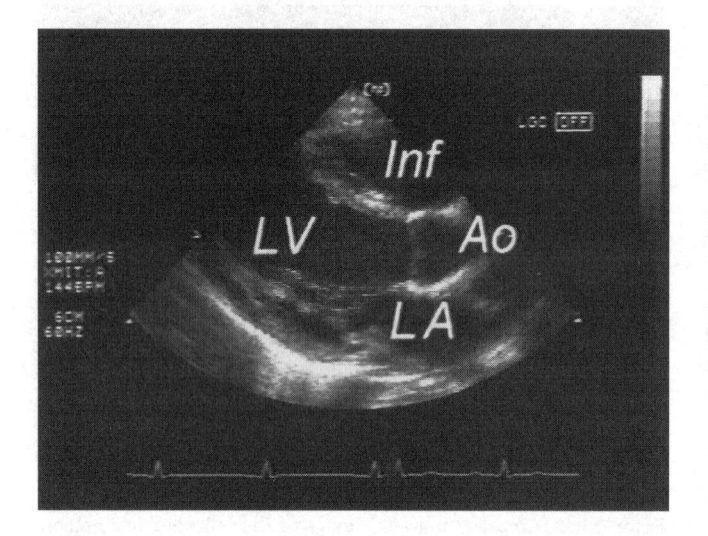

Figure 28.1.10. Parasternal image with the imaging plane aligned with the long axis of the heart. The aortic valve (*Ao*), mitral valve, and left ventricular (*LV*) outflow tract form the center position of this sweep. The right ventricular infundibulum (*Inf*) should also be visible.

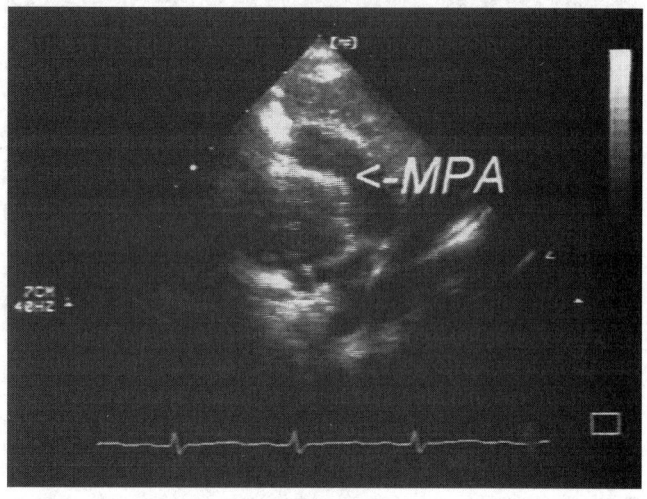

Figure 28.1.12. Parasternal image with the imaging plane aligned with the long axis of the heart. Leftward angulation allows the pulmonary valve, subpulmonary area, and main pulmonary artery (*MPA*) to be imaged.

and use of a small footprint transducer. It is vital that the airway and ventilation be carefully monitored especially during this part of the examination.

Coronal images with the transducer in a right-left orientation imaging through the arch, right pulmonary artery, and left atrium can provide the best access to pulmonary vein connections, particularly in young infants. The innominate vein and right superior vena cava are identified by anterior and rightward angulation, and a left superior vena cava is sought by imaging to the right and anterior to the left pulmonary artery. Imaging in a series of planes during counterclockwise rotation images the left pulmonary artery and left aortic arch in sequence (Fig. 28.1.16).

Measurement of Anatomic Structures

The absolute size of the cardiac valves and the great vessels is often a critical factor in patient management. The resolution which can be achieved with ultrasound is adequate, but consistent and reproducible measurements require attention to certain factors in the imaging process. On-line measurements are generally more accurate than can be obtained during tape review. Most echocardiogram machines have the capacity to capture a sequence of im-

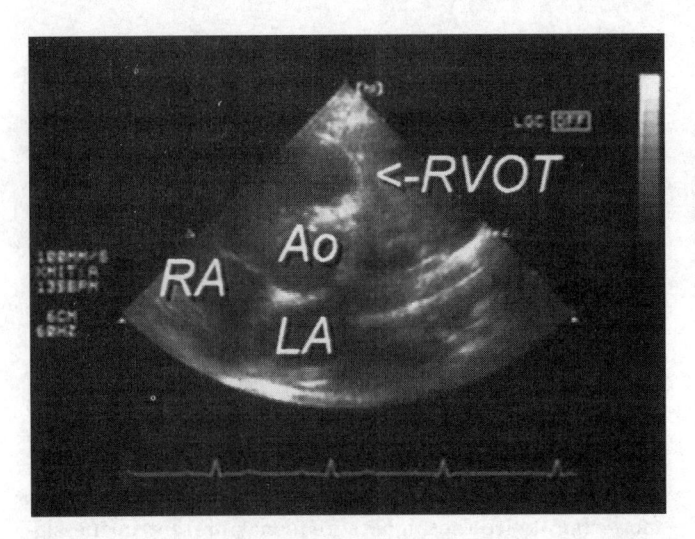

Figure 28.1.13. Parasternal image with the imaging plane aligned with the short axis of the heart. The aortic valve (*Ao*), right (*RA*) and left (*LA*) atria, atrial septum, tricuspid valve, and right ventricular outflow tract (*RVOT*) can be identified.

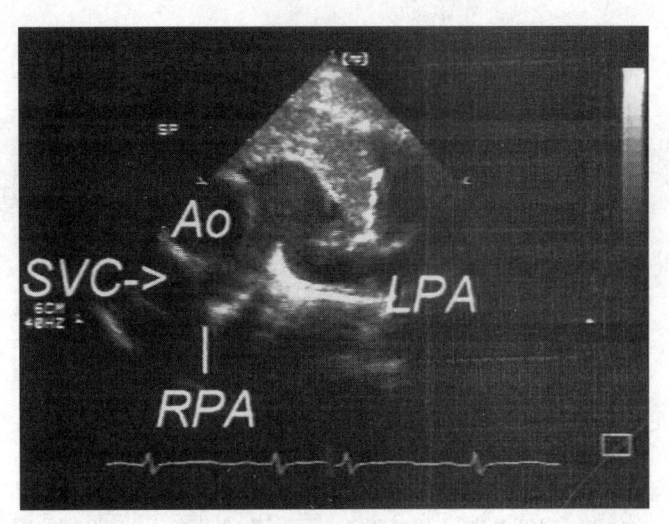

Figure 28.1.15. Parasternal image with the imaging plane aligned with the short axis of the heart. Superior angulation (often with translation of the transducer to a more cephalad intercostal space) displays the pulmonary bifurcation (*RPA*, *LPA*) with the superior vena cava (*SVC*) and ascending aorta (*Ao*) passing anterior to the *RPA*.

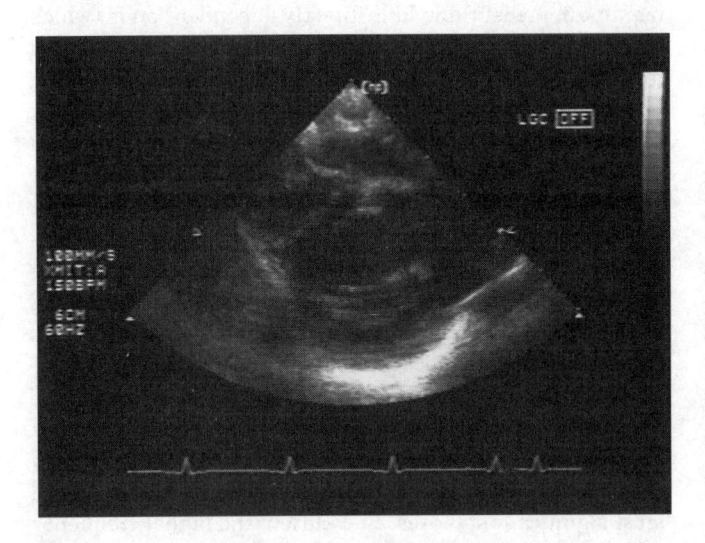

Figure 28.1.14. Parasternal image with the imaging plane aligned with the short axis of the heart. Apical angulation displays the short axis of the left ventricle and cross section of the mitral valve.

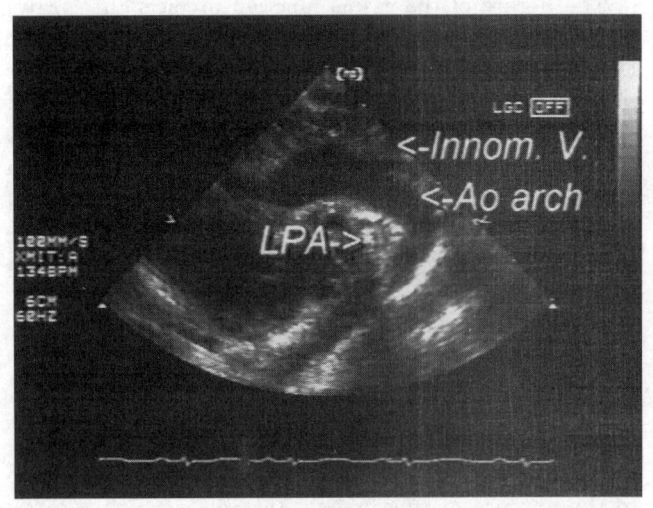

Figure 28.1.16. Suprasternal notch images of a left aortic arch (*Ao arch*) with the origin of the left pulmonary artery (*LPA*). The innominate vein (*Innom V*) passes superior to the arch when present.

ages into active memory for immediate frame-by-frame review at full machine resolution and maximum frame rate, thereby permitting measurements at the correct instant in the cardiac cycle.

DOPPLER ECHOCARDIOGRAPHY

Doppler Principles

When an observer is moving relative to a wave source, the frequency of the wave which he or she detects is different from the emitted frequency. If the direction of movement is toward each other, the frequency is shifted higher, whereas movement away results in a frequency lower than that of the original signal. This observation is known as the **Doppler effect,** named after the Austrian physicist Christian Doppler who described the principle in 1842.

During imaging, ultrasound systems determine the amplitude (or intensity) of reflected sound waves and display this information as a function of the distance of the reflector from the transducer. However, in addition to the information contained within the intensity component of the reflected signal, it is possible to employ spectral analysis to quantify the frequency components of the returned signal. Based on the Doppler effect, during reflection the frequency of the incident signal is shifted in proportion to the velocity of movement of the reflector relative to the transducer. While this information is not useful in the generation of time-position images, it can be used to ascertain the velocity and direction of movement of the reflector. As is readily seen on two-dimensional echocardiographic images, blood is a relatively poor ultrasonic reflector. Nevertheless, with appropriate increase in transmitter power and additional filtering to reduce the intensity of signals generated by the relatively slow-moving cardiac structures, it is possible to measure the frequency shift of ultrasound backscattered by moving red blood cells.

The frequency shift which occurs when a periodic waveform such as ultrasound encounters a moving object is known as the **Doppler frequency shift** (fd) and is related to the transmitted frequency (ft), the velocity of sound in the medium (c = 1,560 m/sec for soft tissue), and the velocity (v) and relative direction of movement (+) of the target by the equation:

$$f_d = \frac{2 \times f_t \times v \times \cos(+)}{c}$$

The nature of the cosine function predicts that travel parallel to the angle of incidence will have the highest Doppler shift whereas targets moving in a perpendicular direction will generate no frequency shift, regardless of their absolute velocity. Due to the angle dependence of the Doppler shift, it is important to position the transmission direction parallel to the direction of flow when quantifying the Doppler shift. The Doppler signals are then sequentially analyzed using Fourier transformation and displayed in a spectral format.

Current Doppler Instrumentation

Continuous Wave Doppler (CWD)

The use of separate transmit and receive elements permits continuous detection of the Doppler shift signal. Due to the absence of time gating, the relation between the time of signal generation and subsequent reception cannot be determined and the Doppler shift signal represents the summation of all reflectors encountered in the path of transmission. This **range ambiguity** represents the principle liability of continuous wave Doppler. The tradeoff for range ambiguity is an improved range of velocity resolution. Thus, CWD is capable of resolving essentially all physiologically relevant velocities, including the relatively high velocities.

Pulsed Wave Doppler (PWD)

By emitting the ultrasonic beam in short pulses followed by a period of listening for the backscatter, it is possible to limit the period of analysis to a predetermined window of time which is calculated for the desired depth of the sampling volume. Thus, velocity of flow can be determined at known positions (**range-gating**) guided by two-dimensional imaging. The velocimeter calculates the Doppler shift from the ultrasound signal by comparing the phase relationships between the transmitted signal and each successive reflected ultrasound pulse. If the target moves more than 1/2 of the wavelength of the transmitted pulse between samples, the phase shift and therefore the velocity will be misrepresented. If the target moves a full wavelength between pulses there will be no phase shift and the target will appear not to have moved.

This misrepresentation of velocity is the Doppler manifestation of the signal processing phenomenon known as **aliasing**. The frequency ambiguity of PWD which results from aliasing is simply an expression of the sampling theorem, which states that it is necessary to sample a signal at more than twice the highest frequency present in the signal to avoid ambiguity. The Doppler pulses are transmitted at a frequency fs to sample a signal of frequency fd. The process of obtaining intermittent samples of a continuous process is a form of analog-to-digital conversion. The maximum measurable fd is directly dependent on fs (which for Doppler is the pulse repetition frequency, for imaging it is the frame rate). According to the sampling theorem, fs must be greater than twice the maximum frequency component of fd for unambiguous frequency recognition, a limit which is known as the **Nyquist frequency** (Fig. 28.1.17). Signals with frequencies above the Nyquist limit are misrepresented as negative velocities until the fs frequency is reached. Although the obvious solution is to increase the fs, there are limits to the maximum sampling frequency for pulsed Doppler. Lower frequency transducers can resolve higher velocities, but spatial resolution diminishes at the longer wavelengths and 2 MHz appears to be the useful lower limit. In any case, there is an upper limit to the frequencies detectable by PWD, and unfortunately this occurs below the level of velocities associated with most significant stenoses. In children, the higher frequency transducers which are preferable for improved image resolution impose even more severe limitations.

Color Flow Mapping (CFM)

This relatively new addition utilizes color mapping to depict flow patterns of vascular and cardiac structures. Ultrasonic image data in general is constructed by the rapid serial interrogation of adjacent radii, combining these lines into a single image for viewing. It is similarly possible to construct a two-dimensional map of the velocity data by establishing a number of individual depth gates along each radius within the sector image, interrogate sequentially for image data and for Doppler shift data at each of the sampling depths, and then to move on to the next radius. This permits a sector scan image to be constructed which contains both image and Doppler data as a function of position. Doppler analysis of signals adds two more dimensions: amplitude of the particular frequency component

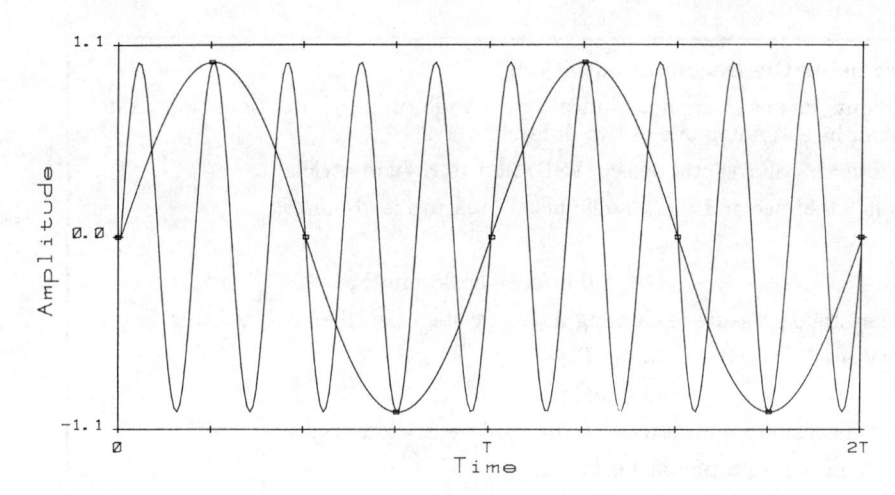

Figure 28.1.17. Illustration of the effect of aliasing on the interpretation of frequencies outside of the Nyquist limit. If samples are obtained at regular intervals of T_4, both sine waves yield the same values, and the higher frequency curve will alias (i.e., it will be misinterpreted as the lower frequency).

(i.e., what portion of the signal was backscattered from targets moving at any given speed) and the frequency shift itself. The frequency shift is represented by hue and the amplitude data is encoded as color intensity. The exact colors selected are arbitrary (by convention—blue for flow away and red for flow towards the transducer), but the move away from gray scale display is necessary because both amplitude and frequency data must be encoded within the color mode.

The simultaneous display of image and spatial distribution of Doppler data such as color flow mapping has represented an enormous advance in the diagnostic utility of ultrasound imaging. However, it should also be kept in mind that color flow mapping has an adverse effect on spatial, temporal, and velocity resolution so that the images are relatively less well-defined. This implies that CFM can be used to define the spatial distribution of Doppler data, but imaging should still be used to define the size of anatomic structures and Doppler techniques used to quantify velocity data. The color image sector should be narrowed and image depth reduced as far as possible to optimize image quality and frame rate. In addition, since Doppler signals are created for the full depth of the two-dimensional image, pulse repetition frequency must be kept low, impairing velocity resolution. It is also important to recall that the Doppler shift is dependent on the angle between the incidence beam and the direction of flow, and therefore flow perpendicular to the beam is invisible.

The Bernoulli Equation: Estimation of Pressure Gradients

Velocity data can be used to estimate the pressure difference between anatomic structures based on a simplification of the Bernoulli formula:

$$\Delta P = 4[(V_2)^2 - (V_1)^2]$$

where V_2 is the downstream velocity and V_1 is the upstream velocity. This simplification is based on two assumptions 1) viscous friction is assumed to be negligible, and 2) the flow acceleration component, which introduces a lag in the velocity curve relative to pressure, is assumed to be small relative to the convective acceleration. (Fig. 28.1.18; see color plate 28.1.18).

Furthermore, for significant stenoses proximal velocity is generally small relative to distal velocity, allowing the proximal velocity to be neglected and the pressure difference can then be estimated from the distal velocity (V) as:

$$\Delta P = 4V^2$$

Although this formula has been shown to be valid in experimental preparations (2–4) and useful for a wide variety of clinical applications, it is worth noting the circumstances under which these assumptions are likely to be invalid. First, in mild stenoses, the velocity proximal to the obstruction is relatively higher in proportion to the distal velocity. Thus, in the presence of smaller gradients such as coarctation, mild aortic stenosis or across atrioventricular valves a greater error is introduced by neglecting the proximal velocity. This is one of the factors involved in the commonly observed poorer correlation of Doppler with invasive measurements in patients with mild aortic stenosis (5). In addition, both in vitro and in vivo experiments have found insignificant viscous losses across discrete orifices greater than 5 mm (6–8). However, smaller orifice diameters or non-discrete stenoses have greater viscous effects which result in underestimation of the actual pressure gradient. This problem can be anticipated particularly in pediatric applications where these smaller orifice diameters may be encountered (for example, in critical valvar stenosis) and where evaluation of long-segment stenoses is desirable (for example, in estimating the gradient across a small tube graft). Lastly, flow acceleration is a significant factor only during the period of valve opening and closure, when flow acceleration is high. This results in an inherent inaccuracy of the simplified formula during the onset and cessation of flow, which is most significant in aortic stenosis.

> **Examples of estimation of pressure using the Bernoulli equation:**
> Doppler estimation of pressure gradients has been applied clinically to a wide range of situations. For example, a right ventricular (RV) pressure can be estimated one of two different ways:
>
> 1) From the velocity of flow across a ventricular septal defect (VSD) (left to right ventricle).
>
> If the velocity of flow across a VSD is 3.0 M/sec and the systolic blood pressure is 96 mmHg,
>
> ΔP (or LV p − RV p) = $4v^2$
> LV p − RV p = $4 \times (3.0 \text{ M/sec})^2$ or 36 mmHg
>
> Since the LV pressure can be aortic systolic pressure (assuming no aortic stenosis), then substituting:
>
> 96 mmHg − RV p = 36 mmHg
> RV p = 60 mmHg
>
> 2) From the velocity of flow of a jet of tricuspid regurgitation (from right ventricle to right atrium).
>
> If the velocity of flow of a jet of tricuspid regurgitation is 4.0 M/sec,
>
> ΔP (or RV p − RA p) = $4v^2$
> RV p − RA p = $4 \times (4.0 \text{ M/sec})^2$ or 64 mmHg
>
> If the measured RA pressure is 6 mmHg, then substituting:
>
> RV p − 6 mmHg = 64 mmHg
> RV p = 70 mmHg

ECHOCARDIOGRAPHIC ASSESSMENT OF VENTRICULAR FUNCTION

General Principles

Echocardiography has evolved into the most important imaging modality for the evaluation of ventricular function in children. Prior to discussion of the capabilities and issues which are unique to echocardiography, it is important to review several general issues surrounding the clinical assessment of ventricular and myocardial mechanics and their interrelationship.

First, echocardiographically-derived indices of systolic and diastolic function are not fundamentally different from the indices derived from other techniques. That is, ejection fraction is an estimate of percent volume change which can be obtained from not just echocardiography, but also angiography, radionuclide angiography, or magnetic resonance imaging. There are differences in factors such as accuracy and time resolution among these methods, but fundamentally each measures the same parameter. Second, the measurements provide data concerning ventricular size and function, whereas the ultimate purpose of these measurements is to assess intrinsic myocardial properties such as contractility and compliance. Although it is possible to directly measure ventricular parameters such as volume, thickness, and pressure, it is not possible to directly measure myofiber parameters such as myofiber length, strain, and stress, which are needed to evaluate the contractile state of the myocardium.

The ventricular parameters are therefore obtained for the purpose of estimating myocardial properties which cannot be measured directly. This process can be divided into four separate steps:

1. Measurement of **ventricular parameters** such as ventricular volume, shape, mass, and pressure
2. Calculation of derived **ventricular indices** such as shortening and ejection fractions, ejection rate, wall stress, time constant of relaxation, and ventricular compliance
3. Estimation of **myocardial behavioral indices** such as myocardial fiber shortening, fiber stress, rate of myocardial relaxation, and myocardial stress-strain relationship
4. Inference of **intrinsic myocardial performance properties** such as contractility or compliance from these indices of myocardial behavior

At each of these steps there are distinct sources of error which must be understood if misinterpretation is to be avoided. This discussion will focus on the technical and physiologic factors which the clinician must consider when applying these methods. The final step in this process, the elucidation of intrinsic myocardial properties, is both complex and controversial, encompassing the entire field of myocardial mechanics.

Shortening fraction is based on M-mode derived measurements of the percent change in ventricular diameter calculated from end-diastolic diameter (D_{ed}) and end-systolic diameter (D_{es}):

$$\text{Shortening Fraction} = \frac{(D_{ed} - D_{es})}{(D_{ed})} \times 100$$

The normal range is 30 to 45%. When the short axis configuration of the ventricle has the normal circular shape, fractional shortening provides a direct estimate of percent circumference change. This is because in a circle there is a fixed mathematical relationship between diameter and circumference. In fact, percent diameter change is mathematically equivalent to percent circumferential fiber shortening, providing the ventricle is circular in the short axis plane. By the same reasoning it is clear that if the short axis plane has any other shape, diameter and circumference will not have the same relationship, and in fact percent diameter change will not accurately reflect circumferential fiber shortening.

$$\text{Ejection Fraction} = \frac{(V_{ed} - V_{es})}{(V_{ed})} \times 100$$

and provides a direct estimate of global percent fiber shortening providing there is a constant and predictable mathematical relationship between volume and surface area. Because the shape of the left ventricle is that of a prolate ellipsoid, the relationship between volume and surface area is more complex than is the relationship of area or diameter to short axis circumference. Nevertheless, if the shape is different from that of the normal left ventricle, the ejection fraction will not have the same relationship to fractional change in surface area, and therefore will not have the same relationship to fiber shortening as that observed in the normal ventricle. Ejection fraction is often incorrectly held up as a means to overcome the geometry dependence of percent fractional shortening. The fallacy of this point is illustrated in Figure 28.1.19.

Unfortunately, abnormal left ventricular shape is a common occurrence in congenital heart disease. Despite the fact that ejection fraction does not provide an accurate estimate of fiber shortening under these circumstances, there is nevertheless a major advantage to ejection fraction over fractional shortening. When the short axis configuration is non-circular, fractional shortening ceases to be reproducible, since each different diameter produces a different fractional shortening. Shortening fraction is therefore no longer a valid index of function under these circumstances and should not be used. Ejection fraction then is a more reproducible measurement and can at least be used to follow patients serially.

Assessment of Systolic Function

The echocardiographically-derived indices of ventricular systolic function such as shortening and ejection fraction provide estimates of **myocardial fiber shortening.** While *circumferential* fiber shortening directly measures change in short axis circumference, *meridional* fiber shortening is measured as change in long axis circumference. The average fiber shortening in both short and long axis directions can therefore be estimated from the systolic reduction in surface area of the endocardium.

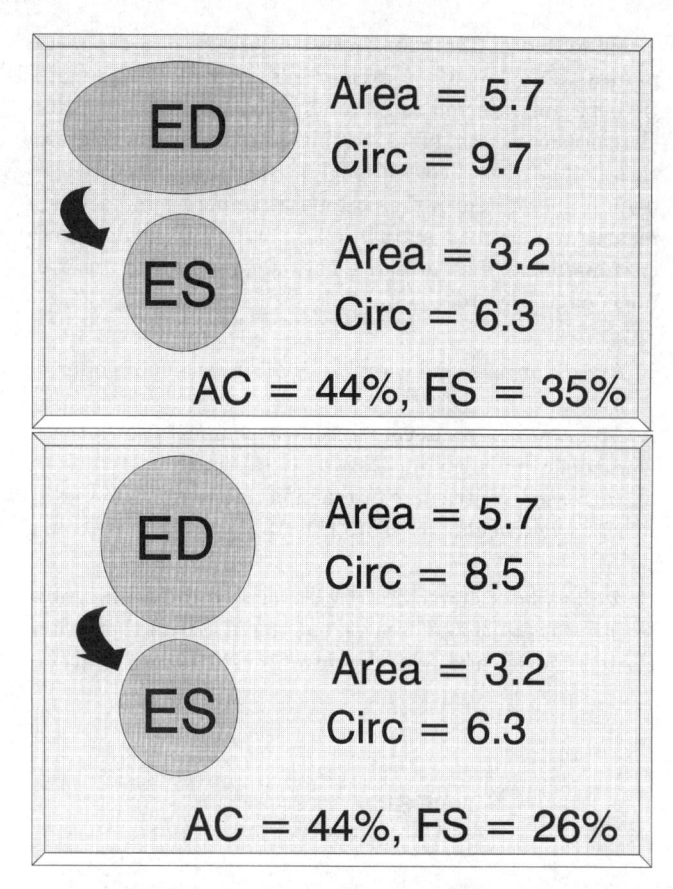

Figure 28.1.19. Diagram of the discrepancy between fiber shortening and percent area change in noncircular ventricles. Although the percent area change (*AC*) in the upper and lower panels is the same, the change in circumference (*Circ*) is substantially different. As a result, the noncircular end-diastolic (*ED*) shape requires a considerably higher fiber shortening (*FS*) to achieve the same end-systolic (*ES*) area.

It is widely understood that fiber shortening is dependent on heart rate, preload, afterload, and contractility. The extent of systolic myocardial fiber shortening is the final outcome of several competing and interacting processes both intrinsic and extrinsic to the myocardium (9). As such, fiber shortening is clinically important since it provides information as to the physiologic balance among these factors. While conceptually straightforward at the fiber level, translation of these properties at the fiber level into their analogous properties at the ventricular level has proved considerably more challenging.

Preload

At the fiber level, preload is best represented by the **end-diastolic fiber length.** There is no means by which this fiber length can be directly measured in the intact ventricle. Although preload in the intact ventricle is often estimated clinically by such parameters as end-diastolic pressure, volume, or wall stress, each of these fails to accurately represent fiber length under certain conditions.

Under normal circumstances, a rise in **end-diastolic pressure** will result in greater end-diastolic fiber length. If there are external constraints such as pericardial effusion or constriction, however, this pressure-length relationship will be disturbed. Although atrial filling pressures are usually monitored in the postoperative period in part as a measure of preload status, it is particularly under these circumstances that pressure may not reflect end-diastolic fiber length due to:

1. Altered myocardial compliance after cardiopulmonary bypass (10)
2. Abnormal external constraint (mechanical ventilation, mediastinal edema, pericardial effusion)
3. Increased ventricular interaction due to elevation in right ventricular pressure (11–13)

End-diastolic volume directly reflects end-diastolic fiber length during acute changes, but the ability of the ventricle to remodel and add new myofibers in series prevents this from being a useful index for comparison between patients or to assess the same patient over longer periods of time. Lastly, **end-diastolic wall stress** provides a measure of the force distending the ventricle, providing true transmural pressure is measured. This is rarely possible in the clinical setting since the presence of any significant external constraint invalidates the use of this index of preload. Numerous conditions (ischemia, fibrosis, drug therapy, or effects of cardiopulmonary bypass) are known to invalidate this assumption.

Afterload

In the isolated muscle preparation, afterload refers to the weight or load which is faced by the contracting muscle, that is, the **force resisting shortening.** Although this force can be readily and directly measured in this experimental situation, it is not directly measurable in the ventricle (14). Frequently, the arterial pressure, resistance, or impedance are used as a measure of afterload (15). These parameters, however, all fail to account for the geometric

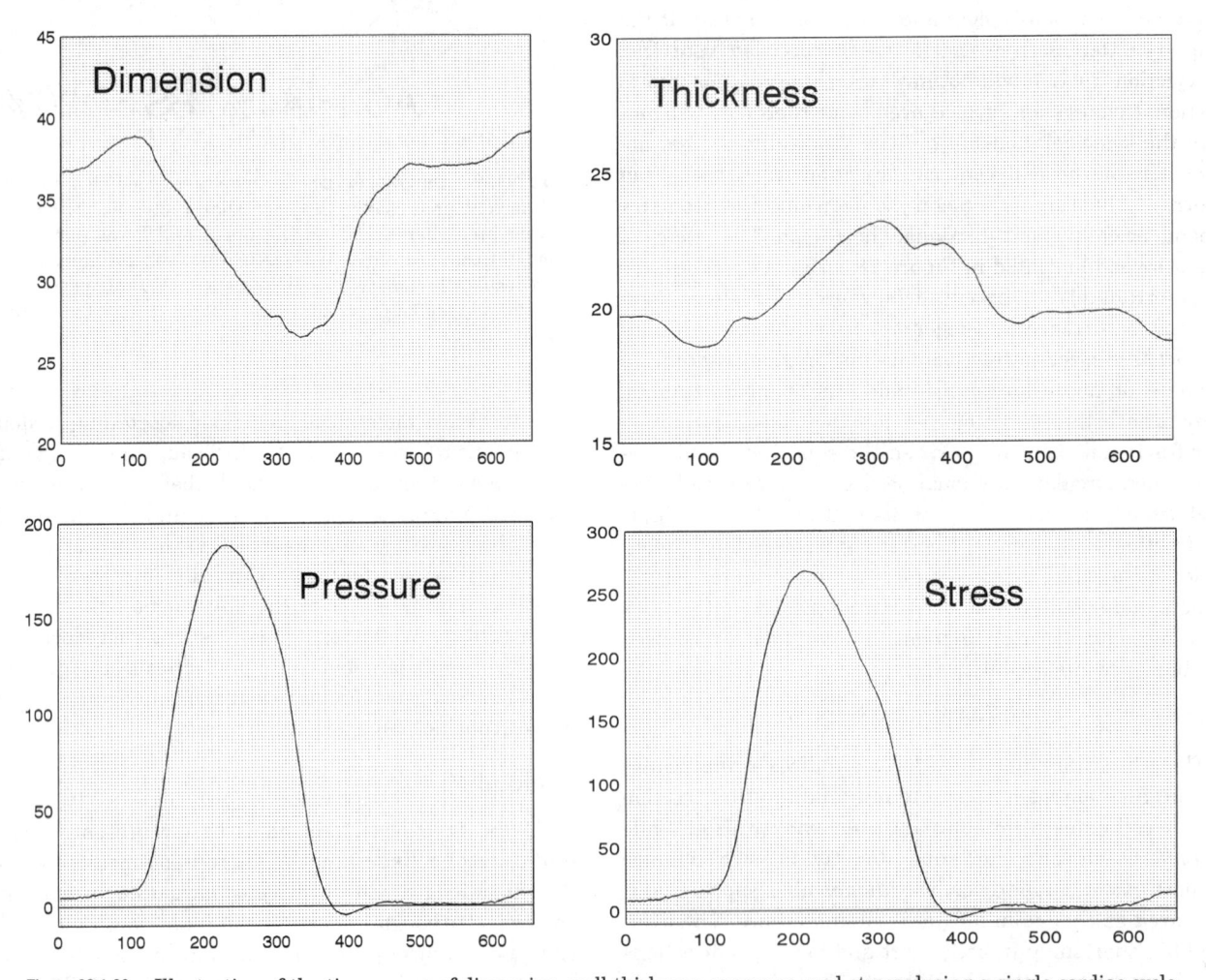

Figure 28.1.20. Illustration of the time course of dimension, wall thickness, pressure, and stress during a single cardiac cycle.

relationship between sarcomere shortening and force generation.

End-systolic wall stress is the force which determines the extent of systolic shortening and is the index of afterload which is the most relevant to the assessment of ventricular function (16–19).

Regardless of which formula is employed, the primary data from which these calculations are performed are transmural pressure, relevant radius of curvature of the wall, and wall thickness. The radius and thickness data can be obtained from any of several modalities including cineangiographic or radionuclide ventriculograms, echocardiograms, or magnetic resonance imaging. Similarly, pressure data can be obtained from either invasive or non-invasive means. Non-invasive aortic pressure can be obtained by recording indirect carotid (or axillary in young children) pulse waveforms calibrated with peripheral blood pressure (20–22).

The transition from the afterload of a constant weight in the isolated muscle preparation to afterload as wall stress in the intact ventricle introduces another level of complexity to the analysis since wall stress is not constant during the course of the cardiac cycle. With the rise and fall of ventricular pressure, the fall in ventricular dimension, and the rise in wall thickness during the contraction phase, wall stress rises rapidly to a peak value in early ejection, falls in a near-linear fashion to end-ejection, and then drops more rapidly to diastolic levels (Fig. 28.1.20). Numerous lines of investigation have documented that the measure of afterload which relates most closely to systolic performance is the stress at end-systole (23–26). That is, end-systolic stress is the force which determines the extent of systolic shortening and is the index of afterload which is most relevant to the assessment of ventricular function.

Contractility

The intrinsic ability of myocardium to shorten against an opposing load is implied by the term contractility. Since the absolute amount of shortening is dependent on both the initial length (preload) and the force which opposes shortening (afterload), indices of fiber shortening provide unreliable means by which to assess contractility. The indices which are known to be relatively load-independent indices of contractility but difficult to apply in a clinical setting include maximum elastance (Fig. 28.1.21), preload-recruitable stroke work (PRSW), and preload-adjusted maximum rate of pressure rise (27–30). The technique which has been found to be more applicable for clinical use in children is described in detail below.

The following is an approach wherein the ejection indices are adjusted for the influence of loading conditions. Mean velocity of shortening (VCF) is calculated as the %FS divided by ejection time. Both percent fractional shortening (%FS) and the VCF are indices of contractility known to be dependent on loading status. The heart rate dependence of this index can be eliminated by correcting ejection time for heart rate in the usual fashion, where rate-corrected ejection time (ETc) equals ejection time divided by the square root of the R-R interval on the electrocardiogram. Rate-corrected mean velocity of fiber shortening (VCFc) is then obtained. When end-systolic stress is used to assess afterload, %FS and VCFc are found to fall in an inversely linear fashion during afterload augmentation (26).

The stress-shortening and **stress-velocity** relationships are sensitive to contractility and thus represent indices of contractility which incorporate afterload as a parameter. Numerous examples of the clinical application of these indices have been reported (31–35). Although these indices permits assessment of contractility independent of afterload effects, it is through the combination of the two that a complete description of the factors influencing cardiac performance can be obtained due to the differential effects of preload on VCFc and %FS.

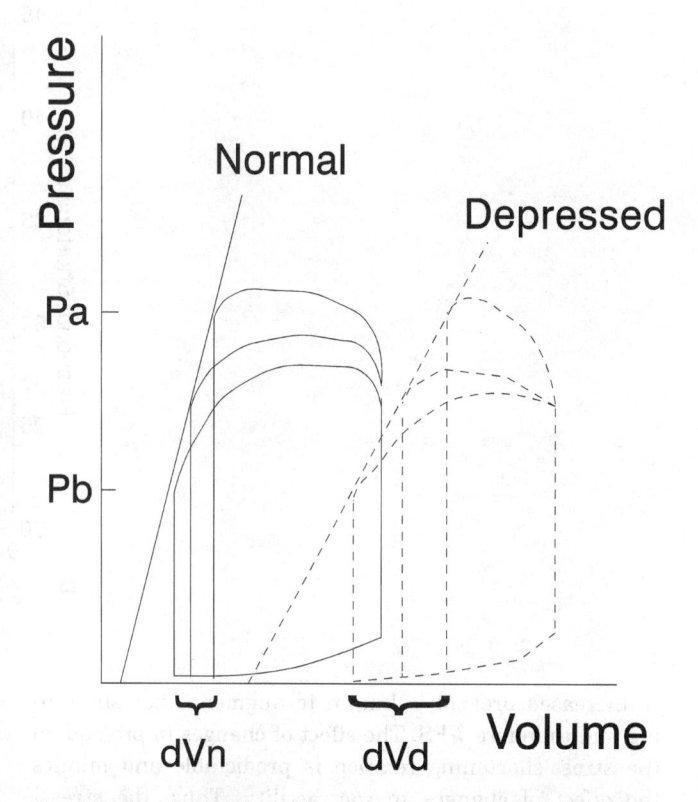

Figure 28.1.21. Derivation of E_{max} from data collected over a range of loading conditions in normal and depressed myocardium. E_{max} is the slope of the end-systolic pressure-volume relationship, derived over a series of variably afterloaded beats at a constant contractile state. E_{max} is shifted rightward and less steep when contractility is depressed. This relationship explains the clinical observation that patients with depressed myocardium are more "afterload sensitive." Reducing end-systolic pressure from P_a to P_b results in a much greater increase in stroke volume in the depressed ventricle (dVd) than in the normal ventricle (dVn).

Figure 28.1.22. Stress-velocity index (*SVI*, relationship of the velocity of circumferential fiber shortening [*VCFc*] to end-systolic stress, *Panel A*) and stress-shortening index (SSI, relationship of fractional fiber shortening to end-systolic stress, *Panel B*), illustrating the method of interpretation of afterload, preload, and contractility from these data. Patient 1 has afterload (end-systolic stress, *ESS*), contractility (*SVI*), and SSI values at the population mean, indicating normal afterload, contractility, and preload. Patient 2 has equivalent reduction of both *SVI* and *SSI*, below the normal range indicated by the *interrupted lines*, indicating depressed contractility but normal preload and afterload. Patient 3 has selective elevation of afterload (ESS), with appropriate and equivalent reduction of both *SVI* and *SSI*, indicating normal contractility and preload despite elevated afterload. Patient 4 has normal *SVI* and *ESS*, indicating normal contractility and afterload. Nevertheless, *SSI* is below normal, indicating a reduced preload state.

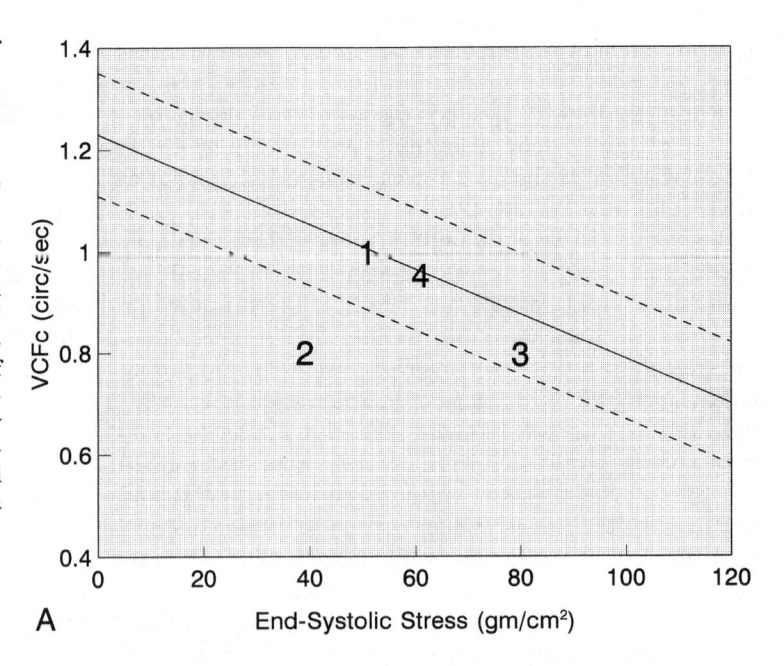

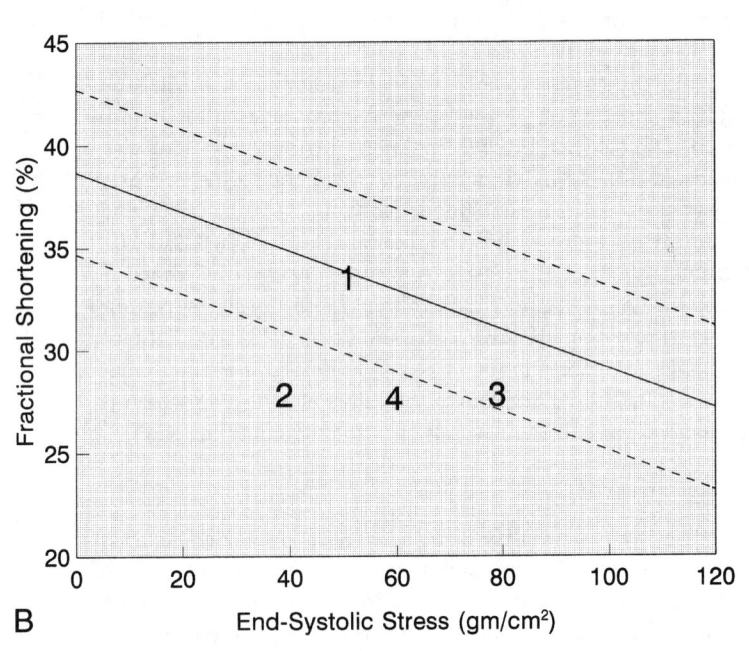

Increased preload is known to augment fiber shortening and therefore %FS. The effect of changes in preload on the stress-shortening relation is predictable and mimics the effect of changes in contractility. Thus, the stress-shortening relation fails to distinguish the effects of altered preload from altered contractility. In contrast, VCFc is not dependent on preload (36–39). Although there are almost certainly limits to the extent of this preload independence, variations in preload within the physiologic range do not significantly alter VCFc. The lack of effect of end-diastolic fiber length on both end-systolic stress and VCFc accounts for the preload-independence of the stress-velocity relation.

When stress-velocity analysis is combined with stress-shortening analysis, abnormalities in fiber shortening which are not related to afterload or contractility (as assessed by the stress-velocity relation) can be recognized as being secondary to preload effects. This analysis is depicted graphically in Figure 28.1.22. The stress-shortening relationship has been used as an index of contractility by a number of authors (40–42) without adjustment for preload effects. Under normal circumstances, the left ventricle operates near the peak of the Frank-Starling mechanism, particularly when measurements are performed in the supine position (43). Thus, the assumption has been made that preload effects are negligible under usual physiological circumstances in humans (44).

Although the data necessary to calculate stress-shortening and stress-velocity indices can be obtained from invasive as well as non-invasive studies, it is the ease with which non-invasive assessment can be performed which allows wide applicability. Non-invasive estimation of end-systolic pressure from the carotid or axillary pulse tracing has been verified against invasive measurements. The calculations for both wall stress and the indices of ventricular function (%FS and VCFc) assume a symmetric ventricular configuration and pattern of contraction (Figure 28.1.22). In the normally shaped ventricle, the radius of curvature of the posterior wall along both the major and minor axes can be measured directly from long and short axis image data. If there are regional abnormalities in shape or movement, or if the ventricle is distorted due to septal displacement (right ventricular pressure or volume overload), then the major and minor axes will not accurately reflect posterior wall radius of curvature and the standard formulae for calculation of wall stress cannot be used.

In addition to data accuracy and value to patient care, the feasibility and ease of performing and repeating a test is a major consideration for clinical utility in the cardiac intensive care unit. The ability to perform this index without disturbing the baseline hemodynamics is an advantage. In addition, data has been collected from hundreds of normal children and this has defined in detail the age-associated variation in contractile performance and hypertrophic response. Thus, the stress-velocity relation represents a preload-independent index of contractility which incorporates afterload.

REFERENCES

1. Fraisse A, Colan SD, Jonas RA, et al. Accuracy of echocardiography for detection of aortic arch obstruction following stage I Norwood procedure. Circulation 1996;94:I-291 Abstract.
2. Holen J, Aaslid R, Landmark K, et al. Determination of effective orifice area in mitral stenosis from non-invasive ultrasound Doppler data and mitral flow rate. Acta Med Scand 1977;201:83-88.
3. Requarth JA, Goldberg SJ, Vasko SD, et al. In vitro verification of Doppler prediction of transvalve pressure gradient and orifice area in stenosis. Am J Cardiol 1984;53:1369-1373.
4. Wong M, Vijayaraghavan G, Bae JH, et al. In vitro study of the pressure-velocity relation across stenotic orifices. Am J Cardiol 1985;56:465-469.
5. Krafchek J, Robertson JH, Radford M, et al. A reconsideration of Doppler assessed gradients in suspected aortic stenosis. Am Heart J 1985;110:765-773.
6. Valdes-Cruz LM, Yoganathan AP, Tamura T, et al. Studies in vitro of the relationship between ultrasound and laser Doppler velocimetry and applicability of the simplified Bernoulli relationship. Circulation 1986;73:300-308.
7. Vasko SD, Goldberg SJ, Requarth JA, et al. Factors affecting accuracy of in vitro valvar pressure gradient estimates by Doppler ultrasound. Am J Cardiol 1984;54:893-896.
8. Teirstein PS, Yock PG, Popp RL. The accuracy of Doppler ultrasound measurement of pressure gradients across irregular, dual, and tunnellike obstructions to blood flow. Circulation 1985;72:577-584.
9. Colan SD. Noninvasive assessment of myocardial mechanics—a review of analysis of stress-shortening and stress-velocity. Cardiology in the Young 1992;2:1-13.
10. Detwiler PW, Nicolosi AC, Weng ZC, et al. Effects of perfusion-induced edema on diastolic stress-strain relations in intact swine papillary muscle. J Thorac Cardiovasc Surg 1994;108:467-476.
11. Sholler GF, Colan SD, Sanders SP. Effect of isolated right ventricular outflow obstruction on left ventricular function in infants. Am J Cardiol 1988;62:778-784.
12. Hoffman D, Sisto D, Frater RWM, et al. Left-to-right ventricular interaction with a noncontracting right ventricle. J Thorac Cardiovasc Surg 1994;107:1496-1502.
13. Beyar R, Dong SJ, Smith ER, et al. Ventricular interaction and septal deformation: A model compared with experimental data. Am J Physiol 1993;265:H2044-H2056.
14. Huisman RM, Elzinga G, Westerhof N, et al. Measurement of left ventricular wall stress. Cardiovasc Res 1980;14:142-153.
15. Lang RM, Borow KM, Neumann A, et al. Systemic vascular resistance: an unreliable index of left ventricular afterload. Circulation 1986;74:1114-1123.
16. Regen DM, Anversa P, Capasso JM. Segmental calculation of left ventricular wall stresses. Am J Physiol 1993;264:H1411-H1421.
17. Mirsky I, Laks MM. A geometric model for the myocardium: biventricular wall stresses in normal and hypertrophied states. Bull Math Biol 1980;42:807-828.
18. Regen DM. Calculation of left ventricular wall stress. Circ Res 1990;67:245-252.
19. Regen DM. Myocardial stress equations: fiberstresses of the prolate spheroid. J Theor Biol 1984;109:191-215.
20. Colan SD, Fujii A, Borow KM, et al. Noninvasive determination of systolic, diastolic and end-systolic blood pressure in neonates, infants and young children: comparison with central aortic pressure measurements. Am J Cardiol 1983;52:867-870.
21. Colan SD, Borow KM, MacPherson D, et al. Use of the indirect axillary pulse tracing for noninvasive determination of ejection time, upstroke time, and left ventricular wall stress throughout ejection in infants and young children. Am J Cardiol 1984;53:1154-1158.
22. Colan SD, Borow KM, Neumann A. Use of the calibrated carotid pulse tracing for calculation of left ventricular pressure and wall stress throughout ejection. Am Heart J 1985;109:1306-1310.
23. Suga H, Kitabatake A, Sagawa K. End-systolic pressure determines stroke volume from fixed end-diastolic volume in the isolated canine left ventricle under a constant contractile state. Circ Res 1979; 44:238-249.
24. Borow KM, Colan SD, Neumann A. Altered left ventricular mechanics in patients with valvular aortic stenosis and coarctation of the aorta: effects on systolic performance and late outcome. Circulation 1985;72:515-522.

25. Borow KM, Green LH, Grossman W, et al. Left ventricular end-systolic stress-shortening and stress-length relations in human. Normal values and sensitivity to inotropic state. Am J Cardiol 1982;50:1301–1308.
26. Colan SD, Borow KM, Neumann A. Left ventricular end-systolic wall stress-velocity of fiber shortening relation: a load-independent index of myocardial contractility. J Am Coll Cardiol 1984;4:715–724.
27. Karunanithi MK, Michniewicz J, Copeland SE, et al. Right ventricular preload recruitable stroke work, end-systolic pressure-volume, and dP/dt$_{max}$-end-diastolic volume relations compared as indexes of right ventricular contractile performance in conscious dogs. Circ Res 1992;70:1169–1179.
28. Little WC, Cheng CP, Mumma M, et al. Comparison of measures of left ventricular contractile performance derived from pressure–volume loops in conscious dogs. Circulation 1989;80:1378–1387.
29. Feneley MP, Skelton TN, Kisslo KB, et al. Comparison of preload recruitable stroke work, end-systolic pressure-volume and dP/dt$_{max}$-end-diastolic volume relations as indexes of left ventricular contractile performance in patients undergoing routine cardiac catheterization. J Am Coll Cardiol 1992;19:1522–1530.
30. Rahko PS. Comparative efficacy of three indexes of left ventricular performance derived from pressure-volume loops in heart failure induced by tachypacing. J Am Coll Cardiol 1994;23:209–218.
31. Colan SD, Sanders SP, Borow KM. Physiologic hypertrophy: effects on left ventricular systolic mechanics in athletes. J Am Coll Cardiol 1987;9:776–783.
32. Colan SD, Trowitzsch E, Wernovsky G, et al. Myocardial performance after arterial switch operation for transposition of the great arteries with intact ventricular septum. Circulation 1988; 78:132–141.
33. Graham TP Jr, Franklin RCG, Wyse RKH, et al. Left ventricular wall stress and contractile function in childhood: normal values and comparison of Fontan repair versus palliation only in patients with tricuspid atresia. Circulation 1986;74: I-61–I-69.
34. Graham TP Jr, Franklin RC, Wyse RK, et al. Left ventricular wall stress and contractile function in transposition of the great arteries after the Rastelli operation. J Thorac Cardiovasc Surg 1987;93:775–784.
35. Rajfer SI, Borow KM, Lang RM, et al. Effects of dopamine on left ventricular afterload and contractile state in heart failure: relation to the activation of beta1-adrenoceptors and dopamine receptors. J Am Coll Cardiol 1988;12:498–506.
36. Quinones MA, Gaasch WH, Alexander JK. Influence of acute changes in preload, afterload, contractile state and heart rate on ejection and isovolumic indices of myocardial contractility in man. Circulation 1976;53:293–302.
37. Mahler F, Ross J, O'Rourke RA, et al. Effects of changes in preload, afterload, and inotropic state on ejection and isovolumic phase measures of contractility in the conscious dog. Am J Cardiol 1975;35:626–634.
38. Nixon JV, Murray RG, Leonard PD, et al. Effect of large variations in preload on left ventricular performance characteristics in normal subjects. Circulation 1982;65:698–703.
39. Quinones MA, Gaasch WH, Cole JS, et al. Echocardiographic determination of left ventricular stress-velocity relations in man. With reference to the effects of loading and contractility. Circulation 1975;51:689–700.
40. Schulman DS, Remetz MS, Elefteriades J, et al. Mild mitral insufficiency is a marker of impaired left ventricular performance in aortic stenosis. J Am Coll Cardiol 1989;13:796–801.
41. Gunther S, Grossman W. Determinants of ventricular function in pressure-overload hypertrophy in man. Circulation 1979;59:679–688.
42. Carabello BA, Green LH, Grossman W, et al. Hemodynamic determinants of prognosis of aortic valve replacement in critical aortic stenosis and advanced congestive heart failure. Circulation 1980;62:42–48.
43. Parker JO, Case RB. Normal left ventricular function. Circulation 1979;60:4–12.
44. Ross JJ. Mechanism of cardiac contraction. What roles for preload, afterload, and inotropic state in heart failure. Eur Heart J 1983;4 Suppl A:19–28.

28.2 Perioperative Echocardiographic Examination in the Intensive Care Setting

Abdul Aldousany, MD, and Barry Marcus, MD

ECHOCARDIOGRAPHIC EVALUATION OF THE PREOPERATIVE PATIENT

Most critically ill children present to the cardiac intensive care unit (ICU) with clinical syndromes of cyanosis or congestive heart failure. With the advent of color Doppler techniques and transesophageal probes, echocardiography can accurately define the complete segmental anatomy and its pathophysiology in most patients admitted to the intensive care setting (1). Transthoracic echocardiography is still the most often used modality of echocardiography with its major limitations being precise definition of certain extracardiac structures and determination of physiologic indices such as pulmonary vascular resistance.

Echocardiographic Evaluation for Cyanosis

In critically ill neonates with cyanosis, preliminary stabilization and pharmacologic therapy (e.g., PGE$_1$ use) and subsequent surgical intervention (e.g., palliation with an aortopulmonary shunt or correction with complete repair) can often be instituted with an accurate echocardiographic survey without cardiac catheterization (2). A brief overview of the impact and specific uses of echocardiography for the more common lesions is presented below with more details discussed in Part B.

Certain lesions are routinely managed with echocardiographic evaluation and without cardiac catheterization. In neonates with D-transposition of the great arteries, diagnosis is usually straightforward in experienced hands, and special attention is paid to coronary artery anatomy (to determine feasibility of arterial switch operation) and to associated lesions (such as left ventricular outflow tract obstruction) (3). In addition, echocardiography is useful in determining the presence of elevated pulmonary vascular resistance in the excessively cyanotic neonate with transposition of the great arteries (4). Lastly, palliative balloon atrial septostomy can be performed under transthoracic (or transesophageal) echocardiographic guidance in the ICU (5). The type of total anomalous pulmonary venous connection and its precise location of venous drainage can be diagnosed accurately by combined two-dimensional and color Doppler flow mapping (6). Transesophageal echocardiography can further improve visualization of the pulmonary venous confluence. Cardiac catheterization may be necessary when echocardiography does not show the drainage location of all of the pulmonary veins, although this procedure should be avoided if at all possible because it has considerable risk in the critically ill neonate. Neonates with truncus arteriosus typically undergo total corrective surgery without catheterization because the anatomy and its associated lesions (e.g., arch obstruction) as well as truncal valve stenosis and regurgitation can usually be clearly defined by echocardiography alone.

Other lesions do warrant a combined echocardiography-catheterization approach to complete the pertinent details of the diagnosis. In infants with pulmonary atresia with intact ventricular septum, for example, although intramyocardial coronary sinusoids can be diagnosed by transthoracic echocardiographic assessment, cardiac catheterization may be necessary to rule out coronary artery stenoses (which would contraindicate right ventricular outflow tract reconstruction with attendant right ventricular decompression and potential coronary artery steal) (7). Patients with tetralogy of Fallot and pulmonary atresia continue to require cardiac catheterization with angiography to define the precise nature of the pulmonary blood supply and to delineate aortopulmonary collaterals (8, 9). In cyanotic infants with tricuspid atresia and other types of single ventricle with ductal-dependent pulmonary blood flow, the major limitation of echocardiography remains the delineation of pulmonary arterial anatomy, especially its more distal portions. Lastly, neonates with Ebstein's anomaly of the tricuspid valve can be accurately diagnosed by transthoracic echocardiography, although cardiac catheterization may be needed to determine whether the pulmonary valve is atretic or severely stenotic.

Transthoracic echocardiography is also useful in managing the neonate with a noncardiac cause of cyanosis. In patients with persistent pulmonary hypertension of the newborn (PPHN), transthoracic echocardiography details normal intracardiac and great vessel anatomy with right-to-left shunting at either the ductal or foramen ovale levels (10). In addition, the rare patient with pulmonary arteriovenous fistulae can be successfully diagnosed with echocardiography and saline contrast study (with the contrast returning to the left atrium almost immediately after it is injected into the systemic venous circulation).

Echocardiographic Evaluation for Congestive Heart Failure

If congestive heart failure is the presenting symptom, transthoracic echocardiography is also the principal diagnostic modality. The cause of congestive heart failure can be broadly categorized into obstruction to systemic blood flow, volume overload, or myocardial dysfunction.

Obstruction to systemic outflow can take the form of interrupted aortic arch, coarctation of the aorta, critical aortic stenosis, or hypoplastic left heart syndrome, all of which can usually be adequately defined by transthoracic echocardiography (11). At diagnosis, intravenous PGE_1 therapy can be immediately initiated and surgical palliation or repair can often follow without cardiac catheterization, except in those neonates deemed candidates for balloon aortic valvotomy for critical aortic stenosis. Lesions with left ventricular inflow obstruction from cor triatriatum, supravalvar mitral stenosis, and congenital mitral stenosis are usually diagnosed accurately by echocardiography without the need for catheterization, unless pulmonary vascular resistance calculation is desired in the older patient (12).

Volume overload lesions such as ventricular septal defect, common atrioventricular canal, patent ductus arteriosus, aortopulmonary window, or severe mitral insufficiency can likewise be diagnosed and surgically treated using transthoracic echocardiography without further studies in the cardiac catheterization laboratory. If pulmonary vascular resistance calculations are deemed vital in the decision for surgical intervention or if certain aspects of the anatomy warrant further investigation (e.g., left ventricular size in variants of common atrioventricular canal), cardiac catheterization can be pursued.

Transthoracic echocardiography is useful to diagnose and serially follow patients with congestive heart failure caused by myocardial dysfunction, whether secondary to myocarditis or cardiomyopathy (13, 14). It is important for echocardiography to rule out the anatomic entity of anomalous left coronary artery from the pulmonary artery in any infant with myocardial dysfunction. M-mode measurement of left ventricular shortening fraction is most commonly used as an index of left ventricular function, but it is a load-dependent index. The relationship of ventricular end-systolic wall stress to the mean velocity of fiber shortening is, however, a load-*independent* index of myocardial contractility (15). Intrinsic contractility changes and response to inotropic or afterload reduction in the intensive care setting can be followed using the latter technique. Lastly, diastolic function can also be assessed and serially followed using a number of specific M-mode and Doppler indices profiling flow across the atrioventricular valves (16).

ECHOCARDIOGRAPHIC EVALUATION OF THE INTRAOPERATIVE PATIENT

Virtually all surgeries for congenital and acquired cardiac anomalies now include intraoperative transesophageal echocardiography (TEE) evaluation. Immediately prior to surgery, TEE is performed to confirm the diagnosis and to gain additional diagnostic information that may have eluded transthoracic imaging. The rates of positive preoperative impact on anatomic diagnosis have varied between 9 and 31% (17–19). Transesophageal echocardiography can add details to atrial septum, subvalvar areas, muscular ventricular septum, right ventricular outflow tract, and more posterior structures (e.g., pulmonary veins and atrioventricular valves).

Transesophageal echocardiography is also used routinely to evaluate specific results of surgery and any potential postoperative residua following separation from cardiopulmonary bypass. Ungerleider et al. demonstrated that intraoperative echocardiography led to a 42% rate of reoperation in patients with residual lesions (versus only a 3% reoperation rate in those without residual defects) (20). In the operating room, TEE can also provide continuous real time data demonstrating ventricular function and volume status from the rewarming phase of cardiopulmonary bypass to sternal closure. These data, combined with the electrocardiogram (ECG) and hemodynamic data, allow for early institution of individualized postoperative care in the operating room prior to transport to the ICU.

ECHOCARDIOGRAPHIC EVALUATION OF THE POSTOPERATIVE PATIENT

In the postoperative patient who has an expectant recovery, frequent routine echocardiographic assessment in the ICU setting is not indicated. When the postoperative course is complicated or protracted and when a cardiac arrest of uncertain cause occurs, echocardiographic evaluation is of paramount importance. In the postoperative patient, transthoracic echocardiographic assessment is initially pursued but TEE should be added as a diagnostic tool if transthoracic acoustic windows are suboptimal. It is important to remember potential hemodynamic, respiratory, and bleeding sequelae with TEE, especially during the probe insertion process. The more common clinical syndromes in postoperative intensive care with relevance to echocardiography are presented below.

Echocardiographic Evaluation for Low Output State

Echocardiographic assessment is useful to delineate the exact cause of low output, which can include (a) hypovolemia, (b) decreased myocardial contractility, (c) myocardial ischemia, (d) excess afterload, (e) pericardial effusion, and most importantly, (f) postoperative residua or previously undiagnosed lesions.

Hypovolemia

Hypovolemia is generally suspected in face of low central venous and left atrial pressures, low systemic arterial blood pressure, and sinus tachycardia. In hypovolemia, the principal echocardiographic finding is empty-appearing ventricular cavities, especially the right ventricle. The other intracardiac and great vessel assessments are normal with normal biventricular function.

Decreased Myocardial Contractility

Decreased myocardial contractility is clinically suspected in the face of elevated central venous and left atrial pressures, low systemic arterial blood pressure, and sinus tachycardia. Echocardiographic imaging of both ventricles can evaluate overall biventricular function. M-mode calculation of left ventricular shortening fraction provides loading condition dependent index of left ventricular performance. If low left ventricular shortening fraction (Fig. 28.2.1; see color plate 28.2.1) is seen in the presence of normal loading conditions, then decreased intrinsic myocardial function is suspected.

Myocardial Ischemia

Modern cardioplegic and myocardial protective techniques during cardiopulmonary bypass generally protect the myocardium from ischemic injury. Surgeries that directly involve manipulation of the coronary arteries (e.g., arterial switch operation for transposition of the great arteries, coronary artery reimplantation for anomalous left coronary artery from the pulmonary artery, or aortic valve replacement with pulmonary autograft valve, or the Ross procedure) place the myocardium at higher risk for ischemia. TEE can directly visualize the coronary artery anastomoses looking for distortion or kinking of these vessels.

In addition, spectral Doppler and color flow mapping can profile coronary flow patterns for turbulence that may be abnormal. Lastly, TEE also evaluates for ventricular function and segmental wall motion abnormalities, and it can be even more sensitive in detecting ischemia than postoperative ECG changes (21).

Excess Afterload

Excess afterload occurs postoperatively when high systemic vascular resistance causes a reduction in cardiac output. This is clinically suspected with peripheral vasoconstriction and a mottled appearance. Hemodynamic profile includes high central venous and left atrial pressures, sinus tachycardia, and systemic arterial blood pressure that can be either normal or high.

Echocardiographic imaging of the left ventricle reveals reduced pumping function and left ventricular shortening fraction. Mitral regurgitation is common in this setting. Loading condition dependent measurements of both left ventricular afterload (wall stress) and intrinsic left ventricular myocardial contractility (velocity of circumferential fiber shortening = VcFc) can be measured to further assess afterload; if wall stress is increased, elevated afterload is diagnosed but if VcFc is reduced, decreased intrinsic myocardial contractility is suspected instead. The relationship of ventricular end-systolic wall stress to the velocity of circumferential fiber shortening can direct therapeutic decision-making regarding the use of inotropic and afterload reduction pharmacologic support (please see previous section).

Pericardial Effusion

Pericardial effusion should be considered in any postoperative patient with low cardiac output, elevated central venous and left atrial pressures, low systemic arterial blood pressure, and sinus tachycardia (see also Chapter 33, *Miscellaneous Topics*). Cardiac tamponade occurs when the pericardial effusion causes right atrial or right ventricular compression, impairing cardiac filling.

Echocardiography is a sensitive and specific noninvasive tool to diagnose and quantify a pericardial effusion rapidly with or without tamponade (Fig. 28.2.2). Occasionally, a large pleural effusion can mimic a pericardial effusion. If pericardiocentesis is indicated, it is generally performed under echocardiographic guidance.

Postoperative Residua or Previously Undiagnosed Lesions

Significant postoperative residua presence can cause low output state via pressure and volume overload (e.g., persistent mitral insufficiency following mitral valve repair [Fig. 28.2.3; color plate 28.2.3]). These findings are now diagnosed intraoperatively by TEE prior to decannulation and sternal closure; return to cardiopulmonary bypass to revise the operation is sometimes necessary prior to sternal closure to assure a smooth postoperative course. It is possible, however, that different loading conditions in the ICU or other mechanical issues (e.g., sutures coming loose or patch being dehisced) can occur following a previously good result based on intraoperative TEE.

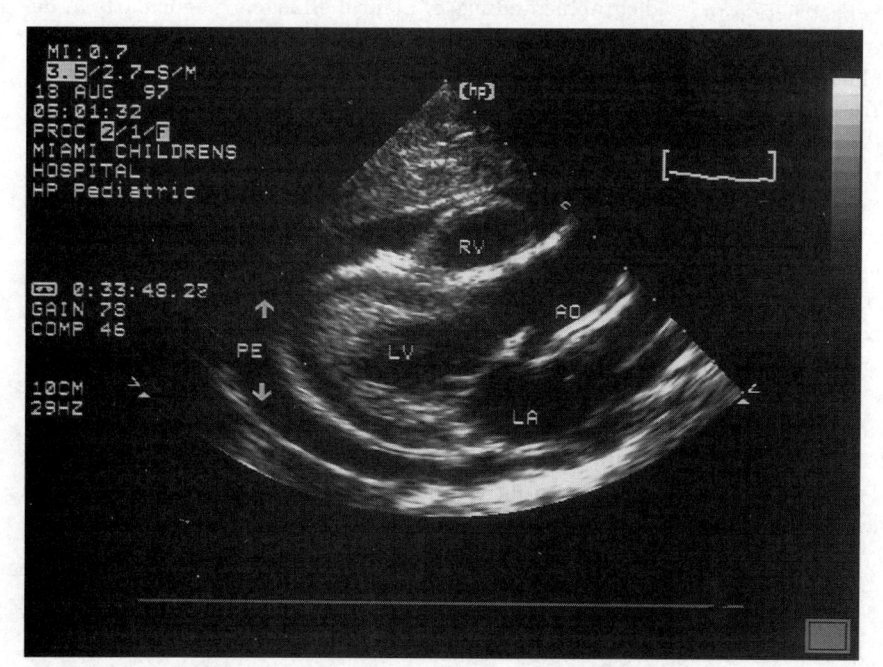

Figure 28.2.2. Pericardial effusion. This parasternal long-axis view demonstrates a circumferential pericardial effusion of about 1 cm (echo-free space with *arrows* and labeled PE). The right ventricle (labeled RV) is collapsed secondary to the pericardial fluid. LA, left atrium; LV, left ventricle; and AO, aorta.

In certain patients, a previously unrecognized lesion can also cause pressure and volume overload and lead to postoperative low output state. Therefore, complete echocardiographic evaluation is always indicated in the postoperative patient with clinical low output state (rather than an evaluation solely directed at the operated segments).

Echocardiographic Evaluation for Hypoxemia

Differential diagnosis of postoperative hypoxemia is extensive, but it can be separated into pulmonary versus cardiac cause. Echocardiography is useful to evaluate for a cardiac cause of postoperative hypoxemia.

The most likely cardiac cause of hypoxemia is intracardiac right-to-left shunting at atrial or ventricular level (Fig. 28.2.4; see color plate 28.2.4). Saline contrast echocardiographic assessment can be even more sensitive for intracardiac right-to-left shunting compared with Doppler color flow mapping (22). In this procedure, a bolus of agitated saline (5–10 mL) is injected quickly into a large bore and preferably central venous catheter to fully opacify the right heart. The appearance of left-sided contrast indicates intracardiac right-to-left shunting. In patients with tetralogy of Fallot and truncus arteriosus after corrective surgery, it is common to have right-to-left shunting at the atrial level because of transient right ventricular dysfunction. In addition, significant postoperative intracardiac ventricular level right-to-left shunting is distinctly abnormal, and it requires a diagnostic explanation to rule out residual ventricular septal defect with elevated pulmonary vascular resistance or right ventricular outflow obstruction (including double-chamber right ventricle).

In single ventricle patients, an important cardiac cause of hypoxemia in the postoperative setting is obstruction to flow through a systemic to pulmonary artery shunt. Echocardiographic evaluation of right or left pulmonary artery flow patterns as well as color Doppler flow from the subclavian artery to the pulmonary artery (Fig. 28.2.5; color plate 28.2.5) can assess whether the shunt is patent. Although echocardiography can usually demonstrate shunt patency, it is not always reliable, and angiography should be pursued if the diagnosis is uncertain. In postoperative Fontan patients, contrast echocardiography is also used to evaluate flow through the lateral tunnel to detect right-to-left shunting across the Fontan fenestration. Contrast medium must be injected from a venous site below the diaphragm so that it flows into the inferior vena cava to opacify the lateral tunnel. Contrast medium injected from above the diaphragm into the superior vena cava will go into the pulmonary circulation, and it may not opacify the lateral tunnel.

Echocardiographic Evaluation for Fever

Differential diagnosis of postoperative fever is extensive, and it is generally not secondary to endocarditis. Evaluation of unexplained or persistent postoperative fever, particularly if a murmur or positive blood cultures are present, should include complete echocardiographic assessment. A history for the presence of indwelling intravascular lines should also increase suspicion for endocarditis and lower the threshold for echocardiographic evaluation.

Echocardiography may be helpful if a vegetation is detected but its sensitivity is limited to 1–2 mm (23) so that a negative echocardiographic evaluation for vegetations does not rule out endocarditis. If a high index of clinical suspicion for endocarditis exists and transthoracic echocardiographic evaluation is negative for vegetations, TEE should be performed because it is more sensitive for vegetations when compared with transthoracic echocardiography (24). Both transthoracic and TEE evaluations of homograft conduits (e.g., right ventricle to pulmonary artery) and prosthetic grafts (e.g., aortic interposition graft for interruption of the aortic arch) are technically difficult to image as the ultrasound beam may not penetrate well within the conduit or graft lumen; magnetic resonance imaging may be helpful in these patients.

Echocardiographic Evaluation for Additional Postoperative Problems

Pleural Effusion

Transthoracic echocardiography is a useful but underutilized tool to diagnose pleural effusion in the postoperative patient (Fig. 28.2.6). A transthoracic sweep above both hemidiaphragms and also laterally, posteriorly, and superiorly of both lungs can detect any significant pleural fluid. This is particularly useful postoperatively when chest radiographic findings of pleural effusions, particularly in neonates, are often inconclusive.

Intracardiac and Great Vessel Thrombi

Echocardiography is the diagnostic modality of choice to evaluate the postoperative patient for clinically suspected thrombi (Fig. 28.2.7). A high index of suspicion and low threshold for evaluation are recommended when a history of long-term indwelling intravascular catheter is present or where low-velocity flow state connections have been established (e.g., postoperative Fontan).

Diaphragmatic Paralysis

In the postoperative patient with a chest radiograph demonstrating an elevated hemidiaphragm, the question of diaphragmatic paresis or paralysis arises. Fluoroscopy can be performed to evaluate diaphragmatic motion but this procedure involves transport of an intensive care patient to the cardiac catheterization laboratory or radiology department. On the other hand, transthoracic echocardiography at the bedside can evaluate movement of each hemi-

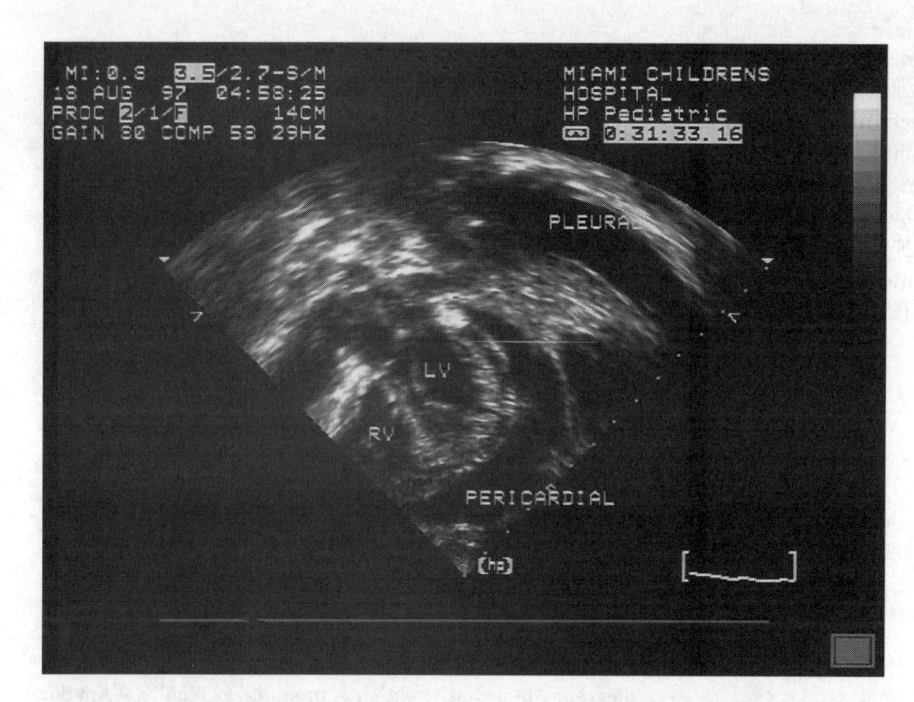

Figure 28.2.6. Pericardial and pleural effusion. This subcostal four-chamber view shows a large pericardial effusion (echo-free space labeled pericardial) as well as a sizable left pleural effusion (labeled pleural) with lung tissue outlined clearly by the pleural fluid. LV, left ventricle; RV, right ventricle.

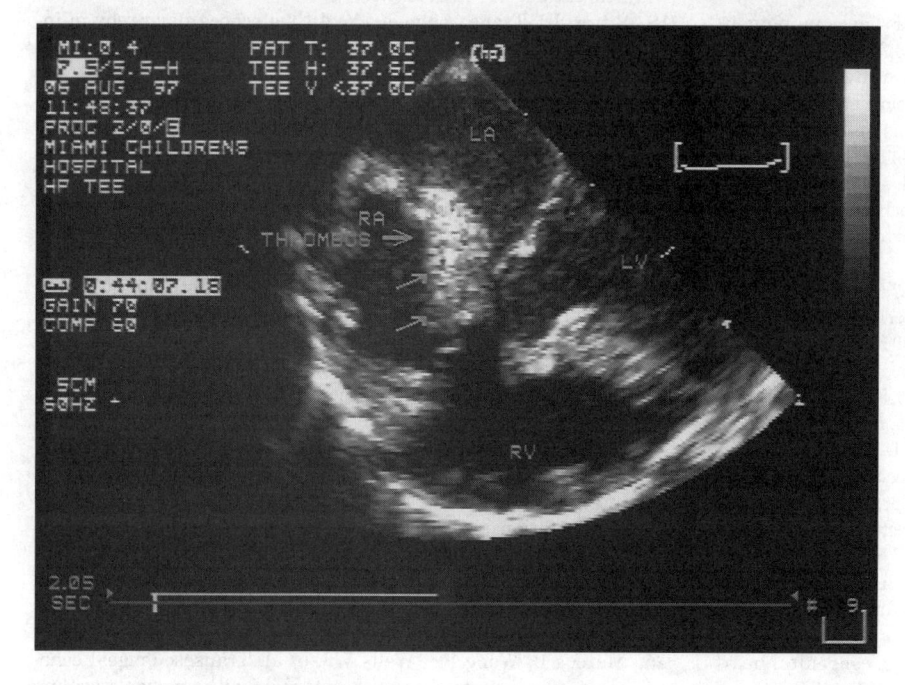

Figure 28.2.7. Right atrial thrombus. Transesophageal echocardiogram illustrating a large thrombus in the right atrium (*arrows*). LA, left atrium; LV, left ventricle; RV, right ventricle.

diaphragm separately and appropriately with spontaneous respirations.

Echocardiographic Evaluation for the Difficult to Image Patient

Open Sternum

In some patients, cardiac edema precludes primary sternal closure and the patient leaves the operating room with a patch covering the sternotomy wound. This situation precludes usual placement of the transthoracic probe for most studies. Therefore, TEE is the modality of choice for patients requiring complete echocardiographic evaluation in this setting (25).

Mechanical Support

Echocardiography is effective to evaluate the postoperative patient requiring extracorporeal membrane oxygenation (ECMO) or ventricular assist device (VAD) support for recovery of a stunned myocardium or cardiopulmonary failure. Intraoperative post-bypass TEE can often recognize myocardial failure necessitating mechanical support in the operating room. In addition, intracavitary or intravascular thromboses, not uncommon complications while these patients are on support, can be followed by echocardiography. Finally, continuous on-line TEE monitoring can direct the timing for weaning from mechanical support and evaluate left ventricle function immediately after removing the support cannulae (26).

High-Frequency Jet Ventilation

When high-frequency jet ventilation is used, transthoracic echocardiographic assessment can be technically difficult because of the rapid chest wall motion and artifact produced by the high-frequency chest oscillation. Transesophageal echocardiography can be used to provide better images.

REFERENCES

1. Ritter SB. Two-dimensional Doppler color flow mapping in congenital heart disease. Clin Cardiol 1986;9:591–599.
2. Stevenson JG, Kawabori I, Bailey WW. Non-invasive evaluation of Blalock-Taussig shunts: determination of patency and differentiation from patent ductus arteriosus by Doppler echocardiography. Am Heart J 1983;106:1121–1129.
3. Pasquini L, Sanders SP, Parness IA, et al. Diagnosis of coronary artery anatomy by two-dimensional echocardiography in patients with transposition of the great arteries. Circulation 1987;75:557–564.
4. Chang AC, Wernovsky G, Kulik T, et al. Management of the neonate with transposition of the great arteries and persistent pulmonary hypertension. Am J Cardiol 1991;68:1253–1255.
5. Steeg CN, Bierman FZ, Hordof AJ, et al. Bedside balloon atrial septostomy in infants with transposition of the great arteries: New concepts using two-dimensional echocardiographic techniques. J Pediatr 1985;107:944–946.
6. Chin AJ, Sanders SP, Sherman F, et al. Accuracy of subcostal two-dimensional echocardiography in prospective diagnosis of total anomalous pulmonary venous connection. Am Heart J 1987;113:1153–1159.
7. Calder AL, Co EE, Sage MD. Coronary arterial abnormalities in pulmonary atresia with intact ventricular septum. Am J Cardiol 1987;59:436–442.
8. Schiller NB, Snider AR. Echocardiography in congenital heart disease: key references. Circulation 1981;63:461–475.
9. Piehler JM, Danielson GK, McGoon DC, et al. Management of pulmonary atresia with ventricular septal defect and hypoplastic pulmonary arteries by right ventricular outflow construction. J Thorac Cardiovasc Surg 1980;80:552–565.
10. Gotteiner NL, Harper WR, Gidding SS, et al. Echocardiographic prediction of neonatal ECMO outcome. Pediatr Cardiol 1997;18:270–275.
11. Huhta JC, Latson LA, Gutgesell HP, et al. Echocardiography in the diagnosis and management of symptomatic aortic valve stenosis in infants. Circulation 1984;70:438–445.
12. Norell MS, Lincoln C, Sutton GC. Two-dimensional echocardiographic diagnosis of cor triatriatum. J Cardiovasc Ultrasonogr 1983;2:369–376.
13. Lewis AB. Prognostic value of echocardiography in children with idiopathic dilated cardiomyopathy. Am Heart J 1994;128:133–136.
14. D'Cruz IA, Daly DP, Shroff SG. Left ventricular shape and size in dilated cardiomyopathy: Quantitative echocardiographic assessment. Echocardiography 1991;8:187–196.
15. Colan SD, Borow KM, Newmann A. Left ventricular end-systolic wall stress-velocity of fiber shortening relation: a load independent index of myocardial contractility. J Am Coll Cardiol 1984;4:715–724.
16. St. Goar FG, Masuyama T, Alderman EL, et al. Left ventricular diastolic dysfunction in end stage dilated cardiomyopathy: Simultaneous Doppler echocardiography and hemodynamic evaluation. J Am Soc Echocardiogr 1991;4:349–356.
17. Lam J, Neirotti RA, Nijveld A, et al. Transesophageal echocardiography in pediatric patients: preliminary results. J Am Soc Echocardiogr 1991;4:43–50.
18. Ritter SB. Transesophageal real-time echocardiography in infants and children with congenital heart disease. J Am Coll Cardiol 1991;18:569–580.
19. Stumper O, Kaulitz R, Elzenga NJ, et al. The value of transesophageal echocardiography in children with congenital heart disease. J Am Soc Echocardiogr 1991;4:164–176.
20. Ungerleider RM, Greeley WJ, Sheikh KH, et al. The use of intraoperative echo with Doppler color flow imaging to predict outcome after repair of congenital cardiac defects. Ann Surg 1989;210:526–534.
21. Smith JS, Cahalan MK, Benefiel DJ, et al. Intraoperative detection of myocardial ischemia in high risk patients: electrocardiography versus two-dimensional transesophageal echocardiography. Circulation 1985;72:1015–1021.
22. Pieroni DR, Varghese PJ, Freedom RM, et al. The sensitivity of contrast echocardiography in detecting intracardiac shunts. Cathet Cardiovasc Diagn 1979;5:19–29.
23. Mugge A, Daniel WG, Frank G, et al. Echocardiography in infective endocarditis: reassessment of prognostic implications of vegetation size determined by the transthoracic and the transesophageal approach. J Am Cardiol 1989;14:631–638.
24. Birmingham GD, Rhako PS, Ballantyne F. Improved detection of infective endocarditis with transesophageal echocardiography. Am Heart J 1992;123:774–782.
25. Marcus B, Wong PC, Wells WJ, et al. Transesophageal echocardiography in the postoperative child with an open sternum. Ann Thorac Surg 1994;58:235–236.
26. Marcus BP, Atkinson J, Wong P, et al. Use of transesophageal echocardiography in infants on extracorporeal membrane oxygenation. J Thorac Cardiovasc Surg 1995;109:846–848.

Cardiac Catheterization in the Critically Ill Cardiac Patient

Jonathan J. Rome, MD, and James E. Lock, MD

Patients recovering from surgery in the intensive care unit may be referred to the catheterization laboratory for diagnostic evaluation, therapeutic intervention, or pharmacologic manipulations. In addition, it is increasingly common for nonoperated patients to require intensive care before or after catheter interventions. This chapter describes current catheter-directed therapies with attention to postprocedure care and complications, and outlines the role of catheterization in diagnosis and treatment of patients after heart surgery.

GENERAL CONSIDERATIONS

Cardiac catheterization can be performed with relatively low risk in even the most unstable of patients. However, this is possible only if the procedure is well planned and expeditiously executed. Timely and effective communication is essential among physicians, surgeons, nurses, and additional personnel involved in catheterization.

Patient Preparation and Transport to the Catheterization Suite

All patients should have a baseline electrocardiogram (ECG) and chest radiograph obtained prior to catheterization. Blood should be available for interventional cases, neonates, and patients with unrepaired tetralogy of Fallot. Choice of access sites used at catheterization can be critical. If indwelling catheters are to be exchanged for the procedure, additional intravenous access should be obtained and infusions switched *before leaving the intensive care unit*. Any additional studies that might be necessary during catheterization (e.g., transesophageal echocardiography, bronchoscopy, or special drug studies) should be coordinated ahead of time. Management of the critically ill patient in the catheterization laboratory is no different from that in the operating room. An appropriately trained physician *not* involved in performing the procedure should be responsible for the patient's medical management from exit from the intensive care unit until return from the catheterization laboratory and stabilization. This individual may be a cardiologist, anesthesiologist, neonatologist, or critical care physician depending on patient needs, institutional expertise, and staffing. In order that transport to the catheterization laboratory be accomplished safely, transport monitors should be used and adequate personnel present to manage the airway, move associated apparatus, and monitor the patient. In some instances (e.g., a child on extracorporeal membrane oxygenation) patient transport can be the riskiest part of the procedure, and it requires careful planning.

Catheterization in the Newborn

Umbilical arterial and venous sites are often used for catheter access in neonates. Before leaving the intensive care unit it is helpful to have umbilical lines available for catheter exchange. It is important to note that infusions given in these catheters will be interrupted during catheterization. An alternative intravenous source of glucose and fluid must be secured, as well as adequate access maintained for inotropic support, prostaglandin E_1 (PGE_1), and so forth. Most newborns, particularly those receiving PGE_1 infusions, should be intubated for catheterization. Prevention of hypothermia during catheterization can be challenging, particularly in the premature infant. Patients should be maintained on warming blankets with their heads covered and the room temperature appropriately adjusted. Radiant warming may also be required in some instances. Ventilatory support often requires adjustment during the procedure because of additional sedation or changes in hemodynamics. Communication between the anesthesiologist or intensivist and the cardiologist performing the procedure must be ongoing: changes made in ventilatory or hemodynamic support can have a profound impact on catheterization data, whereas an optimal response to predictable episodes of blood loss, arrhythmia, or other alterations caused by the procedure requires that the intensivist be able to anticipate such problems.

When a newborn returns to the intensive care unit after catheterization, it is essential that the intensive care team receive a comprehensive report of the procedure. A chest radiograph should be obtained to confirm position of invasive lines and catheters, and an electrocardiogram should be obtained after complex interventions. Repeatedly instrumented umbilical vessels increase the risk for infection. Patients catheterized through umbilical vessels should be closely monitored for evidence of infection. Many centers administer prophylactic antibiotic coverage when umbilical lines have been left in place after catheterization.

THERAPEUTIC CATHETERIZATION

Intensive care is required after therapeutic catheterization in most newborns, in some older patients undergoing complex procedures, and to manage certain postcatheterization complications. Transcatheter treatments also play an increasingly important role in the perioperative care of patients undergoing surgery for complex congenital heart defects. This overview will serve as a brief introduction to transcatheter therapeutics with emphasis on periprocedure patient care. Recent reviews are available for more comprehensive discussions of transcatheter therapies in pediatrics (1, 2).

VALVULOPLASTY

Balloon valvuloplasty is routinely performed for aortic and pulmonary stenosis in all pediatric age groups. Congenital or rheumatic mitral stenosis can also be treated by dilation in many cases (3, 4). Pulmonic stenosis was the first lesion treated by cardiac catheterization and the first valvar lesion treated with inflation balloons (5). Balloon dilation of typical valvar pulmonic stenosis in both infants and adults is technically straightforward, low in risk, and usually curative (6–9). Dilation of aortic stenosis, although generally successful, is a riskier procedure with the potential for significant blood loss, femoral artery injury, and development of aortic insufficiency (10–14). Most patients undergoing routine valvuloplasty of any type do not require intensive care. Newborns are the exception, and their treatment and care will be discussed in greater detail.

Critical Pulmonic Stenosis

Ductal patency must be maintained with PGE_1 infusion in newborns with critical pulmonic stenosis to assure adequate pulmonary blood flow prior to intervention. Catheterization should not be needlessly delayed as complications of PGE_1 therapy (e.g., necrotizing enterocolitis) become more frequent with prolonged medical management. However, patients with superimposed insults (such as infection or posthypoxic end-organ injury) or those with other critical anomalies, should undergo appropriate diagnosis and treatment of these problems prior to catheter intervention. Balloon pulmonary valvuloplasty can be technically challenging, but it is generally well tolerated by the neonate. An umbilical arterial catheter is used for monitoring, whereas diagnostic catheterization and valvuloplasty are generally performed via the femoral vein. Included in the diagnostic evaluation are measurement of right ventricular pressure and angiography to evaluate right ventricular size, tricuspid valve size and function, and pulmonary valve annulus dimension. Rarely, patients with critical pulmonic stenosis have associated coronary fistulae from the right ventricle.

After diagnostic evaluation, the stenotic valve is crossed and a small guidewire advanced either into a distal branch pulmonary artery or preferably through the ductus arteriosus into the descending aorta. Often the valve is predilated with a small balloon to allow passage of the larger definitive valvuloplasty balloon (diameter 120 to 140% the annulus size; Fig. 29.1). The results of dilation are estimated with a pressure pullback from pulmonary artery to right ventricle. Right ventricular pressure typically remains elevated because of the persistent patent ductus as well as the frequent occurrence of dynamic infundibular stenosis after balloon dilation. The pressure, however, should fall approximately to systemic levels (15). Because of significant improvements in balloon technology, the risk of vascular injury after pulmonary valvuloplasty is low in full-term newborns. Although perforation of the right ventricular outflow tract with tamponade has been reported (16), it occurs infrequently.

After completion of valvuloplasty, PGE_1 infusion is discontinued while the patient is carefully observed in the intensive care unit. Right-to-left shunting at atrial level persists for a variable time period because of the poor compliance of the hypertrophied right ventricle. As the ductus closes, patients often become progressively hypoxemic. Severe hypoxemia (Po_2 less than 25 torr) in this setting is rare, and it should prompt evaluation for the presence of persistent right ventricular inflow or outflow obstruction (from tricuspid stenosis, inadequate relief of right ventricular outflow tract [RVOT] obstruction, or hypoplasia of the right ventricle). In general, if RVOT obstruction persists after balloon valvotomy, successful surgical management will require placement of a right ventricular outflow patch. Where anatomic obstructions are absent, reinstitution of PGE_1 for several days may allow time for sufficient remodeling of the right ventricle to permit adequate antegrade flow. In cases where inadequate right ventricular volume or compliance persists, surgical shunt procedures are performed to provide a stable source of pulmonary blood while allowing the remodeling process to occur (16).

Aortic Stenosis

In critical aortic stenosis left ventricular outflow obstruction prevents adequate cardiac output to support the systemic circulation. PGE_1 infusion allows right ventricular output to support systemic blood flow via the ductus arteriosus, thus allowing time for recovery from end-organ injury. Precatheterization diagnostic study of these infants includes full echocardiographic evaluation to determine

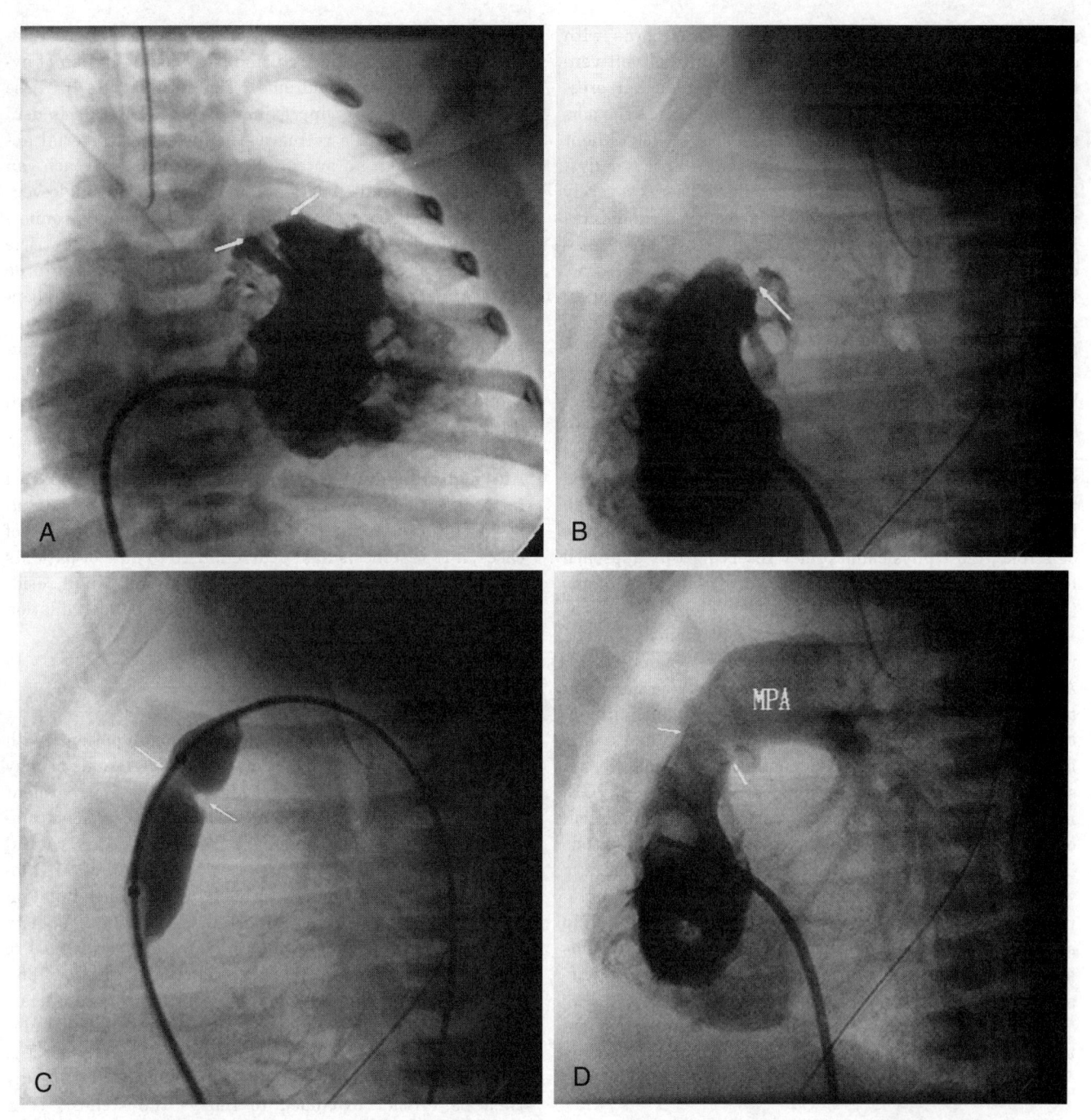

Figure 29.1. Right ventricular angiogram in a patient with critical pulmonic stenosis in (**A**) anteroposterior and (**B**) lateral projections. The ventricle is heavily trabeculated and tricuspid regurgitation is present. A trace of contrast is seen above the level of the pulmonary valve (*arrows*) in the main pulmonary artery. For valvuloplasty the distal wire is positioned through the patent ductus to the descending aorta as seen on lateral projection (**C**). A distinct waist (*arrows*) disappeared with higher pressure inflation. After balloon dilation, lateral projection of a repeat right ventricular angiogram demonstrates antegrade flow through the annulus (*arrows*) with dense opacification of the main pulmonary artery (*MPA*) (**D**).

whether left-sided cardiac anatomy is appropriate for biventricular circulation (17).

Catheterization laboratory management of the newborn with critical aortic stenosis requires assiduous attention to detail: these infants are notoriously fragile. In addition to continuous assessment and therapy to correct hypovolemia, acidosis, or other hemodynamic alterations, malignant arrhythmias must be anticipated and expeditiously treated. A full diagnostic study is performed including left ventriculography to estimate ventricular size, function, and aortic valve annulus size. Although newborns with critical aortic stenosis have markedly diminished left ventricular shortening, measurement of left ventricular pressure generally reveals a significant gradient across the aortic valve. When a left ventricular to aortic systolic gradient is not present, it is more likely that left ventricular dysfunction is irreversible or left ventricular inflow is severely restricted. Such patients should be considered candidates for Norwood procedure (in this instance, preoperative catheter creation of an atrial septal defect may be necessary). Balloon valvuloplasty can be performed either via an antegrade approach (femoral or umbilical vein), or via a retrograde arterial catheter (Fig. 29.2). Retrograde dilation from the femoral artery is better tolerated by the ill newborn, but it risks arterial injury, and whereas the antegrade approach preserves arterial integrity, it generally results in more hemodynamic instability and risks mitral valve injury. A transcarotid approach has been advocated by some for dilation of newborn aortic stenosis (18, 19); however, because of the possibility of carotid artery injury or stroke, most physicians prefer reserving this approach for special circumstances (e.g., the very premature infant) (Fig. 29.2D).

Successful outcome after aortic valvuloplasty in the newborn requires careful postprocedure management. After valve dilation, net ductal flow typically becomes left to right, resulting in a "steal" from the systemic circulation. This can be confirmed by Doppler evaluation, and it is reflected by an increase in postductal arterial oxygen saturation. When this change has been documented, PGE_1 infusion should be discontinued as the ductal shunt will only contribute to congestive heart failure. Intravenous inotropic therapy is continued in patients with evidence of ventricular dysfunction. Afterload reduction may be appropriate, particularly in cases where dilation has resulted in significant aortic insufficiency. As intravenous infusions are weaned, therapy with orally administered agents should be instituted.

Pedal perfusion must be continuously assessed in patients after transfemoral arterial catheterization (see *Iliofemoral Arterial Injury*, discussed below).

ANGIOPLASTY

After experimental studies demonstrated the potential utility of balloon angioplasty in treating nonatherosclerotic arterial stenoses, this procedure has been applied to a large number of vascular obstructions (20).

Coarctation of the Aorta

Both native and postoperative obstructions of the aorta have been treated by balloon angioplasty. Balloon dilation is the accepted primary treatment for patients with *postoperative* arch obstructions (e.g., following repair of coarctation, interrupted aortic arch, and Norwood palliation of hypoplastic left heart syndrome). The success rate in these groups of patients is approximately 80%. Dilation is usually performed via a retrograde transfemoral arterial approach, although an antegrade transvenous approach can be applied in smaller patients or in those with single ventricle heart disease in whom the systemic venous connections still allow passage of a catheter through the ventricle to the distal arch. Patients undergoing this procedure do not routinely require intensive care, however they can benefit from continued observation in an intensive care unit setting, particularly if there is concern of aortic arch aneurysm formation or peripheral vessel damage. The most common reported complication after retrograde aortic arch dilation is femoral artery injury (23, 24).

Dilation for *native* coarctation remains controversial. Although significant gradient reduction has been reported in most patients, failure rates vary from 0 to 12%. Aneurysms after dilation have been reported in 4 to 15% of cases, and restenosis has occurred in 20 to 30% of patients on short-term follow-up (21, 22). In addition, small residual arch gradients are more common after balloon dilation than after surgery.

Branch Pulmonary Artery Stenosis

Pulmonary artery stenoses are common in patients with congenital heart defects, and may be native lesions or may occur after prior surgical procedures. Catheter treatment is the procedure of choice in most instances (25). The complex anatomy of the pulmonary tree necessitates careful angiographic definition of stenoses prior to dilation. Dilation is usually performed with balloons that allow inflation at high pressures (Fig. 29.3). High pressure angioplasty has improved the success rate of the procedure with a 1 to 2% incidence of perforation or aneurysm formation (26). When balloon angioplasty is unsuccessful because of elastic recoil, kinking, or restenosis of the vessel, endovascular stenting has proved effective. A stainless steel stent (Fig. 29.4) is deployed on an angioplasty balloon, and it may then be further expanded to relieve the stenosis (Fig. 29.5) (27).

Patients undergoing pulmonary angioplasty may require intensive care after the procedure under certain circumstances. Most common is the patient who develops, or is at high risk for, segmental pulmonary edema (Fig. 29.6). This process occurs in individuals with systemic or suprasystemic central pulmonary artery pressure in whom dilation or stenting has resulted in massively increased flow and pressure to segments of previously hypoperfused lung ("reperfusion pulmonary edema"). Patients at greatest risk appear to be those in whom persistent pulmonary artery hypertension is present after dilation because of multiple

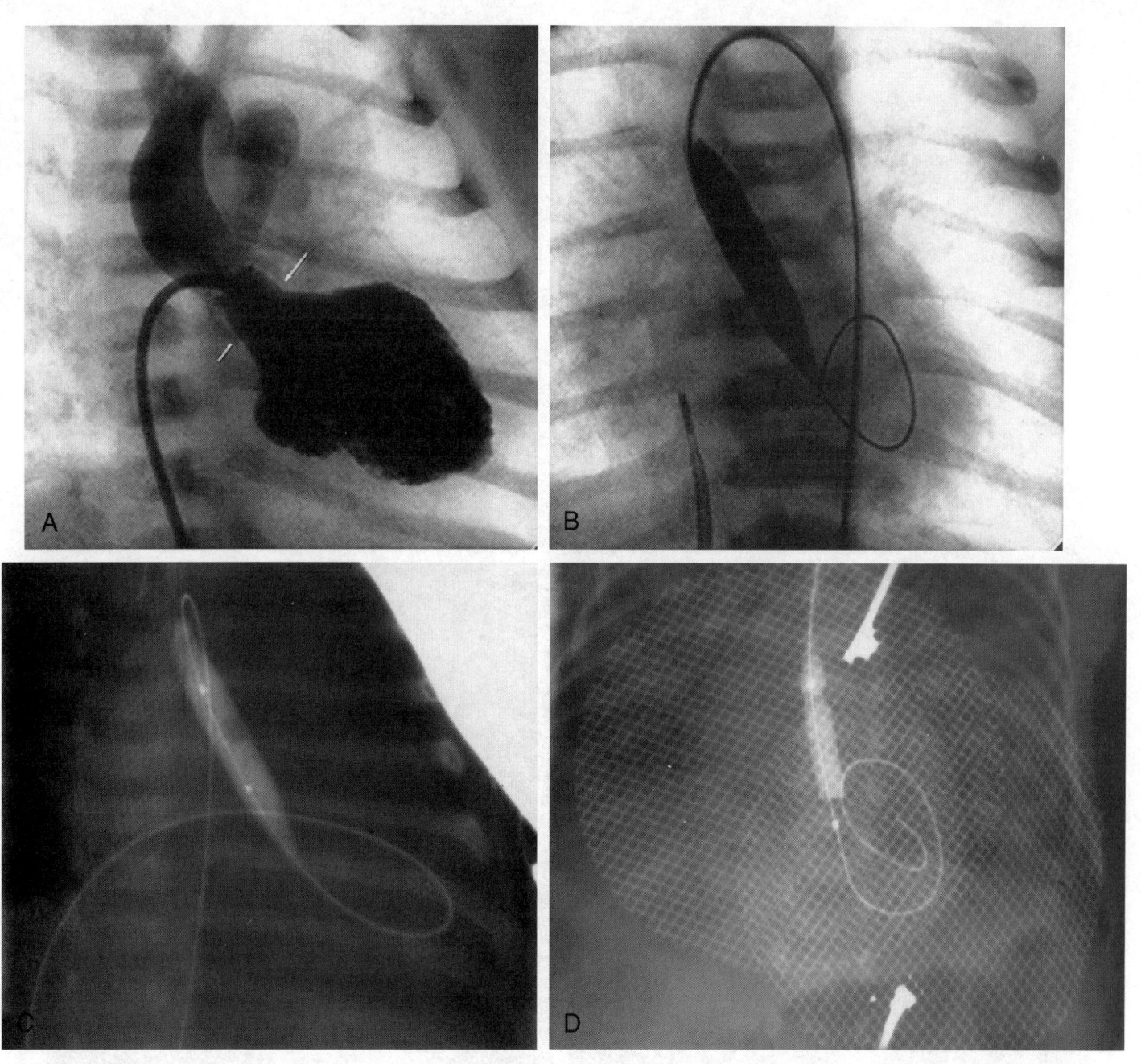

Figure 29.2. **A.** Left ventricular angiogram in a newborn with critical aortic stenosis. The aortic valve leaflets (*arrows*) are thickened and doming. **B.** In this retrograde dilation the valvuloplasty balloon has been advanced over a guidewire via the femoral artery. **C.** Antegrade dilation: the valvuloplasty balloon is inflated across the left ventricular outflow. **D.** Transcarotid retrograde balloon dilation of aortic stenosis in a 1000 g premature infant.

segments of residual stenosis or pulmonary vascular disease. Although the pathophysiology of this phenomenon is not fully understood, it is likely that insufficient capillary density or arteriolar smooth muscle is present in the lung segment to accommodate the sudden elevation in flow and hydrostatic pressure. This process can be life threatening, and it is often difficult to treat. Patients can develop marked ventilation perfusion mismatch with resultant profound hypoxemia. The segmental nature of the process can make mechanical ventilation difficult to manage. Patients at high risk for reperfusion pulmonary edema should be intubated and anesthetized for the procedure and ventilated with positive end expiratory pressure for 24 to 48 hours after it. For those who develop severe hypoxemia unresponsive to such measures, recatheterization for dilation of residual stenoses should be done to allow more even dis-

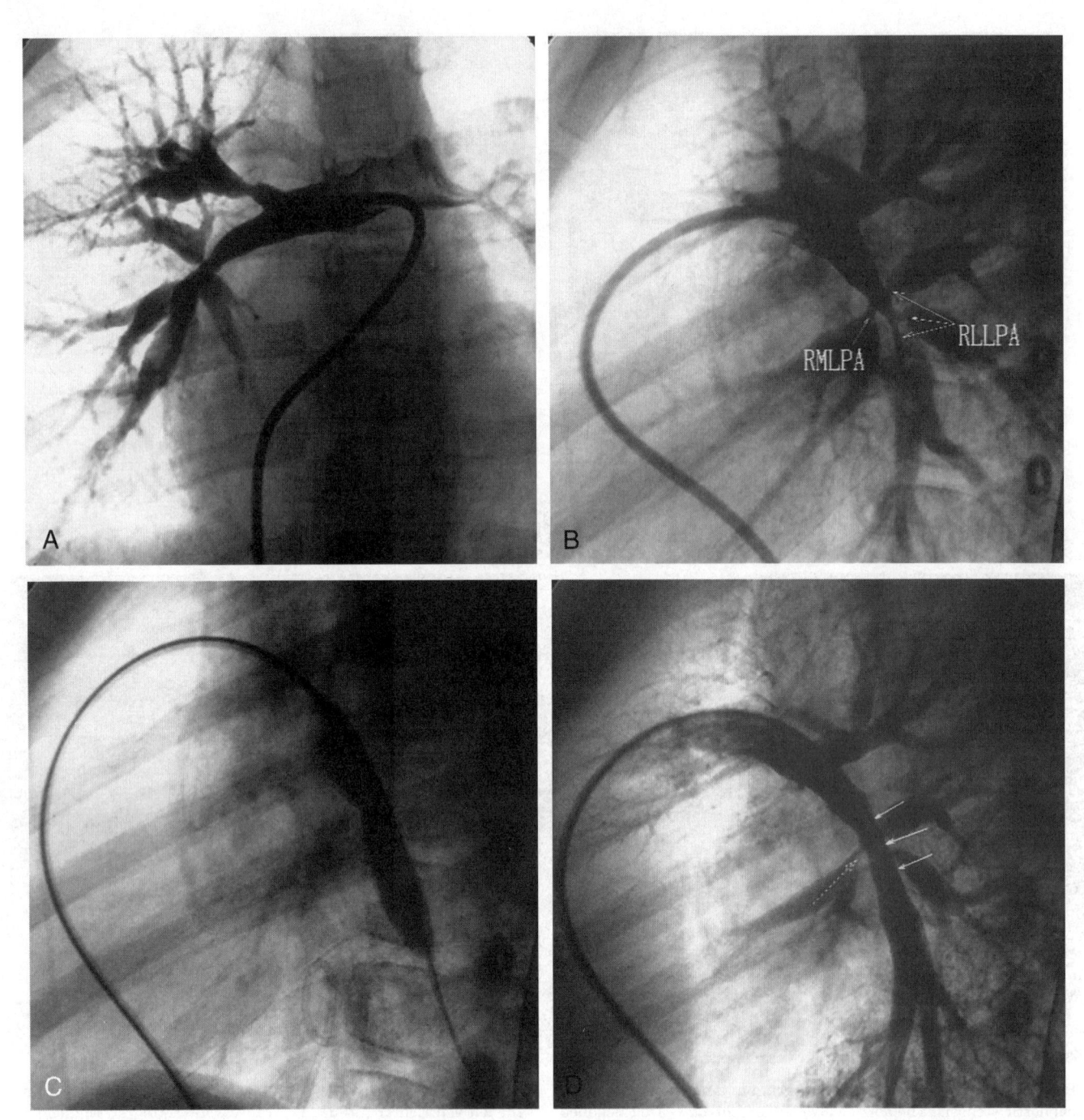

Figure 29.3. **A.** Anteroposterior and (**B**) lateral projections of contrast injection in the right pulmonary artery in a patient with multiple branch pulmonary artery stenoses. Branch stenoses, best seen in the lateral view (**B**), affect origins of the right middle lobe and multiple right lower lobe segmental arteries. **C.** A high-pressure balloon is inflated across one of the lower lobe branches. The waist seen in lateral projection is obliterated at 20 atm pressure. **D.** The lower lobe branch is no longer stenotic postangioplasty (*solid arrows*). The still stenotic middle lobe branch (*dashed arrow*) was treated on subsequent dilation. *RMLPA*, right middle lobe pulmonary artery; *RLLPA*, right lower lobe pulmonary arteries.

tribution of pulmonary blood flow. Despite the hemodynamic and clinical instability high-flow pulmonary edema can cause, it serves as a marker of anatomic success, and typically resolves within 48 hours.

Pulmonary artery perforation or dissection can result in significant hemorrhage after balloon angioplasty. Again, the highest risk patients are those with pulmonary artery hypertension in the affected segment(s). Hemorrhage is usually, but not always, evident in the catheterization laboratory. If a pleural effusion develops on chest radiograph,

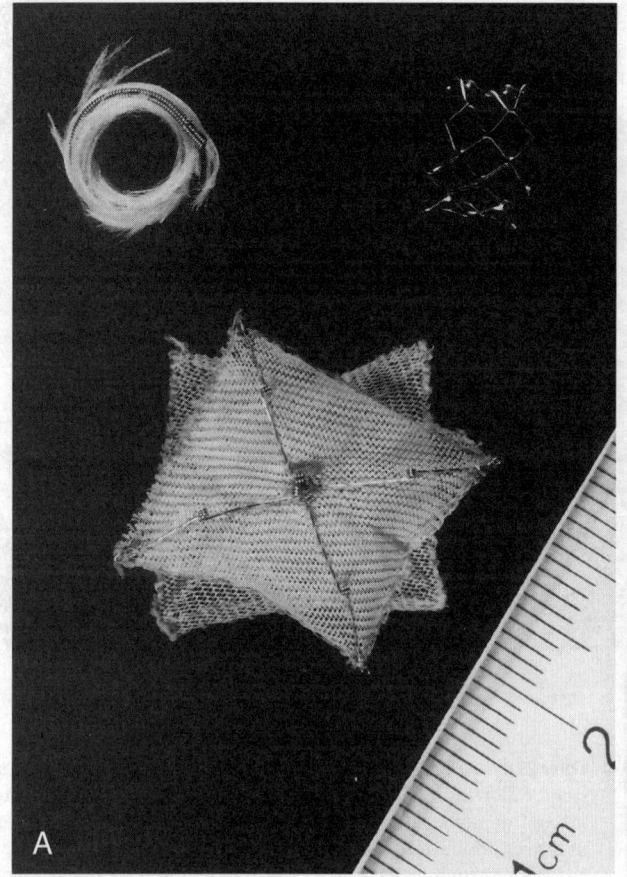

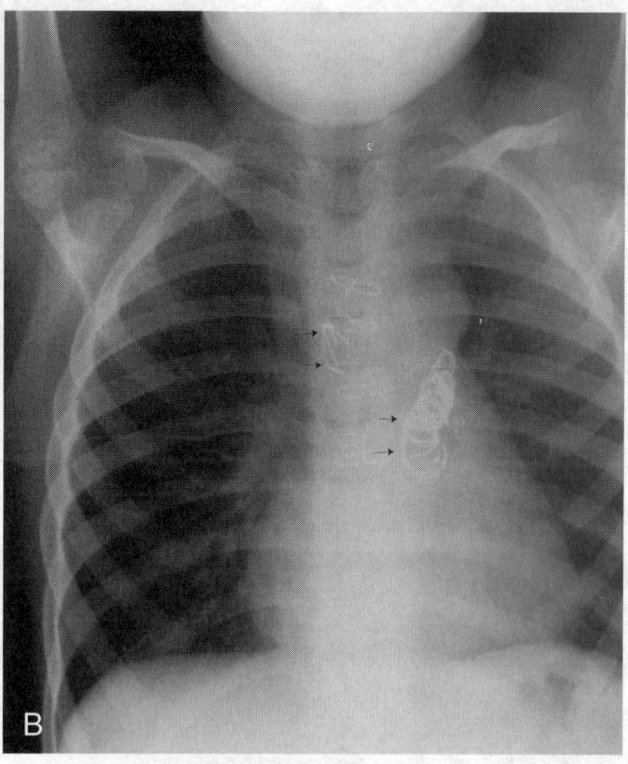

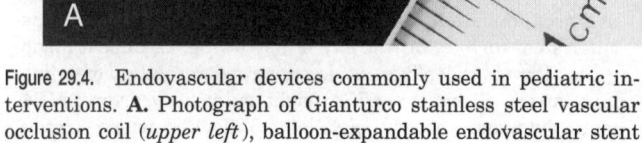

Figure 29.4. Endovascular devices commonly used in pediatric interventions. **A.** Photograph of Gianturco stainless steel vascular occlusion coil (*upper left*), balloon-expandable endovascular stent (*upper right*), and the Clamshell occluder device (*bottom*). **B.** Radiographic appearance of coils occluding right modified Blalock-Taussig shunt and left superior vena cava (*arrows*).

or hemoptysis, hypovolemia, or an unanticipated fall in hematocrit are noted in a patient after pulmonary artery dilation, the interventional cardiologist should be notified immediately while resuscitative measures are instituted.

Iliofemoral Arterial Injury

Arterial injury is more common after left heart dilations performed via the femoral artery because angioplasty balloons have a relatively large exit profile and, therefore, require a large arterial sheath. The spectrum of injury varies from intimal injury with secondary arterial spasm and thrombus formation to major arterial disruption. All patients with evidence of decreased limb perfusion must be carefully and continuously assessed to determine the extent of vascular injury. Patients with occlusion of the *femoral artery* typically have a slightly cooler leg with diminished pedal pulses and delayed capillary refill. Pedal pulses are usually present by Doppler. Limb viability is rarely compromised because of collateral flow via branches of the internal iliac artery. Such patients should receive intravenous heparin infusions with appropriate laboratory and clinical monitoring. Systemic thrombolytic therapy can be instituted after 24 hours if pulses and perfusion have not normalized. Although several agents can be used, the most experience is with urokinase: an initial bolus of 4400 U/kg is given, followed by 4400 U/kg/h for 24 hours (28). Such therapy can be safely used even in neonates; however, risk of intracranial hemorrhage exists, particularly in newborns who have sustained significant injury from shock or are premature (29, 30).

Patients with occlusion of the *common iliac artery* typically have a cold, pallid, pulseless leg. Limb viability compromise has been reported in this group of children. A vascular surgeon should be consulted immediately to permit expeditious diagnostic evaluation and therapy. Surgical management rarely restores normal limb blood flow, but it may be needed to prevent ongoing blood loss.

Major iliofemoral disruptions after catheterization are always associated with evidence of decreased limb perfusion. More limited perforations can result in hemorrhage without decreased pulses, and a high index of suspicion

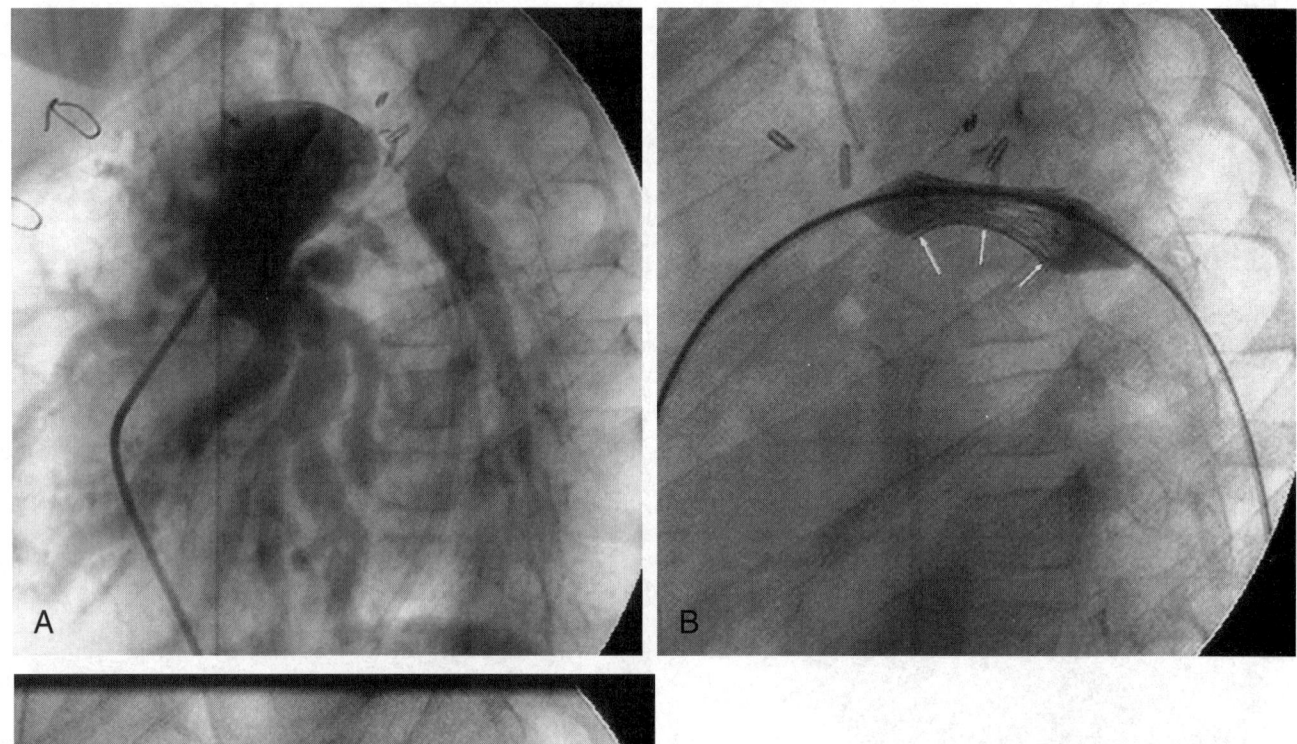

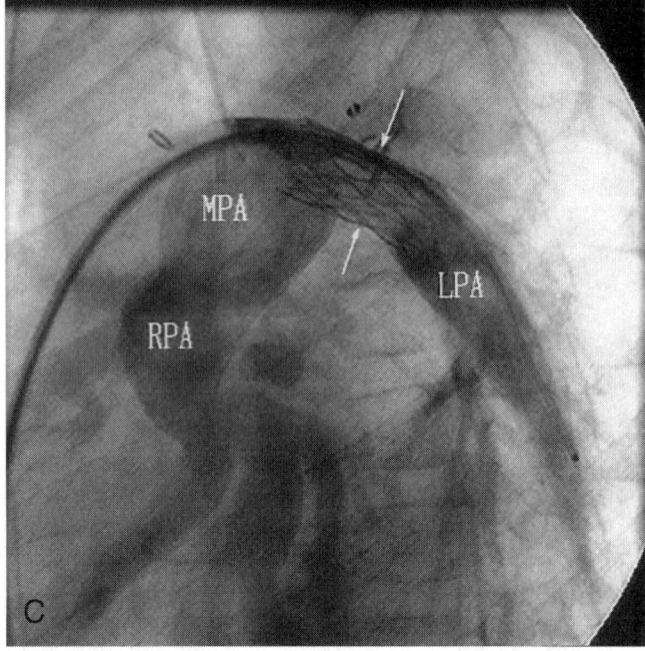

Figure 29.5. **A.** Lateral projection of pulmonary angiogram in patient following repair of tetralogy of Fallot with pulmonary atresia demonstrates severe stenosis of left pulmonary artery at site of prior surgical shunt (*clips*). **B.** Deployment of endovascular stent (*arrows*) at the site of narrowing. **C.** Repeat angiogram after stent deployment demonstrates resolution of pulmonary artery obstruction. RPA, right pulmonary artery; MPA, main pulmonary artery; LPA, left pulmonary artery; *arrows*, stent.

must be maintained. Accurate information regarding blood loss during the procedure as well as any potential concerns about vessel injury must be communicated by the physician performing the procedure to those caring for the patient in the intensive care unit. Patients in whom the hematocrit falls excessively, or evidence of hypovolemia develops, should be thoroughly evaluated with serial chest and abdominal radiographs, noninvasive imaging of the retroperitoneum, and, where appropriate, angiography.

EMBOLIZATION AND CLOSURE PROCEDURES

Metal embolization coils can be used to treat a variety of lesions in patients with congenital heart defects. Coils delivered through a catheter promote thrombus formation with resultant vascular occlusion (Fig. 29.4). A wide variety of lesions including systemic to pulmonary collateral arteries, Blalock-Taussig shunts, venous connections, coronary artery fistulae, and patent ductus arteriosus may be embolized (31, 32).

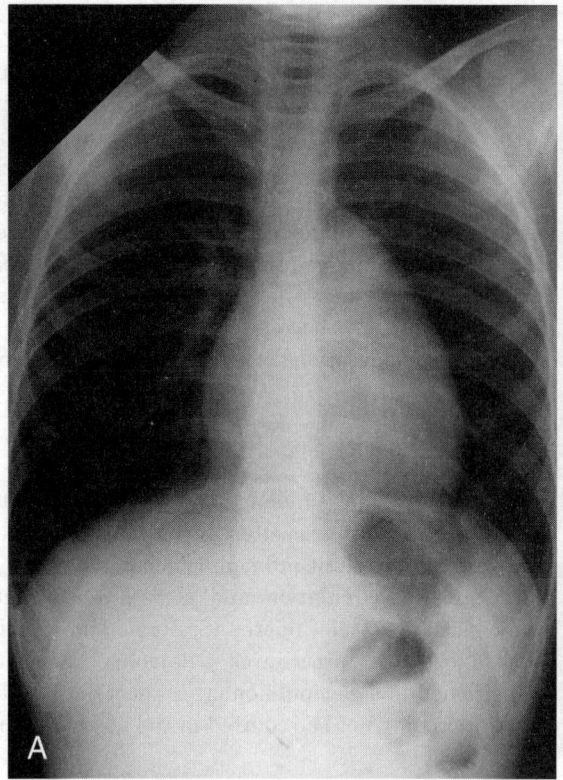

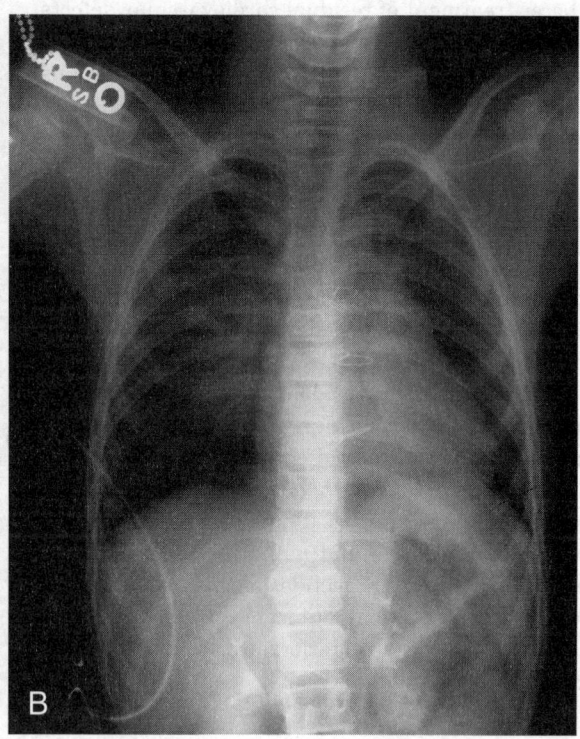

Figure 29.6. Chest radiographs of a child with multiple branch right pulmonary artery stenoses and pulmonary vascular disease in segments of the left pulmonary artery (**A**) before and (**B**) after balloon dilations and placement of endovascular stent in right pulmonary artery. After the procedure the radiograph demonstrates markedly increased blood flow to the right lung with right-sided pulmonary edema.

Since the first report of transcatheter atrial septal defect (ASD) closure in 1976, a variety of devices have been used to close a host of intra and extracardiac defects (2, 33, 34). Although none of these devices has approved applications in the United States, at least two are currently in trials. Umbrella occluders have been successfully used to close atrial communications (ASDs, Mustard and Fontan baffle leaks, and Fontan fenestrations), ventricular septal defects (native and peripatch), paravalvar leaks, and large vascular structures (Fig. 29.4) (34–36). Although patients rarely require intensive care after closure procedures, these techniques can be useful in the postoperative management of patients with complex heart lesions (see below).

SEPTOSTOMY PROCEDURES

The first therapeutic catheter procedure performed for congenital cardiac disease, balloon atrial septostomy, remains an important treatment for newborns with transposition of the great arteries (see Chapter 19.1, *Transposition of the Great Arteries*) and (less commonly) other complex lesions. Although little has changed in the method since the technique was first described, septostomy is now often performed under echocardiographic guidance at the bedside (37). The procedure should probably be performed in the catheterization laboratory when vascular access is difficult or when further diagnostic information is needed. Other techniques for transcatheter creation of interatrial communications include blade atrial septostomy and balloon dilation of the atrial septum. These are often used as part of palliative treatment in children with left or right-sided obstructive lesions, and, in some instances, with severe pulmonary hypertension to improve systemic blood flow (38, 39).

CATHETERIZATION IN THE POSTOPERATIVE PATIENT

Advances in noninvasive imaging, particularly transesophageal echocardiography, have been exceedingly useful in evaluating patients for residual defects in the early postoperative period. Nonetheless, cardiac catheterization remains an essential tool in the diagnosis and treatment of the postoperative patient. Invasive study may be required to delineate anatomy, evaluate hemodynamic consequences of lesions seen on echocardiographic study, or for transcatheter treatment of residual cardiovascular defects. Catheterization in the postoperative patient with unstable hemodynamics is riskier than in other patient populations, but the needed procedures can virtually always be performed with minimal consequences if the approach is well thought out (see *General Considerations* above).

It is important to emphasize that extrapolating the hemodynamic consequences of lesions seen on noninvasive imaging can be misleading. A high index of suspicion should be maintained in patients whose postoperative recovery is unexpectedly prolonged or complicated. The burden of proof is on the caregivers to be absolutely certain that potentially remediable residual cardiovascular defects are not present. This is particularly true in patients whose postoperative course is complicated by low cardiac output, unexplained cyanosis, congestive heart failure, or failure to wean from ventilatory support. Common residual lesions associated with reparative and palliative procedures are described in the appropriate sections of this text. The decision whether to take a given patient to the catheterization laboratory may not be straightforward, and it requires careful analysis of risks and benefits.

Staged Palliation and Repair of Complex Defects

Children with complex congenital defects often require a multistaged approach to treatment involving several operations and catheterizations. Preoperative diagnostic and therapeutic catheterizations are often required in these patients. In addition, catheterization in the immediate postoperative period (planned or unanticipated) is frequently required. All lesions requiring such a staged approach cannot be discussed here; however, the following are among the more commonly encountered lesions and they serve to illustrate considerations in the approach to complex patients.

Single Ventricle (Including Hypoplastic Left Heart Syndrome)

Palliative surgical management of patients with single ventricle heart disease often involves staged operations. Early operations limit pulmonary blood flow from the systemic arterial circulation and assure unobstructed systemic blood flow (see Chapter 18, *Single Ventricle Lesions*). With subsequent procedures pulmonary blood supply is transitioned to a cavopulmonary connection. Routine catheterization may not be required in the newborn period, but

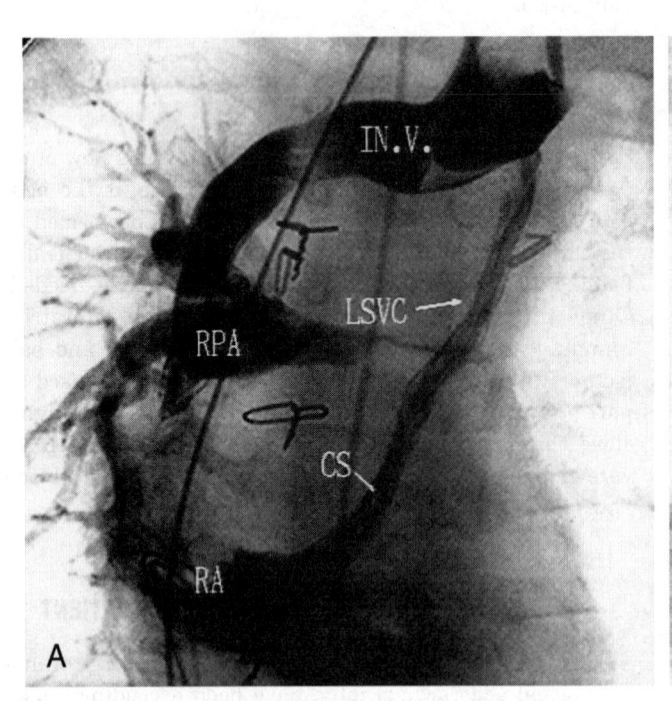

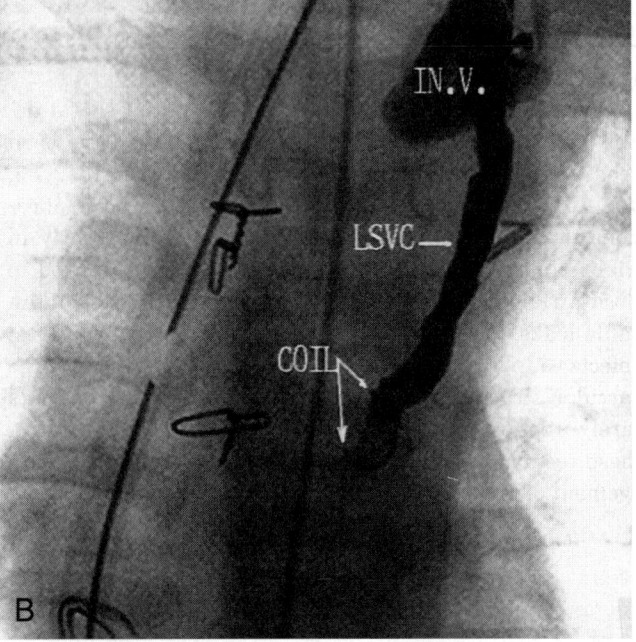

Figure 29.7. A. Angiogram of injection in innominate vein of patient with severe cyanosis 6 hours after right-sided cavopulmonary connection. Contrast is seen filling not only the right pulmonary artery through the cavopulmonary anastomosis, but also decompressing the anastomosis via a left superior vena cava to coronary sinus. **B.** After coil embolization (*arrows*), complete occlusion is seen of flow from the left superior vena cava. *CS*, coronary sinus; *IN. V.*, innominate vein; *LSVC*, left superior vena cava; *RA*, right atrium; *RPA*, right pulmonary artery.

it is performed prior to each subsequent operation to assess ventricular and atrioventricular valve function, and the anatomy and physiology of the pulmonary circulation in particular. Early postoperative catheterization may be required after hemi-Fontan or bidirectional Glenn procedures, typically to investigate severe cyanosis, or excessively high pressure in the superior vena cava. In the cyanotic patient, angiography often reveals an unsuspected connection between the upper venous system and the atrium, typically a previously small vein that has enlarged and "decompresses" the cavopulmonary connection. Most common of these is a persistent left superior vena cava draining either to the coronary sinus or left atrium. Such veins are almost always amenable to transcatheter closure at the time of diagnosis (Fig. 29.7).

Staged surgical approaches to total cavopulmonary repair (40) as well as application of the fenestrated Fontan procedure (41) have dramatically altered the typical postoperative recovery of patients undergoing modified Fontan procedures; uneventful rapid recovery is the rule. Catheterization is usually indicated when this is not the case. Clinical syndromes warranting study include low cardiac output states, persistent pleural or pericardial effusions, and excessive cyanosis. Catheterization is undertaken to determine the cause of the clinical syndrome, and it focuses on treatable lesions. Any obstruction to flow from systemic veins to pulmonary venous atrium results in elevated venous pressure and low systemic output. Anatomic causes include obstruction of the Fontan baffle itself, and pulmonary artery distortion, stenoses, or emboli. Such lesions are often amenable to transcatheter therapy. Pulmonary artery distortion and stenoses can be treated by balloon dilation or endovascular stenting. It must be emphasized that early after surgery pulmonary arteries can be ruptured by the use of oversized balloons generally required for successful balloon angioplasty. If treatment of pulmonary stenoses cannot be delayed 6 to 8 weeks in the postoperative patient to allow for vascular healing, use of smaller balloons and stents can be lifesaving. Pulmonary emboli or thromboses in situ can be amenable to pharmacomechanic thrombolytic treatment (if beyond the immediate postoperative period) (Fig. 29.8) (42).

Persistent systemic arterial sources of pulmonary blood flow in the Fontan-treated patient (patent residual pulmonary outflow, aortopulmonary collateral vessels, residual flow through previously placed surgical shunt) increase venous return to the systemic ventricle, which may lead to diastolic dysfunction with resultant elevation in systemic venous pressures. Such lesions are often amenable to treatment by transcatheter occlusion techniques. Finally, catheterization may reveal atrioventricular valve regurgitation or diastolic ventricular dysfunction without treatable anatomic lesions, and such patients often benefit from medical therapy with afterload reduction.

Cyanosis after Fontan (or excessive cyanosis after fenestrated Fontan) is generally caused by either a venous connection allowing flow from systemic venous system to pulmonary venous atrium, significantly elevated pulmonary vascular resistance (in patients with the anatomic potential for a right-to-left shunt), or additional leaks in the Fontan baffle itself (see Chapter 18). Venous decompressing collaterals are amenable to coil embolization, and

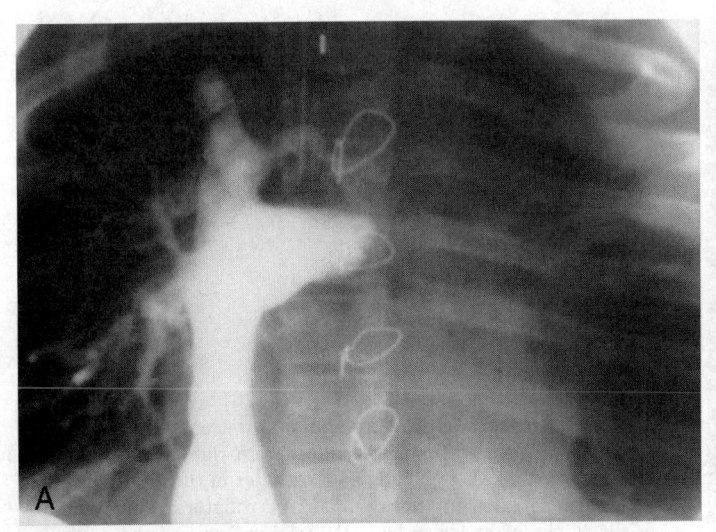

Figure 29.8. **A.** Cineangiogram of pulmonary arteries in patient who has undergone a modified Fontan procedure. The left pulmonary artery is completely occluded from thromboembolism. **B.** Repeat pulmonary arteriogram in same patient after pulse-spray thrombolysis and mechanical disruption of thrombus. Flow has been re-established to the left pulmonary artery.

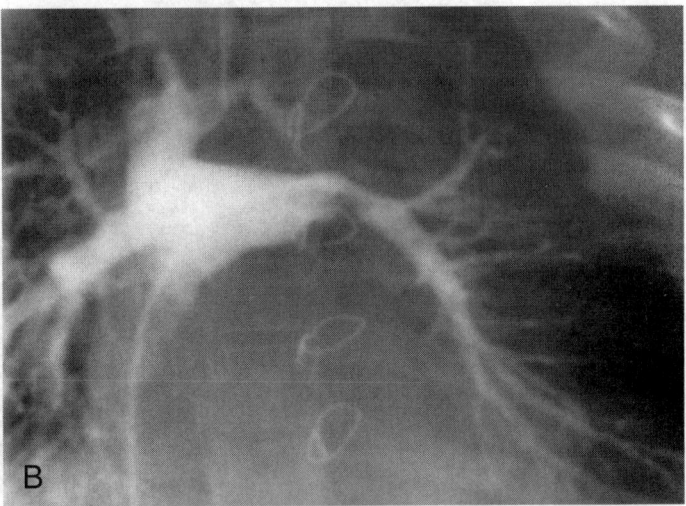

baffle leaks can be treatable by catheter-delivered device closure.

Tetralogy of Fallot with Pulmonary Atresia and Diminutive Pulmonary Arteries

The child with tetralogy of Fallot and diminutive pulmonary arteries (see Chapter 17.1, *Tetralogy of Fallot*) requires multiple catheterizations as part of staged repair. These procedures are usually performed electively between operative stages; however, several situations can arise in the immediate postoperative period where catheterization is required. Institutional approaches to this complex disorder vary. The goal of staged intervention is to reconstruct an adequate pulmonary artery tree to accommodate the entire cardiac output at acceptably low pressures. The first stage operation involves creation of continuity between the right ventricle and pulmonary arteries, with or without unifocalization procedures (43, 44). If the postoperative course is complicated by congestive heart failure or low

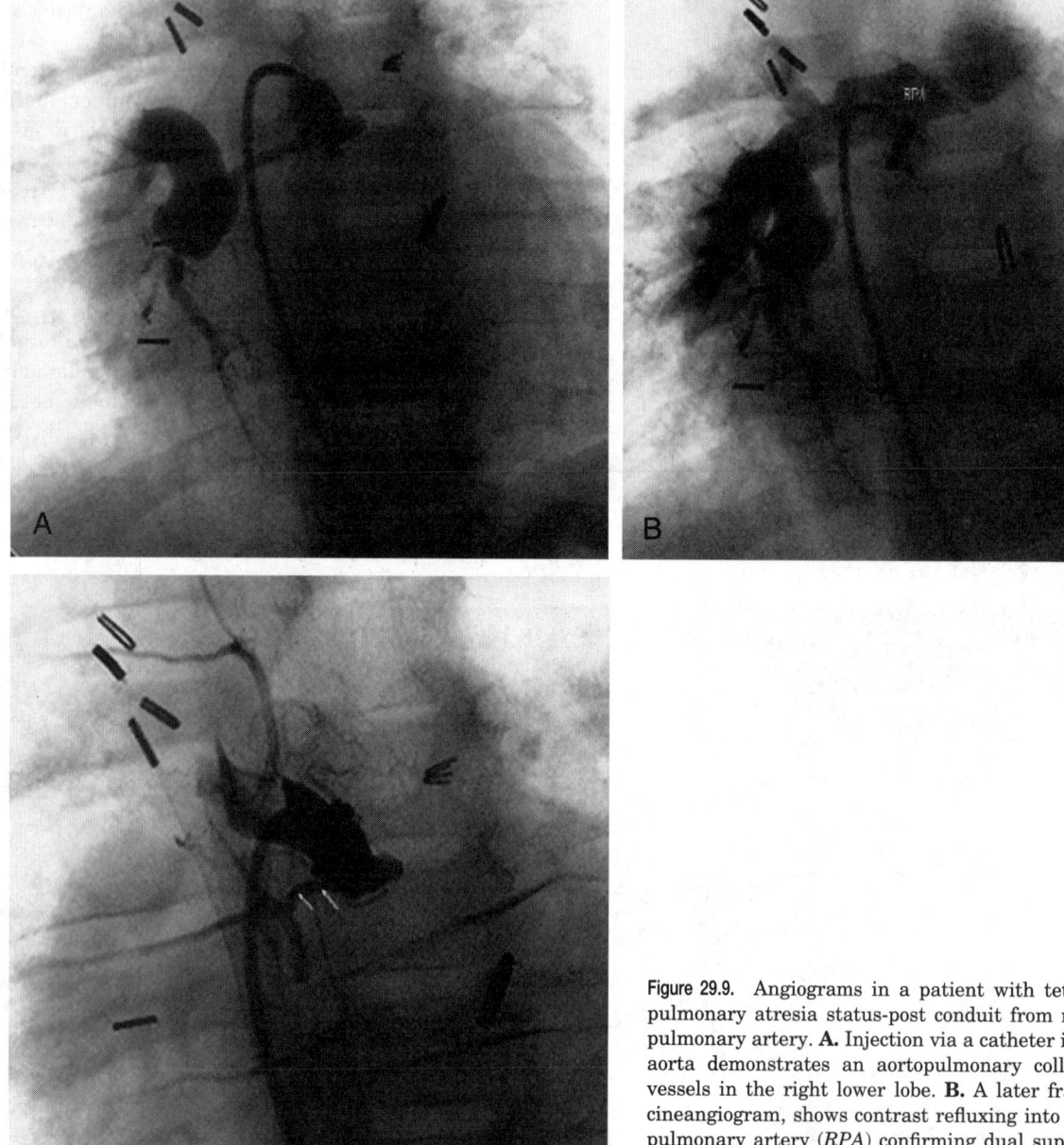

Figure 29.9. Angiograms in a patient with tetralogy of Fallot, pulmonary atresia status-post conduit from right ventricle to pulmonary artery. **A.** Injection via a catheter in the descending aorta demonstrates an aortopulmonary collateral supplying vessels in the right lower lobe. **B.** A later frame of the same cineangiogram, shows contrast refluxing into the central right pulmonary artery (*RPA*) confirming dual supply from the collateral. **C.** After placement of Gianturco coils (*arrows*) the collateral vessel is occluded.

cardiac output, catheterization is required for hemodynamic and angiographic evaluation of pulmonary blood flow. Such patients are often found to have excess pulmonary blood as a result of dual supply from the newly created right ventricle to pulmonary connection with persistent aortopulmonary connections. Excess left-to-right shunt can be treated by transcatheter embolization of aortopulmonary collaterals (Fig. 29.9) (43). Intermediate stages in these patients can involve catheter treatment of pulmonary artery stenoses with angioplasty or stents, embolization of aortopulmonary collaterals, and surgical unifocalization procedures.

At the final operation, patients undergo closure of the ventricular septal defect (VSD). Significant residual hemodynamic lesions in the immediate postoperative period may present with evidence of diminished cardiac output, cyanosis, or congestive failure. Catheterization is required in all such cases. Diagnostic study is focused on evaluation for pulmonary artery obstruction and persistent collateral sources of pulmonary blood flow. The approach to collaterals is usually straightforward (catheter embolization), whereas multiple factors determine the optimal approach to residual pulmonary outflow obstruction. In cases where surgical dissection has spared the pulmonary arteries, pulmonary artery stenoses can be treated with dilation or stents. As noted, the risk of catastrophic vascular disruption with dilation in the immediate postoperative period is significant (25, 26) and reoperation may be necessary for revision of central pulmonary artery distortion. Where invasive evaluation demonstrates marked right ventricular hypertension not amenable to treatment in the postoperative period, reoperation for fenestration of the VSD patch may be necessary to preserve adequate systemic blood flow.

CONCLUSION

Extended indications for complex catheter interventions in sicker patients with more complex lesions continue to increase the number of children receiving care in both the cardiac intensive care unit and the catheterization laboratory. Recent improvements in perioperative monitoring and noninvasive imaging have focused indications for cardiac catheterization in the perioperative period. Appropriate use of invasive studies and catheter-directed therapies will require increasingly sophisticated risk-to-benefit and cost-to-benefit analyses.

REFERENCES

1. Rome JJ, Lock JE. Interventional catheterization in pediatric and congenital heart disease. In: Stark J, De Leval M, eds. Surgery for congenital heart defects. 2nd ed. Philadelphia: WB Saunders, 1993:95–114.
2. Rome JJ. The role of catheter-directed therapies in the treatment of congenital heart disease. Ann Rev Med 1995;46:159–168.
3. Lock JE, Khalilullah M, Shrivastava S, et al. Percutaneous catheter commisurotomy in rheumatic mitral stenosis. N Engl J Med 1985;313:1515–1518.
4. Moore P, Adatia I, Spevak PJ, et al. Severe congenital mitral stenosis in infants. Circulation 1994;89:2099–2106.
5. Kan JS, White RJJ, Mitchell SE, et al. Percutaneous balloon valvuloplasty: a new method for treating congenital pulmonary valve stenosis. N Engl J Med 1982;307:540–542.
6. Stanger P, Cassidy SC, Girod DA, et al. Balloon pulmonary valvuloplasty: results of the valvuloplasty and angioplasty of congenital anomalies registry. Am J Cardiol 1990;65:775–783.
7. McCrindle BW. Independent predictors of long-term results after balloon pulmonary valvuloplasty. Circulation 1994;89:1751–1759.
8. Witsenburg M, Talsma M, Rohmer J, et al. Balloon valvuloplasty for valvular pulmonary stenosis in children over 6 moths of age: initial results and long-term follow-up. Eur Heart J 1993;14:1657–1660.
9. Masura J, Burch M, Deanfield JE, et al. Five-year follow-up after balloon pulmonary valvuloplasty. J Am Coll Cardiol 1993;21:132–136.
10. Sholler GF, Keane JF, Perry SB, et al. Balloon dilation of congenital aortic valve stenosis: results and influence of technical and morphological features on outcome. Circulation 1988;78:351–360.
11. Shaddy RE, Boucek MM, Sturtevant JE, et al. Gradient reduction, aortic valve regurgitation and prolapse after balloon aortic valvuloplasty in 32 consecutive patients with congenital aortic stenosis. J Am Coll Cardiol 1990;16:451–456.
12. O'Connor BK, Beekman RH, Rocchini AP, et al. Intermediate-term effectiveness of balloon valvuloplasty for congenital aortic stenosis. Circulation 1991;84:732–738.
13. Witsenburg M, Cromme-Dijkhuis AH, Frohn-Mulder IME, et al. Short- and midterm results of balloon valvuloplasty for valvular aortic stenosis in children. Am J Cardiol 1992;69:945–951.
14. Rosenfeld HM, Landzberg MJ, Perry SB, et al. Balloon aortic valvuloplasty in the young adult with congenital aortic stenosis. Am J Cardiol 1994;73:1112–1117.
15. Zeevi B, Keane JF, Fellows KE, et al. Balloon dilation of critical pulmonary stenosis in the first week of life. J Am Coll Cardiol 1988;11:821–824.
16. Hanley FL, Sade RM, Freedom RM, et al. Outcomes in critically ill neonates with pulmonary stenosis and intact ventricular septum: a multi-institutional study. J Am Coll Cardiol 1993;22:183–192.
17. Rhodes LA, Colan SD, Perry SB, et al. Predictors of survival in neonates with critical aortic stenosis. Circulation 1991;84:2325–2335.
18. Scleich JM, Rey C, Prat A, et al. Dilatation of critical aortic valve stenosis in infants under 3 months of age. Our experience from 15 cases. Archives des Maladies du Coeur et des Vaisseaux 1993;86:549–554.
19. Asante-Korang A, Fischer DR, Sigfusson G, et al. Carotid approach for balloon valvotomy for critical aortic stenosis in early infancy: medium-term outcome [Abstract]. Circulation 1995;92:I-310.
20. Lock JE, Niemi T, Einzig S, et al. Transvenous angioplasty of experimental branch pulmonary artery stenosis in newborn lambs. Circulation 1981;64:886–893.
21. Shaddy RE, Boueck MM, Sturtevant JE, et al. Comparison of

angioplasty and surgery for unoperated coarctation of the aorta. Circulation 1993;87:793–799.
22. Huggon IC, Qureshi SA, Baker EJ, et al. Effect of introducing balloon dilation of native aortic coarctation on overall outcome in infants and children. Am J Cardiol 1994;73:799–807.
23. Hijazi Z, Fahey JT, Kleinman CS, et al. Balloon angioplasty for recurrent coarctation of aorta. Circulation 1991;84:1150–1156.
24. Hellenbrand WE, Allen HD, Golinko RJ, et al. Balloon angioplasty for aortic recoarctation: results of valvuloplasty and angioplasty of congenital anomalies registry. Am J Cardiol 1990;65:793–797.
25. Rothman A, Perry SB, Keane JF, et al. Early results and follow-up of balloon angioplasty for branch pulmonary artery stenoses. J Am Coll Cardiol 1990;15:1109–1117.
26. Gentiles TL, Lock JE, Perry SB. High pressure balloon angioplasty for branch pulmonary artery stenosis: early experience. J Am Coll Cardiol 1993;22:867–872.
27. O'Laughlin MP, Perry SB, Lock JE, et al. Use of endovascular stents in congenital heart disease. Circulation 1991;83:1923–1939.
28. Wessel DL, Keane JF, Fellows KE, et al. Fibrinolytic therapy for femoral arterial thrombosis after cardiac catheterization in infants and children. Am J Cardiol 1986;58:347–351.
29. Evans DJ, Pizer BL, Moghal NE, et al. Neonatal aortic arch thrombosis. Arch Dis Child 1994;71:F125–127.
30. Dillon PW, Fox PS, Berg CJ, et al. Recombinant tissue plasminogen activator for neonatal and pediatric vascular thrombolytic therapy. J Pediatr Surg 1993;28:1264–1269.
31. Perry SB, Radhke W, Fellows KE, et al. Coil embolization to occlude aortopulmonary collateral vessels and shunts in patients with congenital heart disease. J Am Coll Cardiol 1989;13:100–108.
32. Perry SB, Rome JJ, Keane JF, et al. Transcatheter closure of coronary artery fistulas. J Am Coll Cardiol 1992;20:205.
33. Rome JJ, Keane JF, Perry SB, et al. Double-umbrella closure of atrial defects: initial clinical applications. Circulation 1990;82:751–758.
34. Hourihan M, Keane JF, Perry SB, et al. Transcatheter umbrella closure of valvar and paravalvar leaks. J Am Coll Cardiol 1992;20:1371.
35. van der Velde ME, Sanders SP, Keane JF, et al. Transesophageal echocardiographic guidance of transcatheter ventricular septal defect closure. J Am Coll Cardiol 1994;23:1660–1665.
36. Bridges ND, Perry SB, Keane JF, et al. Preoperative transcatheter closure of congenital muscular ventricular septal defects. N Engl J Med 1991;324:1312–1317.
37. Ashfaq M, Houston AB, Gnanapragasam JP, et al. Balloon atrial septostomy under echocardiographic control: six years' experience and evaluation of the practicability of cannulation via the umbilical vein. Br Heart J 1992;67:205–206.
38. Nihill MR, O'Laughlin MP, Mullins CE. Effects of atrial septostomy in patients with terminal cor pulmonale due to pulmonary vascular disease. Cathet Cardiovasc Diagn 1991;24:166–172.
39. Kerstein D, Levy PS, Hsu DT, et al. Balde balloon atrial septostomy in patients with severe primary pulmonary hypertension. Circulation 1995;91:2028–2035.
40. Bridges ND, Jonas RA, Mayer JE, et al. Bidirectional cavopulmonary anastomosis as interim palliation for high-risk Fontan candidates. Circulation 1990;82:IV-170–IV-176.
41. Bridges ND, Lock JE, Castaneda AR. Baffle fenestration with subsequent transcatheter closure: modification of the Fontan operation for patients at increased risk. Circulation 1990;82:1681–1689.
42. Bookstein JJ, Valji K. Pulse-spray pharmacomechanical thrombolysis. Cardiovasc Intervent Radiol 192;15:228–233.
43. Rome JJ, Mayer JE, Castaneda AR, et al. Tetralogy of Fallot with pulmonary atresia: rehabilitation of diminutive pulmonary arteries. Circulation 1993;88:1691.
44. Shanley CJ, Lupinetti FM, Shah NL, et al. Primary unifocalization for the absence of intrapericardial pulmonary arteries in the neonate. J Thorac Cardiovasc Surg 1993;106:237–247.

Diagnosis and Management of Cardiac Arrhythmias

30

James C. Perry, MD, and Edward P. Walsh, MD

This chapter provides a primer on how to read an electrocardiogram (ECG), and it includes information on the clinical modes of presentation and approaches to therapy for the more commonly encountered cardiac arrhythmias in the intensive care setting. Although the chapter places special emphasis on rhythm abnormalities encountered following surgical intervention for structural congenital cardiac defects, management of the pediatric patient with rhythm disturbances and a structurally normal heart is also presented. Antiarrhythmic drug guidelines with brief descriptions of mechanism of action, metabolism, clinical indications, and adverse effects are also given.

BASIC ELECTROCARDIOGRAPHIC CONSIDERATIONS

Abnormal Q Waves and QRS Axis Deviations

In pediatric patients, abnormal Q waves often represent abnormalities of cardiac chamber position, chamber hypertrophy, or pre-excitation syndromes rather than signs of myocardial infarction. Abnormal Q waves, if unrecognized on preoperative ECG, can lead to unnecessary investigations for postoperative myocardial infarction. Cardiac chamber malposition or inversion, chamber atresia or hypoplasia, and congenital conduction abnormalities often show preoperative patterns of poor R wave progression over the left precordium, left axis deviation, and abnormal Q waves. Conditions such as coronary artery lesions, precedent myocardial resections, or coexisting cardiomyopathy, however, can reflect actual infarction or ischemia, and they should be recognized preoperatively. Lastly, ECG abnormalities make it crucial to obtain preoperative 15-lead ECGs in all patients for comparison against postoperative recordings.

Sinus Bradycardia

Sinus bradycardia can be observed during sleep or vagal maneuvers in normal children. In the preoperative patient, sinus bradycardia observed with congenital heart defects is unusual. Some forms of heterotaxy syndromes (especially polysplenic syndromes) result in bilateral atrial "left-sidedness" (left atrial isomerism) and a true sinus node may be absent.

In the postoperative setting, slow sinus rates can be seen following surgical intervention for specific lesions, including repair of atrial septal defects (especially sinus venosus type), atrioventricular septal defects, complex atrial surgeries such as the Mustard or Senning repair for transposition of the great arteries (1–3), and modifications of the Fontan operation for single ventricle physiology (4). The sinus node is usually a large crescent-shaped structure extending from the superior caval-right atrial junction to the posteroinferior right atrium in the crista terminalis. Each of the surgical procedures mentioned above can damage the sinus node complex and its arterial supply, potentially causing impairment of the resting sinus rate, as well as capacity for chronotropism. In the Mustard procedure, for example, atrial suture lines interrupt the course of the crista terminalis, thereby transecting the lower and upper components of the SA node. Although attempts to protect the node by modifying suture lines and cannulation sites were advocated as helpful in the prevention of bradycardia, slow rhythms have still occurred. In the cardiac intensive care unit, normal increase in chronotropy seen with certain pathophysiologic states (e.g., anemia, fever, hypovolemia, pericardial effusion, and so forth) may be absent in face of sinus node dysfunction and therefore mask the patient's illness severity.

Sinus bradycardia as a secondary phenomenon is not uncommon. This can occur in patients on antiarrhythmic agents (including digoxin, β-adrenergic blockers, calcium-channel blockers, and class IA, IC, and III agents). Additionally, hypoxia, acidosis, hypercalcemia, hypothyroidism, and increased intracranial pressure can also cause bradycardia. In the cardiac intensive care setting, if a patient with bradycardia exhibits signs of low cardiac output (oliguria, decreased perfusion, or metabolic acidosis), the heart rate can be increased either by initiating atrial/atrioventricular pacing or by starting an infusion of isoproterenol.

Bundle Branch Block

Right bundle branch block (RBBB) seen on the ECG of the preoperative patient is unusual, although some patients with right ventricular volume overload lesions (e.g., atrial septal defect or pulmonary anomalous pulmonary venous return) can have partial RBBB pattern on their ECG.

Bundle branch block is a frequent finding after congenital heart surgical procedures. RBBB is the most common finding, and it is seen after repair of ventricular septal defect (VSD), atrioventricular septal defect, tetralogy of Fallot, and truncus arteriosus repairs, and after complex intraventricular procedures such as Rastelli operation for transposition of the great arteries, ventricular septal defect, and pulmonary stenosis.

The cause of postoperative bundle branch block has been investigated most thoroughly in the postoperative tetralogy of Fallot patient with RBBB; it can occur in from 50 to 100% of patients undergoing tetralogy of Fallot repair (5–7). Debate persists whether RBBB is caused by the ventriculotomy incision, damage to the moderator band, the VSD repair itself, or resection of infundibular muscle. Delineation of whether the block is distal or proximal in the right bundle is probably not important, as no adverse prognostic indicators are seen in patients with RBBB after tetralogy repair versus those without RBBB. Left axis deviation of the surface QRS vector ("left anterior hemiblock") can be a concomitant finding in up to 25% of patients with postoperative RBBB (8). The course of the bundle branches varies with the location of the VSD, and it has direct bearing on the incidence of postoperative bundle branch block. Damage to a bundle branch results in delayed activation of the ipsilateral ventricle and results in a late, positive vector on the surface ECG in the leads facing the damaged bundle (Fig. 30.1).

Left bundle branch block (LBBB), which is less common, can be observed in some patients after surgery involving the subaortic area such as resection for subaortic stenosis.

HEART BLOCK

First Degree Atrioventricular Block

Preoperative first degree atrioventricular (AV) block may be seen in the setting of atrial septal defect, total anomalous pulmonary venous return, tricuspid atresia, and Ebstein's anomaly of the tricuspid valve, probably on the basis of slow conduction through a dilated right atrium. With intra-atrial delays, P wave duration tends to be prolonged, and this accounts for most of the increase in PR interval. Patients with l-transposition of the great arteries can also have first degree AV block due to intranodal conduction delays because discontinuities have been demonstrated in nodal architecture at the histologic level. Both atrial and nodal conduction can also be prolonged in patients on antiarrhythmic agents (especially class IA, IC, and III agents).

In the postoperative patient, prolongation of intra-atrial conduction can occur following complex atrial surgeries (see above) because of an interruption of preferential routes of conduction. Corridors of conduction from the upper sinus node complex to the compact atrioventricular node are a primary function of atrial architecture and atrial myocardial fiber orientation. These routes are often damaged or completely interrupted in the course of complex atrial surgery.

Surgeries in and around the AV node can result in prolongation of the PR interval or atrioventricular block. Repair of ventricular septal defects, either isolated or as part of a complex intraventricular repair could potentially result in first or second degree AV block by damage to the more anterior, "fast pathway" components of the AV node (Fig. 30.2). The AV node and His bundle, for most types of ventricular septal defects, run along the posteroinferior rim of the defect. If fast pathway fibers penetrate the node in the usual manner, they can be at greater risk of interruption when sutures are placed close to the defect in the anterosuperior regions of the atrioventricular septum. In addition, the compact node and bundle branches tend to be oriented along a more anterosuperior course in patients with l-transposition of the great arteries. The course of the fast and slow pathways in this defect has not been described, but surgically induced AV block is not uncommon.

Second Degree Atrioventricular Block

Wenckebach type I second degree AV block is relatively uncommon. It is manifested by a progressive prolongation

RIGHT BUNDLE BRANCH BLOCK

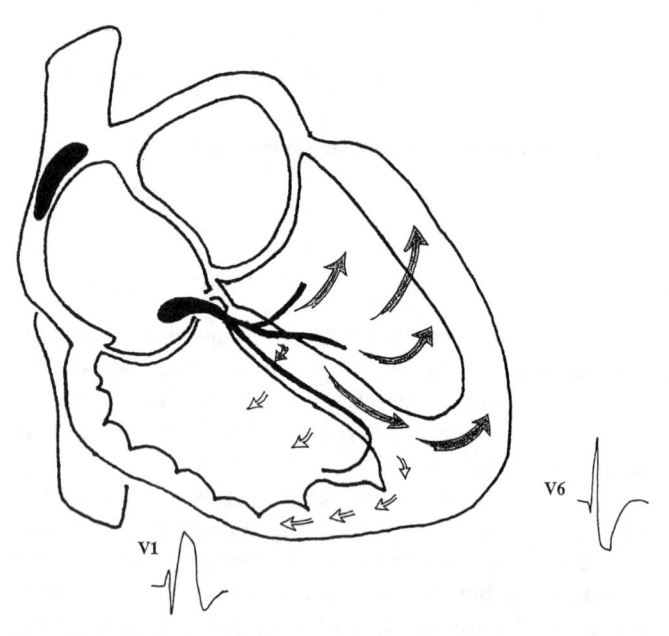

Figure 30.1. Right bundle branch block. With block or delay in the right bundle (*small, white arrows*), the left ventricle is activated first (*large, dark arrows*). Activation of the right ventricle is slow, via myocardial routes outside the His-Purkinje system. Slow, late activation of the right ventricle results in a slow, positive deflection in lead V_1 and slow, negative deflection in V_6.

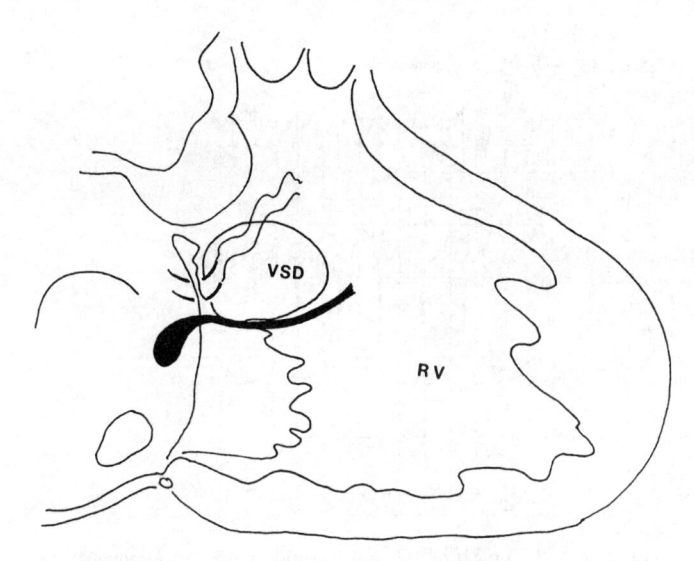

Figure 30.2. Anatomy of ventricular septal defect and the conduction system. Right anterior oblique view of a ventricular septal defect, showing how sutures might interfere with the anterior inputs into the atrioventricular node (*shown in black*). VSD, ventricular septal defect; RV, right ventricle. (Reprinted with permission from Zipes DP, Jalife J, eds. Cardiac electrophysiology. From cell to bedside. 2nd ed. Philadelphia: WB Saunders, 1995.)

of the PR interval leading to a dropped QRS complex. This phenomenon can be observed in the pediatric patient after surgery involving the tricuspid valve annulus and AV junction. A more advanced form, type II second degree block, can occur at relatively long cycle lengths (slow heart rates).

As with sinus bradycardia, if a patient exhibits signs of low cardiac output, heart rate should be increased by initiating appropriate pacing or by starting an infusion of isoproterenol.

Third Degree Atrioventricular Block

The most relevant disorder of atrioventricular conduction in the cardiac intensive care unit involves acquired third degree (complete) AV block. Third degree AV block can occur in the preoperative patient with l-transposition of the great arteries or polysplenia.

Despite an improved knowledge of conduction tissue anatomy in various cardiac malformations (9), surgically induced damage to the AV node or common bundle of His is still encountered. Cardiac lesions most commonly associated with postoperative AV block include VSD, l-transposition of the great arteries, subvalvar aortic obstruction (including the Konno operation), AV canal defects, and tetralogy of Fallot.

Fortunately, postoperative AV block is often a transient phenomenon. In a recent review of a 3-year experience, postoperative complete heart block (lasting longer than 4 hours) was observed in 54 of 2698 (2%) consecutive cardiac surgical patients, with eventual recovery of normal conduction in 63% of those patients (10). Nearly all patients who recovered conduction did so by the tenth postoperative day, so there may be little merit to waiting beyond this time before implanting a permanent pacemaker. Prior to the introduction of reliable pacemaker technology, surgically induced complete heart block had a poor prognosis, with up to 50% mortality rate over the first postoperative year (11). All of the data above prompted the adoption of a strong policy that recommends permanent pacemaker implant in all patients with advanced second degree or third degree block that persisted more than 10 to 14 days after surgery (12).

PRINCIPLES OF TEMPORARY PACING

Placement of temporary atrial and ventricular pacing wires is a standard practice after most cardiac procedures that involve cardiopulmonary bypass. These wires are invaluable tools and can be used for (*a*) support pacing during bradycardia, complete heart block, and atrioventricular dysynchrony, (*b*) rapid overdrive pacing of re-entry tachycardias (see *Rapid Overdrive Pacing* below), and (*c*) diagnostic recording of atrial activity during complex arrhythmias (Fig. 30.3).

Pacemaker Terminology

Pacemaker terminology is as follows: a three-letter code was originally devised to signify cardiac chamber(s) being paced, chamber(s) being sensed, and response to sensing (see Table 30.1). The chamber paced or sensed can be designated as A (atrium), V (ventricle), or D (dual chamber, both A and V). Response can be in terms of the sensed event triggering (T) a pacemaker response (either a paced event or initiation of some of the pacemaker's timing cycles), inhibiting (I) output of the pacemaker, or both types of response (D).

Simple asynchronous AOO or VOO pacemaker mode will pace the atrium or ventricle at the set rate with no regard to sensing. An AAI system would serve as a reliable atrial pacemaker, but it should not be used in the presence of atrioventricular block. The VVI pacing system is a pacing system that paces the ventricle when the sensed ventricular events fall below a set lower rate limit. All sensed rates above this rate will inhibit output of the pacemaker. A DDD pacemaker will pace and sense both atria and ventricles, and it can act in a variety of apparent modes, depending on the underlying rhythm. For example, if AV conduction is intact, but the rate is too slow, the pacemaker may appear as an AAI system, pacing the atrium but allowing AV conduction to result in an intrinsic QRS complex. In the presence of AV block but an adequate atrial rate, the pacemaker can "track" the atrial rate, time out a programmed AV delay in the pacemaker (generally anywhere from 70 to 240 milliseconds), and pace the ventricle when an intrinsic ventricular event is not sensed in the

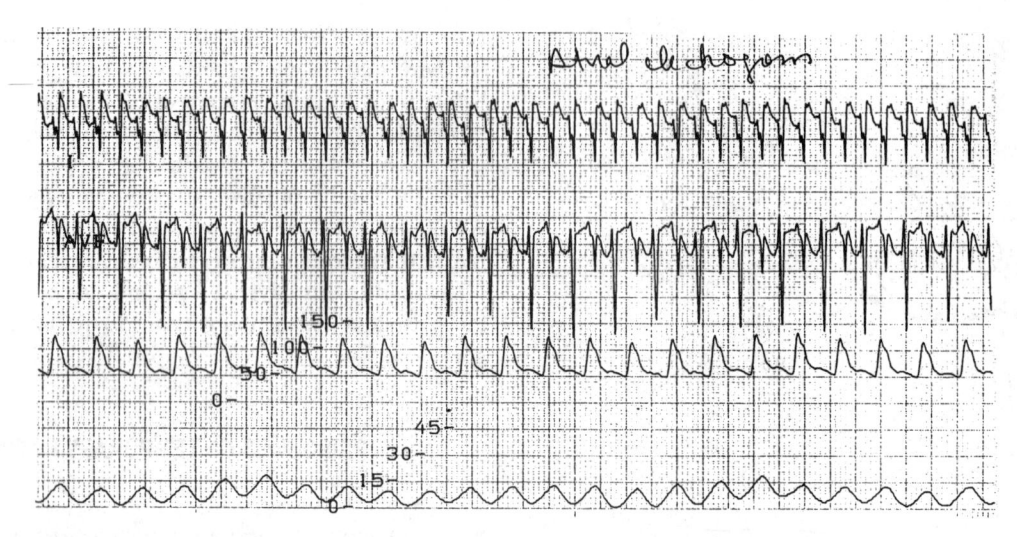

Figure 30.3. Atrial electrocardiogram of an infant after repair of total anomalous pulmonary venous return. Rapid atrial flutter is seen at a cycle length of 160 milliseconds with 2:1 atrioventricular conduction.

Table 30.1. Pacemaker Codes for the ICU[a]

Position	I	II	III
	Chamber paced	Chamber sensed	Response to sensing
	O = None	O = None	O = None
	A = Atrium	A = Atrium	I = Inhibited
	V = Ventricle	V = Ventricle	T = Triggered
	D = Dual (A + V)	D = Dual (A + V)	D = Dual (I + T)

[a] Limited to first three code positions.

allotted AV delay time interval. The DDD pacing mode in atrial flutter or atrial fibrillation can result in a rapid ventricular rate, depending on programmed timing cycles.

Physiology of Pacing

Mechanical contraction of the ventricles is most efficient when depolarization occurs via the normal His-Purkinje system. In a patient with sinus bradycardia and intact AV conduction, for example, atrial pacing is far more efficient than either dual chamber or ventricular pacing. In a patient with AV block, dual chamber pacing that maintains AV synchrony is superior to ventricular pacing alone. Optimal AV delay (PR interval) for dual chamber pacing in a very young pediatric patient tends to be short (70 to 120 milliseconds); longer AV delays can result in atrial cannon waves and elevated filling pressures. It is important to appreciate that benefit of atrioventricular synchrony is often not manifested in increase in blood pressure but rather augmentation in cardiac output (which is often not systematically measured).

Principles of Care

Malfunction of the pacemaker can be secondary to lead-related problems such as fracture or displacement, battery depletion, false sensing, or inappropriate connection or disconnection of leads. Reliable ECG monitoring as well as the defibrillator should be readily available during any manipulation of the pacemaker system.

Pulse Generator

Line-powered equipment should be grounded properly. Other sources that can interfere with the pulse generator function include magnetic resonance imaging equipment, electrosurgical apparatus, or telemetry equipment.

Leads

In unipolar temporary pacing, the heart lead is connected to the negative terminal while the subcutaneously placed lead is connected to the positive terminal. Both heart wires are connected to both terminals in bipolar pacing. Prior to handling the components of the system, the caretaker should touch the patient to avoid discharging static electricity via the leads. In addition, the leads should be separated from the pulse generator during defibrillation because a large current can be discharged via the temporary wires.

Patients with postoperative block who are dependent on temporary wires for rate support need careful checking of pacing wire integrity at least once daily by determining the energy requirement (threshold) for electrical capture. Generally, a pulse width of 2.0 milliseconds and current of 4–6 mA are adequate for atrial capture. Temporary pacing wires are usually reliable for periods of more than 2 weeks, although some fail earlier. If rapid and progressive increases in threshold are noted, new wires (or early implant of a permanent pacemaker) would have to be considered if the patient is pacemaker dependent. It should also be noted that thresholds of pacing wires can be increased in the presence of metabolic acidosis.

In an emergency situation, patients with AV block can also be paced temporarily with transcutaneous units that deliver the energy through special large adhesive electrodes on the chest; prolonged use (beyond 30 minutes) of such devices in infants or neonates, however, can result in serious skin burns. Lastly, an important monitoring concern is that pacing spikes can be detected as if they were QRS complexes on many bedside monitoring systems. In the event of loss of capture, pacing spikes at the programmed pacing rate can be interpreted as a stable heart rate when no heart rate is in fact present (Fig. 30.4). Use of a pulse oximeter, therefore, is advocated in patients being paced.

Battery

Battery life for pacing at 80 beats per minute (bpm), 1 millisecond atrial pulse width, and 2 milliseconds ventricular pulse width with 10 mA (such as the popular default values for the Medtronic Model 5346 temporary pulse generator) is about 7 days. For prolonged pacing, a supply of batteries should be kept handy and notation made on the pacing system of when they were most recently replaced. Batteries should be changed every other day, if possible, while the pulse generator is disconnected from the patient.

Programming the Pacemaker

Rate Programmability

The rate ranges from 30 to 180 bpm. Decreasing the rate gradually (rather than turning the unit off acutely) is the proper method to check the underlying rhythm as abrupt cessation of pacing can lead to asystole. In certain situations, raising the base rate may obliterate either atrial or ventricular arrhythmias. In addition, pacemakers are available with overdrive pacing capability (see below).

Energy Output

Energy output is usually measured in milliamperes (mA) and ranges from 0.1 to 20 mA. Energy output should be about two to two and a half times the energy at which capture is lost. Excessive energy output, which may be necessary in the presence of poor lead contact, can lead to pacing of the diaphragm. Pulse width of the temporary pacemaker is usually 1.0–2.0 milliseconds.

Sensitivity

In the asynchronous mode, the sensitivity setting is set at the lowest number so that no sensing occurs. When the pacemaker is set at maximal sensitivity, it is in the demand mode. Inappropriate sensing of the R or T wave in the atrium or of the P wave or the atrial pacing pulse in the ventricle may need to be managed by decreasing the sensitivity (increasing the numerical millivolt setting). Sensitivity ranges from 0.5 to 15 mV. In addition, when the possibility exists of competition of the patient's rhythm, inappropriate sensing may be the cause.

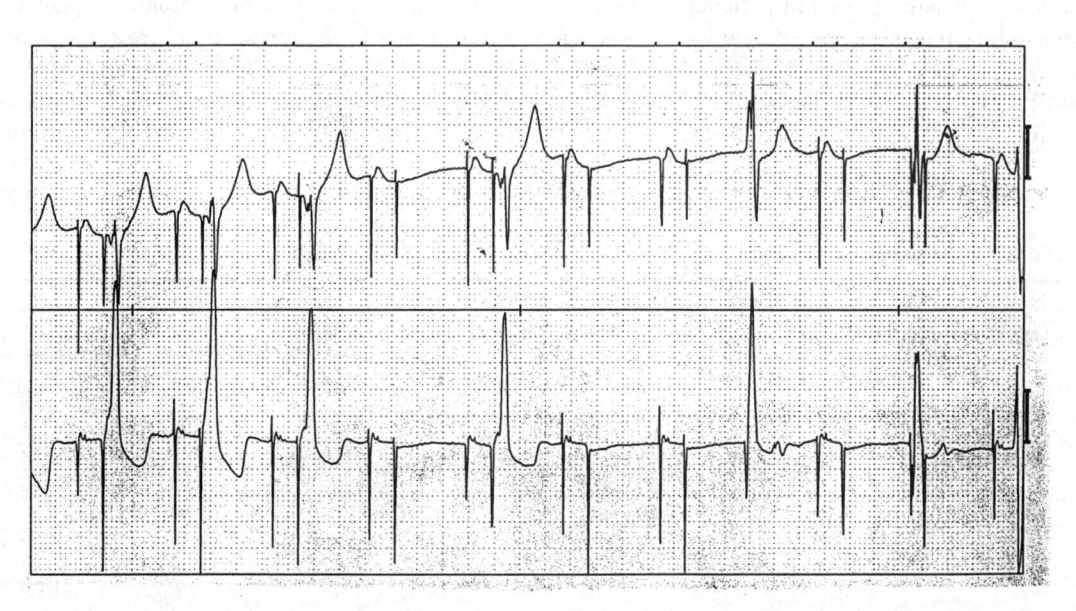

Figure 30.4. Atrioventricular sequential pacing with loss of ventricular capture. The large pacemaker spikes can be detected as *QRS* complexes by monitoring systems, resulting in registration of a heart rate when no ventricular contraction occurs.

Rapid Overdrive Pacing

Rapid overdrive pacing of tachyarrhythmias using temporary wires is an important tool in the postoperative period, where repeated cardioversions or chronic antiarrhythmic drugs should be avoided if possible. This technique is only applicable to re-entrant supraventricular tachycardias (including atrial flutter).

Atrial wires are connected to a special pacing unit capable of high rate pacing, and short (3 to 5 seconds) bursts of pacing are delivered at a rate just slightly (10 to 40 bpm) faster than the tachyarrhythmia. If unsuccessful, both rate and length of the burst can be gradually increased over subsequent trials until the re-entry tachyarrhythmia is terminated. Overdrive pacing rate can be as high as 800 bpm in the Medtronic Model 5346 temporary pulse generator. Rates in excess of 300 bpm are rarely necessary.

Although similar pacing maneuvers can also be used to interrupt some forms of ventricular tachycardia (VT), this should only be attempted by individuals who are experienced with arrhythmia management, because of the risk of accelerating the ventricular rhythm.

Decision for Permanent Pacing

Decisions on the type of permanent pacing system to implant in a child with persistent high grade AV block must take into account patient size, presence or absence of intracardiac shunting, and myocardial performance (see section on third-degree atrioventricular block).

An ideal pacemaker involves a transvenous dual-chamber system, but compromises must often be made. Small infants are often paced with a single chamber ventricular unit, assuming ventricular function is good. In addition, epicardial wires are generally used in patients with right-to-left cardiac shunting to avoid the embolic risk of transvenous wires. Lastly, patients with poor hemodynamics should receive a dual chamber unit regardless of size.

SUPRAVENTRICULAR TACHYCARDIA

An essential requirement for effective management of any supraventricular tachyarrhythmia (SVT) is identification of the precise mechanism. Basically two types of supraventricular tachycardia exist: *re-entry* (with or without an accessory pathway) and *ectopic*. Varieties of supraventricular tachycardia are listed in Table 30.2.

Generally, the more common re-entry tachycardias are characterized by (*a*) paroxysmal onset and termination, with fairly fixed rates, (*b*) reproducible termination with cardioversion and rapid overdrive pacing, and (*c*) predictable response to agents such as adenosine. The less common ectopic tachycardias demonstrate (*a*) gradual "warm-up" and "cool-down" in rates, largely proportional to autonomic tone, (*b*) unresponsiveness to electrical cardioversion and attempts at overdrive pacing, and (*c*) minimal response to conventional antiarrhythmic drugs.

This section focuses on the two most common forms of supraventricular tachycardia in children: accessory pathway-mediated SVT and atrioventricular (AV) node re-entry SVT. A discussion of the mechanisms, natural history, presentation, and therapy for SVT in newborns and young patients with structurally normal hearts will be reviewed, followed by a discussion of the findings of these tachyarrhythmias in patients in the early postoperative period after congenital heart operations.

Re-entry Supraventricular Tachycardia

Patient with a Structurally Normal Heart

The most common mechanism underlying pediatric SVT is that of an accessory pathway participating in "orthodromic" SVT. The term orthodromic implies that the activation wave front during SVT proceeds in an antegrade fashion down the AV node to the ventricles and then retrograde up the accessory pathway back to the atrium. This is in contrast to the rare "antidromic" form of SVT using

Table 30.2. Mechanisms of Supraventricular Tachycardia

Re-entry without an Accessory Pathway	Re-entry with an Accessory Pathway	Automatic
Sinus node re-entry	Orthodromic—WPW	Atrial ectopic
Atrial muscle re-entry/atrial fibrillation	Orthodromic—concealed WPW	Chaotic atrial
Intra-atrial re-entry/atrial flutter	Antidromic	Junctional ectopic
Typical AV node re-entry	Antidromic with more than one pathway	
Atypical AV node re-entry	Permanent junctional reciprocating tachycardia	
His bundle reentry	Mahaim	
	Atrio-His	

AV, atrioventricular; WPW, Wolff-Parkinson-White syndrome.

an accessory connection, wherein the impulse travels antegrade down the accessory pathway to the ventricle and retrograde up the AV node, resulting in a wide QRS tachycardia difficult to distinguish clinically from ventricular tachycardia.

Atrioventricular node re-entry, the next most common form of SVT, uses two functionally and physiologically distinct AV node components, the "slow" and "fast" pathways. "Typical" or slow-fast AV node re-entry, uses the slow pathway in the antegrade direction and fast pathway in the retrograde direction. This is the opposite case in "atypical" AV node re-entry SVT (Fig. 30.5).

The surface electrocardiographic appearance of the two forms of SVT most often allows distinction of one from the other. In narrow QRS (orthodromic) accessory pathway tachycardia, atrial activation occurs via the accessory pathway after ventricular activation. The interval from earliest ventricular activity to earliest atrial activity will be reflected by the RP interval during SVT. Because some time is necessary for activation to proceed from AV node to ventricle to atrium, the RP interval on the ECG tends to be in excess of 80 milliseconds. The retrograde P wave then can be seen either immediately following the QRS complex or buried in the ST or T segments. P waves are higher frequency events than any of these other ECG segments, so a search for rapid deflections in these components can reveal the retrograde atrial activation (Fig. 30.6). In typical AV node re-entry, atria and ventricles are activated nearly simultaneously. The "retrograde" P wave is then buried in the QRS complex and not discernible or, as is often the case, distorts the terminal portion of the QRS complex to some degree.

Mechanisms of SVT in young patients vary with age. A study of this phenomenon from Ko et al. (13) showed the nearly exclusive presence of accessory pathway mediated SVT in fetuses and newborns with a gradual increase in the incidence of AV nodal mechanisms by age 10 years. This phenomenon has direct bearing on therapeutic approaches in both the acute and chronic settings.

A natural history exists for the SVT seen in infants and young children. Of all infants with SVT in the first 2 months of life, 93% will cease having SVT episodes by the eighth month (14). Of the 7% that persist, many are incessant SVTs of the atrial ectopic or permanent junctional re-

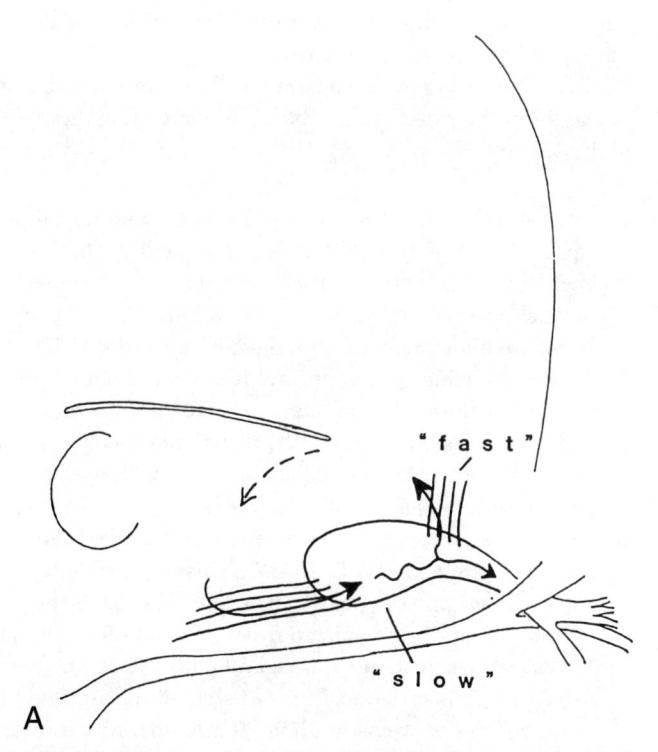

Figure 30.5. AV node re-entry SVT. Schematic drawings of typical (**A**) and atypical (**B**) AV node re-entry SVT. View is from the right, showing the compact AV node above the tricuspid annulus with the mouth of the coronary sinus posteriorly. In typical AV node re-entry (**A**), antegrade conduction in the circuit proceeds down the posterior, slow pathway to the node and retrograde back to the atrium via the anterior, fast pathway. Therefore, nearly simultaneous activation of the atria and ventricles occurs. In atypical AV node re-entry, the circuit is in the opposite direction, antegrade down the fast pathway and retrograde via the slow pathway. Therefore, in atypical AV node re-entry, a long RP interval (slow conduction) is present during tachycardia. AV, atrioventricular; SVT, supraventricular tachycardia.

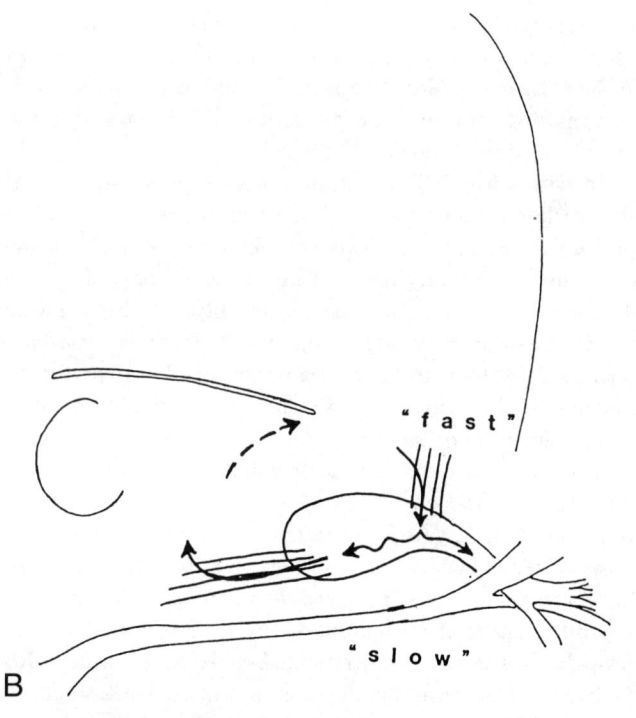

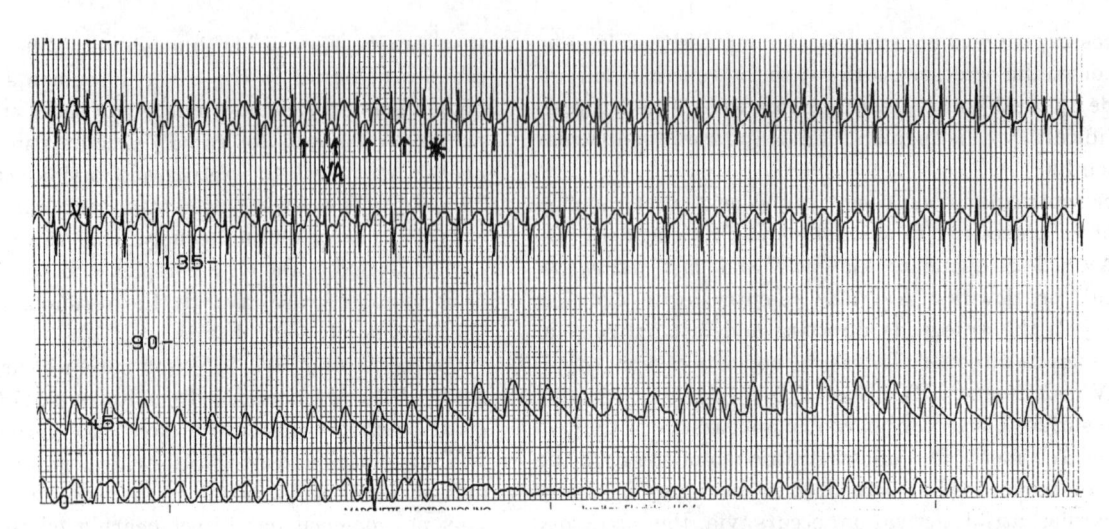

Figure 30.6. Supraventricular tachycardia caused by a concealed accessory pathway. In SVT, there is retrograde activation of the atria, with P waves evident (arrows). The RP interval is approximately 80 milliseconds. Adenosine is given to this patient, blocking SVT in the AV node. The final event of SVT is therefore atrial and the SVT ends with a P wave. No Wolff-Parkinson-White syndrome is evident during the sinus beats. However, SVT resumes, with aberrancy at its onset (Ashman phenomenon). Aberrancy resolves and a narrow QRS SVT is seen. SVT, supraventricular tachycardia.

ciprocating types. In re-examining patients who stop having SVT episodes, nearly one third have an SVT recurrence by a mean of 8 years of age. Children who experience SVT over the age of 5 years will continue having episodes in 78% of the cases. This factor has an influence on the decision making inherent in consideration of catheter ablation versus continued medical therapy.

Infants with SVT are often quite ill, requiring care in the cardiac intensive care setting. Infants with SVT often present in the first 3 to 6 weeks of life and are often discovered only after many hours of rapid rates have led to cardiac decompensation and congestive heart failure. These children can be irritable, diaphoretic, tachypneic, and feed poorly. They tend to have decreased peripheral perfusion and metabolic acidosis in direct relationship to the presumed duration of tachycardia.

The initial approach is to terminate the SVT (see below). Documentation by 12 or 15-lead ECG is helpful prior to conversion, as this is invaluable in confirming the diagnosis of SVT; bedside or transport monitor strips are *not* appropriate for this purpose. A running ECG six-lead rhythm strip is often helpful at the time of conversion to provide additional information. A pattern of wide QRS tachycardia in infants is more often a manifestation of aberrant SVT than ventricular tachycardia. Specifically, a left bundle branch block pattern during SVT is nearly always diagnostic for aberrant SVT in this age group (15).

Treatment for Supraventricular Tachycardia

Initial therapy for SVT depends on the patient's clinical condition. If the infant is in shock, then synchronized cardioversion (using 0.25–1.0 J/kg) should be carried out without delay as first line therapy. The airway should be managed by experienced personnel.

If the infant is not hemodynamically compromised, any of the following strategy can be used (depending on availability).

1. Intravenous (IV) *adenosine* can be used in an initial peripheral dose of 100–200 µg/kg as a rapid push, followed by a flush of crystalloid solution. Adenosine acts to block the AV node briefly (with a half-life of 7 to 10 seconds), allowing resumption of sinus rhythm. The drug is a purinergic agent, and it affects calcium and potassium channel conductance. Sinus bradycardia, which is transient, can result. Ventricular ectopy is not an infrequent result of adenosine administration, resulting in termination of some SVTs.

2. Some experienced centers can perform *transesophageal overdrive pacing of* SVT (16, 17). This is possible because the esophagus passes directly posterior to the left atrium and high pulse duration outputs from a pacing catheter can then capture and pace the atria. Overdrive pacing is often performed using 10 millisecond pulse width durations and 10–20 mA current outputs to pace. These parameters are not possible with most typical bedside DDD or DVI pacing units found in the cardiac intensive care unit. Overdrive pacing at 10 to 20% faster than most SVTs for 5 to 15 seconds is sufficient to break SVT. Alternatively, a protocol using premature impulses placed into paced rhythm may be necessary.

3. In other cases, initial therapy may consist of either so-called "vagal" maneuvers, such as the diving reflex. The diving reflex generally employs a cold washcloth or surgical glove filled with ice chips and water that is placed abruptly over the infant's entire face for 15 to 20 seconds (apnea is probably part of the stimulus). Continue recording the ECG as SVT terminates, as it can quickly reinitiate and the mechanism is again important, particularly if aberrancy is present at the onset. Bradycardia can occur occasionally, and the physician must decide whether an intravenous line is prudent prior to conversion.

Infants are dependent on catecholamine and calcium factors for preservation of cardiac output during SVT. Use of IV β-blockers or calcium-channel blockers should be considered contraindicated in children under 1 year of age as they can result in termination of SVT with subsequent life-threatening hypotension (18).

Intravenous digoxin loading is appropriate for many infants with SVT. This is particularly true in the infant who either does not have sinus rhythm after adenosine or who breaks to sinus rhythm but quickly recurs with SVT. This is a common finding for those patients who have had many hours of SVT before arriving at the hospital. Loading is commonly performed using a total IV dose of 30 μ/kg, given as half the dose, followed 8 hours later by one fourth of the dose, then 8 hours later by the final one fourth dose.

Intravenous procainamide is often helpful as adjunct therapy with digoxin, even if no plans exist to continue this drug. Procainamide is often given as 7–8 mg/kg over 30 to 40 minutes in the patient under 1 year old and 12–15 mg/kg for older patients. An infusion of 40–50 μg/kg/min tends to result in a procainamide level of 3–5 μg/mL within 4 hours of starting the infusion. N-acetylprocainamide (NAPA), the major metabolite of procainamide, needs to be measured as well. NAPA acts as a class III antiarrhythmic agent. Levels of NAPA in the 2–8 μg/mL range are common. Once procainamide has been administered, repeat attempts should be made to convert SVT, with the hope that sustained sinus rhythm will then result.

Although IV amiodarone use is uncommon at present, it may prove a useful agent for resistant cases of SVT in young patients. Based on experience predominantly with postoperative pediatric patients, a dose of 2–3 mg/kg over 5 minutes, repeated to a total of 10 mg/kg if necessary, may prove appropriate (19). An experienced pediatric electrophysiologist should oversee use of this drug when it becomes readily available.

Occasionally, for the infant with long-standing SVT, a high catecholamine state results in persistent episodes of SVT or recurrence. This can be particularly true for the child with an AV node re-entry mechanism. In the sick patient, intubation and sedation may be helpful in breaking the cycle and allowing antiarrhythmic agents time to reach steady state therapeutic levels.

A detailed discussion of chronic antiarrhythmic therapy for pediatric SVTs is beyond the scope of this chapter. Most pediatric cardiologists tend to avoid the use of digoxin if the patient has pre-excitation (Wolff-Parkinson-White syndrome) in sinus rhythm. A β-blocker or class IC agent (flecainide or propafenone) can be used in this setting as initial oral therapy after conversion.

In the Postoperative Patient

The therapeutic approach to SVT caused by either accessory pathway or AV node mechanisms in postoperative patients is similar to that for patients with normal hearts. Some important difference exist in diagnosis and management, however.

From a diagnostic and therapeutic standpoint, transthoracic pacing wires are often in place following surgery, and they provide an invaluable tool for assessing the relationship of atrial and ventricular electrical events. These wires can also be used for pacing for bradycardia or for overdrive pacing therapy for tachyarrhythmias. By attaching one or both of the atrial wires directly to the right and left arm leads of a standard ECG machine, a high-quality atrial electrocardiogram can be recorded, which clarifies atrial timing when the P wave is indistinct or obscured on a surface ECG recording.

In therapeutic interventions, the postoperative patient may be more sensitive to the negative inotropic effects of some drugs. In the treatment of SVT, this is true for the class IA drug, procainamide. This does not mitigate against its use (on the contrary, it is a mainstay of standard therapy), but merely argues for its careful administration, particularly during loading. In addition, renal and hepatic function impairments need to be assessed in the face of antiarrhythmic agent use. Although the classic example of dose reductions in this setting is that for digoxin, the same caution needs to be practiced for the use of all other antiarrhythmics as well, because either the parent compounds or their metabolites generally have renal and/or hepatic metabolism and excretion necessary for elimination.

One of the more important and preventable causes of postoperative SVT is the SVT substrate, which was known to exist preoperatively but persists in the postoperative period. These forms of tachyarrhythmia should be addressed preoperatively for the following reasons: (a) rapid and irregular rhythms in the early postoperative period are hemodynamically poorly tolerated, (b) antiarrhythmic agents often have unwanted negative inotropic effects and can be more proarrhythmic in postoperative hearts both acutely and chronically, and (c) potential catheter cure of these arrhythmias using radiofrequency techniques is often made far more difficult in the postoperative state.

Ebstein's anomaly of the tricuspid valve is frequently associated with accessory pathway-mediated tachycardias, either with overt Wolff-Parkinson-White (WPW) syndrome or via a "concealed" pathway (20). Accessory pathways are nearly all right-sided or septal in location. Complex tricuspid valvuloplasty procedures or tricuspid valve replacement complicates definitive treatment. In l-transposition of the great arteries, the left AV valve may be Ebstein-like in appearance and pathways exist on the left side of the heart. Either preoperative catheter ablation or the addition of a concomitant surgical arrhythmia therapy should be planned. Dysplastic valve tissue can compromise adequate energy delivery to ablate pathways. Lastly, AV node re-entrant tachyarrhythmias can occur in patients who have undergone Mustard or Senning repair for d-transposition of the great arteries. Features of the arrhythmia in this setting are similar to those in the patient with a normal heart. A functional corridor of tissue is created in these procedures between the "baffle" and the tricuspid annulus. This can lead to an increased incidence of AV node re-entry by separating the fast and slow AV node components. If medical therapy is ineffective, transcatheter therapy for slow or fast pathway ablation is possible, but it can be difficult as the preferred slow pathway area for ablation often lies on the pulmonary venous side of the baffle. A "transbaffle" procedure using a Mullins transseptal technique is possible and deflectable catheters could be manipulated to the tricuspid annulus and presumed slow pathway location. Lastly, Fontan operations often result in postoperative atrial tachyarrhythmias; accessory pathway tachycardias and AV node re-entry occur as well.

In the single ventricle patient, serious hemodynamic sequelae result from abnormalities of cardiac rhythm. These patients tend to be more dependent on AV synchrony. Loss of AV synchrony results in lower filling volumes, increased pulmonary venous congestion, and lower cardiac output. Any rhythm disturbance that results in a loss of effective atrial contractility or atrial contraction against a closed AV valve will result in decreased cardiac output. As in the case of atrial tachyarrhythmias, postoperative access to critical parts of tachycardia circuits can be problematic in Fontan procedure patients, by the very nature of redirecting the systemic venous return directly to the pulmonary arteries, and catheter ablation is difficult. A retrograde catheter approach is possible for some forms of SVT.

Atrial Flutter (Intra-atrial Re-entry)/Atrial Fibrillation

Atrial flutter involves a single large circuit of re-entry within atrial muscle, and it is one of the most common forms of tachycardia encountered in children with congenital heart disease (21). Some distinction should probably be made between the classic type of flutter involving a sawtooth pattern of the P wave at 300 bpm, and other varieties of intra-atrial re-entry where the rates can be much slower and the P wave contour can be quite different. The latter are in fact more common in children with heart disease, with the differences in rate and P wave morphology probably caused by the variable location of suture lines and scars within the right atrium and protected zones of slow conduction. Although the term "flutter" can be used practically to describe all these tachycardias, it is important to emphasize that atypical rates and P wave shapes and isoelectric intervals between P waves are the rule rather than the exception in pediatric patients.

Diagnosis of intra-atrial re-entry can usually be made from the surface ECG, demonstrating abrupt onset of a rapid atrial rhythm that remains quite regular over time. The AV conduction pattern is variable, so that the diagnosis can be difficult during times of 1:1 conduction, or during 2:1 conduction when every other flutter wave is obscured by a QRS complex. Adenosine administration during flutter typically causes transient AV block to uncover atrial activity, with rare cases of direct termination. Alternatively, atrial electrical activity can be recorded more directly with an esophageal electrode or from temporary atrial pacing wires (for a postoperative patient) to better define the rhythm (see Fig. 30.3).

Atrial flutter is a cause for significant morbidity and mortality in children with congenital heart disease (21). It can occasionally be seen prior to any operative intervention, but more often it develops after surgical procedures involving extensive atrial suturing (e.g., Mustard, Senning, or Fontan operations). The precise pathophysiology is not fully understood, but it can involve (a) length and location of suture lines, (b) atriotomy and caval cannulation scars, and (c) elevated atrial pressures and/or atrial enlargement. Concomitant sinus node dysfunction is frequently observed in patients with recurrent atrial flutter, producing the clinical picture of "tachy-brady" syndrome. Atrial fibrillation is less common, but it can also occur in the patients mentioned above.

Treatment for Atrial Flutter/Fibrillation

As with other types of SVT (see above), any patient who is severely hemodynamically compromised should be treated promptly with a synchronized cardioversion. Often, an anteroposterior patch or paddle orientation is most effective. In less emergent situations, atrial overdrive pacing (via postoperative pacing wires or an esophageal lead) with short rapid bursts that are faster than the flutter rate can be used to interrupt re-entry (but not atrial fibrillation), and are successful about 70% of the time.

Pharmacologic therapy for acute conversion is seldom efficacious. Digoxin, esmolol, or verapamil can be given to a stable patient in an effort to block the AV node and thereby slow ventricular response, but these agents do little to directly modify the flutter circuit and the latter two can adversely affect ventricular function. Certain class I drugs (e.g., IV procainamide) and class III drugs (e.g., amiodarone) occasionally terminate atrial re-entry, but they should be used only under very close monitoring.

An additional therapeutic challenge with atrial flutter is preventing recurrence. Chronic drug therapy remains suboptimal. The traditional pharmacologic approach can begin with digoxin and a β-blocker, which are largely directed toward preventing a rapid ventricular response in the event of a recurrence. As a second stage, any one of a number of class I (quinidine, procainamide, flecainide, propafenone) or class III (sotalol, amiodarone) agents have been tried. In addition, chronic drugs must be used with caution in patients with tachy-brady syndrome because of the further depression in heart rate that may occur. In patients with an abnormal heart, IC drugs (flecainide, encainide, and propafenone) carry a higher risk of adverse events, such as cardiac arrest and death (22). Pacemaker therapy to prevent bradycardia and flutter initiation has assumed an important role in chronic management of atrial flutter. Automatic atrial antitachycardia pacing has been advocated for some patients (23). Transcatheter radiofrequency ablation of the re-entry circuit is promising, but the rate of acute success (about 70%) is far lower than that seen with ablation for more common varieties of tachycardia.

Ectopic Supraventricular Tachycardia

Ectopic Atrial Tachycardia

A single atrial focus of abnormal automaticity outside of the sinus node is referred to as "ectopic atrial tachycardia" (EAT). This is a relatively rare disorder that occurs in two forms. The first involves a chronic idiopathic tachycardia in children with an otherwise normal heart that can eventually lead to a dilated cardiomyopathy from sustained high rates (24). The second less common form involves what is usually a transient disorder lasting for a few hours or days after congenital heart surgery.

The diagnosis can generally be made from surface ECG recordings that demonstrate an abnormal axis and/or morphology for the P wave, with atrial rates that are excessive for age and physiologic state. Rapid atrial activity can either be incessant or sporadic, but in either case it demonstrates gradual rate acceleration (warm-up) and wide rate fluctuations over time. Intermittent second degree AV block is often noted when the patient is resting or asleep. Cardioversion and pacing techniques have virtually no effect on this arrhythmia to the extent that failure of these maneuvers can be diagnostic.

The idiopathic form of EAT is an important entity to recognize because it represents one of the few potentially reversible causes of cardiomyopathy (24). Not infrequently, young children with long-standing EAT present with poor ventricular function and chronically elevated heart rates in the range of 140–200 bpm, which could initially be misinterpreted as sinus tachycardia. Careful examination of the P wave axis and morphology is required in all such cases to rule out EAT.

Initial therapy can be aimed at slowing the ventricular rate by titrating the degree of AV block with digoxin, although this has minimal effect on the atrial focus itself. Beyond digoxin, therapy choice depends largely on the status of myocardial contractility. For those patients with good ventricular function, trials of a β-blocker, flecainide (25), or amiodarone (26) can be attempted. Fewer than 50% of patients overall respond to chronic drug therapy. More recently, radiofrequency ablation has been successful.

Postoperative EAT following congenital heart surgery is rare. Tachycardia in this setting usually involves sporadic nonsustained bursts rather than an incessant pattern, and it often resolves within a few days of surgery. No large clinical series have critically examined treatment options in postoperative EAT, but the general recommendations involve trials of digoxin, β-blocker, or IV procainamide. Most patients can be managed with these options until the disorder resolves spontaneously. Rarely a postoperative patient may have persistent EAT, in which case amiodarone therapy or an ablation procedure (27) may have to be considered.

Junctional Ectopic Tachycardia

Junctional ectopic tachycardia (JET) is a relatively common (but often under-recognized) tachyarrhythmia that usually occurs in the postoperative patient, and it can be life threatening. This rhythm generally occurs in the first 24 to 48 hours after surgery and may be more commonly seen following surgical intervention for repair of VSD (including AV canal and tetralogy of Fallot), transposition of the great arteries (by arterial switch), total anomalous pulmonary venous connection (TAPVC), and many of the modifications of the Fontan procedure. Because these procedures are performed in younger patients, most patients with this tachyarrhythmia are less than 2 years of age.

Typical electrocardiographic findings in JET usually include AV dissociation with a rapid QRS rate (160–260/min) and a narrow QRS morphology (Fig. 30.7). The QRS rate can be wide in some patients because of rate-related aberrancy (can be variable or constant) or an underlying fixed bundle branch block secondary to the surgical repair. Differentiating JET from ventricular tachycardia is difficult in the face of bundle branch block. Atrial pacing at rates faster than the tachycardia, with capture of the atrium and subsequent AV conduction, can be seen with either JET or VT, but if the QRS morphology remains the same during pacing with intact AV conduction, a diagnosis of JET is most likely. In young patients, the AV node has the capacity to conduct rapid junctional rates in a retrograde fashion (particularly in the presence of inotropic agents) and AV dissociation, therefore, may *not* be present. In this setting, administration of adenosine can result in loss of VA conduction with perpetuation of JET (Fig. 30.8). The combination of loss of AV synchrony and rapid ventricular rates observed in JET is deleterious in any postoperative patient.

The exact mechanism causing JET remains unknown. The rhythm has features of an automatic focus tachycardia, showing warm-up responsiveness to catecholamines

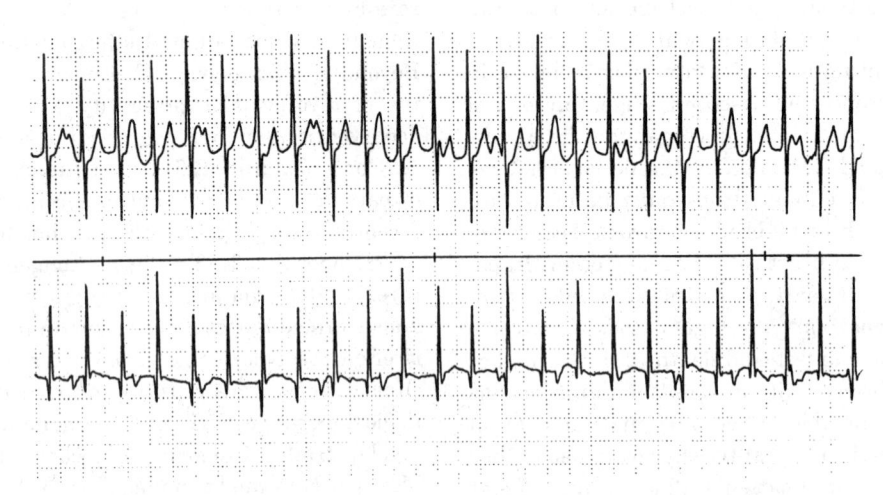

Figure 30.7. Junctional ectopic tachycardia. A narrow QRS tachycardia with atrioventricular dissociation is seen. (Reprinted with permission from Zipes DP, Jalife J, eds. Cardiac electrophysiology. From cell to bedside. 2nd ed. Philadelphia: WB Saunders, 1995.)

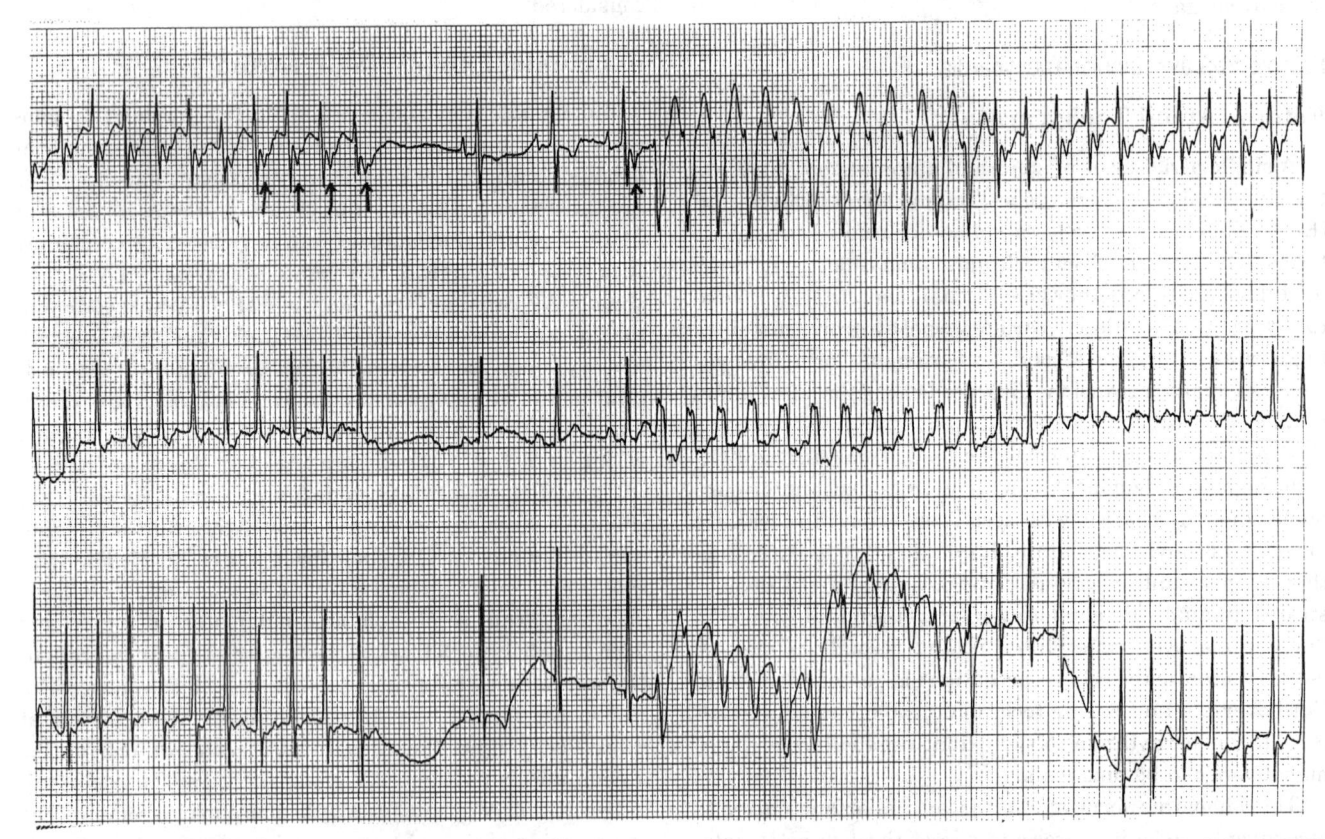

Figure 30.8. Junctional ectopic tachycardia. Administration of adenosine during junctional ectopic tachycardia fails to terminate the arrhythmia. However, in this patient, a 1:1 retrograde activation is seen of the atria (*arrows*) from the junctional focus. With adenosine, a transient retrograde AV node block occurs and the 1:1 relationship is lost, proving the junctional focus.

and overdrive suppression. It is possible that surgeries in the AV junctional area damage components of the AV node or His bundle, causing tissue trauma and changes in cell membrane ionic integrity leading to enhanced automaticity. With JET associated with the arterial switch operation, it is possible that reperfusion of the nodal area (following coronary artery relocation) could result in changes in membrane permeability and thus accelerate the focus of JET. Alternatively, it may be related to closure of the atrial defect (in TAPVC as well) or prior balloon atrial septostomy.

Treatment for Junctional Ectopic Tachycardia

Therapy for JET can be somewhat complex but the overall goal is directed at slowing the ectopic rate to allow restoration of atrioventricular synchrony at a physiologic rate.

Because the AV junctional area is influenced greatly by autonomic factors, rate and hemodynamic effects of JET can be affected by these factors as well. Initial approaches to therapy for JET, therefore, include providing adequate sedation, discontinuing vagolytic agents such as meperidine and pancuronium, and reducing the doses of inotropic agents. Serum calcium and potassium should be normalized.

Core temperature cooling has great value in the infant and small child, generally utilizing cooling blankets to obtain a temperature of approximately 34 to 35°C (28). Shivering should be prevented by use of a muscle relaxant to prevent increases in oxygen consumption.

Anecdotal evidence indicates that IV digoxin loading can help slow the JET rate. This may be of importance for pacing therapy, as discussed below. Intravenous procainamide is used to treat this tachycardia, but it should be administered cautiously; it can accelerate JET and causes hypotension.

Intravenous amiodarone has been found to be useful in patients with JET (19). In a multicenter review of its use in postoperative patients with JET, the drug was successful in either restoring sinus rhythm or slowing the JET to allow atrial pacing (both should be considered successful therapeutic end points) in 11 of 12 patients (29). No deaths or significant adverse events were reported in this group, which is in stark contrast to the high mortality rate reported for JET previously (30, 31). Oral amiodarone use (by nasogastric tube) may suffice, depending on bowel absorption, but this strategy generally requires at least 2 days for the desired electrophysiologic effects to become manifest. Use of IVβ-blockers (such as esmolol) and calcium channel blockers, although having theoretic advantages, generally depresses myocardial contractility significantly in postoperative patients, making their use controversial.

Intravenous class IC agents can also be useful in some instances of postoperative JET, but this pharmacologic intervention has not been studied extensively. Intravenous propafenone was reported in a small series of six patients as terminating or slowing JET in postoperative patients (32). Propafenone is not yet available in the United States and concerns persist regarding its proarrhythmic potential (33). Intravenous flecainide has been used for JET in Europe with some success (34). The presence of a congenital cardiac defect or cardiomyopathy is known to be a risk factor for either sudden death or cardiac arrest in patients taking oral preparations of flecainide (22). Use of the intravenous form in short-term applications (e.g., postoperative JET) may eventually be accepted, but the availability and success of IV amiodarone may obviate its use.

When JET is not eliminated but a reduction in rate is achieved, atrial pacing from atrial wires, transvenous or a transesophageal catheter can be performed, resulting in restoration of AV synchrony and improved cardiac output. Fortunately, JET tends to be limited in duration to 2 to 5 days. If successful hemodynamic stability can be obtained during this time, sinus rhythm tends to recur. In rare resistant cases in which hemodynamic compromise is present, transcatheter radiofrequency ablation or modification of the His bundle may be indicated.

VENTRICULAR ARRHYTHMIAS

Serious ventricular arrhythmias are uncommon in young patients, but they do occur as a late phenomenon in teenage patients and young adults with congenital heart disease (e.g., tetralogy of Fallot [35] and aortic stenosis [36]) or at any age in association with various cardiomyopathies.

This discussion concentrates primarily on evaluation and management of sustained or symptomatic ventricular tachycardia (VT). More benign forms of ventricular ectopy (e.g., isolated premature beats) can be common in the early postoperative setting after congenital heart surgery, but they usually arise from transient problems such as hypokalemia and generally do not require treatment. Sustained VT, however, should be considered unusual in the postoperative setting and suspicion for myocardial ischemia or infarction and postoperative residua should be raised.

Two major categories of ventricular tachycardia can be distinguished based on ECG appearance. Tachycardia that arises from damaged or scarred myocardium typically involves re-entry, and presents an ECG (Fig. 30.9) of a regular wide-QRS rhythm with a single dominant morphology ("monomorphic VT"). This contrasts with another specific type of VT caused by repolarization abnormalities, where the tachycardia has a varying QRS morphology that seems to twist around the isoelectric baseline of the ECG ("torsade de pointes").

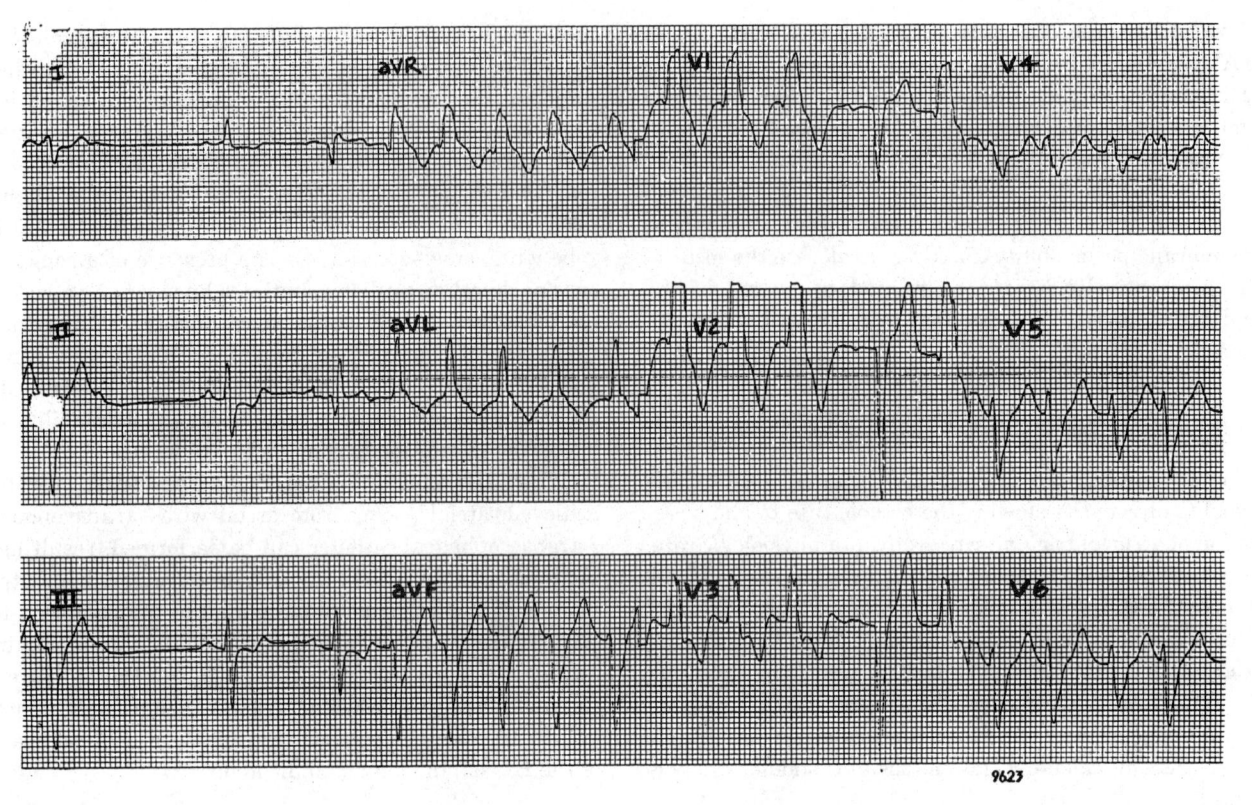

Figure 30.9. Monomorphic ventricular tachycardia seen in a patient following a Konno procedure. Right bundle branch block with left axis morphology is seen. The earliest site of endocardial activation on subsequent catheter mapping was in the left ventricle, near the septal ventricular septal defect patch.

Monomorphic (Re-Entrant) Ventricular Tachycardia

Sustained VT must be treated as an emergency. Although some atypical forms of SVT can mimic VT, any tachycardia at initial presentation with a wide QRS morphology should be approached and treated as VT until definitely proved otherwise. The finding of AV dissociation during the episode will positively identify the rhythm as being of ventricular origin, but P waves may be difficult to see clearly. Although recording from an esophageal electrode or temporary atrial pacing wires can clarify atrial timing, many patients demonstrate passive retrograde conduction to the atrium during VT, so that the presence of AV association does not entirely eliminate the diagnosis of VT. In such cases it can be useful to administer IV adenosine while carefully observing atrial activity. If the tachycardia is truly VT, adenosine should block passive retrograde conduction and uncover AV dissociation. If the tachycardia was SVT, adenosine may well be both diagnostic and therapeutic.

Torsade de Pointes

Torsade de pointes is the typical form of VT encountered in patients with long QT syndrome and in others taking antiarrhythmic drugs (especially class IA and III). It can also be seen in severe central nervous system insults, where central, neural mechanisms bring about a prolongation of cardiac repolarization (Fig. 30.10). In addition, children with long QT syndrome (QT_c more than 450 milliseconds, syncope or near-syncope, and family history) are predisposed to have ventricular arrhythmias. The mechanism is thought to result from early afterdepolarization leading to triggered activity. Torsades can be potentiated by hypokalemia, hypocalcemia, and hypomagnesemia.

The diagnosis of torsades de pointes is easily made from the distinctive ECG appearance. Most often patients have intermittent salvos, which stop after a variable period of time, but the tachycardia can recur frequently or be sustained for long periods with eventual degeneration into ventricular fibrillation. Torsade de pointes typically occurs in the setting of QT prolongation, so the ECG in sinus rhythm demonstrates abnormalities of the T wave and U wave that support the diagnosis.

Treatment for Ventricular Tachycardia

At initial presentation, any compromised patient should be treated immediately with a synchronized cardioversion using energies of 1–2 J/kg.

More stable patients can be treated pharmacologically,

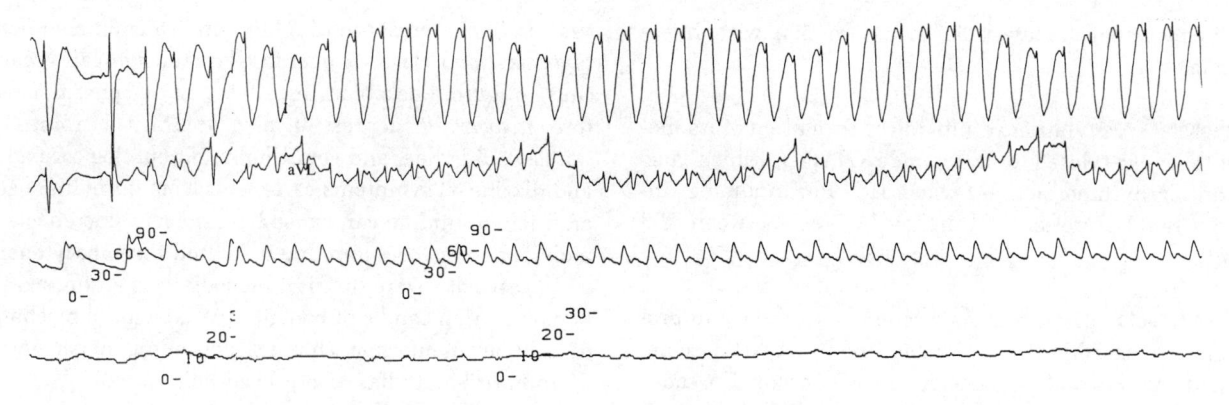

Figure 30.10. Torsade de pointes. The patient had extensive central nervous system injury from trauma. The QT interval was prolonged and salvos of "torsade de pointes" ventricular tachycardia are shown here.

beginning with lidocaine at 1 mg/kg followed by an infusion at 20–50 µg/kg/minute. Intravenous procainamide is a reasonable second choice for re-entry VT followed by an infusion of the drug. Patients who are refractory to these measures may require IV β-blocker, bretylium, or amiodarone.

Torsade de pointes should be treated with electrical cardioversion only if the episode is sustained. Cardioversion is of no benefit in patients with frequent but nonsustained salvos, and it can actually aggravate the situation.

First line medication in this case is magnesium sulfate (37), given at a dose of 25 mg/kg over 5 to 15 minutes. Lidocaine can also be used, but procainamide must be avoided because it prolongs repolarization. For torsade de pointes that occurs in the long QT syndromes, where the trigger for tachycardia relates to catecholamine sensitivity, intravenous β-blocker (e.g., esmolol) is often helpful. By contrast, that seen with certain antiarrhythmic drugs (e.g., quinidine, procainamide, sotalol, and so forth) is generally triggered by abrupt pauses in normal rhythm. Pacing or infused isoproterenol, both of which shorten the QT interval, are more helpful in this setting.

Patients with drug-induced torsade de pointes generally do not require chronic preventive therapy once they are stabilized and the offending agent is eliminated. Those with the congenital form are usually treated with high dose β-blocker as a first stage, but occasionally require more aggressive therapy, including use of implanted defibrillators.

After initial stabilization, most patients with VT should undergo a detailed evaluation of hemodynamics, as well as formal intracardiac electrophysiologic testing. Long-term prevention of symptomatic VT remains a major therapeutic challenge. Options for chronic suppression include (a) medical therapy guided by serial electrophysiologic studies, (b) medical therapy guided by noninvasive monitoring (Holter and exercise testing), (c) implantation of an internal defibrillator, or (d) detailed mapping of the VT circuit with surgical or transcatheter ablation.

Treatment for Ventricular Fibrillation

At initial presentation, the patient should be treated immediately with defibrillation using energies of 2 J/kg. Sedation may not be necessary because the patient usually has become hypotensive with VF. Pharmacologic therapy for ventricular fibrillation includes lidocaine and bretylium use.

ANTIARRHYTHMIC AGENTS

Antiarrhythmic agent use is discussed in the following sections with emphasis on the more frequently used intravenous agents. The classification scheme is based on the individual agent's effects on His-Purkinje tissue.

Class IA Drugs

Class IA agents include procainamide, quinidine, and disopyramide. These agents manifest their electrophysiologic effects by prolonging the effective refractory period and the duration of the action potential via inhibition of the fast sodium current. These agents also have anticholinergic effects secondary to their ability to block potassium channels.

Procainamide

Procainamide slows conduction in the atrium and both QRS and QT_c intervals are prolonged, although procainamide does not prolong the QT interval as much as quinidine. In pre-existing sinoatrial node dysfunction, sinus arrest and exit blocks can occur.

Clinical Indications Procainamide is one of the antiarrhythmic agents most commonly used in the cardiac intensive care setting because of its broad therapeutic spectrum. Indications are supraventricular tachycardia (including atrial flutter or fibrillation) and lidocaine-resistant ventricular tachycardia. Procainamide is also effective against junctional ectopic tachycardia in conjunction with hypothermia.

Metabolism Acetylation results in the formation of its metabolite, N-acetylated procainamide (NAPA), which also has antiarrhythmic activity (class III). Procainamide undergoes renal excretion and the level is kept between 4–8 µg/mL.

Adverse Effects Hypotension is common secondary to procainamide's vasodilating properties, and it may be dose dependent. Myocardial depression can also occur. Torsades de pointes and ventricular arrhythmias are associated with its use (especially when used in combination with class III agents). Lupus-like syndrome and thrombocypotenia are observed with long-term use. For severe cases of toxicity caused by NAPA, hemodialysis can be helpful (38).

Quinidine

Action potential duration and atrial and ventricular effective refractory periods are lengthened with quinidine. In addition, indices of conduction (maximal velocity of phase zero upstroke and action potential amplitude) are affected. Quinidine has effects on anterograde and retrograde limbs of accessory pathways in the form of slowing their conduction. Lastly, quinidine has a vagolytic effect.

Clinical Indications Various types of supraventricular tachycardia including atrial fibrillation and flutter as well as re-entry types respond to quinidine therapy. In addition, ventricular tachycardia can also be treated with quinidine. Ectopic forms of supraventricular tachycardia such as atrial ectopic tachycardia, however, may not be responsive to quinidine.

Metabolism The enteral form of quinidine is usually used. Its metabolism is accomplished by hepatic hydroxylation to an electrophysiologically active metabolite. Quinidine sulfate is more rapidly absorbed than its gluconate congener.

Adverse Effects Many electrophysiologic considerations are related to quinidine use. First, proarrhythmias can occur with administration of quinidine. Second, both QRS and QT intervals can be prolonged, and they are usually monitored closely during its use. Doses are usually reduced if the QRS duration is increased by 50% or more or if the QT interval is greater than 500 milliseconds. Quinidine is contraindicated in patients with long QT syndrome. Torsades de pointes (39) is associated with its use (especially when used in combination with class III agents and with hypokalemia and in patients with structural heart disease). Lastly, atrioventricular block can occur in pre-existing conduction disease.

Quinidine increases serum digoxin levels so that doses of digoxin should be reduced. It also should be used with caution in the presence of β-blockers, calcium channel antagonists, and class IA agents. Hypotension can occur because of quinidine's blocking effects on peripheral α-receptors; myocardial depression also occurs. Gastrointestinal (nausea, diarrhea, and vomiting) and neurologic (headache and dizziness) symptoms can result from quinidine use. In addition, quinidine can cause hematologic side effects (hemolytic anemia and immune-mediated thrombocytopenia).

In cases of severe toxicity, hemodialysis and/or charcoal hemofiltration can be of benefit (40). Given the mechanism of cellular membrane channel poisoning, hypertonic sodium bicarbonate has also proved helpful (40).

Class IB Drugs

Class IB agents inhibit the fast sodium channels but these agents shorten the refractory period and action potential duration. These medications include lidocaine, mexiletine, phenytoin, and tocainide.

Lidocaine

Lidocaine appears to act on ischemic myocardium as it depresses cells with abnormal resting membrane potentials in the presence of potassium. It has minimal effect on QRS and QT_c intervals. Lidocaine slows conduction by delaying phase zero depolarization, and it decreases membrane responsiveness as well as shortens action potential and refractory period of the ventricle.

Clinical Indications Lidocaine is used frequently for ventricular ectopy or ventricular tachycardia. It also can have a role in the prevention of ventricular tachycardia or fibrillation. Hypokalemia should be corrected with its use.

Metabolism Lidocaine's metabolism is via the microsomal enzymes in the liver. It is available only in the parenteral form. Levels should be kept at less than 5 µg/mL.

Adverse Effects Lidocaine has no significant hemodynamic effects. Central nervous system impairment, however, can occur, which includes speech disturbance, lethargy, and seizures.

In cases of severe toxicity, treatment is essentially supportive with hemodialyis or hemofiltration also effective (41).

Mexiletine

Mexiletine is a lidocaine analogue.

Clinical Indications Mexiletine's main indication is for lidocaine-responsive ventricular ectopy or ventricular tachycardia, especially when seen after surgery as it is more effective than with cardiomyopathy (42). Mexiletine also can have a role in the prevention of ventricular tachycardia or fibrillation.

Metabolism The enteral form provides continuation therapy for lidocaine. Metabolism is via the hepatic route.

Adverse Effects As with lidocaine, mexiletine also has frequent central nervous system effects (parasthesia, headaches, and tremor). In addition, gastrointestinal symptoms can occur. Fewer side effects are seen in children (43).

Phenytoin

Phenytoin has little activity in atrial tissue.

Clinical Indications Phenytoin has been demonstrated to be effective in the treatment of ventricular ectopy and ventricular tachycardia in children after cardiac surgery (44). In addition, phenytoin is also used for prolonged QT syndrome to decrease the incidence of sudden death. Lastly, phenytoin is indicated in digoxin-related and tricyclic antidepressant toxicity-related arrhythmias.

Metabolism Phenytoin induces hepatic enzymes.

Adverse Effects Hypotension and bradycardia can occur with rapid administration. Neurologic symptoms such as ataxia and vertigo can be seen.

Class IC Drugs

Class IC agents include flecainide, propafenone, and encainide. As with class IA and IB agents, these agents also inhibit the fast sodium channels, but these agents have no significant effects (prolongation or shortening) on the refractory period. In addition, these agents also shorten the duration of Purkinje action potential and inhibit conduction in the His-Purkinje system.

Flecainide

Flecainide causes prolongation of the QRS and QT_c intervals. Also seen with its use is significant depression of sinoatrial node and delay in conduction through atria, ventricles, AV node, and accessory pathways. It prolongs the effective refractory period in the atria and ventricles (45).

Clinical Indications Flecainide is effective against re-entry supraventricular tachycardia, as well as atrial fibrillation and flutter, ectopic atrial tachycardia, and WPW (46). It is also of purported efficacy in the treatment of permanent form of junctional reciprocating tachycardia (47). Lastly, it is indicated for ventricular tachycardia.

Metabolism Flecainide is metabolized mostly in the liver and eliminated in the kidney.

Adverse Effects Flecainide has negative inotropic effects. In addition, it has a proarrhythmia effect that can be increased with depressed myocardial function or structurally abnormal hearts. Flecainide and encainide have been implicated in an increased risk of death in the post-myocardial infarction patient with premature ventricular contractions (48). These drugs have shown some risk of adverse cardiac events in children as well, but under the specific conditions of the patient with an abnormal heart, particularly with atrial tachycardias (22). Blurred vision and hyperactivity have been reported.

Therapy for overdoses is similar to that for class IA drugs, with gastric emptying and hypertonic sodium bicarbonate solutions (49).

Propafenone

In addition to its class IC effects, propafenone also has β-blocking and weak calcium channel blocking effects. It has marked effects on accessory pathways. Atrial and ventricular effective refractory periods are prolonged.

Clinical Indications Propafenone is effective against re-entry supraventricular tachycardia such as WPW and atrial fibrillation or flutter as well as ectopic atrial tachycardia. Along with amiodarone, it is also effective against chaotic atrial rhythm (50). It is of purported efficacy in the treatment of junctional ectopic tachycardia in the postoperative patient (51). It is also indicated for ventricular tachycardia, although efficacy is uncertain in children with heart defects (52).

Metabolism Propafenone is metabolized mostly in the liver and eliminated in the kidney.

Adverse Effects Hypotension and proarrhythmias can be seen with its administration. Gastrointestinal symptoms are also seen. Combination therapy with amiodarone should be done with extreme caution. Prolongation of QRS interval and elevation of liver enzymes are reported (53).

Class II Drugs

Class II agents differ in terms of their receptor selectivity and intrinsic sympathomimetic activity, but they all decrease sympathetic activity by blocking β-receptors.

Esmolol

Esmolol, because of its short half-life, has recently become a commonly employed β-blocker in the intensive care setting. It inhibits SA and AV node conduction.

Clinical Indications Esmolol is effective against tachyarrhythmias, such as re-entry supraventricular tachycardia, and for ectopic tachycardias. It also has purported efficacy in the treatment of junctional ectopic tachycardia (see above). Lastly, esmolol is also indicated for ventricular tachycardia.

Metabolism Esmolol, with its half-life of 10 minutes, is the shortest acting β-blocker. Esmolol is metabolized by esterases of red blood cells.

Adverse Effects Predominant cardiac manifestations of esmolol are bradycardia, AV block, and hypotension. In severe cases of toxicity, catecholaminergic drugs and glucagon administration, pacing, and either cardiac bypass, ventricular assist, or intra-aortic balloon pumps have all been used (54). In addition, central nervous system side effects (such a headaches, agitation, and dizziness) are also common.

Class III Drugs

The mechanism of action of class III agents is prolongation of the action potential by blocking potassium channels, thereby lengthening the action potential duration and effective refractory period. These agents have significant differences. Overall, these drugs have minimal negative inotropic effects.

Amiodarone

Amiodarone possesses properties of all four classes of antiarrhythmic agents. Amiodarone possesses class I sodium channel blocking properties and therefore depresses conduction in myocardial tissues. Recent animal data suggest that amiodarone can act acutely as a class I antiarrhythmic agent in the newborn heart (55). Amiodarone also has some β-blocking activity and calcium channel antagonism so that SA and AV nodes can be inhibited. PR, QRS, and QT intervals are also prolonged.

Clinical Indications Amiodarone has broad application as an antiarrhythmic agent. Although it has proved efficacy for a variety of supraventricular and ventricular arrhythmias, its adverse effects preclude its use on a routine basis in children (56).

Amiodarone is effective against atrial flutter or fibrillation and re-entry supraventricular tachycardia as well as ectopic atrial tachycardia. In its parenteral form, it is also of purported efficacy in the treatment of junctional ectopic tachycardia (57). Lastly, it is effective against ventricular tachycardia. Amiodarone has also been used with success for hypertrophic cardiomyopathy and cardiac tumors with outflow tract obstruction (58).

Metabolism In its enteral form, amiodarone has a slow onset of action and a long half-life (2 to 4 weeks) because of its lipid solubility and large volume of distribution. Metabolism is via hepatic route and excretion is via the skin, lacrimal and sweat glands, and biliary tract. The parenteral form of amiodarone has recently gained acceptance in the intensive care setting.

Adverse Effects Amiodarone has a myriad of side effects, which constitute a significant disadvantage to its use. Cardiac effects include bradycardia, AV block, and ventricular arrhythmias (59) (including torsade de pointes, which can be seen especially when other antiarrhythmic agents such as class I agents and sotalol are present and/or when hypocalcemia exists). Pacemaker implantation may be indicated if amiodarone is used in patients with sinus node dysfunction.

Other side effects include pulmonary infiltrates and fibrosis (although not yet reported in children), corneal deposits, photosensitivity and grayish discoloration of the skin, alteration of thyroid function, neurologic symptoms (including headaches, peripheral neuropathy), and alteration of hepatic enzymes.

Amiodarone has significant interaction with digoxin and warfarin. It should also be used with caution in the presence of β-blockers and calcium channel antagonists. Intravenous calcium chloride is often helpful for mild hypotensive episodes (60).

Sotalol

Sotalol has β-blocking activity as well as class III action. It also prolongs the effective refractory periods in atrial and ventricular tissues (61) as well as action potential duration of Purkinje fibers (62).

Clinical Indications Sotalol's efficacy as an agent for both supraventricular tachycardia (including atrial flutter) and ventricular tachycardia has been well documented (63, 64).

Metabolism Sotalol is lipid insoluble and therefore not subject to liver metabolism.

Adverse Effects Bradycardia and atrioventricular block are observed. Exacerbation of congestive heart failure can also occur. Torsades de pointes is reported especially with agents that prolong QT interval.

Bretylium

Bretylium is concentrated in the terminal sympathetic neurons. Although its effect is mainly inhibition of norepinephrine release, norepinephrine is initially released and induces a sympathomimetic effect.

Clinical Indications Bretylium's use in the pediatric population is limited. It can be used for ventricular tachycardia or fibrillation unresponsive to lidocaine and cardioversion.

Metabolism No metabolism occurs via the liver. Excretion is through the kidneys by tubular secretion.

Adverse Effects Intravenous bretylium can cause hypotension, which should be addressed with volume expansion and norepinephrine. Gastrointestinal symptoms (nausea and vomiting) also occur.

Class IV Drugs

Class IV agents inhibit the slow inward calcium channels that exist in nodal tissue (especially the AV node).

Verapamil

Verapamil prolongs the conduction time and refractory period of the atrioventricular node (65).

Clinical Indications Verapamil's effectiveness has been shown in the treatment of children with supraventricular tachycardia, especially those that use the AV node as part of the circuit (66). Its use in hypertrophic cardiomyopathy has also been noted.

Metabolism Verapamil is metabolized by the liver.

Adverse Effects Use of verapamil in the infant population should be avoided (67). Verapamil should not be used in the presence of β-blocking agents. Bradycardia and AV block are the most common ECG effects, with hypotension and myocardial depression seen clinically. Lastly, gastrointestinal symptoms can also occur.

Many reports of calcium channel blocker intoxication appear in the literature (68–70). Although no specific antidote is available for calcium channel blockade, calcium and atropine can be useful. Glucagon has been reported as useful for hypotension, in conjunction with amrinone (71). Verapamil is contraindicated as a therapeutic agent for digoxin toxicity.

Miscellaneous Agents

Digoxin

Digoxin activates the parasympathetic system to induce sinus slowing and atrioventricular nodal inhibition. It also slows AV conduction and prolongs the AV refractory period secondary to increasing vagal tone.

Clinical Indications Supraventricular tachycardia, including atrial flutter and fibrillation as well as chaotic atrial tachycardia, can be effectively treated by digoxin. Digoxin is not recommended for patients with WPW re-entrant tachycardia.

Metabolism Digoxin is excreted via the kidneys.

Adverse Effects Digoxin levels are increased with concomitant administration of quinidine, amiodarone, or verapamil. Digoxin is the most thoroughly studied antiarrhythmic agent, and it has the most definitive overdose therapy. Inappropriate administration can result from errors in dosing by misplacing the decimal point in the elixir preparation (e.g., 5.0 mL instead of 0.5 mL), errors in concentration (the elixir is 50 μg/mL and the IV form is 100 μg/mL), or repeated dosing by caretakers unaware of prior drug being given. Cardiac manifestations of digoxin toxicity include nearly every type of arrhythmia–from simple ectopy to ventricular fibrillation–with a predilection for bradycardia and various degrees of AV block being most common. Noncardiac findings include nausea, vomiting, and visual disturbances. Overdose effects are worsened by hypokalemia, hypomagnesemia, hypoxemia, hypothyroidism, and hypercalcemia. These abnormalities need to be corrected at initiation of therapy.

Treatment for Digoxin Toxicity

Therapy consists of emesis, gastric lavage, and charcoal and magnesium citrate for ingestions. Digoxin-specific antibodies (Fab) are effective in lowering serum levels and decreasing toxicity (72). A standard serum level has not been established for use of this agent. Severe arrhythmias and symptoms or a level in excess of 4.0 ng/mL are factors worthy of consideration for Fab therapy. The dose can be determined by giving 60 mg Fab for every 1.0 mg of digoxin absorbed or administered. The body load in milligrams is (level $\times$ 5.6 $\times$ weight in kg)/1000 where 5.6 is the volume of distribution for the drug. Alternatively, the dose can be determined by assessing the number of vials of Fab = (level $\times$ weight in kg)/100, with 40 mg of Fab per vial.

Other therapeutic agents to be considered in digoxin toxicity include phenytoin or lidocaine for ventricular arrhythmias, phenytoin or β-blockers for SVT, and atropine for bradycardia and AV block. Dialysis is generally ineffective. Cardioversion should be avoided when possible because of risk of inducing unresponsive ventricular fibrillation. If the level exceeds 6.0 ng/mL, consideration should be given to placing a temporary pacing catheter.

Adenosine

Adenosine, a purine nucleoside, has become the drug of choice for acute intervention of supraventricular tachycardia, including in the perioperative period (73, 74). Adenosine increases potassium conductance, thereby causing conduction to be impaired in the SA and especially AV node.

Clinical Indications Adenosine serves as an effective therapeutic agent for re-entrant supraventricular tachycardia that involves the AV node. Even if adenosine fails to terminate the tachyarrhythmia, it can also be used diagnostically to delineate the specific type of supraventricular tachycardia as well as to distinguish supraventricular tachycardia from ventricular tachycardia (because the latter can occur as a narrow complex tachycardia).

Metabolism Adenosine's half-life, because of rapid metabolism by erythrocytes and endothelial cells, is short (10 seconds). Adenosine needs to be delivered as a rapid bolus followed by volume. In addition, aminophylline can negate the effects of adenosine.

Adverse Effects Cardiac effects include AV block, ventricular ectopy, sinus bradycardia, and sinus arrest; temporary pacing should be readily available during administration of adenosine. Transient hypotension can also occur. Pulmonary side effects include dyspnea and bronchospasm.

REFERENCES

1. Wittig JH, de Leval MR, Stark J. Intraoperative mapping of atrial activation before, during and after the Mustard operation. J Thor Cardiovasc Surg 1977;73:1.
2. Vetter VL, Tanner CS, Horowitz LN. Inducible atrial flutter after Mustard repair for complete transposition of the great arteries. Am J Cardiol 1988;61:428.
3. Duster M, Bink-Boelkens MTE, Wampler D, et al. Long-term follow-up of dysrhythmias following the Mustard Procedure. Am Heart J 1985;109:1323.
4. Kurer CC, Tanner CS, Norwood WI, et al. Perioperative arrhythmias after Fontan repair. Circulation 1990;82:IV190.
5. Spach MS, Miller MT III, Barr RC, et al. Electrophysiology of the internodal pathways: determining the difference between anisotropic cardiac muscle and a specialized conduction system. In: Little RC, ed. Physiology of atrial pacemakers and connective tissues. Mt. Kisco, NY: Futura Publishing, 1980;367.
6. Vetter VL, Horowitz LN. Electrophysiologic residua and sequelae of surgery for congenital heart defects. Am J Cardiol 1982;50:588.
7. Gelband H, Waldo AL, Kaiser GA, et al. Etiology of right bundle branch block in patients undergoing total correction of tetralogy of Fallot. Circulation 1971;44:1022.
8. Sondheimer HM, Izukawa T, Olley PM, et al. Conduction disturbances after total correction of tetralogy of Fallot. Am Heart J 1976;92:278.
9. Kurosaw H, Becker AE. Atrioventricular conduction in congenital heart disease surgical anatomy. Tokyo: Springer-Verlag, 1987.
10. Weindling SN, Saul JP, Gamble WJ, et al. Duration of complete heart block after congenital heart disease surgery [Abstract]. J Am Coll Cardiol 1994;104A.
11. Squarcia U, Merideth J, McGoon DC, et al. Prognosis of transient atrioventricular conduction disturbances complicating open heart surgery for congenital heart defects. Am J Cardiol 1971;28:648.
12. Drifus LS, Fisch C, Griffin JC, et al. Guidelines for implantation of cardiac pacemakers and antiarrhythmia devices. ACC/AHA Task Force report. J Am Coll Cardiol 1991;18:1.
13. Ko JK, Deal BJ, Strasburger JF, et al. Supraventricular tachycardia mechanisms and their age distribution in pediatric patients. Am J Cardiol 1992;69:1028.
14. Perry JC, Garson A Jr. Supraventricular tachycardia due to Wolff-Parkinson-White in children: early disappearance and late recurrence. J Am Coll Cardiol 1990;16:1215.
15. Cecchin F, Fenrich AL, Friedman RA, et al. Wide QRS tachycardia in infancy: left bundle branch block is common during supraventricular tachycardia [Abstract]. Pediatr Cardiol 1994;15:254.
16. Gallagher JJ, Kasell J, Smith WM, et al. Use of the esophageal lead in the diagnosis of mechanisms of reciprocating tachycardia. PACE 1980;3:440.
17. Pongiglione G, Saul JP, Dunnigan A, et al. Role of transesophageal pacing in evaluation of palpitations in children and adolescents. Am J Cardiol 1988;62:566.
18. Epstein ML, Kiel EA, Victorica BE. Cardiac decompensation following verapamil therapy in infants with supraventricular tachycardia. Pediatrics 1985;75:737.
19. Perry JC, Knilans TK, Marlow D, et al. Intravenous amiodarone for life-threatening tachyarrhythmias in children and young adults. J Am Coll Cardiol 1993;22:95.
20. Oh JK, Homes DR, Hayes DL, et al. Cardiac arrhythmias in patients with surgical repair of Ebstein's anomaly. J Am Coll Cardiol 1985;6:1351.
21. Garson A Jr, Bink-Boelkens M, Hesslein PS, et al. Atrial flutter in the young: a collaborative study of 360 cases. J Am Coll Cardiol 1985;6:871.
22. Fish FA, Gillette PC, Benson DW Jr. Proarrhythmia, cardiac arrest and death in young patients receiving encainide and flecainide. J Am Coll Cardiol 1991;18:356.
23. Gillette PC, Zeigler VL, Case CL, et al. Atrial antitachycardia pacing in children and young adults. Am Heart J 1991;122:844.
24. Gillette PC, Smith RT Jr, Garson A Jr, et al. Chronic supraventricular tachycardia. A curable cause of congestive cardiomyopathy. JAMA 1985;253:391.
25. Perry JC, McQuinn R, Smith RT Jr, et al. Flecainide acetate for resistant arrhythmias in the young: efficacy and pharmacokinetics. J Am Coll Cardiol 1989;14:185.
26. Coumel P, Fidelle J. Amiodarone in the treatment of cardiac arrhythmias in children: one hundred thirty five cases. Am Heart J 1980;100:1063.
27. Walsh EP, Saul JP, Hulse JE, et al. Transcatheter ablation of ectopic atrial tachycardia in young patients using radio frequency current. Circulation 1992;86:1138.
28. Gillette PC. Diagnosis and management of postoperative junctional ectopic tachycardia. Am Heart J 1989;118:192.
29. Perry J, Fenrich A, Hulse JE, et al. and the Pediatric IV Amiodarone Group. Pediatric use of intravenous amiodarone: efficacy and safety in critically ill patients from a multicenter protocol. PACE 1995;18:837.
30. Kurer CC, Tanner CS, Norwood WI, et al. Perioperative arrhythmias after Fontan repair. Circulation 1990;82:IV190.
31. Figa FH, Gow, RM, Hamilton RM, et al. Clinical efficacy and safety of intravenous amiodarone in infants and children. Am J Cardiol 1994;74:573.
32. Garson A Jr, Moak JP, Smith RT, et al. Usefulness of intravenous propafenone for control of postoperative junctional ectopic tachycardia. Am J Cardiol 1987;59:1422.
33. Erickson C, Perry J, Marlow D, et al. Sudden death during propafenone therapy for atrial flutter in young postoperative heart patients [Abstract]. PACE 1993;16:939.
34. Wren C, Campbell RWF. The response of paediatric arrhythmias to intravenous and oral flecainide. Br Heart J 1987;57:171.
35. Chandar JS, Wolff GS, Garson A Jr, et al. Ventricular ar-

rhythmias in postoperative tetralogy of Fallot. Am J Cardiol 1990;65:655.
36. Konishi Y, Matsuda K, Nishiwaki N, et al. Ventricular arrhythmias late after aortic and/or mitral valve replacement. Jpn Circ J 1985;49:576.
37. Tzivoni D, Banai S, Schuger C, et al. Treatment of torsade de pointes with magnesium sulfate. Circulation 1988;77:392.
38. Kar PM, Kellner K, Ing TS, et al. Combined high-efficiency hemodialysis and charcoal hemoperfusion in severe N-acetylprocainamide intoxication. Am J Kidney Dis 1992;20:403.
39. Webb CL, Dick M II, Rocchinin AP, et al. Quinidine syncope in children. J Am Coll Cardiol 1987;9:1031.
40. Kim SY, Benowitz NL. Poisoning due to class IA antiarrhythmic drugs. Quinidine, procainamide and disopyramide. Drug Safety 1990;5:393.
41. Denaro CP, Benowitz NL. Poisoning due to class IB antiarrhythmic drugs. Lignocaine, mexiletine and tocainide. Medical Toxicology and Adverse Drug Experiences 1989;4:412.
42. Moak JP, Smith RT, Garson A. Mexiletine: an effective antiarrhythmic drug for treatment of ventricular arrhythmias in congenital heart disease. J Am Coll Cardiol 1987;10:824.
43. Shakivi JG, Moezzi B. Electrophysiologic effects of mexiletine in children. Jpn Heart J 1982;23:733.
44. Kavey RE, Blackman MS, Sondheimer HM. Phenytoin therapy for ventricular arrhythmias occurring late after surgery for congenital heart disease. Am Heart J 1982;104:794.
45. Musto B, Donofrio A, Cavallaro C, et al. Electrophysiologic effects and clinical efficacy of flecainide in children with recurrent paroxysmal supraventricular tachycardia. Am J Cardiol 1988;62:229.
46. Perry JC, Garson A. Flecainide acetate for treatment of tachyarrhythmias in children: review of world literature on efficacy, safety, and dosing. Am Heart J 1992;124:1614.
47. Chang AC, Zapalla F, Kurer CC, et al. Clinical outcome of children with permanent form of junctional reciprocating tachycardia [Abstract]. J Am Coll Cardiol 1990;15:204.
48. The Cardiac Arrhythmia SuppressionTrial (CAST) Investigators. Increased mortality due to encainide or flecainide in a randomized trial of arrhythmia suppression after myocardial infarction. N Engl J Med 1989;321:406.
49. Winkleman BR, Leinberger H. Life-threatening flecainide toxicity. A pharmacodynamic approach. Ann Int Med 1987;106:807.
50. Dodo H, Gow RM, Hamilton RM, et al. Chaotic atrial rhythm in children. Am Heart J 1995;129:990.
51. Garson A, Moak FP, Smith RT, et al. Usefulness of intravenous propafenone for control of postoperative junctional ectopic tachycardia. Am J Cardiol 1987;59:1422.
52. Heusch A, Kramer HH, Krogmann ON, et al. Clinical experience with propafenone for cardiac arrhythmias in the young. Eur Heart J 1994;15:1050.
53. Janousek J, Paul T, Reimer A, et al. Usefulness of propafenone for supraventricular arrhythmias in infants and children. Am J Cardiol 1993;72:294.
54. Kenyon CJ, Aldinger GE, Joshipura P, et al. Successful resuscitation using external cardiac pacing in beat adrenergic antagonist-induced bradyasystolic arrest. Ann Emerg Med 1988;17:711.
55. Chen F, Wetzel GT, Klitzner TS. Acute effects of amiodarone on sodium currents in isolated neonatal ventricular myocytes. Developmental and Pharmacologic Therapeutics 1992;19:118.
56. Garson A, Gillette PC, McVey P, et al. Amiodarone treatment of critical arrhythmias in children and young adults. J Am Coll Cardiol 1984;4:749.
57. Raja P, Hawker RE, Chaikitpinyo A, et al. Amiodarone management of junctional ectopic tachycardia after cardiac surgery in children. Br Heart J 1994;72:261.
58. Gajarski RJ, Towbin JA. Recent advances in the etiology, diagnosis, and treatment of myocarditis and cardiomyopathies in children. Curr Opin Pediatr 1995;7:587.
59. Pohlgeers A, Villafane J. Ventricular fibrillation in two infants treated with amiodarone hydrochloride. Pediatr Cardiol 1995;16:82.
60. Leatham EW, Holt DW, McKenna WJ. Class III antiarrhythmics in overdose. Presenting features and management principles. Drug Safety 1993;9:450.
61. Houyel L, Fournier A, Ducharme G, et al. Electrophysiologic effects of sotalol on the immature mammalian heart. J Cardiovasc Pharmacol 1992;19:134.
62. Moak J. Developmental cellular electrophysiologic effects of solatol on canine cardiac Purkinje fibers. Pediatr Res 1991;29:104.
63. Pfammatter JP, Paul T, Lehmann C, et al. Efficacy and proarrhythmia of oral sotalol in pediatric patients. J Am Coll Cardiol 1995;29:1002.
64. Maragnes P, Tipple M, Fournier A. Effectiveness of oral sotalol for treatment of pediatric arrhythmias. Am J Cardiol 1992;69:751.
65. Bolens M, Friedli B, Deom A. Electrophysiologic effects of intravenous verapamil in children after operations for congenital heart disease. Am J Cardiol 1987;60:692.
66. Porter CJ, Gillette PC, Garson AJ, et al. Effects of verapamil on supraventricular tachycardia in children. Am J Cardiol 1981;48:487.
67. Epstein ML, Keil EA, Victorica E. Cardiac decompensation following verapamil therapy in infants with supraventricular tachycardia. Pediatrics 1985;75:737.
68. Barrow PM, Houston PL, Wong DT. Overdose of sustained release verapamil. Br J Anaesth 1994;72:361.
69. Leesar MA, Martyn R, Talley JD, et al. Noncardiogenic pulmonary edema complicating massive verapamil overdose. Chest 1994;105:606.
70. Hofer CA, Smith JK, Tenholder MF. Verapamil intoxication: a literature review of overdoses and discussion of therapeutic options. Am J Med 1993;95:431.
71. Wolf LR, Spadafor MP, Otten EJ. Use of amrinone and glucagon in a case of calcium channel blocker overdose. Ann Emerg Med 1993;22(7):1225–1228.
72. Hastreiter AR, van der Horst RL, Chow-Tung E. Digitalis toxicity in infants and children. Pediatr Cardiol 1984;5:131.
73. Till J, Shinebourne EA, Rigby ML, et al. Efficacy and safety of adenosine in the treatment of supraventricular tachycardia in infants and children. Br Heart J 1989;62:204.
74. Rossi AF, Steinberg LG, Kipel G, et al. Use of adenosine in the management of perioperative arrhythmias in the pediatric cardiac intensive care unit. Crit Care Med 1992;20:1107.

Section V. Diagnosis and Management of Acquired and Chronic Heart Disease

The Failing Myocardium

Alan B. Lewis, MD

HEART FAILURE

"Heart failure" has been defined conventionally as a syndrome in which the pump function of the heart is incapable of providing sufficient oxygenated blood to meet the metabolic demands of the tissues. Heart failure can be caused primarily by disorders of the myocardium (e.g., cardiomyopathy or myocarditis) or it can be secondary to abnormal loading conditions. The term "congestive heart failure" (CHF) has been applied to the associated pulmonary congestion and peripheral edema, which develops secondary to salt and water retention. However, this brief definition fails to impart an appreciation of the complex interaction between cardiocirculatory perturbations and neurohormonal activation that accounts for the pathophysiology and symptomatology of the disorder.

Cardiocirculatory Model

Central to the cardiocirculatory concept of heart failure is the progressive development of ventricular dysfunction. Ventricular dysfunction can be caused by increased afterload (severe aortic stenosis or chronic hypertension), increased preload (mitral regurgitation or left-to-right shunts), or intrinsic muscle impairment (myocarditis, dilated cardiomyopathy, or ischemic heart disease). Consequent myocardial remodeling results in myocellular hypertrophy, fibrosis, altered extracellular architecture, slippage of cells, and loss of myocytes (1).

Ventricular Dysfunction

Work of the ventricle can be displayed by the pressure-volume loop (Fig. 31.1A). Contractile (inotropic) function of the heart is represented by the end-systolic pressure-volume relation, the slope of which is an excellent index of contractility (2–4) that incorporates ventricular loading conditions. The relaxation (lusitropic) properties of the myocardium are displayed by the end-diastolic pressure-volume relation. The end-systolic and end-diastolic pressure-volume relations are illustrative of the interaction between the loading conditions on the heart and the inotropic and lusitropic properties of the ventricle (5).

Systolic dysfunction can be depicted by a downward and rightward shift of the end-systolic pressure-volume relation (Fig. 31.1B). Consequently, end-systolic volume is increased and stroke volume is decreased. The left ventricle compensates by increasing end-diastolic volume to restore a more normal stroke volume. *Diastolic or lusitropic dysfunction* is characterized by an upward and leftward shift of the diastolic pressure-volume relation without an alteration of contractility; this phenomenon can be seen in some patients with hypertrophic cardiomyopathy (Fig. 31.1C). End-diastolic pressure is higher at any given end-diastolic volume as a result of the loss of ventricular compliance. In most patients with heart failure, however, both systolic and diastolic dysfunction exist, resulting in symptoms attributable to both a reduction of cardiac output and pulmonary congestion (Fig. 31.1D) (see Chapter 3, *Cardiac Physiology—Selected Topics in Normal Hearts*).

Circulatory Maladaptation

For many years circulatory adaptations engendered by left ventricular dysfunction held center stage in the conceptual framework of the pathophysiology of heart failure and its consequent treatment. Diminished renal blood flow, resulting in impaired sodium and water excretion, was believed to be responsible for the expansion of intravascular volume with consequent peripheral and pulmonary edema. Therapy was directed principally at controlling edema.

As our understanding of the pathophysiology of heart failure evolved, emphasis shifted from intravascular volume expansion to vasoconstriction and increased sympathetic activity. The latter were thought to be essential adaptations that maintained blood pressure and perfusion to vital organs, redistributed intravascular volume, and enhanced cardiac contractility (6). Consequently physicians were hesitant to interfere with these adaptations for fear of worsening the circulatory and clinical condition (7).

Neurohormonal Model

During the past few decades this concept has shifted away from a notion of compensatory adaptations to that of chronic maladaptations, which increase the work of the heart and hasten the progression of heart failure. According to this current view, left ventricular dysfunction leads to activation of adrenergic sympathetic nervous system and several hormonal systems (e.g., renin-angiotensin, atrial natriuretic peptide [ANP], and endothelin-1) (8, 9).

Adrenergic Mechanisms

Plasma norepinephrine levels correlate with the limitation of functional capacity and the magnitude of the hemodynamic disturbance (10). Elevated sympathetic stimula-

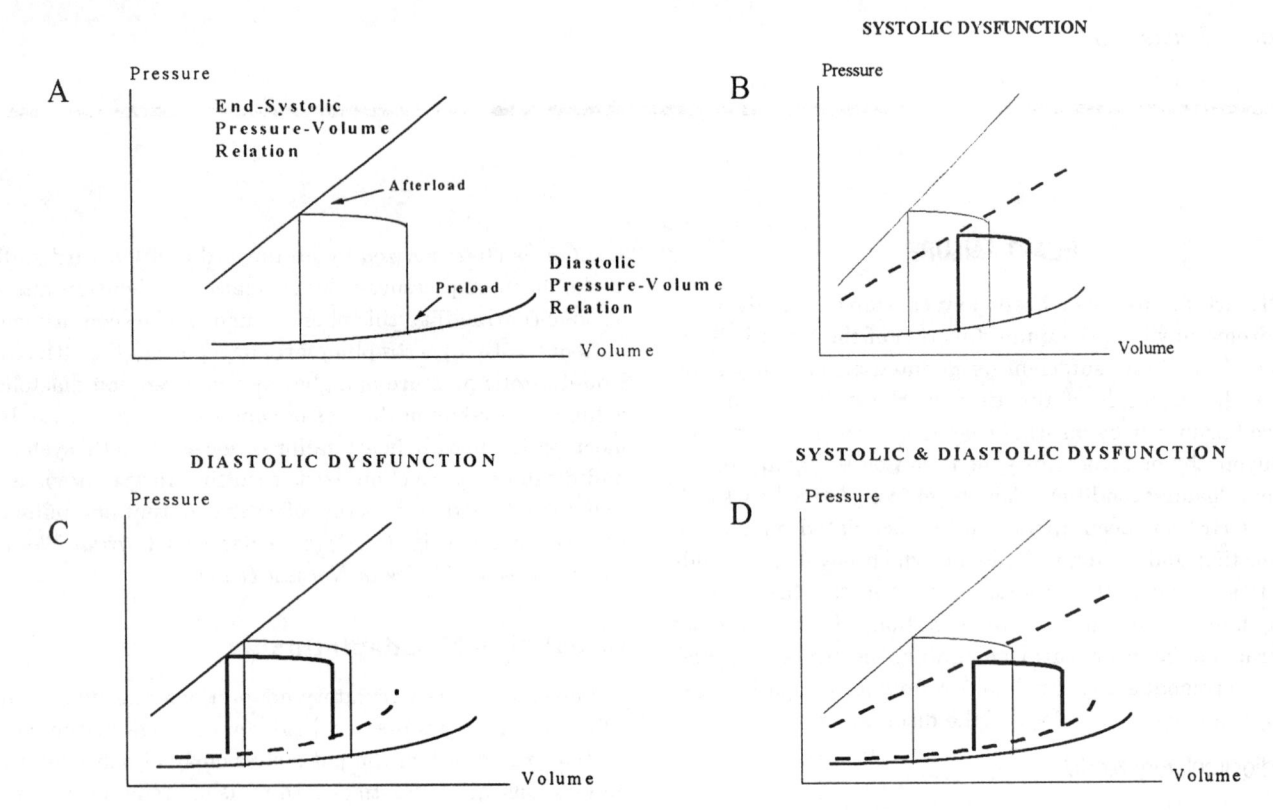

Figure 31.1. Pressure-volume loop of ventricular contraction (see text).

tion results in both decreased β_1-adrenoreceptor density in the myocardium and decreased receptor sensitivity to β-adrenergic stimulation (11, 12). Uncoupling of the receptors from the G protein-adenyl cyclase complex by dysfunction of the G_s proteins and/or increased G_i protein activity results in diminished generation of cyclic adenosine monophosphate (cAMP).

Renin-Angiotensin System

Activation of the renin-angiotensin system is promoted by reduced serum sodium, increased sympathetic tone, and decreased blood pressure (8, 9, 13). Renin, secreted by the kidney, converts angiotensinogen produced by the liver into angiotensin I. Angiotensin I, an inactive decapeptide, is converted to angiotensin II by a converting enzyme that is present ubiquitously in vascular endothelium (14). Angiotensin II is a potent vasoconstrictor that facilitates sympathetic activation, stimulates adrenal release of aldosterone, and contributes to sodium and water retention. In addition to its endocrine function, the renin-angiotensin system has autocrine and paracrine activity in the heart (15, 16). Converting enzyme is synthesized in endothelial cells and angiotensin II receptors exist on myocytes. Angiotensin II has proto-oncogene effects, and it may participate in myocardial remodeling as a growth mediator of myocytes and fibroblasts (17, 18). Early use of angiotensin converting enzyme inhibitors was based on their activity as systemic vasodilators, but recent studies emphasize the effects on myocardial remodeling. Indeed, several important multicenter trials have demonstrated the benefit of converting enzyme inhibition on survival and progression of left ventricular dysfunction in adult patients with both advanced heart failure and asymptomatic left ventricular dysfunction (19, 20).

Other Hormonal Systems

Patients with heart failure exhibit elevated circulating levels of ANP as well as blunted renal response to the hormone (21). ANP is synthesized in atrial myocytes and released from storage granules by atrial distension and elevated pressure. ANP administration results in a prompt increase in sodium and water excretion in healthy subjects, but the response is attenuated in patients with heart failure.

Vascular endothelium performs important regulatory functions including the production of vasoconstrictor (endothelin-1) and vasodilator substances (e.g., endothelial-derived relaxing factor [EDRF]). Endothelin-1 production by the pulmonary vasculature is elevated in patients with heart failure, and it can increase pulmonary and systemic vascular resistance (22, 23). Peripheral vasoconstriction is enhanced by decreased production of EDRF and by blunted responsiveness of vascular smooth muscle to EDRF (24). The net result is increased vasomotor tone from unopposed vasoconstriction. The precise mechanism by which EDRF production is decreased in heart failure has not been elucidated but recent data suggest that nitric oxide synthase mRNA activity may be down-regulated by the low flow state characterized by myocardial failure (25). Alternatively, oxygen-derived free radical superoxide production, which is increased in heart failure, may inactivate EDRF, thereby inhibiting endothelium-dependent vasodilation (26).

MYOCARDITIS

Myocarditis is defined as an inflammatory infiltrate of the myocardium with necrosis and degeneration of adjacent myocytes not caused by coronary artery or other diseases. Lack of standard histologic criteria for establishing the diagnosis of myocarditis had led to surprising reports of the high incidence of myocarditis. These ranged from 4 to 5% in young men dying of trauma (27) to as high as 16 to 21% in an autopsy series of children dying suddenly (28–31).

Pathogenesis

Myocarditis can be caused by a multitude of microorganisms, particularly enteroviruses (Table 31.1). Coxsackie B viruses have been most frequently associated with human myocarditis (32). The pathogenesis of human myocarditis can be studied in a mouse model inoculated with coxsackievirus B_3 (33). Coxsackievirus B_3-induced murine myocarditis is distinguished by an early and late phase. The first histologic abnormalities, appearing 5 days after viral inoculation, consist of focal myocyte necrosis associated with polymorphonuclear and mononuclear cell infiltration (34). Virus can be isolated from the myocardium during the early phase but rapid production of neutralizing antibodies usually results in viral clearance by 2 weeks postinoculation. The late phase begins 7 to 10 days after the onset of infection. Most mouse strains exhibit healing without further inflammation after day 7, but some develop a lymphocytic infiltrate accompanied by foci of myocyte necrosis. Progression to this secondary inflammatory phase is summarized in Figure 31.2.

Diagnosis

Myocarditis should be considered in all patients with recent onset of heart failure and left ventricular dysfunction without other cause. Clinical features are variable, and they can include a history of an antecedent, flulike illness or gastroenteritis and a vague onset of tachypnea, dyspnea, easy fatigability, and general malaise.

Table 31.1. Etiology of Myocarditis

Infectious
  Viral
    Coxsackie A, B
    Echovirus
    Adenovirus
    Epstein-Barr virus
    Influenza
    Human immunodeficiency virus
    Cytomegalovirus
    Rubella
    Measles
    Mumps
    Respiratory syncytial virus
    Parvovirus
  Bacterial
    Streptococcal
    Staphylococcal
    Pneumococcal
    Diphtheria
    Pertussis
    Tetanus
    Tuberculosis
    Typhoid
    Gonococcal
    Brucellosis
  Fungal
    Candida
    Coccidiomycosis
    Cryptococcosis
    Aspergillosis
    Actinomycosis
    Histoplasmosis
  Rickettsial
    Q fever
    Rocky mountain spotted fever
  Protozoal
    Chagas' disease (*Trypanosoma cruzi*)
    Malaria
    Toxoplasmosis
    Leishmaniasis
  Spirochetal
    Syphilis
    Leptospirosis
  Metazoal
    Trichinosis
    Schistosomiasis
    Ascariasis
    Echinococcosis
    Filariasis
    Cysticercosis
Autoimmune
  Systemic lupus erythematosus
  Rheumatoid arthritis
  Sarcoidosis
  Acute rheumatic carditis
  Kawasaki syndrome
  Drug hypersensitivity

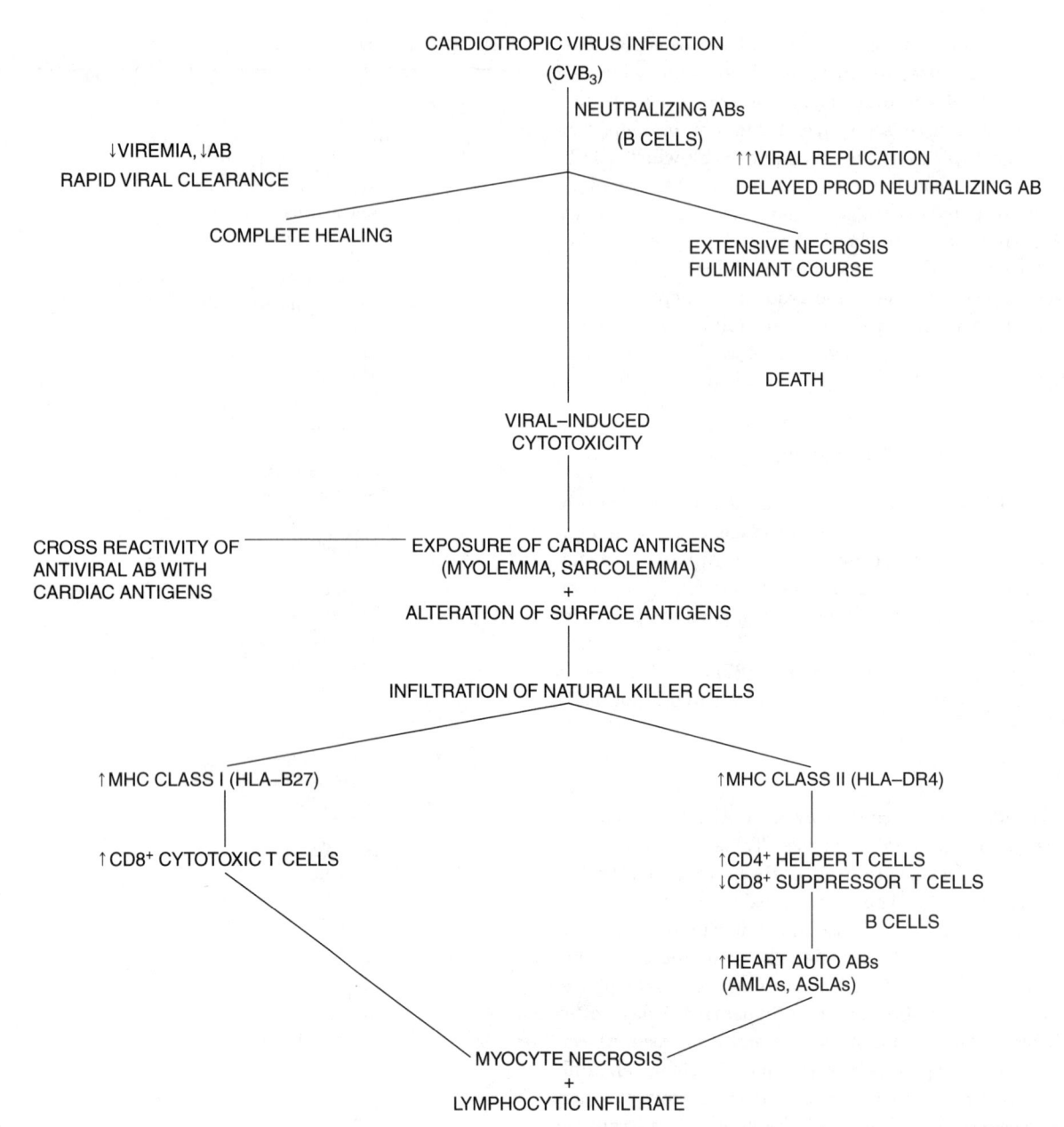

Figure 31.2. Immunomodulation of myocarditis. Susceptibility to the direct viral cytopathic effect during the early phase is related to a genetically determined delay in the production of neutralizing antibodies. Ongoing, active myocarditis appears to be the result of altered immune regulation. Natural killer cells are in the first wave of cell infiltration, and they induce the expression of major histocompatibility complex (*MHC*) antigens. The second wave consist of cytotoxic and helper T cells which lead to ongoing myocyte damage.

Physical examination usually reveals resting tachycardia and respiratory distress. Arrhythmias, particularly ventricular ectopy or tachycardia, and supraventricular tachycardia, can be a presenting features as well. Peripheral pulses may be weak and perfusion poor. Heart sounds are often muffled and gallop rhythms may be prominent. Murmurs, however, are usually absent, although a soft systolic murmur of mitral or tricuspid regurgitation can be auscultated. Jugular venous distention may be observed in older children, but it is difficult to detect in most infants. Pulmonary and systemic venous congestion are manifest by rales and hepatomegaly.

Standard screening tests (Table 31.2) include electrocardiography, chest roentgenogram, echocardiography, and serology; the definitive diagnosis, however, is generally difficult even by routine clinical criteria (35). The electrocardiogram typically demonstrates generalized low amplitude QRS with T wave flattening and/or inversion (Fig. 31.3); anomalous left coronary artery from the pulmonary artery (with deep Q waves in leads I and aVL) must be ruled out. Cardiomegaly is usually present on chest roentgenogram, but it can be absent early in the course of the disease. Pulmonary venous congestion is common. Echocardiography should be performed in all patients suspected of having myocarditis even in the absence of cardiomegaly on the chest roentgenogram. Findings on echocardiogram include ventricular dilation, reduced shortening and ejection fractions, global or regional wall motion abnormalities, mitral or tricuspid valve regurgitation, mural thrombus, and pericardial effusion.

Serologic studies may show elevated serum titers of viral IgM neutralizing antibodies that suggest a viral cause but do not verify causation. Serum should be screened for coxsackie virus, echovirus, adenovirus, and influenza. Erythrocyte sedimentation rate and creatine kinase-MB fraction are variably elevated, depending on the stage of the disease, degree of cardiac failure, and extent of myocellular necrosis. Serum carnitine levels should be measured in all patients to exclude myocardial dysfunction secondary to carnitine deficiency or disorders of fatty acid oxidation (36).

Table 31.2. Diagnostic Evaluation of Myocarditis

Noninvasive Cardiac Screening
  Electrocardiogram
  Chest radiograph
  Echocardiogram
Blood Testing
  Complete blood count with differential
  Erythrocyte sedimentation rate
  Creatine kinase-MB
  Viral IgM antibody titers
  Serum carnitine
    (Circulating anti-heat antibodies)
Invasive Cardiac Testing
  Endomyocardial biopsy

Endomyocardial Biopsy

Endomyocardial biopsy has been considered the "gold standard" for the definitive diagnosis of myocarditis. To minimize subjective discrepancies in interpretation, a standard histopathologic classification of myocarditis, the Dallas criteria, was adopted in 1984 (37). At least four to

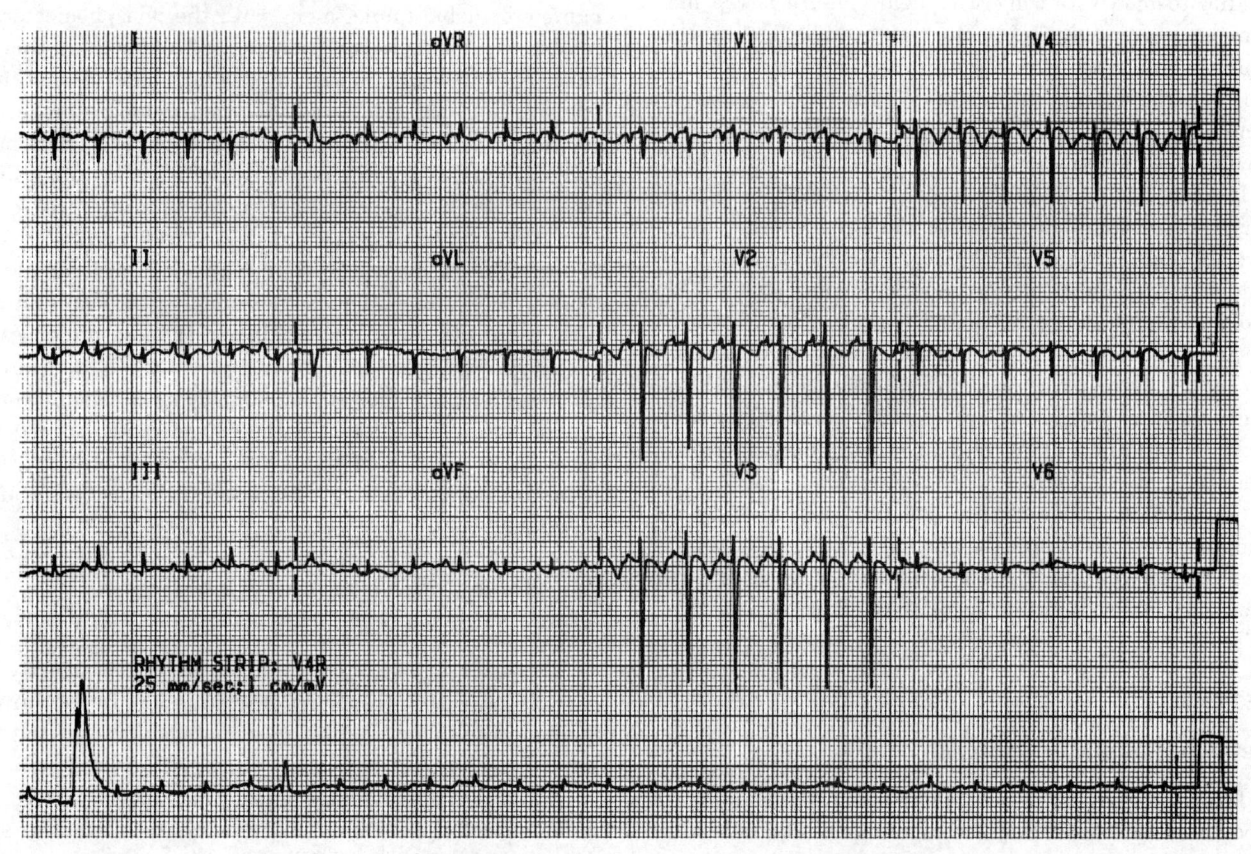

Figure 31.3. Electrocardiogram of a 1-year-old child with biopsy proved myocarditis. Sinus tachycardia is present along with T wave flattening in the left precordial leads.

six biopsy specimens should be submitted for histologic examination because of the focal nature of the process in most cases. Optimal timing of biopsy for acute myocarditis has been suggested to be within 3 to 6 weeks of onset (38). However, many children in whom the presentation and subsequent clinical course are highly suggestive of myocarditis, may have negative biopsies as early as 10 to 14 days following the onset of symptoms. These cases may represent the human counterpart to murine myocarditis, which is limited to the early viral phase without progression to the secondary phase of lymphocytic myocarditis.

Molecular Biology

Molecular biologic techniques have been currently applied to investigate the viral cause of myocarditis and dilated cardiomyopathy. Recent studies utilizing highly sensitive and specific polymerase chain reaction (PCR) gene amplification in children with suspected myocarditis have detected viral genome in 68% (26/38) of endomyocardial biopsy samples (39). Along with enterovirus (40), adenovirus has also been shown by PCR to be an important causative agent in pediatric patients.

Clinical Course

Mild to moderate congestive heart failure is the most common presentation of acute myocarditis. Spontaneous improvement with normalization of ventricular function can be anticipated in most cases within 1 to 3 months. In a minority of patients, recovery is incomplete and left ventricular dysfunction persists.

In about 20 to 30% of the patients, however, cardiac intensive care is necessary because a fulminant onset of myocarditis occurs, which is characterized by the relatively sudden development of pulmonary edema, hypotension, and poor peripheral perfusion. Arrhythmias, both ventricular and supraventricular, can occur, and they are difficult to control. As many as one third of these critically ill patients may die within the first month, whereas persistent heart failure and dilated cardiomyopathy may develop in others.

Occasionally other clinical presentations of non-CHF symptoms can be proved by endomyocardial biopsy to be caused by myocarditis. These include ventricular arrhythmias (41), atrioventricular block, sudden death, and chest pain.

Treatment

General Considerations

Rapid progression of heart failure and worsening of hemodynamic profile are not uncommon and all children admitted to the cardiac intensive care unit warrant a high degree of vigilance. Presence of metabolic acidosis, even mild, should be of concern. Another useful clinical parameter is heart rate; resting sinus tachycardia is ominous. Tachyarrythmias that compromise hemodynamic stability (e.g., ventricular tachycardia) should be aggressively treated with the appropriate antidysrhythmic agents (see Chapter 30, *Diagnosis and Management of Cardiac Arrhythmias*).

Although an arterial monitoring line is often considered necessary, routine placement of a pulmonary artery catheter to monitor cardiac output and pulmonary wedge pressures is probably not warranted, but it can be helpful in the most critically ill child. Urine output should be closely monitored with placement of a Foley catheter.

Inspired oxygen and mechanically assisted ventilation, when indicated, are important adjunct therapies, but endotracheal intubation should be performed with caution because sudden stress from inadequate anesthesia can lead to hemodynamic instability or lethal dysrhythmias.

Inotropic Agents

Treatment of patients with myocarditis should focus on control of congestive heart failure. Intravenous positive inotropic agents are the mainstay of therapy for the short-term management of cardiac failure (see Chapter 5, *Cardiovascular Pharmacology*). Beta-adrenergic agonists, dopamine or dobutamine, along with the phosphodiesterase inhibitors, amrinone or milrinone, are all useful in this regard. The latter can be particularly helpful in view of their peripheral vasodilation and afterload reducing properties as well their lusitropic effects. Recent clinical trials have demonstrated that low doses of digoxin, without digitalization, consistently lessened symptoms and improved exercise tolerance in patients with heart failure (42–44). Use of intravenous digoxin in this clinical setting should be done with caution because the inflamed myocardium can have increased sensitivity to digoxin at the usual doses.

When cardiac failure remains refractory to intravenous inotropic support, mechanical support with extracorporeal membrane oxygenation (ECMO) or ventricular assists devices can be considered along with listing for cardiac transplantation (see Chapter 22, *Mechanical Support of the Myocardium*).

Afterload Reduction and Angiotensin Converting Enzyme Inhibitors

Afterload reduction in the acute setting is usually accomplished with intravenous nitroprusside. In the chronic management of heart failure angiotensin converting enzyme inhibitors (ACEI) (e.g., captopril or enalapril) not only exhibit hemodynamic effects but act to correct the neurohormonal perturbations that characterize the syndrome of heart failure. ACEI have been shown to slow the progression of ventricular dilatation and remodeling (45), improve exercise tolerance (46) and prolong survival (47, 48).

Diuretics

Transition from asymptomatic left ventricular dysfunction to symptomatic congestive heart failure involves the development of sodium and water retention. This has led to the use of diuretics as the most direct way of promoting salt and water excretion. Although some patients may improve with thiazides, most patients with moderate congestive heart failure require more potent loop diuretics (e.g., furosemide). Continuous intravenous infusion of furosemide (0.1–0.4 mg/kg/h) produces a consistent diuresis and it can be used as an alternative to intermittent bolus administration (49). Electrolyte disturbances, particularly hypokalemia, can develop and potassium supplementation or a potassium sparing diuretic (e.g., spironolactone) should be considered. However, ACE inhibitors enhance potassium retention and obviate the need for potassium supplementation or potassium sparing diuretics.

Anticoagulation

Patients with myocarditis or dilated cardiomyopathy, particularly when left ventricle fractional shortening is less than 20%, are at risk for the development of mural thrombi and systemic embolization. Systemic administration of heparin may be warranted in these high-risk patients. In addition, long-term anticoagulation with low dose warfarin can be beneficial in lowering the risk of embolization without exposing the patient to the hemorrhagic complications associated with higher doses of warfarin.

Immunosuppressive Agents

Use of corticosteroids to reduce myocardial inflammation and necrosis remains controversial. Anecdotal reports in adults and children treated with corticosteroids have suggested improvement (50–53) in some cases but no benefit in others (54, 55). The high incidence of spontaneous improvement complicates the analysis of most studies of empiric steroid use. Studies of murine myocarditis have documented the detrimental effects of early administration of corticosteroids (56, 57), cyclophosphamide (58), and cyclosporine (59, 60) on viral replication, myocardial necrosis, and survival. If immunosuppressive agents are to be used, it appears prudent to delay therapy until viral clearance has been completed.

Gamma Globulin

High dose intravenous gamma globulin (IVGG) (2 g/kg) has been associated with both improved recovery of left ventricular function and better survival (61). Polyclonal immunoglobulin reduces the severity of coxsackievirus B_3 murine myocarditis by more than 50% (62). IVGG can contain neutralizing antibodies to the causative virus. Alternatively, IVGG can have immunomodulatory effects that down-regulate cytokines, which depress contractility via nitric oxide-dependent mechanisms or reduce inflammation by preventing induction of new myocellular antigens.

Chronic therapy usually includes digoxin, diuretics, and converting enzyme inhibition. Captopril has been shown to be particularly beneficial in coxsackievirus B_3 murine myocarditis in reducing myocellular necrosis (63).

DILATED CARDIOMYOPATHY

Cardiomyopathies are classified as *dilated, hypertrophic,* or *restrictive* based on clinical, hemodynamic, and structural features with the understanding that considerable overlap often exists, particularly between hypertrophic and restrictive forms (64).

Dilated cardiomyopathy is characterized by ventricular dilation and systolic dysfunction. Heart muscle diseases associated with congenital or acquired structural abnormalities or known systemic disorder are generally excluded.

Epidemiology and Pathogenesis

Dilated cardiomyopathy is the most common cause of congestive heart failure in patients without other known cardiac abnormalities (65). The annual incidence of idiopathic dilated cardiomyopathy (IDC) has been estimated to be approximately 6 to 8 cases per 100,000 population (66). Antecedent myocarditis has been implicated in the pathogenesis of dilated cardiomyopathy. Lymphocytic myocarditis has been reported in 3 to 63% of adults with dilated cardiomyopathy (67), but recent data using the Dallas criteria for histologic classification of right ventricular endomyocardial biopsy specimens (68) and PCR for detection of viral RNA (69) place the incidence lower at 7 to 12%.

Diagnosis

The chest roentgenogram shows cardiomegaly and often pulmonary venous congestion in vast majority of patients. The electrocardiogram shows left ventricular hypertrophy and nonspecific ST and T wave abnormalities. Atrial or ventricular arrhythmias can also be present. In glycogen storage disease IIa (Pompe's disease), a short PR interval, high QRS voltages, and marked left ventricular hypertrophy are typical. As with myocarditis, deep Q waves should be sought (particularly in leads I and aVL) to rule out anomalous left coronary artery from the pulmonary artery.

Echocardiograms demonstrate left atrial and ventricular dilation and decreased fractional shortening and ejection fraction (Fig. 31.4). Wall thickness can be normal or reduced. Deep trabeculations may be observed in patients with so-called "spongy" or noncompaction of the left ven-

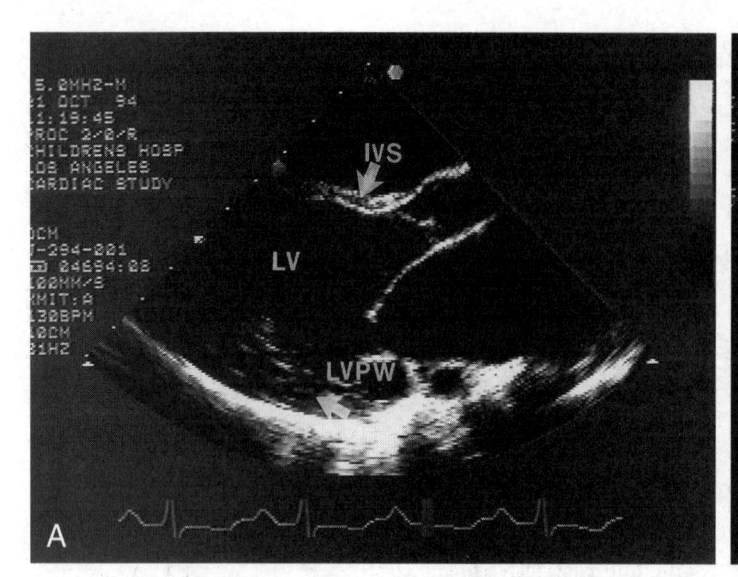

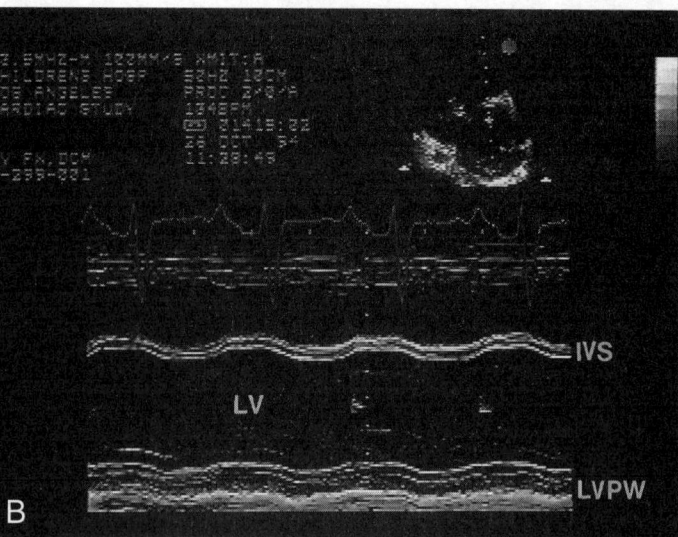

Figure 31.4. Echocardiogram in a child with severe idiopathic dilated cardiomyopathy. Marked ventricular dilatation is seen on two-dimensional imaging (**A**) with diminished shortening evident on the m-mode tracing (**B**). IVS, interventricular septum; LVPW, left ventricular posterior wall.

tricular myocardium (70). Mural thrombi can be detected in a third of patients, with embolization occurring in approximately 10% (71). Mitral and tricuspid regurgitation may be present. Cardiac catheterization can be used to quantitate left ventricular filling pressures and cardiac output, and to demonstrate the coronary arteries in patients in whom echocardiography fails to exclude anomalous origin of the left coronary artery from the pulmonary artery as the cause for ventricular dysfunction. Right ventricular endomyocardial biopsy can be performed to detect myocarditis or specific muscle diseases (72, 73). Patients with IDC demonstrate nonspecific histologic changes including myocyte hypertrophy, nuclear abnormalities, and interstitial fibrosis. Other studies include plasma carnitine levels, which should be obtained on all patients with dilated cardiomyopathy. Free plasma carnitine levels below 20 μmol/L or total carnitine levels below 30 μmol/L are highly suggestive of disorders of carnitine transport or β-oxidation of fatty acids (e.g., medium or long chain acyl-CoA dehydrogenase deficiency). Supplementation of l-carnitine results in dramatic improvement in ventricular function and symptomatology.

Treatment

Except for the use of corticosteroids and gamma-globulins, the strategy for myocardial support is similar to that for the treatment for myocarditis as the mainstay of therapy is supportive in nature.

Natural History and Outcome

Some authors have suggested that children younger than 2 years of age have a better prognosis compared with older children (74). Subsequent reviews of larger numbers of patients indicated no significant relationship between age at presentation and outcome (75, 76). The 1- and 5-year actuarial survival for all children was 75 and 60%, respectively, with the highest mortality rate observed during the initial 6 months. Patients in whom left ventricular fractional shortening remains less than 15% have a 46 and 29% 1- and 5-year survival (77).

Human Immunodeficiency Virus (HIV)-Associated Cardiomyopathy

The first cases of dilated cardiomyopathy in patients with acquired immunodeficiency syndrome (AIDS) were reported in 1986 (78). Subsequent studies have confirmed these observation and have indicated that a significant subgroup of HIV-infected patients may be at risk of developing progressive cardiomyopathy. Prevalence of asymptomatic left ventricular dysfunction is reported to be 14.5% in adult patients and 26% in children, with 2 and 13% developing congestive heart failure, respectively (79, 80). Endomyocardial biopsy or necropsy findings reveal lymphocytic myocarditis in most patients, some of whom may have with opportunistic infections (e.g., cryptococcal myocarditis (77, 81). In situ hybridization studies have revealed HIV ribonucleic acid in 15% of samples and DNA evidence of cytomegalovirus infection in 50% (82).

Anthracycline Cardiomyopathy

Anthracycline antibiotics such as adriamycin and daunomycin have excellent antineoplastic activity, but they are limited by acute and chronic cardiotoxicity (83–85). Myocyte injury seen in patients with anthracycline cardiotoxicity consists of myofibrillar loss and vacuolization caused by sarcoplasmic reticulum swelling within myocytes (82). Dose-dependence of the toxicity has been well documented, and it is usually manifest after a total cumulative dose of more than 450 mg/m^2 (2). Increasing numbers of patients who were successfully treated with anthracyclines for their neoplasm have returned a decade later with cardiomyopathy and heart failure (86). Echocardiography has been particularly helpful in monitoring for anthracycline cardiotoxicity (87). Sequential examination allows identification of subclinical cardiotoxicity, and it can guide modification of subsequent chemotherapy to minimize cumulative myocellular injury (88). A caution has been raised, however, to avoid premature dose reduction or discontinuation of lifesaving chemotherapy based on echocardiographic evidence of asymptomatic left ventricular dysfunction (89).

HYPERTROPHIC CARDIOMYOPATHY

Hypertrophic cardiomyopathy (HCM) is a primary disease of cardiac muscle characterized by left ventricular hypertrophy, principally involving the ventricular septum, without ventricular dilation. It is a leading cause of sudden death in children and young adults. In most patients, asymmetric septal hypertrophy is striking but hypertrophy can be diffuse and involve all segments of the left ventricular wall. Histologic appearance of the myocardium is characterized by cellular disarray and bizarrely shaped myocytes. In addition to the familial form of HCM, other conditions associated with it include Noonan's syndrome and infant of diabetic mother, the latter which regresses over the first few months of life.

Genetics

The estimated prevalence of HCM in the population is 1–10/10,000. The familial nature of HCM has been known for several decades (90, 91). Almost 60% of families will have at least one first degree relative with clinical or echocardiographic evidence of the disease. The pattern of inheritance is most often consistent with autosomal dominant transmission and the remaining 40% are believed to arise as the result of sporadic mutations.

Recent application of molecular genetic techniques has localized the gene for familial HCM to chromosome 14q1 (92, 93). Further studies showed that mutations in the β-myosin heavy chain (β-MHC) gene were responsible for HCM in approximately 50% of families, but at least several other gene defects (on chromosomes 1, 11, and 15) account for the disease in the remainder (94). Over 30 missence point mutations in the β-MHC gene have been described and undoubtedly account for much of the phenotypic heterogeneity of the disorder (95).

Pathophysiology

Pathophysiologic mechanisms underlying HCM probably involve three components: obstruction to left ventricular outflow (occurring in approximately one third of children), diastolic dysfunction, and myocardial ischemia.

Dynamic outflow obstruction is created by the hypertrophied septum and systolic anterior motion (SAM) of the anterior mitral valve leaflet. Degree and duration of the systolic apposition of the anterior mitral leaflet with the ventricular septum correlate with the severity of the hemodynamic obstruction (96).

Exertional dyspnea, fatigue, and chest pain can be present in patients. Infants less than 1 year of age with HCM have a higher incidence of left ventricular outflow obstruction and, unlike older patients, commonly have accompanying right ventricular outflow obstruction. Congestive heart failure is common in this age group, and it is a poor prognostic sign (97).

Diagnosis

Diagnosis of HCM can usually be established by noninvasive screening. The electrocardiogram, although variable, characteristically demonstrates left ventricular hypertrophy, often with ST segment depression and/or T wave inversion. Young infants may also show right ventricular hypertrophy. The chest roentgenogram can be normal or it can reveal cardiomegaly and evidence of pulmonary venous congestion.

The echocardiogram is the principal diagnostic modality, and it has the highest sensitivity and specificity for detecting the disease. The most characteristic finding is asymmetric septal hypertrophy with variable degrees of hypertrophy of other wall segments (Fig. 31.5). Systolic anterior motion of the mitral valve is present in patients with outflow obstruction. Doppler echocardiography is also helpful in quantitating any outflow gradient.

Treatment

Symptoms of pulmonary venous congestion can be treated by judicious use of diuretics. Additional medical therapy of patients with HCM generally includes β-adrenergic blockers and/or calcium channel antagonists. Both classes of drugs have been shown to reduce dynamic left ventricular outflow obstruction. Among β-blockers, propranolol has been the most commonly utilized but newer, long-acting, or cardioselective agents such as atenolol, nadolol, or metoprolol can also be employed. Verapamil is the principal calcium channel blocker used to treat HCM. Although there is paucity of data on intravenous use of calcium channel blocking agents in the pediatric population, chronic administration of verapamil improves exercise capacity as well as symptoms of dyspnea, angina, and syncope (98). The mechanism of action appears to be improve-

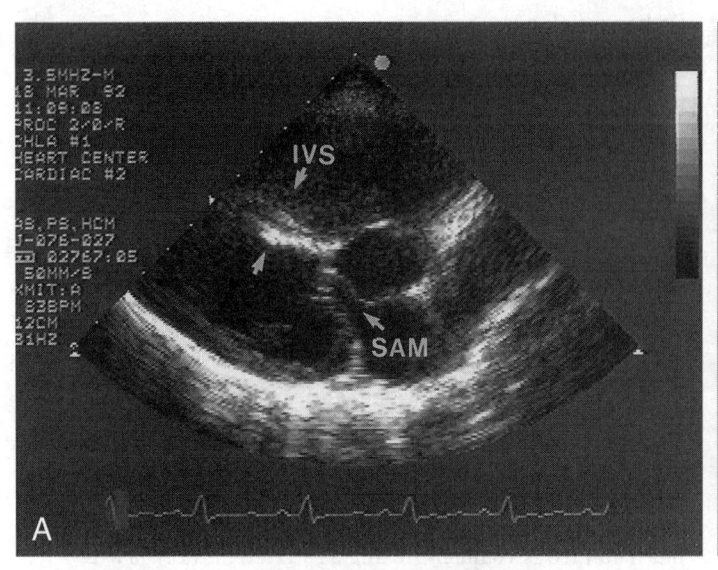

Figure 31.5. Echocardiogram in a child with hypertrophic cardiomyopathy. Asymmetric septal hypertrophy and systolic anterior motion (SAM) of the mitral valve are demonstrated on the two-dimensional (**A**) and m-mode tracings (**B**). IVS, interventricular septum.

ment of diastolic function along with reduction in outflow obstruction (99).

When patients fail to obtain symptomatic relief from either β-adrenergic or calcium channel blockers, then empiric trials of other agents (e.g., disopyramide or amiodarone can be initiated) (100).

Antidysrhythmic agents may be necessary because supraventricular and ventricular dysrhythmias occur in many patients, and they may be a cause of dizziness or syncope. Patients with documented sustained ventricular tachycardia on Holter monitoring or electrophysiologic study are at risk of sudden death (101). Amiodarone has proved to be effective in abolishing arrhythmias and reducing the risk of sudden death (102). Sotalol, a β-adrenergic blocker with class III antiarrhythmic properties, also appears to be effective in suppressing supraventricular and ventricular dysrhythmias and improving exercise capacity (103).

Dual chamber (DDD) pacing is effective in relieving left ventricular outflow tract obstruction and improving symptomatology (104). Pediatric patients treated with DDD pacing have demonstrated significant reduction in outflow gradient, ventricular septal thickness, and left ventricular mass (105).

Surgical septal myotomy-myectomy is generally reserved for patients with severe outflow tract obstruction and symptoms who remain refractory to medical management or DDD pacing. The surgical myotomy-myectomy series from the National Institutes of Health has documented significant reduction or abolition of outflow gradient, increase in exercise capacity, and improvement of symptoms (106). Mitral valve replacement has also been used in some patients as an alternative to myectomy.

Natural History and Outcome

The natural history of HCM is variable depending on the age at presentation, family history of sudden death, and documentation of ventricular arrhythmias. Cumulative mortality rate for infants has been reported to be 40% compared with 19% for older children (107), but may be as high as 82% in infants less than 1 year of age who present with congestive heart failure (103). A 2 to 4% incidence of sudden death is found in patients 10 to 35 years of age (108).

RESTRICTIVE CARDIOMYOPATHY

Restrictive cardiomyopathy (RCM) is the least common of the three primary cardiomyopathies. It is characterized by normal or nearly normal ventricular chamber size and systolic performance with reduced diastolic compliance. Several infiltrative diseases of the myocardium are associated with restrictive physiology, such as amyloidosis, sarcoidosis, hemochromatosis, glycogen storage disease, mucopolysaccharidosis, and endocardial fibrosis. Idiopathic RCM occurs in the absence of other systemic diseases.

Pathophysiology

Diastolic compliance curve is shifted upward (without systolic dysfunction) and thereby causes marked, but unequal, elevation in left and right ventricular end-diastolic pressures. Patients clinically present with dyspnea, decreased exercise tolerance, and signs of congestive heart failure, including pulmonary and systemic venous edema, hepatomegaly, and ascites (109).

Diagnosis

The most consistent electrocardiographic feature is the presence of tall, broad p waves indicating right and/or left atrial enlargement. Evidence of ventricular hypertrophy, ST and T wave abnormalities and conduction disturbances are variable. The chest roentgenogram demonstrates cardiomegaly and pulmonary venous congestion; pleural effusions may also be noted. Echocardiography reveals biatrial enlargement with normal ventricular cavity dimensions and wall thickness. Color Doppler echocardiography may demonstrate tricuspid and mitral regurgitation. Doppler assessment of mitral inflow velocities characteristically reveals increased peak early diastolic (E) velocity but lower velocity following atrial contraction (A), shortened mitral deceleration time (less than 100 milliseconds) and increased pulmonary vein flow reversal (110).

Cardiac catheterization demonstrates marked elevation in ventricular end-diastolic pressures. Left ventricular end-diastolic pressure is typically at least 5–10 torr higher than right ventricular end-diastolic pressure, and it is helpful in differentiating RCM from constrictive pericardial disease. A characteristic early diastolic pressure dip with a rapid rise to a late diastolic plateau ("square root" sign) may be obscured in younger patients with tachycardia. Pulmonary hypertension, occasionally severe, is often present. Endomyocardial biopsy frequently demonstrates interstitial fibrosis, but endocardial sclerosis and myofiber hypertrophy also may be present.

Treatment

Clinical management of RCM is limited because of the lack of specific therapy to improve ventricular compliance. Diuretics are helpful in relieving symptoms of pulmonary and systemic congestion but the effect may be transient. Administration of angiotensin converting enzyme inhibitors such as captopril has been reported to cause systemic hypotension with improving cardiac output (111). Calcium channel blocking agents can have a role in treating selective patients with restrictive cardiomyopathy, particularly if myocardial hypertrophy is present; calcium channel antagonists with significant vasodilating properties, however, should be avoided. Chronic therapy has not been systematically evaluated.

Atrial thrombi are found in a significant number of patients probably as a consequence of the marked atrial dilation; thromboembolism may occur. Anticoagulation with heparin or warfarin should be considered in all patients with RCM.

Natural History and Outcome

Unlike the natural history in adults, RCM in childhood appears to have a more malignant course. Median survival of eight children with RCM who presented with signs of congestive heart failure was only 1.4 years (109). Mortality was nearly 60% within 1.5 years of presentation. In view of the poor outcome, early cardiac transplantation should be considered in patients who remain symptomatic despite maximal medical therapy.

REFERENCES

1. Poole-Wilson PA. Relation of pathophysiologic mechanisms to outcome in heart failure. J Am Coll Cardiol 1992; 22(Suppl A):22A–29A.
2. Suga H, Sagawa K. Instantaneous pressure-volume relationships and their ratio in the excised, supported canine left ventricle. Circ Res 1974;35:117–126.
3. Grossman W, Braunwald E, Mann T, et al. Contractile state of the left ventricle in man as evaluated from the end-systolic pressure-volume relation. Circulation 1977;56:845–852.
4. Suga H, Kitabatake A, Sagawa K. End-systolic pressure determines stroke volume from fixed end-diastolic volume in the isolated left ventricle under a constant contractile state. Circ Res 1979;44:238–249.
5. Katz AM. Influence of altered inotropy and lusitropy on ventricular pressure-volume loops. J Am Coll Cardiol 1988;11: 438–445.
6. Garg R, Packer M, Pitt B, et al. Heart failure in the 1990s: evolution of a major public health problem in cardiovascular medicine. J Am Coll Cardiol 1993;22(Suppl A):3A–5A.
7. Gaffney TE, Braunwald E. Importance of adrenergic nervous system in support of circulatory function in patients with congestive heart failure. Am J Med 1963;34:320–324.
8. Swedberg K, Eneroth P, Kjekshus J, et al for the CONSENSUS Trial Study Group. Hormones regulating cardiovascular function in patients with severe congestive heart failure and their relation to mortality. Circulation 1990; 82:1730–1736.
9. Francis GS, Benedict C, Johnstone DE, et al for the SOLVD Investigators. Comparison of neuroendocrine activation in patients with left ventricular dysfunction with and without congestive heart failure. Circulation 1990;82:1724–1729.
10. Thomas JA, Marks BH. Plasma norepinephrine in congestive heart failure. Am J Cardiol 1987;41:233–243.
11. Bristow MR, Ginsburg R, Fowler M, et al. β_1 and β_2 adrenergic receptor subpopulations in normal and failing human ventricular myocardium. Coupling of both receptor subtypes to muscle contraction and selective β_1 receptor down-regulation in heart failure. Circ Res 1986;59:297–309.
12. Bristow MR. Pathophysiologic and pharmacologic rationales for clinical management of chronic heart failure with beta-blocking agents. Am J Cardiol 1993;71:12C–20C.
13. Curtiss C, Cohn NJ, Vrobel T. Role of the renin-angiotensin system in the systemic vasoconstriction of chronic congestive heart failure. Circulation 1978;58:763–770.
14. Parmley WW. Pathophysiology and current therapy of congestive heart failure. J Am Coll Cardiol 1989;13:771–785.
15. Dzau VJ. Implications of local angiotensin production in cardiovascular physiology and pharmacology. Am J Cardiol 1987;59:59A–65A.

16. Lindpainter K, Ganten D. The cardiac renin-angiotensin system: an appraisal of present experimental and clinical evidence. Circ Res 1991;68:905–921.
17. Lee MA, Bohm M, Paul M, et al. Tissue renin-angiotensin systems. Their role in cardiovascular disease. Circulation 1993;87(Suppl IV):IV-7–IV-13.
18. Dzau VJ. Local contractile and growth modulators in the myocardium. Clin Cardiol 1993;16(Suppl II):II-5–II-9.
19. The CONSENSUS Trial Study Group. Effects of enalapril on mortality in severe congestive heart failure. N Engl J Med 1987;316:1429–1435.
20. The SOLVD Investigators. Effect of enalapril on mortality and the development of heart failure in asymptomatic patients with reduced left ventricular ejection fraction. N Engl J Med 1992;327:685–691.
21. Cody RJ. Atrial natriuretic peptide and the endocrine function of the heart. Primary Cardiology 1991;17:14–24.
22. Steward DJ, Cernacek P, Costello KB, et al. Elevated endothelin-1 in heart failure and loss of normal response to postural change. Circulation 1992;85:510–517.
23. Tsutamoto T, Wada A, Maeda Y, et al. Relation between endothelin-1 spillover in the lungs and pulmonary vascular resistance in patients with chronic heart failure. J Am Coll Cardiol 1994;23:1427–1433.
24. Katz SD, Biasucci L, Sabba C, et al. Impaired endothelium-mediated vasodilation in the peripheral vasculature of patients with congestive heart failure. J Am Coll Cardiol 1992;19:918–925.
25. Treasure CB, Alexander W. The dysfunctional endothelium in heart failure. J Am Coll Cardiol 1993;22(Suppl A):129A–134A.
26. Rubanyi GM, Vanhoutte PM. Superoxide anions and hyperoxia inactivate endothelium-derived relaxing factor. Am J Physiol 1986;250:H822–H827.
27. Stevens PJ, Underwood, Ground KE. Occurrence and significance of myocarditis in trauma. Aerospace Medicine 1970;41:770–780.
28. Woodruff JF. Viral myocarditis—a review. Am J Pathol 1980;101:425–478.
29. Noren GR, Staley NA, Bandt CM, et al. Occurrence of myocarditis in sudden death in children. J Forensic Sci 1977;22:118–196.
30. Molander N. Sudden natural death in later childhood and adolescence. Arch Dis Child 1982;57:572–576.
31. Neuspiel DR, Kuller LH. Sudden and unexpected natural death in childhood and adolescence. JAMA 1985;254:1321–1325.
32. Abelmann WH. Myocarditis. N Engl J Med 1966;275:832–333;944–945.
33. Lerner AM, Wilson FM. Virus myocardiopathy. Prog Med Virol 1973;15:63–91.
34. Herskowitz A, Wolfgram LJ, Rose NR, et al. Coxsackievirus B3 murine myocarditis. A pathologic spectrum of myocarditis in genetically defined inbred strains. J Am Coll Cardiol 1987;9:1311–1319.
35. Dec GW, Palacios IF, Fallon JT, et al. Active myocarditis in the spectrum of acute dilated cardiomyopathies: clinical features, histologic correlates and clinical outcome. N Engl J Med 1985;312:885–890.
36. Ino T, Sherwood G, Benson LN, et al. Cardiac manifestations in disorders of fat and carnitine metabolism in infancy. J Am Coll Cardiol 1988;11:1301–1308.
37. Aretz HT, Billingham ME, Edwards WD, et al. Myocarditis, a histopathologic definition and classification. Am J Cardiovasc Pathol 1986;1:3–14.
38. Billingham ME. Diagnostic criteria of myocarditis by endomyocardial biopsy. Heart Vessels 1985;1(Suppl):133–137.
39. Martin AB, Webber S, Fricker FJ, et al. Acute myocarditis. Rapid diagnosis by PCR in children. Circulation 1994;90:330–339.
40. Jin O, Sole MJ, Butany JW, et al. Detection of enterovirus RNA in myocardial biopsies from patients with myocarditis and cardiomyopathy using gene amplification by polymerase chain reaction. Circulation 1990;82:8–16.
41. Friedman RA, Kearney DL, Moak JP, et al. Persistence of ventricular arrhythmia after resolution of occult myocarditis in children and young adults. J Am Coll Cardiol 1994;24:780–783.
42. Lee DC-S, Johnson RA, Bingham JB, et al. Heart failure in outpatients: a randomized trial of digoxin versus placebo. N Engl J Med 1982;306:699–705.
43. Guyatt GH, Sullivan MJJ, Fallen EL, et al. A controlled trial of digoxin in congestive heart failure. Am J Cardiol 1988;61:371–375.
44. Packer M, Gheorghiade M, Young JB, et al. Withdrawal of digoxin from patients with chronic heart failure treated with angiotensin-converting enzyme inhibitors. N Engl J Med 1993;329:1–7.
45. Sabbah HN, Shimoyama H, Kono T, et al. Effects of long-term monotherapy with enalapril, metoprolol, and digoxin on the progression of left ventricular dysfunction and dilatation in dogs with reduced ejection fraction. Circulation 1994;89:2852–2859.
46. Cody RJ. Clinical and hemodynamic experience with enalapril in congestive heart failure. Am J Cardiol 1985;55:36A–40A.
47. The CONSENSUS Trial Study Group. Effects of enalapril on mortality in severe congestive heart failure: result of the Cooperative North Scandinavian Enalapril Survival Study (CONSENSUS). N Engl J Med 1987;316:1429–1435.
48. Lewis AB, Chabot M. The effect of treatment with angiotensin-converting enzyme inhibitors on survival of pediatric patients with dilated cardiomyopathy. Pediatr Cardiol 1993;14:9–12.
49. Singh NC, Kissoon N, al Mofada S, et al. Comparison of continuous versus intermittent furosemide administration in postoperative pediatric cardiac patients. Crit Care Med 1992;20:17–21.
50. Mason JW, Billingham ME, Ricci DR. Treatment of acute inflammatory myocarditis assisted by endomyocardial biopsy. Am J Cardiol 1980;45:1037–1044.
51. Jones SR, Herskowitz A, Hutchins GM, et al. Effects of immunosuppressive therapy in biopsy-proven myocarditis and borderline myocarditis on left ventricular function. Am J Cardiol 1991;68:370–376.
52. Chan KY, Iwahara M, Benson LN, et al. Immunosuppressive therapy in the management of acute myocarditis in children: a clinical trial. J Am Coll Cardiol 1991;17:458–460.
53. Zales VR, Deal BJ, Pahl E, et al. High-dose steroid therapy for acute myocarditis in pediatric patients. Circulation 1994;90:I-50.
54. Hosenpud JD, McAnulty JH, Niles NR. Lack of objective improvement in ventricular systolic function in patients with myocarditis treatment with azathioprine and prednisone. J Am Coll Cardiol 1985;6:797–801.
55. Fenoglio JJ, Ursell PC, Kellogg CG, et al. Diagnosis and clas-

56. Kilbourne ED, Wilson CB, Perrier D. The induction of gross myocardial lesions by a coxsackie (pleurodynia) virus and cortisone. J Clin Invest 1956;35:362–370.
57. Tomioka N, Kishimoto C, Matsumori A, et al. Effects of prednisolone on acute viral myocarditis in mice. J Am Coll Cardiol 1986;7:868–872.
58. Kishimoto C, Thorp KA, Abelmann WH. Immunosuppression with high doses of cyclophosphamide reduces the severity of myocarditis but increases the mortality in murine coxsackievirus B3 myocarditis. Circulation 1990;82:982–989.
59. O'Connell JB, Reap EA, Robinson JA. The effects of cyclosporine on acute murine coxsackie B3 myocarditis. Circulation 1986;73:353–359.
60. Monrad ES, Matsumori AK, Murphy JC, et al. Therapy with cyclosporine in experimental murine myocarditis with encephalomyocarditis virus. Circulation 1986;73:1058–1064.
61. Drucker NA, Colan SD, Lewis AB, et al. γ-globulin treatment of acute myocarditis in pediatric population. Circulation 1994;89:252–257.
62. Weller AH, Hall M, Huber SA. Polyclonal immunoglobulin therapy protects against cardiac damage in experimental coxsackievirus-induced myocarditis. Eur Heart J 1992;13:115–119.
63. Rezkalla S, Kloner RA, Khatib G, et al. Beneficial effects of captopril in acute coxsackievirus B3 murine myocarditis. Circulation 1990;81:1039–1046.
64. Keren A, Popp RL. Assignment of patients into the classification of cardiomyopathies. Circulation 1992;86:1622–1633.
65. Parmley WW. Pathophysiology and current therapy of congestive heart failure. J Am Coll Cardiol 1989;13:771–785.
66. Manolio TA, Baughman KL, Rodeheffer R, et al. Prevalence and etiology of idiopathic dilated cardiomyopathy (summary of a National Heart, Lung and Blood Institute workshop). Am J Cardiol 1992;69:1458–1566.
67. Zee-Cheng CS, Tsai CC, Palmer DC, et al. High incidence of myocarditis by endomyocardial biopsy in patients with idiopathic congestive cardiomyopathy. J Am Coll Cardiol 1984;3:63–70.
68. Myocarditis Treatment Trial Investigators. Incidence and clinical characteristics of myocarditis [Abstract]. Circulation 1991;84(Suppl II):2.
69. Giacca M, Severini GM, Mestroni L, et al. Low frequency of detection by nested polymerase chain reaction of enterovirus ribonucleic acid in endomyocardial tissue of patients with idiopathic dilated cardiomyopathy. J Am Coll Cardiol 1994;24:1033–1040.
70. Chin TK, Perloff JK, Williams RG, et al. Isolated noncompaction of left ventricular myocardium. A study of eight cases. Circulation 1990;82:507–513.
71. Gottdiener JS, Gay JA, VanVoorhees L, et al. Am J Cardiol 1983;52:1281–1285.
72. Lewis AB, Neustein HB, Takahashi M, et al. Findings on endomyocardial biopsy in infants and children with dilated cardiomyopathy. Am J Cardiol 1985;55:143–145.
73. Yoshizato T, Edwards WD, Alboliras ET, et al. Safety and utility of endomyocardial biopsy in infants, children and adolescents: a review of 66 procedures in 53 patients. J Am Coll Cardiol 1990;15:436–442.
74. Griffin ML, Hernandez A, Martin TC, et al. Dilated cardiomyopathy in infants and children. J Am Coll Cardiol 1988;11:139–144.
75. Lewis AB, Chabot M. Outcome of infants and children with dilated cardiomyopathy. Am J Cardiol 1991;68:365–369.
76. Lewis AB. Prognostic value of echocardiography in children with idiopathic dilated cardiomyopathy. Am Heart J 1994;128:133–136.
77. DeCastro S, D'Amati G, Gallo P, et al. Frequency of development of acute global left ventricular dysfunction in human immunodeficiency virus infection. J Am Coll Cardiol 1994;24:1018–1024.
78. Cohen IS, Anderson DW, Virmani R, et al. Congestive cardiomyopathy in association with the acquired immunodeficiency syndrome. N Engl J Med 1986;315:628–630.
79. Herskowitz A, Vlahov D, Willoughby S, et al. Prevalence and incidence of left ventricular dysfunction in patients with human immunodeficiency virus infection. Am J Cardiol 1993;71:955–958.
80. Lipshultz SE, Chanock S, Sanders SP, et al. Cardiovascular manifestations of human immunodeficiency virus infection in infants and children. Am J Cardiol 1989;63:1489–1497.
81. Herskowitz A, Wu T-C, Willoughby SB, et al. Myocarditis and cardiotropic viral infection associated with severe left ventricular dysfunction in late-stage infection with human immunodeficiency virus. J Am Coll Cardiol 1994;24:1025–1032.
82. Billingham ME, Mason JW, Bristow MR, et al. Anthracycline cardiomyopathy monitored by morphologic changes. Cancer Treatment Reports 1978;62:865.
83. Bristow MR, Billingham ME, Mason JW, et al. Clinical spectrum of anthracycline antibiotic cardiotoxicity. Cancer Treat Rep 1978;62:873–879.
84. Lefrak EA, Pitha J, Rosenheim S, et al. A clinicopathologic analysis of adriamycin cardiotoxicity. Cancer 1973;32:302–314.
85. Gilladoga AC, Manuel C, Tan CTC, et al. The cardiotoxicity of adriamycin and daunomycin in children. Cancer 1976;37:1070–1078.
86. Goorin AM, Chauvenet AR, Perez-Atayde AR, et al. Initial congestive heart failure, six to ten years after doxorubicin chemotherapy for childhood cancer. J Pediatr 1990;116:144–147.
87. Lewis AB, Pilkington R, Takahashi M, et al. Echocardiographic assessment of anthracycline cardiotoxicity in children. Med Pediatr Oncol 1978;5:167–175.
88. Steinherz LJ, Graham T, Hurwitz R, et al. Guidelines for cardiac monitoring of children during and after anthracycline therapy: report of the Cardiology Committee of the Childrens Cancer Study Group. Pediatrics 1992;89:942–949.
89. Lipshultz SE, Sanders SP, Goorin AM, et al. Monitoring for anthracycline cardiotoxicity. Pediatrics 1994;93:433–437.
90. Teare D. Asymmetrical hypertrophy of the heart in young adults. Br Heart J 1958;20:1–8.
91. Frank S, Braunwald E. Idiopathic hypertrophic subaortic stenosis: clinical analysis of 126 patients with emphasis on the natural history. Circulation 1968;37:759–788.
92. Jarcho JA, McKenna W, Pare JAP, et al. Mapping a gene for familial hypertrophic cardiomyopathy to chromosome 14q1. N Engl J Med 1989;321:1372–1378.
93. Hejtmancik JF, Brink PA, Towbin J, et al. Localization of gene for familial hypertrophic cardiomyopathy to chromosome 14q1 in a diverse US population. Circulation 1991;83:1592–1597.
94. Marian AJ, Roberts R. Molecular basis of hypertrophic and dilated cardiomyopathy. Tex Heart Inst J 1994;21:6–15.

95. Watkins H, Rosenzweig A, Hwang D-S, et al. Characteristics and prognostic implications of myosin missense mutations in familial hypertrophic cardiomyopathy. N Engl J Med 1992; 326:1108–1114.
96. Maron BJ, Gottdiener JS, Arce J, et al. Dynamic subaortic obstruction in hypertrophic cardiomyopathy: analysis by pulsed Doppler echocardiography. J Am Coll Cardiol 1985;6: 1–15.
97. Maron BJ, Tajik AJ, Ruttenberg HD, et al. Hypertrophic cardiomyopathy in infants: clinical features and natural history. Circulation 1982;65:7–17.
98. Spicer RL, Rocchini AP, Crowley DC, et al. Chronic verapamil therapy in pediatric and young adult patients with hypertrophic cardiomyopathy. Am J Cardiol 1984;53:1614–1619.
99. Shaffer EM, Rocchini AP, Spicer RL, et al. Effects of verapamil on left ventricular diastolic filling in children with hypertrophic cardiomyopathy. Am J Cardiol 1988;61:413–417.
100. Sherrid M, Delia E, Dwyer E. Oral disopyramide therapy for obstructive hypertrophic cardiomyopathy. Am J Cardiol 1988;62:1085–1088.
101. Fananapazir L, Chang AC, Epstein SE, et al. Prognostic determinants in hypertrophic cardiomyopathy. Prospective evaluation of a therapeutic strategy based on clinical, Holter, hemodynamic and electrophysiological findings. Circulation 1992;86:730–740.
102. McKenna WJ, Harris L, Oakley C, et al. Amiodarone for long-term management of patients with hypertrophic cardiomyopathy. Am J Cardiol 1984;54:802–810.
103. Tendera M, Wycisk A, Schneeweiss A, et al. Effect of sotalol on arrhythmias and exercise tolerance in patients with hypertrophic cardiomyopathy. Cardiology 1993;82:335–341.
104. McAreavey D, Fananapazir L. Altered cardiac hemodynamic and electrical state in normal sinus rhythm after chronic dual-chamber pacing for relief of left ventricular outflow obstruction in hypertrophic cardiomyopathy. Am J Cardiol 1992;70:651–656.
105. Rishi F, Hulse JE, Sharma S, et al. Permanent dual chamber pacing in pediatric patients with hypertrophic obstructive cardiomyopathy. Circulation 1994;90(Part 2):I–98.
106. McIntosh CL, Maron BJ. Current operative treatment of obstructive hypertrophic cardiomyopathy. Circulation 1988;78: 487–495.
107. Romeo F, Cianfrocca C, Pelliccia F, et al. Long-term prognosis in children with hypertrophic cardiomyopathy: an analysis of 37 patients aged ≤14 years at diagnosis. Clin Cardiol 1990;13:101–107.
108. Maron BJ, Roberts WC, Epstein SE. Sudden death in hypertrophic cardiomyopathy: profile of 78 patients. Circulation 1982;65:1388–1394.
109. Lewis AB. Clinical profile and outcome of restrictive cardiomyopathy in children. Am Heart J 1992;123:1589–1593.
110. Appleton CP, Hatle LK, Popp RL. Demonstration of restrictive ventricular physiology by Doppler echocardiography. J Am Coll Cardiol 1988;11:757–768.
111. Bengur AR, Beekman RH, Rocchini AP, et al. Acute hemodynamic effects of captopril in children with a congestive or restrictive cardiomyopathy. Circulation 1991;83:523–527.

Pulmonary Hypertension

Thomas J. Kulik, MD

A variety of reasons are found why the resistance to blood flow through the lungs is of considerable importance: (a) Elevated pulmonary vascular resistance (PVR) increases right ventricular afterload, and hence work, and it may lead to a reduction in cardiac output and heart "failure." (b) In patients with an anatomic connection between the pulmonary and systemic circulations, pulmonary blood flow falls as the ratio of PVR to systemic vascular resistance (SVR) increases, which can cause severe hypoxemia. (c) Conversely, it is possible for PVR to be too low, a situation commonly encountered in neonates with "duct-dependent" circulation (e.g., interruption of the aortic arch) treated with prostaglandin E_1, where such a large fraction of the cardiac output goes to the lungs that the rest of the body suffers from inadequate perfusion. (d) In some patients with lung disease, if only local perfusion of the lung could be better adjusted to local ventilation (via local vasoconstriction), intrapulmonary shunting would be reduced and arterial Po_2 increased. Although our understanding of what regulates PVR and how it does so is rudimentary, more than enough has been learned to help rationalize care for cardiac patients. This chapter is intended to distill this knowledge (and a few of the author's biases) into clinically useful information. Space permits only the most limited excursion into the basic biology, physiology, and pharmacology of the "lesser" circulation; the reader is therefore encouraged to read the classic reviews of Fishman (1–4) to develop a deeper appreciation of this fascinating and important subject.

HOW PVR IS MEASURED OR ESTIMATED

Resistance to blood flow within the lungs is generally calculated as follows: PVR (mm Hg/L/min/m^2) = PAP (mm Hg) − LAP (mm Hg)/Q_P (L/min/m^2), where PAP = mean pulmonary arterial pressure, LAP = mean left atrial pressure, and Q_P = pulmonary blood flow. If resistance in mmHg/L/min (Wood units, U) is multiplied by 80, it is converted to dynes-sec-cm^{-5}. In pediatrics, resistance is usually corrected for body surface area, mmHg/L/min/m^2 (U·m^2). Because calculated PVR is influenced not only by the anatomy of the vascular bed and magnitude of vascular tone but also by Q_P and LAP per se (5), it is an imperfect reflection of pulmonary vascular anatomy and tone, but it is nevertheless the best measure available to the clinician.

In patients in whom Q_P is supplied by restrictive aortopulmonary communication, it is often difficult to measure PAP and Q_P. In these patients a rough estimate of PVR is provided by the arterial oxygen saturation, because this value is partly a function of the ratio of $Q_P:Q_S$ (systemic blood flow) which, in turn, is related to the ratio of PVR:SVR. However, because mixed venous oxygen saturation, pulmonary venous saturation, and hematocrit (as well as SVR) also affect the arterial oxygen saturation in these circumstances, this figure is only tenuously linked to the PVR.

HOW PULMONARY HYPERTENSION IS RELATED TO INCREASED PVR

As is implied by the equation above, *pulmonary hypertension* (mean pulmonary arterial pressure greater than 20 mm Hg after the first few weeks of life) can occur in the setting of increased resistance to blood flow through the lungs, normal resistance with increased pulmonary flow, or a combination of the two. (In addition, increased pulmonary venous pressure can cause pulmonary hypertension without altering PVR.) The distinction between pulmonary hypertension and increased PVR is important, as many patients with congenital heart disease have a large communication between the pulmonary and systemic circulations— and therefore increased pulmonary arterial pressure and flow—but normal calculated PVR, and a functionally nearly normal vascular bed. Increased PVR generally implies a reduction in the number or diameter of pulmonary vessels (see below). Patients with increased PVR are therefore more likely to suffer from pulmonary hypertension immediately following a cardiac operation, and a progressive increase in PVR even after correction of the cardiac lesion, than those with pulmonary hypertension associated with a large left-to-right shunt.

WHAT DETERMINES PVR

Role of Pulmonary Vascular Structure

Pulmonary vascular resistance is primarily a function of the number, length, and diameter of pulmonary blood vessels (discounting the issue of blood viscosity). Whether pathologic changes occur in vessel *length* is unknown, but a reduction in the total *number* of pulmonary arteries can occur as a consequence of congenital heart lesions, and in other circumstances (e.g., congenital diaphragmatic hernia) (6). The *diameter* of small pulmonary blood vessels is determined by the tone of the smooth muscle in their walls (see below) and any narrowing caused by *anatomic pathologic changes* (4). Patients with cardiac defects that increase pulmonary artery pressure (especially) and flow are susceptible to developing these changes, which are also seen in patients with unexplained ("primary") pulmonary hypertension (7). Heath and Edwards detailed and graded these progressive pathologic changes (8). Grade 1 changes consist of medial hypertrophy and extension of smooth muscle into normally nonmuscular arteries. Medial hypertrophy is commonly found even in the first few weeks of life in patients with cardiac lesions associated with increased pulmonary arterial pressure, and it presumably accounts for the increased capacity for pulmonary vasoconstriction in such patients. Medial hypertrophy generally regresses if pulmonary arterial pressure can be reduced to normal. With grade 2 changes there is cellular intimal proliferation. Grade 3 changes include intimal fibrosis, sometimes with early generalized vascular dilation. In grade 4 lesions are found thinning of the media and generalized dilation, and local areas of dilation ("plexiform" lesions). With grade 5, advanced dilation lesions (angiomatoid lesions, and "veinlike" branches of hypertrophied muscular pulmonary arteries), and medial fibrosis are found. Grade 6 indicates the presence of necrotizing arteritis. The term "pulmonary vascular obstructive disease" refers to these pathologic changes, especially those thought to be irreversible (grades 3–6).

Morphometric studies of the lung have better quantified pathologic changes in the muscularization and number of small arteries that occur with congenital heart defects (4): Grade A indicates the appearance of smooth muscle more peripherally than normal, with or without medial hypertrophy in normally muscular vessels. Grade B signifies distal extension of muscle plus medial wall thickness one and a half to two times normal (B mild), or more than two times normal (B severe). Grade C "mild" indicates less than 50% decrease in density of peripheral arteries relative to alveoli, with grade C "severe" being a reduction of more than 50%.

The issue of anatomic pathologic changes is mostly one of prevention (usually through early palliation or correction of the heart lesions that cause these pathologic changes), as at present no means exists of reversing them (save for medial hypertrophy, and perhaps intimal proliferation). Prognostication, too, is an issue vis-à-vis such vascular lesions because a tendency is seen for them to progress, despite correction of the cardiac lesion that initially caused them (9).

ROLE OF PULMONARY VASCULAR SMOOTH MUSCLE TONE

The magnitude of smooth muscle tone in small pulmonary vessels plays the predominant role in determining PVR in patients without anatomic lesions, and it can affect PVR in those with pulmonary vascular obstructive disease as well. Ordinarily *very little tone is found in the normal pulmonary circulation*, but multiple factors are capable of causing constriction in normal and pathologically remodeled vessels. In addition, the lack of endogenously produced vasodilators (e.g., endothelium-derived relaxing factor [EDRF]) can also result in increased tone.

Alveolar Hypoxia

Unlike systemic blood vessels, which dilate with hypoxia, *pulmonary arteries vasoconstrict with alveolar hypoxia*. Why this is so is unclear—especially considering how poorly the normal right ventricle tolerates increased afterload—although it may relate to the fact that hypoxic pulmonary vasoconstriction in utero is a highly adaptive response. Vasoconstriction in hypoxic regions of the lung—thus diverting blood away from regions of reduced alveolar oxygen—improves ventilation-perfusion matching and may therefore also explain this capacity for vasoconstriction with hypoxia. Whereas the Po_2 of pulmonary arterial *blood* can also influence PVR, *alveolar* hypoxia is far more important (10). The mechanism of hypoxic vasoconstriction has yet to be fully elucidated, but it appears to involve inhibition of K^+ channels in pulmonary vascular smooth muscle (11).

Whether alveolar *hyperoxia* (FIO_2 greater than 0.21) causes a reduction in PVR is less clear, as multiple studies in mature humans suggest that it does not (1). Experimental data from lamb studies, however, suggest that hyperoxia decreases PVR (12). Furthermore, in patients with lung disease, enriched inspired O_2 may be necessary to abolish alveolar hypoxia in underventilated regions of the lung.

pH

As is the case with alveolar hypoxia, pH affects the pulmonary circulation in a way opposite to that of the systemic vasculature. Acidosis is a pulmonary vasoconstrictor, and it acts synergistically with alveolar hypoxia to increase PVR (13). Conversely, alkalosis is a pulmonary vasodilator. Many (although not all) experimental studies have shown that *blood pH per se—not* Pco_2—is the operative factor, because alkalosis produced by infusion of base is as effective in decreasing PVR as is respiratory alkalosis. Indeed, some studies suggest that the CO_2 molecule, independent of its effect on pH, is a pulmonary vasodilator (14–17). The mechanism of the effect of pH on pulmonary vascular smooth muscle tone is unclear (18).

Vasoactive Substances

Many substances normally produced in the lungs or circulating in the blood can affect pulmonary vascular tone (Table 32.1). Drugs commonly used to support cardiac patients can also affect PVR (Table 32.2). Merely knowing a compound is generally a "vasodilator" or "vasoconstrictor" is of somewhat limited utility, however, in understanding how these agents actually influence PVR:

1. The action of a substance on the pulmonary circulation is to some extent dependent on the resting tone of the vessels (19) and other factors, making it difficult to generalize about its vasoactive properties. For example, norepinephrine usually acts as a vasoconstrictor, but with elevated PVR it can relax pulmonary arteries (20). Somewhat analogously, vasodilators will have little effect on the maximally vasodilated circulation, and constrictors may not increase PVR in the maximally constricted lung. Endothelial function is also often important in determining the net effect of an agent (v.i.).

2. By and large, it has been difficult to show a cause and effect relationship between production of endogenous vasoactive compounds and a corresponding effect on PVR in vivo. Thus, the precise role of endogenous vasoactive substances in regulating PVR in normal and pathologic states is poorly defined.

3. Aside from the issue of PVR per se, pharmacologic agents are often used in situations where pulmonary blood flow is a function not only of PVR but also of SVR and resistance to flow into the large pulmonary arteries (e.g., a patient with tetralogy of Fallot). In these situations, it is important to consider that the effect of a given agent may depend on its effect on both SVR and PVR, and it may be further constrained by anatomic factors.

Another important generalization that lies at the root of the problem of treating pulmonary hypertension is that excepting the response to hypoxia and pH, pulmonary vascular smooth muscle responds qualitatively to vasoactive agents in the same way as does systemic vascular smooth muscle (i.e., no selective pulmonary vasodilators exist). It is true that in a given patient a given agent can have a greater impact on PVR than SVR, but no pharmacologic agent consistently reduces PVR in excess of SVR. An exception to this generalization—owing to its route of administration and time constant of inactivation—is inhaled nitric oxide (NO) (v.i.).

ROLE OF THE ENDOTHELIUM

For the last 15 years, tremendous attention has been focused on the role of endothelial cells in influencing PVR and SVR. These cells produce a variety of powerful vasoactive substances, a partial list of which includes prostacyclin (prostaglandin I_2), endothelins, and endothelium-

Table 32.1. Partial List of Endogenous Compounds with Pulmonary Vasoactivity

Pulmonary Vasoconstrictors	Pulmonary Vasodilators	Variable Effect on the Pulmonary Circulation
Angiotensin II	Acetylcholine	Epinephrine, norepinephrine
Leukotrienes C_4, D_4, E_4		
	Bradykinin	Endothelins
		Histamine
Prostaglandin $F_2\alpha$		
Thromboxane A_2	Prostaglandin E_1, E_2	Prostaglandin D_2
	Prostaglandin I_2	
Serotonin		
	Nitric oxide	

Table 32.2. Commonly Used Inotropic Drugs for Cardiac Patients

Drug	Effect	Comments
Dopamine	α, β, δ agonist	Data are inconsistent regarding its pulmonary vascular effects. At the usual therapeutic doses it appears to have little effect on PVR or to be a weak vasoconstrictor.
Dobutamine	α, β agonist	Has little effect on PVR.
Isoproterenol	β agonist	A pulmonary vasodilator.
Amrinone	Phosphodiesterase inhibitor	A pulmonary vasodilator, with some data suggesting it may sometimes decrease PVR > SVR.
Epinephrine	α, β agonist	Causes systemic vasoconstriction, but few data exist regarding its effect in the lung, especially in the immature organism. If may be a weak vasoconstrictor, or even a pulmonary vasodilator in the preconstricted circulation.
Norepinephrine	α, β agonist	As for epinephrine, above.

α, β, and δ refer to α and β adrenergic, and dopaminergic receptors, respectively. PVR, pulmonary vascular resistance; SVR, systemic vascular resistance.

derived relaxing factor (EDRF). The latter, which appears at least in part to be accounted for by endothelial production of nitric oxide (NO), is currently under the most intense investigation, both because of the role it may play in normal homeostasis and in the hypertensive lung, and because of its possible therapeutic potential. Current understanding of the physiology and biology of NO in the pulmonary circulation might be summarized:

1. NO is a powerful pulmonary vasodilator (21). It probably relaxes vascular smooth muscle through activation of guanylate cyclase, although alternate mechanisms may be important (22, 23).
2. Some data suggest that NO may partially account for the pulmonary vasodilation that occurs at birth (24), and it modulates the pulmonary vasoconstrictor response to hypoxia and other vasoconstrictors (25).
3. Children with left-to-right shunt lesions (26), and those in the first 24 hours after cardiopulmonary bypass (27), appear to have a reduced capacity for endothelium-dependent pulmonary vasodilation, suggesting that abnormal endothelial function might underlie one or more types of pulmonary vascular pathology.
4. Because NO can reduce vascular smooth muscle proliferation (28) and total protein and connective tissue synthesis (29), it is possible that it can influence normal growth or pathologic vascular remodeling in the lung (30).

ROLE OF THE NERVOUS SYSTEM

Pulmonary blood vessels are innervated by sympathetic and parasympathetic neurons, and they contain both adrenergic and muscarinic receptors, but the role of the autonomic nervous system in influencing PVR is unclear. The autonomic nervous system appears to have little effect on resting PVR, but it is possible that it plays a role in mediating pulmonary vasoconstriction related to endotracheal suctioning and other stimuli.

Pulmonary Venous Hypertension

Vasodilators cause pulmonary arterial pressure to decrease in many patients with left atrial hypertension, indicating that pulmonary venous hypertension can cause active ("reflex") vasoconstriction (31). In addition to vasoconstriction, pulmonary venous hypertension also elicits medial hypertrophy in pulmonary veins and arteries, findings noted even in newborns with obstructed total anomalous pulmonary venous connection. Although increased PVR caused by pulmonary venous hypertension tends to abate following relief of the hypertension, it is sometimes sufficiently persistent to complicate the postoperative course of patients following repair of lesions with increased pulmonary venous pressure (e.g., total anomalous pulmonary venous connection with obstruction).

Effect of Parenchymal Lung Disease

Pneumonia, respiratory distress syndrome, and other acute and chronic pulmonary parenchymal diseases can cause significant elevation in PVR. This increase is likely caused by multiple factors (alveolar hypoxia, locally produced vasoconstrictors, reduced functional residual capacity, and probably others).

Effect of Cardiopulmonary Bypass

It has long been known that cardiopulmonary bypass is sometimes associated with increased PVR. The precise causes for this are unclear. It is possible that increased PVR is somehow related to the generalized inflammatory response caused by cardiopulmonary bypass, and impaired endothelial function might play a role (27).

How Mechanical Ventilation Can Affect PVR

Pulmonary vascular resistance is at a minimum when the lung is inflated to its normal functional residual capacity (FRC), and resistance to flow increases both above and below this value (32). Hence, over or underinflation tends to increase PVR. High levels of positive end-expiratory pressure (PEEP) can also increase PVR, in part by compressing "alveolar" resistance vessels, and perhaps through stimulating vasoconstriction (33). On the other hand, PEEP can be effective in maintaining FRC and alleviating alveolar hypoxia in patients with parenchymal lung disease, and thus even high levels of PEEP in this setting may have little effect on, or even decrease, PVR (34).

PATIENTS AT INCREASED RISK FOR ELEVATED PVR AFTER CARDIAC SURGERY

Anticipating which patient's postoperative course will be complicated by increased PVR is important, as appropriate monitoring and therapy can be instituted early on. The most malignant manifestation of such increased pulmonary vasoactivity is the *pulmonary hypertensive "crises,"* episodic elevations of PVR to the systemic or suprasystemic level (35). Such episodes can cause decreased cardiac output in the patient with two ventricles (or extreme hypoxemia in patients with single ventricle physiology), and they can be fatal. These elevations in PVR usually cannot be linked to any specific perturbation, although they may be caused by endotracheal suctioning. Their cause is unknown. It has often been stated that any patient with increased pulmonary arterial pressure and flow is at increased risk for postoperative pulmonary hypertensive "crises." However, in my experience, patients with ventricular septal defect (VSD) or endocardial cushion defect with a large left-to-right shunt operated in the first months of life are *unlikely* to develop significant pulmonary hypertension in the postoperative period. Patients with tetralogy of Fallot or those with pulmonary atresia previously palliated with an appropriately sized aortopulmonary shunt also appear to be at low risk. Other types of patients are more likely to suffer from postoperative pulmonary hypertension:

1. Babies in the first 1 to 2 days of life. PVR normally falls rapidly in the early neonatal period (to 0.5 or less of systemic pressure within about the first 24 hours), but it continues to decline over the first 2 to 6 weeks in the normal infant (36). PVR is thus somewhat elevated for the first few days, and perhaps what is more important, the PVR seems to be more labile in this early time period. Hence, surgery for correction or palliation of heart lesions (e.g., transposition of the great arteries [TGA] or pulmonary atresia with intact ventricular septum) might be best avoided—stipulating that the patient is medically well-palliated—in approximately the first 24 hours of life.
2. Infants and older children with pulmonary venous hypertension. Excepting the very early neonatal period, most infants in the first few weeks of life are not particularly susceptible to having or developing significantly increased PVR postoperatively, but those with pulmonary venous hypertension (e.g., total anomalous pulmonary venous connection [TAPVC] with obstruction, or hypoplastic left heart syndrome with a highly restrictive atrial septum) are clearly at risk.
3. Infants and older children with *increased* PVR secondary to congenital heart lesions. Infants with certain cardiac lesions (e.g., TGA with VSD, and truncus arteriosus), are susceptible to early (within the first few months of life) development of pulmonary vascular obstructive disease and, therefore, are at increased risk for pulmonary hypertension if operated on beyond the first few weeks of life. Even simple lesions (e.g., VSD) operated after the first year of life are more susceptible to postoperative pulmonary hypertension because of increasing medial hypertrophy and other pathologic vascular changes that evolve as the patient becomes older.
4. Patients with parenchymal lung disease. For obvious reasons, these patients are at greater risk for pulmonary hypertension than those without lung disease.
5. Patients with an unexplained elevation in PVR. An unexplained elevation in PVR can occur in patients without a heart lesion (e.g., persistent pulmonary hypertension of the newborn), or in those with a heart defect (e.g., a 2-month-old patient with a VSD and PVR = SVR). In these rare cases, the risk of postoperative pulmonary hypertension is increased.

PROBLEM OF TOO LITTLE PVR

Because PVR is ordinarily only approximately 20% of SVR, patients with large communication(s) between the systemic and pulmonary circulations (most commonly, patent ductus arteriosus [PDA], VSD, truncus arteriosus, and surgically placed systemic to pulmonary arterial "shunts") may suffer from excessive pulmonary blood flow. Newborns with ductus-dependent cardiac lesions (especially those with left-sided obstructive lesions) palliated with prostaglandin E_1 while awaiting surgery are particularly susceptible to this problem. Increased pulmonary flow and pressure tend to increase lung water and decrease lung compliance, but more importantly, systemic blood flow can be reduced with consequent hypoperfusion of vital organs. Aortopulmonary communications are particularly problematic, as diastolic flow into the lungs diminishes coronary perfusion pressure.

THERAPY FOR INCREASED PVR

The approach to a patient with increased PVR will obviously depend on multiple factors, including the magnitude and impact of the increased PVR on the patient, and the overall context. Because many of the maneuvers available to manipulate PVR carry significant downside risks, it is important to have a clear idea of the precise anatomy and physiology involved in any given patient, and what wants and needs to be achieved. For example, a moderate elevation in pulmonary arterial pressure (e.g., approximately 50% of systemic pressure) in a patient following repair of a large VSD usually warrants *no* acute therapy in the postoperative period, as the increased pressure will have little adverse physiologic effect over the short run.

The following discussion focuses primarily on ways of manipulating PVR, although most patients with increased PVR will require inotropic and other forms of support detailed in other chapters in this book. (Table 32.2 briefly summarizes the pulmonary vascular effects of commonly used inotropic agents.)

Analgesia and Sedation

Patients provided a high level of analgesia and sedation in the postoperative period appear to have less labile, and perhaps lower, PVR. Fentanyl (1–10 µg/kg loading bolus; initial infusion rate = 5–10 µg/kg/h) is the analgesic of choice, being more potent and having fewer systemic vascular effects than morphine. Because fentanyl can cause (especially at high doses and when first administered) chest wall rigidity, neuromuscular blocking agents (e.g., metocurine, pancuronium, vecuronium, or atracurium) should be used concomitantly. Patients become quickly habituated to fentanyl, sometimes necessitating a daily increase in the infusion rate. Because this agent has been shown to blunt the pulmonary (and systemic) vascular responses to endotracheal suctioning (37), additional fentanyl administering can be considered just prior to suctioning in patients known to be highly reactive to this stimulus. For sedation, midazolam, lorazepam, and diazepam are the agents most commonly used in this setting. For patients requiring long-term rather than intermittent sedation, lorazepam or diazepam, by virtue of their longer duration of action, are most appropriate.

Mechanical Ventilation

As noted, it is unclear how effective hyperoxia is as a pulmonary vasodilator in the human, but sufficient anecdotal experience and data exist to justify the use of *enriched inspired oxygen* for patients requiring reduction of PVR, and for patients with lung disease it is mandatory. Because F_{IO_2} greater than approximately 0.60 can cause lung damage, prolonged use of higher concentrations of inspired oxygen should be avoided unless it clearly provides significant salutary effect. Because PVR is minimal when FRC is normal, it is important that the lungs be well, but not over, expanded.

Endotracheal suctioning carries at least two risks relative to the pulmonary circulation. First, it can cause an acute increase in PVR (presumably through a neurally mediated reflex). Second, if performed in conjunction with vigorous bagging with 100% F_{IO_2}, it can cause a precipitous fall in PVR (and therefore systemic hypoperfusion) in patients with an aortopulmonary communication. Because of the adverse effect of tracheal secretions on pulmonary function, however, endotracheal suctioning is nevertheless indicated at intervals appropriate for each individual patient. Measures to reduce the risk of suctioning (e.g., gently bagging the patient with an aortopulmonary shunt, using room air) help reduce the risk of this procedure.

The optimal magnitude of PEEP depends on the patient's lungs: for those with little or no lung disease, PEEP of 2–4 cm/H_2O may be appropriate, whereas patients with considerable pulmonary edema may benefit from a higher level. The notion is widespread that PEEP is either not indicated or it is contraindicated in patients following the "Fontan" operation, given the importance of low PVR in this setting. Whereas a high level of PEEP in a patient with normal lungs may increase PVR, low levels (approximately 2–3 cm/H_2O) help to maintain normal FRC and normal alveolar oxygen levels, and they have little effect on cardiac output in the Fontan patient (38). Furthermore, as noted, with lung disease PEEP may little increase or even decrease PVR. Hence, PEEP of the appropriate magnitude should not be excluded from use in the Fontan patient.

pH

As noted, blood pH has a powerful effect on PVR, and alkalosis (pH generally approximately 7.50–7.60) is routinely applied as therapy for increased PVR. Purely regarding the reduction of vascular tone, it appears largely irrelevant whether alkalosis is achieved via (mechanical) hyperventilation or infusion of base (e.g., sodium bicarbonate or tromethamine [THAM]). However, hyperventilation can be attended by several adverse effects: increased mean airway pressure may itself increase PVR, decrease venous return to the heart (and hence ventricular filling), cause barotrauma, and hypocarbia causes a reduction in cerebral blood flow that might be undesirable. For these reasons, alkalinization should be achieved at least in part via infusion of base, when serum sodium concentration permits.

Intravenous Pharmacologic Agents

A variety of different vasodilators have been used to treat postoperative pulmonary hypertension, but all have suffered from two limitations:

1. The tendency for essentially all vasodilators to relax both systemic and pulmonary blood vessels (causing systemic hypotension).
2. No vasodilator has proved to be consistently effective in dilating the pulmonary circulation. Tolazoline, prostaglandins E_1 and I_2, nitroprusside, isoproterenol, and a variety of other agents have been used (35), but none has been found to be reliably effective in treating acute pulmonary hypertension. This inconsistency, combined with potential complications—especially systemic hypotension—has somewhat dampened enthusiasm for these agents at many centers. Inhaled NO is likely to supplant these agents in the future.

Inhaled Nitric Oxide[1]

Nitric oxide is an endothelium-derived relaxing factor and a gas (22). When inhaled at low concentrations it can relax constricted pulmonary vascular smooth muscle. Hemoglobin rapidly inactivates any NO that crosses the alveolar epithelium and vascular wall to reach the capillary lumen, prompting clinical investigations in diseases where selective pulmonary vasodilation would be beneficial. Early reports demonstrated its usefulness in the perioperative care of the child with congenital heart disease, as well as in the neonate with persistent pulmonary hypertension,

---

[1] This section on nitric oxide was written by DL Wessel, MD.

and the adult with pulmonary hypertension or adult respiratory distress syndrome (27, 39–46).

Inhaled NO has emerged as an important diagnostic and therapeutic agent in the critically ill patient with congenital heart disease. It is a selective pulmonary vasodilator with minimal adverse hemodynamic effects when administered and monitored in a judicious fashion. It has a number of advantages compared with intravenous vasodilators, particularly the absence of systemic hypotension and the salutary effect on intrapulmonary shunt. Its hemodynamic benefit has been demonstrated in patients with pulmonary hypertension associated with total anomalous pulmonary venous connection (47), congenital mitral stenosis (48), postoperative patients with Fontan physiology (49), and those with pre-existing left-to-right shunts and other lesions (27). It can be used in the newborn to help discriminate anatomic obstruction to pulmonary blood flow from pulmonary vasoconstriction (50), and it can be used effectively in the treatment or prevention of pulmonary hypertensive crises after cardiopulmonary bypass (51).

Optimal dosing of NO to maximize pulmonary vascular relaxation without incurring toxic side effects, systemic hypotension, or an increased venous admixture is unclear. Miller showed in 10 infants and children that low and potentially less toxic doses of NO were effective after cardiac surgery, with nearly identical response at two parts per million (ppm) compared with 10 and 20 ppm (52). Day showed little additional value with 60 ppm over 12 ppm in patients with congenital heart disease (53). However, Roberts et al. demonstrated a dose-response relationship up to 80 ppm in a similar population (45).

As an inhaled vasodilator NO has special advantage in the treatment of acute respiratory failure that can arise in conjunction with pulmonary hypertension after bypass. Maximal pulmonary vasodilator response to inhaled NO can occur at a higher dose (80 ppm) than that which produces optimal ventilation perfusion matching in patients with elevated pulmonary artery pressure and severe pulmonary parenchymal disease. By redistributing pulmonary blood flow away from underventilated alveoli toward normally ventilated areas of the lung, inhaled NO in low concentrations may improve intrapulmonary shunt fraction and raise Pa_{O_2}. It has been suggested that this effect can be optimized at doses of inhaled NO that are low (1–10 ppm) although maximal pulmonary vasodilation occurred in the same patients at higher NO doses (10–100 ppm) among 12 adult patients with acute respiratory distress syndrome (ARDS) (54). Improved oxygenation was lost at the higher NO doses in these patients where pulmonary vasodilation was maximized. Presumably this occurred from a "spillover" effect of NO into a poorly ventilated lung with loss of preferential delivery to and vasodilation of better ventilated areas. No data are available for childhood diseases comparing the NO-induced dose response changes in oxygenation simultaneously with changes in PVR. This is especially important in the critically ill population of children with acute severe pulmonary parenchymal disease that complicates their pulmonary hypertensive congenital heart disease. Thus, the desirable dose may depend in part on the severity of the pulmonary artery hypertension versus the severity of intrapulmonary shunting from lung disease. It seems likely that the recommended starting dose of NO for newborns with congenital heart disease falls between 5 and 40 ppm.

Early investigations suggested that this drug improved oxygenation in patients with persistent pulmonary hypertension of the newborn (PPHN) who were administered 6–80 ppm of NO with oxygen (39, 44). Although promising, these initial studies were small case series with physiologic rather than clinical outcomes, and they lacked a control group. Subsequent trials were informative but until recently were still limited by lack of controls, extensive treatment crossover designs, or inherent limitations of multicenter trials with varying definitions of standard clinical practice (55–60). Efficacy of NO in the treatment of PPHN has been recently affirmed in multicenter randomized trials (61, 62).

Concern exists over potential NO-induced cellular injury during exogenous exposure to the drug, as well as the generation of nitrogen dioxide and methemoglobinemia during NO delivery. If the dose of NO is maintained below 40 ppm fewer acute problems have been reported when detailed guidelines of precise delivery and monitoring were followed (63). As with any vasodilator, rebound pulmonary hypertension can complicate drug withdrawal (47).

Potential benefits have been found in chronic, outpatient administration of NO to facilitate growth and beneficial remodeling of the abnormal pulmonary vasculature in unusual forms of idiopathic pulmonary hypertension identified in early infancy. However, none of the purported benefits of inhaled NO in children with congenital heart disease have been studied in a randomized, placebo-controlled manner with convincing demonstration of improved outcomes. This must be borne in mind when evaluating the risks and potential benefits of this new therapy.

Optimal Hematocrit

It is unclear what constitutes the optimal hematocrit for a patient with increased PVR. On the one hand, as the hematocrit increases so does oxygen carrying capacity and therefore oxygen delivery. For patients with right-to-left shunting, increased hematocrit also increases arterial oxygen saturation by virtue of increasing mixed venous oxygen saturation. On the other hand, resistance to blood flow through the lungs increases with hematocrit (and therefore blood viscosity). Lister et al. calculated, based on both empirically derived data and theoretic considerations, that

PVR is 36% greater at a hematocrit of 55% than at a hematocrit of 33% (64). Whether this relationship between hematocrit and PVR is applicable under all circumstances is as yet unclear. Furthermore, the impact of PVR on patient well-being varies considerably depending on the circumstances, making it difficult to assign relative weights to the effects of PVR and oxygen carrying capacity on the physiologic status of the patient. Compare, for example, the postoperative "Fontan" patient with one following simple VSD repair. In the case of the former, relatively small changes in PVR may significantly alter cardiac output, whereas in the latter significantly increased PVR may not affect cardiac output, and oxygen delivery may be influenced more by factors such as hematocrit. Until the crucial question (What is the *net effect* of hematocrit on oxygen delivery, and possibly other relevant variables, in a given patient with increased PVR?) is empirically addressed, it will not be possible to specify an "optimal" hematocrit.

Ensuring Adequate Coronary Perfusion

Compelling studies demonstrating how sensitive the acutely hypertensive right ventricle is to coronary perfusion pressure (65) emphasize the need to maintain adequate aortic diastolic pressure when right ventricular pressure is elevated. Avoiding systemic hypotension is therefore important, as even transient hypotension can rapidly lead to decreased right ventricular function and output in the severely hypertensive right ventricle.

Support Using the Extracorporeal Membrane Oxygenator

Extracorporeal membrane oxygenator (ECMO) is a well-established and generally effective means of supporting neonates with increased PVR until resolution of the primary process occurs. For a variety of reasons, ECMO use in patients following cardiac surgery has generally been less successful than in cases of neonatal lung disease (66), but this modality can be considered for postoperative cardiac patients with life-threatening pulmonary hypertension refractory to other therapy. For obvious reasons, such therapy may not be appropriate for patients thought to be at high risk for having permanently increased PVR.

THERAPY FOR INSUFFICIENT PVR

As noted, patients with aortopulmonary communications can suffer excessive pulmonary blood flow, ultimately related to the ratio of PVR:SVR being too low. Several maneuvers can help (selectively) increase PVR.

1. F_{IO_2} should be approximately 0.21 (presuming little or no lung disease) to avoid pulmonary vasodilation caused by hyperoxia.
2. pH should be kept approximately 7.30–7.40 for the reasons previously outlined. Experience with permissive hypercapnia in patients without cardiac disease suggests that pH considerably lower than 7.30 is well tolerated, but given the adverse effect of acidosis on cardiac contractility, it is unclear whether such levels are prudent in patients with an increased cardiac volume or pressure load. The minimal acceptable pH in patients with cardiac disease has yet to be defined.
3. Increased PEEP is occasionally advocated as a way to increase PVR in this setting. PEEP as high as 8 cm/H_2O generally has little discernible effect on pulmonary blood flow, and given a reluctance to incur possible complications from yet higher levels, I have therefore not found high PEEP to be helpful in this setting.
4. Because alveolar hypoxia is a powerful pulmonary vasoconstrictor, reduction of F_{IO_2} to approximately 0.15–0.17 (using N_2) has been used to increase PVR. Because these patients have some degree of arterial desaturation related to right-to-left shunting on room air, it is necessary to carefully monitor oxygen saturations and to avoid unacceptable hypoxemia.
5. Patients with excessive pulmonary blood flow and systemic hypertension may benefit from vasodilator (such as nitroprusside) use to reduce driving pressure into the pulmonary circuit (and decrease left ventricular afterload) (67). Because PVR is already low in most patients with excess pulmonary flow, if SVR is increased, pharmacologic vasodilators tend to reduce SVR in excess of PVR.
6. It has been reported that the combination of a relatively high minute ventilation combined with exogenously supplied CO_2 enhances hemodynamic stability in patients following "Norwood" palliation for hypoplastic left heart syndrome (68), presumably through limiting pulmonary blood flow. Although a relatively large minute ventilation might increase PVR on a mechanical basis (whereas alkalosis-induced vasodilation is prevented by the addition of CO_2), it is otherwise obscure why this regimen should promote cardiovascular stability in these patients. Insufficient data exist to permit evaluation of this strategy at this time.

REFERENCES

1. Fishman AP. Dynamics of the pulmonary circulation. In: Hamilton WF, Dow P, eds. Handbook of physiology. Vol. II. Washington, DC: American Physiological Society, 1963:1667–1743.
2. Grover RF, Wagner WW Jr, McMurtry IF, et al. Pulmonary circulation. In: Shepherd JT, Abboud FM, eds. Handbook of physiology. Vol. III. Bethesda, MD: American Physiological Society, 1983:103–136.
3. Rudolph AM. Fetal and neonatal pulmonary circulation. Annu Rev Physiol 1979;41:383–395.
4. Rabinovitch M. Pathophysiology of pulmonary hypertension.

In: Emmanoulides GC, Riemenschneider TA, Allen HD, et al., eds. Heart disease in infants, children, and adolescents. Vol 2. Baltimore: Williams & Wilkins, 1995:1659–1695.
5. Kulik TJ, Lock JE. The assessment of pulmonary vascular tone: a review of experimental methodologies. Pediatric Pharmacology 1984;4:73–83.
6. Geggel RL, Reid LM. The structural basis of PPHN. Clin Perinatol 1984;2:525–549.
7. Pietra GG, Edwards WD, Kay JM, et al. Histopathology of primary pulmonary hypertension. A qualitative and quantitative study of pulmonary blood vessels from 58 patients in the National Heart, Lung, and Blood Institute, Primary Pulmonary Hypertension Registry. Circulation 1989;80:1198–1206.
8. Heath D, Edwards JE. The pathology of hypertensive pulmonary vascular disease. Circulation 1958;18:533–547.
9. Friedli B, Kidd BSL, Mustard WT, et al. Ventricular septal defect with increased pulmonary vascular resistance. Am J Cardiol 1974;33:403–409.
10. Bergovsky EH, Hass F, Porcelli R. Determination of the sensitive vascular sites from which hypoxia and hypercapnia elicit rises in pulmonary artery pressure. Federation Proceedings 1968;27:1420–1425.
11. Archer SL, Huang J, Henry T, et al. A redox-based O_2 sensor in rat pulmonary vasculature. Circ Res 1993;73:1100–1112.
12. Custer JR, Hales CA. Influence of alveolar oxygen on pulmonary vasoconstriction in newborn lambs versus sheep. American Review of Respiratory Diseases 1985;132:326–331.
13. Rudolph AM, Yuan S. Response of the pulmonary vasculature to hypoxia and H^+ ion concentration changes. J Clin Invest 1966;45:399–411.
14. Viles PH, Shepherd JT. Evidence for a dilator action of carbon dioxide on the pulmonary vessels of the cat. Circ Res 1968;22:325–332.
15. Barer GR, Shaw JW. Pulmonary vasodilator and vasoconstrictor actions of carbon dioxide. J Physiol 1971;213:633–645.
16. Schreiber MD, Heymann, Soifer SJ. Increased arterial pH, not decreased $Paco_2$, attenuates hypoxia-induced pulmonary vasoconstriction in newborn lambs. Pediatr Res 1986;20:113–117.
17. Brimioulle S, Lejeune P, Vachiery J-L, et al. Effects of acidosis and alkalosis on hypoxic pulmonary vasoconstriction in dogs. Am J Physiol (Heart Circ Physiol) 1990;258:H347–H353.
18. Gordon JB, Martinez FR, Keller PA, et al. Differing effects of acute and prolonged alkalosis on hypoxic pulmonary vasoconstriction. Am Rev Resp Dis 1993;148:1651–1656.
19. Nandiwada PA, Hyman AL, Kadowitz PJ. Pulmonary vasodilator responses to vagal stimulation and acetylcholine in the cat. Circ Res 1983;53:86–95.
20. Silove E, Inoue T, Grover RF. Comparison of hypoxia, pH, and sympathomimetic drugs on the bovine pulmonary vasculature. J Appl Physiol 1986;24:355–365.
21. Frostell C, Fratacci M-D, Wain JC, et al. Inhaled nitric oxide. A selective pulmonary vasodilator reversing hypoxic pulmonary vasoconstriction. Circulation 1991;83:2038–2047.
22. Moncada S, Palmer RMJ, Higgs EA. Nitric oxide: physiology, pathophysiology, and pharmacology. Pharmacol Rev 1991;43:109–142.
23. Bolotina VM, Najibi S, Palacino JJ, et al. Nitric oxide directly activates calcium-dependent potassium channels in vascular smooth muscle. Nature 1994;368:850–853.
24. Moore P, Velvis H, Fineman JR, et al. EDRF inhibition attenuates the increase in pulmonary blood flow due to oxygen ventilation in fetal lambs. J Appl Physiol 1992;73:2151–2157.
25. Fineman JR, Chang R, Soifer SJ. EDRF inhibition augments pulmonary hypertension in intact newborn lambs. Am J Physiol (Heart Circ Physiol) 1992;262:H1365–H1371.
26. Celermajer DS, Cullen S, Deanfield JE. Impairment of endothelium-dependent pulmonary artery relaxation in children with congenital heart disease and abnormal pulmonary hemodynamics. Circulation 1993;87:440–446.
27. Wessel DL, Adatia I, Giglia TM, et al. Use of inhaled nitric oxide and acetylcholine in the evaluation of pulmonary hypertension and endothelial function after cardiopulmonary bypass. Circulation 1993;88:2128–2138.
28. Garg UC, Hassid A. Nitric oxide-generating vasodilators and 8-bromo-cyclic guanosine monophosphate inhibit mitogenesis and proliferation of cultured rat vascular smooth muscle cells. J Clin Invest 1989;83:1774–1777.
29. Kolpakov V, Gordon D, Kulik TJ. Nitric oxide-generating compounds inhibit total protein and collagen synthesis in cultured vascular smooth muscle cells. Circ Res 1995;76:305–309.
30. Roberts JD Jr, Roberts CT, Jones RC, et al. Continuous nitric oxide inhalation reduces pulmonary arterial structural changes, right ventricular hypertrophy, and growth retardation in the hypoxic newborn rat. Circ Res 1995;76:215–222.
31. Adatia I, Perry S, Landzberg M, et al. Inhaled nitric oxide and hemodynamic evaluation of patients with pulmonary hypertension before transplantation. J Am Coll Cardiol 1995;25:1656–1664.
32. Miro AM, Pinsky MR. Cardiopulmonary interactions. In: Fuhrman BP, Zimmerman JJ, eds. Pediatric critical care. St. Louis: Mosby, 1992:251–252.
33. Venkataramen ST, Fuhrman BP, Howland DF, et al. Positive end-expiratory pressure-induced, calcium-channel-mediated increases in pulmonary vascular resistance in neonatal lambs. Crit Care Med 1993;21:1066–1076.
34. Zapol WM, Snider MT. Pulmonary hypertension in severe acute respiratory failure. N Engl J Med 1977;296:476–480.
35. Jones, ODH, Shore DF, Rigby ML, et al. The use of tolazoline hydrochloride as a pulmonary vasodilator in potentially fatal episodes of pulmonary vasoconstriction after cardiac surgery in children. Circulation 1981;64(Suppl II):II-134–II-139.
36. Heymann MA. Control of the pulmonary circulation in the perinatal period. Journal of Developmental Physiology 1984;6:281–290.
37. Hickey PR, Hansen DD, Wessel DL, et al. Blunting of stress responses in the pulmonary circulation of infants by fentanyl. Anesth Analg 1985;64:1137–1142.
38. Williams DB, Kiernan PD, Metke MP, et al. Hemodynamic response to positive end-expiratory pressure following right atrium-pulmonary artery bypass (Fontan procedure). J Thorac Cardiovasc Surg 1984;87:856–861.
39. Kinsella JP, Neish SR, Shaffer E, et al. Low-dose inhalational nitric oxide in persistent pulmonary hypertension of the newborn. Lancet 1992;340:819–820.
40. Pepke-Zaba J, Higenbottam TW, Dinh-Xuan AT, et al. Inhaled nitric oxide as a cause of selective pulmonary vasodilatation in pulmonary hypertension. Lancet 1991;338:1173–1174.
41. Rossaint R, Falke KJ, Lopez F, et al. Inhaled nitric oxide for the adult respiratory distress syndrome. N Engl J Med 1993;328:399–405.
42. Girard C, Lehot JJ, Pannetier JC, et al. Inhaled nitric oxide after mitral valve replacement in patients with chronic pulmonary artery hypertension. Anesthesiology 1992;77:880–883.
43. Adatia I, Thompson J, Landzberg M, et al. Inhaled nitric oxide in chronic obstructive lung disease. Lancet 1993;341:307–308.

44. Roberts JD, Polaner DM, Lang P, et al. Inhaled nitric oxide in persistent pulmonary hypertension of the newborn. Lancet 1992;340:818–819.
45. Roberts JD, Lang P, Bigatello LM, et al. Inhaled nitric oxide in congenital heart disease. Circulation 1993;87:447–453.
46. Wessel DL. Inhaled nitric oxide for the treatment of pulmonary hypertension before and after cardiopulmonary bypass. Crit Care Med 1993;21(Suppl):S344–S345.
47. Atz AM, Adatia I, Wessel DL. Rebound pulmonary hypertension after inhalation of nitric oxide. Ann Thorac Surg 1996;62:1759–1764.
48. Atz AM, Adatia I, Jonas RA, et al. Inhaled nitric oxide in children with pulmonary hypertension and congenital mitral stenosis. Am J Cardiol 1996;77:316–319.
49. Goldman AP, Delius RE, Deanfield JE, et al. Pharmacologic control of pulmonary blood flow with inhaled nitric oxide after the fenestrated Fontan operation. Circulation 1996;94(Suppl II):II-44–II-48.
50. Adatia I, Atz AM, Jonas RA, et al. Diagnostic use of inhaled nitric oxide after neonatal cardiac operations. J Thorac Cardiovasc Surg 1996;112:1403–1405.
51. Journois D, Pouard P, Mauriat P, et al. Inhaled nitric oxide as a therapy for pulmonary hypertension after operations for congenital heart defects. J Thorac Cardiovasc Surg 1994;107:1129–1135.
52. Miller OI, Celermajer DS, Deanfield JE, et al. Very low dose inhaled nitric oxide: a selective pulmonary vasodilator after operations for congenital heart disease. J Thorac Cardiovasc Surg 1994;108:487–494.
53. Day R, Lynch J, Shaddy R, et al. Pulmonary vasodilatory effects of 12 and 60 parts per million inhaled nitric oxide in children with ventricular septal defect. Am J Cardiol 1995;75:196–198.
54. Gerlach H, Rossaint D, Pappert D, et al. Time-course and dose-response of nitric oxide inhalation for systemic oxygenation and pulmonary hypertension in patients with adult respiratory distress syndrome. Eur J Clin Invest 1993;23:499–502.
55. Kinsella JP, Neish SR, Ivy DD, et al. Clinical responses to prolonged treatment of persistent pulmonary hypertension of the newborn with low doses of inhaled nitric oxide. J Pediatr 1993;123:103–108.
56. Barefield ES, Karle VA, Philips JB, et al. Inhaled nitric oxide in term infants with hypoxemic respiratory failure. J Pediatr 1996;129:279–286.
57. Finer NN, Etches PC, Kamstra B, et al. Inhaled nitric oxide in infants referred for extracorporeal membrane oxygenation. dose response. J Pediatr 1994;124:302–308.
58. Day R, Lynch J, White K, et al. Acute response to inhaled nitric oxide in newborns with respiratory failure and pulmonary hypertension. Pediatrics 1996;98:698–705.
59. Goldman A, Tasker R, Haworth S, et al. Four patterns of response to inhaled nitric oxide for persistent pulmonary hypertension of the newborn. Pediatrics 1996;98:706–713.
60. Turbow R, Waffarn L, Yang L, et al. Variable oxygenation response to inhaled nitric oxide in severe persistent pulmonary hypertension of the newborn. Acta Paediatr 1995;84:1305–1308.
61. The Neonatal Inhaled Nitric Oxide Study Group. Inhaled nitric oxide in full-term and nearly full-term infants with hypoxic respiratory failure. N Engl J Med 1997;336:597–604.
62. Roberts JD, Fineman JR, Morin FC, Inhaled nitric oxide and persistent pulmonary hypertension of the newborn. N Engl J Med 1997;336:605–610.
63. Atz AM, Wessel DL. Delivery and monitoring of inhaled nitric oxide. Current Opinion in Critical Care 1997;3:243–249.
64. Lister G, Hellenbrand WE, Kleinman CS, et al. Physiologic effects of increasing hemoglobin concentration in left-to-right shunting in infants with ventricular septal defect. N Engl J Med 1982;306:502–506.
65. Vlahakes GJ, Turley K, Hoffman JI. The pathophysiology of failure in acute right ventricular hypertension: hemodynamic and biochemical correlations. Circulation 1981;63:87–95.
66. Kulik TJ, Moler FW, Palmisano JM, et al. Outcome-associated factors in pediatric patients treated with extracorporeal membrane oxygenator after cardiac surgery. Circulation 1996;94(Suppl II):II-63–II-68.
67. Rossi AF, Sommer RJ, Lotvin A, et al. Usefulness of intermittent monitoring of mixed venous oxygen saturation after stage 1 palliation for hypoplastic left heart syndrome. Am J Cardiol 1994;73:1118–1123.
68. Jobes DR, Nicolson SC, Steven JM, et al. Carbon dioxide prevents pulmonary overcirculation in hypoplastic left heart syndrome. Ann Thorac Surg 1992;54:150–151.

Miscellaneous Topics

Henry J. Issenberg, MD

CARDIAC TRAUMA

Accidents are the leading cause of death in the United States for children in the 1- to 14-year-old age range with about 50% being transportation-related injuries (vehicular, bicycle, or pedestrian) (1). In a study of 551 trauma deaths, 24% of these involved traumatic rupture of the aorta (2). The most severe cases of cardiac trauma are usually evaluated and stabilized at the accident site or the emergency department, with the most critical requiring immediate surgical intervention with an open thoracotomy; unfortunately, few of these children survive (3). Most of the remaining cases are usually more stable on admission to the intensive care setting, sometimes having only required thoracostomy tube drainage of blood, and they are admitted for further evaluation and observation. Frequently, this involves a short 1- to 2-day period that does not reveal any significant myocardial injury (4). Type and degree of cardiac insult can initially be underestimated or even unrecognized in a child with multiple trauma, because the evaluation of the central nervous system, abdomen, neck and extremities is usually more thorough.

Types of Thoracic Injury

The two mechanisms of thoracic injury are penetrating and nonpenetrating, with the nonpenetrating type being more common and the predominant type in the preadolescent aged patient. Beyond this age, accidents from gunshot wounds and stabbings begin to increase, especially in the subgroup of adolescent urban males.

Penetrating Type

Penetrating wounds are conventionally from gunshot or sharp objects. An increasing number of injuries, however, are occurring during interventional cardiac catheterization or the placement of intravascular lines (5). Gunshot wounds are frequently fatal because a large volume of blood loss flowing into the pleural space through a pericardial opening along with direct tissue destruction. More than 50% of children injured by knife wounds survive with sufficient time to reach treatment. A knife laceration of the myocardium and pericardium may seal (especially if through the thicker left ventricle), creating pericardial hemorrhage and tamponade, which can be effectively treated with drainage and surgery only if needed. Retention of the foreign body within the heart can be well tolerated with no ill effect or it can erode into the cavity creating a nidus for endocarditis, thromboembolism, and potential migration into the pulmonary or aortic vessels. The same concerns are present for foreign bodies that may erode into a large peripheral vein or artery and embolize a considerable distance into distal organs. The decision for surgical foreign body removal has to be individualized based on the risks of local tissue damage and embolization.

After immediate stabilization, further treatment requires a more comprehensive evaluation of cardiac structure and function (see Table 33.1). A chest roentgenogram should be obtained to delineate any retained radiopaque foreign body. An electrocardiogram (ECG) should be obtained to rule out obvious ischemia or infarction. Transthoracic echocardiogram may have limited visualization because of chest tubes and subcutaneous emphysema, making transesophageal echocardiogram an acceptable alternative (6, 7). Intracardiac defects such as atrial and ventricular septal defects or valve leaflet, chorda, and cuspal damage should be readily apparent on echocardiogram with immediate surgical treatment if the patient is hemodynamically compromised. Other lesions such as coronary cameral fistulas and ventricular aneurysms are less common, and they can present late, occasionally requiring further diagnostic evaluation with cardiac catheterization and selective angiography. Complications from infection, arrhythmias, and pericarditis should also be suspected. A form of post-pericardiotomy syndrome is seen in approximately 20% of children with recurrent sterile effusions and chest pain requiring appropriate treatment.

Nonpenetrating Type

Nonpenetrating or blunt trauma to the chest creates a high level of anxiety during initial evaluation, but because of a child's thoracic cage resiliency, it frequently requires only vigilant observation (see Table 33.2). Because of the flexibility and elasticity of the child's chest wall, however, higher amounts of energy are dissipated to the internal organs, rather than being absorbed within fracturing ribs. More than 50% of these children have multiple organ system injury, which must be sought. In addition, absence of obvious cutaneous trauma or rib fractures does not preclude significant intrathoracic damage. It is estimated that myocardial contusion occurs in approximately 25% of chil-

Table 33.1. Penetrating Cardiac Wounds

Pericardium
  Laceration
  Hemopericardium and tamponade
  Pneumopericardium
  Pericarditis—postpericardiotomy or infectious
Myocardium
  Laceration
  Penetration
  Retained foreign body
  Aneurysm
Intracardial defect
  Atrial septal defect
  Ventricular septal defect
  Valvar damage—laceration, leaflet, and subvalvar
Coronary artery
  Laceration—without myocardial infarction
  Thrombosis
  Coronary—cameral fistula
  Aneurysm
Embolism
  Foreign body
  Thrombosis
Infectious endocarditis
Rhythm—conduction disturbances

Table 33.2. Nonpenetrating Cardiac Wounds

Pericardium
  Disruption—herniation
  Hemopericardium and tamponade
  Pericarditis—postpericardiotomy
Myocardium
  Concussion
  Contusion
  Thrombembolism
  Compression and rupture
  Septal perforation
  Myocardial pump failure
  Late aneurysm—true and pseudo
Valvar damage (regurgitation)
Coronary arteries
  Contusion and thrombosis—with or without myocardial infarction
  Arteriovenous fistula
  Laceration
Great vessel injury
  Rupture—at isthmus or aortic root
  Aneurysm—true or pseudo
  Aortic–cameral fistula
  Thrombosis
Venae caval
Electrocardiographic changes
  Atrial or ventricular ectopy
  Atrioventricular block
  Bundle branch block
  ST-T wave abnormality
  Injury or infarction

(Modified from Liedtke AJ, Demuth WE. Non-penetrating cardiac injuries: a collective review. Am Heart J 1973;86:687–697.)

dren who sustain severe thoracic blunt trauma, and it is distinguished from a myocardial concussion, which does not create any visible myocardial damage (8). Cardiac concussion (commotion cordia) from a ball hitting the chest is the most common cause of traumatic death in youth baseball in the United States (9).

Aortic rupture can occur from rapid deceleration injuries such as falls or pedestrian trauma. Ascending and descending thoracic aorta are rigidly fixed in position relative to the heart, which is free to swing in the pericardial sac. The points of maximal fixation, the aortic isthmus at the ligamentum arteriosum and the intrapericardial portion of the ascending aorta, are most vulnerable to shearing and rupture. Complete disruption leads to hemorrhage and immediate death, but lesser degrees of wall damage frequently occur with intimal tears that can lead to branch vessel occlusion or aortic dissection. Tears through the media that are being limited by a thin layer of structurally weak adventitia can create a pseudoaneurysm that requires surgical repair. Rupture at the aortic root leads to pericardial tamponade.

Similar to the penetrating type of thoracic injury, initial diagnostic evaluation must be complete and it can include myocardial enzymes (10). A radiographic review of the chest should determine bony fractures, pneumothorax, hemothorax, widened cardiothymic silhouette, widened mediastinum, or obliteration of the aortic knob. An electrocardiogram should be performed for ST-T wave abnormalities, arrhythmias, or conduction abnormalities that can indicate cardiac contusion. ST-T wave abnormalities should be interpreted serially, as they are often nonspecific; progressive changes can be from evolving pericardial injury or coronary artery trauma that can lead to an ischemic pattern. Laboratory studies should include fractionated creatinine kinase (CK) to determine if the MB isoenzyme is elevated to greater than 5% of the total, which should prompt further cardiac diagnostic studies. On the other hand, a single negative MB fraction does not totally preclude a myocardial contusion because this test has limited reliability in children. These tests are better obtained and interpreted serially in these patients.

Echocardiography and radionucleotide-gated blood pool studies are useful in evaluating wall motion abnormalities after blunt trauma where up to two thirds of the patients can show some dysfunction in either the right or left ventricles. Transthoracic echocardiogram is often difficult to obtain after blunt trauma because of subcutaneous air, pneumothorax, drainage tubes, and so forth. Transesophageal echocardiography may be preferable, and it can be safely performed after the neck and esophagus have been evaluated for injury. Besides wall motion abnormalities, pericardial fluid, intracardiac thrombi, torn chordae with valvar insufficiency, myocardial hematomas, and aortic tears should be ruled out.

Therapy

Supportive therapy and intervention strategy for both penetrating and nonpenetrating injury are similar. Acute chest pain can be either angina-like or pericardial in origin, and it can be treated with analgesics, because vasodilators and coronary nitrates are usually ineffective. If the cardiac function is depressed from contusion, supportive care with appropriate intravenous (IV) inotropic agents and volume expansion may be needed. Constant ECG monitoring with prompt treatment of arrhythmias is also advocated. If a contusion is documented, daily echocardiographic evaluation should be done for the development of intracardiac thrombi, although the controversy over the risks versus benefits of anticoagulation has not been resolved. In this setting, myocardial hemorrhage within the contusion has the theoretic potential of extension.

Late evaluation should first be performed 1 to 2 weeks later as the region of contusion can necrose and rupture leading to an atrial septal defect (ASD), ventricular septal defect (VSD), or pseudoaneurysm requiring surgical repair. A dyskinetic area of true aneurysm may warrant surgical resection if significant hemodynamic compromise is seen. As a general rule, serial echocardiographic follow-up should continue for 6 to 12 months.

AORTIC DISSECTION

In contrast with adults with aortic dissection in which most is caused by a complication of long-standing atherosclerotic disease, aortic dissection in the pediatric age group occurs with two main clinical situations: trauma and connective tissue disorders.

Trauma can be either accidental or iatrogenic, as a consequence of cardiac catheterization and balloon angioplasty (especially coarctation of the aorta). Abnormalities in the ultrastructure of elastin (seen in Marfan's syndrome patients) can lead to cystic medial necrosis, with subsequent medial weakening, aneurysm formation, intimal tearing, and aortic dissection. Systemic arterial hypertension will increase sheer forces and hasten the pathophysiologic process, thus enlarging the dissection. A hematoma can rupture through the adventitia, creating a periaortic collection, or into the left thorax, with a pleural effusion or hemopericardium, leading to tamponade (11).

The natural history of aneurysm growth in Marfan syndrome is predictable, and dissection is rarely seen before the second decade. It can be followed noninvasively, with echocardiography, computed tomography (CT), or magnetic resonance imaging (MRI), until reaching a certain diameter after which the risk of dissection or rupture dramatically increases, or when symptoms of dysphagia, hoarseness, chest, or back pain herald an early dissection (12, 13). Pain can evolve from a low grade to a more severe sharp pain with exacerbations with coughing and Valsalva maneuver, indicating further tearing or rupture and bleeding. Obstruction of other major branches can lead to syncope or mesenteric ischemia. These phenomena can also involve the aortic root with coronary ostial occlusion or dissection extending into the proximal coronary artery or into the aortic valve, creating aortic insufficiency.

Evaluation

Blood pressure measurement of four extremities should be performed because if the dissection extends over aortic arch branches, pulses can be lost or blood pressure gradients will occur (from arteries proximal to distal to the dissection). In addition, neurologic and abdominal examinations should be thorough to rule out vascular occlusion. The plain chest radiograph can reveal the aneurysmal dilation of the aortic segment affected, but it usually does not confirm the presence of dissection or rupture.

Noninvasively, the aortic wall and lumen can be imaged by echocardiography, CT, or MRI. Transesophageal echocardiography has extended the field of view from the proximal ascending aorta, which is usually seen transthoracically, into the arch and descending thoracic aorta to the diaphragm. Intimal flaps are more easily distinguished and the proximal lumen can be defined with color flow through the dissecting false lumen, unless it is filled with clot. The procedure can be quickly and safely performed in the emergency room as an initial screen with CT, MRI, and aortic angiography reserved for greater diagnostic clarity. Cardiac catheterization is useful only to define other associated diseases (such as coronary artery stenosis, atherosclerosis, or peculiar coronary ostial anatomy) in preparation for surgical intervention (14, 15).

Therapy

Emergency medical therapy should be directed at controlling any systolic hypertension to diminish the sheer stress imposed on the aorta. Whereas sodium nitroprusside can decrease afterload by vasodilation, it reflexly increases the left ventricular contraction index, dP/dt, and this reflex needs to be blocked with a β-antagonist such as IV propranolol or esmolol. The nitroprusside and β-antagonist combination seems to be the most efficacious in controlling hypertension as well as decreasing the likelihood of dissection. Alternatively, labetalol with its combined α- and β-adrenergic blocking effects can also be used as a single drug infusion. In addition, the pain of acute dissection can be severe, and it will exacerbate catecholamine release with wild fluctuations in blood pressure. Pain relief with a parenteral narcotic such as morphine can act both as a primary analgesic and a secondary vasodilator.

Uncomplicated dissections distal to the aortic isthmus can be successfully treated medically, whereas those involving the proximal ascending aorta and arch require urgent surgery after stabilization and diagnosis (16). An acute stroke in progress is an absolute contraindication to repair because heparinization and low perioperative carotid flow will lead to stroke extension. In Marfan syndrome patients with severe aneurysmal ascending aorta and root dilation with aortic insufficiency, a composite graft that extends from the root to the innominate artery, with an aortic valve prosthesis and coronary artery reimplantation, provides the best long-term results for the combination of problems.

Postoperatively, bleeding from long suture lines in friable aortic tissue poses an immediate problem and requires aggressive correction of clotting abnormalities with volume and blood resuscitation.

PERICARDIAL EFFUSION

Accumulation of fluid in the pericardial space can occur from a myriad of conditions, and it becomes important in the critical care unit in two contexts: (a) What is the diagnostic significance of the fluid and (b) is it impeding cardiovascular function and leading to tamponade?

Pericardial space is formed between the parietal (external) and visceral (internal) pericardial layers, and it contains between 15–50 mL (less than 1 mL/kg) of a clear, plasma ultra filtrate. This small, normal fluid volume can occasionally be visualized on echocardiography, especially posterior to the left ventricle and apically. Pericardial pressure is subatmospheric and equal to the pleural pressure, which is in turn a few millimeters of mercury less than the atrial pressures, creating a compliant space that does not restrict cardiac filling. As this space fills with fluid, it can enlarge with minimal pressure change until its distensibility becomes limited and after which the pressure can *acutely* rise. The steep portion of the pressure-volume relationship is often underappreciated, and this represents "tamponade," which restricts diastolic filling and diminishes cardiac output (17, 18) (see Fig. 33.1). A slowly accumulating effusion may allow the pericardium to distend at little change in pressure, whereas a relatively small volume collecting rapidly can create acute tamponade with hemodynamic collapse. This is particularly apparent during iatrogenic perforations at cardiac catheterization, or from chest trauma, when a high index of suspicion should prevail if there is an abrupt deterioration of vital signs, associated with a rapid rise in the central venous pressure (if monitoring is available).

Evaluation

Fluid can accumulate from pericarditis, heart failure, or trauma. The differential diagnosis of pericarditis is lengthy because frequently the fluid is formed secondary to a sys-

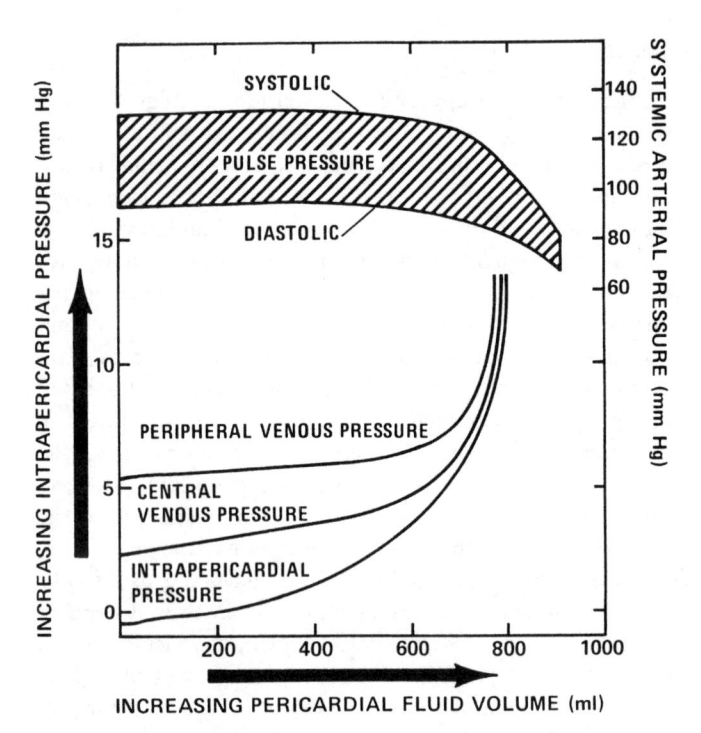

Figure 33.1. Pericardial effusion. (Reprinted with permission from Hancock EW. Cardiac tamponade. Philadelphia: WB Saunders, 1979:63(1)).

temic illness (Table 33.3). In older children, the physical examination usually includes an elevated jugular venous pulse, muffled heart sounds, or pericardial friction rub, whereas in neonates and infants, tachycardia may be the only sign. Pulsus paradoxus, which is the pronounced fall (more than 10 mm Hg) of the inspiratory systolic blood pressure, can be present and it demands immediate attention (19–21).

The chest radiograph usually reveals an increased cardiothymic silhouette, although the increase in size can be less than impressive in some patients. Transthoracic echocardiography is extremely sensitive and specific for defining fluid amount and location. The size of the effusion can have a poor correlation to hemodynamic embarrassment and tamponade. Impending tamponade physiology can be diagnosed echocardiographically by looking for diastolic collapse of the right atrium and right ventricle, allowing prompt treatment prior to the deterioration of cardiac output (22). The echocardiogram can also be helpful in defining the underlying cause of the effusion because any associated intracardiac finding such as thrombi or valve regurgitation can be additional clues to the diagnosis of systemic diseases. Lastly, echocardiography can delineate other similar pathophysiologic states, such as restrictive cardiomyopathy.

If the decision is made to evacuate the pericardial fluid, it should be sent for appropriate chemistry, culture, and histologic examinations.

Table 33.3. Pericarditis

Infectious
  Bacterial
    Staphylococcus aureus
    Meningococcus
    Hemophilus influenza
      —Pneumocococcal, streptococcal, gram negative
  Viral
    Coxsackie B5, B6
    Echo virus
    Adeno virus
    Epstein-Barr
    Influenza
    Human immunodeficiency virus
    Tuberculous
  Fungal—histoplasmosis,
    aspergillosis, parasitic,
    amebiasis, echinococcal
  Rickettsial
Rheumatic Fever
Congestive Heart Failure
Collagen Vascular
  Lupus erythematosus
  Juvenile rheumatoid arthritis
  Scleroderma
  Dermatomyositis
Sarcoid
Uremic
Myxedema—Hypothyroid
Tumors
  Malignant
    Lymphoma
      Hodgkins and non-Hodgkins
      Leukemia
    Metastatic
  Benign
    Hemangioma, teratoma, pericardial and thymic cyst,
    rhabdomyosarcoma
Kawasaki's—Mucocutaneous
Lymph Node Syndrome
Radiation
Trauma or Chest Wall Injury
  Hickman indwelling lines
  Cardiac catheterization
  Crush
  Penetrating
  Dissection
Postpericardiotomy
Postperfusion Syndrome
  Cytomegalovirus
Myocardial Infarction
  Dressler's syndrome
Constrictive
Drug-Induced
  Procainamide
  Hydralazine
  Methysergide
  Minoxidil

Therapy

Supportive therapy before any attempted evacuation involves appropriate fluid resuscitation with the caveat that a higher filling pressure (more than 10 mm Hg) is needed to maintain hemodynamic stability in these patients. Pressor support can also be useful, but it is usually not desirable because tachycardia can occur, and it is not necessary if fluid resuscitation is adequate. Use of vasodilators, diuretics, and preload reducers are contraindicated. The patients should also not be given fluids enterally in anticipation of potential anesthesia. Blood should be typed and cross-matched for availability. Ambient oxygen is recommended, but extreme caution should be exercised in instituting mechanical ventilation and using elevated inspiratory or end-expiratory pressures, which by increasing the intrathoracic pressure will further impede cardiac output.

Definitive treatment consists of pericardial fluid drainage via pericardiocentesis (usually with simultaneous echocardiographic imaging) or surgical pericardiotomy if deemed necessary. A drainage tube should always be placed on low pressure suction to measure the rate of fluid accumulation; it can be removed when the daily volume is substantially less. Purulent pericardial fluid should prompt immediate antibiotic treatment with vancomycin and ampicillin for staphylococcal and hemophilus influenza coverage. Fluid analysis, cultures, and sensitivities will govern later antibiotic adjustments (23).

MYOCARDIAL INFARCTION

Myocardial infarction in infants and children is a relatively uncommon clinical problem with many pathophysiologic or anatomic causes. Among the more common causes are anomalous left main coronary artery arising from the main pulmonary artery (Bland-Garland-White disease), Kawasaki disease, myocarditis, and asphyxia. Rarely, a postoperative patient can also have coronary supply deficits. Unfortunately, drug usage, especially cocaine and amphetamines, has become a more frequent cause of myocardial ischemia, infarction, and sudden death in an otherwise healthy teenager without a cardiac disease history.

Evaluation

Symptoms and physical findings, which are often nonspecific, include vomiting, sweating, or inconsolable crying. Anginal chest pain can easily go unrecognized. On physical examination, gallop rhythms or a mitral regurgitation murmur may be detected. The 12-lead ECG is widely used as an initial screening test. Based on clinicopathologic correlation, Towbin developed criteria that include wide notched or unnotched Q waves of more than 35 milliseconds, ST segment elevation more than 2 mm, and prolongation of the corrected QT interval more than 440 milliseconds accompanied by Q waves (24). Serial ECGs should be performed during the acute period, along with constant monitoring for arrhythmias. Those with an anomalous left main coronary artery arising from the main pulmonary artery have the characteristic pattern of an anterolateral infarction with prominent Q waves in leads 1, aVL, V_5, and V_6. These changes may become minimal postoperatively or even return to normal on a resting ECG (Fig. 33.2).

Cardiac isoenzymes (creatinine kinase, lactate dehydrogenase, and glutamic oxaloacetic transferase [GOT]) are usually measured serially, but frequently are difficult to

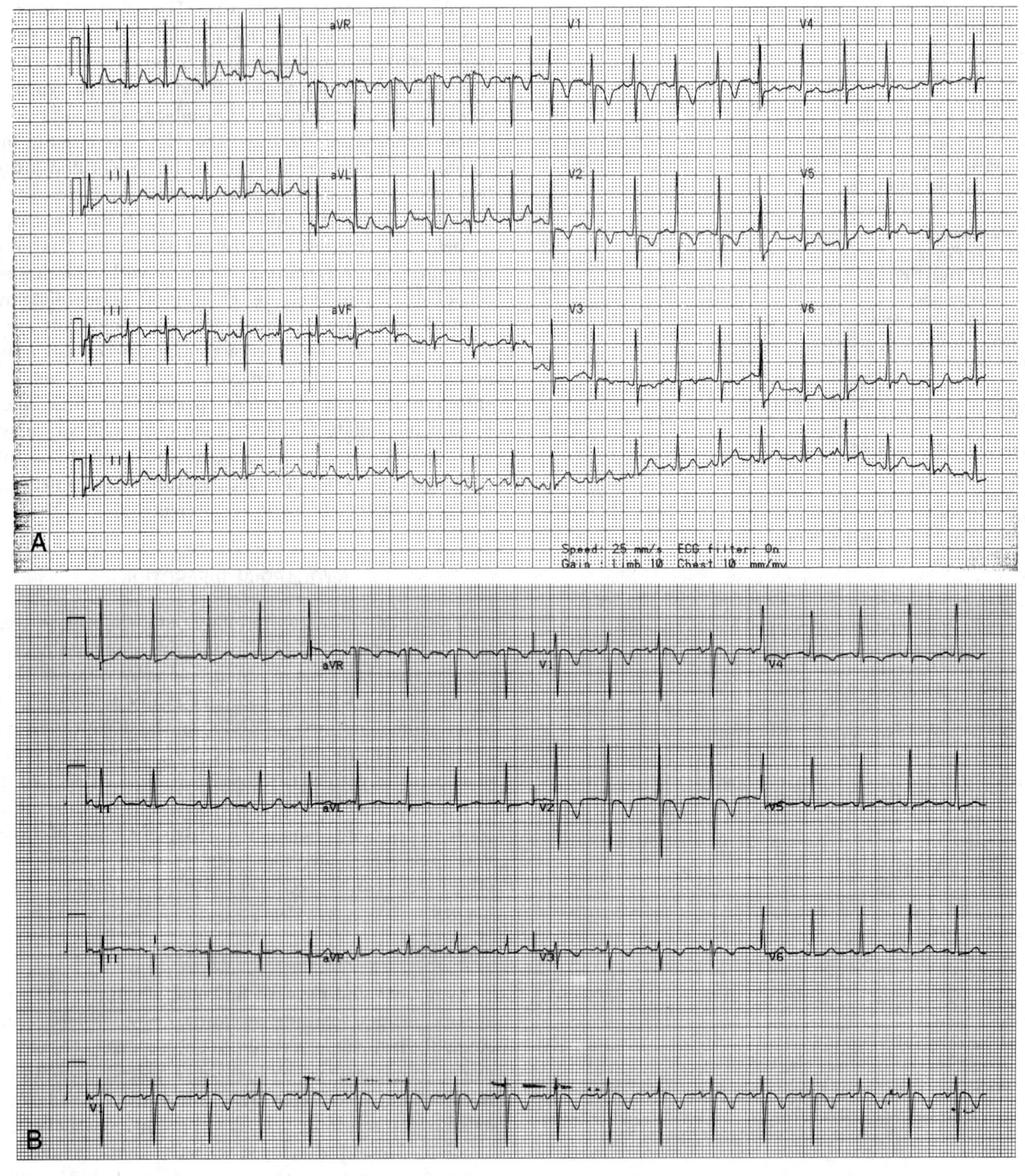

Figure 33.2. **A.** Myocardial infarction. A 3-month-old infant with acute anterolateral myocardial infarction from an anomalous left coronary artery arising from the main pulmonary artery. Note the Q waves in I and aVL on the electrocardiogram. **B.** Same patient 2-year status after revascularization. Note normalization of the ECG.

interpret in infants or small children. A creatinine kinase MB fraction more than 5% is suggestive, and it warrants serial studies and further diagnostic evaluations (25). The MB fraction peak will occur 24 to 48 hours after acute myocardial infarction, to be followed by GOT at 48 hours, and the lactate dehydrogenase at 5 days. Serum and urine toxicology for cocaine and amphetamines should be obtained on admission (26).

Echocardiography can delineate ventricular function, wall motion abnormality, coronary aneurysm formation, artrioventricular (AV) valve regurgitation, and intramural thrombus. The coronary ostial origins, arterial course, aneurysms, and color Doppler flow pattern can be evaluated to determine whether an anomalous left coronary system or other anomalies exist. Thallium imaging is useful to confirm the extent of infarction and differentiate potentially "stunned" myocardium from that which may be viable. Dipyridamole or adenosine infusion can be used as a potent coronary vasodilator, in place of exercise, for unmasking limited coronary reserve and mimicking stress-induced ischemia in the uncooperative child and infant (27).

If the anatomy is in doubt, cardiac catheterization with selective coronary angiograms will more clearly define the arterial anatomy and elucidate the pathophysiology by separating spasm, embolism, and thrombosis from arteriosclerotic narrowing. Early cardiac catheterization with selective coronary angiography is indicated when surgical revascularization is being considered to prevent further infarction; it should also be seriously considered if the cause is unclear. Localized stenosis can be bypassed with a native arterial conduit (i.e., internal mammary or radial), which has a higher long-term patency rate than saphenous venous grafts. In addition, if myocarditis is suspected, an endomyocardial biopsy can be obtained from the right or left ventricle.

Therapy

After a tentative diagnosis is made, acute therapy is tailored to the diagnosis, but it is generally focused at myocardial preservation to prevent further ischemic damage. The peri-infarct region of myocardium may be "stunned" and noncontractile, but still salvageable, and can return to normal function if coronary blood flow can be improved through either revascularizing the obstructed artery or developing collateral flow (28).

Constant electrocardiography, pulse oximetry, and blood pressure monitoring or telemetry are best accomplished in an intensive care setting with staff experienced with rhythm and ST segment interpretation. Transvenous pacing must be available to pace the heart if atrioventricular block and bradycardia ensue. Management of ventricular ectopy is best accomplished with lidocaine infusion, which is frequently started prophylactically. Defibrillation equipment should be easily accessible.

Acute stabilization also includes sedation, usually with an opiate, to diminish pain and limit increased stress from activity and crying. Supplemental inspired oxygen (with or without mechanical ventilation) may improve local O_2 tissue delivery and overcome any intrapulmonary shunt from pulmonary edema and left ventricular dysfunction.

Hypotension that develops from congestive heart failure with poor ventricular function or severe atrioventricular valve regurgitation may require volume expansion and judicious inotropic support. The balance between maintaining an adequate arterial perfusion pressure at the lowest possible left ventricular wall stress and myocardial O_2 consumption requires constant vigilance. Nitroglycerin, either sublingual, cutaneous, or intravenous, can further decrease myocardial O_2 requirements. β-blockade can decrease myocardial O_2 consumption and suppress ectopy, but it is contraindicated with severe pump failure. Calcium antagonists and angiotensin-converting enzyme inhibitors for afterload reduction have not been evaluated in children, but they have shown selective benefits in adults.

Anticoagulation with heparin is sometimes used in the acute phase if not contraindicated. Heparin has to be continued to prevent early rethrombosis with the partial thromboplastin time adjusted to one and a half to two times control until ambulation occurs (29–33). This is followed by early institution of antiplatelet agents, which will be continued into the convalescent phase. Thrombolytic agents, such as streptokinase or tPA (tissue thromboplastin activator) are administered parenterally within the first 6 to 12 hours during the ischemic phase to be effective. Thrombin time and fibrinogen level have to be measured with a prolongation of the thrombin time indicating fibrinolytic activity. Those with ventricular aneurysm, large anterior infarction, or akinetic ventricles are at high risk to develop mural thrombi, and they should be maintained on coumadin for 3 to 6 months.

SEPSIS

Septic shock, as with anaphylaxis or toxic shock syndrome, is a form of distributive shock. It is caused primarily by bacteremia, but it can also be seen in viremia and fungemia. Early recognition and treatment are essential to lessen the high mortality and morbidity rates.

Clinically, two distinct phases may be seen. Initially, in "warm shock," cardiac output is elevated with a hyperdynamic circulation, low filling pressures, and diminished peripheral vascular resistance. Peripheral perfusion is usually not diminished. This phase is followed by "cold shock," with myocardial depression and diminished cardiac output as well as extravascular transudation and elevated peripheral vascular resistance; peripheral perfusion is poor and the extremities cool (34, 35). It can be difficult to differentiate this shock from low cardiac output after cardiac surgery but recent research shows that circulating endotoxins are present in both (36, 37).

Evaluation

Initial evaluation of these patients should include all appropriate cultures, electrolytes, renal and liver function tests, arterial blood gas, blood count and clotting studies, along with close hemodynamic monitoring. A Swan-Ganz thermodilution catheter and arterial pressure line are essential to guide fluid and pressor therapy. An echocardiogram will help to assess pump function.

Therapy

Initially, crystalloid fluid resuscitation will often normalize blood pressure, and further fluid administration should be governed by hemodynamic monitoring. Hemorrhage from abnormalities in platelet number and function along with clotting deficiencies requires correction with blood products, clotting factors, and/or fresh frozen plasma. These large volumes of infused colloid will replace the ongoing losses that are being "third-spaced" because of capillary hyperpermeability.

Broad-spectrum antibiotic coverage should be empirically chosen to cover suspected pathogens with regard to common resistances, pending culture and sensitivity results. In postoperative patients, nosocomial infection from *Staphylococcus aureus* is frequently seen requiring vancomycin along with a third generation cephalosporin.

In the "cold shock" phase, hypoxia and ventilatory failure are frequently encountered, requiring mechanical ventilation. A low-grade metabolic acidosis unresponsive to volume indicates poor vascular perfusion and oxygen delivery, and it portends multiorgan ischemia, with resultant abnormalities in renal, hepatic, and central nervous system function. Profound metabolic acidosis with a lactate acidemia may warrant sodium bicarbonate administration to maintain pressor efficacy.

If poor ventricular shortening is seen by echocardiography, inotropic support should be initiated and higher doses (more than 10–15 μg/kg/min) may be necessary to achieve adequate vasoconstriction. Occasionally, norepinephrine, a potent α-agonist with less chronotropic and inotropic response, is effective in raising the systemic vascular resistance.

INTRACARDIAC MASSES

Detection of an intracardiac mass is most often in the setting of a larger diagnostic workup, such as endocarditis, acute pulmonary embolus, cerebrovascular event, or congestive cardiomyopathy (Table 33.4).

One frequent cause is thrombi from long-standing indwelling central venous lines for chemotherapy that terminate in the proximal superior vena cava or extend into the right atrium. As a foreign body, these catheters collect platelets and fibrin and the thrombogenicity can be further exacerbated by the pharmacologic infusions. These thrombi can become infected (most commonly with *S. aureus* or *Candida* organisms), friable, and embolize distally as well as obstruct the superior vena cava or interfere with right atrial filling and tricuspid valve function (38).

Evaluation

Blood cultures, obtained from a site other than the indwelling catheter being evaluated, are crucial to determine if the mass is infected, either as a primary vegetation or secondarily.

Echocardiography is the primary imaging modality used to detect intracardiac masses. Size, attachments, consistency, and texture of these masses can be useful in the characterization (Fig. 33.3). Sensitivity has been enhanced

Table 33.4. Intracardiac Masses

Neoplastic
  Malignant
    Wilms—Extension via inferior vena cava
    Melanoma—Metastatic
  Benign
    Rhabdomyoma—Tuberous sclerosis
    Myxoma
Thrombi
  Vegetations
    Endocarditis
  Systemic Venous Baffles
    Mustard, Senning, Fontan
  Foreign Body
  Prosthetic Valves
    Mechanical
  Catheters
    Pacemaker (permanent)
    Hickman, Broviac
    Diagnostic (temporary)
Coagulopathy
  Protein C,S and antithrombin III deficiency
  Polycythemia
  Thrombocytosis
Collagen Vascular
  Lupus erythematosus
  Periarteritis nodosa
Stasis
  Congestive cardiomyopathy
  Ventricular aneurysm
  Myocardial infarction
  "Giant atrium"
    Mitral stenosis
  Atrial fibrillation
Trauma
  Myocardial contusion
  Penetrating wounds
Artifact
  Trabeculations—false tendons

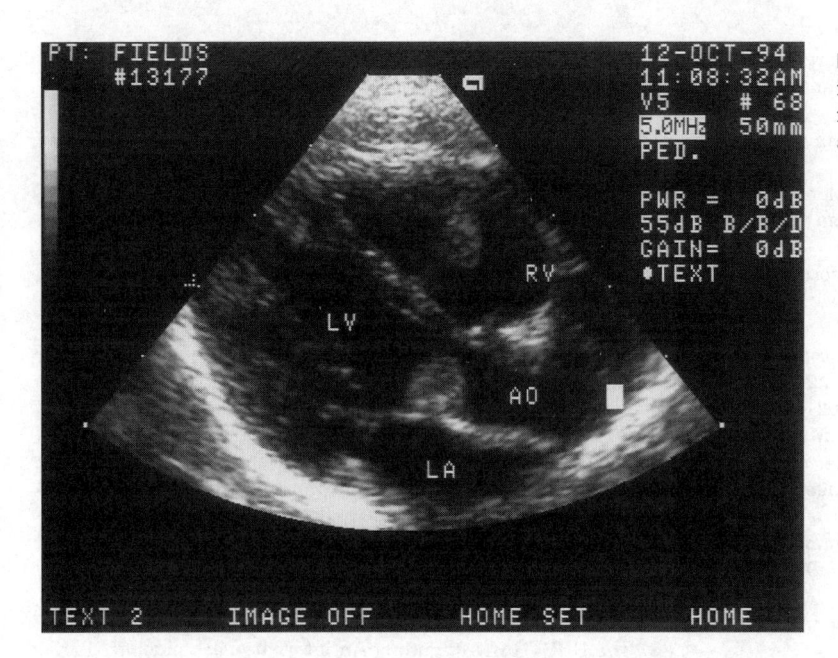

Figure 33.3. Intracardiac masses. Two rhabdomyomas in right ventricular and left ventricular outflow tracts in a 3-week-old infant with tuberous sclerosis. Ao, aorta; LA, left atrium.

by transesophageal echocardiography in selected cases, especially when imaging of the left and right atrial appendages is needed prior to cardioversion to prevent systemic embolization. Thrombi on foreign bodies (prosthetic valves and catheters) can be difficult to separate from the highly reflective plastic or metal unless they are sessile and move within the cardiac cavity.

Distal embolization of these masses should be investigated. Pulmonary emboli can be silent if small, or lead to dyspnea, hypoxia, chest pain, hypotension, and hemoptysis if large. The chest radiograph may demonstrate an infiltrate or elevated hemidiaphragm; the ECG can show acute signs of cor pulmonale with right atrial enlargement, right ventricular hypertrophy, or arrhythmias. Ventilation-perfusion scintigraphy and pulmonary angiography are sometimes necessary to confirm the diagnosis. Arterial embolization, either from a thrombus or paradoxic embolization across a patent foramen ovale, can lead to a downstream infarction. Altered mental status or seizures would suggest a cerebrovascular accident, necessitating a head CT or MRI. This should be performed prior to anticoagulation, which may not be advisable, because it could lead to further extension of a hemorrhagic infarct.

Therapy

An organized thrombus adherent to the endocardium, found incidentally on echocardiography, may not require any further attention or therapy as the risk of embolization is relatively low. It can either slowly fibrinolyse or calcify over time. Those masses with a higher risk of embolization may require IV heparinization followed by coumadin; an unchanged echocardiographic appearance of an intracardiac mass after a few months of follow-up may indicate a low risk for embolization or obstruction and may not justify the risks of indefinite anticoagulation therapy (39).

Sterilization of an infected catheter or prosthesis requires prolonged antibiotic therapy. If signs of infection or positive blood cultures persist, the foreign material should probably be removed. Catheters with large thrombi and masses are best removed surgically to prevent the mass from being embolized. Alternative causes of occult infection (e.g., phlebitis, myocardial abscess, brain abscess, immunodeficiency, and so forth) should be sought (38).

Thrombolysis can be used with freshly clotted material, and it is best delivered locally into the mass, often through the clotted catheter. Streptokinase can be injected through catheter or peripheral vein, and it will frequently dissolve the mass within 24 to 48 hours. Thrombin time is maintained at one and a half to two and a half times control. Recent surgery (within 2 months), bleeding, and allergy to streptococcal antigen are contraindications to its use (40, 41). The most frequent side effect is oozing at the catheter insertion site and puncture wounds, which can be controlled with pressure occlusion (42). Alternatively, urokinase is used in some institutions (43, 44). Certain anatomic masses (e.g., ones with sessile bases, larger sizes, or associated with flow disturbances or obstructions) may warrant surgical resection.

REFERENCES

1. Division of Injury Control, Center for Environmental Health and Injury Control, Centers for Disease Control. Childhood injuries in the United States. Am J Dis Child 1990;144: 627–646.
2. Templeton JM. Thoracic aorta and great vessel injuries. In: Fleisher GR, Ludwig S, eds. Textbook of pediatric emergency medicine. Baltimore: Williams & Wilkins, 1993:1160–1165.

3. Rothenberg SS, Moore EE, Moore FA, et al. Emergency department thoracotomy in children—a critical analysis. J Trauma 1989;29:1322–1325.
4. Meller JL, Little AG, Shermeta. Thoracic trauma in children. Pediatrics 1984;74:813–819.
5. Golladay ES, Donahoo JS, Haller JA. Special problems of cardiac injuries in infants and children. J Trauma 1979;19:526–531.
6. Nagy KK, Lohmann C, Kim DO, et al. Role of echocardiography in the diagnosis of occult penetrating cardiac injury. J Trauma 1995;38:859–862.
7. Meyer DM, Jessen ME, Grayburn PA. Use of echocardiography to detect occult cardiac injury after penetrating thoracic trauma: a prospective study. J Trauma 1995;39:902–909.
8. Fabian TC, Mangiante EC, Patterson CR, et al. Myocardial contusion in blunt trauma: clinical characteristics, means of diagnosis, and implications for patient management. J Trauma 1988;28:50–57.
9. Abrunzo TJ. Commotio cordis: the single most common cause of traumatic death in youth baseball. Am J Dis Child 1991;145:1279–1282.
10. Liedtke AJ, DeMuth WE. Non-penetrating cardiac injuries: a collective review. Am Heart J 1973;86:687–697.
11. Slater EE, DeSanctis RW. Dissection of the aorta. Med Clin N Am 1979;63:141–153.
12. Roman MJ, Rosen SE, Kramer-Fox R, et al. Prognostic significance of the pattern of aortic root dilation in the Marfan syndrome. J Am Coll Cardiol 1993;22:1470–1476.
13. Salim MA, Alpert BS, Ward JC, et al. Effect of beta-adrenergic blockade on aortic root rate dilation in the Marfan syndrome. Am J Cardiol 1994;74:629–633.
14. Nienaber CA, von Kodolitsch Y, Nicolas V, et al. The diagnosis of thoracic aortic dissection by noninvasive imaging procedures. N Engl J Med 1993;328:1–9.
15. Cigarroa JE, Isselbacher EM, DeSanctis RW, et al. Diagnostic imaging in the evaluation of suspected aortic dissection- old standards and new directions. N Engl J Med 1993;328:35–43.
16. DeSanctis RW, Doroghazi RM, Austen WG, et al. Aortic dissection. N Engl J Med 1987;317:1060–1067.
17. Hancock EW. Cardiac tamponade. Med Clin N Am 1979;63:223–237.
18. Freeman GL, LeWinter M. Pericardial adaptations during chronic cardiac dilation in dogs. Circ Res 1984;54:294–300.
19. Shabetai R. Diseases of the pericardium. In: Hurst JW, ed. The heart. New York: McGraw-Hill, 1990;1348–1374.
20. Fowler NO. Physiology of cardiac tamponade and pulsus paradoxus. II. Physiology, circulatory, and pharmacological responses in cardiac tamponade. Mod Concepts in Cardiovascular Disease 1978;47:115–118.
21. Brown J, MacKinnon D, King A, et al. Elevated arterial blood pressure in cardiac tamponade. N Engl J Med 1992;327:463–466.
22. Pinsky WW, Friedman RA. Pericarditis. In: Garson A, Bricker JT, McNamara DG, eds. The science and practice of pediatric cardiology. Philadelphia: Lea & Febiger, 1990;1590–1599.
23. Dupuis C, Gonnier P, Kachaner J, et al. Bacterial pericarditis in infancy and childhood. Am J Cardiol 1994;74:807–809.
24. Towbin JA. Myocardial infarction in childhood. In: Garson A, Bricker JT, McNamara DG, eds. The science and practice of pediatric cardiology. Philadelphia: Lea & Febiger, 1990;1684–1722.
25. Ingwall JS, Kramer MF, Fifer MA, et al. The creatine kinase system in normal and diseased human myocardium. N Engl J Med 1985;313:1050–1054.
26. Mathias DW. Cocaine associated myocardial ischemia: review of clinical and angiographic findings. Am J Med 1986;675–678.
27. Schelbert HR. Current status and prospects of new radionuclides and radiopharmaceuticals for cardiovascular nuclear medicine. Semin Nucl Med 1987;17:145–181.
28. Jeroudi MO, Cheirif J, Habib G, et al. Prolonged wall motion abnormalities after chest pain at rest in patients with unstable angina: a possible manifestation of myocardial stunning. Am Heart J 1994;127:1241–1250.
29. The TIMI IIIB investigators. Effects of tissue plasminogen activator and a comparison of early invasive and conservative strategies in unstable angina and non-Q-wave myocardial infarction. Circulation 1994;89:1545–1556.
30. White HD, Rivers JT, Maslowski AH, et al. Effect of intravenous streptokinase as compared with that of tissue plasminogen activator on left ventricular function after first myocardial infarction. N Engl J Med 1989;320:817–821.
31. Bleich SD, Richard R, Teichman S. Effect of heparin on coronary arterial patency after thrombolysis with tissue plasminogen activator in acute myocardial infarction. Am J Cardiol 1990;66:1412–1417.
32. The GUSTO investigators. An international randomized trial comparing four thrombolytic strategies for acute myocardial infarction. N Engl J Med 1993;329:673–682.
33. The GUSTO angiographic investigators. The effects of tissue plasminogen activator, streptokinase, or both on coronary arterial patency, ventricular function, and survival after acute myocardial infarction. N Engl J Med 1993;329:673–682.
34. Voyce SJ, Becker RC. Adaptive and maladaptive cardiovascular responses in human sepsis. Am Heart J 1991;122:1441–1448.
35. Vincent JL, Gris P, Coffernils M, et al. Myocardial depression characterizes the fatal course of septic shock. Surgery 1992;111:660–667.
36. Casey WF, Hauser GJ, Hannallah RS, et al. Circulating endotoxin and tumor necrosis factor during pediatric cardiac surgery. Crit Care Med 1992;20:1090–1096.
37. Jansen NJG, van Oeveren W, Gu YJ, et al. Endotoxin release and tumor necrosis factor formation during cardiopulmonary bypass. Ann Thorac Surg 1992;54:744–748.
38. King DR, Komer M, Hoffman J, et al. Broviac catheter sepsis: the natural history of an iatrogenic infection. J Pediatr Surg 1985;20:728–733.
39. Prince A, Heller B, Levy J, et al. Management of fever in patients with ventral vein catheters. Pediatr Infect Dis 1986;5:20–24.
40. Wang EEL, Prober CG, Ford-Jones L. The management of central intravenous catheter infections. Pediatr Infect Dis 1984;3:110–113.
41. Nahata MC, King DR, Powell DW, et al. Management of catheter-related infections in pediatric patients. JPEN 1988;12:58–59.
42. Wessel DL, Keane JF, Fellows KE, et al. Fibrinolytic therapy for femoral arterial thrombosis after cardiac catheterization in infants and children. Am J Cardiol 1986;58:347–351.
43. Bagnall HA, Gomperts E, Atkinson, JB. Continuous infusion of low-dose urokinase in the treatment on central venous catheter thrombosis in infants and children. Pediatrics 1989;83:963–966.
44. Delaplane D, Scott JP, Riggs TW, et al. Urokinase therapy for a catheter-related right atrial thrombus. J Pediatr 1982;100:149–152.

Section VI.

Issues in Cardiac Intensive Care

Nursing Perspective in the Cardiac Intensive Care Unit

Patricia Hickey, MS RN, and Teresa Atz, BSN RN

For critical care nurses involved in the care of infants and children with congenital heart disease, these are exciting times. A wonderful opportunity exists to provide leadership to the reshaping of the delivery of patient services and to strengthen the scope of the nurse's role as a direct care provider and collaborator.

This chapter describes innovative nursing roles and practices that can be implemented in cardiac intensive care units (CICUs). In successful practice environments, a genuine mutual respect and collegiality exists between CICU nurses and their medical and surgical associates. This contributes to optimal patient outcomes and satisfied patients and families who feel supported during one of the most stressful experiences of their lives. The impact of such collaborative spirit and passionate commitment to common goals cannot be underestimated in a pediatric critical care environment.

PROFESSIONAL PRACTICE MODEL: SHARED GOVERNANCE

The successful professional practice model in the CICU is a unit-based governance system in which staff nurses are empowered and have accountability for all aspects of their practice. Peer review is a well-established evaluation process. Individual nurses are accountable to peers for collaboration, communication, and commitment and to the director or nurse manager of the CICU for overall productivity and performance.

Cardiac ICU nurses maintain accountability for clinical practice standards, quality of care, assurance of peer competency, and the continuing education and development of peers by participating in unit-based councils that are chaired by senior staff nurses. These unit-based councils include (a) practice, (b) education, (c) peer review, and (d) leadership. The nursing director or nurse manager's role is one of involvement with issues that provide support for practice such as staffing, resources use, and finance. In a shared governance model, the manager's role is one of integration, facilitation, and coordination. The manager supports peer review and provides the necessary resources for the clinical nurse to practice and develop professionally.

PROFESSIONAL ADVANCEMENT

Many professional advancement programs are based on the work of Benner, who describes the advancement of nurses from novice to expert using the Dreyfus Model of Skill Acquisition. Benner explains how, through experience, a nurse attains increasing levels of clinical expertise and scope of practice. The practitioner advances through five phases: novice, advanced beginner, competent, proficient, and expert and moves from a focus of self-development (novice) to one that influences change and the development of the profession as a whole (expert) (1). Three levels of nurses practice in the CICU at Children's Hospital, Boston. These levels of practice are categorized as follows:

Staff Nurse Level I: Competent

Staff Nurse Level II: Proficient

Staff Nurse Level III: Expert

Differentiated levels of practice allow each nurse to be evaluated by objective standards appropriate to current level of practice. Each level describes practice in four domains: (a) clinical practice, (b) leadership, (c) professional growth, and (d) quality improvement.

UNIT-BASED INTERDISCIPLINARY PRACTICE

Because of the critical patient focused nature of the work, CICU nurses at every level collaborate with physicians and other members of the team to provide quality patient outcomes through interdisciplinary care plans. Patient-focused policies, procedures, and standards of practice are developed jointly by these nurses and physicians. In successful programs is found an interdisciplinary structure to all components of the care process, including patient care rounds, team conferences, morbidity and mortality conferences, and quality improvement and cost containment efforts.

RESTRICTED PRACTICES

A successful interdisciplinary effort to certify proficient and expert level nurses to discontinue intracardiac monitoring catheters, perform right ventricular-pulmonary arterial pressure gradient measurements when pulmonary arterial catheters are withdrawn, and to remove chest tubes was implemented in the early 1990's in the CICU at Children's Hospital, Boston. These nurses received education from their physician colleagues about correct technique, interpretation of chest x-rays, and analysis of hemodynamic waveforms to competently perform the procedures. Every CICU nurse who advances to the proficient level receives this education. Each year the nurses are recertified by demonstrating competence in knowledge and skill for these restricted practices. Prior to the inception of this practice, one nurse clinician was responsible for discontinuing all intracardiac monitoring catheters, chest tubes, and performing right ventricular-pulmonary artery pressure gradient measurements. This collaborative endeavor has demonstrated that properly trained critical care nurses can achieve the same low complication rate as physicians or nurse clinicians. To determine the complication rate when nurses removed the monitoring catheters, the quality improvement (QI) coordinator kept detailed records on every line nurses pulled during a 1-year period. Data in this prospective study cover 461 pulmonary artery lines, 316 left atrial lines, and 431 right atrial lines (2) (Table 34.1).

Another restricted practice for proficient and expert level staff nurses in the CICU is the role of charge nurse. As part of their leadership responsibilities at the proficient and expert level, the charge nurse works collaboratively with the attending CICU physician to manage patient flow and the daily operations of the CICU.

EXPANDED STAFF NURSE ROLES

Several creative roles can be designed for CICU expert staff nurses to support the work of the CICU and also to influence practice and patient outcomes throughout the entire continuum of a cardiovascular program. These roles are successful because they are performed by expert staff nurses who remain engaged in the "real work" of continuing to take care of patients at least 50% of the time.

Education Coordinator

Education coordinator is the role designed for an expert CICU staff nurse who has completed a master's degree program. In addition to clinical and leadership responsibilities, 50% of the time in this position is spent developing, implementing, and evaluating professional staff nurse orientation, inservices, and continuing education programs for the CICU. The educational coordinator also provides the appropriate orientation competencies and education for the clinical assistants in the CICU.

Cross-Training Program

The education coordinator also assumes responsibility for the cross-training program, which enables CICU nurses to routinely rotate into the cardiac catheterization laboratory as well as voluntary rotation to the cardiac inpatient ward and clinic. A cadre of cardiac inpatient nurses can also be trained to work in the CICU.

Quality Improvement Coordinator

This expert level CICU staff nurse, the quality improvement (QI) coordinator, co-chairs the cardiovascular program QI committee with a CICU attending physician. Together, they coordinate all QI efforts in the CICU and across the cardiovascular program.

Clinical Practice Guidelines Coordinator

Clinical practice guidelines (CPG) coordinator is the role designed for a masters degree-prepared expert staff nurse. In addition to clinical and leadership responsibilities within the program, 50% of the time the position involves coordinating the CPG effort. The CPG coordinator is responsible for educating all the nurses and physicians within the program about the CPG process, as well as collecting and reporting case and mix data for the CPG committee, designing the actual CPG, monitoring variances, chairing the cardiovascular program CPG committee, and representing the cardiovascular program on the hospital CPG committee.

FAMILY-CENTERED CARE

Admission of a critically ill infant or child to the CICU is one of the greatest stressors for any family, especially if the admission is unplanned. Anxiety, fear, helplessness, and hopelessness are common feelings experienced by family members. Fear of death is the most common one, cou-

Table 34.1. Intracardiac Line Removal by Cardiac Intensive Care Unit Nurses

Line	N	Complications: N(%)	N(%)
PA	461	Bleeding: 7(1.5)	10(2.1)
		Transient hemodynamic instability: 2(0.4)	
		Tamponade: 1(0.2)	
LA	316	Entrapment: 6(1.9)	6(1.9)
RA	431	Entrapment: 3(0.7)	5(1.2)
		Bleeding: 2(0.5)	
TOTAL	1208		21(1.2)

PA, Pulmonary artery; LA, Left atrial; RA, Right atrial; N, Number; N(%), Percentage of complications.

pled with fear of possible brain damage. The strange environment, equipment tubes, sights, and sounds in the CICU are common fears as well. Parents may be unnerved by their child's behaviors and emotional responses. Studies show that most parents feel information is the most important factor in lessening anxiety (3). Other factors are trusting care givers, being recognized as important to their child's recovery, being able to help care for the child, having friends and family nearby, and being given reassurance and hope. Despite all of the fears parents face, research studies suggest difficult stressors are feelings of separation and role deprivation (3). It is the nurse's responsibility to facilitate trust by providing information, assisting parents to cope, and facilitating in the re-establishment of parental roles. Ongoing assessments of families and their vulnerabilities and strengths allow nurses to devise effective strategies that focus on minimizing stress and enhancing coping skills (3). A reliable method of accomplishing this is giving parents what is most important to them—information.

PRENATAL PROGRAM

Because parents are the most important resources nurses have in reducing the anxiety of a child, it is important that they are prepared adequately for their child's hospitalization (3). This preparation can begin as early as in the prenatal period. At the cardiovascular program at Children's Hospital in Boston, a prenatal program has been designed for families with an unborn child diagnosed by fetal echocardiogram with a congenital heart defect. This program was designed to:

- reduce parental anxiety by providing accurate and appropriate information about their baby's defect and the anticipated course of treatment for the baby after birth
- introduce the parents to the care environment (CICU)
- establish a liaison person with whom the parents can communicate throughout the remainder of the prenatal course and birth

This program is voluntary, and it is introduced to the parents following initial diagnosis. It is at this time that the parent-professional relationship is established. Parents begin to make many important decisions and changes. Some mothers are encouraged to deliver at a high-risk tertiary care center. Some parents choose not to continue the pregnancy. Whatever the decision, an interdisciplinary team of cardiovascular physicians, nurses, and social workers attempts to help the families through this difficult and emotional time. Parents receive a telephone call within a week of the diagnosis from the liaison nurse and usually an appointment is made to meet with the family on the day of the next echocardiogram. Parents are encouraged to write down questions in preparation for the meeting.

The meeting, which is held in a quiet area in the CICU, includes general discussions regarding the baby's defect and the parent's expectations and questions. A brief tour of the CICU and ward is conducted, followed by a return to the meeting place for further discussions of any questions. Handouts are given that include information regarding breast-feeding, blood donation, CICU parent information booklet, and the nurse's business card. It is not unusual for parents to make subsequent visits. If they request a parent to parent contact, every effort is made to honor the request. The program is currently being evaluated after its first year, and the feedback received from families thus far has been positive.

A similar program is in place for children and families who are preparing for cardiac surgery. Verbal preoperative teaching begins immediately on admission to the ward or on clinic visits if the child is a same day of surgery admission. Families, and children if appropriate, are offered a tour of the CICU. They are shown an infant who has had surgery that day. Ventilators and monitors are explained as well as chest tubes, intracardiac monitoring catheters, incision, and overall appearance of the child. Parents are informed about what they can expect as far as visiting, procedures, and sleeping and waiting areas. This is generally an emotional time for families. The tour and information are tailored to each individual family. Although every attempt is made to prepare parents for their stay in the CICU, they often state that they are never prepared for the sight of their own child postoperatively. Nurses take the time to cover the incision, tubes, and any blood, and encourage parents to bring in a favorite blanket or toys for the child to hold. The literature is replete with studies that show that excellent physical care of a child is the cornerstone of developing parental trust, which is integral to coping (3).

PARENT INFORMATION GROUP

The cardiovascular program at Children's Hospital in Boston also has a parent information group meeting every week. The group is led by a CICU nurse and cardiovascular social worker. It is a forum where parents can share their experience with other parents and draw strength from others' experiences. As families' support systems are often unavailable, it is crucial that families receive the support they need from alternative sources (4).

This program was initiated during the mid-1980s by a core group of CICU nurses. The name has recently been changed from "Parent Support Group" to "Parent Information Group" to encourage participation. The term "support" can be viewed in a negative or threatening way, implying a need for psychotherapy (5). Each week the group meets for 1 hour. The time is usually in the mid-afternoon, a time when most parents are waiting to visit their children postoperatively. The time is posted weekly in both the parents' waiting room and at each child's bedside. Parents introduce themselves, and they are encouraged to talk about their child and share experiences and feelings with the group. Parents generally are supportive of each other as they can relate to each other's experiences.

Feedback from parents has been positive. A questionnaire given out after the meeting asks for evaluations and suggestions. Nurses, as well, have given positive feedback. It is important to communicate with parents away from the stress at the bedside, and to be able to participate in such family-centered care.

CARDIOPULMONARY RESUSCITATION CLASSES

Cardiopulmonary resuscitation (CPR) classes have been known to boost parents' confidence in caring for their child (6). Some may feel the stress created by the hospitalization of a critically ill child is too distracting for an appropriate learning process. However, studies have shown that these families generally can learn despite their anxiety level (7). Many CICUs now include parent CPR classes for infants and children in their program.

Weekly classes are led by a core group of CICU and ward nurses. Pamphlets with step-by-step instructions for CPR are given out prior to the class for the parents to study. This is an informal class lasting at least an hour or until everyone is comfortable performing their skills. Feedback has been positive and parents state that they feel more confident about caring for their children at home.

TRANSITIONAL FAMILY CARE

When a child is well enough to transfer from the CICU to the ward, parents can feel anxious and afraid instead of relieved. Families have just begun to familiarize themselves and be comfortable with the CICU environment and the nurses and physicians. Now, families are faced with new staff and new routines. The nurse:patient ratio may now be 1:4 or 1:5 instead of 1:1 or 1:2. Knowing that nurses will not always be in the rooms creates feelings of frustration and abandonment for some parents. It is the responsibility of the nurse to devise a plan of care to facilitate this transition (8).

On admission to the CICU or the ward, a family education plan of care is initiated and communicated to all of the nurses caring for the child. This facilitates consistency of care and education. An information packet is given to parents before or during admission. This helps familiarize parents with both the CICU and ward by showing pictures and explaining routines. If the family and the child have been in the hospital long term, frequent interdisciplinary team meetings are planned, including staff from both the CICU and the ward, to maintain continuity of care. Families are often included in these meetings. CICU nurses prepare families for the ward by discussing the different routines they may encounter. This is all documented and discussed with the inpatient ward nurses on transfer. It is not unusual for the CICU nurse to arrange for a group of inpatient ward nurses to care for a patient, especially if the patient has been in the CICU for a long period of time. Follow-up visits by the CICU nurses continue until discharge.

BEREAVEMENT PROGRAM

No greater loss may occur than the parent's loss of a child. Grief experienced by parents is particularly severe, long-lasting, and devastating (9). Often such a sense of yearning for the child exists that it can heighten feelings of loneliness, helplessness, anger, and despair. During this time parents are at risk for major physical symptoms that can fluctuate over a long period of time. The death of a child is particularly devastating to parents because of the lack of previous knowledge and experience from which to draw strength or resources. Potential for negative family coping is a great risk at this time (10).

Many factors hinder effective family coping. Guilt is a normal part of the grief process. Although it is common, it can be devastating. Feelings of guilt can occur if parents blame themselves for the cause of death. They may blame others exhibiting displacement or projection of blame. Parents can even desperately want to punish themselves for the child's suffering. Detaching themselves from the pain by removing themselves from the situation or from others can be harmful, because they can be detaching themselves from their only support systems. Refusing to talk to anyone about the death frequently potentiates feelings of guilt and loneliness (4).

Nurses in the CICU inevitably experience the death of a patient and are actively involved in the dying process of children (11). Nurses are an integral part of the parents' support system. The CICU nurse intervenes by focusing on the family as a whole and by being present both physically and emotionally (4). Helping parents to cope with the grieving process is one of the greatest privileges of being a CICU nurse.

Goals of a CICU bereavement program are to support and educate the family of a child before and after death to facilitate grieving. The nurse caring for the child assists parents with all of the potentially overwhelming decisions they need to make, for example, funeral arrangements and family contacts. Parents are allowed to hold their child if they wish. The child's personal effects are given to the parents before they leave as well as the phone number of the CICU and the nurse's name. A follow-up phone call to parents is made about 2 weeks after the child's death. The nurse also sends the parents a card along with bereavement information, including names of support groups in their area, and information on how to talk to siblings and other family members about the death. Parents know that they can always call the CICU with questions as they can feel uncomfortable talking about the death of their child with others who they perceive may not understand. The nurse can assist families in making contacts with bereavement workshops, mental health practitioners, and other families, as appropriate.

CONCLUSION

Enormous privileges accrue to practice with critically ill infants and children. Caring for children with cardiac disease at this time in their illness is a special challenge. Care is provided for the family as a whole at a time of true crisis. It is the wholeness of expert nursing and medical practice in a collegial and risk willing environment that creates the optimal advantage for these patients and their families.

REFERENCES

1. Benner P. From novice to expert. Am J Nurs 1982;82:402–407.
2. Barker S. Nurses remove transthoracic intracardiac lines safely. CV Nurse: Trends in Cardiovascular Care 1993;6:8.
3. Miles MS, Mathes M. Preparation of parents for the ICU experience. Children's Health Care 1991;20:132–137.
4. Heiney SP, Hasan L, Price K. Developing and implementing a bereavement program for a children's hospital. J Pediatr Nurs 1993;8:385–391.
5. McClelland M. Our unit has a bereavement program. Am J Nurs 1993;93:62–66.
6. Donaher-Wagner BM, Braun DH. Infant cardiopulmonary resuscitation for expectant and new parents. Matern Child Nurs J 1992;17:27–29.
7. Sigsbee M. Effects of anxiety on family members of patients with cardiac disease learning cardiopulmonary resuscitation. Heart Lung 1990;19:662–665.
8. Braun R, St Clair C. Transitional family care: PICU to pediatrics. Crit Care Nurse 1994;14:65–68.
9. Stutzer CA. Developing a bereavement follow-up program for families of children who die of cancer. J Pediatr Oncol Nurs 1991;8:69.
10. Miles MS, Perry K. Parental responses to sudden accidental death of a child. Crit Care Quart 1985;8:73–84.
11. de Groot-Bollujt W, Mourik M. Bereavement: role of the nurse in the care of terminally ill and dying children in the pediatric intensive care unit. Crit Care Med 1993;21:391–392.

The Role of the Advanced Practice Nurse 35

Leslie Schoenberg, RN, MN, CPNP, and Barbara P. Gross, RN, MSN

Advances in the surgical and medical management of infants and children with congenital heart disease have led to an increase in the acuity of patients in the cardiac intensive care unit (CICU). External forces in the marketplace make cost reduction a critical imperative, resulting in closer scrutiny of how patients are managed while hospitalized. Along with this, resident education has changed focus from specialty care to primary care, which in turn lowers the number of residents available for intensive care management (1). In response to these changes in health care, the role of the advanced practice nurse (APN) is evolving to meet the needs in critical care.

Advanced practice nurses are those with a graduate degree in nursing, and they include clinical nurse specialists (CNS) and nurse practitioners (NP) (2). Nurses in advanced clinical practice function in an expanded nursing role by conducting comprehensive health assessments and diagnosing and treating responses to intricate health problems (3). Graduate level curriculum for the APN includes advanced physical assessment, pathophysiology, patient management strategies, research, and education techniques. Acute care practitioners have completed internships during their training in the intensive care unit (ICU) setting. Highly skilled APNs are innovators; they are able to analyze complex clinical problems to effect system changes. These competencies allow the APN to function as an independent practitioner, in collaboration with the multidisciplinary team, to manage and coordinate care for critically ill children and their families (2). APNs are responsible for keeping updated on current practice in their fields through continuing education and involvement in professional organizations.

In one model, APNs evaluate patients each morning, review their clinical course and current management, perform a physical assessment, and consult with the team to determine necessary changes in the treatment plan. Written protocols are used to manage changes in the patient's condition. These protocols specify problems that the APN can manage independently versus those requiring physician consultation. Other responsibilities include daily notes, follow-up of laboratory studies, coordination with consult services, admission and discharge orders, and performance of other necessary procedures (e.g., removing intracardiac lines and chest tubes, inserting arterial and central lines, intubating patients, pulling pacer wires).

In this chapter, we discuss the role of the APN as patient manager, educator, researcher, community liaison, and case manager, as well as future trends for APNs in critical care.

THE ROLE OF THE ADVANCED PRACTICE NURSE IN PATIENT MANAGEMENT

Dramatic changes are taking place in health care systems which influence the roles of all health care workers. The creation of the role of the APN in the critical care setting evolved in response to these changes. It is a role that merges and extends many of the functions of the CNS and NP. APNs are now being utilized as direct patient managers as a result of the decreased number of residents available in specialty settings.

In many pediatric institutions, house staff have traditionally been responsible for patient care in the ICU. Recently, however, resident education focus has shifted to primary care. Training programs are assessing the amount of tertiary experience required and moving residents out of the ICUs to ambulatory sites (1). This gap created by this refocusing is being filled by NPs and specialty fellows who are stable, experienced care givers rather than rotating residents who may have less knowledge of pediatric care (4).

For many years, primary care NPs have worked in a collaborative practice model with physician colleagues in the primary care setting. This paradigm can be transferred to the critical care setting. Collaborative practice involves jointly determining relationships between the nurses and physicians to integrate care regimens into a single comprehensive approach to meet patient's needs (5).

EDUCATION

Educational background enables the APN to assess the learning needs of and create educational programs for staff, patients, families, and the community (6). Formal and informal education include orientation classes, ongoing inservice education and impromptu teaching sessions, and conferences. Patient and family education is an essential component of the APN's role that often is accomplished by equipping staff nurses to educate families along with providing direct patient teaching. The APN is also responsible for overseeing the development and evaluation of educational materials used for patients and families. Through role modeling, staff empowerment, and development of educational materials, the APN can have a positive impact on patients and staff alike (7).

RESEARCH

The APN is the staff nurse's link to using research findings to improve patient care (8). APNs can use research methods to advance overall practice (9). Research can be transferred into the clinical setting for bedside care givers in several ways: through regular journal club meetings, by maintaining an archive of current literature in the ICU, and by circulating specific articles related to current clinical situations.

Many cardiac surgery programs use data bases to assist with collecting research information. These can contain detailed information about patients' diagnoses, surgery, length of hospitalization, and postoperative course. Data gathered about large numbers of patients with similar diagnoses can be analyzed by the APN to detect trends and track complications to improve clinical care.

The APN can participate in clinical research in the CICU as a primary investigator or in collaboration with other researchers. The APN should have knowledge of all clinical studies or protocols that impact on patient care in the CICU. Involvement in these studies can include identifying research problems, developing research protocols, educating the staff providing care, collecting and analyzing data, and publishing results.

CASE MANAGEMENT

Increased acuity of hospitalized patients coupled with the mandatory reduction in health care costs led to the development of a systematic approach to managing patient care now referred to as "case management." Case management is defined by the American Nurses Association as a system of health care delivery that facilitates achievement of expected patient outcomes within an appropriate length of stay (10). Case management goals include providing quality health care throughout the hospital course, minimizing fragmentation of care across settings, and efficiently utilizing resources (11).

The APN in the critical care unit is in an ideal position to provide case management by coordinating each patient's treatment plan to ensure the delivery of quality, cost-effective care. This involves creating systems and procuring the resources needed by each patient and family to achieve optimal outcomes within an appropriate time frame.

Critical pathways were developed in conjunction with case management. An example of critical pathways at Childrens Hospital Los Angeles, Multidisciplinary Action Plans (MAPs), is shown in Figure 35.1. These plans identify key events from preadmission through discharge that must occur in a timely manner to achieve an appropriate length of stay. Essential treatments, laboratory tests, medications, and nursing care are outlined for each day of care (12). Patient outcomes are identified and tracked; deviations from the pathway are monitored closely so that any changes required in the patient's care or in the care delivery system can be identified and addressed. MAPs are effective in streamlining care for children who have surgical procedures with highly patternable postoperative courses, but they can be less applicable for congenital lesions with heterogeneous presentations or expected recovery.

As an integral part of the multidisciplinary team, the APN coordinates the development and implementation of appropriate MAPs for pediatric cardiac patients and is a consultant and resource to the direct care givers. The APN has the advanced assessment skills necessary to determine variations in the critical pathway, anticipate potential problems, and implement interventions aimed at preventing the occurrence of these problems (12).

Many CICU patients present with unique problems that do not lend themselves to management via a critical pathway. These patients require individualized case management. The APN's clinical expertise enables him or her to identify optimal outcomes, develop a personalized plan of care, and mobilize appropriate resources to implement this plan (13). The APN can shorten hospital stays by attending to important details such as ensuring optimal nutrition, managing respiratory support, preventing infections by early removal of invasive lines, carefully monitoring fluid and electrolyte status, and overseeing medications management in consultation with the physician.

Several studies have demonstrated the advantages of case management models. Nugent described increased patient satisfaction, enhanced nurse satisfaction, and reduced health care costs when case management was utilized (12). Thompson reported a decreased length of stay and cost savings for premature infants managed via a critical pathway (14); and Schull et al. found that utilization of APNs (specifically CNSs) as case managers resulted in impressive improvements in outcomes, increased compliance with follow-up appointments, lower hospital charges, and decreased lengths of stay (15).

Financial Implications

The health care environment has become increasingly competitive. Fee-for-service providers are less common, and the proliferating managed care providers are demanding lower costs. They are attempting to control costs for some disease processes by contracting for a specific overall payment for the episode of illness rather than paying on a per diem basis. This has led to the development of case rates, or packaged fees, for certain groups of patients.

Multidisciplinary action plans facilitate the formation of

Case Type: Surgical Repair of Patent Ductus Arteriosus (≥ 12 months)
Excludes premature infants and patients with pulmonary hypertension, bronchopulmonary dysplasia, pulmonary disease, uncontrolled congestive heart failure, and associated cardiac anomalies

UNIT:	Surgical Admitting	OR to PACU to 6 West	6 West–Discharge POD #1
DATE:			
PROCESS:	Pre-Admit	Day 1 Day of Admit	Day 2 (Begins 12 AM)
1. Lab Dx Evaluation	10 Hemogram, Type & Screen optional: Electrolytes if on diuretics	11	12
2. Radiology Dx Evaluation	20 CXR – PA view (if one not done within past 6 week period &/or not available)	21	22
3. Other Dx Evaluation	30 History and Physical Exam done by Cardio-thoracic service	31	32
4. Medications	40	41 Antibiotics (Ancef) in OR and q 8 hr × 2 doses Pain Management: Morphine intermittent or PCA Morphine 30 min prior to chest tube removal Acetaminophen for temp ≥ 38.5 or mild pain	42 Pain management DC Morphine PO pain med prn ———————→
5. Treatment	50	51 Surgical Procedure Extubate in OR Cardiorespiratory and continuous pulse ox monitoring × 12 hr VS per PACU then q 4 hr Chest tube to 15 cm suction, monitor drainage q 2 hr × 2 then q 4 hr DC chest tube and dressing in pm if no air leak and drainage < 5 cc/kg/hr Oxygen per NC, wean keeping O₂ sat > 95% Chest physiotherapy or incentive spirometry as indicated Strict I & O	52 VS q 4 hr Continue to wean oxygen, then DC, keeping O₂ sat > 92 ———————→ ———————→
6. Consults	60 Anesthesiology evaluation	61	62
7. Nutrition	70	71 IVF full maintenance NPO advance diet as tolerated when bowel sounds present Heplock IV when tolerating clears	72 Regular diet for age (PO fluids ad lib) DC IV heplock
8. Activity	80	81 Turn q 4 hr until OOB OOB to chair in pm	82 Full ambulation (age dependent) or up ad lib
9. Psychosocial/Spiritual	90 Assess level of anxiety, provide support	91 ———————→	92 ———————→

10. Patient problems	100 Refer to Standard of Care for Heart Surgery & Pre-Op Care N-II027 Cardiovascular/ respiratory assessment with VS	101 ⟶ Dressing check with VS	102 ⟶ Incision check with VS
11. Teaching	110 Pre-op teaching: Surgical procedure Review "Pre-op Cardiac Teaching Book" with pt/family Pain Management Discuss "Pre-op letter"	111 Update family re progress Include family in care giving Instruct family re home care Review "Caring for your Child after Heart Surgery," "Endocarditis Prophylaxis" Reinforce cough/deep breathing/spirometry	112 Final review of home care instructions Review F/U appointments
12. Discharge Plan	120 Discuss anticipated length of stay	121 Notify family of probable discharge Arrange F/U appointments, discuss with family MD to write Rx for meds if indicated	122 Assess readiness for discharge
13. Outcomes	130 Pre-op evaluation, labs completed Pt/family prepared for surgery Discharge planning initiated	131 To OR per schedule VS stable Transferred to general floor Chest tube removed in pm	132 VS stable Afebrile Incision without signs of infection Tolerating oral feeds Pt/family verbalizes knowledge per "Education Discharge Planning" form Discharge home
Variation from MAP	☐ Yes* ☐ No	☐ Yes* ☐ No	☐ Yes* ☐ No

*Document intervention and assign variance code
This MAP is designed as a tool for patient care coordination and as a guideline for clinical care. This does not represent a standard of care. The plan of care may be modified according to individual patient's needs.

Figure 35.1. Childrens Hospital Los Angeles: Multidisciplinary Action Plan (MAP).

case rates for patients undergoing cardiac surgery because required treatments and staffing are specified, making cost determination easy. The APN is then responsible for managing available resources to ensure that the desired patient outcome is achieved within the case rate fee structure.

REFERRAL LIAISON

Cardiovascular programs are dependent on referrals from community and hospital-based physicians and managed care providers. A key role as the liaison for all referral sources is filled by APNs who assist with patient transfers into the hospital, provide a communication link during the patient's hospitalization, and transition patients back to their referral source. This is achieved by maintaining frequent telephone contact and sending updates, operative reports, and discharge summaries in a timely manner. Open communication with referring physicians, other advanced care practitioners, and case managers is essential for enhancing continuity of care. Feedback from referring physicians also helps to improve systems to meet the needs of patients and physicians.

CURRENT ISSUES FACING APNS

Several education, legislative, and reimbursement issues related to nurses functioning in advanced practice roles are currently being addressed at a national level, including the following:

1. Nursing schools are creating graduate core curriculums that focus on the critical care environment. These programs must provide a well-rounded theory and research-based education along with adequate practicum experience (3).

2. Present regulatory statutes restrict an APN's prescriptive authority and reimbursement practices, and limit productivity. Each state has its own nursing practice act that defines nursing practice. With the advent of APNs, several states are now including specific regulations related to the practice of APNs in the nursing practice act. This situation makes it difficult to standardize the role of the APN nationwide. APNs are responsible for understanding their state's specific laws and must work together to eliminate impediments to practice and seek uniform national standards.
3. Reimbursement issues must be addressed in the context of a managed care environment. As traditional fee-for-service reimbursements are slowly disappearing, it is difficult for the APN to bill directly for services rendered in the critical care setting. Although it has been demonstrated that in some settings nurses functioning in advanced roles are more cost-effective than physicians (16), this has not been proven in critical care.

CONCLUSION

An exciting future is seen for APNs in the critical care setting. Clearly it is a role that must meet the demands of the changing health care system by remaining flexible and collaborating with the health care team in direct patient management, education, research, and community outreach. This emerging system can improve patient care and enhance program marketability dramatically because APNs are in an ideal position to provide access to high quality health care at a reasonable cost (17).

REFERENCES

1. Schwartz A, Ginsburg PB, LeRoy LB. Reforming graduate medical education: summary report of the physician payment review commission. JAMA 1993;270(9):1079–1082.
2. Keefe MR, Biester DJ. Advanced practice in pediatric nursing. J Pediatr Nurs 1988;(4):263–264.
3. Mirr MP. Advanced clinical practice: a reconceptualized role. AACN Clinical Issues in Critical Care Nursing 1993;4(4):599–602.
4. The National Joint Practice Commission. Guidelines for establishing joint or collaborative practice in hospitals. Chicago: The commission, 1981.
5. Keane A, Richmond T, Kaiser L. Critical care nurse practitioner: evolution of the advanced practice nursing role. Am J Crit Care 1994;3(3):232–237.
6. Keckeisen M. The critical care clinical nurse specialist in critical care staff education. In: Gawlinski A, Kern LS, eds. The clinical nurse specialist role in critical care. Philadelphia: WB Saunders, 1994:99–119.
7. Weilitz PB. The critical care clinical nurse specialist role in patient education. In: Gawlinski A, Kern LS, eds. The clinical nurse specialist role in critical care. Philadelphia: WB Saunders, 1994:120–132.
8. Herrin DM. Linking management and advanced practice at the department level: a collaborative leadership model. Aspen's Advisor for Nurse Executives 1994;9(11):6–8.
9. Askin DF, Bennett K, Shapiro C. The clinical nurse specialist and the research process. J Obstet Gynecol Neonatal Nurs 1994;23(4):336–340.
10. American Nurses' Association. Standards of practice for the primary health care nurse practitioner. Kansas City, MO: ANA, 1986; NP-71.
11. Uzark K, LeRoy S, Callow L, et al. The pediatric nurse practitioner as case manager in the delivery of services to children with heart disease. Journal of Pediatric Health Care 1994;8(2):74–78.
12. Nugent KE. The clinical specialist as case manager in a collaborative practice model: bridging the gap between quality and cost of care. Clinical Nurse Specialist 1992;6(2):106–111.
13. DeZeil A, Corneau E, Zander K. Nursing case management: managed care via the nursing case management model. Patients and purse strings II. New York: National League for Nursing, 1988.
14. Thompson DG. Critical pathways in the intensive care and intermediate care nurseries. Matern Child Nurs J 1994;19(1):29–32.
15. Schull DE, Tosch P, Wood M. Clinical nurse specialist as collaborative care managers. Nursing Management 1992;32(3):30–33.
16. Fenton MV, Brykczynski KA. Qualitative distinctions and similarities in the practice of clinical nurse specialists and nurse practitioners. J Prof Nurs 1993;9(6):313–326.
17. Moore SM. Promoting advanced practice nursing. AACN Clinical Issues in Critical Care Nursing 1993;4(4):603–608.

Ethical and Legal Issues

36

Robert D. Truog, MD

The fact that a textbook on critical care medicine would include a chapter on ethics is a telling example of how much more importance is given to this topic in recent years. Indeed, the need for more ethical consideration and analysis is largely the result of the tremendous developments that have occurred in critical care medicine itself. The technologies of the intensive care unit (ICU) are now recognized as being two-edged swords, possessing not only the power to achieve cures never before thought possible, but also the power to prolong life long past the time when any hope for benefit or recovery exists. This chapter presents an overview of the approaches taken by ethicists in thinking about moral dilemmas in critical care, and then reviews some key issues that frequently arise around informed consent and decision-making at the end of life.

HOW DO WE REASON ABOUT ETHICAL PROBLEMS?

The difficult part in an argument is not to defend one's opinion, but rather to know it. André Maurois (1885–1967), French author and critic (1).

Physicians are often frustrated by ethical dilemmas. Many clinicians believe that ethical debates are just a matter of one person's opinion versus that of another. With other types of medical problems, physicians can take a scientific approach to determining the right answer, either by consulting the literature or by designing experiments and clinical trials to shed light on unanswered questions. By contrast, ethical dilemmas are not amenable to this mode of linear reasoning. Nevertheless, clinicians should recognize that ethics is not simply a matter of individual opinion, without any basis in principle or fact. Indeed, scholars have been addressing the problems of ethics for a lot longer than physicians have been doing medical research, and this philosophical literature has much that is relevant to the ethical dilemmas that arise in the cardiac ICU. One of the most valuable contributions of this ethical theory to modern medicine is that it offers clinicians the possibility of actually "knowing" their opinions, by helping them to gain understanding and insight into the assumptions and presumptions that lie behind their ethical views. The potential benefit of this knowledge is the possibility of elevating ethical discussion and debate to a level above that of mere opinion, so that varying views on an issue can be resolved by reasoning rather than by simple rhetoric or emotional persuasion.

Consequentialism Versus Deontology

One of the most important distinctions in moral reasoning is between consequentialist approaches and deontologic views (2). Simply put, a consequentialist evaluates the rightness of an act solely in terms of its consequences, whereas a deontologist believes that certain acts are always wrong, regardless of the consequences. Some deontologists base their beliefs on a religious perspective (the Ten Commandments are a typical list of deontologic principles), whereas others derive a set of duties and obligations from theoretic analysis.

Current debate about euthanasia illustrates the differences between these approaches. Consequentialists may argue, for example, that when a terminally ill patient requests to be killed, the consequences of complying with that request are favorable for everyone concerned. The patient's desires are satisfied, the physician can rest assured that the act was in the patient's best interest (as defined by the patient), and even society may benefit by not incurring the expenses associated with a prolonged dying process. Deontologists, on the other hand, feel differently. For a deontologist, the prohibition against killing should stop us from taking the life of another, regardless of the consequences. Under this approach, euthanasia is always wrong, even if we are convinced that doing so does not harm anyone's interest.

As this example illustrates, deontologists are generally concerned with identifying relevant rules of conduct, whereas consequentialists tend to evaluate each case solely in terms of the expected outcome. Nevertheless, even consequentialists usually agree that rules have an important place in ethics, if only because of the inherent difficulties involved in predicting the consequences of our actions. To use the euthanasia example again, a deontologist might claim that even when performing euthanasia does not appear to harm anyone's interest, the long-term consequences of permitting this act might be to diminish our respect for human life, and it could eventually work to erode the core values of the medical profession. This would be a reason to oppose euthanasia, even by the consequentialist standard.

In reality, few people are pure deontologists or consequentialists. Most of us blend these two perspectives in our reasoning about ethical issues. Nevertheless, when analyzing our own opinions or evaluating the views of others, an understanding of the assumptions that underlie these opinions is generally helpful.

Principle-Based Reasoning Versus Other Approaches

Another important controversy in bioethics concerns the role of "principles" in thinking about ethical issues. In their classic textbook on bioethics, Beauchamp and Childress articulate four principles that they believe should serve as guideposts in ethical analysis (2). They are respect for autonomy (self-determination), beneficence (doing good), nonmaleficence (avoiding harm), and justice (fair distribution). Analysis of ethical dilemmas in terms of these four principles is seldom sufficient in determining the "correct" answer, but it is often useful in helping to identify the salient issues that are at stake.

More recently, several alternatives to the principle-based mode of analysis have been proposed and developed. Proponents of "case-based reasoning," or casuistic analysis, argue that the four principles of Beauchamp and Childress are too indeterminate and abstract to be of much help with real-life dilemmas (3, 4). They advocate instead for the use of "paradigmatic cases," that is, real cases about which a consensus currently exists. As new cases arise, they are analyzed in terms of the ways that they are similar to or different from the paradigmatic cases. This has been referred to as "moral triangulation." For example, since the "Baby Doe" episode in 1984, general agreement is found in medicine, law, and ethics that babies with Down syndrome and correctable surgical anomalies should undergo surgical repair of their conditions, and not be allowed to die from them (5). Similarly, general agreement is also found that babies with trisomy 13 or 18 who have potentially lethal congenital defects need not be offered life-prolonging therapies, but may ethically be treated with only comfort care. When faced with the problem of how to treat a newborn with congenital anomalies intermediate between those of trisomy 21 and 13 or 18, a proponent of the case-based approach might attempt to address the question by first exploring the ways in which the child is more like an infant with Down syndrome or more like an infant with trisomy 13 or 18. In combination with factors such as the severity of the defects and the preferences of the family, this approach would attempt to "triangulate" toward the most reasonable solution.

As the field of bioethics has continued to develop, still other ways of thinking about difficult cases have emerged. An alternative that has arisen from the feminist movement is an approach based on the primacy of "caring" (6). In its more radical form, this perspective minimizes the importance of ethical theory and principles, and seeks resolutions to difficult cases that best preserve the relationships involved. As opposed to a principle-based approach, this perspective is less concerned with maintaining internal consistency and with the observance of formal rules. When confronted with a case about whether to allow a small child to donate a kidney to a sibling, for example, a proponent of the "caring" approach would ask which of the alternative options would best promote the well-being of the relationships between the family and others involved.

Finally, a perspective that has developed within the fields of literature and the humanities focuses on the value of "narrative" (7). Unlike the terse case-histories that tend to be favored in the busy hospital setting, this approach emphasizes the importance of understanding cases in all of their detail and complexity. Rather than attempting to "shrink" cases to their essential elements, and then applying a specific rule or principle, the proponent of the narrative approach will insist that only by analyzing cases in all of their richness and texture can we hope to arrive at solutions that are sufficiently nuanced and sophisticated. Indeed, this approach hearkens back to the admonitions of many of the great medical clinicians who emphasized the overriding importance of careful history taking. These giants of medicine would undoubtedly be just as critical of our over-reliance on "catheter data" and imaging studies as the proponent of narrative is critical of principles.

Ethics and the Law

> A society that is based on the letter of the law and never reaches any higher is taking small advantage of the high level of human possibilities. The letter of the law is too cold and formal to have a beneficial influence on society. Whenever the tissue of life is woven of legalistic relations, there is an atmosphere of mediocrity, paralyzing man's noblest impulses.
> Solzhenitsyn A, 1978 (8).

Many clinicians fail to see the importance of ethics to medical practice. "Just tell me what's legal. All I care about is not being sued," they may say. The relationship of law to ethics is complicated, but in simple terms the law can be thought of as the floor below which we should not fall, whereas ethics often points toward the ceiling for which we should aspire. At a deeper level, it is helpful to remember that creation of the law is a very human enterprise, undertaken by judges when they decide on cases and by legislators when they develop legislation. And when judges and legislators struggle with what should be the correct decision in a case or what should be the law of the land, they, of course, are asking questions about ethics.

DECISION-MAKING FOR CHILDREN

Case: Hypoplastic Left Heart Syndrome

A full-term 3.5 kg baby is born to a 35-year-old primiparous woman following several years of fertility counseling and treatment. Although the baby initially appears to be healthy, he is noted to be somewhat pale and mottled by the nurses in the well-baby nursery. A pediatrician is called, and subsequent evaluation reveals that the child has hypoplastic left heart syndrome (HLHS). A pediatric cardiologist is consulted to discuss treatment options with the baby's parents, including the Norwood Procedure, a heart transplant, or comfort care. In preparing for this discussion, the cardiologist must address issues concerning informed consent, the best interests of the child, and the role of parents in medical decision-making.

Informed Consent

Perhaps the greatest impact of the "bioethics movement" on the practice of medicine has been on the process of informed consent. From the times of Hippocrates until the very recent past, medical decision-making has been driven almost solely by the opinions and perspective of the physician. This approach has acquired the pejorative label of "paternalism," but this does not imply that the physicians of the past were unethical in their practice of medicine. For the most part, these physicians were acting in good faith to promote their patient's health and welfare as they perceived it. Indeed, respected bioethicists continue to maintain that this beneficent approach to the practice of medicine and the patient-doctor relationship has many features that we should try to preserve (9).

Nevertheless, over the past several decades a sea change has arisen in our approach to informed consent, with a much greater emphasis now being placed on patient autonomy and the right to self-determination (10). This transformation has not been limited to the realm of medicine, but it is reflective of a greater shift within our society toward individualism and an emphasis on human rights more generally. For physicians, this change has meant that they can no longer assume that they can determine the optimal therapy for their patients on medical grounds alone, but that they must take into account nonmedical factors as well, such as the values and attitudes of their patients and their families.

Substituted Judgment and Best Interest

This shift from sole reliance on the expertise of the physician to an emphasis on patient self-determination has been most easily implemented in the care of competent adults making decisions for themselves. Application of these principles to the practice of pediatrics has been much more difficult, because it is impossible to know the current or future preferences of a newborn or young child. Even in the case of decision-making for elderly patients who have become demented, it is possible to ask what the patient would have wanted done if he or she were still competent, based on opinions and views expressed by the patient earlier in life. This approach is known as "substituted judgment," and it is the usual strategy employed in decision-making for once-competent individuals. In the case of children, however, we lack even these clues to what the patient would want, because newborns and young children have not had the opportunity to form any opinions or preferences. In these cases, we cannot rely on "substituted judgment," but must rather make decisions based on the child's "best interest."

The Role of Parents in Decision-Making for Children

Broad societal consensus proposes that parents are the preferred decision makers for their children (11, 12). When a child is too young to have formed any clear preferences regarding treatment, it is generally left to the parents to decide what is in the best interests of the child based on an assessment of the benefits and burdens of the proposed therapy.

Nevertheless, at times it is appropriate to question the decisions that parents make on behalf of their children. The threshold for overriding the parents' wishes depends on an objective assessment of the risks to the child. In general, if the circumstances do not involve life-threatening choices, and no certain risks are seen of substantial harm to the child, physicians are obligated to respect the decisions of the parents, even when they strongly disagree with the choice. In some jurisdictions, for example, parents are permitted the right to refuse standard immunizations for religious reasons (11).

It is only as the threat to the child increases, and the benefits of treatment are more certain, that actions to override parental choices are not only legally supportable, but in most jurisdictions required. Numerous court opinions have upheld the notion, first articulated in the famous 1944 case of *Prince* v. *Massachusetts*, that a parent may make a martyr of himself because of religious convictions, "but he is not free to make a martyr of his child" (13). In numerous decisions since then, courts have upheld the right of physicians to override parental refusal of transfusions or other accepted therapy when the child's life is at risk (11).

In many medical situations, however, knowing what is in the child's best interest is not as clear. The case of the child with HLHS is an excellent example. The generally accepted approach to these questions is to give the child's parents primary responsibility for deciding on the child's best interest. Several reasons are found why this should be considered the preferred approach. First, the vast majority of parents have a profound love for and commitment to their children, and they can be trusted to be acting in good faith for the child's best interest. Second, it is reasonable to assume that children will grow up to share many of the same values as their parents and family. In other words, we approximate what a child would choose for him or herself later in life by asking the parents what they believe is best for the child, based on their personal values and attitudes. Third, it is the parents who will primarily shoulder the burden of whatever choices are made on behalf of the child. This is not to say that it is appropriate for the child's parents to make decisions based solely on the financial or social consequences of those choices for themselves, but it is to recognize that these decisions will often have a profound impact on the child's parents and family, and that their views and preferences therefore deserve serious consideration and have moral weight.

For all of these reasons, parental decisions about medical treatment for their children should be questioned only in rare situations. In these circumstances, great care should be taken to ensure that the parental opinions are clearly unreasonable. Most institutions now have Ethics Committees that can serve as initial forums for discussions of ethically difficult cases. Often the process of ethics consultation is itself sufficient to generate an agreement between the family and care team about an appropriate course of action. Only when all avenues of alternative resolution have failed should caregivers turn to the courts for a solution. Because parents generally have the legal right to approve or refuse medical treatment on behalf of their child, judicial intervention is usually necessary if the caregivers believe it is imperative to override the parental decision. Again, however, the need for such intervention should be exceedingly rare, and the frequent need for judicial involvement could indicate an institutional failure of internal methods for dispute resolution.

The "Mature Minor"

Although parents generally take full responsibility for decision-making for newborns and young children, this should not be the case for older children and adolescents. The legal age of majority (18 years of age in most jurisdictions) is an oversimplification of the maturational and developmental process in children. Children as young as 6 or 7 are often able to have reasoned opinions about certain aspects of their care, and most adolescents have views and perspectives that deserve serious consideration. The fact that parents must give legal consent for medical treatments performed on minor children does not mean that the opinions of the children and adolescents should be considered irrelevant or ignored.

Many states have recognized this developmental continuum in the law (14). In some jurisdictions, case law has precedents for minors (usually adolescents) being allowed to make independent decisions about their care. Other jurisdictions have "mature minor" statutes that give certain rights to minors who are able to contribute to decision-making about proposed medical treatments. Although the legal requirements can vary, a generally accepted ethical principle is that children at the very least should always be evaluated for their ability to "assent" to treatment. In other words, although children may not have the cognitive or emotional skills to fully understand all of the implications of various treatment choices, even young children often have the capacity for a general understanding of the proposed course of treatment and what they should expect. Furthermore, children should be given the opportunity to "assent" to this treatment ("consent" being reserved for those situations in which the patient can fully understand the benefits, risks, and alternatives for the proposed treatment). If the child refuses to assent, considerable effort should be taken to explore the child's feelings and to seek strategies for accommodating these views and preferences. Only in unusual circumstances should children not be apprised of a proposed treatment plan, or should their refusal to assent be categorically overridden.

Adequately Informing Patients and Families

Against this background, the case of the newborn with HLHS can be seen to be a matter of determining the baby's best interest. Furthermore, this is a case where medical factors alone are insufficient to fully determine the best course of action. In this situation, deference should be given to the parents as the primary decision-makers for passing judgment on the child's best interest. To make an informed choice, however, the parents need to be educated about the implications of the various alternatives.

Unfortunately, this is an area where the parents' choice can often be intentionally or unwittingly manipulated by the views of the caregivers. For example, in a series of classic studies by Wennberg et al. in the 1970s, the performance of procedures like hysterectomies, tonsillectomies, and prostatectomies was shown to vary substantially among communities, with no evidence of differences that could account for these variations (15–18). For example, men with benign prostatic hypertrophy who were referred to urologists were more likely to have a surgical procedure than men who were referred to internists.

Investigators in this study followed up on their findings with an interesting intervention (19–21). They developed a videodisc presentation in which the various treatment options for this condition were presented by recognized experts in the field. In addition, patients were interviewed on the videodisc about why they made the choices they did and their satisfaction with the outcome. By incorporating information about the patient's clinical condition and personal values into the software, a much more individualized choice for the patient could be suggested.

The investigators then enrolled a number of urologists and internists into a program to give the videodisc to patients who were newly diagnosed with prostatic hypertrophy. Not surprisingly, patients who had the opportunity to view the videodisc were much more likely to make their choice between surgery or medical treatment independent of the specialist to whom they were initially referred. It therefore appeared that these patients made their choice more on the basis of their own preferences and values and less on the basis of their physician's opinions and biases.

This study has obvious implications for the management of newborns with HLHS, because management of these children is heavily influenced by the biases of the centers and physicians that make the diagnosis and counsel the parents. Clearly, the "right" choice for a family should not depend primarily on which medical center is closest to their home, and yet this would appear to be the major determinant of how the child is actually managed. For example, whether the parents of a newborn with HLHS are offered the option of surgery depends heavily on the attitudes of the physician and institution about the appropriateness of the procedure. In addition, the shift toward a managed care environment has placed increased pressure on physicians to limit referrals to specialists outside of the managed care system. If the surgical experience with HLHS within a particular system has not been favorable, a cardiologist may be reluctant both to recommend the procedure within the system as well as to refer the patient to another surgeon outside of the system. All of these factors can limit parents' ability to make the best choice for their child, or even to be fully aware of what choices are available.

From an ethical perspective, this would therefore seem to be an ideal situation for an approach analogous to that adopted for the management of benign prostatic hypertrophy. Leading centers with different approaches to HLHS could cooperate in the development of a videodisc, with proponents of each approach reviewing the pros and cons of their preferred option. In addition, volunteer parents could be interviewed, and they could explain why they made the choices that they did on behalf of their child and their satisfaction with the outcome. This videodisc could then be distributed around the country and used by pediatric cardiologists in counseling the parents of children with HLHS. This type of approach is now receiving substantial encouragement from organizations with an interest in improving decision-making in health care (such as the Agency for Health Care Policy and Research), and it could be a significant advance in improving decision-making for infants with this condition.

LIMITATIONS OF LIFE-SUSTAINING TREATMENTS

Case: Do-Not-Resuscitate Orders

A newborn is referred from a nearby nursery with poor perfusion and metabolic acidosis. Evaluation reveals coarctation of the aorta. A prostaglandin infusion is begun, and the acidosis improves. The coarctation is repaired the following morning. The child does well in the immediate postoperative period, but then has recurrence of the acidosis with abdominal distention and thrombocytopenia. Abdominal x-rays reveal dilated loops of bowel with pneumatosis intestinales. A presumptive diagnosis of necrotizing enterocolitis is made. Despite antibiotic and other supportive therapy, the child's condition worsens. Surgical intervention is not thought to be feasible. The pediatric cardiologist meets with the family to discuss the appropriateness of a do not resuscitate (DNR) order. What ethical principles should guide the discussion?

Do Not Resuscitate Orders

Until 1976, no hospital in the United States publicly acknowledged that they ever provided care that was not solely intended to prolong and preserve life. In that year, both the Massachusetts General Hospital and Boston's Beth Israel Hospital acknowledged their use of "do-not-resuscitate" orders in the *New England Journal of Medicine*

(22, 23). Over the past 20 years, DNR orders have become increasingly accepted and have undergone numerous modifications. More recently, however, evidence is found that the complexity of decision-making around terminally ill patients has progressed to the point where the philosophy behind DNR orders is no longer sufficient. Alternatives to the traditional DNR order will be discussed below.

Procedure-Specific Do Not Resuscitate Orders

In most hospitals, DNR orders are written by the attending physician in the Doctor's Orders Sheets. These orders are often vague, and they can leave substantial opportunity for miscommunication and error. Does "resuscitation" refer to treatment of an acute cardiac arrest (intubation and ventilation, chest compressions, cardioversion, and medications), or does it also mean "do-not-intubate" for conditions such as respiratory failure from pneumonia? Should patients with DNR orders receive suctioning for airway secretions, be treated with antibiotics, or be given tube feedings? Should they be excluded from the ICU, or denied palliative surgery? The answers to these questions are almost never clear in the interpretation of a simple "DNR order."

In response to these concerns, many institutions have now adopted "Procedure-Specific DNR Orders." This approach is intended to reduce much of the ambiguity surrounding these orders. The form currently used at one children's hospital is shown in Figure 36.1. This page appears at the beginning of the "Doctor's Orders" section of the patient's chart, so that it is readily available at all times in a place easily identified by physicians and other caregivers who may not be familiar with the details of the patient's care at the time of an arrest. The form first specifies whether a "code blue" should be called in the event of cardiorespiratory arrest, and then provides a checklist of exactly which procedures are to be performed or withheld. A section is provided for identifying special instructions, and then lines for the signatures of both the attending physician and the bedside nurse, with a requirement for renewal every 7 days. Finally, a section is to be completed if the patient or family rescind the DNR order. A recent study showed that use of procedure-specific DNR forms reduces the uncertainty and confusion that often accompany the decision not to resuscitate (24).

"Cardiopulmonary Resuscitation-Not-Indicated" Orders

Is it necessary for the patient or family to consent to a DNR order (25–30)? Some states (e.g., New York) have laws that generally require the consent of the patient or family before a DNR order is written, and many hospitals have this requirement in their internal policies (31). Recently, however, some hospitals have adopted policies that permit physicians to write DNR orders without the permission (or sometimes, without even the knowledge) of the patient or family. The presumption behind this approach is the view that cardiopulmonary resuscitation (CPR) is a medical therapy, and that physicians are uniquely qualified to determine whether and when a medical therapy is indicated. These policies are therefore often referred to as "CPR-not-indicated" policies.

The belief of many physicians that they should have the authority to determine when CPR is appropriate is understandable. Many patients and families are unable to accept the fact that they or a loved one is terminally ill and about to die. In these situations, patients or families may maintain an irrational belief that CPR can offer them a meaningful extension in the quality or duration of their life. Under these circumstances, caregivers often feel that they are doing CPR to "treat the family," and that performing this procedure when it can offer no real benefit to the patient is a violation of their professional integrity.

On the other hand, this development in DNR orders should be viewed with great caution. As noted in the discussion of informed consent, physicians have a long history of seeing complex situations from a uniquely medical perspective, ignoring important factors related to the patient's values and preferences. Rarely is the question of whether or not to do CPR purely a medical issue. Often the patient's or family's denial of impending death can be overcome by proper counseling, whereas simply using the physician's authority to overrule the family's wishes can be profoundly destructive to the patient-physician relationship. Although this debate over the legitimacy of "CPR-not-indicated" orders is far from resolved, little doubt remains that this approach should be used only under the most conservative and well-defined circumstances.

Redirection of Care and Comfort Policies

Do not resuscitate orders are unique. They are the only physician's order that is focused exclusively on what *will not* be done, rather than what *will* be done. Not surprisingly, patients with DNR orders often feel that they have been abandoned by their caregivers. Indeed, studies have shown that physicians do in fact spend less time caring for patients who have DNR orders. This is not always appropriate, because patients with DNR orders often need more attention in terms of aggressive palliative care than patients who are not imminently dying.

In addition, DNR orders tend to be concerned with only a small fraction of the issues that arise with dying patients. Often the question of whether or not a patient should be resuscitated is actually peripheral to the more important questions surrounding the use of less dramatic interventions. Should the patient be intubated and venti-

Ethical and Legal Issues 537

Children's Hospital

PHYSICIAN'S ORDERS: DO-NOT-RESUSCITATE

USE PLATE OR PRINT

MR. NO. _____ DATE _____

PT. NAME _____

DATE OF BIRTH _____

This order sheet will appear first in the Physician's Orders Section. Do-Not-Resuscitate Orders must be renewed weekly. See the House Officer's Manual for additional information.

In case of cardiopulmonary arrest: Call a code ☐ Yes ☐ No

Regarding the following interventions (mark all that apply)
- ____ No supplemental oxygen
- ____ No oral airway
- ____ No intubation
- ____ No needle thoracentesis
- ____ No venipuncture
- ____ No arterial puncture
- ____ No deep suctioning
- ____ No bag and mask ventilation
- ____ No chest compressions
- ____ No chest tube
- ____ No electrical cardioversion
- ____ No arrest medications (epi, atropine, NaHCO$_3$, calcium, fluid boluses)

Additional Instructions:

Attending Physician Signature _____ Date/Time _____   RN Signature _____ Date/Time _____
Attending Physician _____ (Print Name)

Renewal: Attending Signature _____ Date/Time _____   RN Signature _____ Date/Time _____
Attending Physician _____ (Print Name)

Renewal: Attending Signature _____ Date/Time _____   RN Signature _____ Date/Time _____
Attending Physician _____ (Print Name)

Renewal: Attending Signature _____ Date/Time _____   RN Signature _____ Date/Time _____
Attending Physician _____ (Print Name)

Discontinuation: Specify date and time this order is rescinded:

Attending Physician Signature _____ Date/Time _____   RN Signature _____ Date/Time _____

Figure 36.1 The Do-Not-Resuscitate Form used at Children's Hospital in Boston.

lated for the next episode of pneumonia? Should the patient receive antibiotics? Should the patient receive opioids to relieve the sensation of dyspnea, although the respiratory depression from the opioids could hasten death? Should the patient be fed only as much as can be personally consumed, realizing that this could lead to death from gradual dehydration and malnutrition, or should the patient be given a gastrostomy tube to optimize nutrition and hydration?

These questions are not adequately addressed by the traditional DNR order. Hospitals are therefore increasingly developing more global policies that are more responsive to the variety of issues posed by end-of-life decision-making than narrow DNR policies. The Joint Commission on Accreditation of Hospitals Organization (JCAHO) has indicated that it will soon require hospitals to have policies of this type.

WITHDRAWING LIFE-SUSTAINING TREATMENTS

Case: Escalating and Withdrawing Therapy

A 2-year-old child is admitted to the cardiac intensive care unit following surgical repair of complex cardiac disease. The child had difficulty weaning from cardiac bypass following the procedure, and is now rapidly developing myocardial failure. Options at this point include placing the child on extracorporeal membrane oxygenation (ECMO) or another ventricular assist device, or continuing conventional support with the expectation that the child will not survive. If the latter course is chosen, then questions about the withdrawal of life-support and the provision of analgesics and sedatives during the dying process must be addressed. What are the ethical principles that should guide this decision-making?

The Ordinary or Extraordinary Distinction

One of the most commonly used justifications for withholding "high-tech" therapy from patients is the belief that "extraordinary" treatments are not ethically mandatory. For example, a recent survey showed that 74% of physicians and nurses think that the distinction between ordinary and extraordinary is helpful in resolving ethical dilemmas (32). In the case described above, for instance, if the cardiologists and surgeons believe that ECMO or a ventricular assist device will not offer the child a reasonable chance of survival, they might argue that such treatment would be "extraordinary," and therefore should not be done. Although this terminology is still used in the writings of some religious traditions, clinicians should understand that the distinction between ordinary and extraordinary treatments is not considered to be helpful when trying to reason about the ethical aspects of difficult decisions.

To illustrate why this is so, consider two alternative interpretations of the ordinary or extraordinary distinction. One interpretation would be that ordinary treatments are customarily performed, whereas extraordinary treatments are not. The cardiologists in the case described above might argue, for example, that ECMO would be extraordinary in the case because they do not customarily perform ECMO for children in this condition. Clearly, however, a simple appeal to what is customary cannot suffice as a justification for what is morally required. In addition, from a legal perspective, the courts have explicitly rejected the view that any relationship exists between what is "customary" and what is "legal."

Another interpretation of the ordinary or extraordinary distinction would hold that ordinary treatments are morally required, whereas extraordinary treatments are morally optional. But this is essentially a circular argument, because it claims that ordinary treatments are morally required because they are ordinary, and extraordinary treatments are morally optional because they are extraordinary. Words cannot substitute for moral reasoning.

As an example of this fallacy in the literature, pediatricians were asked about their views on repair of duodenal atresia in healthy babies and in babies with Down syndrome (33). Most pediatricians said that duodenal atresia was an "ordinary" procedure in the case of healthy infants, but an "extraordinary" procedure in the case of babies with Down syndrome. Again, the use of this terminology hides the lack of any moral reasoning or ethical justification.

A much more legitimate and useful approach to thinking about whether a procedure is ethically required is to inquire about the balance of the benefits versus the burdens for a particular procedure in a particular patient. In other words, instead of relying on terminology such as ordinary and extraordinary to decide whether a treatment should be offered, consider instead whether the proposed benefits exceed the burdens. If the child described in the case above is very unlikely to survive despite treatment with ECMO, then the burdens of that therapy clearly exceed the benefits. On the other hand, physicians and society now generally agree that the benefits of repairing a duodenal atresia in patients with Down syndrome exceed the burdens, and thus the procedure is morally required.

The Withholding or Withdrawing Distinction

Is there a difference between stopping a treatment once it is started, and not starting it in the first place? In other words, is there an ethical difference between deciding not to intubate a patient because we do not think recovery is possible, and extubating a patient who has failed to recover despite a period of ventilation? Surveys have repeatedly shown that physicians do believe a difference exists. For example, one recent study reported that 66% of physicians and nurses think that an ethical difference is seen between withdrawing and withholding treatment, and nearly half agreed with the statement "there is an emerging consensus that withdrawing a treatment is ethically different from withholding or not starting it" (32). In another survey of 360 attending physicians, housestaff, and medical students, 73% felt that withdrawing is different from withholding (34). These reports all indicate that physicians are much more comfortable withholding treatments than in withdrawing them.

This issue is particularly interesting in light of the fact that this opinion among clinicians is strikingly at odds with the prevailing views among ethicists and judges. Legal scholars and judges have been consistent in expressing the opinion that doctors should not differentiate between decisions to withhold or withdraw medical treatments. In the landmark Cruzan case, for example, justices from the US Supreme Court wrote that doctors should consider decisions to withhold and withdraw as equivalent to assure that patients receive adequate trials of therapy (35–37). In the case described above, for instance, the physicians involved might claim that they are reluctant to begin ECMO therapy for this patient, even though they think it might offer a benefit, because they are concerned that once they start the therapy they will not feel that they can ethically stop it. Because they do not want to commit to an indefinite course of ECMO on a patient who might not survive, they would rather not start the therapy in the first place. Justices from the Supreme Court would reject this reasoning, and insist that a better approach would be to give the child a trial of therapy with ECMO, with the understanding that ECMO would be discontinued in a timely manner if the child did not respond.

Philosophers have also been strong advocates of the position that we should not differentiate between withholding and withdrawing life-sustaining treatments. Unlike the legal scholars, however, they have argued more from a logical perspective. If a physician makes a decision to stop treating a patient with dialysis, for example, should we say that the patient has been withdrawn from a series of dialysis treatments, or should we say simply that the next treatment has been withheld? Philosophers claim that either description is factually accurate. If either description is accurate, then how can there be a moral difference between the two? In other words, how can there be a moral difference between withholding and withdrawing? This analogy can be extended. If a physician decides to take a patient off of mechanical ventilation, should we say that the patient has been withdrawn from a series of mechanical breaths, or should we simply say that the next breath has been withheld? Again, the argument can be made that either description is true; that describing the action as either a withholding or as a withdrawing is an accurate account of the situation. If this is the case, then how can a moral distinction between withholding and withdrawing exist?

Despite these opinions from law and philosophy, clinicians persist in believing that there is a difference between these two actions. Part of the reason is clearly psychological. Physicians feel more responsible for the death of a patient when it results from the withdrawal of a therapy than they do when it results from the withholding of a therapy. This psychological distinction is important, and it cannot be made to disappear by legal or philosophical reasoning, no matter how persuasive. Nevertheless, when confronted with these situations, physicians should consider the perspectives from law and philosophy, because in many cases adoption of these views will lead to better clinical decision-making.

Another reason that clinicians are reluctant to withdraw life-sustaining therapy is their fear of legal liability, both civil and criminal. In this case, however, many clinicians are simply misinformed. In a review by David Orentlicher from the American Medical Association's Council on Judicial and Ethical Affairs, he concludes that "No person has ever been found liable for withdrawing life-sustaining treatment without court permission" (35). This is a strong statement, and it should be reassuring to physicians who are concerned about this issue.

On the other hand, physicians often believe that they have no legal liability if they refuse to terminate life-sustaining treatments at the request of a patient or family, as long as they always act to preserve life. This is also a serious misconception. Orentlicher notes that "The risk of liability may be significant, however, when a physician refuses to honor a request to have life-sustaining treatment withdrawn" (35). He cites two successful suits against physicians who refused to withdraw care at the request of a patient or surrogate. In other words, the commonly held view among physicians that they can be at legal risk if they withdraw life-support but are legally immune if they always act to prolong life can be seen to be exactly backward!

Sedatives and Analgesics in the Care of the Dying

Unfortunately, physicians who care for patients in the cardiac intensive care unit will frequently be called on to discontinue life-support from a dying patient. As in the case described above, the question then becomes how best to manage the patient during the dying process. Some erroneously believe that no sedatives or analgesics should be given in these situations, because they believe that it is important both ethically and legally that the patient die from the underlying disease, without any contribution from the respiratory or cardiac depression that is frequently a side-effect of these medications.

The reluctance of many physicians to aggressively treat the pain and suffering often experienced by the terminally ill has been one of the most powerful forces driving the movement in favor of euthanasia and physician-assisted suicide over the last several years (38–40). Individuals who have watched loved ones die without adequate pain relief have spearheaded this movement with the belief that patients should have the opportunity to commit suicide if their suffering is unbearable, particularly because physicians seem unwilling to do whatever is necessary to control that suffering. This is unfortunate, particularly because nothing found in the law, ethics, or any of the major religious traditions should preclude physicians from aggressively treating the pain and suffering of the terminally ill, even when such treatment may hasten a patient's death. Nevertheless, a recent survey showed that as many as 40% of doctors and nurses give inadequate pain medication mostly out of fear of hastening a patient's death (32).

The ethical principle that is relevant to this question is the Doctrine of Double Effect, originally developed within the Catholic tradition but now widely acknowledged in other religious traditions as well as law and philosophy (2). The doctrine states that when an action has two effects, one of which is inherently good and the other of which is inherently bad, it can be justified if certain conditions are met. For example, administering morphine to a dying patient has both a good effect (relief of pain and suffering) and the potential for a bad effect (hastening the patient's death through respiratory depression). The conditions that must be satisfied for the action to be justified are:

1. The action in itself must be good or at least morally indifferent. (Administration of the morphine itself is morally indifferent.)
2. The agent must intend only the good effect and not the evil effect. The evil effect is foreseen, not intended. It is allowed, not sought. (In the case of administering morphine to a terminally ill patient, the physician must intend only the relief of the patient's pain and suffering. Respiratory depression and the potential for an earlier death is a foreseen complication, but it is not sought.)
3. The evil effect cannot be a means to the good effect. (If the physician administers a bolus of potassium chloride instead of morphine, this condition would be violated. By administering potassium chloride, the evil effect [death] becomes the means to the good effect [relief from suffering]. By contrast, morphine does not depend on the side effect of death to effectively relieve pain.)
4. The good intended must outweigh the evil permitted. (In the case of an imminently dying patient, the benefit of pain relief clearly outweighs the risk of death. This would not be true if the patient was not terminally ill. For example, if an otherwise healthy patient required so much morphine for pain control that serious respiratory depression developed, the patient should be placed on a ventilator, not allowed to die.)

SUMMARY

In summary, despite the beliefs of many clinicians, no moral, legal, or religious reasons are found for withholding adequate pain relief from dying patients. Pain and suffering should always be adequately treated, even if the treatment results in a foreseen but unintended hastening of death.

What is the difference between currently accepted practice and the performance of euthanasia? The key difference lies in the *intention* of the physician. As long as the physician's intention is treatment of the patient's pain and suffering, the administration of analgesics and sedatives is noncontroversial. When the physician's intention is to kill the patient, then the line between accepted practice and euthanasia has been crossed. This distinction is observed within the law as well as within ethics. Physicians should be reassured that as long as they act with the intention of relieving a patient's pain and suffering, the risk of legal liability is exceedingly small. In a recent review by Larry Gostin, then the Executive Director of the American Society of Law and Medicine, he wrote, "In a search of reported decisions, *no case* was found in which a health care professional was convicted of causing, inducing, or assisting in the death of her patient" (41).

Medical Nutrition and Hydration

Should techniques for providing medical nutrition and hydration (intravenous fluids, parenteral nutrition, tube feedings, and so forth) be considered medical treatments? If so, can they then be ethically withdrawn by the same process and criteria that are used for other types of medical treatment? In other words, if it is ethically acceptable to withdraw a ventilator from a terminally ill patient, is it also ethically acceptable to withdraw medically provided nutrition and hydration? (Note that this question does not propose withholding oral feedings from patients who want to eat or drink.)

The last decade has seen a gradually emerging consensus in both law and ethics that answers the questions on medical nutrition and hydration posed above in the affirmative (42, 43). A large number of court decisions, including the decision of the US Supreme Court in Cruzan, have now concluded that medically provided nutrition and hydration should be considered medical treatments, and that patients or their surrogates should have the right to refuse them (35–37). The decision of whether or not to administer this therapy should be based on the same criteria outlined above for other treatments, that is, an analysis of the balance between the benefits and burdens of providing the therapy.

Many clinicians have been reluctant to accept this approach, at least in part because "feeding" seems to be such a basic and fundamental aspect of the care that they provide to their patients. In the terminology of the distinction discussed above, it seems so "ordinary." This provides yet another example of the inadequacies of the ordinary or extraordinary distinction, however, because for certain patients, particularly those who are permanently unconscious or imminently dying, medically administered feedings can no longer provide any benefit.

Pediatricians have been particularly slow to acknowledge this emerging consensus (44). The reasons for this reluctance are several. First, prognoses are often more uncertain in children, given their remarkable ability to recover from injury. Second, even normal newborns need assistance with feedings, so pediatricians are less likely to see artificial feedings as a "medical" treatment. Third, whereas the hospice experience shows that refusal of food and water is frequently seen in elderly patients dying a natural death, the death of a child is never a "natural" event, and there is a reluctance to accept it with apparent passivity. Nevertheless, the principles that have evolved governing the administration or withdrawal of medically provided feedings in adults are equally applicable in children, and no justifiable reason is found to treat the pediatric population any differently.

REFERENCES

1. Maurois A. The Columbia dictionary of quotations. New York: Columbia University Press, 1993.
2. Beauchamp TL, Childress JF. Principles of biomedical ethics. New York: Oxford University Press, 1994.
3. Jonsen AR, Toulmin S. The abuse of casuistry. Los Angeles: University of California Press, 1988.
4. Toulmin S. The tyranny of principles. Hastings Cent Rep 1981;11:31–39.
5. Lantos JD. Baby Doe five years later. Implications for child health. N Engl J Med 1987;317:444–447.
6. Carse AL. The "voice of care": implications for bioethical education. J Med Philos 1991;16:5–28.
7. Coles R. The call of stories: teaching and the moral imagination. Boston: Houghton Mifflin, 1989.
8. Solzhenitsyn A. The exhausted west. Harvard Magazine 1978; Jul/Aug:22.
9. Pellegrino ED, Thomasma DC. For the patient's good: the restoration of beneficence in health care. New York: Oxford University Press, 1988.
10. Katz J. The silent world of doctor and patient. New York: Free Press, 1984.
11. Holder AR. Legal issues in pediatrics and adolescent medicine. New Haven: Yale University Press, 1985.
12. Buchanan AE, Brock DW. Deciding for others: the ethics of surrogate decision making. Cambridge: Cambridge University Press, 1989.
13. Prince v. Commonwealth of Massachusetts. 321 U.S. 158 (1944).
14. Sigman GS, O'Connor C. Exploration for physicians of the mature minor doctrine. J Pediatr 1991;119:520–525.
15. Wennberg JE, Gittelsohn AM. Small area variations in health care delivery. Science 1973;183:1102–1108.
16. Wennberg JE, Mulley AG, Hanley D, et al. An assessment of prostatectomy for benign urinary tract obstruction. Geographic variations and the evaluation of medical care outcomes. JAMA 1988;259:3027–3030.
17. Wennberg JE, Freeman JL, Shelton RM, et al. Hospital use and mortality among Medicare beneficiaries in Boston and New Haven. N Engl J Med 1989;321:1168–1173.
18. Wennberg JE, Gittelsohn A. Variations in medical care among small areas. Sci Am 1982;246:120–134.
19. Kasper JF, Mulley AG, Wennberg JE. Developing shared decision-making programs to improve the quality of health care. Quality Review Bulletin 1992;18:182–190.
20. Randall T. Producers of videodisc programs strive to expand patient's role in medical decision-making process. JAMA 1993;270:160–162.
21. Kasper JF, Fowler FJ. Responding to the challenge: a status report on shared decision-making programs. HMO Practice 1993;7:176–181.
22. Rabkin MT, Gillerman G, Rice NR. Orders not to resuscitate. N Engl J Med 1976;295:364–366.
23. Optimum care for hopelessly ill patients. A report of the Clinical Care Committee of the Massachusetts General Hospital. N Engl J Med 1976;295:362–364.
24. Mittelberger JA, Lo B, Martin D, et al. Impact of a procedure-specific do not resuscitate order form on documentation of do not resuscitate orders. Arch Intern Med 1993;153:228–232.
25. Murphy DJ, Finucane TE. New do-not-resuscitate policies: a first step in cost control. Arch Intern Med 1993;153:1641–1648.
26. Snider GL. The do-not-resuscitate order: ethical and legal imperative or medical decision. Am Rev Respir Dis 1991;143:665–674.
27. Hackler JC, Hiller FC. Family consent to orders not to resuscitate: reconsidering hospital policy. JAMA 1990;264:1281–1283.
28. Tomlinson T, Brody H. Futility and the ethics of resuscitation. JAMA 1990;264:1276–1280.
29. Blackhall LJ. Must we always use CPR? N Engl J Med 1987; 317:1281–1285.

30. Waisel DB, Truog RD. The cardiopulmonary resuscitation-not-indicated order: futility revisited. Ann Intern Med 1995; 122:304–308.
31. McClung JA, Kamer RS. Legislating ethics: implications of New York's do-not-resuscitate law. N Engl J Med 1990;323: 270–272.
32. Solomon MZ, O'Donnell L, Jennings B, et al. Decisions near the end of life: professional views on life-sustaining treatments [see comments]. Am J Public Health 1993;83:14–23.
33. Shaw A, Randolph JG, Manard B. Ethical issues in pediatric surgery: a national survey of pediatricians and pediatric surgeons. Pediatrics 1977;60:588–599.
34. Caralis PV, Hammond JS. Attitudes of medical students, housestaff, and faculty physicians toward euthanasia and termination of life-sustaining treatment. Crit Care Med 1992; 20:683–690.
35. Orentlicher D. From the Office of the General Counsel. Cruzan v. Director of Missouri Department of Health: an ethical and legal perspective. JAMA 1989;262:2928–2930.
36. Bioethicists' statement on the U.S. Supreme Court's Cruzan decision. N Engl J Med 1990;323:686–687.
37. Annas GJ. Nancy Cruzan and the right to die. N Engl J Med 1990;323:670–673.
38. Angell M. The quality of mercy. N Engl J Med 1982;306: 98–99.
39. Foley KM. The relationship of pain and symptom management to patient requests for physician-assisted suicide. J Pain Symptom Manage 1991;6:289–297.
40. Truog RD, Berde CB. Pain, euthanasia, and anesthesiologists. Anesthesiology 1993;78:353–360.
41. Gostin LO. Drawing a line between killing and letting die: the law, and law reform, on medically assisted dying. Journal of Law, Medicine, and Ethics 1993;21:94–101.
42. McCann RM, Hall WJ, Groth-Juncker A. Comfort care for terminally ill patients: the appropriate use of nutrition and hydration. JAMA 1994;272:1263–1266.
43. Lynn J, ed. By no extraordinary means. Bloomington: Indiana University Press, 1989.
44. Frader J. Forgoing life-sustaining food and water: newborns. In: Lynn J, ed. By no extraordinary means: the choice to forgo life-sustaining food and water. Bloomington: Indiana University Press, 1989:180–185.

Appendix: Drugs

	Drug	Dosage	Bolus Dose	Infusion Dose	Levels
RESUSCITATION					
	Atropine	0.01–0.03 mg/kg (maximum 2 mg)			
	Calcium chloride	0.1–0.3 mL/kg			
	Epinephrine (1:10000)	0.1 mL/kg			
	Lidocaine	1 mg/kg			
	Sodium bicarbonate	1–2 mEq/kg			
CARDIAC MEDICATIONS					
Inotropic Agents					
	Digoxin	10 µg/kg/d ÷ BID			< 2 ng/mL
	Dopamine			2–20 µg/kg/min	
	Dobutamine			2–20 µg/kg/min	
	Epinephrine			0.05–1.0 µg/kg/min	
	Isoproterenol			0.05–1.5 µg/kg/min	
	Norepinephrine			0.05–1.0 µg/kg/min	
Vasodilators					
	Hydralazine	0.1–0.4 mg/kg IV Q 4–6 h			
	Nitroglycerine			0.3–5.0 µg/kg/min	
	Nitroprusside			0.3–10.0 µg/kg/min	Thiocyanate < 12 mg/L

	Drug	Dosage	Bolus Dose	Infusion Dose	Levels
Phosphodiesterase Inhibitors					
	Amrinone (Inocor)		1–3 mg/kg	3–20 µg/kg/min	
	Milrinone (Primacor)		50 µg/kg	0.25–0.75 µg/kg/min	
Diuretic Agents					
	Acetazolamide (Diamox)	5 mg/kg QD			
	Bumetamide (Bumex)	0.01–0.1 mg/kg QD			
	Ethacrynic acid (Edecrin)	1 mg/kg			
	Furosemide (Lasix)	1 mg/kg Q 6–12 h	0.1 mg/kg	0.1–0.4 mg/kg/h	
	Spironolactone	1–3.5 mg/kg/d QD–QID			
β-Blockers					
	Esmolol		500 µg/kg	50–250 µg/kg/min	
	Labetolol	0.2–0.5 mg/kg			
	Propranolol	0.01–0.1 mg/kg			
Angiotensin-Converting Enzyme Inhibitors					
	Captopril (Capoten)	0.1–1.0 mg/kg/d ÷ TID			
	Enalapril (Vasotec)	0.1–0.5 mg/kg/d QD			
Antidysrhythmic Agents					
	Adenosine	50–200 µg/kg			
	Amiodarone		10–15 mg/kg/d QD–BID	5 mg/kg/d QD–BID	
	Bretylium	5 mg/kg			

	Drug	Dosage	Bolus Dose	Infusion Dose	Levels
Antidysrhythmic Agents (cont.)					
	Lidocaine	1 mg/kg		20–50 µg/kg/min	1.5–5.0 µg/L
	Procainamide		2–6 mg/kg	20–80 µg/kg/min	4–10 mg/L; 10–30 mg/L (if combined with NAPA)
	Quinidine	6 mg/kg Q 4–6 h			
	Verapamil	0.05–0.3 mg/kg			
Ductal Manipulation					
	Indomethacin (Indocin)	0.1–0.25 mg/kg			
	Prostaglandin E_1			0.01–0.2 µg/kg/min	
Miscellaneous					
	Immune globulin	1–4 g/kg			
	Nifedipine (Procardia)	0.25–0.50 mg/kg/dose Q 6–8 h			
	Nitric oxide			2–80 ppm	Nitrogen dioxide < 2 ppm
	Phenylephrine	10–100 µg/kg	0.1–0.5 µg/kg/min		
	Tromethamine (THAM)	3.5–6 mL/kg/dose			

	Drug	Dosage	Bolus Dose	Infusion Dose	Levels
NONCARDIAC MEDICATIONS					
Anticoagulants					
	Aspirin	5–10 mg/kg/d			
	Heparin		50–100 U/kg	10–25 U/kg/h	
	Streptokinase		1000–4000 U/kg	1000–1500 U/kg/h	
	Tissue plasminogen activator		1.25 mg/kg	0.1–0.5 mg/kg/h	
	Urokinase		4400 U/kg	4400 U/kg/h	
	Warfarin (Coumadin)	0.1–0.3 mg/kg QD			
Sedatives					
	Chloral hydrate	25–50 mg/kg Q 4–8 h			
	Lorazepam (Ativan)	0.05 mg/kg Q 4–8 h			
	Midazolam (Versed)	0.03–0.1 mg/kg Q 1–2 h		0.1 mg/kg/h	
Analgesics					
	Fentanyl	1–5 µg/kg Q 1–2 h		1–10 µg/kg/min	
	Methadone	0.1 mg/kg Q 6–12 h			
	Morphine	0.1–0.2 mg/kg Q 2–4 h			
Muscle Relaxants					
	Atracurium	0.3–0.5 mg/kg			
	Vecuronium (Norcuron)	0.1 mg/kg Q 1 h	0.05–0.2 mg/kg	0.05–0.1 mg/kg/h	

	Drug	Dosage	Bolus Dose	Infusion Dose	Levels
Miscellaneous					
	Aminophylline		5–7 mg/kg	0.7–1.4 mg/kg/h	10–20 µg/mL
	Dexamethasone	0.3–2.0 mg/kg/d ÷ Q 6 h			
	Naloxone	0.01–0.1 mg/kg			
	Phenobarbital	3–5 mg/kg/d BID-TID	10–20 mg/kg		10–20 µg/mL

BID, twice daily; IV, intravenous; NAPA, *N*-acetylated procainamide; PPM, parts per million; Q, every; QD, every day; QID, four times daily; TID, three times daily.

Compiled by Dr. Ana Maria Rosales and Dr. Anthony C. Chang

Index

Page numbers in *italics* denote figures; those followed by "t" denote tables.

Abdominal radiography, 415–417, *416*
ABG. *See* Arterial blood gas analysis
Absent pulmonary valve syndrome, *xxii*, 357
Absorption of drug, 45
ACE inhibitors. *See* Angiotensin-converting enzyme inhibitors
Acetazolamide, 544
N-Acetylprocainamide (NAPA), 469, 476
Acid-base balance
    cardiac output and, 178
    intraoperative management of, 370–371
    postoperative, 167
    pulmonary vascular effects of, 498, 502
Acrocyanosis, 155
Active compression-decompression CPR, 134
Acute renal failure, postoperative, 388
Acute respiratory distress syndrome (ARDS), 360–361, 419–420
    clinical stages of, 361
    continuous positive airway pressure for, 119
    definition of, 360
    due to respiratory syncytial virus infection, 360
    effects of PEEP on right ventricular function in, 117–119
    management of, 361
Acyl-CoA dehydrogenase deficiency, 490
Adenosine, 479–480
    adverse effects of, 480
    dosage of, 544
    effects in junctional ectopic tachycardia, 472, *472*
    indications for, 479–480
        monomorphic ventricular tachycardia, 474
        supraventricular tachycardia, 468
    metabolism of, 480
ADH. *See* Antidiuretic hormone
Adjustment disorders, post-transplant, 338
Adrenergic agonists, 129–130
Adrenocorticotropic hormone, 380
Adriamycin-induced cardiomyopathy, 490–491
Advanced practice nurse, 525–529
    critical pathways and case management, role of, 526, *527–528*
    current issues related to, 528–529
    education of, 525–526
    financial implications of, 526–528
    patient management by, 525
    as referral liaison, 528
    research by, 526
Afterload, 25–26
    definition of, 23, 436
    fetal, 17–18, 23
    increased postoperative, 181, 443
    indices of, 436–437
    neonatal, 23
    reduction of
        for myocarditis, 488–489
        sodium nitroprusside for, 55
        after surgery for D-transposition of great arteries, 296
α-Agonists, 129–130
Airway edema, 71
Airway management, 95–104, 155–156
    in child with absent pulmonary valve, 357
    extubation, 103–104, 104t
    intubation, 95–96, 128
        complications of, 358
    mechanical ventilation, 96–103
    postoperative, 165
        radiographic assessment for, 419
    for resuscitation, 128
    in transplant recipients, 335–336
Airway obstruction, upper, 357–359
Airway reactivity, 71
Airway resistance, 70–71, *71*
Alagille's syndrome, 159, 160t, 414
Aliasing, 432, *433*
α receptors, 47, 48t
Aluminum intoxication, 388
Alveolar carbon dioxide equation, 74
Alveolar dead space, 73
Alveolar gas equation, 74
Alveolar hypoxia, 498
Alveolar pressure, 68, *75*, 76
Alveolar ventilation, 73–74
Aminophylline, 546
Amiodarone, 478
    adverse effects of, 478
    dosage of, 544
    drug interactions with, 478
    indications for, 478
        atrial flutter/atrial fibrillation, 471
        ectopic atrial tachycardia, 471
        hypertrophic cardiomyopathy, 492
        junctional ectopic tachycardia, 473
        supraventricular tachycardia, 469
    metabolism of, 478
Amrinone, 48t, 52
    adverse effects of, 52
    dosage of, 544
    guidelines for clinical use of, 52
    metabolism of, 52
    for myocarditis, 488
    pulmonary vascular effects of, 499t
Analgesics, 88–90. *See also* Sedation and analgesia
    assessing need for, 86
    dosages of, 87t, 546
    indications for, 85–86
        dying patients, 540
        mechanical ventilation, 86
        postoperative, 85–86
        preoperative, 85
        procedures in cardiac intensive care unit, 86
        stress response attenuation, 85–86
    ketamine, 90
    opioids, 88–90
    post-transplant, 338
Anatomy, cardiac, 3–15
    anatomical diagnosis, *14*, 14–15
    diagram for cardiac catheterization, *30*
    morphologic, 3–10
        left atrium, *5*, 5–6
        left ventricle, 8–10, *9*, 112
        right atrium, 3–5, *4*
        right ventricle, 6–8, *7*, 108–109, 111–112
    segmental, 10–14
    types of conus, 10, *13*, 14

Anatomy, cardiac—*Continued*
    types of ventricular situs, 10, *11, 12*
    types of visceroatrial situs, 10, *10*
Anemia, 40
Anesthetic agents, 87t, 90–91
    barbiturates, 90
    etomidate, 91
    propofol, 90–91
Aneurysm
    of atrial septum, 208
    postoperative mediastinal, 421–422
ANF. *See* Atrial natriuretic factor
Angiography in graft coronary artery disease, 338–339
Angioplasty, 450–454
    for branch pulmonary artery stenosis, 450–453, *452–455*
    for coarctation of aorta, 250, 251, 450
    iliofemoral arterial injury and, 453–454
    subclavian flap, 251
Angiotensin I and II, 484
Angiotensin-converting enzyme (ACE) inhibitors, 56–57, 544
    captopril, 56–57, 544
    enalapril, 57, 544
    mechanism of action of, 56
    for myocardial infarction, 513
    for myocarditis, 488–489
    postoperative administration of, 184
    for restrictive cardiomyopathy, 493
    for transplant recipients, 335
Anomalies, extracardiac, 158–161, 160t
Anomalous origin of left coronary artery from pulmonary artery, 312–315, 511
    anatomy of, 312–313, *313*
    clinical course of, 313
    pathophysiology of, 313
    postoperative management of, 315
    postoperative problems associated with, 315
        low cardiac output, 315
        ventricular dysrhythmias, 315
    preoperative evaluation of, 313
    surgical procedures for, 313–315
        direct reimplantation of left coronary artery, 315
        ligation of anomalous coronary artery, 314
        subclavian artery turndown, 314–315
        Takeuchi operation, *314,* 315
Anomalous pulmonary venous connection, *xix,* 223–227
    anatomy of, 223–224
    clinical course of, 224–225
    definition of, 223
    lesions associated with, 224
    mixed drainage patterns, 224
    obstructed vs. nonobstructed, 224
    partial, 224
    pathophysiology of, 224
    postoperative management of, 227
    postoperative problems associated with, 227
        low cardiac output, 227
        perioperative dysrhythmias, 227
        pulmonary hypertension, 227
        respiratory insufficiency, 227
    preoperative evaluation of, 225, 441
    scimitar syndrome, 226
    surgical procedures for, 225–227, *226*
    types of, 223–224
        infracardiac, 224, 226
        intracardiac, 224, 226
        supracardiac, 223, *224,* 225, *226*
Antacids, 401
    for patients with acute renal failure, 388
Anthracycline-induced cardiomyopathy, 490–491
Antiarrhythmic agents, 475–480, 544–545. *See also* specific drugs
    adenosine, 479–480
    for atrial flutter/atrial fibrillation, 470–471
    class IA, 475–476
    class IB, 476–477
    class IC, 477
    class II, 477–478
    class III, 478–479
    class IV, 479
    digoxin, 479
    for ectopic atrial tachycardia, 473
    for junctional ectopic tachycardia, 473
    for supraventricular tachycardia, 468–469
    for ventricular tachycardia, 474–475
Antibiotics, 155
    anthracycline-induced cardiomyopathy, 490–491
    for sepsis, 514
Anticoagulants, 60, 545
    aspirin, 60
    during cardiopulmonary bypass, 196–197
    heparin, 60
    for myocardial infarction, 513
    for myocarditis, 489
    for patient on myocardial mechanical support, 348
    postoperative, 399
    for restrictive cardiomyopathy, 493
    warfarin, 60
Anticonvulsants, 375, 376t, 381
Antidiuretic hormone (ADH), 387
Antifibrinolytic therapy, 399
Antihypertensive agents, for transplant recipients, 335
Antileukocyte adhesion molecules, 371
Antithymocyte globulin (ATG), 333, 334t
Aorta
    coarctation of, 247–254 (*See also* Coarctation of aorta)
    cross-clamping of, 190, *191*
    in D-transposition of great arteries, 289–290, *290*
    in L-transposition of great arteries, *297,* 297–298
    pulmonary artery-aortic anastomosis, 276
Aortic arch
    definitions of segments of, 247
    double, 322–324
        anatomy of, 322, *322*
        repair of, *323,* 323–324
    interrupted, 243–245 (*See also* Interrupted aortic arch)
    right, with aberrant left subclavian artery, 322
    in situs solitus or inversus states, 410
Aortic atresia, 272t
Aortic dissection, 509–510
    causes of, 509
    evaluation of, 509
    iatrogenic, 509
    therapy for, 509–510
Aortic insufficiency, 233, 238
Aortic sinuses of Valsalva, 290, *291*
Aortic stenosis, *xxi,* 38, 233–238. *See also* Subaortic stenosis
    anatomy of, 233
    balloon valvuloplasty for, 234, 448–450, *451*
    clinical course of, 233
    echocardiographic evaluation of, 441
    lesions associated with, 233
    pathophysiology of, 233
    postoperative management of, 235
    postoperative problems associated with, 238
        aortic insufficiency, 238
        low cardiac output, 238
    preoperative evaluation of, 233–234
    preoperative management of, 234
    supravalvar, 240–242
        anatomy of, 240
        clinical course of, 240
        lesions associated with, 240
        pathophysiology of, 240
        postoperative management of, 242

Index 551

postoperative problems associated with, 242
  preoperative evaluation of, 241–242
  surgical procedure for, 241, 242
  types of, 240
surgical procedures for, 234–235, 235–237
Aortic valve, 4
  replacement of, 235, 236–237
Aorticopulmonary window, 38, 201–202
  anatomy of, 201, 201
  clinical course of, 201
  lesions associated with, 201
  pathophysiology of, 201
  postoperative management of, 202
  preoperative evaluation of, 201
  surgical procedure for, 202, 202
Aortoplasty, 251
Aortoventriculoplasty, 235, 237
Apnea, prostaglandin E_1-induced, 157
Aprotinin, 399
ARDS. See Acute respiratory distress syndrome
Arrhythmias, 152, 461–480. See also Electrocardiogram
  associated with traumatic injury, 508, 508t
  atrioventricular block, 462–463, 463
  bundle branch block, 461–462, 462
  dilated cardiomyopathy and, 489
  drug therapy for, 475–480, 544–545
  fetal, 153
  hyperkalemia and, 176
  hypertrophic cardiomyopathy and, 492
  hypokalemia and, 174–175
  myocarditis and, 486
  perioperative
    anomalous pulmonary venous connection and, 227
    after Fontan procedure, 283, 470
    supraventricular tachycardia, 469–470
    after surgery for anomalous origin of left coronary artery
      from pulmonary artery, 315
    after surgery for D-transposition of great arteries, 296, 470
    after surgery for Ebstein's anomaly, 320, 470
    tetralogy of Fallot and, 261
    in transplant recipients, 335
    truncus arteriosus and, 232
  sinus bradycardia, 461
  supraventricular tachycardia, 466–473
  temporary pacing for, 463–466 (See also Pacing)
  ventricular, 473–475
    monomorphic (re-entrant) ventricular tachycardia, 474, 474
    torsade de pointes, 474, 475
    treatment of, 474–475
    ventricular fibrillation, 475
Arterial access, 140–141
  radial artery cannulation, 141
  umbilical artery cannulation, 140, 141, 155, 447
Arterial blood gas (ABG) analysis
  during CPR, 132
  postoperative, 166–167
Arterial switch procedure, 294, 295
  cardiac index after, 181
  echocardiographic evaluation for, 294, 294, 441
  heart transplantation after failure of, 328
  mortality from, 294–296
Arteriovenous malformation, 38
ASD. See Atrial septal defect
Asphyxia, 23, 127
Aspirin, 60, 399, 545
Asplenia, 409, 410–411
Atelectasis, 410, 419
Atenolol, 491
ATG. See Antithymocyte globulin
Ativan. See Lorazepam
Atracurium, 87t, 92–93, 502, 546
Atrial anatomy, 3–6, 4, 5. See also Left atrium; Right atrium

Atrial appendage
  left, 5
  right, 3–5
Atrial flutter/atrial fibrillation, 5, 470–471
  atrial septal defect and, 209
  diagnosis of, 470
  postoperative, 464, 470
  treatment of, 470–471
Atrial isomerism, 10
Atrial natriuretic factor (ANF), 387, 484
Atrial septal defect (ASD), 207–211
  anatomy of, 207–208
    aneurysm of atrial septum, 208
    common atrium, 208
    patent foramen ovale, 208
  clinical course of, 208–209
  due to cardiac trauma, 507–509
  epidemiology of, 207
  lesions associated with, 208
  occluder devices for, 453, 455
  pathophysiology of, 208
  postoperative management of, 210–211
  postoperative problems associated with, 210–211
    atrioventricular block, 211
    cyanosis, 211
    left ventricular dysfunction, 211
    postpericardiotomy syndrome, 210
    pulmonary hypertension, 211
    residual atrial septal defect, 211
    sinoatrial node dysfunction, 210
    venous obstruction, 211
  preoperative evaluation of, 209
  restrictive vs. nonrestrictive, 208
  surgical procedure for, 209, 210
  types of, 207–208, 208
    coronary sinus, 217–218
    ostium primum, 217–222, 218
    ostium secundum, xix, 6, 207
    sinus venosus, 217
Atriopulmonary connections, 278
Atrioventricular (AV) block, 462–463
  first degree, 462, 463
  postoperative, 462–463
    after repair of atrial septal defect, 211
    after repair of common atrioventricular canal, 222
    after repair of subaortic stenosis, 240
    after repair of tetralogy of Fallot, 261
    after repair of ventricular septal defect, 216, 462, 463
    after tricuspid valve replacement, 320
  second degree, 462–463
    Wenckebach type I, 462–463
    Wenckebach type II, 463
  third degree, 463
Atrioventricular (AV) canal, 5, 8, 9
  common, 217–222 (See also Common atrioventricular canal)
  defects of, 152
  malaligned, with hypoplastic left or right ventricle, 272t
Atrioventricular (AV) dissociation, 474
Atrioventricular (AV) node, 5, 41
Atrioventricular (AV) valves, xx
  borderline hypoplasia of, 271
  left (See Mitral valve)
  right (See Tricuspid valve)
Atropine, 131, 543
Auscultation of heart, 39–40
Autonomic effects on pulmonary vascular resistance, 500
Autonomy of patients, 532
Azathioprine, 333, 334t

"Baby Doe" case, 532
Baclofen, 380

BAEPs. *See* Brainstem auditory evoked potentials
BAL. *See* Bronchoalveolar lavage
Balloon angioplasty, 450–454
　for branch pulmonary artery stenosis, 450–453, *452–455*
　for coarctation of aorta, 250, 450
　iliofemoral arterial injury and, 453–454
Balloon atrial septostomy, 293, 441, 455
Balloon valvuloplasty, 448–450
　for aortic stenosis, 234, 448–450, *451*
　for mitral stenosis, 308, 448
　for pulmonary stenosis, *268,* 269, 448, *449*
Band(s)
　limbic, 3–4
　moderator, 6, 8
　parietal (conal septum), 6–8
　septal, 6, 8
Barbiturates, 90, 380
Basal ganglia lesions, *372*
Beer Lambert law, 138
Benzodiazepines, 87t, 87–88, 380, 502
Bereavement program, 522–523
Bernoulli equation, 433–434
"Best interest" principle, 532
β-Blockers, 58–59, 469, 544
　for atrial flutter, 471
　for ectopic atrial tachycardia, 471
　esmolol, 58–59, 544
　for hypertrophic cardiomyopathy, 491
　labetalol, 59, 544
　for myocardial infarction, 513
　for patient with aortic dissection, 509
　for torsade de pointes, 475
β receptors, 47, 48t
Bidirectional Glenn/hemi-Fontan procedure, *278,* 278–281, *279*
　physiology and indications for, 278–280
　postoperative issues related to, 280–281
　pulmonary arteriovenous fistulae and, 412, *413*
Bioavailability of drug, 45
Bioethics. *See* Ethical and legal issues
Blalock-Taussig shunt, *xxi,* 61, 168, 173, 174, 181, 266–267, *267,* 275, *275,* 361, 417
Bland-White-Garland syndrome. *See* Anomalous origin of left coronary artery from pulmonary artery
Bleeding
　gastrointestinal, 401
　postoperative, 206, 397–399, 398t
　　in patient on mechanical support, 348
　　risk factors for, 397–399
　　treatment of, 399
Blood flow. *See also* Circulation
　calculation in catheterization laboratory, 31–32, *32*
　cerebral
　　during CPR, 128, 132–133
　　recovery after deep hypothermia with circulatory arrest, 195
　during CPR, 128–129
　fetal, 17, *18*
　pulmonary (*See* Pulmonary blood flow)
Blood pressure. *See also* Hypertension
　measurement in neonate with suspected congenital heart disease, 154
　monitoring of, 137, *138*
　　Doppler ultrasound, 137
　　historical methods, 137, *138*
　　oscillometric method, 137
　neonatal, 151
Blood transfusion, 399
Blood urea nitrogen (BUN), 178
Blunt cardiac injury, 507–508, 508t
Bohr equation, 74
Bony thorax, 414
Bounding pulses, 39

Bowel obstruction, 416–417
Brachial plexus lesions, *372*
Bradycardia
　cardiac output and, 178, 181
　after cavopulmonary shunt, 280
　fetal, 22, 153
　isoproterenol for, 130
　sinus, 39, 181, 461
Brain death, 381
Brain resuscitation, 132–133
Brain ultrasound, 369–370, 374t
Brainstem auditory evoked potentials (BAEPs), 373t
Breathing, 96–98, *98.* *See also* Respiratory physiology; Ventilation
　in child with cardiac arrest, 128
　hemodynamic changes with, 107–121 (*See also* Cardiopulmonary interactions)
　paradoxic, 352
　work of, 72
Bretylium, 478–479
　adverse effects of, 479
　dosage of, 544
　indications for, 478
　metabolism of, 478
Brockenbrough atrial septostomy, 3
Bronchiolitis
　due to respiratory syncytial virus, 360
　obliterative, after lung transplantation, 327, 339
Bronchoalveolar lavage (BAL), 336, 354–355
Bronchomalacia, 360
Bronchopleural fistula, 362
Bronchopulmonary dysplasia (BPD), 359–360
　definition of, 359
　pathology of, 359
　perioperative management of, 360
Bronchoscopy, 354–355
　complications of, 355
　indications for, 354–355, 355t
　instruments for, 354, *354*
　in neonate, 355
　sedation for, 354
Bubble oxygenators, 193
Bumetanide (Bumex), 544
BUN. *See* Blood urea nitrogen
Butterfly vertebrae, 414
Butyrophenones, 380

Calcifications on chest radiography, 413, *414*
Calcium, 176–177
　hypercalcemia, 175t
　hypocalcemia, 175t, 177
　management during cardiopulmonary bypass, 196
　normal serum levels of, 176
　postoperative levels of, 176–177
　for resuscitation, 130, 543
　role in cell death, 132
　role in ischemia-reperfusion process, 196
　role in myocardial contractility, 46
Calcium antagonists, 56, 469
　effects in infants, 22
　for hypertrophic cardiomyopathy, 491–492
　for myocardial infarction, 513
　neuroprotective effect of, 133, 371
　nifedipine, 56
　for restrictive cardiomyopathy, 493
　verapamil, 56
Calcium chloride, 130, 543
　for hyperkalemia, 176
　for hypocalcemia, 177
Calcium gluconate, 130
　for hyperkalemia, 176
　for hypocalcemia, 177

Captopril (Capoten), 48t, 56–57
  adverse effects of, 57
  dosage of, 544
  guidelines for clinical use of, 56–57
  mechanism of action of, 56
  metabolism of, 56
  for myocarditis, 488–489
  postoperative administration of, 184
  for restrictive cardiomyopathy, 493
  for transplant recipients, 335
Carbamazepine, 380
Carbon dioxide
  elimination from pulmonary capillary blood, 74
  measurements during CPR, 132
Carboxyhemoglobin, 139
Cardiac catheterization, 29–32, 447–459
  for angioplasty procedures, 450–454
  choice of access sites for, 447
  diagnostic, 158
    anomalous origin of left coronary artery from pulmonary artery, 313
    anomalous pulmonary venous connection, 225
    aortic stenosis, 234
      supravalvar, 242
    aorticopulmonary window, 201
    atrial septal defect, 209
    coarctation of aorta, 249
    common atrioventricular canal, 219
    dilated cardiomyopathy, 490
    Ebstein's anomaly, 318
    interrupted aortic arch, 245
    mitral valve disease, 307–308
    myocardial infarction, 513
    patent ductus arteriosus, 204
    pulmonary atresia with intact ventricular septum, 266
    restrictive cardiomyopathy, 493
    subaortic stenosis, 239
    tetralogy of Fallot, 258–259
    transposition of great arteries, 294, 298
    truncus arteriosus, 230
    vascular rings and slings, 323
    ventricular septal defect, 214
  echocardiography and, 441
  for embolization and closure procedures, 454–455
  hemodynamic calculations from, 31–32, *32*
  indications for, 29
  intubation for, 447
  of left atrium, 3
  to measure oxygen saturation, 30–31
  in newborn, 159t, 447–448
  patient preparation and transport for, 447
  physiologic diagram for, 30, *30*
  postoperative, 345, 455–456
  for pressure measurements, 31
  preventing hypothermia during, 447
  radiographic assessment after, 414–415, *415*
  for septostomy procedures, 455
  for staged palliation and repair of complex defects, 456
    single ventricle, 456–457, *456–457*
    tetralogy of Fallot with pulmonary atresia and diminutive pulmonary arteries, 11–13, *12*
  therapeutic, 448–450
    aortic stenosis, 448–450, *451*
    critical pulmonic stenosis, 448, *449*
    valvuloplasty, 448
Cardiac impulse, 178
Cardiac index (CI), 177
Cardiac isoenzymes, 512–513
Cardiac loop formation, 10, *11*, *12*
Cardiac massage, 128–129
  closed chest, 128–129
  open chest, 128–129

Cardiac output (CO), 25
  cellular basis for manipulation of, 46–47, *47*
  definition of, 177
  determinants of, 22–23, 25, 177–178
  determination of, 145
    based on Fick principle, 31, 145–146, 179
    bedside measurements, 178–179
    echocardiography, 178
    thermodilution method, *179*, 179–180, 180t
  fetal, 17
  increase at birth, 21, 23
  low-output cardiac failure, 45–46
  maintained by cardiac massage, 128–129
  neonatal, 22–23
  postoperative, 177–180, 345
    causes of low cardiac output, 180
    echocardiographic evaluation of low output states, 442–444
      decreased myocardial contractility, 442
      excess afterload, 443
      hypovolemia, 442
      myocardial ischemia, 442–443
      pericardial effusion, 443, *443*
      postoperative residua or previously undiagnosed lesions, 443–444
    after Fontan procedure, 283, 283t
    after mitral valve surgery, 309–311
    after Norwood or Damus-Kaye-Stansel procedure for single ventricle lesions, 277
    after repair of anomalous pulmonary venous connection, 227
    after repair of aortic stenosis, 238
    after repair of coarctation of aorta, 254
    after repair of common atrioventricular canal, 222
    after repair of pulmonary atresia with intact ventricular septum, 268
    after repair of truncus arteriosus, 231
    after surgery for anomalous origin of left coronary artery from pulmonary artery, 315
    after surgery for D-transposition of great arteries, 296
    after surgery for Ebstein's anomaly, 320
  provided by mechanical support, 347–348
  related to age, 177
  related to body surface area, 177
  signs of inadequacy of, 178
Cardiac physiology, 25–35
  cardiac catheterization, 29–32, *30*
  cardiac output, 25
  diastolic mechanics, 26
  myocardial oxygen physiology, 32–35
  pressure-volume analyses, *27*, 27–28, *28*
    over changing load, 28–29, *29*
  systolic mechanics, 25–26
Cardiac silhouette, 411, 420, 455
Cardiac tumors, 514–515, *515*
Cardiomegaly, *410*, *412*, *421*
  anomalous origin of left coronary artery from pulmonary artery and, 313
  coarctation of aorta and, 249
  dilated cardiomyopathy and, 489
  myocarditis and, 487
Cardiomyopathy, 489–493
  anthracycline-induced, 490–491
  dilated, 489–490, *490*
  heart transplantation for, 328
  HIV-associated, 490
  hypertrophic, 491–492, *492*
  restrictive, 492–493
Cardioplegia solution, 190–191, *191*
Cardiopulmonary bypass (CPB), 189–198
  acid-base management during, 370–371
  aortic cross-clamping for, 190, *191*
  cannulation for, 189–190
  cardioplegia solution for, 190–191, *191*

Cardiopulmonary bypass (CPB)—*Continued*
  cardiotomy suction devices for, 189–190
  components of system for, 189, *190*
  de-airing heart at completion of, 191
  definition of, 189
  extracorporeal circulation and circulatory arrest during, 190–191
  fluid and electrolyte status/management after, 173–174, 387–388
  function of, 189
  hypothermia for, 190, 191, *192*, 194–195, 370–371
  inflammatory response to, 197, 387
  partial, 191
  pathophysiology of, 387
  problems resulting from, 192–198
    bleeding, 397–399, 398t
    cerebrovascular accident, 376–377
    circulation, 192–193
    electrolyte and glucose composition, 196
    hematocrit and oncotic pressure, 195–196, 393
    myocardial protection, 197–198
    pharmacologic manipulations, 196–197
    respiration, 193–194, 356
    temperature, 194–195
  pulmonary vascular effects of, 500
  renal effects of, 387
  safety of, 189
  sequence of events for, 190
  temporary pacing after, 463–466 (*See also* Pacing)
  total, 190–191
  ultrafiltration during, 393–395, *393–395*
  vent catheters for, 191
  weaning from, 191–192
Cardiopulmonary interactions, 67, 107–121
  description of cardiopulmonary circulation, 107, *108*
  left ventricle, 112–114, *113*
  positive intrathoracic pressure and cardiac function in normal heart, *116*, 116–117
  positive pressure ventilation and PEEP in cardiopulmonary disease, 117–120
    left ventricle, 119–120, *121*
    right ventricle, 117–119
  pulmonary vascular bed, 110
  right ventricle, 111–112
  right ventricular output, 108–110
  spontaneous respiration and abnormal heart function, 114–115
    congenital heart disease, 115
    left ventricular failure, 114–115
  venous return (preload), 107–108, *109*
  ventricular interdependence, 107, 111–112
    intraventricular septum, 111–112
    pericardium, 112
Cardiopulmonary resuscitation (CPR), 127–134
  ABC algorithm for, 127
  adrenergic agonists, 129–130
  airway and breathing, 128
  assessment before initiation of, 127
  brain resuscitation, 132–133
  circulatory support, 128–129
  cough CPR, 119
  definition of, 127
  do-not-resuscitate orders, 535–538, *537*
  drugs for, 130–131, 543
  establishing protocols for, 127
  management of acidosis, 130–131
  monitoring during, 131–132
    hemodynamic, 131–132
    neurologic, 132
    respiratory, 132
  new techniques for, 133–134
    active compression-decompression, 134
    extracorporeal circulation, 134
    pneumatic vest CPR, 133–134
    simultaneous compression-ventilation, 133
  postresuscitation stabilization, 132
  teaching parents procedure for, 522
  vascular access, 129
Cardiorespiratory arrest, 127
  causes of, 127, 128t
  management of, 128–134
  neurologic impairment in survivors of, 127, 132
  prevention of, 127
  prognosis for, 127
  recognition/management of impending arrest, 127–128
Cardiothoracic ratio, 411
Cardiotomy suction devices, 189–190
Cardioversion, 468, 470, 475
Carnitine levels in dilated cardiomyopathy, 490
Case management, 526–528
  advantages of, 526
  critical pathways for, 526, *527–528*
  definition of, 526
  financial implications of, 526–528
  goals of, 526
Casuistic analysis, 532
Catecholamines, 47–51
  adverse effects of, 48
  definition of, 47
  digoxin, 51
  dobutamine, 50–51
  dopamine, 49–50
  endogenous, 47, *48*
  epinephrine, 48–49
  isoproterenol, 51
  norepinephrine, 49
  receptors for, 47, 48t
  sites of action and hemodynamic effects of, 48t
Catheter sepsis, 402
Cat's eye syndrome, 38t
CAVH. *See* Continuous arteriovenous hemofiltration
Cavopulmonary connections, 173, 277–284
  bidirectional Glenn/hemi-Fontan procedure, *278*, 278–281, *279*
  Fontan operation, *281–282*, 281–284
CC. *See* Closing capacity
Central venous access, 141, *142*
Cerebral blood flow
  during CPR, 128, 132–133
  recovery after deep hypothermia with circulatory arrest, 195
Cerebral hyperthermia, 133
Cerebral hypothermia, 133
Cerebral lesions, *372*
Cerebral protection strategies, 370–371
Cerebral reperfusion injury, 132–133
Cerebroplegia, 371
Cerebrovascular accident, postoperative, 376–378
  atrial septal defect and, 209
  cardiopulmonary bypass and, 376–377
  factors predisposing to, 377
  hemorrhagic transformation of, 378
  incidence of, 376
  infective endocarditis and, 378
  management of, 377–378
  mechanisms of, 376–377, *377*, *378*
  presentation of, 377
  prevention of, 377–378
CHARGE, 159, 160t
CHD. *See* Congenital heart disease
Chest compressions, 128–129
Chest radiography, 407–422
  to assess thoracoabdominal situs, 410–411, *411*
  bony thorax on, 414
  calcifications on, 413, *414*
  before cardiac catheterization, 414–415, *415*, 447
  cardiac silhouette on, 411

to confirm placement of tubes and catheters, 407–409, *408–409*, 447
after CPR, 132
findings associated with cardiac output, 178
findings associated with radiographic contrast media, 407
lungs on, 411–413, *412–414*
postoperative, 166, *166*, 415–422
    airway and lungs, 419–420, *420*
    cardiac size and blood volume, 415
    heart and great vessels, 420, *421*
    mediastinum, 420–422, *421*
    thorax, 417–418, *417–419*
preoperative, 410
projections for, 410
in specific disorders
    anomalous origin of left coronary artery from pulmonary artery, 313
    anomalous pulmonary venous connection, 225
    aortic stenosis, 234
        supravalvar, 242
    atrial septal defect, 209
    coarctation of aorta, 249
    common atrioventricular canal, 219
    dilated cardiomyopathy, 489
    Ebstein's anomaly, 317–318
    hypertrophic cardiomyopathy, 491
    interrupted aortic arch, 245
    mitral regurgitation, 307
    mitral stenosis, 307
    patent ductus arteriosus, 204
    pericardial effusion, 510
    pulmonary artery sling, 323
    pulmonary atresia with intact ventricular septum, 266
    restrictive cardiomyopathy, 493
    subaortic stenosis, 238
    tetralogy of Fallot, 257–258
    truncus arteriosus, 230
    vascular rings, 323
    ventricular septal defect, 214
systematic approach to, 407–409, 408t
technical considerations for, 409–410
Chest tubes for pneumothorax, 362
Chloral hydrate, 86–87, 87t, 380, 546
Chlorothiazide, 174
Chordae tendineae, 305
Choreoathetosis, postoperative, 379–380
Chromosomal abnormalities, 158–159, 160t
Chylothorax, 363, 418
CI. *See* Cardiac index
Circulation
    cardiopulmonary, 107, *108* (*See also* Cardiopulmonary interactions)
    changes at birth, 20, *20–22*
    coronary, 33, *33*
    extracorporeal, 134, 190–191
    fetal, 17–20, *18, 19*
    intercirculatory mixing in D-transposition of great arteries, 291–293, *293*
    problems during cardiopulmonary bypass, 192–193
    pulmonary, 74–78, 353–354 (*See also* Pulmonary blood flow)
    in single ventricle lesions, 271–274
    transitional, 37, 151, 272
Circulatory collapse
    aortic stenosis and, 233
    Ebstein's anomaly and, 317
Circulatory support, 128–129
Cisatracurium, 87t, 93
C_L. *See* Pulmonary compliance
Clinical nurse specialists. *See* Nursing roles and responsibilities
Clinical practice guidelines coordinator, 520
Clonazepam, 380

Closed chest cardiac massage, 128–129
Closing capacity (CC), 67, *68*
CMV. *See* Cytomegalovirus
CO. *See* Cardiac output
Coagulation cascade, 397, *398*
Coanda effect, 31, 241
Coarctation of aorta, *xx*, 38, 247–254
    anatomy of, 247, *248*
    clinical course of, 248–249
    definition of, 247
    lesions associated with, 247–248
    management of, 250–251
        balloon angioplasty, 250, 450
        surgical procedures, 250–251, *252–253*
    pathophysiology of, 248
    postoperative management of, 251
    postoperative problems associated with, 251, 254
        injury to structures near aortic arch, 254
        low cardiac output, 254
        paradoxical hypertension, 251
        postcoarctectomy syndrome, 251, 254
        residual coarctation, 254
        residual ventricular septal defect, 254
        spinal cord ischemia, 254
    preoperative evaluation of, 249–250
    preoperative management of, 250
    in Shone's syndrome, 247, 271
Colloid solutions, 388
Color flow mapping, 432–433
Coma, 381
Common atrioventricular canal, 217–222
    anatomy of, 217–218
    clinical course of, 219
    complete, 217–218, *218*
        tetralogy of Fallot with, 263–264
    lesions associated with, 218
    partial, 217, *218*
    pathophysiology of, 219
    postoperative management of, 222
    postoperative problems associated with, 222
        elevated left atrial pressure, 222
        heart block, 222
        junctional ectopic tachycardia, 222
        low cardiac output, 222
        pulmonary hypertension, 222
        residual ventricular septal defect, 222
    preoperative evaluation of, 219, *220*
    Rastelli classification of, 218, *218*
    surgical procedures for, 219–222, *220–221*
    transitional, 217
Common atrium, 208
Complement system activation during cardiopulmonary bypass, 197
Computed tomography (CT), 407
    brain, *xxii*, 374t, *377*, 379
Conduction system, 41–42
    correlation with papillary musculature, 8
    left bundle branch, 8
    right bundle branch, 7–8
Congenital extracardiac anomalies, 158–161, 160t
Congenital heart disease (CHD)
    clinical presentations in neonate, 152, 153t
    diagnosed by fetal echocardiography, 152–154, 153t
    evaluation for, 154
    extracardiac manifestations of, 158–161, 160t–161t
    heart transplantation for, 327–329, 329t
    mechanism of pulmonary compromise in, 355–356, *356*
    neurologic complications of, 369–382
    pulmonary disorders and, 355–363
    shunt lesions, 201–232
    spontaneous respiration and, 115

Congestive heart failure (CHF), 38t, 152, 483. *See also* Heart failure
  aortic stenosis and, 233
  aorticopulmonary window and, 201
  atrial septal defect and, 208
  coarctation of aorta and, 248–249
  definition of, 483
  Ebstein's anomaly and, 317
  echocardiographic evaluation of, 441–442
  interrupted aortic arch and, 244
  L-transposition of great arteries and, 298
  patent ductus arteriosus and, 204
  single ventricle lesions and, 274
  tetralogy of Fallot and, 257
Consent for treatment, 533–534
Consequentialism, 531–532
Continuous arteriovenous hemofiltration (CAVH), 391–393
Continuous positive airway pressure (CPAP), 119
Continuous wave Doppler, 432
Conus, 10, 14
  absent or deficient, 10, *13*, 14
  bilateral, 10, *13*, 14
  subaortic, 10, *13*, 14
  subpulmonary, 6–7, 10, *13*, 14
Cor pulmonale, 360, 515
Cor triatriatum, 305, 441
Coronary arteries
  anomalous origin of left coronary artery from pulmonary artery, 312–315
  graft coronary artery disease, 338–339
  in hearts with transposition of great arteries, 290–291, *292*
  right
    acute marginal branch of, 6
    epicardial branches of, 6
  supplying sinoatrial node, 3
  traumatic injury of, 507–508, 508t
Coronary circulatory physiology, 33, *33*
Coronary perfusion pressure, 128
  pulmonary hypertension and, 504
Coronary sinus
  defect of, *208*, 217
  ostium of, 3, 5
Corticosteroids
  for bronchopulmonary dysplasia, 360
  before cardiopulmonary bypass, 197
  for myocarditis, 489
  for respiratory syncytial virus infection, 360
  for transplant recipient, 333, 334t
Cough CPR, 119
Coumadin. *See* Warfarin
Coxsackie B virus-induced myocarditis, 485
CPB. *See* Cardiopulmonary bypass
CPR. *See* Cardiopulmonary resuscitation
Cranial ultrasound, 369–370, 374t
Creatinine
  cardiac output and, 178
  postoperative clearance of, 388
Crista terminalis, 3, 4
Critical care nursing. *See* Nursing roles and responsibilities
Critical pathways, 526, *527–528*
Croup, 358–359
Crystalloid solutions, 173
CT. *See* Computed tomography
Cyanosis, 37, 137–138, 152
  acrocyanosis, 155
  atrial septal defect and, 209, 211
  definition of, 154
  diagnostic evaluation of, 40–41
    echocardiography, 440–441
    in neonate, 154–155
  differential, 40
  differential diagnosis in neonate, 155, 156t

Ebstein's anomaly and, 317
after Fontan procedure, 283–284
hyperoxia test for, 41, 154, 155t
after Norwood or Damus-Kaye-Stansel procedure for single ventricle lesions, 277
after repair of truncus arteriosus, 231–232
reverse differential, 40–41
in tetralogy of Fallot, 257
Cyclic adenosine monophosphate (cAMP), 46, 52
Cyclophosphamide, for myocarditis, 489
Cyclosporine, 333, 334t, 335
  for myocarditis, 489
Cytokines, elevation during cardiopulmonary bypass, 197
Cytomegalovirus (CMV), post-transplant, 337

DAG. *See* Diacyl glycerol
Damus-Kaye-Stansel procedure, 276
Daunomycin-induced cardiomyopathy, 490–491
Dead space ventilation, 73–74
De-airing of heart, 191
Deep hypothermia with circulatory arrest (DHCA), 191, *192*, 194–195, 370–371
Deontology, 531–532
Depolarization, 41
Depression, post-transplant, 338
Dexamethasone, 546
Dextrocardia, 410
Diacyl glycerol (DAG), 46
Diagnostic evaluation, 37–43
  anatomic diagnosis, *14*, 14–15
  cardiovascular anomalies associated with pediatric syndromes, 38t
  confirming the diagnosis, 158
  electrocardiogram findings, 41–43
  hyperoxia test, 41, 154, 155t
  implications of transitional circulation, 37
  indications for, 37
  physical examination, 37–41
  signs and symptoms, 37, 38t
Dialysis, 389–393
  continuous hemofiltration, 391–393, *392*
  indications for, 389
  intermittent hemodialysis, 390
  peritoneal, 389t, 389–390
Diamox. *See* Acetazolamide
Diaphragmatic hernia, 159
Diaphragmatic paralysis, 352, 361–362, 419, *420*
  postoperative echocardiographic evaluation of, 444–445
Diastolic function, 26, 483
Diazepam, 87, 87t, 502
Diet and nutrition
  for chylothorax, 363
  enteral nutrition, 400
  goals of nutritional support, 400
  medical nutrition and hydration for dying patient, 540–541
  perioperative, 399–400
  total parenteral nutrition, 400
  for transplant recipients, 337–338
Diffusion of gas, 73
DiGeorge syndrome, 38t, 232, 246
Digoxin, 48t, 51, 479, 543
  adverse effects of, 51, 479
  drug interactions with, 479
  efficacy of, 51
  guidelines for clinical use of, 51
  indications for, 479
    atrial flutter/atrial fibrillation, 470–471
    ectopic atrial tachycardia, 471
    junctional ectopic tachycardia, 473
    myocarditis, 488
    supraventricular tachycardia, 469
  metabolism of, 51, 479

postoperative administration of, 184
   treatment of toxicity, 479
Dilated cardiomyopathy, 489–490
   diagnosis of, 489–490, *490*
   epidemiology of, 489
   natural history and outcome of, 490
   pathogenesis of, 489
   treatment of, 490
Diphenhydramine, 380
Dipyridamole, 197, 399
Disopyramide, for hypertrophic cardiomyopathy, 492
Distribution of drug, 45
Diuretics, 57–58, 544
   for bronchopulmonary dysplasia, 360
   electrolyte imbalances due to, 174
   furosemide, 57–58, 544
   for hyperkalemia, 176
   for hypertrophic cardiomyopathy, 491
   for myocarditis, 489
   postoperative, 173, 174
   for restrictive cardiomyopathy, 493
   sites of action of, *58*
Diving reflex, 469
D-loop ventricles, 10, *11–13*, 14
DNR. *See* Do-not-resuscitate orders
Dobutamine, 48t, 50–51, 157
   dosage of, 157, 543
   guidelines for clinical use of, 50–51
   mechanism of action of, 50, 157
   metabolism of, 50
   for myocarditis, 488
   postoperative administration of, *182,* 183
   pulmonary vascular effects of, 499t
   for transplant recipients, 333
   use in neonates, 157
Doctrine of Double Effect, 540
DOLV. *See* Double-outlet left ventricle
Do-not-resuscitate (DNR) orders, 535–538
   limitations of, 536–538
   parental consent for, 536
   procedure-specific, 536, *537*
L-Dopa, 380
Dopamine, 48t, 49–50, 157
   dosage of, 157, 543
   guidelines for clinical use of, 50
   mechanism of action of, 49–50, 157
   metabolism of, 50
   for myocarditis, 488
   postoperative, *182,* 183
      for oliguric patient, 388
      for transplant recipients, 333
   pulmonary vascular effects of, 499t
   "renal dose," 174
   use in neonates, 157
Dopamine receptor blockers, 380
Dopamine receptors, 47, 48t, 49–50
Doppler ultrasound, 431–434. *See also* Echocardiography
   Bernoulli equation, 433–434
   color flow mapping, 432–433
   continuous wave, 432
   Doppler effect, 431
   Doppler frequency shift, 432
   to measure blood pressure, 137
   principles of, 431–432
   pulsed wave, 432, *433*
DORV. *See* Double-outlet right ventricle
Double aortic arch, 322–324
   anatomy of, 322, *322*
   repair of, *323,* 323–324
Double switch procedure, *299*
Double-inlet left ventricle, 272t
Double-outlet left ventricle (DOLV), 10, *13,* 14

Double-outlet right ventricle (DORV), *14,* 272t, 289
   with remote ventricular septal defect, 271
   variations in conotruncal anatomy with, 10, *13*
Down syndrome, 38t, 158, 160t, 217, 358, 417, 419, 532
Drug abuse, 511
Drug interactions
   with amiodarone, 478
   with digoxin, 479
   with quinidine, 476
Drugs, 45–61, 543–546. *See also* specific drugs and classes
   α-agonists, 129–130
   analgesics, 88–90, 546
   angiotensin-converting enzyme inhibitors, 56–57, 544
   antiarrhythmic agents, 475–480, 544–545
   anticoagulants, 60, 545
   anticonvulsants, 375, 376t, 381
   antihypertensive agents, 335
   β-blockers, 58–59, 544
   calcium antagonists, 56
   catecholamines, 47–51, *48,* 48t
   diuretics, 57–58, *58,* 544
   for ductal manipulation, 59–60, 545
   inotropic agents, 47–51, 48t, 543
   miscellaneous, 545, 546
   muscle relaxants, 91–93, 546
   phosphodiesterase inhibitors, 52–53, 544
   principles of pharmacology, 45–47
      cellular basis for manipulation of cardiac output, 46–47, *47*
      drug bioavailability, 45
      pharmacotherapy of heart failure, 45–46
   for resuscitation, 130–131, 543
   sedatives, 86–88, 546
   sites of action and hemodynamic effects of cardiac drugs, 48t
   thrombolytic agents, 60–61, 545
   vasodilators, 53–57, 543
Ductal manipulation, drugs for, 59–60, 545
Ductus arteriosus
   closure of, 21, 203
   in coarctation of aorta, 249
   maintaining patency before surgery for D-transposition of great arteries, 293
   patent (*See* Patent ductus arteriosus)
Dye dilution curves, 32, *32,* 139
Dying patients
   do-not-resuscitate orders, 535–538, *537*
   sedatives and analgesics for, 540
   withdrawal of life-sustaining treatments from, 538–541
Dyskinesias, 378–381. *See also* Movement disorders

EACA. *See* Epsilon aminocaproic acid
EAT. *See* Ectopic atrial tachycardia
Ebstein's anomaly, 316–321
   anatomy of, 316, *317*
   clinical course of, 317
   lesions associated with, 316
   pathophysiology of, 316–317
   postoperative management of, 319–321
   postoperative problems associated with, 320
      dysrhythmias, 320, 470
      low cardiac output, 320
      pulmonary insufficiency, 320
      residual tricuspid regurgitation, 320
   preoperative evaluation of, 317–318, *318,* 441
   preoperative management of, 318–319
      correct metabolic acidosis, 319
      fluid management, 319
      inotropic agents, 319
      lower pulmonary vascular resistance, 318
      prostaglandin E_1, 318
   surgical procedures for, 319
      Fontan operation, 319
      heart transplantation, 319, 328

Ebstein's anomaly—*Continued*
    palliative surgery, 319
        systemic-to-pulmonary shunt, 319
        tricuspid valvuloplasty or replacement, 319, *320*
ECG. *See* Electrocardiogram
Echocardiography, *xix–xxi*, 425–446
    avoiding artifacts and errors in, 426–427
    in cardiac ICU, 164
    during and after CPR, 132
    to determine cardiac output, 178, 180
    diagnostic, 158
        anomalous origin of left coronary artery from pulmonary artery, 313
        anomalous pulmonary venous connection, *xix*, 225, 441
        aortic dissection, 509
        aortic stenosis, *xxi*, 234
            supravalvar, 242
        aorticopulmonary window, 201, 441
        atrial septal defect, *xix*, 209
        coarctation of aorta, *xx*, 249
        common atrioventricular canal, 219, *220*, 441
        dilated cardiomyopathy, 490, *490*
        Ebstein's anomaly, 318, *318*
        hypertrophic cardiomyopathy, 491, *492*
        interrupted aortic arch, 245, *245*, 441
        intracardiac masses, 514–515, *515*
        mitral regurgitation, *xx*, 307
        mitral stenosis, 307, 441
        myocardial infarction, 513
        myocarditis, 487
        patent ductus arteriosus, *xix*, 204, 441
        pericardial effusion, 510
        pulmonary artery sling, 323
        pulmonary atresia with intact ventricular septum, 266
        restrictive cardiomyopathy, 493
        subaortic stenosis, 238–239, *239*
        tetralogy of Fallot, *xxi*, 258, *258*
        after thoracic trauma, 507, 508
        transposition of great arteries, 294, *294*, 298, 441
        truncus arteriosus, 230
        vascular rings, 323
        ventricular septal defect, *xix*, 214, 441
    Doppler ultrasound, 431–434
    to evaluate ventricular function, 436–442
        afterload, 436–437
        contractility, 437–439
        estimation of fiber shortening, 434–435, *435*
        preload, 435–436
        principles of, 434–435
        steps in, 434
        stress-velocity analysis, 437–439, *438*
        systolic function, 435
    examination techniques, 427–431
        apical views, 427–428, *429–430*
        measurement of anatomic structures, 430–431
        parasternal views, 428–429, *430–431*
        subxiphoid views, 427, *428–429*
        suprasternal notch and high parasternal views, 429–430, *431*
    fetal, 152–154, 153t
    instrumentation for, 425
    intraoperative, 442
    limitations of, 426–427
    M-mode, 425
    physics of, 425
    postoperative, 442–446
        to evaluate diaphragmatic paralysis, 444–445
        to evaluate fever, 444
        to evaluate hypoxemia, 444
        to evaluate intracardiac and great vessel thrombi, 444, *445*
        to evaluate low output states, 442–446
        to evaluate pleural effusion, 444, *445*
        in patient requiring high-frequency jet ventilation, 446
        in patient requiring mechanical support, 445–446
        in patient with open sternum, 445
    preoperative, 152–154, 440–442
        to evaluate congestive heart failure, 441–442
        to evaluate cyanosis, 440–441
    two-dimensional, 425–426
        interference, 426
        penetration, 425–426
        resolution, 426
ECMO. *See* Extracorporeal membrane oxygenation
Ectopic atrial tachycardia (EAT), 471
Edecrin. *See* Ethacrynic acid
Edema, 39
    airway, 71
    pulmonary, 77–78, 353, *413*
        on chest films, *413*, 419
        noncardiogenic, 360–361
        reperfusion, 450–452
    subglottic, 358–359
EDRF. *See* Endothelial-derived relaxing factor
Education coordinator, nurse as, 520
Edward's syndrome, 38t, 158, 160t, 532
EEG. *See* Electroencephalogram
Effusions
    chylous, 363, 418
    after Fontan procedure, 284
    pericardial, 335, 420, 443, *443*, *445*, 510, 510–511
    pleural, 362–363, *410*, 418, *418–419*, 444, *445*
Eisenmenger's syndrome, 214, 330
Ejection fraction, 434–435
Elastance, 26
    maximal, 437, *437*
Elastase during cardiopulmonary bypass, 197
Electrocardiogram (ECG), 41–43. *See also* Arrhythmias
    abnormal Q waves and QRS axis deviations on, 461
    atrial flutter on, *464*
    atrioventricular block on, 462–463, *463*
    bundle branch block on, 461–462, *462*
    before cardiac catheterization, 447
    cardiac output and, 178
    changes associated with traumatic injury, 508, 508t
    interpretation of, 41
    junctional ectopic tachycardia on, 471, *472*
    maturational changes in, 42
    monomorphic ventricular tachycardia on, 474, *474*
    normal, 41–42
    postoperative, 166, *167*
    preoperative, 461
    re-entry supraventricular tachycardia on, 467, 468, *468*
    sinus bradycardia, 39, 181, 461
    in specific disorders
        anomalous origin of left coronary artery from pulmonary artery, 313
        anomalous pulmonary venous connection, 225
        aortic stenosis, 234
            supravalvar, 242
        atrial septal defect, 209
        coarctation of aorta, 249
        common atrioventricular canal, 219
        dilated cardiomyopathy, 489
        Ebstein's anomaly, 318
        hyperkalemia, 176, *176*
        hypertrophic cardiomyopathy, 491
        hypokalemia, 174
        interrupted aortic arch, 245
        mitral regurgitation, 307
        mitral stenosis, 307
        myocardial infarction, 511–512, *512*
        myocardial ischemia, 43
        myocarditis, 486–487, *487*
        patent ductus arteriosus, 204

pulmonary atresia with intact ventricular septum, 266
restrictive cardiomyopathy, 493
right and left atrial enlargement, 42
subaortic stenosis, 238
tetralogy of Fallot, 257
truncus arteriosus, 230
ventricular hypertrophy, 42–43
ventricular septal defect, 214
torsade de pointes on, 474, 475
Electroencephalogram (EEG), 132, 373t, 374
Electrolyte status
cardiac output and, 178
during cardiopulmonary bypass, 196
postoperative, 168, 172–177
Electromechanical dissociation (EMD), 131
Electromyography (EMG), 373t
Elimination of drug, 45
Ellis-van Creveld syndrome, 158, 160t
Embolization coils, 453, 454–455, 456
EMD. See Electromechanical dissociation
EMG. See Electromyography
Enalapril, 57
dosage of, 544
for myocarditis, 488–489
postoperative, 184
for transplant recipients, 335
Encainide, 471
End-diastolic fiber length, 435
End-diastolic pressure, 436, 483
End-diastolic volume, 436, 483
End-diastolic wall stress, 436
Endocardial cushion defect. See Common atrioventricular canal
Endocardial cushions, 217
Endocarditis, infective
atrial septal defect and, 209
cerebrovascular complications of, 378
Endothelial-derived relaxing factor (EDRF), 484–485, 499–500
Endothelin-1, 484
Endotracheal suctioning, pulmonary vascular effects of, 502
Endovascular devices, 453, 455, 456
End-systolic volume, 483
End-systolic wall stress, 437
Enoximone, 48t, 53
Enteral nutrition, 400
Epinephrine, 48t, 48–49, 157
dosage of, 157, 543
endotracheal administration of, 129
guidelines for clinical use of, 49
metabolism of, 49
postoperative administration of, 182, 183
pulmonary vascular effects of, 499t
racemic, 358
for resuscitation, 128, 130, 543
use in neonates, 157
Epsilon aminocaproic acid (EACA), 399
Equipment in cardiac ICU, 163–164, 164t
Esmolol, 58–59, 477–478
adverse effects of, 478
dosage of, 544
indications for, 477
atrial flutter/atrial fibrillation, 470
torsade de pointes, 475
metabolism of, 478
use in patient with aortic dissection, 509
Ethacrynic acid, 544
Ethical and legal issues, 531–541
ethics and the law, 532–535
adequately informing parents and families, 534–535
informed consent, 533
"mature minor" statutes, 534
role of parents in decision-making for children, 533–534
substituted judgment and best interest, 533

limitations of life-sustaining treatments, 535–538
do-not-resuscitate orders, 535–536, 537
redirection of care and comfort policies, 536–538
reasoning about ethical problems, 531
consequentialism vs. deontology, 531–532
principle-based reasoning vs. other approaches, 532
withdrawing life-sustaining treatments, 538–541
medical nutrition and hydration, 540–541
ordinary or extraordinary distinction, 538–539
sedatives and analgesics in care of the dying, 540
withholding or withdrawing distinction, 539–540
Etomidate, 87t, 91
Eustachian valve, 4
Euthanasia, 540–541
Excitotoxin antagonists, 371
Extracorporeal membrane oxygenation (ECMO), 134, 182, 190–191, 345–348, 415. See also Myocardial mechanical support
for acute respiratory distress syndrome, 361
choosing between ventricular assist device and, 346, 346, 347t
ethical issues regarding, 538–539
management of patients on, 347–348
mechanics of, 347
for myocarditis, 488
outcome of, 348
postoperative echocardiography in patient on, 445–446
for pulmonary hypertension, 504
for respiratory syncytial virus infection, 360
Extubation, 103–104, 104t

Family-centered care, 520–521
transitional care, 522
Femoral vein catheterization, 141–142
Fentanyl, 87t, 89, 501–502, 546
Fetal circulation, 17–20
blood flow patterns, 17, 18
pulmonary vascular resistance, 18–20, 19
vascular pressure, 17–18
Fetal echocardiography, 152–154, 153t
Fetal interventions, 153–154
Fever, postoperative, 444
Fibrinolytic system, 397
Fick's principle, 31, 73, 145–146, 179
Fistula
bronchopleural, 362
pulmonary arteriovenous, 412, 413, 441
transesophageal, 159
FK506, 334t, 335
Flecainide, 477
adverse effects of, 477
indications for, 477
atrial flutter/atrial fibrillation, 471
ectopic atrial tachycardia, 471
junctional ectopic tachycardia, 473
metabolism of, 477
Fluid management
for acute respiratory distress syndrome, 361
for brain injury, 133
after cardiopulmonary bypass, 387–388
for Ebstein's anomaly, 319
postoperative, 165, 172–174
during prostaglandin E_1 administration, 157
for septic shock, 514
for transplant recipients, 337
Fontan procedure, 4, 173, 181, 281–282, 281–284, 461
cerebrovascular accidents and, 377–378, 378
for Ebstein's anomaly, 319
heart transplantation after failure of, 328
modifications of, 281–282
postoperative issues related to, 283–284
arrhythmias, 283, 470
cyanosis, 283–284

Fontan procedure—*Continued*
  low cardiac output, 283, 283t
  mechanical ventilation, 283
  pleural and pericardial effusions, 284
  thrombosis, 284
Foramen ovale, 3, 6, 17
  closure of, 21
  patent, 6, 208
Forced vital capacity (FVC), 353
Foreign body in heart, 507
Fossa ovalis, 6
Frank-Starling mechanism, 22, 181
FRC. *See* Functional residual capacity
Free radicals
  inhibitors and scavengers of, 371
  produced during cardiopulmonary bypass, 197
Fresh frozen plasma transfusions, 399
Functional residual capacity (FRC), 67–69, *68*, 353, 500
Furosemide, 57–58
  adverse effects of, 58
  dosage of, 544
  guidelines for clinical use of, 58
  for hyperkalemia, 176
  metabolism of, 57
  for myocarditis, 489
  postoperative, 174
    for oliguric patient, 388
FVC. *See* Forced vital capacity

G proteins, 484
Gas exchange, 67, 70–78, 96–97, 351–354
  abnormalities in congenital heart disease, 79
  during cardiopulmonary bypass, 193–194
  dynamic mechanisms of gas flow, 70–72
    airway reactivity, 71
    airway resistance, 70–71, *71*
    flow-volume relationships and expiratory flow limitation, *71*, 71–72, *72*
    work of breathing, 72
  lung fluid balance and, 77–78
  perfluorocarbon-associated, 361
  pulmonary circulation and distribution of pulmonary blood flow, 74–78
    alveolar pressure effects, 76
    hypoxic pulmonary vasoconstriction and pulmonary vasoreactivity, 77
    lung fluid balance, 77–78
    lung volume effects, 76, *76*
    pulmonary pressure-flow relationships, 74–75, *75*
    regional pulmonary blood flows, *76*, 76–77
  ventilation, 73–74
    alveolar gas equation, 74
    carbon dioxide elimination, 74
    dead space and alveolar ventilation, 73–74
    diffusion, 73
    gas properties, 73
Gastrointestinal issues, 399–401
  anomalies, 161
  bowel obstruction, 416–417
  bronchopulmonary dysplasia and gastroesophageal reflux, 360
  cardiac procedures associated with gastrointestinal complications, 400
  complications of cardiothoracic surgery, 415
  gastric motility after transplantation, 338
  gastric pH, 45, 401
  gastric ulcers and bleeding, 401
  gastroschisis, 159
  gut ischemia, 400–401
  necrotizing enterocolitis, 161, 407, 415–416, *416*, 420
  perioperative nutrition, 399–400
GCAD. *See* Graft coronary artery disease
Genetic disorders, 158–159, 160t

Glomerular filtration rate (GFR)
  during cardiopulmonary bypass, 387
  neonatal, 173
Glucose
  during cardiopulmonary bypass, 196
  for hyperkalemia, 176
  during resuscitation, 131
Goldenhar syndrome, 38t
Graft coronary artery disease (GCAD), 338–339
Graft rejection, 332–333
  acute, 332
  chronic, 332
  hyperacute, 332
  immunosuppression for prevention of, 333, 334t
  intensive care management of, 333
  signs and symptoms of, 332–333
Granulocyte activation during cardiopulmonary bypass, 197
Gunshot wounds, 507

Half-life of drug, 45
Haloperidol, 380
Hammock mitral valve, 306
HCM. *See* Hypertrophic cardiomyopathy
Heart and lung transplantation, 327–339
  contraindications to, 327, 328t
  donor and recipient considerations for, 330–331
  indications for heart transplantation, 327–329
    cardiomyopathy, 328
    congenital heart disease, 328–329, 329t
    Ebstein's anomaly, 319, 328
    pulmonary vascular resistance and, 327–328
  indications for lung and heart-lung transplantation, 329t, 329–330
  long-term follow-up of, 338–339
    graft coronary artery disease, 338–339
    obliterative bronchiolitis, 339
    post-transplant lymphoproliferative disease, 339
    pulmonary function tests, 339
  patient selection for, 327
    pretransplant testing, 328t
    status I and status II patients, 327
  postoperative care for, 332–338
    cardiovascular management, 333–335
    fluid and renal management, 337
    graft rejection and immunosuppression, 332–333, 334t
    infectious disease management, 336–337, 337t
    neurologic management, 338
    nutritional and gastrointestinal management, 337–338
    pulmonary and ventilatory management, 335–336
  preoperative care for, 330
  survival after, 327, 338
  techniques for, 331–332
    heart transplantation, 331, *331*
    lung and heart-lung transplantation, 331–332
  waiting period for, 327
Heart block. *See* Atrioventricular block
Heart failure, 483–493
  cardiocirculatory model of, 483
    circulatory maladaptation, 483
    ventricular dysfunction, 483, *484*
  congestive (*See* Congestive heart failure)
  definition of, 483
  due to myocardial disorders, 485–493
    dilated cardiomyopathy, 489–491
    hypertrophic cardiomyopathy, 491–492
    myocarditis, 485–489
    restrictive cardiomyopathy, 492–493
  neurohormonal model of, 483–485
    adrenergic mechanisms, 483–484
    other hormonal systems, 484–485
    renin-angiotensin system, 484

Heart murmurs, 152
　in aortic stenosis, 233–234
　in coarctation of aorta, 249
　in mitral regurgitation, 307
　in mitral stenosis, 307
　in subaortic stenosis, 238
　in tetralogy of Fallot, 257
Heart rate, 25
　assessment of, 39
　neonatal, 22, 39
Heart size, 411, 415, 420
Heart sounds, 39–40
Hematocrit, 154
　during cardiopulmonary bypass, 195–196, 393
　optimal, for patient with pulmonary hypertension, 503–504
Hematologic issues, 397–399
　coagulation cascade, 397, *398*
　postoperative anticoagulation, 399
　postoperative bleeding, 397–399, 398t
Hematuria, 395
Hemi-Fontan procedure. *See* Bidirectional Glenn/hemi-Fontan procedure
Hemodialysis
　continuous hemofiltration, 391–393
　　advantages of, 391
　　complications of, 393
　　indications for, 391
　　principles of, 391
　　techniques for, 391–393, *392*
　disadvantages of, 390
　for hyperkalemia, 176
　indications for, 390
　intermittent, 390
Hemodynamic monitoring during CPR, 131–132
"Hemodynamic vise," 224
Hemoglobin
　cyanosis and, 154–155
　oxygen saturation of, 138–139
Hemoglobinuria, 395
Hemostasis, 397, *398*
Heparin, 60, 399
　during cardiopulmonary bypass, 196–197
　during continuous hemofiltration, 391
　dosage of, 545
　for myocardial infarction, 513
　for myocarditis, 489
　for patient on myocardial mechanical support, 348
　protamine reversal of, 192, 197
　for restrictive cardiomyopathy, 493
Heparin cofactor, 196
Hepatic drug metabolism, 45
Hepatic dysfunction
　postoperative bleeding and, 397–398
　in transplant recipients, 338
Hepatomegaly, 178
Hering-Breuer reflex, 353
Heterotaxy syndromes, 272t, 410, 461
High frequency ventilation, 101–103
Hirschsprung's disease, 159
His bundle, 5, 41–42
HLHS. *See* Hypoplastic left heart syndrome
"Holmes heart," 272t
Holt-Oram syndrome, 38t, 158, 160t
Hoover's sign, 362
Human immunodeficiency virus-associated cardiomyopathy, 490
Hydralazine, 55–56
　adverse effects of, 55–56
　dosage of, 543
　guidelines for clinical use of, 55
　metabolism of, 55
Hydration for dying patient, 540–541
Hydrogen peroxide, 197

Hydrops fetalis, 22, 154
Hypercalcemia, postoperative, 175t
Hypercapnia, permissive, 360
Hyperglycemia, 131, 133
　associated with peritoneal dialysis, 390
　after cardiopulmonary bypass, 173
Hyperkalemia, 175–176
　electrocardiogram in, 176, *176*
　postoperative, 175t, 175–176, 388
　treatment of, 176, 388
Hypermagnesemia, postoperative, 175t, 177
Hyperoxia, 139
Hyperoxia test, 41, 154, 155t
Hypertension
　after cavopulmonary shunt, 280
　coarctation of aorta and, 249, 251
　after CPR, 133
　management in transplant recipients, 335
　pulmonary (*See* Pulmonary hypertension)
Hyperthermia, cardiac output and, 178
Hypertrophic cardiomyopathy (HCM), 491–492
　diagnosis of, 491, *492*
　genetics of, 491
　natural history and outcome of, 492
　pathophysiology of, 491
　prevalence of, 491
　treatment of, 491–492
Hyperuricemia, 388
Hypocalcemia
　ionized, 130
　postoperative, 175t, 177
Hypochloremia, diuretic-induced, 174
Hypoglycemia, 131, 133, 155
Hypokalemia, 174–175
　cardiac effects of, 174–175
　diuretic-induced, 174
　postoperative, 174–175, 175t
　treatment of, 175
Hypomagnesemia, postoperative, 175t, 177
Hyponatremia, diuretic-induced, 174
Hypoplastic left heart syndrome (HLHS), 37, 38, 271, 272t
　anatomy of, *273*
　echocardiography in, *273*, 441
　ethics of discussion with parents about, 533–535
　heart transplantation for, 329, 330
　multiple catheterizations as part of staged repair of, 456–457
　Norwood procedure for, 166, 168, 180, 276, *276*, 329
Hypoplastic right heart syndrome, 265
Hypoproteinemia, 390
Hypotension
　cardiac output and, 178
　myocardial infarction and, 513
　neonatal, 158
　postoperative treatment of, 181–184, *182–183*
Hypothermia
　during cardiopulmonary bypass, 190, 191, *192*, 194–195
　deep hypothermia with circulatory arrest, 191, *192*, 194–195, 370–371, 379
　fluid sequestration in tissues associated with, 195
　importance of hemodilution during, 195–196
　movement disorders and, 379–380
　respiratory management during, 193–194
　tissue protective effects of, 194, 370
Hypovolemia, 442
Hypoxemia, 127, 154
　associated with single ventricle lesions, 272–274
　after balloon valvuloplasty for pulmonic stenosis, 448
　after cavopulmonary shunt, 280–281
　diagnostic evaluation of, 40–41
　management in neonates with transposition of great arteries, 293–294
　myocardial effects of, 23

Hypoxemia—Continued
    postoperative echocardiographic evaluation of, 444
    pulse oximetry for detection of, 137–139
    in tetralogy of Fallot, 257
        with absent pulmonary valve, 263
    from ventilation-perfusion mismatch, 358
Hypoxic-ischemic encephalopathy, 381

IABP. See Intra-aortic balloon pump
Ibuprofen, 203
"Ice-pick" view of heart, 425
IE. See Infective endocarditis
Iliofemoral arterial injury, 453–454
Iloprost, 197
Immune globulin, 545
Immunosuppressive agents
    for myocarditis, 489
    for transplant recipients, 333, 334t
Imperforate anus, 159
IMV. See Intermittent mandatory ventilation
Indocin. See Indomethacin
Indocyanine green dye, 139
Indomethacin, 59–60
    adverse effects of, 60
    dosage of, 545
    for patent ductus arteriosus, 203
Infections, 401–403
    catheter-related, 402
    diagnosis of, 401–402
    echocardiographic evaluation of postoperative fever, 444
    mediastinitis, 403
    myocarditis associated with, 485, 485t
    nosocomial, 401
    pericarditis associated with, 511t
    pneumonitis, 402
    respiratory syncytial virus, 360
    sepsis, 513–514
    in transplant recipients, 336–337, 337t
    urinary tract, 402
Infective endocarditis (IE)
    atrial septal defect and, 209
    cerebrovascular complications of, 378
Inferior vena cava (IVC), 3, 4
Inflammatory response to cardiopulmonary bypass, 197, 387
Informed consent, 533
Inocor. See Amrinone
Inositol 1,4,5-triphosphate (IP$_3$), 46
Inotropic agents, 47–51, 48t, 543
    after CPR, 132
    for myocarditis, 488
    for neonates, 23, 157–158
    postoperative administration of, 181–184, 182–183
    pulmonary vascular effects of, 499, 499t
    for sepsis, 514
    before surgery for Ebstein's anomaly, 319
    for transplant recipients, 333–335
Inspection, 37–38
Insulin for hyperkalemia, 176
Intercirculatory mixing in transposition of great arteries, 291–293, 293
Interleukin-8 during cardiopulmonary bypass, 197
Intermittent mandatory ventilation (IMV), 98
Internal jugular vein catheterization, 142–143, 144
Interrupted aortic arch, 243–245
    anatomy of, 243, 244
    clinical course of, 244
    lesions associated with, 244
        truncus arteriosus, 229, 230, 232
    pathophysiology of, 244
    postoperative management of, 246
    postoperative problems associated with, 246

hyperinflation of left lung, 246
pulmonary hypertension, 246
related to DiGeorge syndrome, 246
residual obstruction, 246
residual ventricular septal defect, 246
preoperative evaluation of, 244–245, 245, 441
surgical procedures for, 245, 246
types of, 243–244, 244
Intestinal atresia, 159
Intestinal malrotation, 159
Intraabdominal pressure during respiratory cycle, 108
Intra-aortic balloon pump (IABP), 330, 345
Intracardiac drug administration, 129
Intracardiac masses, 514–515
    evaluation of, 514–515, 515
    therapy for, 515
    types of, 514t
Intracranial hemorrhage, 369–370
    incidence of, 369
    indications for perioperative cranial ultrasound, 369–370
    risk factors for, 369
    timing and management of cardiac surgery in infants with, 370
Intraosseous infusion, 129
Intrapericardial pressure, 112
Intraperitoneal air, 416
Intraperitoneal fluid, 416
Intrathoracic pressure, 107–121
Intravenous gamma globulin (IVGG), 489
Intraventricular septum, 111–112
Intubation, 95–96, 128
    complications of, 358
    endotracheal tube size for upper airway obstruction, 359, 359t
Inverse ratio ventilation (IRV), 101
IP$_3$. See Inositol 1,4,5-triphosphate
IRV. See Inverse ratio ventilation
Isoproterenol, 48t, 51, 157
    for bradycardia, 130
    dosage of, 157, 543
    guidelines for clinical use of, 51
    mechanism of action of, 157
    metabolism of, 51
    postoperative administration of, 184, 227
    pulmonary vascular effects of, 499t
    during resuscitation, 130
    for transplant recipients, 335
    use in neonates, 157
IVC. See Inferior vena cava
IVGG. See Intravenous gamma globulin

Jamshidi bone marrow needle, 129
Junctional ectopic tachycardia (JET), 471–473
    on electrocardiogram, 471, 472
    mechanism of, 472–473
    postoperative, 471
        after repair of common atrioventricular canal, 222
        after repair of tetralogy of Fallot, 261
        after repair of ventricular septal defect, 216
    treatment of, 473

Kawasaki disease, 61, 511
Kerley B lines, 412, 419
Ketamine, 87t, 90
Knife wounds, 507
Konno procedure, 235, 239, 474

LA. See Left atrium
Labetalol, 59
    dosage of, 544
    for patient with aortic dissection, 509
Lactoferrin, 197

LAp. *See* Left atrial pressure
Laplace's law, 69
Laryngeal nerve palsy, 206
Laryngoscopy, 95
Laryngotracheitis, 358–359
Lasix. *See* Furosemide
LBBB. *See* Left bundle branch block
Lecompte maneuver, 294
Left atrial pressure (LAp), 26, 271, 497
 cardiac output and, 178
 causes of elevation or reduction of, 168t
 changes at birth, 21
 fetal, 17
 postoperative, 168–169
  elevation after mitral valve surgery, 311
  elevation after repair of common atrioventricular canal, 222
Left atrium (LA)
 catheterization of, 3
 compliance of, 6
 hypoplasia of, 169
 morphologic anatomy of, *5*, 5–6
Left bundle branch, 8
Left bundle branch block (LBBB), 462
 after repair of subaortic stenosis, 239–240
 during supraventricular tachycardia, 468
Left ventricle (LV)
 D-loop and L-loop, 10
  variations in conotruncal anatomy with, *13*, 14
 double-inlet, 272t
 double-outlet, *14*
  variations in conotruncal anatomy with, 10, *13*
 dysfunction of
  circulatory adaptations to, 483
  coarctation of aorta and, 249
  after repair of atrial septal defect, 211
  spontaneous respiration and, 114–115
  after surgery for D-transposition of great arteries, 296
 effects of positive pressure ventilation and PEEP on function of
  in cardiopulmonary disease, 119–120
  in normal heart, 116–117
 morphologic anatomy of, 8–10, *9*, 112
 passive stiffness of, 26
 phylogenetics of, 9
 during respiration, 112–114, *113*
 single, 272t
Left ventricular hypertrophy (LVH)
 aortic stenosis and, 233, 234
 on electrocardiogram, 42–43
Left ventricular outflow tract obstruction, 233–254
 aortic stenosis, 233–238
  supravalvar, 240–242
 coarctation of aorta, 247–254
 interrupted aortic arch, 243–245
 subaortic stenosis, 238–240
 surgery for D-transposition of great arteries, ventricular septal defect and, 296–297
  anatomic considerations, 296
  postoperative management, 297
  Rastelli procedure, 296
  REV procedure, 296–297
Left ventriculotomy, 8
Left-to-right shunting, 6, 21
 anomalous pulmonary venous connection and, 224
 aorticopulmonary window and, 201
 atrial septal defect and, *xix*, 208
 coarctation of aorta and, 249
 common atrioventricular canal and, 219
 D-transposition of great arteries and, 291–293, *293*
 hyperinflated lungs and, 411
 patent ductus arteriosus and, 203
 pulmonary blood flow and, 74
 radiographic signs of, 411, *412*
 respiratory mechanics and, 355, *356*
 transitional circulation and, 37
 ventricular septal defect and, *xix*, 213–214
Legal issues. *See* Ethical and legal issues
Lidocaine, 476
 adverse effects of, 475
 dosage of, 543, 545
 indications for, 476
  ventricular tachycardia, 475
 metabolism of, 475
Lidoflazine, 133
Life-sustaining treatments, 535–541
 do-not-resuscitate orders, 535–538, *537*
 withdrawal of, 538–541
  medical nutrition and hydration, 540–541
  ordinary or extraordinary distinction, 538–539
  sedatives and analgesics in care of dying patients, 540
  withholding or withdrawing distinction, 539–540
Ligamentum arteriosum, 203, 322
Limbic bands, 3–4
Limbic ledge, 3
L-loop ventricles, 10, *11*, *12*
Long QT syndrome, 474, 475, *475*
Lorazepam, 87t, 88, 502, 546
Lung fluid balance, 77–78
Lung transplantation. *See also* Heart and lung transplantation
 donor and recipient considerations for, 331
 indications for, 329t, 329–330
 lobar, 330
 obliterative bronchiolitis after, 327, 339
 pulmonary function tests after, 339
 pulmonary management after, 336
 signs of graft rejection after, 332–333
 single lung, 330, 331
 technique for, 331–332
Lung volumes, 67, *68*
 effects on pulmonary vascular resistance, 76, *76*
LV. *See* Left ventricle
LVH. *See* Left ventricular hypertrophy

Magnesium, 177
 antacids containing, 388
 cardiovascular functions of, 177
 hypermagnesemia, 175t, 177
 hypomagnesemia, 175t, 177
Magnesium sulfate, 177
Magnetic resonance imaging (MRI), 159, 374t, 379, 407
Managed care, 526–528
Mannitol
 during cardiopulmonary bypass, 197
 postoperative, 174
Marfan's syndrome, 509
"Mature minor" statutes, 534
Maximal elastance (E_{max}), 437, *437*
Maximal expiratory flow-volume (MEFV) curves, 353
Mechanical ventilation, 96–103
 for acute respiratory distress syndrome, 361
 analgesia and sedation for, 86
 effects of positive pressure ventilation and PEEP on cardiac function, 116–120
  in cardiopulmonary disease, 117–120, *121*
  in normal heart, *116*, 116–117
 indications for positive-pressure ventilation, 98, 98t
 initiation of, 99t
 instituting before surgical correction of coarctation of aorta, 250
 modes of, 99–103
  advantages and disadvantages of, 103t
  high frequency ventilation, 101–103
  inverse ratio ventilation, 101

Mechanical ventilation—*Continued*
    liquid ventilation, 103
    pressure control, 99–100, *101*
    pressure control plus pressure support, 100–101, *102*
    pressure regulated plus volume control, 101
    pressure support ventilation, 100, *102*
    volume control, 99, *100*
    volume control plus pressure support, 100, *102*
  permissive hypercapnia and, 361
  postoperative, 165
    after Fontan procedure, 283
    after repair of truncus arteriosus, 231
    for transplant recipients, 335–336
  postoperative echocardiography and high-frequency jet ventilation, 446
  pulmonary vascular effects of, 500, 502
  for respiratory syncytial virus infection, 360
  technical features of ventilators, 97t
  triggers to, 98–99
  weaning from, in bronchopulmonary dysplasia, 360
Mediastinal assessment, postoperative radiographic, 420–422
Mediastinal cart, 164
Mediastinitis, 403
MEFV. *See* Maximal expiratory flow-volume curves
Mental status, cardiac output and, 178
Mesocardia, 410
Metabolic acidosis
  correcting before surgery for coarctation of aorta, 250
  diuretic-induced hypochloremic, 174
  Ebstein's anomaly and, 317, 319
  effect on pulmonary circulation, 498
  management during CPR, 130–131
  postoperative, 167, 388
Metabolism of drug, 45
Methadone, 87t, 89–90, 546
Methemoglobinemia, 139
Methohexital, 87t
Methoxamine, 130
Methylene blue, 139
Metocurine, 87t, 92, 502
Metolazone, postoperative, 174
Metoprolol for hypertrophic cardiomyopathy, 492
Mexiletine, 476–477
  adverse effects of, 477
  indications for, 476
  metabolism of, 477
Meyer procedure, 314–315
Midazolam, 87t, 87–88, 380, 502, 546
Milrinone, 48t, 52–53, *54*
  adverse effects of, 53
  dosage of, 544
  guidelines for clinical use of, 53
  mechanism of action of, 53
  metabolism of, 53
  for myocarditis, 488
  for transplant recipients, 333
Minimally invasive surgery for mitral valve disease, 308–309
Minute volume, 74
Mitral annulus, 305
Mitral valve anatomy, *xx*, 4, 8, 305
Mitral valve disease, *xx–xxi*, 305–311
  clinical course of, 306–307
  lesions associated with, 306
  medical management of, 307
  mitral regurgitation, *xx–xxi*
    coarctation of aorta and, 249
    types of, 306
  mitral stenosis, 272t, 305–306
    balloon valvuloplasty for, 308, 448
    echocardiographic evaluation of, 307, 441
    subvalvar, 305–306
      absence of papillary muscles, 306
      hammock mitral valve, 306
      parachute mitral valve, 306
    supravalvar, 305
      cor triatriatum, 305
      supravalvar mitral ring, 305
    valvar, 305
      commissural fusion, 305
  pathophysiology of, 306
  postoperative management of, 309–311
  postoperative problems associated with, 309–311
    elevated left atrial pressure, 311
    low cardiac output, 309–311
    prosthetic valve problems, 311
    pulmonary hypertension, 311
  preoperative evaluation of, 307–308, 441
  surgical procedures for, *xxi*, 308–309
    minimally invasive surgery, 308–309
    mitral valve repair, 308, *309*
    mitral valve replacement, 308, *310*
      bileaflet valve, 308
      bioprosthetic valves, 308
      heterograft valves, 308
      for hypertrophic cardiomyopathy, 492
    operative approach, 308
Mivacurium, 87t, 92
M-mode echocardiography, 425. *See also* Echocardiography
Molecular biology
  of hypertrophic cardiomyopathy, 492
  of myocarditis, 488
Monitoring, 137–146
  during CPR, 131–132
  invasive, 140–146
    arterial access, 140–141
    central venous access, 141, *142*
    inserting intravascular monitoring lines, 140, *140*
    internal jugular and subclavian vein catheterization, 142–143, *144*
    percutaneous femoral vein catheterization, 141–142
    pericardiocentesis, 146
    pulmonary artery catheterization, 143t, 143–146, *145*
  noninvasive, 137–139
    blood pressure, 137, *138*
    pulse oximetry, 137–139
  of patient on myocardial mechanical support, 347
  specialized equipment for, 163–164, 164t
Monosomy X (Turner's syndrome), 38t, 39, 158, 160t
Moral reasoning, 531–532. *See also* Ethical and legal issues
"Moral triangulation," 532
Morphine, 87t, 88–89, 509, 546
Movement disorders, postoperative, 378–381
  clinical course of, 379
  incidence of, 378–379
  management of, 380, 380t
  mechanisms of, 379–380
  outcome of, 380–381
MRI. *See* Magnetic resonance imaging
Mucopolysaccharidoses, 38t
Multidisciplinary action plans, 526, *527–528*
Murmurs, 37, 40
Muscle lesions, *372*
Muscle of Lancisi, 7
Muscle relaxants, 87t, 91–93, 502, 546
  depolarizing, 91
  for intubation, 96
  nondepolarizing, 91–93
Mustard procedure, 4, 299, 328, 461, 470
Mycophenolate mofetil, 333
Myeloperoxidase, 197
Myocardial contractility, 25–26, 46
  decreased postoperative, 181, 442
  definition of, 25, 437
  fetal, 22

fiber shortening, 435, *435*
indices of, *437*, 437–439
stress-velocity analysis, 437–438, *438*
neonatal, 22–23
Myocardial infarction, 511–513
causes in children, 511
electrocardiogram findings in, 511–512, *512*
evaluation of, 511–512
signs and symptoms of, 511
therapy for, 513
Myocardial mechanical support, 345–348
application of device for, 346–347
complications of, 348
extracorporeal membrane oxygenation vs. ventricular assist devices for, 346, *346*, 347t
indications for, 345–346
management of patients on, 347–348
methods of, 345, 346t
outcome of, 348
postoperative monitoring of patients on, 347
troubleshooting guidelines for, 348t
weaning from, 348
Myocarditis, 485–489
clinical course of, 488
definition of, 485
diagnosis of, 485–488, 487t
electrocardiogram, 486–487, *487*
endomyocardial biopsy, 487–488
molecular biology, 488
etiology and pathogenesis of, 485, 485t, *486*
incidence of, 485
treatment of, 488–489
afterload reduction and angiotensin-converting enzyme inhibitors, 488–489
anticoagulation, 489
diuretics, 489
gamma globulin, 489
immunosuppressive agents, 489
inotropic agents, 488
Myocardium
blood flow during CPR, 128
failure of, 483–493
function in neonate, 22–23
oxygen physiology of, 32–35, *34*
postoperative ischemia, 442–443
postoperative support of, 180–184, *182–183*
protection during cardiopulmonary bypass, 197–198
traumatic injury of, 507–508, 508t

Nadolol for hypertrophic cardiomyopathy, 491
Naloxone, 546
NAPA. *See* N-Acetylprocainamide
NCV. *See* Nerve conduction velocity
Necrotizing enterocolitis (NEC), 161, 407, 415–416, *416*, 420
Neonate
bronchoscopy in, 355
cardiac catheterization in, 159t, 447–448
circulation of, *20*, 20–22, 37, 151
clinical presentations of congenital heart disease in, 152
cyanotic, 154–155
evaluation for suspected congenital heart disease, 154
glomerular filtration rate in, 173
hypoxia tolerance in, 151
intracranial hemorrhage in, 369–370
myocardial function of, 22–23
neurologic plasticity in, 151
preoperative assessment/care of, 151–152
stabilization and transport of, 155–158
Neoplasms, intracardiac, 514–515, *515*
Neostigmine, 87t
Nephron structure and function, *58*
Nerve conduction velocity (NCV), 373t

Neural tube defects, 159
Neurologic disorders, 159, 369–382
intraoperative injury, 370–371
etiology and mechanisms of, 370
strategies for protection against, 370–371
neonatal intracranial hemorrhage, 369–370
postoperative, 371–381
brain death, 381
cerebrovascular accidents, 376–378, *377*, *378*
movement disorders, 378–381, 380t
neuroaxis levels of injury, 371–373, *372*
in patient on myocardial mechanical support, 348
seizures, 373–376, 376t
techniques for diagnosis of, 373, 373t–375t
in transplant recipients, 338
preoperative, 369
Neurologic evaluation
during CPR, 132, 133
of patient on myocardial mechanical support, 348
Neuromuscular junction lesions, *372*
Nifedipine, 56
dosage of, 545
for transplant recipients, 335
Nissen fundoplication procedure, 360
Nitric oxide (NO), 164
for acute respiratory distress syndrome, 361
dosage of, 503, 545
inhaled, for pulmonary hypertension, 502–503
pulmonary vascular effects of, 500, 502–503
for respiratory syncytial virus infection, 360
Nitroglycerin, 48t, 53–55
adverse effects of, 54–55
dosage of, 543
guidelines for clinical use of, 54
mechanism of action of, 53
metabolism of, 53–54
for myocardial infarction, 513
NO. *See* Nitric oxide
Nonpenetrating cardiac injury, 507–508, 508t
Noonan syndrome, 38t, 39, 158, 160t
Norcuron. *See* Vecuronium
Norepinephrine, 48t, 49
dosage of, 543
guidelines for clinical use of, 49
heart failure and, 483
metabolism of, 49
postoperative administration of, *182*, 183–184
pulmonary vascular effects of, 499t
during resuscitation, 130
Norwood procedure, 166, 168, 180, 276, *276*, 329
heart transplantation after failure of, 328
mediastinum after, 421
Nursing roles and responsibilities, 519–523
advanced practice nurse, 525–529
case management and critical pathways, 526, *527–528*
current issues, 528–529
education, 525–526
financial implications, 526–528
patient management, 525
referral liaison, 528
research, 526
bereavement program, 522–523
cardiopulmonary resuscitation classes, 522
expanded staff nurse roles, 520
clinical practice guidelines coordinator, 520
cross-training program, 520
education coordinator, 520
quality improvement coordinator, 520
family-centered care, 520–521
parent information group, 521–522
prenatal program, 521
professional advancement, 519

Nursing roles and responsibilities—*Continued*
  professional practice model of shared governance, 519
  restricted practices, 520, 520t
  transitional family care, 522
  unit-based interdisciplinary practice, 519
Nutrition. *See* Diet and nutrition
Nyquist frequency, 432, *433*

Occluder devices, *453*, 455, *456*
Oculogyric crisis, postoperative, 379
OKT3, 333, 334t
Oliguria, postoperative, 388
Omphalocele, 159
Oncotic pressure during cardiopulmonary bypass, 195–196
Open chest cardiac massage, 128–129
Ophthalmoplegia, supranuclear, 379
Opioid analgesics, 88–90
  dependence on, 88
  epidural, 88
  fentanyl, 89, 546
  methadone, 89–90, 546
  morphine, 88–89, 546
  patient-controlled analgesia, 88
  respiratory depression from, 88
  sufentanil, 89
Oral clefts, 159
Oscillometric blood pressure measurement, 137
Ostium primum defect, *208*, 217–222, *218*
Ostium secundum defect, *xix*, 6, 207, *208*
Oxygen consumption
  calculation in catheterization laboratory, 31–32
  definition of, 31
  myocardial, 34–35
    double product as estimate of, 34
    pressure-volume area and, 34, *34*
  neonatal, 151
Oxygen free radicals
  inhibitors and scavengers of, 371
  produced during cardiopulmonary bypass, 197
Oxygen saturation, 30–31, 138–139, 154–155, 271. *See also* Hypoxemia and cyanosis
  cardiac output and, 178
  after Norwood or Damus-Kaye-Stansel procedure for single ventricle lesions, 277
  postoperative interpretation of data from intravascular catheters, 170–172, 171t
  in tetralogy of Fallot, 257
  ventilation-perfusion inequality and mixed venous oxygen content, 78
Oxygen therapy, 79, 155–156
"Oxygen wasting effect," 34
Oxyhemoglobin, 138–139

P waves, 41, *42*
  in atrial flutter, 470
  in first degree atrioventricular block, 462
  "himalayan," 318
  in re-entry supraventricular tachycardia, 467, *468*
Pacing, cardiac, 164, 463–466
  for atrial flutter/fibrillation, 471
  in cardiac ICU, 164
  causes of pacemaker malfunction, 464
  during/after surgery for L-transposition of great arteries, 299
  after Fontan procedure, 283
  for hypertrophic cardiomyopathy, 492
  for junctional ectopic tachycardia, 473
  pacemaker programming, 465–466
    energy output, 465
    rapid overdrive pacing, 466
    rate programmability, 465
    sensitivity, 465
  pacemaker terminology, 463–464, 464t
  permanent, 466
  physiology of, 464
  principles of care, 464–465
    battery, 465
    leads, 464–465, *465*
    pulse generator, 464
  transesophageal overdrive pacing for supraventricular tachycardia, 468
Pain management. *See* Analgesics
Pancreatitis, post-transplant, 338
Pancuronium, 87t, 93, 502
PAp. *See* Pulmonary artery pressure
Papillary muscles
  absence of, 306
  anterior, 8
  anterolateral, 8
  of conus, 7
  correlation with conduction system, 8
  of left ventricle, 8
  mitral valve attachment to, 305
  posteromedial, 8
  of right ventricle, 8
  of tricuspid valve, 6
Parachute mitral valve, 271, 305, 306
Parent information group, 521–522
Parental medical decision-making, 533–535
  adequately informing parents and families, 534–535
  "mature minor" statutes, 534
Parkinsonism, postoperative, 379
Patau's syndrome, 38t, 158, 160t
Patch aortoplasty, 251
Patent ductus arteriosus, *xix*, 21, 30, 38, 59, 155, 156, 203–206, 412
  anatomy of, 203, *204*
  clinical course of, 204
  incidence of, 203
  lesions associated with, 203
  medical management of, 203
  multidisciplinary action plan for, *527–528*
  pathophysiology of, 203
  postoperative complications associated with, 206
    bleeding, 206
    mediastinal problems, 206
    related to adjacent structures, 206
  postoperative management of, 206
  preoperative evaluation of, 204
  surgical procedure for, 204–206, *205*
Paternalism, 532
Patient-controlled analgesia, 88
PBF. *See* Pulmonary blood flow
PDE inhibitors. *See* Phosphodiesterase inhibitors
Pectinate muscles
  of left atrium, 5
  of right atrium, 4–5
PEEP. *See* Positive end-expiratory pressure
Penetrating cardiac injury, 507, 508t
Pentobarbital, 87t
Pericardial effusions, 420, 510–511
  causes of, 510
  evaluation of, 510
  after Fontan procedure, 284
  pathophysiology of, 510, *510*
  pericarditis and, 510, 511t
  postoperative, 443, *443*
  therapy for, 511
  in transplant recipients, 335
Pericardial pressure, 510
Pericardial tamponade, 510
Pericardiocentesis, 146, 511
  complications of, 146

indications for, 146
procedure for, 146
Pericarditis, 510, 511t
Pericardium
    traumatic injury of, 507–508, 508t
    ventricular interdependence and, 107, 112
Peripheral nerve lesions, 372
Peripheral perfusion
    assessment of, 38–39
    cardiac output and, 178
Peristalsis, 45
Peritoneal dialysis, 389–390
    advantages of, 389
    catheter insertion for, 389, 389t
    complications of, 390
        catheter-related, 390
        hyperglycemia, 390
        hypoproteinemia, 390
        peritonitis, 390
    contraindications to, 389
    for hyperkalemia, 176
    solutions for, 389–390
    technique for, 389–390
Persistent pulmonary hypertension of the newborn (PPHN), 21, 40, 441
Pharmacology. See Drugs
Phasic high intrathoracic pressure support ventilation (PHIPS), 119–120
Phenobarbital, 375, 546
Phenothiazines, 380
Phenylephrine, 59
    dosage of, 545
    nebulized, 358
Phenytoin, 375, 380, 477
    adverse effects of, 477
    indications for, 477
    metabolism of, 477
PHIPS. See Phasic high intrathoracic pressure support ventilation
Phosphodiesterase (PDE) inhibitors, 52–53, 231, 544
    advantages of, 52
    amrinone, 52, 544
    enoximone, 53
    hemodynamic effects of, 52
    milrinone, 52–53, 54, 544
    for myocarditis, 488
Phosphorylation, 46
Phrenic nerve lesions, 361–362
Phylogenetics, 9–10
Physical examination, 37–41
    assessment of peripheral perfusion, 38–39, 39t
    cardiac auscultation, 39–40
    cyanosis, 40–41
    edema, 39
    heart rate, 39
    indications for emergent echocardiography, 40t
    inspection, 37–38
    respiratory effort, 39
Physiology
    cardiac, 25–35
    respiratory, 67–79, 351–354
Plasmalyte A, 173
Platelet effects of cardiopulmonary bypass, 196–197
Platelet plug formation, 397
Platelet transfusion, 399
Pleural effusions, 362–363, 410
    after Fontan procedure, 284
    postoperative echocardiographic evaluation of, 444, 445
Pleural pressure, 68, 70, 107–110, 109
Pneumatic vest CPR, 133–134
Pneumatosis intestinalis, 416, 416

Pneumomediastinum, 420–421, 421
Pneumonia, 419
Pneumonitis, 402
Pneumopericardium, 420, 421
Pneumothorax, 362, 417–418, 418, 421
Poiseuille's law, 70, 97
Polycythemia, 40, 154, 173
Polysplenia, 408, 410–411, 411, 461
Pompe's disease, 38t, 489
Positive end-expiratory pressure (PEEP), 78, 98
    for acute respiratory distress syndrome, 361
    effects in cardiopulmonary disease, 117–120
        left ventricle, 119–120, 121
        right ventricle, 117–119
    effects on function of normal heart, 117
    pulmonary vascular effects of, 500, 502
    for tetralogy of Fallot with absent pulmonary valve, 263
Positive pressure ventilation
    effects in cardiopulmonary disease, 117–120
        left ventricle, 119–120, 121
        right ventricle, 117–119
    effects on function of normal heart, 107, 115, 115–116
Postcoarctectomy syndrome, 251, 254
Postoperative care, 163–184
    cardiac output assessment, 177–180, 180t
    environment and specialized equipment in cardiac ICU, 163–164, 164t
    fluid and electrolyte management, 172–177, 175t
    interpretation of oxygen saturation data from intravascular catheters, 170–172, 171t
    interpretation of pressure data from intravascular catheters, 168–170
        left atrial pressure, 168t, 168–169
        pulmonary artery pressure, 169–170, 170t
        right atrial pressure, 169, 169t
    knowledge required for, 163
    myocardial support, 180–184, 182–183
    transition from operating room to ICU and initial postoperative assessment, 164–168, 165t
        airway management and mechanical ventilation, 165
        arterial blood gas analysis, 166–167
        chest radiography, 166, 166
        electrocardiography, 166, 167
        fluid management, 165
        laboratory evaluation, 166
        metabolic acidosis, 167
        serum electrolytes, 167
Postpericardiotomy syndrome, 210, 507
Post-transplant lymphoproliferative disease (PTLD), 339
Potassium, 174–176
    hyperkalemia, 175–176
    hypokalemia, 174–175
Potassium chloride, 175
Potts shunt, 275
PR interval, 41
    in AV node re-entry supraventricular tachycardia, 467, 468
    in dilated cardiomyopathy, 489
    in first degree atrioventricular block, 462
    prolonged postoperative, 462
Preload, 25–26, 107–108
    decreased postoperative, 181
    fetal, 18, 22
    indices of, 435–436
    neonatal, 22
Preload-recruitable stroke work (PRSW), 437
Prenatal program for parents, 521
Preoperative care, 151–161
    chest films, 410
    confirming the diagnosis, 158
    considerations in neonate, 151–152
    echocardiography, 440–442

Preoperative care—*Continued*
  evaluation of additional organ systems, 158–161
    central nervous system, 159
    gastrointestinal, 161
    genetic disorders, 158–159, 160t
    renal, 159
  evaluation of cyanotic neonate, 154–155
  evaluation of neonate with suspected congenital heart disease, 154
    hyperoxia test, 41, 154, 155t
    fetal echocardiography, 152–154, 153t
    stabilization and transport, 155–158
      airway management and supplemental oxygen, 95–104, 155–156
      initial resuscitation, 127–134, 155
      inotropic agents, 157–158
      prostaglandin E_1, 37, 59, 156–157
      transport, 158
  timing and type of surgery, 161
Pressure-volume area (PVA), 34, *34*
Primacor. *See* Milrinone
Principle-based reasoning, 532
Procainamide, 475–476
  active metabolite of, 469, 476
  adverse effects of, 476, *476*
  dosage of, 545
  indications for, 475–476
    atrial flutter/atrial fibrillation, 471
    ectopic atrial tachycardia, 471
    supraventricular tachycardia, 469
  metabolism of, 476
Procardia. *See* Nifedipine
Propafenone, 477
  adverse effects of, 477
  indications for, 477
    atrial flutter/atrial fibrillation, 471
    junctional ectopic tachycardia, 473
  metabolism of, 477
Propofol, 87t, 90–91
Propranolol
  dosage of, 544
  for hypertrophic cardiomyopathy, 491
  for patient with aortic dissection, 509
Prostacyclin, 197, 499
Prostaglandin E_1, 37, 59, 156–157, 441, 447, 448
  adverse effects of, 59, 157, 449
  clinical deterioration after initiation of, 157
  dosage of, 157, 545
  peripheral vasodilation due to, 157
  before surgery for coarctation of aorta, 250
  before surgery for D-transposition of great arteries, 293
  before surgery for Ebstein's anomaly, 318
Prostaglandin E_2, 21
Protamine, 192, 197
Protein binding, 45
Pseudoaneurysms, postoperative mediastinal, 421–422
PTLD. *See* Post-transplant lymphoproliferative disease
Pulmonary arteries
  alveolar hypoxia-induced vasoconstriction of, 357
  aneurysmal dilation in infants with absent pulmonary valves, 357
  anomalous origin of left coronary artery from pulmonary artery, 312–315
  in D-transposition of great arteries, 289–290, *290*
  fetal, 18
  in L-transposition of great arteries, *297*, 297–298
  pulmonary artery sling, 322–324 (*See also* Vascular rings and slings)
    anatomy of, 322, *322*
    repair of, 324, *324*
  pulmonary artery-aortic anastomosis, 276
  stenosis of, 411, *412*
    balloon angioplasty for, 450–453, *452–455*
  systemic-pulmonary artery shunt, 275, *275*
Pulmonary arteriovenous fistula, 412, *413*, 441
Pulmonary artery banding
  for common atrioventricular canal, 221–222
  for single ventricle lesions, *275*, 275–276
  for ventricular septal defect, 215
Pulmonary artery capillary wedge pressure, 145, 145t
Pulmonary artery catheterization, 143–146, *145*
  complications of, 143t
  to determine cardiac output, 145–146
  indications for, 143t
  to measure pulmonary artery capillary wedge pressure, 145, 145t
  procedure for, 144–145
Pulmonary artery pressure (PAp), 110, 497
  causes of elevation or reduction of, 170t
  postoperative, 169–170
Pulmonary atresia, 271, *413*
  with intact ventricular septum, 265–269
    anatomy of, 265, *266*
    pathophysiology of, 265–266
    postoperative management of, *268*, 268–269
    preoperative evaluation of, 266
    surgical procedure for, 266–268, *267*
  preoperative evaluation of, 441
  tetralogy of Fallot with, 261–263, 272t (*See also* Tetralogy of Fallot)
Pulmonary blood flow (PBF), 74–78, 271, 353–354, 497
  abnormalities in congenital heart disease, 79
  alveolar pressure effects on, *75*, 76
  calculation of, 30–31
  cardiac lesions associated with increases in, 355
  effects of hypoxic pulmonary vasoconstriction and pulmonary vasoreactivity, 77
  lung volume effects on, *76*, 76
  obstruction to, 271
    transposition of great arteries and, 289–290
  pressure-flow relationships, 74–75, *75*
  radiographic evaluation of, 412–413, *414*
  regional, *76*, 76–77
  in single ventricle lesions, 74, 271–274
    congestive heart failure, 274
    hypoxemia, 272–274
Pulmonary compliance (C_L), 67–68
Pulmonary disorders, 355–363
  absent pulmonary valves, 357
  acute respiratory distress syndrome, 360–361, 419–420
  bronchopulmonary dysplasia, 359–360
  on chest films, 411–413, *412–414*, 419–420, *420*
  chylothorax, 363, 418
  effect of parenchymal lung disease on pulmonary vascular resistance, 500
  hyperinflated lungs due to left-to-right shunting, 411
  mechanism of pulmonary compromise in congenital heart disease, 355–356, *356*
  noncardiogenic pulmonary edema, 360–361
  phrenic nerve lesions and, 361–362
  pleural effusions, 362–363, 418, *418–419*
  pneumothorax, 362, *417–418*, 418
  pulmonary insufficiency after surgery for Ebstein's anomaly, 320
  residual lung disease after surgery for vascular rings, 324
  respiratory insufficiency after repair of anomalous pulmonary venous connection, 227
  respiratory syncytial virus infection, 360
  upper airway obstruction, 357t, 357–359, *359*, 359t
  vascular rings, 357
Pulmonary edema, 77–78, 353
  on chest films, *413*, 419
  noncardiogenic, 360–361
  reperfusion, 450–452

Pulmonary emboli, 515
Pulmonary function tests, 352
  post-transplant, 339
Pulmonary hypertension, 497–504. *See also* Pulmonary vascular resistance
  anomalous pulmonary venous connection and, 227
  aorticopulmonary window and, 201, 202
  atrial septal defect and, 208, 211
  bronchopulmonary dysplasia and, 360
  common atrioventricular canal and, 222
  interrupted aortic arch and, 246
  mitral stenosis and, 306
  after mitral valve surgery, 311
  persistent pulmonary hypertension of the newborn, 21, 40, 441
  relation to increased pulmonary vascular resistance, 75, *75,* 497
  significance of, 497
  stress response attenuation for patients with, 85–86
  therapy for, 501–504
    alkalosis, 502
    analgesia and sedation, 501–502
    ensuring adequate coronary perfusion, 504
    extracorporeal membrane oxygenation, 504
    inhaled nitric oxide, 502–503
    intravenous vasodilators, 502
    maintaining optimal hematocrit, 503–504
    mechanical ventilation, 502
    in transplant recipients, 335
  truncus arteriosus and, 231
  ventricular septal defect and, 216
Pulmonary physiology. *See* Respiratory physiology
Pulmonary valve, 4
  absent, *xxii,* 357
    tetralogy of Fallot with, 263, *263, 264*
  stenosis of, *268–269,* 269, 271
    anatomy of, *268*
    balloon valvuloplasty for, *268,* 269, 448, *449*
Pulmonary vascular resistance (PVR), 497–504
  calculation of, 75, 497
    in catheterization laboratory, 32
  changes at birth, *20,* 20–21, 272
  determinants of, 497–500
    alveolar hypoxia, 77, 498
    alveolar pressure, 76
    autonomic nervous system, 500
    cardiopulmonary bypass, 500
    endothelial cells, 499–500
    lung volume, 76, *76*
    mechanical ventilation, 500
    parenchymal lung disease, 500
    pH, 498
    pulmonary vascular smooth muscle tone, 498
    pulmonary vascular structure, 497–498
    pulmonary venous hypertension, 75, *75,* 500
    vasoactive substances, 499, 499t
  effect of respiration on, 110
  elevation of (*See also* Pulmonary hypertension)
    heart transplantation and, 327–328
    hypoxemia due to, 272–274
    patients at increased risk for after cardiac surgery, 500–501
    relation to pulmonary hypertension, 497
    right ventricle in diseases associated with, 109–110
    therapy for, 501–504
  fetal, 18–20, *19*
  insufficient, 497, 501
    in patients with single ventricle lesions, 274
    therapy for, 274, 504
  neonatal, 151
    in newborns with large communications at ventricular or great vessel level, 21
    in persistent pulmonary hypertension of the newborn, 21

Pulmonary vasculature, 110. *See also* Pulmonary arteries; Pulmonary veins
  pulmonary vascular resistance and structure of, 497–498
  radiographic assessment of, 411–413, *412*
  redistribution of, 411, *412*
  unilateral prominence of, 412
Pulmonary veins, 5
  anomalous pulmonary venous connection, *xix,* 223–227, *224, 226*
  confluence of, 223
Pulse oximetry, 40, 137–139
  during CPR, 132
  limitations and pitfalls of, 139
    effects of ambient lighting, 139
    effects of dyes and pigments, 139
    effects of motion, 139
    hyperoxia, 139
    hypoxemia, 139
    methemoglobinemia, 139
  principles of, 138–139
Pulse patterns, 38–39, 39t
Pulsed wave Doppler, 432, *433*
Pulsus paradoxus, 358
PVA. *See* Pressure-volume area
PVR. *See* Pulmonary vascular resistance

Q waves, 461
  in anomalous origin of left coronary artery from pulmonary artery, 313
  in dilated cardiomyopathy, 489
  in myocardial infarction, 511–512, *512*
  in myocarditis, 487
QRS complex, 461
  in dilated cardiomyopathy, 489
  in junctional ectopic tachycardia, 471
  maturational changes in, 42
  in myocarditis, 487
QT prolongation, 474, 475, *475*
Quality improvement nurse coordinator, 520
Quinidine, 476
  adverse effects of, 476
  dosage of, 545
  drug interactions with, 476
  indications for, 476
    atrial flutter/atrial fibrillation, 471
  metabolism of, 476

RA. *See* Right atrium
Radial artery cannulation, 141
RAp. *See* Right atrial pressure
Rapamycin, 333
Rastelli procedure, 181, 271, 296, *299*
RBBB. *See* Right bundle branch block
RCM. *See* Restrictive cardiomyopathy
Receptors, 47–50
  α and β, 47, 48t
  dopamine, 47, 48t, 49–50
Referral liaison nurse, 528
Relaxation characteristics of heart, 26
Renal issues, 387–396
  anomalies, 159
  dialysis, 389–393
  effects of cardiopulmonary bypass, 387
  hemoglobinuria and hematuria, 395
  postoperative acute renal failure, 388
  postoperative fluid management, 387–388
  postoperative oliguria, 388
  radiographic findings, 407
  renal drug excretion, 45
  renal dysfunction in transplant recipients, 337
  ultrafiltration, 393–395, *393–395*
Renin-angiotensin system, 56, 484

Reperfusion effects
  cerebral injury, 132–133
  pulmonary edema, 450–452
Reserpine, 380
Residual volume, 67, 68
Respiration. See Ventilation
Respiratory effort, 39
Respiratory physiology, 67–79, 351–354
  assessment of pulmonary function, 352
  causes of respiratory compromise in cardiac patients, 352t
  dynamic mechanisms of gas flow, 70–72
    airway reactivity, 71
    airway resistance, 70–71, 71
    flow-volume relationships and expiratory flow limitation, 71, 71–72, 72
    work of breathing, 72
  functional residual capacity, 353
  gas exchange in lung, 72–78 (See also Gas exchange)
    pulmonary circulation and distribution of pulmonary blood flow, 74–78
    ventilation, 73–74
  lung volumes, 67, 68
  maximal expiratory flow-volume curves, 353
  pressure-volume relations of lung and chest wall, 68, 68–69
  pulmonary compliance, 67–68
  pulmonary diffusing capacity and pulmonary blood flow, 353–354
  pulmonary mechanics, 67–72, 352–353
  regional lung compliance and ventilation, 70, 70
  surface tension and surfactant, 69–70
  thoracoabdominal asynchrony, 352
  ventilation-perfusion relationships, 78–79
    mixed-venous oxygen content, 78
    therapies to improve inequality, 78–79
    ventilation-perfusion inequality, 78
Respiratory syncytial virus (RSV) infection, 360
Restrictive cardiomyopathy (RCM), 492–493
  conditions associated with, 492
  diagnosis of, 493
  natural history and outcome of, 493
  pathophysiology of, 492–493
  treatment of, 493
REV procedure, 296–297
Rhabdomyoma, intracardiac, 515
Rib notching, 249, 414
Ribavirin, 360
Right atrial pressure (RAp)
  cardiac output and, 178
  causes of elevation or reduction of, 169t
  changes at birth, 21
  fetal, 17
  postoperative, 169
  during respiratory cycle, 108, 109
Right atrium (RA)
  compliance of, 6
  morphologic anatomy of, 3–5, 4
Right bundle branch, 7–8
Right bundle branch block (RBBB), 461–462, 462
  Ebstein's anomaly and, 318
  after Konno procedure, 474
  after repair of tetralogy of Fallot, 261, 462
Right ventricle (RV)
  D-loop and L-loop, 10, 12
    variations in conotruncal anatomy with, 13, 14
  "double chamber," 213
  double-outlet, 14, 272t
    variations in conotruncal anatomy with, 10, 13
  dysfunction after repair of tetralogy of Fallot, 261
  effects of positive pressure ventilation and PEEP on function of, 116–119
    in cardiopulmonary disease, 117–119
    in normal heart, 116–117
  function of, 108–110
  morphologic anatomy of, 6–8, 7, 108–109, 111–112
  output of, 108–110
  phylogenetics of, 9
  single, 272t
Right ventricular hypertrophy (RVH)
  aortic stenosis and, 234
  coarctation of aorta and, 249
  on electrocardiogram, 42
  interrupted aortic arch and, 245
Right ventricular outflow tract obstruction, 257–269
  after balloon valvuloplasty for pulmonic stenosis, 448
  pulmonary atresia with intact ventricular septum, 265–269
  pulmonary stenosis, 269
  tetralogy of Fallot, 257–264
Right ventriculotomy, 6
Right-to-left shunting, 6, 21
  anomalous pulmonary venous connection and, 224
  bronchopulmonary dysplasia and, 359
  D-transposition of great arteries and, 291–293, 293
  Ebstein's anomaly and, 316, 318
  tetralogy of Fallot and, 257
Rocuronium, 87t, 92
Ross procedure, 235, 236
Ross-Konno procedure, 235, 237, 239
RSV. See Respiratory syncytial virus infection
RV. See Right ventricle
RVH. See Right ventricular hypertrophy

"Sail sign," 421
Scimitar syndrome, 226
SCUF. See Slow continuous ultrafiltration
Sedation and analgesia, 85–93
  analgesics, 88–90, 546
  anesthetic agents, 90–91
  assessing need for, 86
  drug dosages for, 87t
  indications for, 85–86
    dying patients, 540
    intubation, 96
    mechanical ventilation, 86
    postoperative analgesia and anxiolysis, 85
    postoperative control of pulmonary vascular resistance, 501–502
    preoperative, 85
    procedures in cardiac intensive care unit, 86
    stress response attenuation, 85–86
  muscle relaxants, 91–93, 546
  sedatives, 86–88, 546
Seizures, postoperative, 373–376
  associated with stroke, 375
  incidence of, 373
  management of, 374–375, 376t
  mechanisms of, 373
  outcome of, 376
  postpump, 373–376
  presentation of, 373–374
  in transplant recipients, 338
Self-determination, 532
Senning procedure, 299, 299, 328, 461, 470
Sepsis, 155
Septal myotomy-myectomy for hypertrophic cardiomyopathy, 492
Septic shock, 513–514
  evaluation of, 514
  therapy for, 514
  "warm" vs. "cold," 513
Septum
  aortopulmonary, 7
  conal (parietal band), 6–8
  intraventricular, 111–112
  primum, 3–4
  secundum, 3–4

Shock, 127, 152
  septic, 513–514
Shone complex, 169, 247, 271, 305
Shortening fraction, *xxi*, 434–435
Shunt lesions, 201–232. *See also* Left-to-right shunting; Right-to-left shunting
  anomalous pulmonary venous connection, 223–227, *224, 226*
  aorticopulmonary window, 201–202, *201–202*
  atrial septal defect, 207–211, *208, 210*
  common atrioventricular canal, 217–222, *218, 220*
  patent ductus arteriosus, 203–206, *204–205*
  truncus arteriosus, 228–232, *229, 231*
  ventricular septal defect, 212–216, *213, 215*
SIADH. *See* Syndrome of inappropriate secretion of antidiuretic hormone
Sick sinus syndrome, 4
Signs and symptoms of heart disease, 37, 38t
Simultaneous compression-ventilation CPR, 133
Single photon emission computed tomography (SPECT), *xxii*, 379
Single ventricle lesions, 271–284
  anatomic lesions associated with, 271, 272t, *273*
  balancing circulation in, 271–274
    excessive pulmonary blood flow, 274
    inadequate pulmonary blood flow, 272–274
    transitional circulation, 37, 151, 272
  physiology of, 271
  postoperative catheterization as part of staged repair of, 456–457, *456–457*
  surgical management in newborn, 274–284 (*See also* specific procedures)
    immediate postoperative management, 277
      cyanosis, 277
      elevated oxygen saturations, 277
      low cardiac output, 277
    principles of, 274
    pulmonary artery banding, *275*, 275–276
    pulmonary artery-aortic anastomosis, 276
    separating the circulation, 277–284
      bidirectional Glenn/hemi-Fontan procedure, *278,* 278–281, *279*
      Fontan operation, *281–282,* 281–284
      general principles, 277–278
    stage I Norwood procedure, 276, *276*
    systemic-pulmonary artery shunt, *275*, 275
Sinoatrial nodal artery thrombosis, 4
Sinoatrial (SA) node, 3, 41
  dysfunction of, 209, 210
Sinus bradycardia, 39, 181, 461
Sinus tachycardia, 39, 181
Sinus venosus, 3, 5
  defect of, *208*, 217
Situs
  ambiguus, 10, *10*, 410
  inversus, 3, 4, 10, *10*, 410
  solitus, 3, 4, 10, *10*, 410
  thoracoabdominal, 410–411, *411*
  ventricular, 10, *11, 12*
  visceroatrial, 10, *10*
Slow continuous ultrafiltration (SCUF), 391–393, *392*
Sodium bicarbonate, 388
  dosage of, 543
  for hyperkalemia, 176
  for resuscitation, 130–131, 543
Sodium carbonate, 131
Sodium nitroprusside, 48t, 55
  adverse effects of, 55
  dosage of, 543
  guidelines for clinical use of, 55
  mechanism of action of, 55
  metabolism of, 55
  for patient with aortic dissection, 509
Sodium overload, postoperative, 173

Sodium polystyrene sulfonate, 176
Somatosensory evoked potentials (SSEPs), 373t
Sotalol, 478
  adverse effects of, 478
  indications for, 478
    atrial flutter/atrial fibrillation, 471
  metabolism of, 478
Sphygmomanometer, 137
Spinal cord
  ischemia after repair of coarctation of aorta, 254
  lesions of, *372*
Spirometry, 67
Spironolactone, 544
"Square root" sign, 493
SSEPs. *See* Somatosensory evoked potentials
Starling's law, 77, 107
Status epilepticus, 374
Sternotomy in cardiac ICU, 164
Streptokinase, 60–61, 513, 515, 545
Stress response attenuation, 85–86
  after complex repairs, 86
  for patients with labile pulmonary hypertension, 85–86
  for patients with limited myocardial reserve, 85
Stress-velocity analysis, 437–438, *438*
Stridor, 357–359
  causes of, 357t
  due to vascular rings, 357
  inspiratory, 357–358
  postextubation, 358–359, *359*
Stroke. *See* Cerebrovascular accident
Subaortic stenosis, 238–240
  clinical course of, 238
  lesions associated with, 238
  pathophysiology of, 238
  postoperative management of, 239
  postoperative problems associated with, 239–240
  preoperative evaluation of, 238–239, *239*
  in Shone's syndrome, 271
  surgical procedure for, 239, *240*
  types of, 238
    discrete membranous, 238
    fibromuscular tunnel, 238
    hypertrophic, 238
Subclavian artery
  aberrant left, right aortic arch with, 322
  turndown procedure for anomalous origin of left coronary artery from pulmonary artery, 314–315
Subclavian flap angioplasty, 251
Subclavian steal syndrome, 244
Subclavian vein catheterization, 142–143, *144*
Subglottic edema, 358–359
Substance abuse, 511
"Substituted judgment" principle, 532
Succinylcholine, 91
Sucralfate, 401
Sufentanil, 87t, 89
Sulcus terminalis (sinoatrial), 3
Superior vena cava (SVC), 3, 4
Supranuclear ophthalmoplegia, 379
Surfactant, 69–70, 361
Suxamethonium, 87t
SVC. *See* Superior vena cava
SVR. *See* Systemic vascular resistance
SVT. *See* Tachycardia, supraventricular
Swan Ganz catheter. *See* Pulmonary artery catheterization
Sympathomimetic amines, 48–51, 157–158
Syndrome of inappropriate secretion of antidiuretic hormone (SIADH), 173
Systemic vascular resistance (SVR), 107, 497
  calculation in catheterization laboratory, 32
  changes at birth, 22
  treating elevation of, 181–183, *183*

Systemic-pulmonary artery shunt, 275, *275*
Systolic function, 25–26, 435–439, 483

T waves
  in aortic stenosis, 234
    supravalvar, 242
  in dilated cardiomyopathy, 489
  in hypertrophic cardiomyopathy, 491
  maturational changes in, 42
  in myocarditis, 487
  in restrictive cardiomyopathy, 493
  in subaortic stenosis, 238
  in tetralogy of Fallot, 257
  in torsade de pointes, 474
TA. *See* Tranexamic acid
Tachy-brady syndrome, 471
Tachycardia, 39
  cardiac output and, 178, 181
  fetal, 22, 153
  sinus, 181
  supraventricular (SVT), 466–473
    atrial flutter (intra-atrial re-entry)/atrial fibrillation, 470–471
    characteristics of, 466
    Ebstein's anomaly and, 317, 320
    ectopic, 466, 466t, 471–473
      ectopic atrial tachycardia, 471
      junctional ectopic tachycardia, 471–473, *472*
    mechanisms of, 466, 466t
    postoperative, 469–470
    recurrent, 469
    re-entry, 466t, 466–468
      with accessory pathway, 466t, 466–467
      age-related variations in, 467
      AV node, 467, *467*
      diagnosis of, 468
      on electrocardiogram, 467, *468*
      natural history of, 467–468
      orthodromic vs. antidromic, 466–467
      in patient with structurally normal heart, 466–468
    treatment of, 468–469
  ventricular (VT), 473–475
    monomorphic (re-entrant) VT, 474, *474*
    after surgery for Ebstein's anomaly, 320
    torsade de pointes, 474, *475*
    treatment of, 474–475
Tachypnea, cardiac output and, 178
Tacrolimus, 334t, 335
Takeuchi operation, *314*, 315
TAPVC. *See* Anomalous pulmonary venous connection
TAR. *See* Thrombocytopenia-absent radius syndrome
Taussig-Bing anomaly, 289
Tendon of Todaro, 5
Tetrabenazine, 380
Tetralogy of Fallot (TOF), *xxi*, 257–264, 271, *414*
  with absent pulmonary valve, 263
    anatomy of, 263, *263*
    pathophysiology of, 263
    surgical procedure for, 263, *264*
  anatomy of, 257, *258*
  with complete atrioventricular canal, 263–264
  lesions associated with, 257
  pathophysiology of, 257
    hypercyanotic spells, 257
  postoperative management of, 259, 261, *421*, 422
  postoperative problems associated with, 259–261
    electrophysiologic abnormalities, 261
    residual or previously undiagnosed ventricular septal defect, 259
    residual right ventricular outflow tract obstruction, 259–261

right bundle branch block, 261, 462
right ventricular dysfunction, 261
preoperative management of, 257–259, *258*, 441
with pulmonary atresia, 261–263, 272t
  anatomy of, 261
  postoperative catheterization as part of staged repair of, 457–459, *458*
  surgical procedures for, 261–263, *262*
surgical procedure for, 259, *260*
TGA. *See* Transposition of great arteries
THAM. *See* Tromethamine
Thebesian valve, 4, 5
Thermodilution method for measuring cardiac output, *179*, 179–180, 180t
Thiopental, 87t
Thiopentone, 133
Thoracoabdominal situs, 410–411, *411*
Thorax
  radiographic evaluation of, 414 (*See also* Chest radiography)
    postoperative, 417–418, *417–419*
  traumatic injury of, 507–508
"3" sign, 249
Thrombocytopenia-absent radius (TAR) syndrome, 159, 160t
Thrombolytic therapy, 60–61, 545
  contraindications to, 60
  for intracardiac thrombi, 515
  for myocardial infarction, 513
  streptokinase, 60–61
  tissue-type plasminogen activator, 61
  urokinase, 61
Thrombosis
  echocardiographic evaluation for, 444, *445*
  after Fontan procedure, 284
  intracardiac, 514–515
  intravascular lines and, 140
  prevention during cardiopulmonary bypass, 196–197
Tidal volume (V_T), 67, *68*
Timing of surgery, 161
Tinea sagittalis, 4
Tissue-type plasminogen activator (tPA), 61, 513, 545
TLC. *See* Total lung capacity
TLV. *See* Total liquid ventilation
TOF. *See* Tetralogy of Fallot
Torsade de pointes, 474, *475*
Total anomalous pulmonary venous connection. *See* Anomalous pulmonary venous connection
Total artificial heart, 330, 345, 346
Total liquid ventilation (TLV), 103
Total lung capacity (TLC), 67–69, *68*
Total parenteral nutrition, 400
tPA. *See* Tissue-type plasminogen activator
Trabeculae carneae
  of left ventricle, 8
  of right ventricle, 6
Tracheomalacia, 324, 357, 359
Tracheostomy for bronchopulmonary dysplasia, 360
Tranexamic acid (TA), 399
Transesophageal fistula, 159
Transfusion, 399
Transitional family care, 522
Transmural pressure, *68*, 68–69
Transplantation. *See* Heart and lung transplantation
Transport of patient, 158
  to catheterization suite, 447
Transposition of great arteries (TGA), 4, *14*, 151
  cardiac index after repair of, 181
  "corrected," 297, *297*
  definition of, 289
  D-transposition, 289–297
    anatomy of, 289–291, *290, 291*
    arterial switch procedure for, 294–296, *295*

coronary artery variations in, 290–291, *292*
with intact ventricular septum, 289–290
management of profound hypoxemia in, 293–294
pathophysiology of, 291–293, *293*
postoperative management of, 296
postoperative problems associated with, 296, 470
preoperative evaluation of, 294, *294*
pulmonary blood flow obstruction and, 289–290
surgery for left ventricular outflow tract obstruction, ventricular septal defect and, 296–297
   anatomic considerations, 296
   postoperative management, 297
   Rastelli operation, 296
   REV procedure, 296–297
ventricular septal defect and, 271, 289
echocardiography in, 294, *294,* 298, 441
epidemiology of, 289
incidence of, 289
L-transposition, 297–300
  anatomy of, *297,* 297–298
  pathophysiology of, 298
  postoperative management of, 300, 470
  preoperative evaluation of, 298
  surgical procedures for, *298–299,* 298–300
mortality from, 289
relationship between ventricular work load and ventricular mass in, 23
variations in conotruncal anatomy with, 10, *13*
Transpulmonary pressure, 68–70, *70*
Trauma
  aortic dissection due to, 509–510
  cardiac, 507–509
    nonpenetrating, 507–508
    penetrating, 507, 508t
  therapy for, 509
Triangle of Koch, 5
Tricuspid valve, 4, 5
  anatomy of, *xx,* 6
  atresia of, 272t, *273*
  chordae, 271
  Ebstein's anomaly of, 316–321 (*See also* Ebstein's anomaly)
  number of leaflets of, 6
  papillary muscles of, 6
  valvuloplasty or replacement of, 319, *320*
Trisomy 13, 38t, 158, 160t, 532
Trisomy 18, 38t, 158, 160t, 532
Trisomy 21, 38t, 158, 160t, 217, 358, 417, 419, 532
Tromethamine (THAM), 131, 388, 545
Truncus arteriosus, 152, 228–232, 272t
  anatomy of, 228–229, *229*
  classification of, 228, *229*
  clinical course of, 229–230
  definition of, 228
  lesions associated with, 228, 229
    interrupted aortic arch, 229, 230, 232
    ventricular septal defect, 228, 232
  pathophysiology of, 229
  postoperative management of, 231–232
  postoperative problems associated with, 231–232
    cyanosis, 231–232
    dysrhythmias, 232
    low cardiac output, 231
    neoaortic (truncal) valve stenosis/regurgitation, 232
    pulmonary hypertensive crisis, 231
    related to interrupted aortic arch, 232
    residual ventricular septal defect, 232
  preoperative evaluation of, 230
  surgical procedures for, 230–231, *231*
Tuberous sclerosis, 38t, *515*
Tumors, intracardiac, 514–515, *515*
Turner's syndrome (Monosomy X), 38t, 39, 158, 160t

Two-dimensional echocardiography, 425–436. *See also* Echocardiography
Ultrafiltration during cardiopulmonary bypass, 393–395
  conventional, *393,* 393–394
  modified, 394–395, *394–395*
Ultrasound, 407
  brain, 159, 369–370, 374t
  cardiac, 425–446 (*See also* Echocardiography)
Umbilical artery cannulation, 140, 141, 155, 447
Umbilical vein cannulation, 140, 155, 447
Urinary tract infection, 402
Urine output
  cardiac output and, 178
  after cardiopulmonary bypass, 173, 174, 388
Urokinase, 61, 515, 545

VACTERL association, 159, 160t, 414
VADs. *See* Ventricular assist devices
Valproic acid, 380
Valsalva's maneuver, 116
Valves, cardiac, 4. *See also* specific valves
Vascular access, 140–146, 155
  arterial, 140–141
  central venous, 141, *142*
  choice of sites for cardiac catheterization, 447
  during CPR, 129
  inserting intravascular lines, 140, *140*
  internal jugular vein catheterization, 142–143, *144*
  percutaneous femoral vein catheterization, 141–142
  pulmonary artery catheterization, 143–146, *145*
  removal of lines by nurses, 520, 520t
  subclavian vein catheterization, 142–143, *144*
  thrombosis and, 140
Vascular pressures
  fetal, 17–18
  measurement in catheterization laboratory, 31
Vascular rings and slings, 322–324, 357, 411
  anatomy of, 322
    double aortic arch, 322, *322*
    pulmonary artery sling, 322, *322*
    right aortic arch with aberrant left subclavian artery, 322
  clinical course of, 323
  lesions associated with, 322
  pathophysiology of, 322–323
  postoperative management of, 324
  postoperative problems associated with, 324
    mediastinal complications, 324
    residual lung disease, 324
  preoperative evaluation of, 323
  surgical procedures for, 323–324
    pulmonary artery sling, 324, *324*
    vascular rings, *323,* 323–324
Vascular smooth muscle, 46–47
Vasoconstrictors, 499, 499t
Vasodilators, 53–57, 543
  angiotensin-converting enzyme inhibitors, 56–57, 544
    captopril, 56–57, 544
    enalapril, 57, 544
  calcium antagonists, 56
    nifedipine, 56
    verapamil, 56
  effect on pulmonary vascular resistance, 499, 499t, 502
  hydralazine, 55–56, 543
  nitroglycerin, 53–55, 543
  sites of action and hemodynamic effects of, 48t
  sodium nitroprusside, 55, 543
Vasopressin, 387
Vasotec. *See* Enalapril
Vecuronium, 87t, 92, 502, 546

Velocardiofacial syndrome, 159
Vent catheters, 191
Ventilation, 73–74, 96–98, *98,* 351–354. *See also* Breathing; Respiratory physiology
  alveolar gas equation, 74
  carbon dioxide elimination, 74
  during cardiopulmonary bypass, 193–194, 356
  dead space and alveolar ventilation, 73–74
  diffusion, 73
  gas properties, 73
  mechanical, 96–103 (*See also* Mechanical ventilation)
Ventilation-perfusion mismatch, 78–79, 97, 355, 358
  causes of, 78
  estimating extent of, 78
  therapies for, 78–79
Ventilation-perfusion ratio, 78
Ventricle(s). *See also* Left ventricle; Right ventricle
  D-loop and L-loop, 10, *11, 12*
    variations in conotruncal anatomy with, *13,* 14
  echocardiographic assessment of function of, 434–439
  interdependence of, 107, 111–112
  mass of, 23
  morphologic anatomy of, 6–10, *7, 9,* 111–112
  output of, 271
  single, 271–284, 456–457 (*See also* Single ventricle lesions)
Ventricular assist devices (VADs), 330, 345–348. *See also* Myocardial mechanical support
  choosing between extracorporeal membrane oxygenation and, 346, *346,* 347t
  complications of, 348
  for myocarditis, 488
  outcome of, 348
  postoperative echocardiography in patient with, 445–446
  troubleshooting guidelines for, 348, 348t
  weaning from, 348
Ventricular fibrillation, 127, 131, 475
  effects of cough CPR in, 119
  after surgery for Ebstein's anomaly, 320
Ventricular hypertrophy, 23, 42–43
  left
    aortic stenosis and, 233, 234
    on electrocardiogram, 42–43
  right
    aortic stenosis and, 234
    coarctation of aorta and, 249
    on electrocardiogram, 42
    interrupted aortic arch and, 245
Ventricular pressure-volume loop, 27–29, *27–29,* 483, *484*
Ventricular septal defect (VSD), 151, 212–216
  anatomy of, 212
  chest film after repair of, *408*
  clinical course of, 214
  due to cardiac trauma, 507–509
  lesions associated with, 212, 213
    transposition of great arteries, 271, 289, 298
    truncus arteriosus, 228, 232
  pathophysiology of, 213–214
  postoperative management of, 216
  postoperative problems associated with, 216
    heart block, 216, 462, *463*
    junctional ectopic tachycardia, 216
    pulmonary hypertension, 216
    residual ventricular septal defect, 216
  preoperative evaluation of, 214
  restrictive vs. nonrestrictive, 213
  spontaneous closure of, 214
  surgical procedures for, 214–215, *215*
  tetralogy of Fallot and, 259
  types of, 212–213, *213*
    canal type, 213, 215
    malalignment type, 212–213, 215
    muscular type, 212, 215
    perimembranous type, *xix,* 212, 214–215
    subpulmonary type, 212, 215
  umbrella occluders for, 455
Ventriculotomy
  left, 8
  right, 6
VEPs. *See* Visual evoked potentials
Verapamil, 56, 479
  adverse effects of, 479
  dosage of, 545
  indications for, 479
    atrial flutter/atrial fibrillation, 470
    hypertrophic cardiomyopathy, 491
  mechanism of action of, 491–492
  metabolism of, 479
Versed. *See* Midazolam
Vertebral defects, 414
Via dextra, 3
Via sinistra, 3
Visual evoked potentials (VEPs), 373t
Vocal cord paralysis, 206, 358
Volume expansion, 388
Volume of distribution of drug, 45
von Willebrand factor, 397
VSD. *See* Ventricular septal defect
V_T. *See* Tidal volume

Warfarin, 60, 308, 399, 493, 545
Waterston shunt, 275
Wenckebach types I and II atrioventricular block, 462–463
West syndrome, 376
Williams syndrome, 38t, 159, 160t, 240
Wolff-Parkinson-White syndrome, 318, 469, 470

WHEN MINUTES COUNT, 3 References to Help Improve Patient Outcomes.

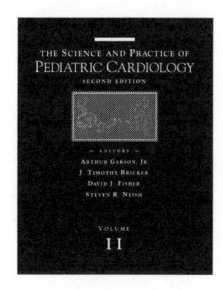

The Science and Practice of Pediatric Cardiology
2nd EDITION
Arthur Garson, Jr., MD, J. Timothy Bricker, MD, David J. Fisher, MD, and Steven R. Neish, MD
1998/3,072 pages/0-683-03417-0

Harness breakthroughs in pediatric cardiology and you can improve your patients' quality of life and help ensure their survival. Here's a new and innovative reference that helps you master both the basic and clinical science issues that shape your management decisions.

Major advances in molecular cardiology have helped drive much of the progress in your specialty, and these are highlighted throughout the text. Key topics include: • fetal medicine • therapeutic catheterization • radiofrequency therapy of arrhythmias • transplantation • pharmacologic treatment of heart failure • positron emission tomography • transesophageal echocardiography • three-dimensional image reconstruction.

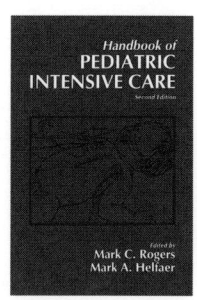

Handbook of Pediatric Intensive Care
2nd EDITION
Mark C. Rogers, MD and Mark A. Helfaer, MD
1994/873 pages/104 illustrations/0-683-07326-5

Organized by organ system and designed for easy bedside consultation, here is a compact, practical guide to patient management emphasizing problems frequently encountered in the ICU. A synopsis of the clinical chapters of **Textbook of Pediatric Intensive Care**, this latest edition features many more line drawings, tables and graphs for fast referral, more coverage of procedures, a new chapter on postoperative management of cardiac surgical patients, and a new chapter on liver transplantation.

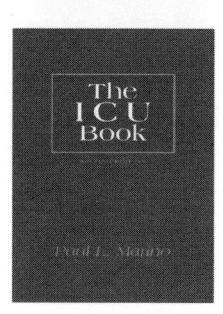

The ICU Book
2nd EDITION
Paul L. Marino, MD, PhD
1997/972 pages/439 illustrations/0-683-05565-8

This heavily revised edition provides the basic technical skills needed to solve the common problems confronted in any intensive care unit. Offering a problem-solving approach, the focus is on the fundamental principles generic to all intensive care functions and on duplicating the actual approach to patient care in the ICU. Clinical pearls are included to provide the techniques, calculations, treatments, indications, drug dosages, and clinical insights that all critical care professionals need to survive in the ICU.

New chapters in this edition provide specific clinical coverage of neurologic crises, myocardial infarction, AIDS and the important issue of post-operative management.

Yes! I'd like to add these pediatric references to my library!
Phone orders accepted 24 hours a day, 7 days a week (US only).

From the US:
Call: 1-800-638-0672

From Canada:
Call: 1-800-665-1148

INTERNET:
E-mail: custserv@wwilkins.com
Home page: www.wwilkins.com

PEDBIA   S8B929

Williams & Wilkins
A Waverly Company
351 West Camden Street
Baltimore, Maryland 21201-2436